Emergency Care

12th Edition

BRADY

Emergency
Care
12th Edition

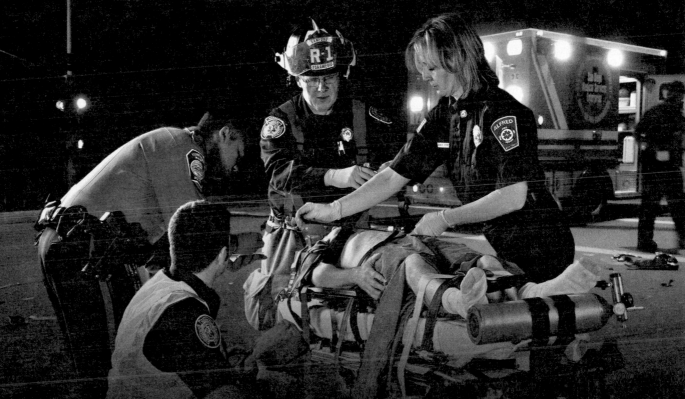

DANIEL LIMMER | MICHAEL F. O'KEEFE

MEDICAL EDITOR

EDWARD T. DICKINSON, MD, FACEP

LEGACY AUTHORS

Harvey D. Grant | Robert H. Murray, Jr. | J. David Bergeron

Brady is an imprint of Pearson

Boston Columbus Indianapolis New York San Francisco Upper Saddle River
Amsterdam Cape Town Dubai London Madrid Milan Munich Paris Montréal Toronto
Delhi Mexico City São Paulo Sydney Hong Kong Seoul Singapore Taipei Tokyo

Library of Congress Cataloging-in-Publication Data

Emergency care. — 12th ed. / Daniel Limmer, Michael F. O'Keefe
; medical editor, Edward T. Dickinson ; legacy authors, Harvey D.
Grant, Robert H. Murray, Jr., J. David Bergeron.
    p. ; cm.
  Includes index.
  ISBN-13: 978-0-13-254380-4
  ISBN-10: 0-13-254380-X
  1. Emergency medicine. 2. First aid in illness and injury. 3.
Rescue work. 4. Emergency medical personnel. I. Limmer, Daniel. II.
O'Keefe, Michael F. III. Dickinson, Edward T.
  [DNLM: 1. Emergency Medical Services—methods. 2. Emergencies. 3.
Emergency Medical Technicians. 4. Emergency Treatment—methods. WX
215]
  RC86.7.B68 2012
  616.02'5—dc22   2010046129

Publisher: Julie Levin Alexander
Publisher's Assistant: Regina Bruno
Editor-in-Chief: Marlene McHugh Pratt
Acquisitions Editor: Sladjana Repic
Senior Managing Editor for Development: Lois Berlowitz
Project Manager: Sandra Breuer
Editorial Assistant: Jonathan Cheung
Director of Marketing: David Gesell
Executive Marketing Manager: Katrin Beacom
Marketing Manager: Brian Hoehl
Marketing Coordinator: Michael Sirinides
Managing Editor for Production: Patrick Walsh
Production Liaison: Faye Gemmellaro/Yagnesh Jani
Production Editor: Heather Willison, S4Carlisle Publishing
Services
Manufacturing Manager: Alan Fischer
Manager of Design Development: John Christiana
Cover and Interior Design: John Christiana
Cover Photography: foreground image, Michal Heron for
Pearson Education; background image, © Daniel Limmer
Managing Photography Editor: Michal Heron
Photographers: Nathan Eldridge, Michael Gallitelli, Michal
Heron, Ray Kemp/911 Imaging, Richard Logan
Editorial Media Manager: Amy Peltier
Media Project Manager: Lorena Cerisano
Composition: S4Carlisle Publishing Services
Printer/Binder: RR Donnelley/Willard
Cover Printer: Lehigh-Phoenix Color/Hagerstown

NOTICE ON CARE PROCEDURES

It is the intent of the authors and publisher that this textbook be used as part of a formal Emergency Medical Technician (EMT) education program taught by qualified instructors and supervised by a licensed physician. The procedures described in this textbook are based upon consultation with EMT and medical authorities. The authors and publisher have taken care to make certain that these procedures reflect currently accepted clinical practice; however, they cannot be considered absolute recommendations.

The material in this textbook contains the most current information available at the time of publication. However, federal, state, and local guidelines concerning clinical practices, including (without limitation) those governing infection control and universal precautions, change rapidly. The reader should note, therefore, that the new regulations may require changes in some procedures.

It is the reader's responsibility to familiarize himself or herself with the policies and procedures set by federal, state, and local agencies as well as the institution or agency where the reader is employed. The authors and the publisher of this textbook and the supplements written to accompany it disclaim any liability, loss, or risk resulting directly or indirectly from the suggested procedures and theory, from any undetected errors, or from the reader's misunderstanding of the text. It is the reader's responsibility to stay informed of any new changes or recommendations made by any federal, state, or local agency as well as by his or her employing institution or agency.

NOTICE ON GENDER USAGE

The English language has historically given preference to the male gender. Among many words, the pronouns *he* and *his* are commonly used to describe both genders. Society evolves faster than language, and the male pronouns still predominate in our speech. The authors have made great effort to treat the two genders equally, recognizing that a significant percentage of EMTs are female. However, in some instances, male pronouns may be used to describe both males and females solely for the purpose of brevity. This is not intended to offend any readers of the female gender.

NOTICE RE "STREET SCENES" AND "SCENARIOS"

The names used and situations depicted in the Street Scenes and Scenarios throughout this text are fictitious.

NOTICE ON MEDICATIONS

The authors and the publisher of this book have taken care to make certain that the equipment, doses of drugs, and schedules of treatment are correct and compatible with the standards generally accepted at the time of publication. Nevertheless, as new information becomes available, changes in treatment and in the use of equipment and drugs become necessary. The reader is advised to carefully consult the instruction and information material included in the page insert of each drug or therapeutic agent, piece of equipment, or device before administration. This advice is especially important when using new or infrequently used drugs. Prehospital care providers are warned that use of any drugs or techniques must be authorized by their Medical Director, in accord with local laws and regulations. The publisher disclaims any liability, loss, injury, or damage incurred as a consequence, directly or indirectly, of the use and application of any of the contents of this book.

Brady
is an imprint of

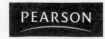

Pearson Health Science
Upper Saddle River, NJ 07458
www.bradybooks.com

10 9 8 7 6 5 4 3 2 1
ISBN-10 0-13-254380-X
ISBN-13 978-0-13-254380-4

BRIEF CONTENTS

DETAILED CONTENTS

SECTION 4 — Medical Emergencies 423

Chapter 18 • General Pharmacology 424

Chapter 19 • Respiratory Emergencies 443

Chapter 20 • Cardiac Emergencies 469

Chapter 36 • Geriatric Emergencies — 930

Chapter 37 • Emergencies for Patients with Special Challenges — 949

SECTION 7 | Operations — 973

Chapter 38 • EMS Operations — 974

PHOTO SCANS

VISUAL GUIDES

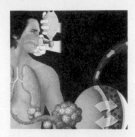
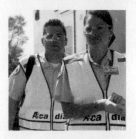
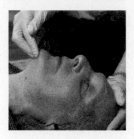
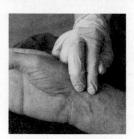
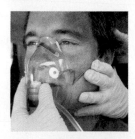
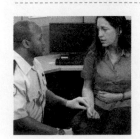
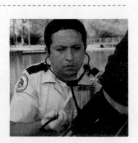

LETTER TO STUDENTS

BRADY

Dear Student:

You are beginning your EMT education at a pivotal time in EMS. The course you are taking is based on new EMS Education Standards that have changed the way you will learn and practice EMS. This course contains more science knowledge than previous courses and expects you, the EMT, to practice at a level of knowledge, skills, and clinical thinking unlike ever before in EMS.

We believe our book, Emergency Care, will provide you with the best possible resources to take you through class and into the field. The hallmark of this text— over generations of EMTs—has been a combination of readability, practicality, and the information you need to know to pass your exam.

This edition has many features to help you learn. We are particularly proud of the way we integrated scientific principles in an easy to understand manner. No other text out there helps you to think like an EMT more than Emergency Care. You will find multiple critical thinking and decision-based features throughout this text to help you integrate the need-to-know material of the classroom with the reality of being an EMT on the street.

Your author team has been working together on Emergency Care for six consecutive editions and more than 20 years. With more than 120 combined years of experience in EMS, firefighting, law enforcement, and education, we still practice EMS and emergency medicine to ensure the book you will use is as current and practical as possible.

We are proud of our book and pleased you will use it in your studies to become an EMT. Our email addresses are in the book. If we may ever be of service to answer a question about EMS or anything in this text, please contact us.

Our best wishes go out to you for a wonderful course, and for safe, rewarding experiences on the street.

Daniel Limmer,
EMT-P
danlimmer@mac.com

Michael F. O'Keefe,
MS, EMT-P
MikeOKVT@aol.com

Edward T. Dickinson,
MD, FACEP
edward.dickinson@uphs.upenn.edu

PREFACE

EMERGENCY CARE has set the standard for EMT training for over 30 years. We strive to stay current with new research and developments in EMS, and this new edition is no exception. We've updated the text to meet 2010 American Heart Association guidelines for CPR and ECC to prepare your students for testing and practice in the year 2011 and beyond.

The foundation of *Emergency Care* is the National EMS Education Standards. While using the Standards as our base, *Emergency Care*, 12th edition, has been written to go beyond the Standards to provide the most current reflection of EMS practice and show readers what EMS systems and EMTs are actually doing around the country today. The caveat "follow local protocols," of course, appears frequently—whenever the equipment or practice described has been adopted in some—but not all—systems.

In addition, the text and the accompanying Resource Central were developed taking into account the years of experience that the authors, with the input of countless instructors and students, have had with EMS curricula and practice. The result is a proven text with outstanding readability and a level of detail that instructors have found more appropriate for their classrooms than any other.

The content of the 12th edition is summarized in the following text, with emphasis on "what's new" in each section of this edition.

SECTION 1 • FOUNDATIONS: CHAPTERS 1–7

The first section sets a framework for all the sections that follow by introducing some essential concepts, information, and skills. The section introduces the EMS system and the EMT's role within the system. The section then covers issues of EMT safety and well-being, including safe techniques of lifting and moving patients. Legal and ethical issues are then discussed. Basic medical terminology, anatomy, physiology, and pathophysiology, as well as life span development, round out this first section.

What's New in the Foundations Section?

- In Chapter 1, "Introduction to Emergency Medical Care," we've added a section on the **role of research in EMS** (including its influence on the development of **evidence-based practices**). We also included a new section on the **EMS role in Public Health**.

- In Chapter 2, "The Well-Being of the EMT," there is a new emphasis on **long-term prevention and well-being**, while still including the traditional and necessary short-term safety precautions.

- Chapter 3, "Lifting and Moving Patients," now emphasizes the **power stretcher**, and there is added information and illustration of **bariatric devices**.

- Chapter 5, "Medical Terminology and Anatomy and Physiology," now begins with a new section on **medical terminology**. Many new **high-quality illustrations** accompany the text on anatomy and physiology.

- Chapter 6, "Principles of Pathophysiology," is a new chapter in the 12th edition, reflecting the emphasis on pathophysiology in the new EMS Standards. Rather than being a full course in pathophysiology, Chapter 6 focuses on **pathophysiology of the cardiopulmonary system** with additional information on disruptions that may occur to **fluid balance** and the **nervous system**.

- Chapter 7, "Life Span Development," now follows a girl named **Jamie through the entire course of her life**.

SECTION 2 • AIRWAY MANAGEMENT, RESPIRATION, AND ARTIFICIAL VENTILATION: CHAPTERS 8–9

There are only two chapters in Section 2, but it may be the most important section in the text, because no patient will survive without an adequate airway, adequate respiration, and adequate ventilation.

The chapters in this section and throughout the text have been updated to conform to the *2010 American Heart Association Guidelines for Cardiopulmonary Resuscitation and Emergency Cardiovascular Care.*

What's New in the Airway Management, Respiration, and Artificial Ventilation Section?

- Chapter 8, "Airway Management," is **entirely devoted to airway issues**.
- Chapter 9, "Respiration and Artificial Ventilation," places an emphasis on **cardiopulmonary pathophysiology**. A new section on **CPAP/BiPAP** has been added to the more **traditional techniques for assisting respiration and ventilation**.

SECTION 3 • PATIENT ASSESSMENT: CHAPTERS 10–17

Key elements of the EMT's job are the ability to perform a thorough and accurate assessment, treat for life-threatening conditions, and initiate transport to the hospital within optimum time limits. This section explains and illustrates all of the assessment steps and their application to different types of trauma and medical patients. In addition, it focuses on the skills of measuring vital signs, using monitoring devices, taking a patient history, communicating, and documenting.

All chapters in the Patient Assessment section—and throughout the text—have been revised to use current terminology for the assessment steps (**primary assessment, secondary assessment**—with secondary assessment defined as "everything after the primary assessment," including history, physical exam, vital signs, and use of monitoring devices) and the **history (history of the present illness [HPI]** and **past medical history [PMH])**. This section describes the traditional **anatomical approach** (head to toe) to assessment, and in Chapter 14, "Assessment of the Medical Patient," it adds the **body systems approach**, in which the physical exam is tailored to chief complaints associated with specific body systems, including the respiratory, cardiovascular, neurologic, and gastrointestinal systems.

What's New in the Patient Assessment Section?

- In Chapter 10, "Scene Size-Up," there are new emphases on **protective apparel**, on **temperature/weather protection**, on **unstable conditions and secondary collapse**, and on **following the Incident Command system** at the scene.
- Chapter 11, "The Primary Assessment," includes new information on **classifying patients as stable, potentially unstable, or unstable**.
- Chapter 12, "Vital Signs and Monitoring Devices," has added **temperature** to the vital signs. The use of **monitoring devices** is now emphasized, including automatic blood pressure monitors, CO-oximeters, and blood glucose monitors.

- Chapter 13, "Assessment of the Trauma Patient," has been revised to **incorporate all body regions into the rapid trauma assessment** (similar to the exam formerly termed "detailed physical exam"), with the difference between the rapid trauma assessment and the detailed physical exam now being chiefly the speed with which they are performed.

 The mnemonic DCAP-BTLS is no longer used, replaced instead with a simpler list of what to look for during the physical exam: **wounds, tenderness, and deformities**. The **field triage criteria** (for significant mechanisms of injury warranting transport to a trauma center) have been updated in accordance with current Centers for Disease Control (CDC) guidelines.

- Chapter 14, "Assessment of the Medical Patient," now places more **emphasis on oxygen saturation**. As already noted, a **body systems approach** has been added to the traditional **anatomical (head to toe) approach** for physical examination of a medical patient.
- Chapter 15, "Reassessment," is mostly unchanged from the prior edition except for the change in terminology from ongoing assessment to **reassessment**.
- Chapter 16, "Critical Thinking and Decision Making," a **new chapter** in the 12th edition, teaches how the EMT can apply lessons from experienced physicians to learn how to use **critical thinking/decision-making skills** to reach a **field diagnosis**.
- Chapter 17, "Communication and Documentation," now emphasizes, in addition to the preparation of traditional paper reports, the preparation of **electronic prehospital care reports**.

SECTION 4 • MEDICAL EMERGENCIES: CHAPTERS 18–26

The Medical Emergencies section begins with a chapter on pharmacology that introduces the medications the EMT can administer or assist with under the 1994 curriculum. The section continues with chapters on respiratory, cardiac, diabetic/altered mental status (including seizure and stroke), allergic, poisoning/overdose, abdominal, behavioral/psychiatric, and hematology/nephrology emergencies.

What's New in the Medical Emergencies Section?

- Chapter 18, "General Pharmacology," adds **aspirin** as a medication carried on the ambulance, and deemphasizes activated charcoal. The chapter contains expanded information on routes of administration with a new section on the **intraosseous route**. There is a new note on **force protection medications**, such as an atropine auto-injector, that can be used to treat EMS personnel in the event of a terrorist-type chemical attack. The ALS-assist skill, **assisting with IV therapy**, has been added to the chapter.
- Chapter 19, "Respiratory Emergencies," now includes a discussion and photo scan on the use of **CPAP** in EMS to relieve breathing difficulty. The discussion of specific res-

piratory conditions, in addition to **COPD** and **asthma**, now includes **pulmonary edema**, **pneumonia**, **spontaneous pneumothorax**, **pulmonary embolism**, **epiglottitis**, **pertussis**, **cystic fibrosis**, and **viral respiratory infections**.

- Chapter 20, "Cardiac Emergencies," has been entirely revised to conform to the *2010 American Heart Association Guidelines for Cardiopulmonary Resuscitation and Emergency Cardiovascular Care*.

- Chapter 21, "Diabetic Emergencies and Altered Mental Status," discusses **diabetic emergencies** and other causes of altered mental status, including **seizure**, **stroke**, **dizziness**, and **syncope**. This chapter includes an expanded emphasis on the **pathophysiology** associated with these causes of altered mental status.

- Chapter 22, "Allergic Reaction," includes new text and a new table summarizing **when to give and when not to give epinephrine**. There is an increased emphasis on **pathophysiology** throughout the chapter.

- In Chapter 23, "Poisoning and Overdose Emergencies," we have revised the section on **syrup of ipecac** to meet new Standards, added a section on **detergent suicides**, and updated the tables **Common Ingested Poisons** and **Commonly Abused Drugs**.

- Chapter 24, "Abdominal Emergencies," includes a new section on **history specific to female patients**.

- Chapter 25, "Behavioral and Psychiatric Emergencies and Suicide," differentiates behavior from psychiatric emergencies, including **definitions of psychiatric disorders** consistent with those published by the National Institute of Mental Health, and distinguishes between **mental and physical causes for behavioral emergencies**.

- Chapter 26, "Hematologic and Renal Emergencies," is a new chapter that focuses on blood disorders (hematology), especially **anemia** and **sickle cell anemia**, as well as kidney/renal disorders (nephrology), focusing on **renal failure**, **end-stage renal disease**, and **dialysis**.

SECTION 5 • TRAUMA EMERGENCIES: CHAPTERS 27–33

The Trauma Emergencies section begins with a chapter on bleeding and shock and continues with chapters on soft-tissue trauma; chest and abdominal trauma; musculoskeletal trauma; trauma to the head, neck, and spine; multisystem trauma; and environmental emergencies.

What's New in the Trauma Emergencies Section?

- Chapter 27, "Bleeding and Shock," includes a new focus on the latest guidelines for **tourniquet use** and **hemostatic agents** as the major techniques for bleeding control.

- Chapter 28, "Soft-Tissue Trauma," includes a new section on **blast injuries**, based on current CDC guidelines. The chapter also features a new section on **genital trauma**.

- Chapter 29, "Chest and Abdominal Trauma," includes new sections on *commotio cordis* (heart dysrhythmia caused by a blow to the chest) and on **blunt trauma affecting one or more abdominal organs**.

- Chapter 30, "Musculoskeletal Trauma," includes an increased emphasis on signs of, and care for, **pelvic trauma**.

- Chapter 31, "Trauma to the Head, Neck, and Spine," features added information on **increased intracranial pressure (ICP)** and **when and how to hyperventilate** in the presence of ICP.

- Chapter 32, "Multisystem Trauma," emphasizes the **effects of trauma on body systems**, such as the cardiovascular and pulmonary systems, and the importance of supporting body system function while managing the specific trauma. The chapter includes and discusses the **Centers for Disease Control (CDC) criteria for determining patient severity**. A final section discusses managing the patient with multiple or multisystem trauma, including **key decisions on transport and destination priorities**.

- In Chapter 33, "Environmental Emergencies," the category regarding heat emergencies, "Patient with Hot, Dry, or Moist Skin," has been reworded as "Patient with Hot Skin, whether Dry or Moist" to emphasize **hot skin** as the criterion regardless of dryness or moisture. To conform to the new EMS Standards, this chapter, which was formerly grouped with Medical Emergencies, now appears in the **Trauma Emergencies** section.

SECTION 6 • SPECIAL POPULATIONS: CHAPTERS 34–37

Special populations discussed in this section include those with emergencies related to the female reproductive system, pregnancy, or childbirth; pediatric patients; geriatric patients; and patients with certain disabilities, as well as those who rely on advanced medical devices at home. The chapters in this section emphasize how to serve all of these patients by applying the basics of patient assessment and care that the student has already learned.

What's New in the Special Populations Section?

- Chapter 34, "Obstetric and Gynecologic Emergencies," Chapter 35, "Pediatric Emergencies," and Chapter 36, "Geriatric Emergencies," are updated throughout, with special attention to the **latest American Heart Association guidelines**, but with basically the same content as in the 11th edition.

- Chapter 37, "Emergencies for Patients with Special Challenges," has a new opening section/overview of patients with special challenges, including such issues as **disability**, **terminal illness**, **obesity**, and **homelessness/poverty**. The sections on general considerations, diseases, and advanced medical devices are generally unchanged from the 11th edition. However, we have added a new section on **abuse and neglect** and a new section on **autism** to the chapter.

SECTION 7 • OPERATIONS: CHAPTERS 38–41

This section deals with nonmedical operations and special situations, including EMS operations, hazardous materials, multiple-casualty incidents and incident management, highway safety, vehicle extrication, and the EMS response to terrorism.

What's New in the Operations Section?

- Chapter 38, "EMS Operations," has been revised to list the **equipment required** on an ambulance as recommended **by the following: American College of Surgeons, Committee on Trauma; American College of Emergency Physicians; National Association of EMS Physicians; American Academy of Pediatrics**; and **2009 Required Equipment for Basic Life Support Ambulances**.

    There is a new section, "**Getting There: Navigating to the Scene**," with information on using maps and **GPS equipment**. There is also new information on **scene safety** and on **safety in the ambulance**.

- Chapter 39, "Hazardous Materials, Multiple-Casualty Incidents, and Incident Management," and Chapter 40, "Highway Safety and Vehicle Extrication," have numerous small revisions and updates. In Chapter 40, there is a major new section on **how to operate safely at the scene of a highway incident**.

- Chapter 41, "EMS Response to Terrorism," has been updated to include information about the growing **radicalization of some American citizens** and the increasing **ability of rogue nations to acquire and sell nuclear technology**. Information has been added about the four categories of **blast injury**, as defined by the CDC, **and blast injury patterns** to the lungs, ears, abdomen, and brain. The chapter introduces the mnemonic **SLUDGEM** to help readers remember the signs and symptoms of nerve agent poisoning. There is still an important emphasis on **how EMS personnel can protect themselves** when responding to a terrorist incident.

APPENDICES AND REFERENCES

Appendices in this edition include a practice examination, a basic cardiac life support review, and an article on research. References include anatomy and physiology illustrations, an article on medical terminology, the answer key, glossary, and index.

What's New in the Appendices?

- Appendix A, "Practice Examination," has been added to this edition to help you prepare for your NREMT or Sate exam.

- Appendix B, "Basic Cardiac Life Support Review," has been updated to reflect the 2010 AHA guidelines. A section on assisting with placement of ECG leads and a section on post-cardiac-arrest care are newly added to this appendix.

- Appendix C, "Research in EMS," has been added to this edition to offer guidance in appreciating the importance of research, interpreting research, and participating in research studies in EMS.

What's New in the References?

Reference sections in this edition are those that have been included in prior editions but are updated for this edition: The Anatomy and Physiology Illustrations are entirely new for this edition. "Medical Terminology," listed as an appendix in the prior edition, is included in the Reference section this time. The Answer Key, Glossary, and Index are all revised and updated for the current edition.

OUR GOAL: IMPROVING FUTURE TRAINING AND EDUCATION

Some of the best ideas for better training and education methods come from instructors who can tell us what areas of study caused their students the most trouble. Other sound ideas come from practicing EMTs who let us know what problems they faced in the field. We welcome any of your suggestions. If you are an EMS instructor who has an idea on how to improve this book, the companion CD, the Companion web site, or EMT training in general, please write to us at:

Brady/Pearson Health Sciences
c/o EMS Editor
Pearson Education
One Lake Street
Upper Saddle River, NJ 07458

You can also reach the authors through the following email addresses:

danlimmer@mac.com
MikeOKVT@aol.com

Visit Brady's web site:

http://www.bradybooks.com

ABOUT THE PEOPLE

Content Contributors

Becoming an EMT requires study in a number of content areas ranging from airway to medical and trauma emergencies to pediatrics and rescue. To ensure that each area is covered accurately and in the most up-to-date manner, we have enlisted the help of several expert contributors. We are grateful for the time and energy each has put into his or her contribution.

Melissa Alexander, EdD, NREMT-P
University of New Mexico
Albuquerque, NM

Dan Batsie, BA, NREMT
Education Coordinator
Northeast Maine EMS
Bangor, ME

Edward T. Dickinson, MD, NREMT-P, FACEP
Associate Professor
Department of Emergency Medicine
University of Pennsylvania School of Medicine

Bruce Evans, MPA, NREMT-P
EMS Chief
North Las Vegas Fire Department
North Las Vegas, NV

Jonathan Politis, MPA, NREMT-P
EMS Chief
Colonie EMS Department
Colonie, NY
We would also like to acknowledge Dean R. Kelble, Jr., EMT-P, for the information he provided on autism from his article "The ABCs of Autism."

Reviewers

We wish to thank the following reviewers for providing invaluable feedback and suggestions in preparation of the 12th edition of *Emergency Care*.

Chris Bearb, AAS, NREMT-P
Basic Program Coordinator
National EMS Academy
Lake Charles, LA

John L. Beckman, AA, BS, FF/EMT-P, EMS Instructor
Fire Science Instructor
Addison Fire Protection District/Technology Center of DuPage
Addison, IL

Anthony M. Caliguire, EMT-P, AS
Paramedic Instructor/Coordinator
Hudson Valley Community College Cardio-Respiratory and Pre-Hospital Emergency Medicine Program
Troy, NY

Joshua Chan, BA, NREMT-P
EMS Educator
Cuyuna Regional Medical Center
Crosby, MN

Lyndal M. Curry, MA, NREMT-P
EMS Degree Program Director
University of Southern Alabama
Mobile, AL

Kenneth J. Feldman, EMT-CC, PhD, FACHE
Dean
SUNY Empire State College
Regional EMS Faculty
NYS Department of Health
Old Westbury, NY

Robert H. Finger Jr., BS, FF/EMT-P, RRT
Medical Training Officer
Manlius Fire Department
Manlius, NY

Sheldon Guenther, BS, DC, NREMT-P
Associate Professor of EMS
Kansas City Kansas Community College
Kansas City, KS

Lt. Christian M. Hartley
Medical Officer and Training Officer
Houston (Alaska) Fire Department
Houston, AK

Dave Hunt, BS, NREMT-P
EMS Program Developer
Kirkwood Community College
Cedar Rapids, IA

Sharon A. Ingram, NREMT-P
Training Officer
Stone Ambulance Service, Inc.
Stuart, VA

William Justiz, BS, NREMT-P
Coordinator Emergency Medical Technology & Emergency Management
Triton Community College
River Grove, IL
Firefighter/Paramedic: Chicago Fire Department, Chicago, IL
Firefighter/Paramedic/Fire Investigator: River Grove Fire Department, River Grove, IL

Deb Kaye, BS, NREMT
Coordinator/Instructor/EMT
Dakota County Technical College
Sunburg Ambulance/Lakes Area Rural Responders
Rosemount, MN

Jordan J. Khoury, REMT-B I/C
BOD for RAC
Rehoboth Ambulance Committee, Inc.
Rehoboth, MA

Mark Komins, BSEMS, Paramedic
Lead Instructor/Clinical Direction
Moorpark College
Moorpark, CA

Lawrence Linder, PhD(c), NREMT-P
EMS Faculty
Hillsborough Community College EMS Programs
South Shore Campus
Ruskin, FL

Russell Malone
EMT Training Supervisor
Salt Lake Community College
Salt Lake City, UT

Steve McGraw, MHSA, NREMT-P
ALS Training Specialist
Prince William County Department of Fire & Rescue
Nokesville, VA

Dean C. Meenach, AAS, RN, BSN, CEN, CCRN, EMT-P
Director of EMS Education
Mineral Area College
Park Hills, MO

Lawrence Boogie Molina, BS, NREMT-P, CCEMTP
Lecturer (CC)
Dept. of Emergency Medical Services
Kapi'olani Community College
University of Hawaii
Honolulu, HI

Nicholas J. Montelauro, AAS, NREMT-P, NCEE
Training Officer/Primary Instructor
Trans-Care Ambulance
Terre Haute, IN

Ron Mrochko, NREMT-P
Paramedic
Trans-Med Ambulance, Inc.
Forty Fort, PA

Mark Podgwaite, NREMT-I, NECEMS I/C
Training Coordinator
VT EMS District 6
Berlin, VT

Perry Putnam, BA/BS SEI
Lead Instructor, EMT Program
Everett Community College
Everett, WA

Lt. Douglas Rohn, EMT-B
Lieutenant
Madison Fire Department
Madison, WI

Kimberly Schilling, NREMT-P, BS
EMT Coordinator (retired)
Orlando, FL

Marjorie O. Smith, Esq., EMT
South Orange Rescue Squad
South Orange, NJ

Janet M. Spellman, MS, RN, CEN, EMT-P
Adjunct Faculty/Clinical Coordinator
Northeastern University Institute for EMS
Burlington, MA

David J. Turner, NREMT-P, IC
EMS Educator
University of New Mexico School of Medicine
Emergency Medical Services Academy
Albuquerque, NM

Wayne D. Turner, EMT-P, EMSI
EMS Lab Manager/EMS Instructor
Cincinnati State Technical and Community College
Cincinnati, OH

Carolyn Vining, MS, BS, NREMT-P, EMSI
Field Service Instructor Paramedic Program
University of Cincinnati Clermont College
Batavia, OH

Tracey Welchert, NREMT-P
Paramedic Instructor Rescue Training Inc.
Savannah, GA

Jeannien Wentworth, EMT-P, MPA
Lead EMT, Pmrt. Clinical Instructor
Palm Beach State College
Lake Worth, FL

Steve White, BS, NREMT-P
Program Director
Pensacola State College
Pensacola, FL

Brittany Ann Williams, MS, RRT, NREMT-P
Associate Professor
Santa Fe College
Gainesville, FL

Photo Advisors and Sources

All photographs not credited adjacent to the photograph or in the photo credit section that follows were photographed on assignment for Brady Prentice Hall Pearson Education.

Photos in Voices Feature, by chapter:

© Daniel Limmer: 6, 11, 15, 16, 21, 24, 28, 29, 33, 35, 36, 38

© Edward T. Dickinson, MD: 31, 32

© Kevin Link: 18, 39, 40, 41

© Mark C. Ide: 34

Photos in Point of View Features, by chapter:

© Edward T. Dickinson, MD: 29

Photos in Section Openers, by chapter:

© Daniel Limmer: 2, 5, 6, 7

Photos in Text, by figure number:

Kevin Link for Pearson Education: 34-5, 34-7, 34-10a, 34-10b, 34-11, 34-13, 34-14, 34-8, 37-5a, 37-5b, 37-10

Ray Kemp/911 Imaging for Pearson Education: 12-11, 17-1, 17-12, 17-13, 23-2

Organizations

We wish to thank the following organizations for their assistance in creating the photo program for the 12th edition:

In Louisiana:

Keith Simon, VP of PR & Marketing
Acadian Ambulance Service
Lafayette, LA

Gifford Saravia, AAS, NREMT-P
Director, National EMS Academy
Lafayette, LA

Richard Belle, BS, NREMT-P
Continuing Education Manager
National EMS Academy
Lafayette, LA

In Maine:

Kenneth MacDonald, Director of Support Services
North East Mobile Health Services
Scarborough, ME

Chief Jeffery H Rowe
Sanford Fire Department
Sanford, ME

Technical Advisors

Thank you to the following people for providing technical support during the photo shoots for the 12th edition:

In Louisiana:

Richard Belle, BS, NREMT-P
Continuing Education Manager
National EMS Academy

Craig A. Hamilton, NREMT-P

Mary C. Hamilton, BSN, RN, NREMT-P

Gifford Saravia, AAS, NREMT-P
Director of National EMS Academy

Keith Simon
VP of PR & Marketing
Acadian Ambulance Service

Brandy Trahan, EMT-Basic

In Maine:

Carl W. French, EMT-P

Locations

Thank you to the following people who provided locations for our photography:

In Louisiana:

Acadian Ambulance Service

Mr. E.J. Beadle
Production Enhancement Systems LLC

Mr. John E. Hebert and Mrs. Madeline K. Hebert

Chief Chad Leger
Scott Police Department

Mr. Eddie Leger and Mrs. Nellie Leger

Chief Troy Lopez
Judice Volunteer Fire Department

Mr. Huey Miller and Mrs. Mary Ann Miller

National EMS Academy

Mr. Danny Smith
(Owner) Louisiana IceGators

In Maine:

Steve Adams

Models

In Louisiana:

Ryan Andrews	Mary Ann Miller
Pat Benoit	Matt Miller
Whitney Broussard	Jenni Morrow
Michael Burley	Ariel Morvant
Desiree Coméaux	Terrence Mouton
Tracy M. Doré	David Mowry
Lara Dunn	James M. Olivier
Laura Duplantis	Kathy Olivier
Molli Early	Gabriella Payne
Diego D. Escandon	Nicole Payne
Michael Godeaux	Jeremy Percle
Oscar Goodie, Sr.	Krystal Pulles
John R. Hamilton	Joshua D. Reed
Mary Hamilton	Eddie Robinson
Earl Herbert	Victor Rodriguez
Jacob Iden	Ashley Rooneem
Kayla Iden	Mark Rooneem
Logan Iden	Lauren Saravia
Sherrie Johnson	Cindy Smith
Bill Kavanagh	Dustin Soileau
John Keef	Jerry Sonier
Kenneth C. Landor	Kevin Stelly
Kevin Larriviere	Jesse Toney
Ryan LeBlanc	Heath Tyler
Eddie Leger	Kim Tyler
Nellie Leger	Kelli Venable
Troy Lopez	Pablo Yocupicio
Seth Mayeaux	Kendra Young

ABOUT THE AUTHORS

DANIEL LIMMER | AUTHOR

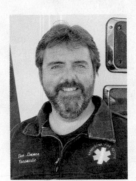

Began EMS in 1978. Became an EMT in 1980 and a paramedic in 1981.

Is Lead Paramedic Instructor and Adjunct Instructor for two national college/university-level paramedic programs. Enjoys especially teaching patient assessment and believes critical thinking and decision-making skills are the key to successful clinical practice of EMS.

Works part-time as a freelance photojournalist and is working on a documentary project photographing EMS people and agencies throughout the United States.

Is an avid blogger. His EMS blog can be seen on www.bradybooks.com.

In addition to his EMS experience, was a dispatcher and police officer in upstate New York.

Lives in Maine, where he is married to Stephanie and has two daughters, Sarah and Margo.

Is a Jimmy Buffett fan (Parrothead) who attends at least one concert each year.

MICHAEL F. O'KEEFE | AUTHOR

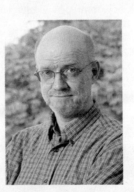

EMT Provider Level Leader for National EMS Education Standards.

Expert writer for 1994 revision of EMT-Basic curriculum.

EMS volunteer since college in 1976.

Member of development group for the National EMS *Education Agenda for the Future: A Systems Approach* and *The National EMS Scope of Practice Model.*

Has a special interest in EMS research, and got a master's degree in biostatistics.

Past chairperson of the National Council of State EMS Training Coordinators.

Interests include science fiction, travel, foreign languages, and stained glass.

EDWARD T. DICKINSON | MEDICAL EDITOR

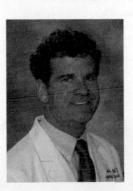

In 1985, was the first volunteer firefighter to receive the top award from *Firehouse Magazine* for heroism for the rescue of two elderly women trapped in a house fire.

Is the Medical Director of the Malvern and Berwyn Fire Companies, and the Haverford Township Paramedics in Pennsylvania.

Has been continuously certified as a National Registry Paramedic since 1983.

First certified as an EMT in 1979 in upstate New York.

Has a full-time academic emergency medicine practice at the Hospital of the University of Pennsylvania in Philadelphia.

Has served as medical editor for numerous Brady EMT and First Responder texts.

Lives with his wife and two sons in suburban Chester County outside of Philadelphia.

■ CORE CONCEPTS

Highlights the key points addressed in each chapter. The topics not only help students anticipate chapter content, but also guides their studies through the textbook and supplements.

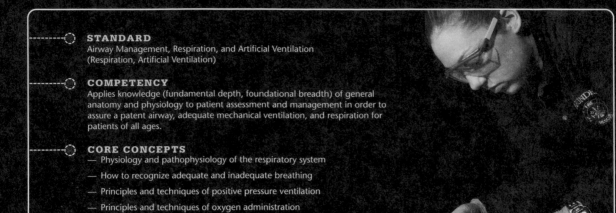

○ **STANDARD**
Airway Management, Respiration, and Artificial Ventilation
(Respiration, Artificial Ventilation)

○ **COMPETENCY**
Applies knowledge (fundamental depth, foundational breadth) of general anatomy and physiology to patient assessment and management in order to assure a patent airway, adequate mechanical ventilation, and respiration for patients of all ages.

○ **CORE CONCEPTS**
— Physiology and pathophysiology of the respiratory system
— How to recognize adequate and inadequate breathing
— Principles and techniques of positive pressure ventilation
— Principles and techniques of oxygen administration

EXPLORE Resource Central

To access Resource Central, follow directions on the Student Access Card provided with this text. If there is no card, go to **www.bradybooks.com** and follow the Resource Central link to Buy Access from there. Under Media Resources, you will find:

▶ **Effective BVM Ventilations**
Learn how to give effective BVM ventilations, how to properly position a patient's head and why it is important to have the proper mask size.

▶ **Oxygen Delivery Devices**
See a video on different types of oxygen delivery devices. Who knew there were so many choices? Learn the flow rates and oxygen delivery amounts associated with each device as well as the pros and cons of these devices.

▶ **King Airway Insertion**
Watch this video to learn how to insert a King airway and what you should do directly after insertion of this device.

■ RESOURCE CENTRAL

NEW! At the beginning of each chapter, students are prompted to visit Resource Central to view weblinks, animations, or video presentations around material described in the chapter.

■ OBJECTIVES

NEW! Objectives form the basis of each chapter and were developed around the Education Standards and Instructional Guidelines.

OBJECTIVES

After reading this chapter you should be able to:

9.1 Define key terms introduced in this chapter.

9.2 Explain the physiological relationship between assessing and maintaining an open airway, assessing and ensuring adequate ventilation, and assessing and maintaining adequate circulation. (pp. 198–201)

9.3 Describe the mechanics of ventilation. (pp. 198–199)

9.4 Explain mechanisms that control the depth and rate of ventilation. (pp. 198–199)

9.5 Explain the relationships between tidal volume, respiratory rate, minute volume, dead air space, and alveolar ventilation. (pp. 198–199)

9.6 Describe the physiology of external and internal respiration. (p. 199)

■ INSIDE/OUTSIDE

*Calls out relevant pathophysiology for a condition or series of conditions.
Helps students understand disease presentation and treatment.*

Inside/Outside

RESPIRATORY DISTRESS TO RESPIRATORY FAILURE

Respiratory failure occurs when the mechanisms of respiratory compensation can no longer keep up with a respiratory challenge. To illustrate this process, let's review the progression of a patient having an asthma attack.

Patients with asthma have episodic attacks where their bronchiole tubes spasm and constrict. This leads to decreased air flow and decreased tidal volume. As minute volume and alveolar ventilation decrease, the body senses increased levels of carbon dioxide and slight hypoxia. The brain responds with an increased stimulus to breathe and activation of the sympathetic nervous system.

Inside the body, the respiratory system compensates. Respiratory rate and depth are increased in an attempt to increase alveolar ventilation. The heart pumps faster and harder in an attempt to move oxygen and carbon dioxide more quickly. Blood vessels constrict as the "fight-or-flight" response engages.

Outside the body, the patient may notice a sensation of

Unfortunately, the asthma attack continues. Inside the body, the patient's bronchiole tubes get narrower as they begin to swell in response to the attack. Tidal volume and alveolar ventilation decrease even more, and the brain now lacks sufficient oxygen. Carbon dioxide also has been building up and is beginning to interfere with normal function. As you reassess this patient, you notice he is beginning to get anxious, maybe even a bit combative, as hypoxia increases and affects his brain. You notice it is harder to hear air moving when you listen to his chest. His wheezes have become "tighter." His fingernails are now turning blue, and you notice a similar discoloration in his lips and around his eyes. *Respiratory failure* has begun. Compensation can no longer keep up with his needs.

As the attack continues, tidal volume and alveolar ventilation decrease even further. Hypoxia is now profound. The patient's body has become acidotic from the retention of

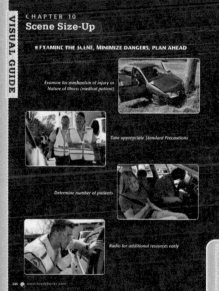

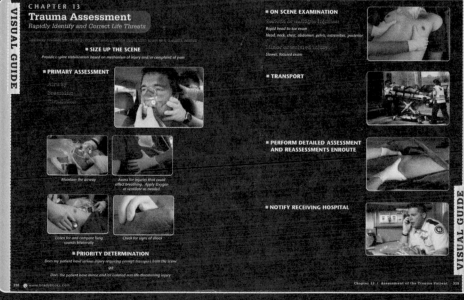

■ VISUAL GUIDES

Visually presents patient assessment in a series of flow charts.

■ DECISION POINTS

Found within the patient assessment/patient care feature in the book, these call out key decisions that are made during assessment and care of a patient.

■ Providing supplemental oxygen to the breathing patient

These procedures are discussed next and on the following pages.

Decision Point

When Do I Intervene?

It can sometimes be difficult to determine when a patient needs your intervention. Often patients in respiratory failure will be breathing and conscious. It is important, however, to identify not just the presence of breathing but the adequacy of breathing. Even though the patient may still be breathing, if he is displaying the signs of inadequate breathing, he absolutely needs your intervention. Keep in mind that what the patient is doing on his own is not meeting his needs. If left unchecked, his condition will progress to respiratory arrest. In general, it is better to be too aggressive than not aggressive enough. If the patient will allow you to intervene with a bag-valve mask, it generally means he needs it.

CRITICAL DECISION MAKING

Oxygen or Ventilation?

You have learned several methods to administer supplemental oxygen and to provide ventilations to a patient. It has been said that the decision on when to provide supplemental oxygen (e.g., nonrebreather mask or cannula) or to ventilate (e.g., BVM, FROPVD) is one of the most important decisions you will make.

For each of the following patients, decide whether you would administer oxygen or ventilate the patient.

1. A patient who was found on the floor by a relative. He has no pulse or respirations.
2. A 14-year-old patient who has a broken femur. She is alert; pulse 110, strong and regular; respirations 28, rapid and deep.
3. A 64-year-old male with chest pain. He is alert; pulse 56; respirations 18 and normal.
4. A 78-year-old patient with COPD. He has had increasing difficulty breathing over the past few days. He responds verbally but is not oriented. His pulse is 124; respirations 36 and shallow.

■ CRITICAL DECISION MAKING

A scenario-based feature that offers practice in making critical decisions.

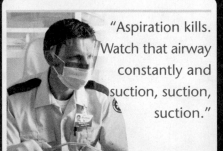

"Aspiration kills. Watch that airway constantly and suction, suction, suction."

■ VOICES

Insights or facts from EMTs in the field.

■ POINT OF VIEW

Tells stories of EMS care from the patient's perspective and includes photos that illustrate the patient's viewpoint.

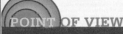

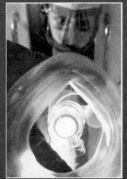

"I still can't tell you why I didn't know it was coming on. I didn't feel right for a few days. Then it hit me. I couldn't move without feeling like I would suffocate. I just couldn't breathe. Couldn't catch my breath. I could tell it was serious when the EMTs came in. It showed in their faces.

"I think I must've started getting even worse, because I remember feeling like I was losing it. I remember them trying to calm me down, but I really felt like I was going to have to be peeled off the ceiling of that ambulance.

"When they tried to put that big mask on my face I felt like it was going to kill me. To take away all my air. I fought it. The EMTs kept calming me and putting that mask on my face. Somehow I calmed down a little and they gave me air or oxygen or something. I made it to the hospital. The doctor told me that the EMTs may have saved my life.

"I appreciate that more than I can say—even if that mask felt pretty intimidating at the time."

CHAPTER REVIEW

Key Facts and Concepts

- Respiratory failure is the result of inadequate breathing, breathing that is insufficient to support life.
- A patient in respiratory failure or respiratory arrest must receive artificial ventilations.
- Oxygen can be delivered to the nonbreathing patient as a supplement to artificial ventilation.
- Oxygen can also be administered as therapy to the breathing patient whose breathing is inadequate or who is cyanotic, cool and clammy, short of breath, suffering chest pain, suffering severe injuries, or displaying an altered mental status.

Key Decisions

- Is the patient breathing? Is the patient breathing adequately (ventilating *and* oxygenating)? Does the patient need supplemental oxygen?
- Is there a need to initiate artificial ventilation?
- Are my artificial ventilations adequate (proper rate and volume)?

■ CHAPTER REVIEW

NEW! Includes a summary of key points, key terms and definitions, review questions, critical thinking exercises that asks students to apply knowledge, case studies, and more!

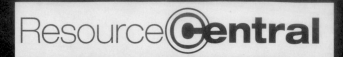

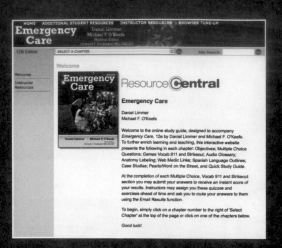

Resource Central provides a one-stop shop for online chapter support materials and resources. Students can prepare for class and exams with skills and objectives checklists, multiple-choice questions, case study activities, web links, animations, study aids, audio glossary, trauma gallery, chapter summary in Spanish, and more! To access Resource Central, please visit www.bradybooks.com. A few key components are described here...

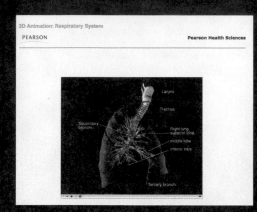

VIRTUAL TOURS

3D animations, including a Heart and Airway virtual tour, offer a deeper under-standing and graphical view of difficult concepts.

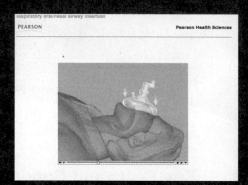

ANIMATIONS, VIDEOS, AND INTERACTIVITIES

Highly visual exercises enhance and reinforce anatomy, physiology, and specific processes.

AUDIO GLOSSARY

This interactive, indexed glossary contains the definitions and audio pronunciations of the key terms presented in the student text.

ANATOMY LABELING EXERCISES

Drag-and-drop activities test knowledge of human anatomy.

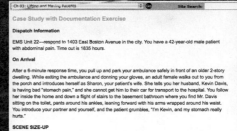

CHAPTER QUIZZES

Chapter-specific multiple-choice quizzes test and reinforce knowledge.

CASE STUDY WITH DOCUMENTATION EXERCISE

Designed to develop critical thinking, each case study offers questions that help to hone students' assessment skills.

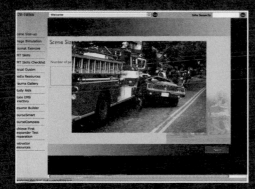

SCENE SIZE-UP

Tests students' ability by flashing scenes on screen and asking questions regarding number of patients, resource determination, BSI precautions, scene safety, and mechanism of injury.

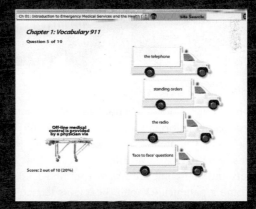

GAMES AND PUZZLES

Strikeout and Vocab911 make learning terminology easy and fun.

ADDITIONAL STUDENT RESOURCE

WORKBOOK FOR EMERGENCY CARE, 12TH EDITION

This self-paced workbook contains matching exercises, multiple-choice questions, short-answer questions, street-scene questions, labeling exercises, case studies, case-study questions, and skill performance checklists. This workbook is available for purchase at www.bradybooks.com.

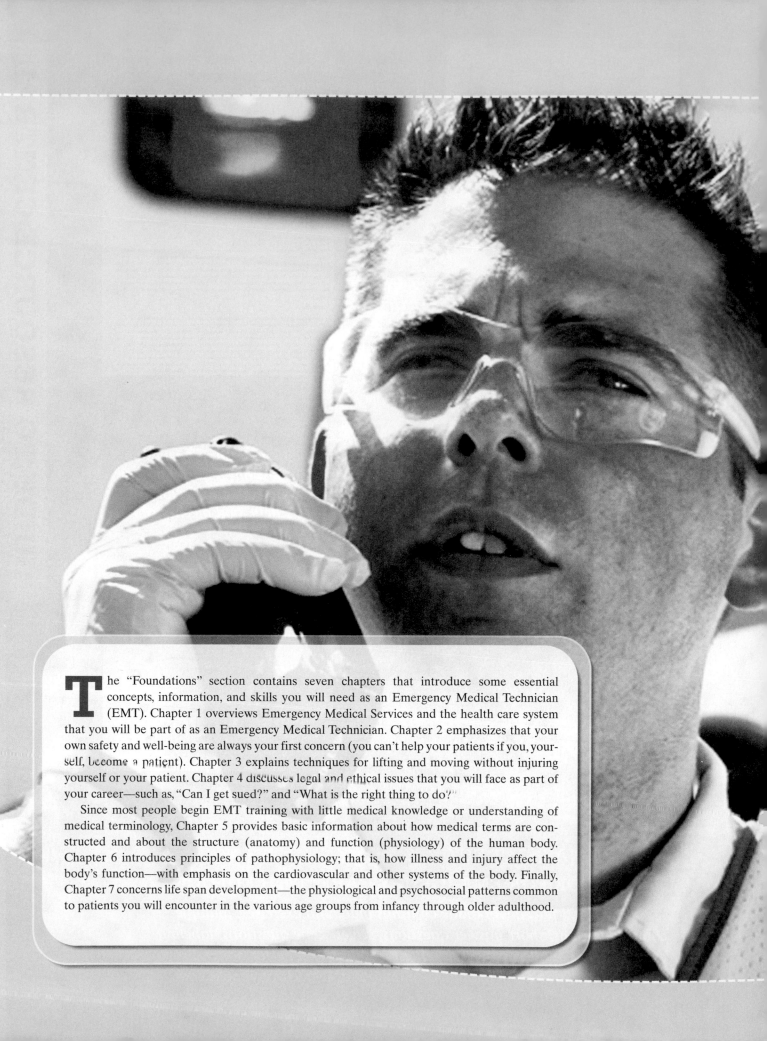

The "Foundations" section contains seven chapters that introduce some essential concepts, information, and skills you will need as an Emergency Medical Technician (EMT). Chapter 1 overviews Emergency Medical Services and the health care system that you will be part of as an Emergency Medical Technician. Chapter 2 emphasizes that your own safety and well-being are always your first concern (you can't help your patients if you, yourself, become a patient). Chapter 3 explains techniques for lifting and moving without injuring yourself or your patient. Chapter 4 discusses legal and ethical issues that you will face as part of your career—such as, "Can I get sued?" and "What is the right thing to do?"

Since most people begin EMT training with little medical knowledge or understanding of medical terminology, Chapter 5 provides basic information about how medical terms are constructed and about the structure (anatomy) and function (physiology) of the human body. Chapter 6 introduces principles of pathophysiology; that is, how illness and injury affect the body's function—with emphasis on the cardiovascular and other systems of the body. Finally, Chapter 7 concerns life span development—the physiological and psychosocial patterns common to patients you will encounter in the various age groups from infancy through older adulthood.

Foundations

1

Introduction to Emergency Medical Care

⭘ **STANDARD**
Preparatory (EMS Systems; Research); Public Health

⭘ **COMPETENCY**
Applies fundamental knowledge of the EMS system, safety/well-being of the EMT, medical/legal and ethical issues to the provision of emergency care.

⭘ **CORE CONCEPTS**
— The chain of human resources that forms the EMS system

— How the public activates the EMS system

— Your roles and responsibilities as an EMT

— The process of EMS quality improvement (QI)

EXPLORE Resource**C**entral

To access Resource Central, follow directions on the Student Access Card provided with this text. If there is no card, go to **www.bradybooks.com** and follow the Resource Central link to Buy Access from there. Under Media Resources, you will find:

▶ **EMT Occupational Overview**
Read all about it! Everything you want to know about the profession can be found here, including nature of the work, job qualifications, and employment opportunities.

▶ **The Winding Road of EMS**
Discover how this exciting and important profession came to be, its progression throughout history and possible future advancements!

▶ **EMS, the Community, and Children**
Watch a video on how most communities access emergency services and how EMS responds to the specific needs of children.

OBJECTIVES

After reading this chapter you should be able to:

1.1 Define key terms introduced in this chapter.

1.2 Give an overview of the historical events leading to the development of modern emergency medical services (EMS). (pp. 5–7)

1.3 Describe the importance of each of the National Highway Traffic Safety Administration standards for assessing EMS systems. (pp. 6–7)

1.4 Describe the components of an EMS system that must be in place for a patient to receive emergency medical care. (pp. 7–18)

1.5 Compare and contrast the training and responsibilities of EMRs, EMTs, AEMTs, and Paramedics. (pp. 8–9)

1.6 Explain each of the specific areas of responsibility for the EMT. (p. 10)

1.7 Give examples of the physical and personality traits that are desirable for EMTs. (pp. 11–12)

1.8 Describe various job settings that may be available to EMTs. (p. 12)

1.9 Describe the purpose of the National Registry of Emergency Medical Technicians. (p. 13)

KEY TERMS

designated agent, *p. 16*
evidence-based, *p. 16*
medical direction, *p. 15*

Medical Director, *p. 15*
911 system, *p. 8*

patient outcomes, *p. 16*
protocols, *p. 15*

quality improvement, *p. 13*
standing orders, *p. 16*

When a person is injured or becomes ill, it rarely happens in a hospital with doctors and nurses standing by. In fact, some time usually passes between the onset of the injury or illness and the patient's arrival at the hospital, time in which the patient's condition may deteriorate, time in which the patient may even die. The modern Emergency Medical Services (EMS) system has been developed to provide what is known as *prehospital* or *out-of-hospital* care. Its purpose is to get trained personnel to the patient as quickly as possible and to provide emergency care on the scene, en route to the hospital, and at the hospital until care is assumed by the hospital staff. The Emergency Medical Technician (EMT) is a key member of the EMS team.

As you begin to study for a career as an EMT, you will want to answer some basic questions, such as: What is the EMS system? How did it develop? And what will be your role in the system? This chapter will help you begin to answer these questions.

THE EMERGENCY MEDICAL SERVICES SYSTEM

How It Began

In the 1790s, the French began to transport wounded soldiers away from the scene of battle so they could be cared for by physicians. This is the earliest documented emergency medical service. However, no medical care was provided for the wounded on the battlefield. The idea was simply to carry the victim from the scene to a place where medical care was available.

Other wars inspired similar emergency services. For example, during the American Civil War, Clara Barton began such a service for the wounded and later helped establish the American Red Cross. During World War I, many volunteers joined battlefield ambulance corps. And during the Korean Conflict and the Vietnam War, medical teams produced further advances in field care, many of which led to advances in the civilian sector, including specialized emergency medical centers devoted to the treatment of trauma (injuries).

Nonmilitary ambulance services began in some major American cities in the early 1900s—again as transport services only, offering little or no emergency care. Smaller communities did not develop ambulance services until the late 1940s, after World War II. Often the local undertaker provided a hearse for ambulance transport. In locations where emergency care was offered along with transport to the hospital, the fire service often was the responsible agency.

The importance of providing hospital-quality care at the emergency scene—that is, beginning care at the scene and continuing it, uninterrupted, during transport to the hospital—soon became apparent. The need to organize systems for such emergency prehospital care and to train personnel to provide it also was recognized.

EMS Today

During the 1960s, the development of the modern EMS system began. In 1966 the National Highway Safety Act charged the United States Department of Transportation (DOT) with developing EMS standards and assisting the states to upgrade the quality of their prehospital emergency care. Most EMT courses today are based on models developed by the DOT.

In 1970, the National Registry of Emergency Medical Technicians was founded to establish professional standards. In 1973, Congress passed the National Emergency Medical Services Systems Act as the cornerstone of a federal effort to implement and improve EMS systems across the United States.

Since then, the states have gained more control over their EMS systems, although the federal government continues to provide guidance and support. For example, the National Highway Traffic Safety Administration (NHTSA) Technical Assistance Program has established an assessment program with a set of standards for EMS systems. The categories and standards set forth by NHTSA, summarized in the following list, will be discussed in more detail throughout this chapter and the rest of this textbook.

- **Regulation and policy.** Each state EMS system must have in place enabling legislation (laws that allow the system to exist), a lead EMS agency, a funding mechanism, regulations, policies, and procedures.

- **Resource management.** There must be centralized coordination of resources so that all victims of trauma or medical emergencies have equal access to basic emergency care and transport by certified personnel, in a licensed and equipped ambulance, to an appropriate facility.

- **Human resources and training.** At a minimum, all those transporting prehospital personnel (those who ride the ambulances) should be trained to the EMT level using a standardized curriculum taught by qualified instructors.

- **Transportation.** Safe, reliable ambulance transportation is a critical component. Most patients can be effectively transported by ground ambulances. Other patients require rapid transportation, or transportation from remote areas, by helicopter or airplane.

- **Facilities.** The seriously ill or injured patient must be delivered in a timely manner to the closest appropriate facility.

- **Communications.** There must be an effective communications system, beginning with the universal system access number (911), dispatch-to-ambulance, ambulance-to-ambulance, ambulance-to-hospital, and hospital-to-hospital communications.

- **Public information and education.** EMS personnel may participate in efforts to educate the public about their role in the system, their ability to access the system, and prevention of injuries.

- **Medical direction.** Each EMS system must have a physician as a Medical Director accountable for the activities of EMS personnel within that system. The Medical Director delegates medical practice to nonphysician providers (such as EMTs) and must be involved in all aspects of the patient care system.

- **Trauma systems.** In each state, enabling legislation must exist to develop a trauma system including one or more trauma centers, triage and transfer guidelines for trauma patients, rehabilitation programs, data collection, mandatory autopsies (examination of bodies to determine cause of death), and means for managing and ensuring the quality of the system.

FIGURE 1-1 Out of hospital care can take many forms. Here, EMTs stand by to provide help as needed at a walkathon. *(© Philip Gould)*

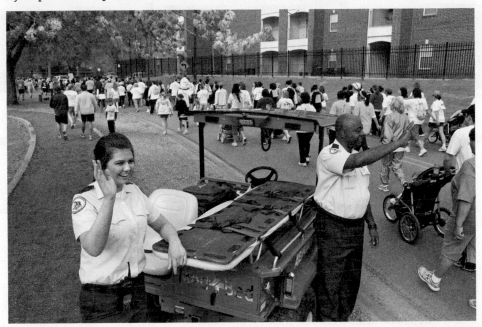

FIGURE 1-1 Out of hospital care can take many forms. Here, EMTs stand by to provide help as needed at a walkathon. *(© Philip Gould)*

- **Evaluation.** Each state must have a program for evaluating and improving the effectiveness of the EMS system, known as a quality improvement (QI) program, a quality assurance (QA) program, or total quality management (TQM).

With the development of the modern EMS system, the concept of ambulance service as a means merely for transporting the sick and injured passed into oblivion. No longer could ambulance personnel be viewed as people with little more than the strength to lift a patient into and out of an ambulance. The hospital emergency department was extended, through the EMS system, to reach the sick and injured at the emergency scene. "Victims" became patients, receiving prehospital assessment and emergency care from highly trained professionals. The "ambulance attendant" was replaced by the Emergency Medical Technician (EMT).

A current development in some areas is use of the term *out-of-hospital care,* rather than *prehospital care,* as EMS personnel begin to provide primary care for some conditions and in some circumstances without transport to a hospital (Figure 1-1). However, the term *prehospital care* will be used in the remainder of this text.

COMPONENTS OF THE EMS SYSTEM

To understand the EMS system, you must look at it from the patient's viewpoint rather than from that of the EMT (Figure 1-2). For the patient, care begins with the initial phone call to the Emergency Medical Dispatcher (EMD). The EMS system responds to the call for help by sending to the scene available responders, including Emergency Medical Responders, EMTs, and advanced life support providers (Advanced EMTs and Paramedics). An ambulance will transport the patient to the hospital.

From the ambulance, the patient is received by the emergency department. There, the patient receives laboratory tests, diagnosis, and further treatment. The emergency department serves as the gateway for the rest of the services offered by the hospital. If a patient is brought to the emergency department with serious injuries, care is given to stabilize the patient, and the operating room is readied to provide further lifesaving measures.

Some hospitals handle all routine and emergency cases but have a specialty that sets them apart from other hospitals. One specialty hospital is the trauma center. In some hospitals, a surgery team may not be available at all times. In a trauma center, surgery teams capable of the comprehensive treatment of trauma patients are available 24 hours a day.

CORE CONCEPT ●
The chain of human resources that forms the EMS system

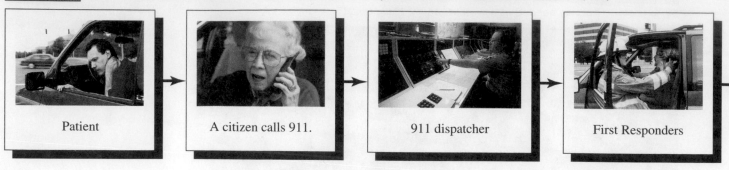

| Patient | A citizen calls 911. | 911 dispatcher | First Responders |

In addition to trauma centers, there are also hospitals that specialize in the care of certain conditions and patients, such as burn centers, pediatric centers, cardiac centers, and stroke centers.

As an EMT, you will become familiar with the hospital resources available in your area. Many EMS regions have specific criteria for transporting patients with special needs. Choosing the right hospital may actually be a lifesaving decision. Of course, it is important to weigh the patient's condition against the additional transport time that may be required to take him to a specialized facility. On-line medical direction (discussed later) may be available to help with this decision.

Dispatchers and EMTs are key members of the prehospital EMS team. (The levels of EMS training will be discussed later in the chapter.) Many others make up the hospital portion of the EMS system. They include physicians, nurses, physician's assistants, respiratory and physical therapists, technicians, aides, and others.

Accessing the EMS System

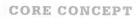

CORE CONCEPT

How the public activates the EMS system

911 system
a system for telephone access to report emergencies. A dispatcher takes the information and alerts EMS or the fire or police departments as needed. *Enhanced 911* has the additional capability of automatically identifying the caller's phone number and location.

Most localities have a ***911 system*** for telephone access to report emergencies. A dispatcher answers the call, takes the information, and alerts EMS or the fire or police departments as needed. Since the number 911 is designed to be a national emergency number, there will be a time when someone may dial 911 from any phone in the country and be connected to the appropriate emergency center.

Many communications centers have *enhanced 911*. This system has the capability of automatically identifying the caller's phone number and location. If the phone is disconnected or the patient loses consciousness, the dispatcher will still be able to send emergency personnel to the scene.

There are still a few communities that do not have 911 systems. In these locations, a standard seven-digit telephone number must be dialed to reach ambulance, fire, or police services. Dialing 911 where a 911 system is not in operation will usually connect the caller to an operator who will attempt to route the call to the appropriate dispatch center. This adds an extra step and extra time to the process, so it is important to make sure that the emergency numbers in use in a local area are prominently displayed on all telephones.

Another development in the communication and dispatch portion of the EMS system is the training and certification of EMDs. These specially trained dispatchers not only obtain the appropriate information from callers, but they also provide medical instructions for emergency care. These include instructions for CPR, artificial ventilation, bleeding control, and more. Research has consistently pointed to the importance of early access and prompt initiation of emergency care and CPR. The EMD is one example of the EMS system providing emergency care at the earliest possible moment.

Levels of EMS Training

There are four general levels of EMS training and certification (described in the following list). These levels vary from place to place. Your instructor will explain any variations that may exist in your region or state.

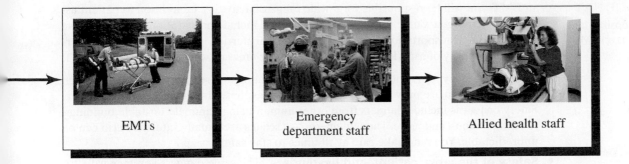

EMTs   Emergency department staff   Allied health staff

- *Emergency Medical Responder (EMR) (previously called First Responder).* This level of training is designed for the person who is often first at the scene. Many police officers, firefighters, and industrial health personnel function in this capacity. The emphasis is on activating the EMS system and providing immediate care for life-threatening injuries, controlling the scene, and preparing for the arrival of the ambulance.

- *Emergency Medical Technician (EMT) (previously called EMT-Basic).* In most areas, the EMT is considered the minimum level of certification for ambulance personnel. EMTs provide basic-level medical and trauma care and transportation to a medical facility.

- *Advanced Emergency Medical Technician (AEMT) (previously called EMT-Intermediate).* The AEMT, like the EMT, provides basic-level care and transportation as well as some advanced-level care, including use of advanced airway devices, monitoring of blood glucose levels, and administration of some medications, which may include intravenous and intraosseous administration.

- *Paramedic (previously sometimes called EMT-Paramedic).* The paramedic performs all of the skills of the EMT and AEMT plus advanced-level skills. The paramedic provides the most advanced level of prehospital care.

CRITICAL DECISION MAKING

A Key Concept

Critical decision making is a very important concept. It essentially means that an EMT takes in information from the scene, the patient assessment, and other sources and makes appropriate decisions after synthesizing—or interpreting all of—the information. There are times when the information you obtain initially won't be enough to be a basis for decision making, so you will need to ask more questions and perform additional examinations to get everything you need to make a decision.

It may be difficult to see how this all fits together now. Before long, however, you'll be learning and practicing patient assessment and care. Some examples of critical decision making that will be a part of the assessment and care you will perform include:

1. **Deciding which hospital to transport someone to.** Should you take your patient to the closest hospital or to a more distant specialty hospital?

2. **Deciding whether you should administer a medication to a patient.** Will it help the patient's current condition? Could it make the condition worse?

When you begin to work with more experienced EMTs, you will come across many who are smart and know what to do and how to treat patients (both clinically and personally). These are the EMTs you would want to take care of you or your family should EMS be needed. These EMTs are good critical decision makers.

Roles and Responsibilities of the EMT

● CORE CONCEPT

Your roles and responsibilities
as an EMT

As an EMT, you will be responsible for a wide range of activities. In addition to patient assessment and emergency care, your responsibilities will include preparation, a safe response to the scene, safe transportation to the hospital, and transferring the patient to hospital personnel for continuity of care. The following are specific areas of responsibility for the EMT.

- **Personal safety.** It is not possible to help a patient if you are injured before you reach him or while you are providing care, so your first responsibility is to keep yourself safe. Safety concerns include dangers from other human beings, animals, unstable buildings, fires, explosions, and more. Though emergency scenes are usually safe, they also can be unpredictable. You must take care at all times to stay safe.

- **Safety of the crew, patient, and bystanders.** The same dangers you face will also be faced by others at the scene. As a professional, you must be concerned with their safety as well as your own.

- **Patient assessment.** As an EMT, one of your most important functions will be assessment of your patient, or finding out enough about what is wrong with your patient to be able to provide the appropriate emergency care. Assessment always precedes emergency care.

- **Patient care.** The actual care required for an individual patient may range from simple emotional support to lifesaving CPR and defibrillation. Based on your assessment findings, patient care is an action or series of actions that your training will prepare you to take in order to help the patient deal with and survive his illness or injury.

- **Lifting and moving.** Since EMTs are usually involved in transporting patients to the hospital, lifting and moving patients are important tasks. You must perform them without injury to yourself and without aggravating or adding to the patient's existing injuries.

- **Transport.** It is a serious responsibility to operate an ambulance at any time, but even more so when there is a patient on board. Safe operation of the ambulance, as well as securing and caring for the patient in the ambulance, will be important parts of your job as an EMT.

- **Transfer of care.** Upon arrival at the hospital, you will turn the patient over to hospital personnel. You will provide information on the patient's condition, your observations of the scene, and other pertinent data so that there will be continuity in the patient's care. Although this part of patient care comes at the end of the call, it is very important. You must never abandon care of the patient at the hospital until transfer to hospital personnel has been properly completed.

- **Patient advocacy.** As an EMT, you are there for your patient. You are an advocate, the person who speaks up for your patient and pleads his cause. It is your responsibility to address the patient's needs and to bring any of his concerns to the attention of the hospital staff. You will have developed a rapport with the patient during your brief but very important time together, a rapport that gives you an understanding of his condition and needs. As an advocate, you will do your best to transmit this knowledge in order to help the patient continue through the EMS and hospital system. In your role as an advocate, you may perform a task as important as reporting information that will enable the hospital staff to save the patient's life—or as simple as making sure a relative of the patient is notified. Acts that may seem minor to you may often provide major comfort to your patient.

EMTs may also be involved in community health initiatives such as injury prevention. The EMT is in a position to observe situations where injuries are possible and help correct them before injuries, or further injuries, are sustained. Hospital personnel do not see the scene and cannot offer this information. An example might be a call to the residence of a senior citizen who has fallen. You make observations about improper railings or slippery throw rugs or shoes and bring this to the attention of the patient and his family. Another place where injury prevention may be beneficial is with children. If you respond to a residence where there are small children and you observe potential for injury (e.g., poisons the child can access or unsafe conditions such as a loose railing), your interventions can make a difference. These community health issues are discussed throughout the book and can be found in Chapter 23, "Poisoning and Overdose Emergencies," Chapter 35, "Pediatric Emergencies," and Chapter 36, "Geriatric Emergencies."

Traits of a Good EMT

Certain physical traits and aspects of personality are desirable for an EMT.

Physical Traits

Physically, you should be in good health and fit to carry out your duties. If you are unable to provide needed care because you cannot bend over or catch your breath, then all your training may be worthless to the patient who is in need of your help.

You should be able to lift and carry up to 125 pounds. Practice with other EMTs is essential so that you can learn how to carry your share of the combined weight of the patient, stretcher, linens, blankets, and portable oxygen equipment. For such moves, coordination and dexterity are needed, as well as strength. You will have to perform basic rescue procedures, lower stretchers and patients from upper levels, and negotiate fire escapes and stairways while carrying patients.

Your eyesight is very important in performing your EMT duties. Make certain that you can clearly see distant objects as well as those close at hand. Both types of vision are needed for patient assessment, reading labels, controlling emergency scenes, and driving. Should you have any eyesight problems, they must be corrected with prescription eyeglasses or contact lenses.

Be aware of any problems you may have with color vision. Not only is this important to driving, but it could also be critical for patient assessment. Color of the patient's skin, lips, and nail beds often provides valuable clues to the patient's condition.

You should be able to give and receive oral and written instructions and communicate with the patient, bystanders, and other members of the EMS system. Eyesight, hearing, and speech are important to the EMT; thus, any significant problems must be corrected if you are going to be an EMT.

Personal Traits

Good personal traits are very important to the EMT. You should be:

- *Pleasant* to inspire confidence and help to calm the sick and injured.
- *Sincere* to be able to convey an understanding of the situation and the patient's feelings.
- *Cooperative* to allow for faster and better care, establish better coordination with other members of the EMS system, and bolster the confidence of patients and bystanders.
- *Resourceful* to be able to adapt a tool or technique to fit an unusual situation.
- *A self-starter* to show initiative and accomplish what must be done without having to depend on someone else to start procedures.
- *Emotionally stable* to help overcome the unpleasant aspects of an emergency so that needed care may be rendered and any uneasy feelings that exist afterward may be resolved.
- *Able to lead* in order to take the steps necessary to control a scene, organize bystanders, deliver emergency care, and, when necessary, take charge.
- *Neat and clean* to promote confidence in both patients and bystanders and to reduce the possibility of contamination (Figure 1-3).
- *Of good moral character and respectful of others* to allow for trust in situations when the patient cannot protect his own body or valuables and so that all information relayed is truthful and reliable.
- *In control of personal habits* to reduce the possibility of rendering improper care and to prevent patient discomfort. This includes never consuming alcohol within eight hours of duty and not smoking when providing care. (Remember: Smoking can contaminate wounds and is dangerous around oxygen delivery systems.)
- *Controlled in conversation and able to communicate properly* in order to inspire confidence and avoid inappropriate conversation that may upset or anger the patient or bystanders or violate patient confidentiality.
- *Able to listen to others* to be compassionate and empathetic, to be accurate with interviews, and to inspire confidence.

FIGURE 1-3 A professional appearance inspires confidence.

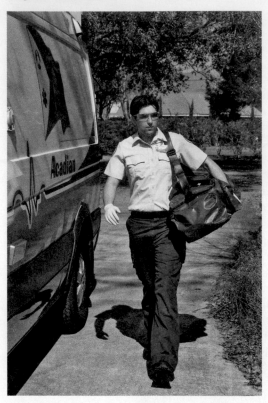

FIGURE 1-4 Your patients may come from a wide variety of cultures. As an example, Muslims such as this woman from Afghanistan have standards of modesty that may require examination by an EMT of the same sex.

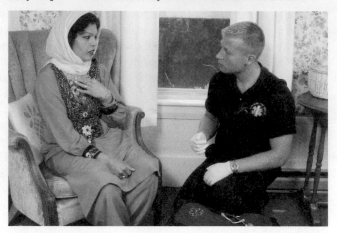

- *Nonjudgmental and fair,* treating all patients equally regardless of race, religion, or culture. There are many cultural differences you will encounter among patients. Figure 1-4 highlights one example of the cultures you may encounter in EMS. You will find additional features involving cultural issues throughout the book.

Education

An EMT must also maintain up-to-date knowledge and skills. Since ongoing research in emergency care causes occasional changes in procedure, some of the information you receive while you are studying to become an EMT will become outdated during your career.

There are many ways to stay current. One way is through refresher training. Most areas require recertification at regular intervals. Refresher courses present material to the EMT who has already been through a full course but needs to receive updated information. Refresher courses, which are usually shorter than original courses, are required at 2- to 4-year intervals.

Continuing education is another way to stay current. This type of training supplements the EMT's original course. It should not take the place of original training. For example, you may wish to learn more about pediatric or trauma skills or driving techniques. You can obtain this education in conferences and seminars and through lectures, classes, videos, or demonstrations.

It is important for you to realize that education is a constant process that extends long past your original EMT course.

Where Will You Become a Provider?

As an EMT, you will have a wide variety of opportunities to use the skills you will learn in class. EMTs are employed in public and private settings, such as fire departments, ambulance services, and rural/wilderness or urban/industrial settings (Figure 1-5). In fact, many fire departments require their firefighters to be cross-trained as both firefighters and EMTs.

You may be taking this course to volunteer. A large portion of the United States is served by volunteer fire and emergency medical services. Your willingness to participate in training to help others is both necessary for and appreciated by your community.

FIGURE 1-5 There is a wide variety of career opportunities for EMTs, including work in (A) urban/industrial settings and (B) rural/wilderness settings. *(Photo B: © Kevin Link)*

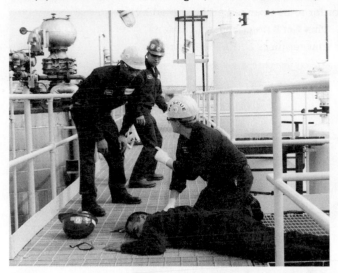

(A)

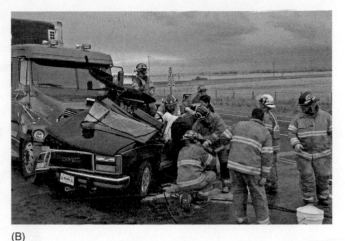

(B)

National Registry of Emergency Medical Technicians

The National Registry of Emergency Medical Technicians (NREMT), as part of its effort to establish and maintain national standards for EMTs, provides registration to EMRs, EMTs, AEMTs, and Paramedics. Registration is obtained by successfully completing NREMT practical and computer-based knowledge examinations. Holding an NREMT registration may help in reciprocity (transferring to another state or region). It is usually considered favorably when you apply for employment, even in areas where NREMT registration is not required (Figure 1-6).

Many states use the National Registry examinations as their certification exams. If your state or region does not use the registry exam, ask your instructor how you can sit for the examination. Upon passing the exam and obtaining registry, you will be entitled to wear the NREMT patch.

The National Registry is also active in EMS curriculum development and other issues that affect EMS today. For information, contact:

National Registry of Emergency Medical Technicians
6610 Busch Boulevard
P.O. Box 29233
Columbus, OH 43229
614-888-4484
www.nremt.org

Quality Improvement

Quality improvement, an important concept in EMS, consists of continuous self-review with the purpose of identifying aspects of the system that require improvement. Once a problem is identified, a plan is developed and implemented to prevent further occurrences of the same problem. As implied by the name, quality improvement is designed and performed to ensure that the public receives the highest quality prehospital care.

A sample quality improvement review might go as follows:

As part of a continuous review of calls, the Quality Improvement (QI) committee has reviewed all of your squad's run reports that involve trauma during one particular month. The committee has noted that the time spent at the scene of serious trauma calls was excessive. (You will learn later that time at the scene of serious trauma should be kept to a minimum, because the injured patient must be transported to the hospital for care that cannot be provided in the field.)

CORE CONCEPT ●-----

The process of EMS quality improvement (QI)

quality improvement
a process of continuous self-review with the purpose of identifying and correcting aspects of the system that require improvement.

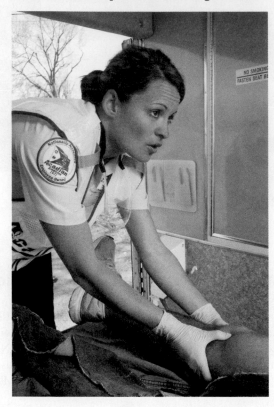

In many states, an EMT candidate must have passed the NREMT exam in order to be licensed and certified by the state. This EMT practices in Louisiana, one state that requires NREMT registration.

The QI committee has brought this fact to the attention of the Medical Director and the leadership of the ambulance squad. As a result, better protocols have been instituted. Monthly squad training is developed that covers topics such as how to identify serious trauma patients and then requires skill practice to reinforce techniques of trauma care. (Later in the year, the QI committee will review the same criteria to ensure that the extra training has been effective in improving the areas that were found to be deficient.)

During the review, the QI committee has also identified calls during which the crews followed procedures and performed well. A letter has been sent to these EMTs commending them for their efforts.

As an EMT, you will have a role in the quality improvement process. In fact, a dedication to quality can be one of the strongest assets of an EMT. There are several ways you can work toward quality care. These include:

- **Preparing carefully written documentation.** Call reviews are based on the prehospital care reports that you and other crew members write. If a report is incomplete, it is difficult for a QI team to assess the events of a call. If you are ever involved in a lawsuit, an inaccurate or incomplete report may also be a cause for liability. Be sure the reports you write are neat, complete, and accurate.

- **Becoming involved in the quality process.** As you gain experience, you may wish to volunteer for assignment to the QI committee. In addition, quality improvement has a place on every call. An individual ambulance crew can perform a critique after each call to determine things that went well and others that may need improvement. Have another EMT or advanced EMT look over your report before turning it in to ensure that it is accurate and complete.

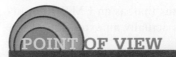
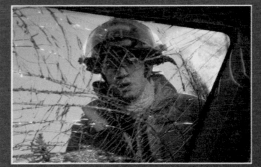

"I was driving along, not a care in the world, when all of a sudden this car pulled out from a side street—and pulled right in front of me. I couldn't brake in time. I couldn't steer in time. The crash made thunder seem like a whisper. I didn't just hear it. I felt it. The next thing I knew I was sitting in my car and it was smoky. I thought it was on fire. Then I noticed the air bag, which must've gone off. People were running up to my window to ask if I was OK. I felt so foggy I didn't even know what to say.

"A fireman came up to my window and asked how I was doing. By then I had a minute to think and compose myself. It felt like I'd cry if I opened my mouth to say anything. The ambulance came in and the EMTs and firefighters worked to get me out of the car. The fireman who came to my window must've climbed into the back seat. I could feel hands alongside my head.

"The collar felt like it was going to choke me. The board was uncomfortable. And everything was so, so loud. But what I remember most, more than the crash or the hospital or the bills, were the kind words the fireman said from behind me. In spite of everything going on that day, his reassuring, kind voice is my best memory from the whole miserable day. It was like an angel being there for me."

As you begin your training as an EMT you will learn many clinical skills. For this patient, you will perform an assessment, immobilize the neck and spine, take vital signs, and transport the patient—perhaps to a trauma center.

You will also provide emotional reassurance and support in this time of crisis. It has been said that you should treat your patients as you would want your family to be treated. This is a good rule.

"Point of View" features like this one will appear throughout the text. Their purpose is to present an emergency from the *patient's* perspective, or point of view, because understanding how the patient feels is a critical element in developing people skills. The clinical skills you learn are vital to your success in becoming an EMT. However, people skills are essential for you to thrive as an EMT.

- **Obtaining feedback from patients and the hospital staff.** This may be done informally or, in some cases, formally. Your organization may send a letter to patients that asks for comments on the care they were given while under your care. Hospital staff may be able to provide information that will help strengthen your caregiving skills.

- **Maintaining your equipment.** It will be difficult to provide quality care with substandard, damaged, or missing equipment. Although the ingenuity of EMTs should never be underestimated, it would be impossible to administer oxygen or provide cardiac defibrillation without proper, functional equipment. Check and maintain equipment regularly.

- **Continuing your education.** An EMT who was certified several years ago and has never attended subsequent training will have a problem providing quality care. Seldom-used skills deteriorate without practice. Procedures change. Without some form of regular continuing education, it will be difficult to maintain standards of quality.

Quality improvement is another name for providing the care that you would want to have provided to you or a loved one in a time of emergency. That is the best care possible. Maintaining continuous high quality is not easy; it requires constant attention and a sense of pride and obligation. Striving for quality—both in the care you personally give to patients and as a collective part of an ambulance squad—is to uphold the highest standards of the EMS system.

Medical Direction

Each EMS service or agency has a *Medical Director*, a physician who assumes the ultimate responsibility for *medical direction*, or oversight of the patient-care aspects of the EMS system. The Medical Director also oversees training, develops *protocols* (lists of steps for assessment and interventions to be performed in different situations), and is a crucial part of the quality improvement process. An EMT at a basic or advanced level is

Medical Director
a physician who assumes ultimate responsibility for the patient-care aspects of the EMS system.

medical direction
oversight of the patient-care aspects of an EMS system by the Medical Director.

protocols
lists of steps, such as assessments and interventions, to be taken in different situations. Protocols are developed by the Medical Director of an EMS system.

operating as a *designated agent* of the physician. This means that, as an EMT, your authority to give medications and provide emergency care is actually an extension of the Medical Director's license to practice medicine.

The physician obviously cannot physically be at every call. This is why EMS systems develop *standing orders*. The physician issues a policy or protocol that authorizes EMTs and others to perform particular skills in certain situations. An example may be the administration of glucose. Glucose is very beneficial to certain diabetic patients who are experiencing a medical emergency. The Medical Director issues a standing order that allows EMTs to give glucose in certain circumstances without speaking to the Medical Director or another physician. This kind of "behind the scenes" medical direction is called **off-line medical direction**.

Certain other procedures that are not covered by standing orders or protocols require the EMT to contact the on-duty physician by radio or telephone prior to performing a skill or administering a medication. For example, EMTs carry aspirin, which is beneficial to many—but not all—patients who have possible cardiac symptoms. Prior to administering aspirin, you may be required to consult with the on-duty physician. You would use a radio or cell phone from the ambulance to provide patient information to the physician. After receiving your information, the physician would instruct you on whether and how to administer the aspirin. Orders from the on-duty physician given by radio or phone are called **on-line medical direction**. On-line medical direction may be requested at any time you feel that medical advice would be beneficial to patient care.

Protocols and procedures for on-line and off-line medical direction vary from system to system. Your instructor will inform you what your local policies are. Always follow your local protocols.

Research

Medicine is based on research. Some of the procedures you will be trained to perform have been developed as a result of research—but not all. If you believe this should be changed you are not alone. Experts universally agree that research must play a greater role in EMS for it to continue to evolve as a respected profession. Many of the things we do are based on tradition—simply stated, because that is how we have always done them. Many other techniques were developed from hospital procedures and applied to the field.

Although teaching how to perform or even interpret research is beyond the scope of your EMT class, it is important for you to know the importance of research and how it will shape the future of EMS.

Two ways research impacts EMS is through a focus on improving *patient outcomes* and through *evidence-based* techniques.

Although our concern may seem to be whether patients make it to the hospital alive, we must remember that EMS is part of a larger system. What we do also affects the patient's long-term survival. If something appears to help in the short term but has no effect in the long term it is not useful. This research into long-term results (patient outcomes) allows us to make the best decisions for the patient's overall care.

Evidence-based decision making means that the procedures and knowledge we use in determining what care works is based on scientific evidence. A scenario involving evidence-based decision making might go like this:

> You are at the ambulance bay when an experienced member of your crew is talking with your Medical Director about adding a new medication to the EMT scope of practice. This member has heard that the new drug has been successful in other local squads and has seen it in magazines for EMS providers.
>
> Your Medical Director finds it interesting but asks the member for evidence. "Check the literature," he says. "If we can find evidence that this makes a difference in outcomes and doesn't have a significant risk, we'll take a look at it."

The evidence-based process here demonstrates the general procedures needed to make these decisions. It includes:

• **Forming a hypothesis.** In this case, the experienced provider felt that a new medication would be safe to use and beneficial.

FIGURE 1-7 Read and evaluate research.

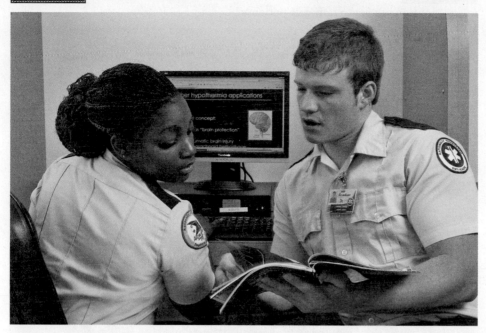

- **Reviewing literature.** The provider goes to the local college library and searches medical literature to determine if the new medication has been studied—especially for use by EMTs (Figure 1-7).

- **Evaluating the evidence.** The provider meets with the Medical Director to review the literature. If there was no literature they could decide to create a research project to study it in the organization or region.

- **Adopting the practice if evidence supports it.** It turns out that the medication has been studied and appears safe. The Medical Director is convinced that the medication should be brought into the EMT scope of practice. Training sessions are scheduled prior to implementation.

The EMS Role in Public Health

From clean drinking water and sewage systems to the decline of infectious diseases through vaccination, we have reaped the benefits of public health. Although public health has many definitions, it is considered the system by which the medical community oversees the basic health of a population. Additional efforts by the public health system include prenatal care, reducing injury in children and geriatric patients, and campaigns to reduce the use of tobacco.

EMS has a role in many public safety issues including:

- **Injury prevention for geriatric patients.** When on calls to a patient's home, the EMT can identify things that may cause falls such as footwear or rugs (Figure 1-8). EMS may also run blood pressure clinics and offer methods for the elderly to present medications and medical history to EMTs in the event of emergency (e.g., file of life).

- **Injury prevention for youth.** EMS is frequently involved in child safety seat clinics, distribution of bicycle helmets, and other programs for youth.

- **Public vaccination programs.** More and more EMS providers are being trained and allowed to provide vaccination clinics for the public. Seasonal flu and variations such as H1N1 are examples of vaccinations that are frequently offered by EMS providers. Some regions are beginning to allow specially trained EMS providers to take routine vaccinations (e.g., routine childhood vaccinations) out to the public—especially in areas where many children do not have routine well care and are at risk.

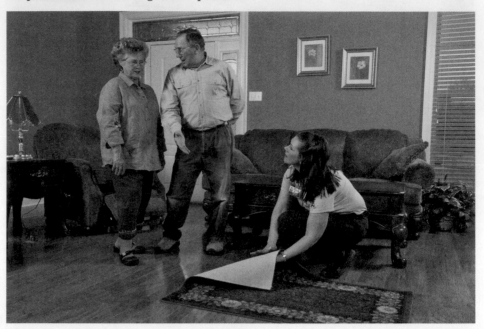

FIGURE 1-8 EMTs play important roles in public safety issues such as providing fall-prevention advice to geriatric patients.

- **Disease surveillance.** At the front lines EMS reports may serve as an indication that a trend in injury or disease is beginning. This may range from flu to violence to terrorist attacks.

Programs are developing around the country that utilize EMS providers in different and innovative public health roles. Unlike hospital or office-based medicine, EMS is always in the field, in patient's homes, and in the public eye. This visibility and access is vital to getting health services at the point they are needed and to identify areas where injuries and disease may be prevented.

One thing is certain—EMS does more than just respond to emergencies. In your future as an EMT you will likely take an even greater role in public health.

Special Issues

EMTs are people and people make mistakes. You may have seen in your local news about errors that have occurred in the hospital and have resulted in lawsuits. All of medicine—including EMS—recognizes this as a serious issue. Chapter 4, "Medical, Legal, and Ethical Issues," will cover this topic in detail.

In the coming weeks and through the chapters that follow in this textbook, you will be studying to become an EMT. As part of your course, your instructor will advise you on local issues and administrative matters, such as a course description, class meeting times, and criteria including physical and mental requirements for certification as an EMT, as well as specific statutes and regulations regarding EMS in your state, region, or locality.

The Americans with Disabilities Act (ADA) has set strict guidelines preserving the rights of Americans with disabilities. If you have a disability or have questions about the ADA, ask your instructor for more information.

CHAPTER REVIEW

Key Facts and Concepts

The EMS system has been developed to provide prehospital as well as hospital emergency care.

- The EMS system includes 911 or another emergency access system, dispatchers, EMTs, the hospital emergency department, physicians, nurses, physician's assistants, and other health professionals.
- The EMT's responsibilities include safety; patient assessment and care; lifting, moving, and transporting patients; transfer of care; and patient advocacy.

- An EMT must have certain personal and physical traits to ensure the ability to do the job.
- Education (including refresher training and continuing education), quality improvement procedures, and medical direction are all essential to maintaining high standards of EMS care.

Key Decisions

Making accurate decisions in patient care is the hallmark of a competent EMT. This feature will be used throughout this text to help you identify these important decisions and relate their importance in emergency care.

Since this is a nonclinical chapter, picture yourself applying for a job or being interviewed for membership in a volunteer squad. How would you answer the following questions asked in the interview?

- Do you think EMS makes a difference? Why?
- If EMS is about helping people, how do you anticipate helping people as an EMT?
- Can EMS have a role in injury prevention or public health?
- How will EMS look in the future?

Chapter Glossary

designated agent an EMT or other person authorized by a Medical Director to give medications and provide emergency care. The transfer of such authorization to a designated agent is an extension of the Medical Director's license to practice medicine.

evidence-based description of medical techniques or practices that are supported by scientific evidence of their safety and efficacy, rather than merely by supposition and tradition..

medical direction oversight of the patient-care aspects of an EMS system by the Medical Director. **Off-line medical direction** consists of standing orders issued by the Medical Director that allow EMTs to give certain medications or perform certain procedures without speaking to the Medical Director or another physician. **On-line medical direction** consists of orders given directly by the on-duty physician to an EMT in the field by radio or telephone.

Medical Director a physician who assumes ultimate responsibility for the patient-care aspects of the EMS system.

911 system a system for telephone access to report emergencies. A dispatcher takes the information and alerts EMS or the fire or police departments as needed. *Enhanced 911* has the additional capability of automatically identifying the caller's phone number and location.

patient outcomes the long-term survival of patients.

protocols lists of steps, such as assessments and interventions, to be taken in different situations. Protocols are developed by the Medical Director of an EMS system.

quality improvement a process of continuous self-review with the purpose of identifying and correcting aspects of the system that require improvement.

standing orders a policy or protocol issued by a Medical Director that authorizes EMTs and others to perform particular skills in certain situations.

Preparation for Your Examination and Practice

Short Answer

1. What are the components of the Emergency Medical Services system?

2. What are some of the special designations that hospitals may have? List them. Then name the special centers you have in your region.

3. What are the four national levels of EMS training and certification?

4. What are the roles and responsibilities of the EMT?

5. What are desirable personal and physical attributes of the EMT?

6. What is the definition of the term *quality improvement*?

7. What is the difference between on-line and off-line medical direction?

Critical Thinking Exercises

Of course you want to be the best EMT you can be. The purpose of this exercise will be to consider some ways to accomplish that goal.

1. What qualities would you like to see in an EMT who is caring for you? How can you come closer to being this kind of EMT?

2. You are devoting a considerable amount of time to becoming an EMT. How do you plan to refresh your knowledge and stay current once you are out of the classroom?

Street Scenes

As a new EMT, you are assigned to Station 2 to ride with Susan Miller, a seasoned EMS veteran with 7 years on the job. You have heard that she is a good EMT, and you remember that she helped teach some of your skill sessions. She was a good instructor—patient, understanding, and considerate.

When you arrive at the station, you find out she has been delayed and you will be riding with Chuck Hartley instead. When you are introduced to Chuck, you see that his uniform is unkempt. He tells you to sit until he needs you.

Your first call of the day is a 70-year-old female with abdominal pain. As you approach the ambulance, Chuck tells you to get in the back. He'll let you know when you can help. At the scene, after ensuring scene safety, you both enter the patient's home. Chuck doesn't bother to introduce himself and proceeds to ask the patient, "What's wrong, Hon?" She describes her symptoms. Chuck tells you to put her on a nasal cannula. As you hook up the O_2, Chuck says in a loud voice, "Didn't you learn anything in EMT class? That liter flow rate is too high."

As the patient is being loaded onto the stretcher, she tries to tell Chuck something that she obviously believes is urgent. Chuck tells her that if it's that important, she can tell the doctor at the hospital.

Street Scene Questions

1. What would have been a more appropriate action for Chuck when the shift started?

2. What behavior characteristics of Chuck's would be considered unprofessional?

3. What would you expect from someone providing initial field training?

When you return to the station, Susan Miller has arrived. This time, when you are introduced, you notice that her uniform is pressed and neat. She asks you about your background and when you finished training. She remembers you from class, she says. Then she tells you there are some things you both need to do. "First, let's go to the ambulance and check the equipment. Next, I want to explain how we operate on calls. You need to know what equipment we always take to the patient and responsibilities of the crew members."

Just as you are completing your orientation, a call comes in for a 55-year-old male with chest pain. While en route, Susan briefly goes over the routine that she and her partner use. She asks you to take the automatic defibrillator. When you enter the patient's house, Susan introduces herself and the members of the crew. She asks the patient: "Sir, why did you call 911?" He tells you that he had chest pain but he took a nitroglycerin tablet and now most of the pain is gone. He apologizes for calling.

While you get the vital signs, Susan tells the patient that he did just the right thing by calling EMS. He is reassured and agrees to be transported for further evaluation.

Street Scene Questions

4. What did Susan Miller do that was appropriate and professional?

5. How was Susan's behavior beneficial to you as a new EMT?

6. What personal traits are the professional standards for EMTs?

During the trip to the hospital Susan continues to reassure the patient. In fact, she tells you to talk to the patient about his medical history. When you arrive at the hospital, Susan sees that the oxygen tank is getting low, so she asks you to switch "bottles" before moving the patient, but you forget to turn off the tank being replaced. Susan turns it off, sets it aside, looks you in the eyes, and gives you a smile. You both know that you will not forget the next time.

After the call, Susan gives a short critique and discusses the prehospital care report. When you call back in service, you realize that to be a good EMT you not only need to have good technical skills but, just as important, you also must act as a professional with your patients and with your colleagues.

The Well-Being of the EMT

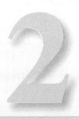

STANDARD ○------
Preparatory (Workforce Safety and Wellness)

COMPETENCY ○------
Uses fundamental knowledge of the EMS system, safety/well-being of the EMT, medical/legal and ethical issues to the provision of emergency care.

CORE CONCEPTS ○------
— Standard Precautions, or how to protect yourself from transmitted diseases

— The kinds of stress caused by involvement in EMS and how they can affect you, your fellow EMTs, and your family and friends

— The impact that dying patients have on you and others

— How to identify potential hazards and maintain scene safety

EXPLORE Resource Central

To access Resource Central, follow directions on the Student Access Card provided with this text. If there is no card, go to **www.bradybooks.com** and follow the Resource Central link to Buy Access from there. Under Media Resources, you will find:

▸ **Putting on Gloves**
View a video on putting on gloves. There's a right way and wrong way to do things, so pay attention and keep yourself safe. You don't want to miss the part on how to properly remove contaminated gloves!

▸ **Stress Management**
Explore your options! Massage, yoga, and even effective time management can help relieve stress. How? Click on the links to find out. Don't think you need any help? Read about the effects of stress on an EMT and expand your mind!

▸ **Hepatitis B and the Health Care Worker**
Read and discuss why EMS professionals should receive the hepatitis B vaccination and what steps you should take if you are exposed.

OBJECTIVES

After reading this chapter you should be able to:

2.1 Define key terms introduced in this chapter.

2.2 Describe health habits that promote physical and mental well-being. (pp. 22–23)

2.3 Given an example of a patient-care situation, determine the appropriate personal protective equipment to prevent exposure to infectious disease. (pp. 23–28)

2.4 Describe proper procedures for hand washing and using alcohol-based hand cleaners. (p. 26)

2.5 Discuss the health concerns related to exposure to hepatitis B, hepatitis C, tuberculosis, and AIDS. (pp. 28–30)

2.6 Access the Centers for Disease Control web site to obtain the latest information on diseases of concern to EMS providers. (p. 30)

2.7 Explain the essential provisions of OSHA, the CDC, and the Ryan White CARE Act as they relate to infection control in EMS. (pp. 30–35)

2.8 Describe the indications for use of an N-95 or HEPA respirator. (p. 35)

(continued)

KEY TERMS

Learning how to safeguard your well-being as an EMT is critical. To do this, you will make several important decisions on each call—decisions such as determining if the scene is safe from a variety of hazards and which precautions you should take to avoid danger and protect yourself from disease.

This chapter will also teach you about stress. During your EMS career, you will be exposed to all kinds of stress, including that which accompanies death and dying.

Remember: If the EMT becomes a patient, he is of little or no use to a patient and even may put other rescuers in jeopardy. Most EMS calls are safe. This chapter will help you deal safely and appropriately with the ones that aren't.

>>>>>> WELL-BEING

Prevention is a hot topic. Our physicians stress this when we see them. Eat right, lose weight, exercise. This advice—and this chapter—are designed to promote your overall well-being. This section begins the well-being chapter with some important concepts designed to help you obtain and maintain a state of well-being.

If you were faced with a dangerous situation, would you respond better if you were in shape? If you were faced with a challenging situation where you had to drag or carry a patient several hundred feet to safety, would you do better if you were in shape? If you were faced with a call that hit you hard emotionally, would you get through it better if you were in a better physical and mental place?

The answer to all these questions is yes. And the concepts of well-being aren't difficult if you start and maintain some healthy habits. These include:

- **Maintaining solid personal relationships.** If you have a difficult call, you will do better dealing with it if you have a support system. Family, EMS colleagues, and friends who are there for you every day and in difficult times are vital for well-being.

- **Exercise.** An exercise program helps you in many ways. A well-designed program helps you build strength and improve flexibility and also promotes cardiovascular fitness. An exercise regime is also an important part of a weight-loss program.

- **Sleep.** Rest is important. Lack of sleep can be a significant factor in medical errors and improper decision making. Fatigue also increases the potential for motor-vehicle collisions, harms personal relationships, and can lead to frequent illnesses by decreasing immune system function.

- **Eat right.** Eating provides fuel for the body—especially during long EMS shifts and with strenuous activities. Eating the right foods rather than wolfing down junk foods is critical.

- **Limit alcohol and caffeine intake.** Although alcohol may be enjoyable in moderation, excess intake reduces performance and brings on personal, medical, and social issues. Caffeine may seem like a pick-me-up at the moment, but as the saying goes, what goes up must come down. Your body will take only so much artificial stimulation before it crashes. Plus, even though you feel more awake when jazzed on caffeine, your decision making and reaction times can still be impaired.

- **See your physician regularly and keep up-to-date on vaccines.** Bringing this well-being section full circle: Regular check-ups help ensure we are well—and can help prevent or catch any serious issues before they arise.

The topics that follow in this book involve safety and response to danger, decision making, lifting and moving, and others—all of which will be better performed if you are well and, if well performed, can help keep you well. The section in dealing with stress lists all of the items just listed as ways to deal with stress. It is reasonable to expect that practicing wellness daily would eliminate or significantly reduce stress. Why not do it now?

PERSONAL PROTECTION

Standard Precautions

Diseases are caused by *pathogens*, organisms that cause infection, such as viruses and bacteria. Pathogens may be spread through the air or by contact with blood and other body fluids. *Bloodborne pathogens* can be contracted by exposure to the patient's blood and sometimes other body fluids, especially when they come in contact with an open wound or sore on the EMT's hands, face, or other exposed parts including mucous membranes, such as those in the nose, mouth, or eyes. Even minor breaks in the skin, such as those found around fingernails, can be enough for a pathogen to enter your body. *Airborne pathogens* are spread by tiny droplets sprayed during breathing, coughing, or sneezing. These particles can be absorbed through your eyes or when you inhale.

Since it is impossible for an EMT or other health care professional to identify patients who carry infectious diseases just by looking at them, all body fluids must be considered infectious, and appropriate precautions taken for all patients at all times.

Equipment and procedures that protect you from the blood and body fluids of the patient—and protect the patient from your blood and body fluids as well—are referred to as **Standard Precautions**, also known as body substance isolation (BSI) precautions or infection control. For each situation you encounter, it is important to apply the appropriate precautions. Taking too few will clearly increase your risk of exposure to disease. Too many can potentially alienate the patient and reduce your effectiveness.

Your selection of which Standard Precautions to use is one of the most important decisions you will make on any call. You will make this decision initially upon seeing the patient and reconsider it throughout the call as the patient's condition changes.

CORE CONCEPT ●
Standard Precautions, or how to protect yourself from transmitted diseases

pathogens
the organisms that cause infection, such as viruses and bacteria.

Standard Precautions
a strict form of infection control that is based on the assumption that all blood and other body fluids are infectious.

CRITICAL DECISION MAKING

Standard Precautions

Although you may be thinking that the most important decisions you will make as an EMT have to do with clinical situations affecting your patient, some of the most important decisions you will make actually have to do with routine things such as Standard Precautions.

Be sure you always carry gloves on your person and have face protection immediately available in kits (e.g., first-in bags) and suction units. Your decision about the level of precautions to take will initially be determined as part of the scene size-up (the first part of the patient assessment process you will learn about in Chapter 10, "Scene Size-Up"). Take precautions against anything you see *or anything you reasonably expect to encounter.* Some examples include:

1. When called to a motor-vehicle collision where you observe broken glass, you should expect broken skin and the potential for contact with blood—even if you don't see wounds. Wearing nonlatex gloves to protect you from blood as well as heavy-duty gloves to protect you from the broken glass is prudent.

2. When called to a nursing home for an interfacility transfer, you must reach under the patient to move the person to your stretcher. Because of the possibility of contact with urine, feces, or bed sores, you should wear nonlatex gloves.

3. You are called to a patient with a sprained ankle. There are no open wounds. Guidelines indicate that no precautions are necessary, although many routinely wear gloves on all calls.

4. You are working with an advanced life support crew treating a patient with chest pain. Although there are no open wounds, the paramedic started an IV and some blood is present on the patient's forearm from the IV start. In addition, a small amount is seen on the IV tubing. Gloves are required.

Your decisions about Standard Precautions do not end at the scene size-up. In fact, you should be alert for changes throughout the call. For example:

5. You are treating a patient with chest pain who suddenly becomes unresponsive. The patient requires suction. In addition to the gloves you may already be wearing, you will now need to protect your face from spatter encountered in airway and suction procedures.

---

personal protective equipment (PPE)

equipment that protects the EMS worker from infection and/or exposure to the dangers of rescue operations.

The Occupational Safety and Health Administration (OSHA) has issued strict guidelines about precautions against exposure to bloodborne pathogens. Under the OSHA guidelines, employers and employees share responsibility for these precautions. Employers must develop a written exposure control plan and must provide emergency care providers with training, immunizations, and proper *personal protective equipment (PPE)* to prevent transmission of disease. (Volunteer organizations are also required to provide these services for their members.) The employee's responsibility is to participate in the training and to follow the exposure control plan.

There is also a requirement for all agencies to have a written policy in place in the event of an exposure to infectious substances. Any contact such as a needlestick or contact with a potentially infectious fluid must be documented. Refer to your local policy's guidelines for reporting an exposure incident. Most plans call for baseline testing of the exposed person immediately following the exposure and periodic follow-up testing. Additionally, federal legislation has made it possible for emergency care providers to be notified if a patient with whom they have had potentially infectious contact turns out to be infected by a disease or virus such as tuberculosis (TB), hepatitis B, or HIV (the virus associated with AIDS).

Although deciding on and taking Standard Precautions may seem intimidating—especially if you are just beginning your training—remember that it is possible, by following the proper precautions, to have a long and safe career in EMS free from infection and disease.

FIGURE 2-1 Always wear personal protective equipment to prevent exposure to contagious diseases.

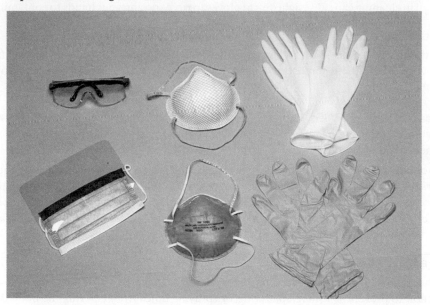

Personal Protective Equipment

Protect yourself from all possible routes of *contamination*, or introduction of disease or infectious materials. Follow Standard Precaution guidelines and wear the appropriate personal protective equipment on every call (Figure 2-1).

Protective Gloves

Vinyl or other nonlatex gloves should be used whenever there is the potential for contact with blood and other body fluids. This includes actions such as controlling bleeding, suctioning, artificial ventilation, and CPR. Make sure that you have the gloves on or available before you come in contact with a patient. Otherwise, you might get distracted and forget the gloves and may accidentally become contaminated. Be sure to change gloves between patients.

In many years of using latex in health care—in both hospital and prehospital environments—many patients and providers developed allergies to latex. The gloves you will see in the ambulance are now latex-free, as are oxygen delivery devices and other supplies.

contamination
the introduction of dangerous chemicals, disease, or infectious materials.

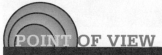

POINT OF VIEW

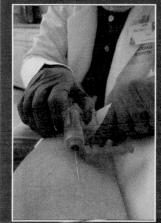

"I consider myself careful. I wear gloves on every call. But here I am getting blood drawn because I had an exposure to a patient's blood.

"I'm really not sure when or how it happened. I guess I put on gloves and then was on autopilot. I didn't notice they had a rip in them. Making things worse, I had a cut on my finger. Murphy's Law—the cut was right near the tear in the glove. It didn't even seem like a lot of blood at the scene. I looked at my glove. Saw the tear. Took off the glove and saw the blood on my open skin. My heart sank.

"Now the nurse will draw blood. Then I have to talk with a counselor. I'll get more blood drawn every so often. I already dread waiting to get the results—wondering if I'll get sick.

"Trust me. Never take Standard Precautions lightly. Think about them during the call. If I did, I would've seen that tear in my gloves. And my life would be very different. I'd give anything not to be sitting here right now."

A different type of glove must be worn when you clean the ambulance and soiled equipment. This glove should be heavyweight and tear-resistant. The force and type of movements involved in cleaning can cause lightweight gloves to rip, exposing your hands to contamination.

Hand Washing

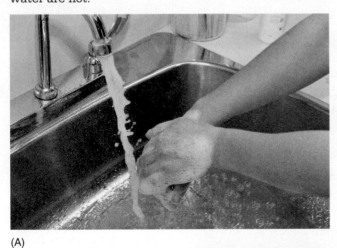

"Everyone thinks to wear gloves. Remember to protect your eyes and face as well."

Even though you wear gloves when assessing and caring for patients, you must still wash your hands after patient contacts when gloves are removed. There are two methods of hand cleaning (Figure 2-2):

- **Hand washing.** When soap and water are available, vigorous hand washing is recommended. Wash your hands after each patient contact (even if you were wearing gloves) and whenever they become visibly soiled.
- **Alcohol-based hand cleaners.** These cleaners are considered effective by the Centers for Disease Control (CDC)—except when hands are visibly soiled or when anthrax is present—and are often available when soap and water are not. The alcohol helps kill microorganisms. Place the amount of hand cleaner recommended by the manufacturer in one palm and rub it so it covers your hands. Rub until dry.

Eye and Face Protection

The mucous membranes surrounding the eyes are capable of absorbing fluids. Wear eye protection to prevent splashing, spattering, or spraying fluids from entering the body through these membranes. Protective eyewear should provide protection from the front and the sides.

FIGURE 2-2 (A) Careful, methodical hand washing is effective in reducing exposure to contagious disease. (B) Use a paper towel to turn off the faucet. (C) Alcohol-based hand cleaners are effective and often available when soap and water are not.

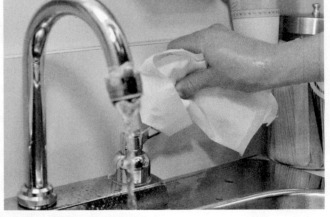

(A)

(B)

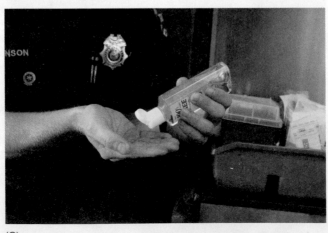

(C)

FIGURE 2-3 Wear a NIOSH-approved respirator when you suspect a patient may have tuberculosis.

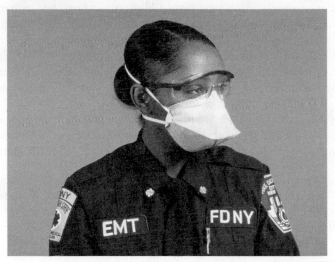

Various types of eyewear are on the market. If you wear prescription eyeglasses, clip-on side protectors are available. Some companies offer protective eyewear that resembles eyeglasses.

Masks

In cases where there will be blood or fluid spatter, wear a surgical-type mask. In cases where tuberculosis (a disease that is carried by fine particles in the air) is suspected, an N-95 or a high efficiency particulate air (HEPA) respirator approved by the National Institute for Occupational Safety and Health (NIOSH) is the standard (Figure 2-3). Face shields offer protection of the entire face by use of a mask with an attached see-through shield that covers the eyes (Figure 2-4).

In some jurisdictions, when a patient is suspected of having an infection spread by droplets (such as flu or measles), a surgical-type mask may be placed on the patient if he is alert and cooperative.

NOTE: *When you cover a patient's mouth and nose with a mask of any kind, use caution. The mask reduces your ability to visualize and protect the airway. Monitor respirations and be prepared to remove the mask and use suction to clear the airway if necessary (see Chapter 8, "Airway Management," and Chapter 9, "Respiration and Artificial Ventilation").*

FIGURE 2-4 Wear a protective mask and face shield when suctioning a patient.

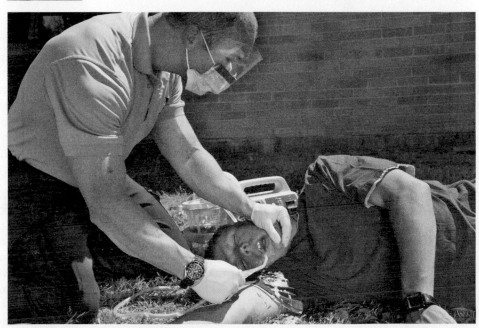

Gowns

A gown is worn to protect clothing and bare skin from spilled or splashed fluids. Arterial (spurting) bleeding is an indication for a gown. Childbirth and patients with multiple injuries also often produce considerable amounts of blood. Any situation that would call for the use of a gown would also require gloves, eye protection, and a mask.

It is a good idea not only to use personal protective equipment yourself but also to be an advocate for its use; that is, to encourage members of your crew and others to use appropriate protective equipment. In addition to the moral and ethical obligation to do so, you will be helping to keep your crew in good health.

Always properly remove and discard protective garments after use, carry out disinfection and cleaning operations, and complete all reporting documentation regarding infection control. You will learn more about these procedures in Chapter 38, "EMS Operations."

NOTE: *When you finish your EMT training and begin in the field, you will observe differences in the methods and levels of Standard Precautions taken by those around you. You will likely notice that some EMTs don gloves and protective eyewear before exiting the ambulance and wear them throughout the call. Others will go through an entire call without even wearing gloves.*

In the 1980s an increased emphasis was placed on body substance isolation. Diseases such as AIDS and hepatitis brought a startling reality to the health care profession. As a result, gloves, protective eyewear, and masks were used with increasing frequency. These items were worn as a "precaution," even when not technically necessary.

Today, providers have a more realistic attitude about Standard Precautions. Think back to your last physical examination, for example. Your physician most likely examined your eyes and ears, palpated your abdomen, and performed other examinations without gloves. Why is this? Because it is not necessary to wear gloves if your skin and the skin of your patient is intact. Additionally, wearing gloves while you exit the ambulance, carry equipment, and enter a scene may cause the gloves to rip before you reach the patient, rendering them ineffective.

Common sense should be the rule. To protect yourself from disease:

- *Follow Standard Precaution guidelines as outlined in this chapter and in the rules and policies of your organization.*

- *Always have personal protective equipment immediately available on your person and in kits.*

- *Carry two sets of gloves—one to put on when you encounter infectious substances and another in the event your gloves tear or become soiled.*

- *If in doubt, take Standard Precautions.*

DISEASES OF CONCERN

The communicable diseases we are most concerned with are caused by bloodborne and airborne pathogens such as viruses, bacteria, and other harmful organisms. Bloodborne pathogens are contracted by exposure to an infected patient's blood, especially exposure through breaks in the noninfected person's skin. Airborne pathogens are spread by tiny droplets sprayed when a patient breathes, coughs, or sneezes. These droplets are inhaled or are absorbed through the noninfected person's eyes, mouth, or nose.

Although there are many communicable diseases (Table 2-1), four are of particular concern: hepatitis B, hepatitis C, tuberculosis, and HIV/AIDS.

- *Hepatitis*, an infection that causes an inflammation of the liver, comes in several forms, including hepatitis A, B, C, and other strains. Hepatitis A is acquired primarily through contact with food or water contaminated by stool (feces). The other forms are acquired through contact with blood and other body fluids. The virus that causes hepatitis is especially hardy. Hepatitis B has been found to live for many days in dried blood spills, posing a risk of transmission long after many other viruses would have died. For this reason, it is critical for you to assume that any body fluid in any form, dried or otherwise, is infectious until proven otherwise. Hepatitis B can be deadly. Before hepatitis B vaccine was available, the virus (HBV) killed hundreds of health care

Table 2-1 Communicable Diseases

DISEASE	MODE OF TRANSMISSION	INCUBATION
AIDS (acquired immune deficiency syndrome)	HIV-infected blood via intravenous drug use, unprotected sexual contact, blood transfusions, or (rarely) accidental needlesticks. Mothers also may pass HIV to their unborn children.	Several months or years
Chicken pox (varicella)	Airborne droplets. Can also be spread by contact with open sores.	11 to 21 days
German measles (rubella)	Airborne droplets. Mothers may pass the disease to unborn children.	10 to 12 days
H1N1 (flu)	Respiratory droplet.	1 to 7 days
Hepatitis	Blood, stool, or other body fluids, or contaminated objects.	Weeks to months, depending on type
Meningitis, bacterial	Oral and nasal secretions.	2 to 10 days
Mumps	Droplets of saliva or objects contaminated by saliva.	14 to 24 days
Pneumonia, bacterial and viral	Oral and nasal droplets and secretions.	Several days
Staphylococcal skin infections	Direct contact with infected wounds or sores or with contaminated objects.	Several days
Tuberculosis (TB)	Respiratory secretions, airborne or on contaminated objects.	2 to 6 weeks
Whooping cough (pertussis)	Respiratory secretions or airborne droplets.	6 to 20 days

workers every year in the United States, more than any other occupationally acquired infectious disease. There is no cure, but an effective vaccine that prevents contracting HBV is available. (See "Immunizations" in this chapter.) Today, hepatitis C infects many EMS providers in the same way as hepatitis B, yet there is no vaccine against hepatitis C.

- *Tuberculosis (TB)* is an infection that sometimes settles in the lungs and that in some cases can be fatal. It was once thought to be largely eradicated, but in the late 1980s it made a comeback. TB is highly contagious. Unlike many other infectious diseases, it can spread through the air. Health care workers and others can become infected even without any direct contact with a carrier. Because it is impossible for the EMT to determine why a patient has a productive cough, it is safest to assume that it could be the result of TB and that you should take the necessary respiratory precautions. This is especially true in institutions such as nursing homes, correctional facilities, or homeless shelters where there is an increased risk of TB.

- *AIDS (acquired immune deficiency syndrome)* is a set of conditions that results when the immune system has been attacked by HIV (human immunodeficiency virus) and rendered unable to combat certain infections adequately. Although advances are being made in the treatment of HIV/AIDS, no cure has been discovered at the time of publication of this text. However, HIV/AIDS presents far less risk to health care workers than hepatitis and TB, because the virus does not survive well outside the human body. This limits the routes of exposure to direct contact with blood by way of open wounds, intravenous drug use, unprotected sexual contact, or blood transfusions. Puncture wounds into which HIV is introduced, such as with an accidental needlestick, are also potential routes of infection. However, less than half of 1 percent of such incidents result in infection, according to the U.S. Occupational Safety and Health Administration (OSHA), compared to 30 percent for the hepatitis B virus (HBV). The difference is due to the quantity and strength of HBV compared to HIV.

Hepatitis B, hepatitis C, TB, and HIV/AIDS are the communicable diseases of greatest concern because they are potentially life threatening. However, there are many communicable diseases to which emergency response and other health care personnel may be exposed. Table 2-1 lists common communicable diseases, their modes of transmission, and their incubation periods (the time between contact and the first appearance of symptoms).

Emerging Diseases and Conditions

In recent years, some diseases have worsened and new ones have been discovered. West Nile virus, which originally was limited to Europe and Africa, has spread throughout the United States by mosquitoes, causing flu-like symptoms in mild cases and infections of the brain and meninges in severe cases.

Severe acute respiratory syndrome (SARS) has caused concern worldwide. SARS appears to be spread through respiratory droplets, by coughing, sneezing, or touching something contaminated and then touching your nose or eyes. It is a respiratory virus with symptoms that include fever, dry cough, and difficulty breathing. Protection against SARS in a patient-care setting includes frequent hand washing and the use of gloves, gowns, eye protection, and an N-95 respirator.

Avian flu is a disease found in poultry that can also affect humans. Outbreaks have been seen in Asia, the Near East, and Africa and have been fatal in about half the reported cases. The virus has not shown to be easily transmissible from human to human. Symptoms include traditional flu-like symptoms that progress to more severe conditions such as pneumonia and acute respiratory distress syndrome. Precautions against this condition are the same as those just listed for SARS.

Influenza has been around for hundreds of years. The influenza pandemic of 1918 killed between 30 and 50 million people around the world. There are many strains of flu including each year's seasonal flu. Recently the H1N1 (swine flu) virus has caused widespread illness and even greater panic. You will likely be called to treat and transport patients who have the flu or flu-like symptoms. Take Standard Precautions for respiratory diseases and treat the patient as you will be trained to do during your course.

One additional effect of the H1N1 flu has been to quicken the pace at which EMS becomes involved in public health endeavors. EMS is on the front lines of flu care, responding to many calls for flu and flu-like symptoms. EMTs can help prevent the spread of flu by recognizing flu symptoms and placing a mask on any potential flu patient before entering the hospital. The Centers for Disease Control, state and local health agencies, and hospitals routinely communicate with EMS agencies to provide updates and advice on preventing the spread of flu and flu-care updates.

Many states have passed legislation that allows EMS providers to be more involved in public health efforts including administering vaccinations to the public (as will be discussed later in this chapter).

Interestingly, some diseases are also on the decline. For example, vaccines have significantly reduced the number of cases of chicken pox and epiglottitis in children.

Diseases of concern will change during the time you are an EMT. Your county or state health agencies will issue warnings and advisories on these diseases. You can also look for information from the Centers for Disease Control at www.cdc.gov.

Infection Control and the Law

Scientists have identified the main culprits in the transmission of many deadly infectious diseases: blood and body fluids. EMTs and other health care workers have been recognized as having a higher-than-usual exposure and, therefore, a higher risk of contracting these unwanted infections.

Congress and federal agencies have responded by taking several steps to ensure the safety of people who are in high-risk positions. In particular, the Occupational Safety and Health Administration (OSHA) of the U.S. Department of Labor and the Centers for Disease Control and Prevention (CDC) of the U.S. Department of Health and Human Services have issued standards and guidelines for the protection of workers whose jobs may expose them to infectious diseases. The Ryan White CARE Act establishes procedures by which emergency response workers may find out if they have been exposed to life-threatening infectious diseases. These legal protections are described in more detail in the next sections.

Occupational Exposure to Bloodborne Pathogens

In 1992, the OSHA standard on bloodborne pathogens took effect. It mandates employers of emergency responders must take certain measures to protect employees who are likely to be exposed to blood and other body fluids. One of the basic principles behind the standard is that infection control is a joint responsibility between employer and employee. The employer must provide training, protective equipment, and vaccinations to employees who are subject to exposure in their jobs. In return, employees must participate in an infection exposure control plan that includes training and proper workplace practices.

Without the active participation of both the employer and the employee, any workplace infection control program is destined to fail. Be sure your system has an active and up-to-date infection exposure control plan and that you and your fellow EMTs follow it carefully at all times. Consult with your state OSHA representative to make sure that specific hazards are identified and corrected.

Contact the U.S. Department of Labor to request the booklet *Occupational Exposure to Bloodborne Pathogens: Precautions for Emergency Responders—OSHA 3106 1998*, an overview of the standard. For details regarding how to develop an infection control plan, request Title 29 Code of Federal Regulation 1910.1030 for the complete text of the standard and all requirements regarding occupational exposure to bloodborne pathogens. Critical elements of the standard are summarized in the following list:

- **Infection exposure control plan.** Each emergency response employer must develop a plan that identifies and documents job classifications and tasks in which there is the possibility of exposure to potentially infectious body fluids. The plan must outline a schedule of how and when the bloodborne pathogen standards will be implemented. It also must include identification of the methods used for communicating hazards to employees, postexposure evaluation, and follow-up.

- **Adequate education and training.** EMTs must be provided with training that includes general explanations of how diseases are transmitted, uses and limitations of practices that reduce or prevent exposure, and procedures to follow if exposure occurs.

- **Hepatitis B vaccination.** Employers must make the hepatitis B vaccination series available free of charge and at a reasonable time and place.

- **Personal protective equipment.** This equipment must be of a quality that will not permit blood or other infectious materials to pass through or reach an EMT's work clothes, street clothes, undergarments, skin, eyes, mouth, or other mucous membranes. This equipment must be provided by the employer to the EMT at no cost and includes, but is not limited to, protective gloves, face shields, masks, protective eyewear, gowns, and aprons, plus bag-valve masks, pocket masks, and other ventilation devices.

- **Methods of control.** Engineering controls remove potential infectious disease hazards or separate the EMT from exposure. Examples include pocket masks, disposable airway equipment, and puncture-resistant needle containers. Work practice controls improve the manner in which a task is performed to reduce risk of exposure. Examples include the proper and safe use of personal protective equipment; proper handling, labeling, and disposal of contaminated materials; and proper washing and decontamination practices.

- **Housekeeping.** The EMT and the employer are both responsible for maintaining clean and sanitary conditions of the emergency response vehicles and work sites. Procedures include the proper handling and proper decontamination of work surfaces, equipment, laundry, and other materials.

- **Labeling.** The standard requires labeling of containers used to store, transport, or ship blood and other potentially infectious materials, including the use of the biohazard symbol (Figure 2-5).

- **Postexposure evaluation and follow-up.** EMTs must immediately report suspected exposure incidents—including mucous membrane or broken-skin contact with blood or other potentially infectious materials—that result from the performance of an employee's duties. (See Figure 2-6 for a model plan based on the Ryan White CARE Act, which is described next.)

FIGURE 2-5 The biohazard symbol must be included with warning labels for containers used to ship blood or other potentially infectious materials.

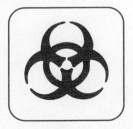

FIGURE 2-6 Under the Ryan White CARE Act, there is a procedure for finding out and following up if you have been exposed to a life-threatening disease.

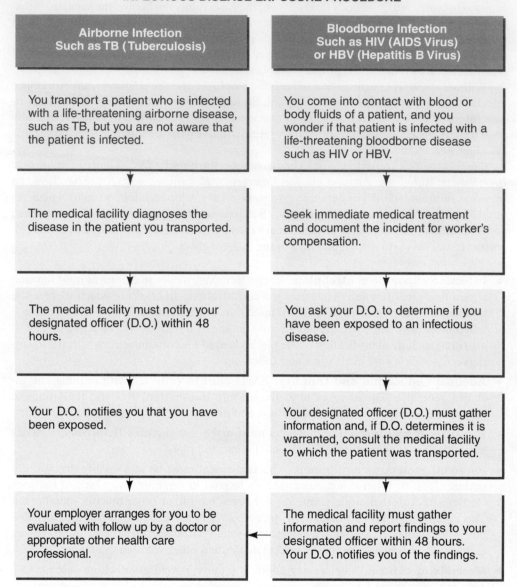

INFECTIOUS DISEASE EXPOSURE PROCEDURE

Airborne Infection Such as TB (Tuberculosis)	Bloodborne Infection Such as HIV (AIDS Virus) or HBV (Hepatitis B Virus)
You transport a patient who is infected with a life-threatening airborne disease, such as TB, but you are not aware that the patient is infected.	You come into contact with blood or body fluids of a patient, and you wonder if that patient is infected with a life-threatening bloodborne disease such as HIV or HBV.
The medical facility diagnoses the disease in the patient you transported.	Seek immediate medical treatment and document the incident for worker's compensation.
The medical facility must notify your designated officer (D.O.) within 48 hours.	You ask your D.O. to determine if you have been exposed to an infectious disease.
Your D.O. notifies you that you have been exposed.	Your designated officer (D.O.) must gather information and, if D.O. determines it is warranted, consult the medical facility to which the patient was transported.
Your employer arranges for you to be evaluated with follow up by a doctor or appropriate other health care professional.	The medical facility must gather information and report findings to your designated officer within 48 hours. Your D.O. notifies you of the findings.

Ryan White CARE Act

In 1994, the CDC issued the final notice for the Ryan White Comprehensive AIDS Resources Emergency (CARE) Act Regarding Emergency Response Employees. This federal act, which applies to all 50 states, mandates a procedure by which emergency response personnel can seek to find out if they have been exposed to potentially life-threatening diseases while providing patient care. Emergency response personnel referred to in this act include firefighters, law enforcement officers, EMTs, and other individuals who provide emergency aid on behalf of a legally recognized volunteer organization.

The CDC has published a list of potentially life-threatening infectious and communicable diseases to which emergency response personnel can be exposed. The list includes airborne diseases such as TB, bloodborne diseases such as hepatitis B and HIV/AIDS, and uncommon or rare diseases such as diphtheria and rabies.

The Ryan White CARE Act requires every state's public health officer to designate an official within every emergency response organization to act as a "designated officer." The designated officer is responsible for gathering facts surrounding possible emergency responder airborne or bloodborne infectious disease exposures. Take time to learn who is the designated officer within your organization.

Two different notification systems for infectious disease exposure are defined in the act:

- **Airborne disease exposure.** You will be notified by your designated officer when you have been exposed to an airborne disease.
- **Bloodborne or other infectious disease exposure.** You may submit a request for a determination as to whether or not you were exposed to bloodborne or other infectious disease.

The difference between the two procedures results from the differences in how an exposure is most likely to be detected. With an airborne disease such as TB, you may not realize that the patient you have cared for and transported was infected. However, a disease like TB will be diagnosed at the hospital. Therefore, the Ryan White CARE Act states that for airborne diseases like TB, the hospital will notify the designated officer, who will notify you.

A bloodborne disease such as hepatitis B or HIV/AIDS may or may not be diagnosed at the hospital, but you will know if you have had contact with a patient's blood or body fluids. If so, you can submit a request to your designated officer who will gather the information necessary to request a determination from the hospital on whether you have been exposed and then will notify you of the result.

In either case, once you have been notified of an exposure, your employer will refer you to a doctor or other health care professional for evaluation and follow-up (Figure 2-7).

Consider how the Ryan White CARE Act would apply in the following example of exposure to an airborne pathogen.

As an EMT, you treat and transport a patient who complains of weakness, fever, and chronic cough. The next day you receive a phone call from your organization's designated officer, who informs you that you have been exposed to a patient with TB. The designated

FIGURE 2-7 Once you have been notified of an exposure, your employer will refer you to a doctor or other health care professional for evaluation and follow-up.

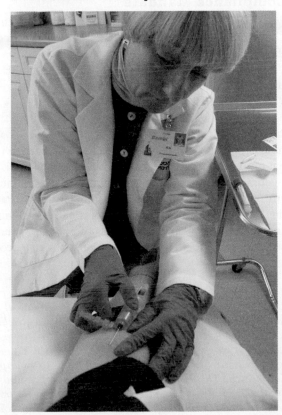

officer helps you arrange an appointment with a doctor who can determine if you have contracted the disease and arrange for early treatment if you have.

According to CDC guidelines, exposure to airborne pathogens may occur when you share "air space" with a tuberculosis patient. So, if a medical facility diagnoses that patient as having the airborne infectious disease, it must notify the designated officer within 48 hours. The designated officer must then notify the emergency care workers of disease exposure. Finally, the employer must schedule a postexposure evaluation and follow-up.

Consider a possible exposure to a bloodborne pathogen.

As an EMT, you are called to treat an unconscious woman. Pink, frothy sputum trickles from her mouth. Her breathing is labored. A hypodermic needle lies beside her. While you are suctioning the patient, your eye shield slips and fluids from her mouth splash into your eyes. You report the incident immediately after the call is completed. Your designated officer follows up, and you learn that you have not been exposed to a life-threatening bloodborne disease.

Under CDC guidelines, after contact with the blood or body fluids of a patient you have transported, you may submit a request for a determination to your designated officer. The designated officer must then gather information about the possible exposure. If the information indicates a possible exposure, the officer forwards the information to the medical facility where the patient is being treated. If the patient can be identified, medical records are reviewed to determine if the patient has a life-threatening disease. The medical facility then must notify your designated officer of their findings in writing within 48 hours after receiving the officer's request. The designated officer must notify you, and you will be directed by your employer to a health care professional for a postexposure evaluation and follow-up as appropriate.

It is important to note that the Ryan White CARE Act does not empower hospitals to test patients for bloodborne diseases at the request of the emergency worker or designated officer. Rather, they can only review the patient's medical records to see if evidence of a bloodborne or other disease exists. Thus, a patient could be infected, but if the records reveal no testing or known indication of the presence of such an infection, the hospital can only report that "no evidence of bloodborne infection could be detected."

Tuberculosis Compliance Mandate

Thousands of new cases of TB are reported in the United States each year. Hundreds of health care workers have been infected or exposed. Of particular concern is multidrug resistant TB (MDR-TB), which does not respond to the usual medications. In 1994, the CDC issued guidelines for treating a suspected or confirmed TB patient. OSHA has announced it will enforce those guidelines as if they were OSHA rules and will also require employers of health care workers to follow OSHA's respiratory standard (1910.134). This standard describes the selection and proper use of different kinds of respirators including those classified as N-95 or HEPA.

Study the guidelines as summarized in the following text. Learn to recognize situations in which the potential of exposure to TB exists. Those at greatest risk of contracting and transmitting TB are people who have suppressed immune systems, including people with HIV/AIDS and elderly patients such as those living in nursing homes. Patients who have TB may have the following signs and symptoms: productive cough (coughing up mucus or other fluid) and/or coughing up blood, weight loss and loss of appetite, lethargy and weakness, night sweats, and fever. It is safest to assume that any person with a productive cough may be infected with TB.

NOTE: *If you are actually exposed to a bloodborne pathogen (e.g., by a needlestick or splashing of fluids to a mucous membrane), you must seek medical attention immediately. It is important that you receive care for the wound, obtain baseline blood work including determining hepatitis B immunity, evaluate the need for a tetanus shot, and document the incident for worker's compensation or insurance. You may also be asked to consider taking an antiviral drug or combination of drugs to attempt to counteract the effects of HIV if it is present. This is a personal issue and a very serious decision. It is important to know that current research indicates that waiting 48 hours for the requested Ryan White information to determine if the patient whose blood you were exposed to may be HIV-infected may reduce the effectiveness of the drugs. Even a few hours may make a significant difference in treatment outcome. Do not delay seeking care. Each situation is different. You will wish to seek the advice of the attending physician where you are being treated as well as that of your Medical Director.*

When the potential exists for exposure to exhaled air of a person with suspected or confirmed TB, OSHA requires that you wear a NIOSH-approved N-95 or high efficiency particulate air (HEPA) respirator. You are required to wear an N-95 or HEPA respirator when you are:

- Caring for patients suspected of having TB. High-risk areas include correctional institutions, homeless shelters, long-term care facilities for the elderly, and drug treatment centers.

- Transporting an individual from such a setting in a closed vehicle. If possible, keep the windows of the ambulance open and set the heating and air conditioning system on the nonrecirculating cycle.

- Performing high-risk procedures such as endotracheal suctioning and intubation.

Remember to take all recommended infection control precautions, including hand washing and using personal protective equipment and barrier devices such as pocket masks or bag-valve masks for rescue breathing. Properly dispose of contaminated equipment and materials, and decontaminate all surfaces, clothing, and equipment.

Immunizations

Immunizations against many diseases are available. Most people receive tetanus immunizations either routinely or after certain injuries. There is currently an immunization available to prevent hepatitis B. It will be provided by your EMS agency, usually through a local physician or your Medical Director.

Although there is no immunization against tuberculosis used in the United States, a tuberculin skin test (TST) can detect exposure. (The Centers for Disease Control and Prevention now uses the term *tuberculin skin test (TST)* rather than the older but synonymous term, *purified protein derivative (PPD) test*.) EMTs are often given this test during routine or employment screening physicals. If the test determines that you have been exposed to tuberculosis, seek treatment and follow-up from a doctor or other health care professional. EMS workers should be checked for exposure to TB on a regular basis (usually yearly).

Some EMS agencies and medical facilities may require immunizations for measles and other common communicable diseases. Consult your instructor, your Medical Director, or your personal physician for more information on your current status and local protocols for immunizations.

EMOTION AND STRESS

CORE CONCEPT ●------------
The kinds of stress caused by involvement in EMS and how they can affect you, your fellow EMTs, and your family and friends

Take a minute to think about the last time you told someone that you felt "stressed out." How did you feel? Did you feel tense, as if every muscle was tight, every nerve on edge? Were your palms sweaty and your stomach in knots? Was your heart pounding and did you have a lump in your throat? Did you have trouble sleeping or always feel exhausted no matter how much sleep you had the previous night? What was going on in your life at that time? Were you preparing for a big exam? Was a family member's illness causing you to worry? Did you feel torn between the demands of family, work, and school? Were you worried about your financial state, wondering how you would cover some large unexpected expense? Were you about to change jobs or were you going through a divorce? How you manage these and other stressors is critical to your well-being.

Physiologic Aspects of Stress

During the Middle Ages and for much of the next 200 or 300 years, people viewed the mind and body as separate entities. In the last third of the twentieth century, however, medical science began to give increasing scrutiny to how the mind and body work together and influence each other. In fact, today it would be hard to find anyone who denies that there is a connection between mind and body or that stress plays a role in illness.

Stress is a widely used term in today's society. It is derived from a word used in the 1600s (*stresse*, a variation of *distresse*), which meant acute anxiety, pain, or sorrow. Today, doctors and psychologists generally define stress as a state of physical and/or psychological arousal to a stimulus. Any stimulus is capable of being a stressor for someone, and stressors vary from individual to individual and from time to time.

Many agree that stress poses a potential hazard for EMS personnel. However, it is important to recognize that stress is a normal part of life and, when managed appropriately, does not have to pose a threat to your well-being. As an EMT you will be routinely exposed to stress-producing agents or situations. These stressors may be environmental factors (e.g., noise, inclement weather, unstable wreckage), your dealings with other people (e.g., unpleasant family or work relationships, abusive patients or bystanders), or your own self-image or performance expectations (e.g., worry over your expertise at specific skills or guilt over poor patient outcomes).

Ironically, these stress-causing factors may be some of the same things that first attracted you to EMS, such as an atypical work environment, an unpredictable but varied work load, dealing with people in crisis, or the opportunity to work somewhat independently. How you manage these stressors is critical to your survival as an EMS provider as well as in life.

Dr. Hans Selye (a Canadian physician and educator who was born in Austria) did a great deal of research in this area and found that the body's response to stress (*general adaptation syndrome*) has three stages.

During the first stage (*alarm reaction*), your sympathetic nervous system increases its activity in what is known as the "fight-or-flight" syndrome. Your pupils dilate, your heart rate increases, and your bronchial passages dilate. In addition, your blood sugar increases, your digestive system slows, your blood pressure rises, and blood flow to your skeletal muscles increases. At the same time, the endocrine system produces more cortisol, a hormone that influences your metabolism and your immune response. Cortisol is critical to your body's ability to adapt to and cope with stress.

In the second stage (*stage of resistance*), your body systems return to normal functioning. The physiologic effects of sympathetic nervous system stimulation and the excess cortisol are gone. You have adapted to the stimulus and it no longer produces stress for you. You are coping. Many factors contribute to your ability to cope; these include your physical and mental health, education, experiences, and support systems, such as family, friends, and coworkers.

Exhaustion, the third stage of the general adaptation syndrome, occurs when exposure to a stressor is prolonged or the stressor is particularly severe. During this stage, the physiologic effects described by Selye include what he called the stress triad: enlargement (hypertrophy) of the adrenal glands, which produce adrenaline; wasting (atrophy) of lymph nodes; and bleeding gastric ulcers. At this point the individual has lost the ability to resist or adapt to the stressor and may become seriously ill as a consequence. Fortunately, most individuals do not reach this stage.

Types of Stress Reactions

Three types of stress reactions are commonly encountered: acute stress reactions, delayed stress reactions, and cumulative stress reactions. Any of these may occur as a result of a *critical incident*, which is any situation that triggers a strong emotional response. An *acute stress reaction* occurs simultaneously with or shortly after the critical incident. A *delayed stress reaction* (also known as posttraumatic stress disorder) may occur at any time, days to years, following a critical incident. A *cumulative stress reaction* (also known as *burnout*) occurs as a result of prolonged recurring stressors in our work or private lives.

Acute Stress Reaction

Acute stress reactions are often linked to catastrophes, such as a large-scale natural disaster, a plane crash, or a coworker's line-of-duty death or injury. Signs and symptoms of an acute stress reaction will develop simultaneously or within a very short time following the incident. They may involve any one or a combination of the following areas of function: physical, cognitive (the ability to think), emotional, or behavioral. These are signs that this particular situation is overwhelming your usual ability to cope and to perform effectively. It is important to keep in mind that they are ordinary reactions to extraordinary situations. They reflect the process of adapting to challenge. They are normal and are not a sign of weakness or mental illness.

Some of these signs and symptoms require immediate intervention from a physician or mental health professional, whereas others do not. As a rule, any sign or symptom that indicates an acute medical problem (such as chest pain, difficulty breathing, or abnormal heart rhythms) or an acute psychological problem (such as uncontrollable crying, inappropriate behavior, or a disruption in normal, rational thinking) are the kinds of problems that demand immediate corrective action. These are the same kinds of problems that alert us to a potentially dangerous situation when we see them in a patient, and they should trigger the same response when exhibited by us or our coworkers. Helping people is not just about taking care of your patient; it is also always about taking care of each other and yourself.

As previously mentioned, some signs and symptoms associated with an acute stress reaction may not require intervention. For instance, you may feel nauseated, tremulous, or numb after working a cardiopulmonary arrest, particularly if your patient is close to your age. You may feel confused or have trouble concentrating or difficulty sleeping after working at a particularly bloody crash scene or a prolonged extrication. You may find that you have no appetite for food or cannot get enough to eat. If not too severe or long-lasting, these responses are uncomfortable but probably not dangerous, since they pose no immediate threat to your health, safety, or well-being.

Remember that you are not losing your mind if you exhibit signs and symptoms of stress after a critical incident. You are merely reacting to an extraordinary situation. Remember, too, that there is nothing wrong with you if you do *not* experience any symptoms after such an incident. This, too, is common. In other words, a wide range of responses is normal and to be expected.

Delayed Stress Reaction

Like an acute stress reaction, a delayed stress reaction, also known as posttraumatic stress disorder (PTSD), can be triggered by a specific incident; however, the signs and symptoms may not become evident until days, months, or even years later. This delay in presentation may make it harder to deal with the stress reaction since the individual has seemingly put the incident behind him and moved on with his life. Signs and symptoms may include flashbacks, nightmares, feelings of detachment, irritability, sleep difficulties, or problems with concentration or interpersonal relationships.

It is not uncommon for persons suffering from PTSD to seek solace through drug and alcohol abuse. Because of the delay and the apparent disconnect between the triggering event and the response, the patient with PTSD may not understand what is causing the problems. PTSD requires intervention by a mental health professional.

Cumulative Stress Reaction

Cumulative stress reaction, or burnout, is not triggered by a single critical incident, but instead results from sustained, recurring low-level stressors—possibly in more than one aspect of one's life—and develops over a period of years.

The earliest signs are subtle. They may present as a vague anxiety, progressing to boredom and apathy, and a feeling of emotional exhaustion. If problems are not identified and managed at this point, the progression will continue. Now the individual will develop physical complaints (such as headaches or stomach ailments), significant sleep disturbances, loss of emotional control, irritability, withdrawal from others, and increasing depression. Without appropriate intervention, the person's physical, emotional, and behavioral condition will continue to deteriorate, with manifestations such as migraines, increased smoking or alcohol intake, loss of sexual drive, poor interpersonal relationships, deterioration in work performance, limited self-control, and significant depression.

At its worst, cumulative stress may present as physical illness, uncontrollable emotions, overwhelming physical and emotional fatigue, severe withdrawal, paranoia, or suicidal thoughts. Long-term psychological intervention is critical at this stage if the individual is to recover.

The ultimate key to preventing or managing cumulative stress lies in seeking balance in our lives.

Causes of Stress

Emergencies are stressful by nature. Although most EMS calls are considered "routine," some calls seem to have a higher potential for causing excess stress on EMS providers (Figure 2-8). They include the following:

- **Multiple-casualty incidents.** A *multiple-casualty incident (MCI)* is a single incident in which there are multiple patients. Examples range from a motor-vehicle crash in which two drivers and a passenger are injured to a hurricane that causes injuries to hundreds of people.

- **Calls involving infants and children.** Involving anything from a serious injury to sudden infant death syndrome (SIDS), these calls are known to be particularly stressful to all health care providers.

- **Severe injuries.** Expect a stress reaction when your call involves injuries that cause major trauma or distortion to the human body. Examples include amputations, deformed bones, deep wounds, and violent death.

- **Abuse and neglect.** Cases of abuse and neglect occur in all social and economic levels of society. You may be called to treat infant, child, adult, or elder abuse victims.

- **Death of a coworker.** A bond is formed among members of the public services. The death of another public-safety worker—even if you do not know that person—can cause a stress response.

Stress may be caused by a single event or it may be the cumulative result of several incidents. Remember that any incident may affect you and your coworkers differently. Two EMTs on the same call may have opposite responses. Try never to make negative judgments about another person's reaction.

Stress may also stem from a combination of factors, including problems in your personal life. One common cause of stress is people who "just don't understand" the job. For example, your EMS organization may require you to work on weekends and holidays. Time spent on call may be frustrating to friends and family members. They may not understand why you cannot participate in certain social activities or why you cannot leave a certain area. You might get frustrated, too, because you cannot plan around the unpredictable nature of emergencies. Then, after a very trying or exciting call, for instance, you may wish to share your feelings with a friend or someone you love. You find instead that the person does not understand your emotions. This can lead to feelings of separation and rejection, which are highly stressful.

Signs and Symptoms of Stress

There are two types of stress: eustress and distress. *Eustress* is a positive form of stress that helps people work under pressure and respond effectively. *Distress* is negative. It can happen when the stress of a scene becomes overwhelming. As a result, your response to the

FIGURE 2-8 Emergencies are often stressful for EMS providers. (© *Mark C. Ide*)

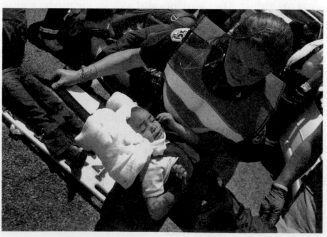

emergency will not be effective. Distress also can cause immediate and long-term problems with your health and well-being.

The signs and symptoms of stress include irritability with family, friends, and coworkers; inability to concentrate; changes in daily activities, such as difficulty sleeping or nightmares, loss of appetite, and loss of interest in sexual activity; anxiety; indecisiveness; guilt; isolation; and loss of interest in work.

Dealing with Stress

Lifestyle Changes

There are several ways to deal with stress. They are called *lifestyle changes* and offer a benefit in both preventing stress and dealing with it when stress occurs. They include:

- **Develop more healthful and positive dietary habits.** Avoid fatty foods and increase your carbohydrate intake. Also reduce your consumption of alcohol and caffeine, which can have negative effects, including an increase in stress and anxiety and disturbance of sleep patterns.

- **Exercise.** When performed safely and properly, exercise helps to "burn off" stress. It also helps you deal with the physical aspects of your responsibilities, such as carrying equipment and performing physically demanding emergency procedures.

- **Devote time to relaxing.** Try relaxation techniques, too. These techniques, which include deep-breathing exercises and meditation, are valuable stress reducers.

In addition to the changes you can make in your personal life to help reduce and prevent stress, there also are changes you can make in your professional life. If you are in an organization with varied shifts and locations, consider requesting a change to a different location that offers a lighter call volume or different types of calls. You may also want to change your shift to one that allows more time with family and friends.

Critical Incident Stress Management

Critical incident stress management (CISM) is a comprehensive system that includes education and resources to both prevent stress and to deal with stress appropriately when it does occur. EMS systems and organizations have different systems for dealing with stress prevention, critical incident stress, and chronic stress, including wellness incentives, professional counseling, and peer support.

Medical professionals and EMS leaders agree that the best course of action for an EMT who is experiencing significant stress from a serious call or experience is to seek help from a mental health professional who is experienced in treating these issues.

Everyone responds to these stresses differently. Some may go on the most serious calls and seemingly be unaffected whereas others have deep emotional reactions to such calls. Most important, remember that seeking care is not a sign of weakness. Many professionals can help you deal with stress, and much of the care may be covered by health insurance policies or employee assistance programs.

The critical incident stress debriefing (CISD) model is a process in which a team of trained peer counselors and mental health professionals meet with rescuers and health care providers who have been involved in a major incident. The meetings are generally held within 24 to 72 hours after the incident. The goal is to assist emergency-care workers in dealing with the stress related to that incident.

Sometimes a "defusing session" is held within the first few hours after a critical incident. Although CISD includes all personnel involved in the incident, a defusing session is usually limited to the people who were most directly involved with the most stressful aspects. It provides them an opportunity to vent feelings and receive information before the larger group meets.

The CISD (debriefing/defusing) model is now used less frequently and is not recommended by many in EMS and mental health professions.

critical incident stress management (CISM)
a comprehensive system that includes education and resources to both prevent stress and to deal with stress appropriately when it occurs.

Understanding Reactions to Death and Dying

As an EMT, you will undoubtedly be called to patients who are in various stages of a terminal illness. Understanding what the families and the patients go through can help you deal with the stress they feel as well as your own.

CORE CONCEPT
The impact that dying patients have on you and others

When a patient finds out that he is dying, he goes through emotional stages, each varying in duration and magnitude. These sometimes overlap, and all affect both the patient and the family.

- **Denial or "Not me."** The patient denies that he is dying. This puts off dealing with the inevitable end of the process.

- **Anger or "Why me?"** The patient becomes angry at his situation. This anger is commonly vented upon family members and EMS personnel.

- **Bargaining or "Okay, but first let me. . . ."** In the mind of the patient, bargaining seems to postpone death, even for a short time.

- **Depression or "Okay, but I haven't. . . ."** The patient is sad, depressed, and despairing, often mourning things not accomplished and dreams that will not come true. He retreats into a world of his own, and is unwilling to communicate with others.

- **Acceptance or "Okay, I'm not afraid."** The patient may come to accept death, although he does not welcome it. Often, the patient may come to accept the situation before family members do. At this stage, the family may need more support than the patient.

Not all patients go through all these stages. Some may seem to be in more than one stage at the same time. Some reactions may not seem to fit any of the described stages. Those who die rapidly are likely not to have such a predictable response to their own mortality. However, a general understanding of the process can help you to communicate with patients and families effectively.

As an EMT, you will also encounter sudden, unexpected death; for example, as a result of a motor-vehicle collision. In cases of sudden death, family members are likely to react with a wide range of emotion.

You can take several steps or approaches in dealing with the patient and family members confronted with death or dying:

- **Recognize the patient's needs.** Treat the patient with respect and do everything you can to preserve the patient's dignity and sense of control. For example, talk directly to the patient. Avoid talking about the patient to family members in the patient's presence as if the patient were incompetent or no longer living. Be sensitive to how the patient seems to want to handle the situation. For example, allow or encourage the patient to share feelings and needs, rather than cutting off such communications because of your own embarrassment or discomfort. Respect the patient's privacy if he does not want to communicate personal feelings.

- **Be tolerant of angry reactions from the patient or family members.** There may be feelings of helpless rage about the death or prospect of death. The anger is not personal. It would be directed at anyone in your position.

- **Listen empathetically.** Although you cannot "fix" the situation, just listening with understanding and patience will be very helpful.

- **Do not falsely reassure.** Avoid saying things like "Everything will be all right," which you, the patient, and the family all know is not true. Offering false reassurance will only be irritating or convey the impression that you do not really understand.

- **Offer as much comfort as you realistically can.** Comfort both the patient and the family. Let them know that you will do everything you can to help or to get them whatever help is available from other sources. Use a gentle tone of voice and a reassuring touch, if appropriate.

SCENE SAFETY

CORE CONCEPT
How to identify potential hazards and maintain scene safety

Scene safety is perhaps the most important concept in your EMT training—and the most important decision you will make on a call. Unless you stay safe, you will not be able to help your patient and you may suffer serious injury—or die.

Fortunately EMS is safe, especially when care is taken on every call to avoid hazards and danger. Television has given us false information on what the dangers actually are. Based on

Table 2-2	Causes of EMS Provider Deaths			
	2004	**2005**	**2006**	**2007**
Air-medical crash	17	8	3	21
Heart attack/medical	3	0	3	10
Motor-vehicle collision	3	10	3	10
Violence	3	0	0	0
9/11/2001 complications	0	2	1	1
Rescue	1	0	1	1
Other	0	1	0	2

this you may visualize criminals and drug-crazed people being the most frequent hazard. You may, in fact, see these people. But in most places, these are not the most common EMS hazards.

In a review of EMS provider deaths over the past several years, few EMS providers were killed by violence. Heart attack, motor-vehicle collisions, and air-medical crashes are a greater risk by far. Table 2-2 lists causes of provider deaths for the most recent years available.

The remainder of this chapter will discuss several ways to remain safe in EMS. You will learn more on safety in Chapter 10, "Scene Size-Up."

Hazardous Material Incidents

Many chemicals are capable of causing death or lifelong complications even if they are only briefly inhaled or in contact with a person's body. Many of these materials are commercially transported, often by truck or rail. Such materials are also often stored in warehouses and used in industry. When there is an accident or when containers begin to leak, a *hazardous material incident* may occur, which will pose serious dangers for you as an EMT as well as for others who are in the vicinity. When you face an emergency involving such materials, remember—you will not be able to help anyone if you are injured. Exercise caution.

hazardous material incident
the release of a harmful substance into the environment.

The primary rule is to maintain a safe distance from the source of the hazardous material. Make sure your ambulance or other emergency vehicle is equipped with binoculars. They will help you identify placards, which are placed on vehicles, structures, and storage containers when they hold hazardous materials (Figure 2-9). These placards use coded colors and identification numbers that are listed in the *Emergency Response Guidebook* developed by the U.S. Department of Transportation, Transport Canada, and the Secretariat of

FIGURE 2-9 Placards with coded colors and identification numbers must be used on vehicles and containers to identify hazardous materials.

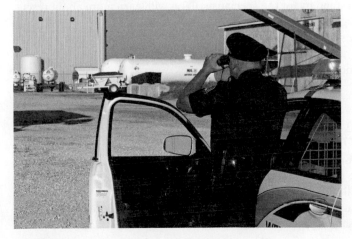
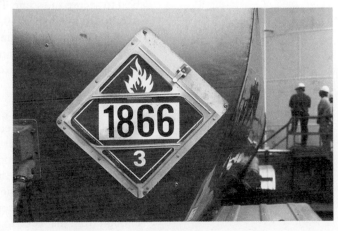

Communications and Transportation of Mexico. This reference book should be placed in every vehicle that responds to, or may respond to, a hazardous material incident. It provides important information about the properties of the dangerous substance as well as information on safe distances, emergency care, and suggested procedures in the event of spills or fire. The *Emergency Response Guidebook* is available online from the U.S. Department of Transportation Pipeline and Hazardous Materials Safety Administration at www.phmsa.dot.gov.

Your most important roles at the scene of a hazardous material incident are recognizing potential problems, taking initial actions for your personal safety and the safety of others, and notifying an appropriately trained hazardous material response team. Do not take any actions other than those aimed at protecting yourself, patients, and bystanders at the scene. An incorrect action can cause a bigger problem than the one that already exists.

The hazardous material response team is made up of specially trained technicians who will coordinate the safe approach and resolution of the incident. Each wears a special suit that protects the skin. A self-contained breathing apparatus (SCBA) is also required because of the strong potential for poisonous gases, dust, and fumes at a hazardous material incident. You will generally not be required to wear personal protective equipment of this sort unless you have been specially trained to be part of a hazardous material response team. Instead, you will remain at a distance until the team has made the scene safe.

As an EMT, you should not be treating patients until after they have undergone *decontamination* (cleansing of dangerous chemicals and other materials). If you take a contaminated patient into your ambulance, it will be considered contaminated and cannot be used again until it is thoroughly decontaminated. Furthermore, should you bring a contaminated patient to the emergency department of a hospital, you could effectively close that hospital down. (See Chapter 39, "Hazardous Materials, Multiple-Casualty Incidents, and Incident Management," for more information on hazardous material incidents.)

Terrorist Incidents

As an EMT, you may be called to respond to a terrorist incident. This incident may be small or large in scale and may include chemical agents, biological agents, radiation, and/or explosive devices. Although these topics are covered in other areas of this text—including Chapter 41, "EMS Response to Terrorism"—it is important to consider this type of incident and its effect on your personal safety in the general context of scene safety.

As part of your initial and subsequent training, you will likely be made aware of any specific threats or targets in your area in addition to any specific protocols relating to potential chemical, biological, nuclear, or explosive incidents.

Rescue Operations

Rescue operations include rescuing or disentangling victims from fires, auto collisions, explosions, electrocutions, and more. As with hazardous materials, it is important to evaluate each situation and ensure that appropriate assistance is requested early in the call. Depending on the emergency, you may need the police, fire department, power company, or other specialized personnel. Never perform acts that you are not properly trained to do. Do your best to secure the scene. Then stand by for the specialists. (You will learn more about rescue operations in Chapter 40, "Highway Safety and Vehicle Extrication.")

As you work in rescue operations or on patients during a rescue operation, you will need personal protective equipment that includes turnout gear (coat, pants, and boots), protective eyewear, helmet, and puncture-proof gloves.

Violence

As an EMT, you will be called to scenes involving violence. Your first priority—even before patient care—is to be certain that the scene is safe. Dangerous persons or pets, people with weapons, intoxicated people, and others may present problems you are not prepared to handle. Learn to recognize those occasions. If the dispatcher knows that violence is or potentially may be present, he will advise you not to approach the scene until it is safe. The dispatcher may name a certain location where you should wait, or stage, a location that is far enough from the scene to be safe but near enough that you can respond as soon as the scene

decontamination
the removal or cleansing of dangerous chemicals and other dangerous or infectious materials.

has been secured. Remember, it is the responsibility of the police to secure a scene and make it safe for you to perform your EMS duties.

Three words sum up the actions required to respond to danger: *plan, observe,* and *react*.

Plan

Many EMTs work together to prevent dangerous accidents and know what to do as a team when danger strikes. Scene safety begins long before the actual emergency. Plan to be as safe as possible under all circumstances. The following factors should be addressed:

- **Wear safe clothing.** Nonslip shoes and practical clothing will not only help you provide emergency care more efficiently, but they also help you to respond to danger without unnecessary restrictions. For personal protection, have reflective clothing available if you will be near traffic or in areas where it is important for you to be visible. Some EMTs wear body armor (bulletproof vests) when working in high-risk areas or situations.

- **Prepare your equipment so it is not cumbersome.** You will be carrying your first-response kit into emergencies. If it is too heavy or bulky, it will take your attention away from the careful observation of the scene as you approach and slow you down if retreat becomes necessary. Many practical containers of reasonable size and weight are available.

- **Carry a portable radio whenever possible.** A radio allows you to call for help if you are separated from your vehicle.

- **Decide on safety roles.** If there will be more than one EMT on any call, tasks should be split up. For example, one EMT can obtain vital signs while another applies oxygen. One role that is frequently underused is that of observer. The EMT directly involved in patient care should always be aware of, but will have trouble constantly monitoring, the surroundings. The EMT who is not directly involved with patient care will be better able to actively observe for such things as weapons, mechanisms of injury, medications, and other important information.

Observe

Remember that it is always better to prevent a dangerous situation than to deal with one. If you observe or suspect danger, call the police. Do not enter the scene until they have secured it.

Observation begins early in the call. Observe the neighborhood as you look for house or building numbers. As you near the scene, turn off your lights and sirens to avoid broadcasting your arrival and attracting a crowd.

As you approach an emergency scene, notice what is going on. Emergencies are very active events. In situations where you notice an unusual silence, a certain amount of caution is advisable (Figure 2-10). In addition, observe for the following:

- **Violence.** Any indication that violence has occurred or may take place is significant. Signs include broken glass or overturned furniture, arguing, threats, or other violent behavior.

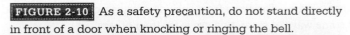
FIGURE 2-10 As a safety precaution, do not stand directly in front of a door when knocking or ringing the bell.

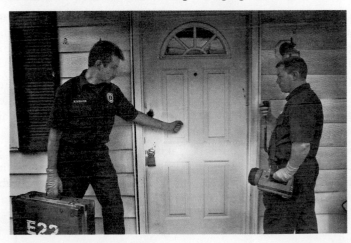

- **Crime scenes.** Try not to disturb a crime scene except as necessary for patient care. Make every effort to preserve evidence. You will learn more about these aspects of emergency care at a crime scene in Chapter 4, "Medical, Legal, and Ethical Issues."

- **Alcohol or drug use.** When people are under the influence of alcohol and other drugs, their behavior may be unpredictable. You also may be mistaken for the police because you drove up in a vehicle with lights and sirens.

- **Weapons.** If anyone at the scene (other than the police) is in possession of a weapon, your safety is in danger. Even weapons that are only in view of a hostile person are a potential problem. Remember that almost any item may be used as a weapon. Weapons are not limited to knives and guns. If you observe or suspect the presence of any kind of weapon, notify the police immediately.

- **Family members.** Emotional or overwrought family members are often capable of violence or unpredictable behavior. Even though you are there to take care of a loved one, the violence may be directed at you.

- **Bystanders.** Many people gather at the scene of a collision (or anywhere an emergency vehicle parks). Sometimes you will find a bystander or group of bystanders beginning to show aggressive behavior. If this happens, call for the police. In some settings, it may be necessary to place the patient in the ambulance and leave the scene rather than wait for the police.

- **Perpetrators.** A perpetrator of a crime may still be on the scene—in sight or in hiding. Do not enter a crime scene or a scene of violence until police have secured it and told you it is safe to do so.

- **Pets.** Although most domestic animals are not dangerous in ordinary circumstances, the presence of an animal at the emergency scene poses problems. Even friendly animals may become defensive when you begin to treat the owner. Animals also can be very distracting, interfere with patient care, and cause falls while you are lifting and moving the patient. No matter what the pet owner says ("He won't hurt you. He's very friendly."), it is usually best to have pets placed securely in another room.

Keep in mind that the vast majority of EMS calls will go by uneventfully. As an EMT, you are a vital part of the EMS system. Nothing in this text is intended to create fear or paranoia. However, when a call does pose some kind of threat, you must be prepared to recognize the subtle and not-so-subtle signs that can warn you before danger strikes.

React to Danger

Observation has provided the critical information needed about the danger. The next step involves knowing how to react. The three Rs of reacting to danger are retreat, radio, and reevaluate.

It is not part of your responsibilities as an EMT to subdue a violent person or wrestle a weapon away from anyone. To *retreat* from such dangers is a clear and justified course of action. Note that some ways of retreating are safer than others:

- **Flee.** Get far enough away so you will have time to react should the danger begin to move toward your new position. Place two major obstacles between you and the danger. If the dangerous person gets through one of the obstacles, you have a built-in buffer with the second.

- **Get rid of any cumbersome equipment.** In the event you must flee from the scene, do not get bogged down by your equipment. Discard all of it if this will enhance your ability to get away. Use equipment to your benefit. For example, if you are being pursued, wedge your stretcher in a doorway to slow down the aggressor.

- **Take cover and conceal yourself.** Taking cover means finding a position that protects your body from projectiles, such as behind a brick wall. Concealing yourself is hiding your body behind an object that cannot protect you, such as a shrub. Find a position that will both conceal and protect you (Figure 2-11).

FIGURE 2-11 (A) Concealing yourself is placing your body behind an object that can hide you from view. (B) Taking cover is finding a position that both hides you and protects your body from projectiles.

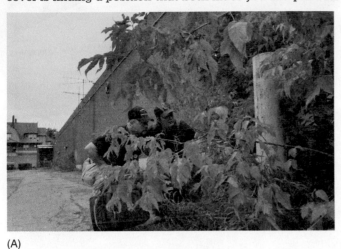

(A)

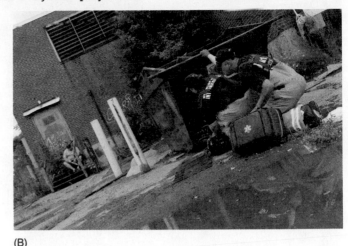

(B)

When fleeing danger, your best option is to use distance, cover, and concealment to protect yourself. Do not return to the scene until the police have secured it.

The second R of reacting to danger is *radio*. The portable radio is an important piece of safety equipment. Use it to call for police assistance and to warn other responding units of the danger. Speak into it clearly and slowly. Advise the dispatcher of the exact nature and location of the problem. Specify how many people are involved and whether or not weapons were observed. Remember, the information you have about the scene must be shared as soon as possible to prevent others from encountering the same danger.

Finally, the third R of reacting to danger is *reevaluate*. Do not reenter a scene until it has been secured by the police (Figure 2-12). Even then, be aware that where violence has been, it may begin again. Emergencies are situations packed with stress for families, patients, responders, and bystanders. Maintain a level of alert observation throughout the call. Occasionally you may find weapons or drugs while you are assessing the patient. If that happens, stop what you are doing and radio the police immediately. After the call, document the situation on your run report. Occasionally, the danger may cause delays in reaching the patient. Courts have held this delay acceptable, provided there has been a real and documented danger.

FIGURE 2-12 Never enter a scene that is potentially violent until the police have secured it and told you it is safe. *(©Craig Jackson/In the Dark Photography)*

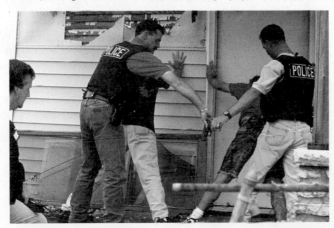

CHAPTER REVIEW

Key Facts and Concepts

- Your well-being is an important concept. This chapter has provided several ways to protect and maintain it.

- You should never take safety or Standard Precautions lightly. Each is an important decision you will make at least once at each scene you respond to—always.

- Protect yourself from violence and scene hazards at all costs.

- Protect yourself from disease. Do not be paranoid about catching a disease, but take appropriate precautions.

- Stress may be an immediate reaction from a particular call or cumulative from a combination of life and EMS. Both are bad for you. Seek help if you need to.

- You will see death and reaction to death. Each is very personal to those involved. The stages of death are denial, anger, bargaining, depression, and acceptance.

- Treat people who are under stress fairly and compassionately, even if it is difficult to do so.

Key Decisions

- Is the scene safe? Should I enter—or not?

- What Standard Precautions must I take? What PPE should I use?

- Is stress getting the best of me? Is it hurting me, my work, or my family and friends?

Chapter Glossary

contamination the introduction of dangerous chemicals, disease, or infectious materials.

critical incident stress management (CISM) a comprehensive system that includes education and resources to both prevent stress and to deal with stress appropriately when it occurs.

decontamination the removal or cleansing of dangerous chemicals and other dangerous or infectious materials.

hazardous material incident the release of a harmful substance into the environment.

multiple-casualty incident (MCI) an emergency involving multiple patients.

pathogens the organisms that cause infection, such as viruses and bacteria.

personal protective equipment (PPE) equipment that protects the EMS worker from infection and/or exposure to the dangers of rescue operations.

Standard Precautions a strict form of infection control that is based on the assumption that all blood and other body fluids are infectious.

stress a state of physical and/or psychological arousal to a stimulus.

Preparation for Your Examination and Practice

Short Answer

1. Name some of the causes of stress for an EMT and explain some ways the EMT can alleviate job-related stress.

2. Describe the purpose and process of a critical incident stress debriefing (CISD).

3. What are the stages of grief? How should the EMT deal with these emotions?

4. List the types of personal protective equipment used in Standard Precautions. Identify a condition or patient with which each one should be used.

Thinking and Linking

Body substance isolation is an important concept to protect you from disease. Linking with the roles and responsibilities of an EMT in Chapter 1, "Introduction to Emergency Medical Services and the Health Care System," and the material covered in this chapter, list the type of Standard Precautions you would use in each of the following circumstances:

1. A patient who has severe bleeding from his arm

2. A patient who is vomiting

3. A patient who is spitting up blood

Critical Thinking Exercises

Many emergency calls pose dangers to EMS personnel. The purpose of this exercise will be to consider actions you should take at a dangerous scene.

- You are called to an unknown emergency at a tavern. As you approach the scene, you see a man lying supine in the parking lot, apparently bleeding profusely. Two other men are scuffling, and one seems to have a gun. What actions must you take?

Pathophysiology to Practice

The following questions are designed to assist you in gathering relevant clinical information and making accurate decisions in the field.

1. How do you think you caught your last cold or stomach "bug?"
2. What is your body's response to stress? What does it do to your pulse, respiration, and blood pressure?
3. How is "good stress" different than "bad stress" to your body?

Street Scenes

While you are en route to a motor-vehicle collision, the dispatcher gives your responding ambulance an update. "Ambulance Charlie 7, you have one patient with bad facial injuries." After judging the scene safe to enter, you immediately start to assess the patient. Just as you open the airway and your partner provides oxygen, the paramedic unit arrives and takes over care of the patient.

As you are finishing loading the patient into the back of the paramedic's ambulance, one of them asks where your gloves are. You don't think much of it and start to clean up your equipment. As you get into the ambulance, your partner tells you that not only is it against the ambulance service's standard operating procedure for you not to wear gloves on this type of call, but it is foolish. You reluctantly agree to tell your supervisor.

Later, you enter the supervisor's office, describe the call and the amount of blood, and then tell her that you did not wear any protective gloves. You also point out that you may have had a partially healed cut on your hand. She tells you that you are out-of-service.

Street Scene Questions

1. Why wear protective gloves on this type of call?
2. What is the impact of an occupational exposure on you, your family, and your fellow EMS workers?
3. What can you expect after exposure?

Your supervisor explains that you need to go to the emergency department for an occupational evaluation. There is a prearrangement with the hospital, and they will have a member of their infection control staff go through your evaluation and counseling.

When you get to the hospital, the infection control nurse interviews you and asks many specific questions about the call, your health, and what type of immunizations you have had. She examines your hands for breaks in the skin, and a number are identified. When the interview is over she recommends that you get some baseline blood tests; one is for HIV. All of a sudden you realize the seriousness of this situation. She recommends that you take some medications, and gives you information on precautions that you need to take when having intimate relations with your spouse. It hits you again how serious this has become.

Street Scene Questions

4. How will stress be a factor in your life for the next few months?
5. How important is hand washing?
6. What type of Standard Precautions should EMTs always be ready to use on all EMS calls?

You try to take your mind off the situation, but you can't. It affects your sleep. You are irritable around your family. When you try to talk to your partner, you find you're too embarrassed.

Quite some time later, the infection control nurse tells you that your latest blood tests are back. They're all negative. A personal tragedy has been avoided. As you start to leave her office, the nurse tells you to remember—gloves and hand washing are very important. With a big smile, you look back and say: "I GET IT!"

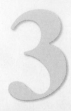

3 Lifting and Moving Patients

⭘ **STANDARD**
Preparatory (Workforce Safety and Wellness)

⭘ **COMPETENCY**
Uses fundamental knowledge of the EMS system, safety/well-being of the EMT, medical/legal and ethical issues to the provision of emergency care.

⭘ **CORE CONCEPTS**
— How using body mechanics to lift and move patients can help prevent injury

— When it is proper to move a patient, and how to do so safely

— The various devices used to immobilize, move, and carry patients

EXPLORE Resource**Central**

To access Resource Central, follow directions on the Student Access Card provided with this text. If there is no card, go to **www.bradybooks.com** and follow the Resource Central link to Buy Access from there. Under Media Resources, you will find:

▶ **Prehospital Lifting of Patients**
View a video describing the EMT's role of lifting and moving patients in the prehospital environment, when you would need to use an emergency move, and different types of equipment that can be used to move patients. One, two, three, lift!

▶ **Proper Body Mechanics When Moving a Patient**
Watch this video and learn the five rules of body mechanics, the challenges associated with moving patients, and why you should have a plan for safely transferring a patient. Don't you love it when a plan comes together?

▶ **Lifting Bariatric Patients**
Learn about the challenges faced by the EMT when lifting and moving a bariatric patient, considerations that should be taken into account and equipment that can be used to help lift and move these patients.

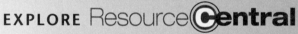

OBJECTIVES

After reading this chapter you should be able to:

3.1 Define key terms introduced in this chapter.

3.2 Describe the factors that you must consider before lifting any patient. (pp. 49–50)

3.3 Use principles of proper body mechanics when lifting and moving patients and other heavy objects. (pp. 49–51)

3.4 Demonstrate the power lift and power grip when lifting a patient-carrying device. (pp. 50–51)

3.5 Follow principles of good body mechanics when reaching, pushing, and pulling. (p. 51)

3.6 Give examples of situations that require emergency, urgent, and non-urgent patient moves. (pp. 51–70)

3.7 Demonstrate emergency, urgent, and non-urgent moves. (pp. 53–70)

3.8 Given several scenarios, select the best patient-lifting and moving devices for each situation. (pp. 56–64)

3.9 Demonstrate proper use of patient-lifting and carrying devices. (pp. 56–70)

3.10 Differentiate between devices to be used to lift and carry patients with and without suspected spinal injuries. (pp. 60–69)

3.11 Identify with the feelings of a patient EMS personnel are lifting or carrying. (pp. 51–70)

KEY TERMS

peed is a major objective on many of the calls you will make as an EMT. At dangerous scenes, for example, you must rapidly move the patient to a safe place. When the patient has a life-threatening medical problem or a serious injury, getting him to a hospital quickly can mean the difference between life and death.

Doing things fast, however, can mean doing them wrong. You can be so focused on the need to hurry as you lift and carry the patient that you make careless moves. These can injure your patient. They can also injure you. Back injuries are serious and have the potential to end an EMS career as well as cause lifelong problems. With the proper techniques, however, you can lift and move patients safely. Proper lifting and moving must be practiced on every call.

PROTECTING YOURSELF: BODY MECHANICS

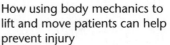

Body mechanics refers to the proper use of your body to prevent injury and to facilitate lifting and moving. Consider the following before lifting any patient:

- **The object.** What is the weight of the object? Will you require additional help in lifting?

- **Your limitations.** What are your physical characteristics? Do you (or your partner) have any physical limitations that would make lifting difficult? Although it may not always be possible to arrange, EMTs of similar strength and height can lift and carry together more easily.

- **Communication.** Make a plan. Then communicate the plan for lifting and carrying to your partner. Continue to communicate throughout the process to make the move comfortable for the patient and safe for the EMTs.

When it comes time to do the lifting, there are rules that must be followed to prevent injury:

- **Position your feet properly.** They should be on a firm, level surface and positioned shoulder-width apart.

- **Use your legs.** Do not use your back to do the lifting.

- **Never turn or twist.** Attempts to make any other moves while you are lifting are a major cause of injury.

CORE CONCEPT
How using body mechanics to lift and move patients can help prevent injury

body mechanics
the proper use of the body to facilitate lifting and moving and prevent injury.

- **Do not compensate when lifting with one hand.** Avoid leaning to either side. Keep your back straight and locked.
- **Keep the weight close to your body, or as close as possible.** This allows you to use your legs rather than your back while lifting. The farther the weight is from your body, the greater your chance of injury.
- **Use a stair chair when carrying a patient on stairs whenever possible.** Keep your back straight. Flex your knees and lean forward from the hips, not the waist. If you are walking backward down stairs, ask a helper to steady your back (Figure 3-1).

There are many kinds of patient-carrying devices, including stretchers, backboards, and stair chairs. (Specifics are offered later in this chapter.) When possible, it is almost always safer, as well as more efficient, to move patients over distances on a wheeled device such as a wheeled stretcher or a stair chair. These devices allow the patient to be rolled along instead of carried.

When lifting a patient-carrying device, it is best to use an even number of people. For a stretcher or backboard, one EMT lifts from the end near the patient's head, the other from the feet. If there are four rescuers available, one person can take each corner of a stretcher or board. If there are only three people available, however, never allow the third person to assist by lifting one side. This can cause the device to be thrown off balance, resulting in the stretcher tipping over and injuring the patient.

To prevent injury when lifting a patient-carrying device, the general rules of body mechanics mentioned earlier apply. Two more methods also can help to prevent injury. The first is the **power lift** (Figure 3-2A), so named because it is used by power weight lifters. It is also known as the *squat-lift* position. In this position, you will squat rather than bend at the waist, and you will keep the weight close to your body, even straddling it if possible. When rising, your feet should be a comfortable distance apart, flat on the ground, with the weight primarily on the balls of the feet or just behind them. Your back should be locked-in. Be sure to raise your upper body before your hips. When you are lowering a patient, use the reverse order of this procedure.

The second method is the **power grip** (Figure 3-2B). Remember that your hands are often the only portion of your body actually in contact with the object you are lifting, making your grip a very important element in the process. As great an area of your fingers and palms as possible should be in contact with the object. All of your fingers should be bent at the same angle. When possible, keep your hands at least 10 inches apart.

There are situations in which you will find yourself reaching for patients or using a considerable amount of effort to push and pull a weight. These are moves that must be performed carefully to prevent injury. In general:

---

power lift

a lift from a squatting position with weight to be lifted close to the body, feet apart and flat on the ground, body weight on or just behind the balls of the feet, and the back locked-in. The upper body is raised before the hips. Also called the *squat-lift position*.

power grip

gripping with as much hand surface as possible in contact with the object being lifted, all fingers bent at the same angle, and hands at least 10 inches apart.

FIGURE 3-1 Moving a stair chair down steps.

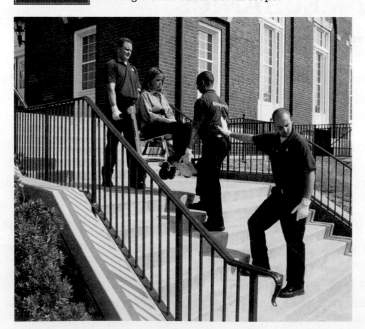

FIGURE 3-2 (A) The power lift and (B) the power grip.

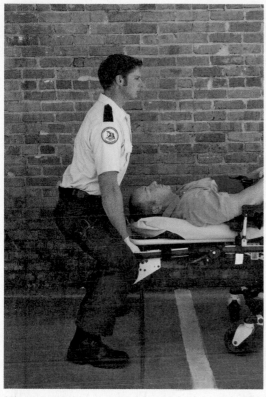

(A)

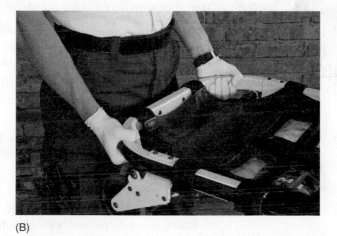

(B)

When reaching:

- Keep your back in a locked-in position.
- Avoid twisting while reaching.
- Avoid reaching more than 15 to 20 inches in front of your body.
- Avoid prolonged reaching when strenuous effort is required.

When pushing or pulling:

- Push, rather than pull, whenever possible.
- Keep your back locked-in.
- Keep the line of pull through the center of your body by bending your knees.
- Keep the weight close to your body.
- If the weight is below your waist level, push or pull from a kneeling position.
- Avoid pushing or pulling overhead.
- Keep your elbows bent and arms close to your sides.

PROTECTING YOUR PATIENT: EMERGENCY, URGENT, AND NON-URGENT MOVES

How quickly should you move a patient? Must you complete your assessment before moving him? How much time should you spend on spinal precautions and other patient-safety measures? The answer is: It depends on the circumstances.

If the patient is in a building that is in danger of collapse or a car that is on fire, speed is the overriding concern. The patient must be moved to a safe place, probably before you have

CORE CONCEPT ●

When it is proper to move a patient, and how to do so safely

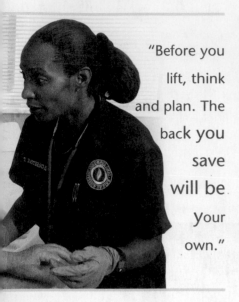

time to begin or complete an assessment, immobilize the patient's spine, or move a stretcher into position. In this situation, you would use what is known as an *emergency move*.

Sometimes the situation is such that you have time to carry out an abbreviated version of assessment and spinal immobilization. For example, consider the patient who has been trapped in wreckage, possibly incurring serious injuries. When the patient is extricated, you would place him on a spine board, working quickly to perform the proper assessments and patient care. That move to the spine board is called an *urgent move*.

Most of the time, you will be able to complete your on-scene assessment and care procedures and then move the patient onto a stretcher or other device in the normal way. This would be called a *non-urgent move*.

Emergency Moves

Three situations may require the use of an emergency move:

- **The scene is hazardous.** Hazards may make it necessary to move a patient quickly in order to protect you and the patient. This may occur when there is uncontrolled traffic, fire or threat of fire, possible explosions, electrical hazards, toxic gases, or radiation.

- **Care of life-threatening conditions requires repositioning.** You may have to move a patient to a hard, flat surface to provide CPR, or you may have to move a patient to reach life-threatening bleeding.

- **You must reach other patients.** When there are patients at the scene requiring care for life-threatening problems, you may have to move another patient to access them.

The greatest danger to the patient in an emergency move is that a spine injury may be aggravated. Since the move must be made immediately to protect the patient's life, full spinal precautions will not be possible. Therefore, to minimize or prevent aggravation of the injury, *move the patient in the direction of the long axis of the body when possible.* The long axis is the line that runs down the center of the body from the top of the head and along the spine.

There are several rapid moves called drags. In this type of move, the patient is dragged by the clothes, the feet, the shoulders, or a blanket. These moves are reserved only for emergencies, because they do not provide protection for the neck and spine. Most commonly, a long-axis drag is made from the area of the shoulders. This causes the remainder of the body to fall into its natural anatomical position, with the spine and all limbs in normal alignment.

Drags and other emergency moves known as carries and assists are illustrated in Scans 3-1, 3-2, and 3-3.

Urgent Moves

Urgent moves are required when the patient must be moved quickly for treatment of an immediate threat to life. However, unlike emergency moves, urgent moves are performed with precautions for spinal injury. Examples in which urgent moves may be required include the following:

- **The required treatment can only be performed if the patient is moved.** A patient must be moved in order to support inadequate breathing or to treat for shock or altered mental status.

- **Factors at the scene cause patient decline.** If a patient is rapidly declining because of heat or cold, for example, he may have to be moved.

Moving a patient onto a long spine board, also called a *backboard*, is an urgent move used when there is an immediate threat to life and suspicion of spine injury. If the patient is supine on the ground, a log-roll maneuver must be performed to move him onto his side. The spine board is then placed next to the patient's body, and he is log-rolled onto the board. After the patient is secured and immobilized on the spine board, the board and patient are lifted together onto a stretcher, the board is secured to the stretcher, and the stretcher with spine board and patient firmly secured are loaded into the ambulance. (When reaching across the patient to perform a log roll, remember the principles of body mechanics: Keep your back straight, lean from the hips, and use your shoulder muscles to help with the roll.

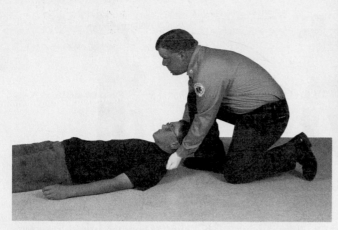

CLOTHES DRAG.

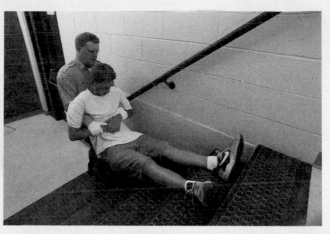

INCLINE DRAG. *Always* head first.

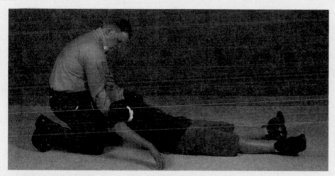

SHOULDER DRAG.

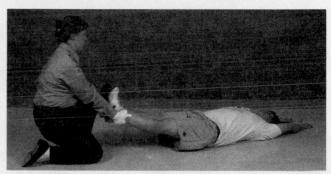

FOOT DRAG. Do not bump the patient's head.

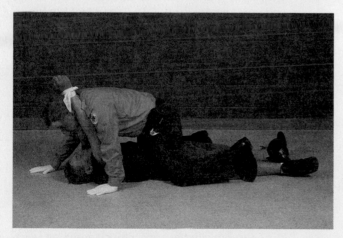

FIREFIGHTER'S DRAG. Place patient on his back and tie his hands together. Straddle him, crouch, and pass your head through his trussed arms. Raise your body, and crawl on your hands and knees. Keep the patient's head as low as possible.

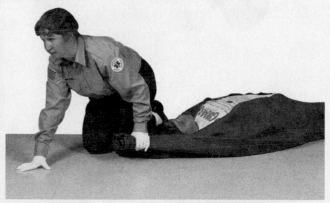

BLANKET DRAG. Gather half of the blanket material up against the patient's side. Roll him toward your knees, place the blanket under him, and gently roll him onto the blanket. During the drag, keep the patient's head as low as possible.

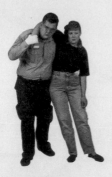

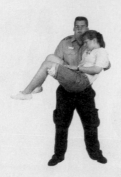

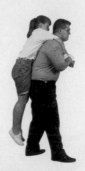

ONE-RESCUER ASSIST. Place the patient's arm around your neck, grasping her hand in yours. Place your other arm around the patient's waist. Help the patient walk to safety. Be prepared to change your movement technique if the level of danger increases. Be sure to communicate with the patient about obstacles, uneven terrain, and so on.

CRADLE CARRY. Place one arm across the patient's back with your hand under her arm. Place your other arm under her knees and lift. If the patient is conscious, have her place her near arm over your shoulder.

> **NOTE:** *This carry places a lot of weight on the carrier's back. It is usually appropriate only for very light patients.*

PACK STRAP CARRY. Have the patient stand. Turn your back to her, bringing her arms over your shoulders to cross your chest. Keep her arms as straight as possible, with her armpits over your shoulders. Hold the patient's wrists, bend, and pull her onto your back.

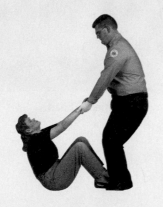

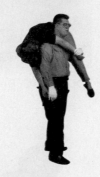

FIREFIGHTER'S CARRY. Place your feet against the patient's feet and pull her toward you. Bend at your waist and flex your knees. Duck and pull her across your shoulder, keeping hold of one of her wrists. Use your free arm to reach between her legs and grasp her thigh. This way, the weight of the patient falls onto your shoulders. Stand up. Transfer your grip on her thigh to the patient's wrist.

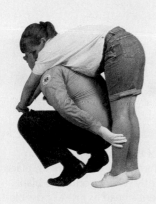

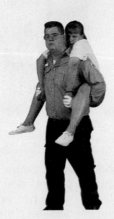

PIGGYBACK CARRY. Assist the patient to stand. Place her arms over your shoulder so they cross your chest. Bend over and lift the patient. While she holds on with her arms, crouch and grasp each leg. Use a lifting motion to move her onto your back. Pass your forearms under her knees and grasp her wrists.

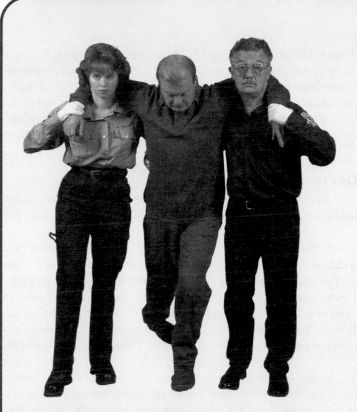

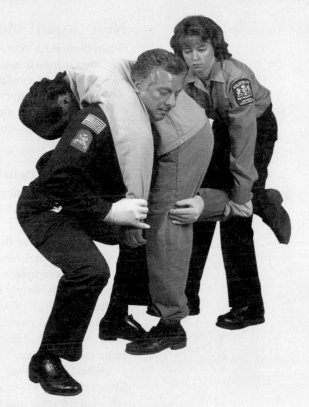

TWO-RESCUER ASSIST. Place the patient's arms around the shoulders of both rescuers. They each grip a hand, place their free arms around the patient's waist, and then help him walk to safety.

FIREFIGHTER'S CARRY WITH ASSIST. Have someone lift the patient. The second rescuer helps to position the patient.

See Figure 3-3.) Log rolls and immobilization on a long spine board will be discussed in Chapter 31, "Trauma to the Head, Neck, and Spine."

Another example of an urgent move is the rapid extrication procedure from a vehicle. If the patient has critical injuries, taking the time to immobilize him with a short backboard or vest while he is still in the car may cause a deadly delay. During a rapid extrication, EMTs use

FIGURE 3-3 When doing a log roll, keep your back straight, lean from the hips, and use your shoulder muscles.

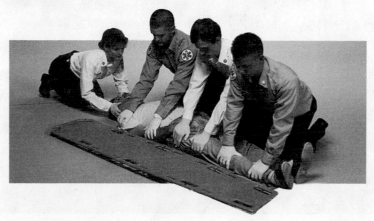

a quicker procedure: They stabilize the spine manually as they move the patient from the car onto a long spine board. Rapid extrication will also be discussed in Chapter 31.

Non-Urgent Moves

When there is no immediate threat to life, the patient should be moved when ready for transportation, using a non-urgent move. On-scene assessment and any needed on-scene treatments, such as splinting, should be completed first. Non-urgent moves should be carried out in such a way as to prevent injury or additional injury to the patient and to avoid discomfort and pain.

In a non-urgent move, the patient is moved from the site of on-scene assessment and treatment (perhaps a bed or sofa, perhaps the floor or the ground outdoors) onto a patient-carrying device.

Patient-Carrying Devices

● CORE CONCEPT
The various devices used to immobilize, move, and carry patients

A patient-carrying device is a stretcher or other device designed to carry the patient safely to the ambulance and/or to the hospital. Devices described on the following pages are pictured in Scan 3-4.

Patient-carrying devices are mechanical devices, and all EMTs must be familiar with how to use them. Errors in the use of these devices may result in injuries to the patient and to you. For example, a stretcher that is not locked in position may collapse, and untended stretchers may simply roll away. Such incidents may be cause for a lawsuit if the patient is injured as a result of improper practices or faulty equipment. The devices must be regularly maintained and inspected. You should know the rating of each piece of equipment (how much weight it will hold safely). Have alternatives available if the patient is too heavy or too large for any device.

Wheeled Stretcher   This device—commonly referred to simply as the stretcher, cot, or litter (Figure 3-4)—is in the back of all ambulances. There are many brands and types of wheeled stretcher, but their purpose is the same: to safely transport a patient from one place to another, usually in a reclining position. The head of the stretcher can be elevated, which will be beneficial for some patients, including cardiac patients, who have no suspected neck or spinal injuries.

Depending on the model, the stretcher will have variable levels. When moving the patient, the safest level is closest to the ground. Wheeling the stretcher in the elevated position raises the center of gravity, making it easier for the stretcher to tip over. The stretcher is ideal for level surfaces. Rough terrain and uneven surfaces may cause the stretcher to tip.

FIGURE 3-4 A wheeled stretcher is carried on every ambulance.

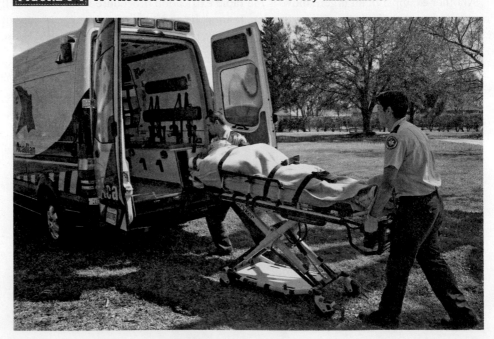

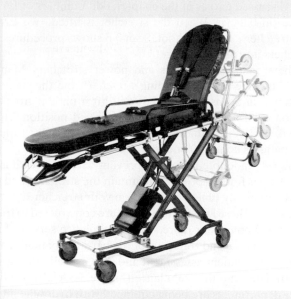

Power stretcher. *(© Ferno Corporation)*

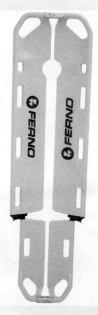

Scoop (orthopedic) stretcher. *(© Ferno Corporation)*

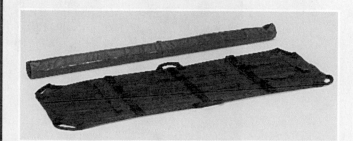

Flexible stretcher.

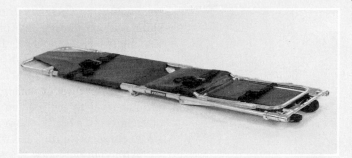

Portable stretcher.

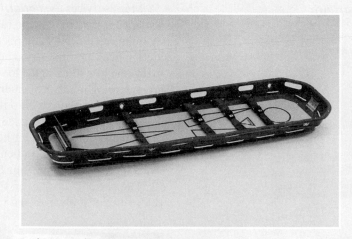

Basket stretcher. *(© Ferno Corporation)*

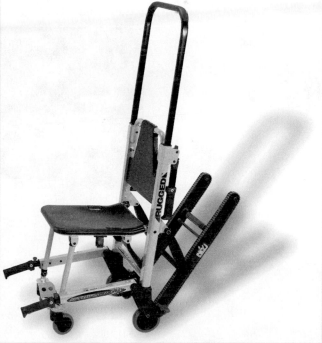

Stair chair. *(Stryker)*

Make sure to use proper body mechanics while placing the stretcher into or taking it out of the ambulance. Proper body mechanics are also important while wheeling the stretcher from place to place. Remember, as discussed earlier in the chapter, odd numbers of EMTs may cause the stretcher to become off-balance. When the stretcher is lifted, two EMTs should lift at opposite ends of the stretcher—head and foot. Scan 3-5 shows procedures for loading two types of wheeled stretchers into an ambulance.

There are two types of stretchers: manual stretchers and power stretchers. Manual stretchers are lifted by EMTs. These include the "self-loading stretcher" and the standard stretcher. A power stretcher (as shown in Scans 3-4 and 3-5) will lift a patient from the ground level to the loading position or lower a patient from the raised position. These stretchers use a battery-powered hydraulic system that manufacturers state will lift patients on 20 consecutive runs and will lift patients up to 700 pounds.

Although these power stretchers will undoubtedly help to prevent back injuries, it is vital to follow the manufacturer's guidelines for use, properly maintain the stretcher, and use safe techniques as discussed in this chapter any time a patient is on your stretcher.

Many services use **bariatric** stretchers. These are stretchers that are constructed to transport obese patients—some rated for 800 pounds or more. Many ambulance services have ambulances specially equipped for the loading and transport of the bariatric patient. These ambulances have oversized equipment for patient assessment and care as well as ramps or hydraulic lifts to raise the loaded stretcher into the ambulance (Figure 3-5A). In addition, an increasing number of emergency departments are being equipped with hydraulic lifts to transfer obese patients onto the hospital cot (Figure 3-5B).

A stretcher can be carried by four EMTs, one at each corner. This method can be useful on rough terrain because it helps keep the wheels from touching the ground and provides greater stability. It is also beneficial when carrying a patient a long distance because it divides the weight among four EMTs instead of two.

The patient will stay on the stretcher during transport to the hospital. Make sure that the stretcher is always used in accordance with manufacturer's recommendations. Secure

bariatric
having to do with patients who are significantly overweight or obese.

FIGURE 3-5 (A) Many EMS services are now equipped with specially constructed stretchers and loading equipment for obese patients. (B) An increasing number of emergency departments are being equipped with hydraulic lifts to transfer obese patients onto the hospital cot. *(Photo B: © Edward T. Dickinson, MD)*

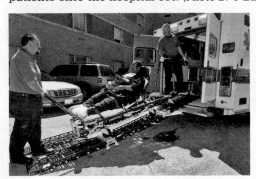

(A)

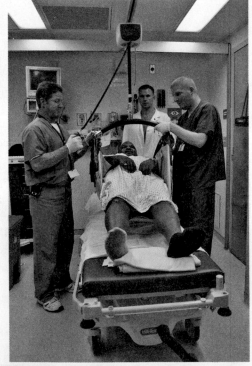

(B)

SELF-LOADING STRETCHER

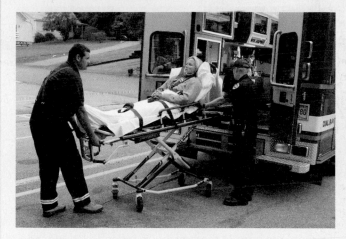

1 Position the wheels closest to the patient's head securely on the inside floor of the ambulance.

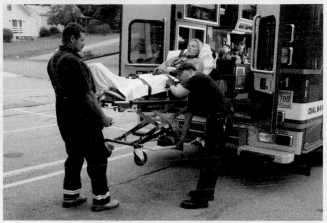

2 Once the wheels are securely on the ambulance floor, the rescuer at the rear of the stretcher activates the lever to release the wheels. (This may require a slight lift to get weight off the wheels.) The second rescuer should guide the collapsing carriage, if necessary.

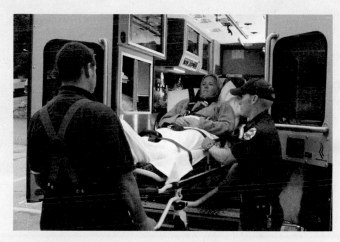

3 Move the stretcher into the securing device and secure the stretcher in the front and rear.

(continued)

the patient to the stretcher before lifting or moving. After placing the patient into the ambulance, secure the stretcher to the ambulance. Ambulances have installed hardware for keeping the stretcher secured while the ambulance is moving. Failure to secure the stretcher properly will allow it to shift during transit, causing an unsafe condition for the EMTs as well as the patient.

Stair Chair The stair chair has many benefits for moving patients from the scene to the stretcher. The first benefit, as the name implies, is that it is excellent for use on stairs. Large stretchers often cannot be carried around tight corners and up or down narrow staircases. The stair chair transports the patient in a sitting position, which greatly reduces the length of patient and device, allowing the EMT to maneuver around corners and through narrow spaces. It also has a set of wheels that allow the device to be rolled like a wheelchair over flat surfaces, lessening the strain on the EMT.

POWER STRETCHER

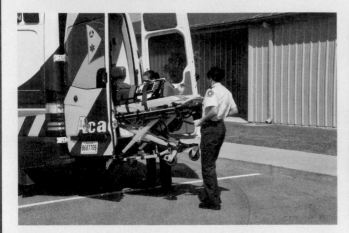

1 Remove the power stretcher from the ambulance. Equipment that will be needed is loaded atop the stretcher.

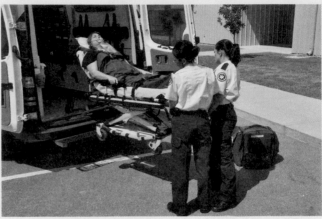

2 Once the head of the stretcher is supported inside the ambulance, raise the stretcher legs.

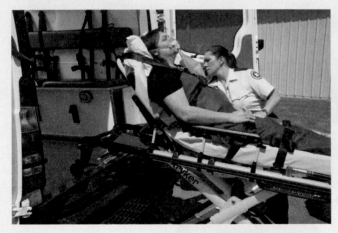

3 Check that the stretcher is properly supported as the patient is loaded into the ambulance.

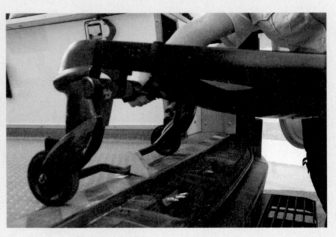

4 Make sure the locking mechanism is secured.

Another type of stair chair has come into wide use in EMS. This chair has wheels to roll the patient along a floor or level ground but also has a tracklike system that allows EMTs to gently slide the patient down a staircase instead of lifting him (Figure 3-6). The patient's weight increases the friction along the track, which helps to control the rate of descent.

As with older stair chair models, two rescuers are necessary, and a third as a spotter is preferred when available. Indications and contraindications for this stair chair are the same as for older models.

As with all devices in this chapter, there are times when the stair chair should be used and times when it should not. The device is often ideal for patients with difficulty breathing. These patients usually find that they must sit up to breathe more easily, which the stair chair allows them to do. The stair chair must not be used for patients with neck or spine injury, because these patients must be immobilized supine on a backboard to prevent further injury. Unresponsive patients, those with a severely altered mental status, or patients who require airway care may not be transported on the stair chair.

Spine Boards There are two types of spine boards, or backboards: short and long (Scan 3-6). They are used for patients who are found lying down or standing and who must be immobilized. These devices are available in traditional wood as well as in plastic versions that resist splintering. (Splintered boards absorb body fluids, which may harbor infection.)

FIGURE 3-6 (A) A modern stair chair has wheels to roll the patient along a floor or level ground. (B) It also has a track that can be lowered that (C and D) allows EMTs to gently slide the patient down a staircase.

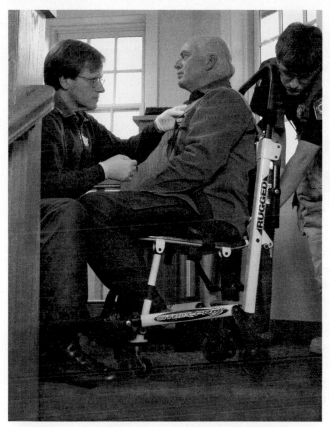

(A)

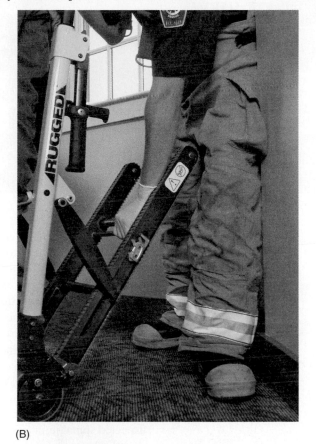

(B)

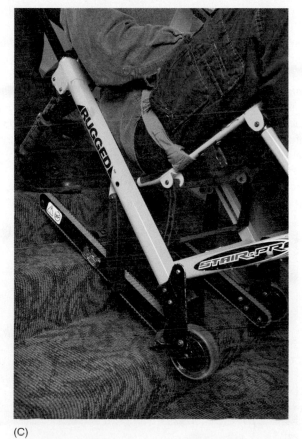

(C)

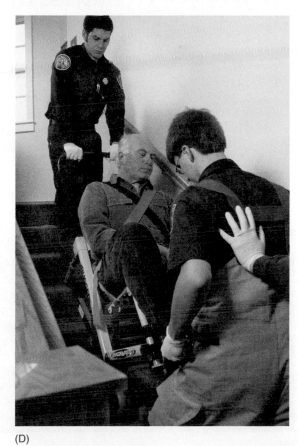

(D)

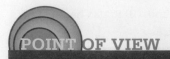
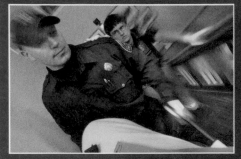
Short spine boards are used primarily for removing patients from vehicles when a neck or spine injury is suspected. A short spine board can slide between the patient's back and seat back. Once secured to the short spine board and wearing a rigid cervical collar, the patient can be moved from a sitting position in the vehicle to a supine position on a long spine board. Often, a vest-type extrication device is used in place of a short spine board. You will learn more about extrication using short spine boards and vests in Chapter 31, "Trauma to the Head, Neck, and Spine."

Other Types of Stretchers The portable stretcher, or folding stretcher, may be beneficial in multiple-casualty incidents (incidents with many patients). These stretchers may be canvas, aluminum, or heavy plastic and usually fold or collapse.

The *scoop stretcher*, or orthopedic stretcher, splits into two pieces vertically, allowing the patient to be "scooped" by pushing the halves together under him. The scoop stretcher does not offer any support directly under the spine, so it is not recommended for patients with suspected spinal injury. Follow your local protocols on the use of this device.

A *basket stretcher*, or Stokes stretcher, can be used to move a patient from one level to another or over rough terrain. The basket should be lined with a blanket before positioning the patient.

A *flexible stretcher*, or Reeves stretcher, is made of canvas or some other rubberized or flexible material, often with wooden slats sewn into pockets and three carrying handles on each side. Because of its flexibility, it can be useful in restricted areas or narrow hallways.

Some services now use a *vacuum mattress* when transporting patients (Figure 3-7). The patient is placed on the device and air is withdrawn by means of a pump. The mattress then becomes rigid and conforming, padding voids naturally for greater comfort. Vacuum mattresses reduce some of the discomfort associated with rigid backboards. In later chapters, you will see vacuum splints that use the same principle.

FIGURE 3-7 (A) A vacuum mattress may be used to transport a patient. (B) When the patient is placed on the device and air is withdrawn, the mattress becomes rigid and conforming, automatically padding voids.

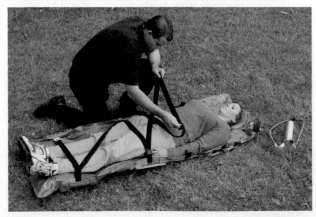

(A)

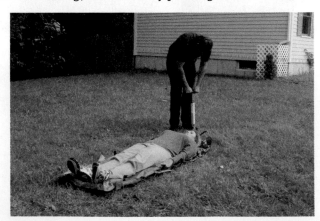

(B)

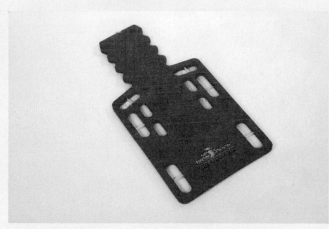

Short spine board.

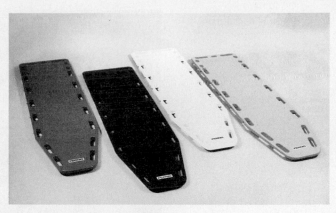

Long spine board.

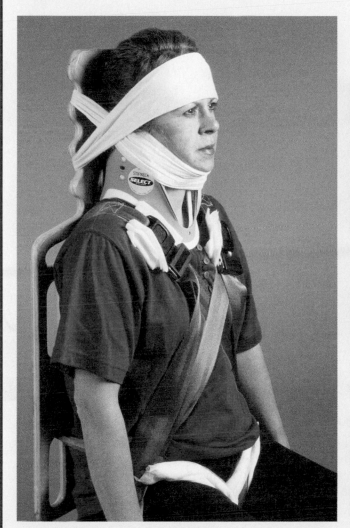

Patient properly secured to short spine board.

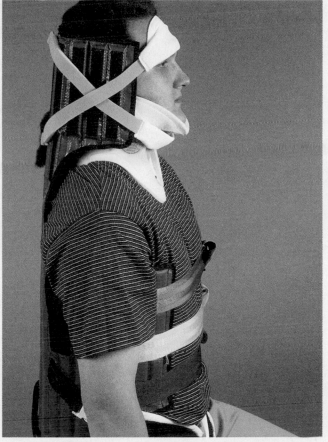

Patient properly secured to vest-type extrication device.

(continued)

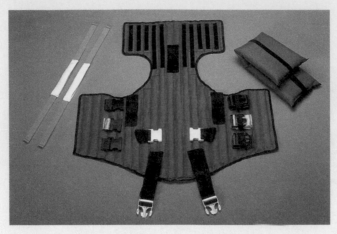

Vest-type extrication device.

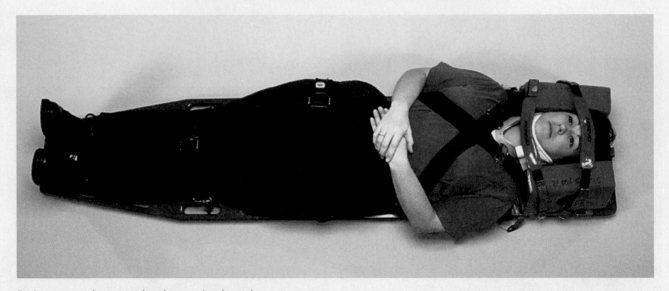

Patient properly secured to long spine board.

CRITICAL DECISION MAKING

Choosing a Patient-Carrying Device

The process of lifting and moving patients requires more than just muscles. Decisions made in patient transportation have a significant impact on the patient's condition—and the EMTs' well-being. For each of the following patients, choose a carrying device to get the patient from the scene to the ambulance stretcher:

1. A patient complaining of severe respiratory distress who is in an upstairs back bedroom

2. A patient thrown from an ATV several hundred yards into the woods

3. A patient who fell down several stairs from the back deck to the concrete landing who complains of neck and back pain

4. An unresponsive medical patient found down a narrow hallway on the first floor

Moving Patients onto Carrying Devices

There are several ways to move a patient onto a carrying device. Choose a move based on the position the patient is in when it is time to move him to a carrying device and whether or not the patient is suspected of having a spine injury.

Patient with Suspected Spine Injury   A patient with suspected spine injury must have his head, neck, and spine immobilized before being moved. Perform manual stabilization, place a rigid cervical collar, and maintain manual stabilization until the patient is immobilized to a spine board. If he is seated in a vehicle, you will next immobilize him with a short spine board or vest and then on a long spine board (unless it is an urgent situation and you substitute the rapid extrication procedure described earlier under "Urgent Moves").

If the patient is lying down or standing, move him directly to a long spine board. The long spine board will then be placed on a wheeled ambulance stretcher for transport to the hospital. You will learn more about manual stabilization in Chapter 11, "The Primary Assessment"; about cervical collars in Chapter 13, "Assessment of the Trauma Patient"; and about immobilization for possible spine injury in Chapter 31, "Trauma to the Head, Neck, and Spine."

Remember that immobilization is mandatory for any patient who has any possibility of a spine injury.

Patient with No Suspected Spine Injury   The extremity lift, direct ground lift, draw-sheet method, and direct carry, described in the following list, are methods of moving a patient to a stretcher. All are appropriate only for a patient with no suspected spine injury. See Scan 3-7 for pictures and detailed descriptions of these methods.

- An *extremity lift* is used to carry a patient with no suspected spine or extremity injuries to a stretcher or a stair chair. It can be used to lift a patient from the ground or from a sitting position.

- A *direct ground lift* is performed when a patient with no suspected spine injury needs to be lifted from the ground to a stretcher.

- The *draw-sheet method* is one of two methods (along with the direct carry method) that is performed during transfers between hospitals and nursing homes, or when a patient must be moved from a bed at home to a stretcher. It is used for a patient with no suspected spine injury.

- A *direct carry* is performed to move a patient with no suspected spine injury from a bed or from a bed-level position to a stretcher.

Patient Positioning

Positioning the patient during transfer to the ambulance and during transportation is a very important part of your care. Lifting, moving, and transport must be performed as an integral part of your total patient-care plan. The position in which the patient is transported depends on his medical condition and the device best designed to help this condition.

Unresponsive patients with no suspected spine injury should be placed in the recovery position (Figure 3-8). The patient should be on his side to aid drainage from his mouth and,

extremity lift
a method of lifting and carrying a patient during which one rescuer slips hands under the patient's armpits and grasps the wrists, while another rescuer grasps the patient's knees.

direct ground lift
a method of lifting and carrying a patient from ground level to a stretcher in which two or more rescuers kneel, curl the patient to their chests, stand, then reverse the process to lower the patient to the stretcher.

draw-sheet method
a method of transferring a patient from bed to stretcher by grasping and pulling the loosened bottom sheet of the bed.

direct carry
a method of transferring a patient from bed to stretcher, during which two or more rescuers curl the patient to their chests, then reverse the process to lower the patient to the stretcher.

FIGURE 3-8 A patient in the recovery position.

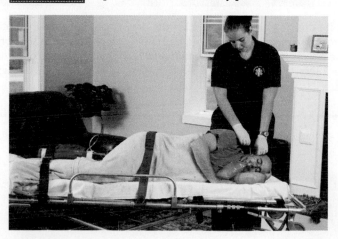

EXTREMITY CARRY

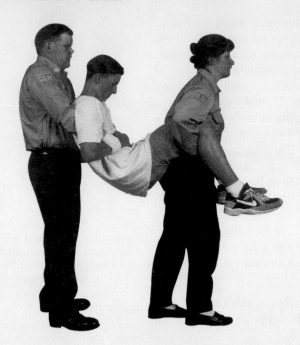

The extremity carry may be used as an emergency move or a non-urgent move for patients with no suspected spine injury.

Place the patient on his back with knees flexed. Kneel at the patient's head. Place your hands under his shoulders. The second EMT kneels at the patient's feet, grasps the patient's wrists, and lifts the patient forward. At the same time, slip your arms under the patient's armpits and grasp his wrists. The second EMT can grasp the patient's knees while facing, or facing away from, the patient. Direct the second EMT, so you both move to a crouch, and then stand at the same time. Move as a unit when carrying a patient.

If the patient is found sitting, crouch and slip your arms under the patient's armpits and grasp his wrists. The second EMT crouches, then grasps the patient's knees. Lift the patient as a unit.

DRAW-SHEET METHOD

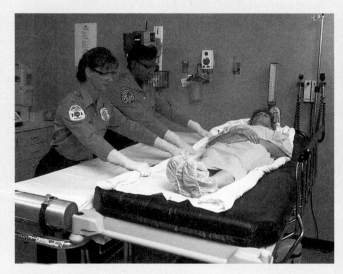

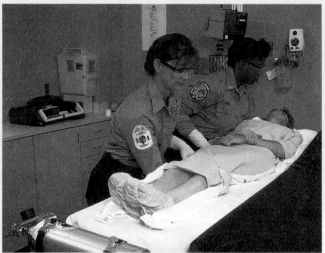

❶ Loosen the bottom sheet of the bed and roll It from both sides toward the patient. Place the stretcher, rails lowered, parallel to the bed and touching the side of the bed. EMTs use their bodies and feet to lock the stretcher against the bed.

❷ EMTs pull on the draw sheet to move the patient to the side of the bed. Both use one hand to support the patient while they reach under him to grasp the draw sheet. Then they simultaneously draw the patient onto the stretcher.

DIRECT GROUND LIFT

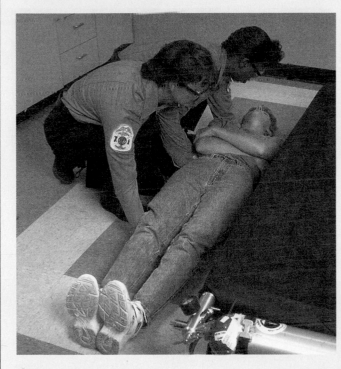

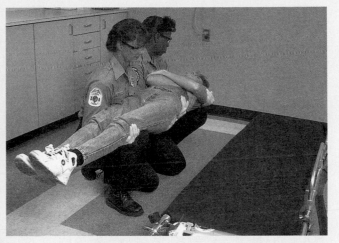

❷ On signal, the EMTs lift the patient to their knees.

❶ The stretcher is set in its lowest position and placed on the opposite side of the patient. The EMTs face the patient, drop to one knee, and, if possible, place the patient's arms on his chest. The head-end EMT cradles the patient's head and neck by sliding one arm under the neck to grasp the shoulder, moving the other arm under the patient's back. The foot-end EMT slides one arm under the patient's knees and the other arm under the patient above the buttocks.

NOTE: *If a third rescuer is available, he should place both arms under the patient's waist while the other two slide their arms up to the mid-back or down to the buttocks, as appropriate.*

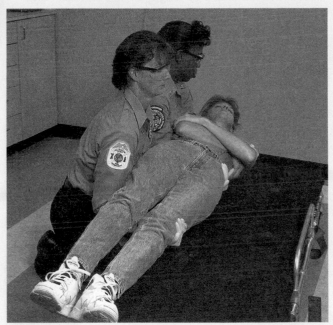

❸ On signal, the EMTs stand and carry the patient to the stretcher, drop to one knee, and roll forward to place him onto the mattress.

(continued)

DIRECT CARRY

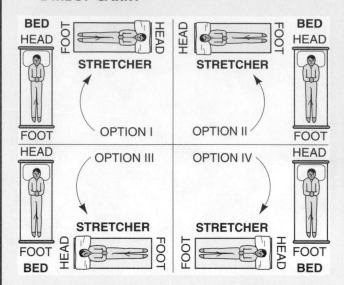

Place the stretcher at a 90° angle to the bed, depending on the room configuration. Prepare the stretcher by lowering the rails, unbuckling straps, and removing other items. Both EMTs stand between the stretcher and bed, facing the patient.

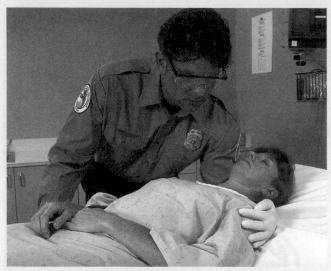

❶ The head-end EMT cradles the patient's head and neck by sliding one arm under the patient's neck to grasp the shoulder.

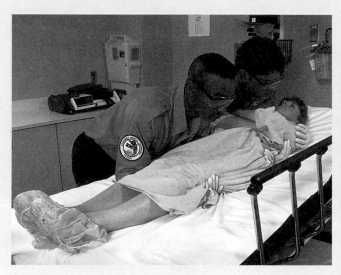

❷ The foot-end EMT slides a hand under the patient's hip and lifts slightly. The head-end EMT slides the other arm under the patient's back. The foot-end EMT places arms under the patient's hips and calves.

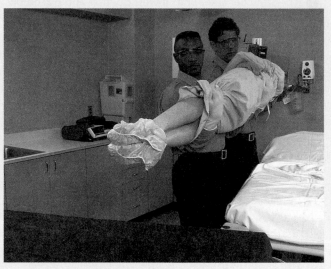

❸ EMTs slide the patient to the edge of the bed and bend toward her with their knees slightly bent. They lift and curl the patient to their chests and return to a standing position. They rotate, then slide the patient gently onto the stretcher.

FIGURE 3-9 For many patients, the position of comfort is a semi-sitting position.

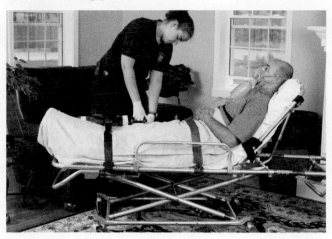

if he vomits, to help prevent his breathing the vomitus into his lungs. This can be accomplished on a wheeled stretcher. You should avoid transporting the unresponsive patient in a chair-type device since the airway cannot be properly maintained.

Many patients who have no suspected spine injuries may be transported in a position of comfort. This includes many patients with medical complaints such as chest pain, nausea, or difficulty breathing. In this situation, allow the patient to choose a position he feels comfortable in. Breathing is often aided by raising the back of the stretcher so that the patient is in a semi-sitting position, also called the Fowler or semi-Fowler position (Figure 3-9). The position must be safe and not prohibit the proper use of any transportation device. The position of comfort must be used cautiously in case the patient vomits. Always monitor the patient's airway and level of responsiveness. Place the patient in the recovery position at the first sign of a decreased level of responsiveness.

Positioning for Shock   Patients who are believed to be in shock are placed in a supine position. This allows maximum blood flow throughout the body with minimal resistance from gravity. It is important that all parts of the body—especially vital organs such as the brain—remain perfused.

Patients who have experienced trauma (injury) are placed on a spine board and immobilized to prevent further injury. These patients should remain in a supine and level position on the backboard. Do not lower the head (which may cause difficulty breathing) or raise the legs (which may aggravate injury and make transportation more difficult). In this case, the risks of raising the legs outweigh the benefits. Recent research has shown there is minimal or no benefit to elevating the legs.

Transferring the Patient to a Hospital Stretcher

When you arrive at the hospital, you will move the patient from the ambulance stretcher to the hospital stretcher. You will probably use a modified draw-sheet method to transfer the patient (Scan 3-8).

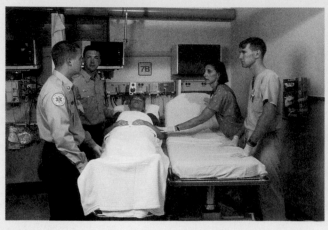

1 Position the raised ambulance cot next to the hospital stretcher. Hospital personnel then adjust the stretcher (raise or lower the head) to receive the patient.

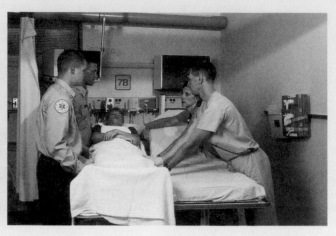

2 You and the hospital personnel gather the sheet on either side of the patient and pull it taut in order to transfer the patient securely.

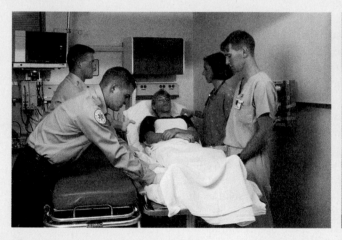

3 Holding the gathered sheet at support points near the patient's shoulders, mid-torso, hips, and knees, you and the hospital personnel slide the patient in one motion onto the hospital stretcher.

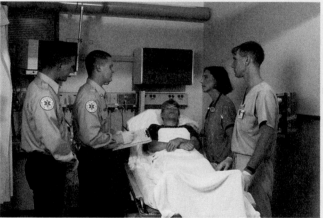

4 Make sure the patient is centered on the stretcher and the stretcher rails are raised before turning him over to the emergency department staff.

CHAPTER REVIEW

Key Facts and Concepts

- The process of lifting and moving patients is a task that requires planning, proper equipment, and careful attention to body mechanics in order to prevent injury to your patient and to yourself.

- The most important rule in lifting is to lift with your legs, not your back. Keep your feet shoulder-width apart and keep your knees bent. Rules for lifting are for patients as well as equipment.

- Emergency moves are those that may aggravate spine injuries and, therefore, are reserved for life-threatening situations.

- Urgent moves are used when the patient must be moved quickly but there is time to provide quick, temporary spinal stabilization.

- Non-urgent moves are normal ways of moving a patient to a stretcher after performing a complete on-scene assessment and completing any needed spinal stabilization and immobilization.

- Positioning the patient for transport should take into account the patient's comfort, medical needs, and safety.

- Remember the importance of correct lifting and moving techniques on every call. Protect your patient and protect yourself from injury to maintain a long and positive EMS experience.

Key Decisions

- How quickly must I move this patient?
- Is the patient at risk where he is?
- Do I need to move this patient to provide care?
- Will moving the patient cause further harm?

- Is there a way to move or position the patient that will help his current condition?
- Can I move this patient with the personnel and equipment available on-scene?

Chapter Glossary

bariatric having to do with patients who are significantly overweight or obese.

body mechanics the proper use of the body to facilitate lifting and moving and prevent injury.

direct carry a method of transferring a patient from bed to stretcher, during which two or more rescuers curl the patient to their chests, then reverse the process to lower the patient to the stretcher.

direct ground lift a method of lifting and carrying a patient from ground level to a stretcher in which two or more rescuers kneel, curl the patient to their chests, stand, then reverse the process to lower the patient to the stretcher.

draw-sheet method a method of transferring a patient from bed to stretcher by grasping and pulling the loosened bottom sheet of the bed.

extremity lift a method of lifting and carrying a patient during which one rescuer slips hands under the patient's armpits and grasps the wrists, while another rescuer grasps the patient's knees.

power grip gripping with as much hand surface as possible in contact with the object being lifted, all fingers bent at the same angle, and hands at least 10 inches apart.

power lift a lift from a squatting position with weight to be lifted close to the body, feet apart and flat on the ground, body weight on or just behind the balls of the feet, and the back locked-in. The upper body is raised before the hips. Also called the *squat-lift position*.

Preparation for Your Examination and Practice

Short Answer

1. Define the term *body mechanics*. Then describe several principles of body mechanics related to safe lifting and moving.

2. List several situations that may require an emergency move of a patient.

3. Describe several lifts and drags.

4. Define a long-axis drag and explain its importance.

Thinking and Linking

Use your knowledge from Chapter 2, "The Well-Being of the EMT," along with the material learned in this chapter to answer the following question.

1. How could infectious diseases be spread to patients and/or EMTs while using the following devices or procedures?

   One-rescuer assist

   Firefighter's carry

   Transporting the patient on the wheeled stretcher

   Applying a vest-type extrication device

Critical Thinking Exercises

For each of the following patients, use the knowledge gained in this chapter to identify the appropriate procedure or device for lifting and moving that patient:

1. A patient who has fallen 18 feet and has suspected spinal injuries

2. A patient with chest pain (with no spine injury) who lives on the fifth floor of a building with no elevator

3. A patient who is found in an environment with a risk of immediate explosion

Street Scenes

You are having a discussion with a group of your EMS colleagues about the role of the EMT. You focus on direct patient care and the need to do thorough assessments. Another person argues that EMS focuses on doing airway, breathing, and circulation care really well. Kim, an EMT who has been doing EMS for more time than anyone else in the room, says that EMTs must know how to do all those things well "but don't forget that moving and transporting patients is significant, too." When you hear that, you silently disagree. "That's really not an important part of patient care," you say.

Well, the discussion ends—at least for you—when dispatch sends you and your partner to a single-occupant motor-vehicle crash. When you reach the scene, the police tell you that the patient is conscious and alert but is complaining of neck pain, that the crash appears to be low impact with significant front-end damage, and that the patient was wearing a lap belt only.

You introduce yourself to the patient, who is still sitting in the driver's seat of her car, and begin your assessment. The patient states that she ran into a parked car. At impact, her head hit the steering wheel, but she denies any loss of consciousness. You continue with the primary assessment and determine the patient is alert and having no difficulty breathing. You observe no signs of bleeding.

Street Scene Questions

1. What device should be used to remove the patient from the vehicle?

2. What patient-care issues are important when using an extrication device?

3. What is the next thing to consider when actually moving the patient from the vehicle?

   Your local protocol requires that a patient with this mechanism of injury—a car crash resulting in the head impacting the steering wheel—gets a cervical collar and a short immobilization device. Your partner, who has been stabilizing the patient's head and neck since shortly after making contact, asks the Emergency Medical Responder unit from the fire department for assistance and suggests to you that a quick neuro exam should be done to check for pulses, motor function, and sensation in all extremities. After the neuro exam, you size a cervical collar and apply it to the patient. You ask the patient if it is causing any additional pain, and she responds that it is uncomfortable but "no additional pain." Next, while your partner still maintains manual stabilization, you position a vest-type extrication device behind her. As you tighten the straps to secure it in place, you ask if it is causing any difficulty with breathing. The patient responds again, "No." You then perform another quick neuro exam. Once completed, the long backboard is positioned and the patient is rotated onto it, with head and neck stabilization still being maintained. The patient is then lowered to the ground.

Street Scene Questions

4. What emergency-care equipment was used for this patient? Why?
5. What is the next step before moving this patient again?
6. What other safety considerations should be considered when moving the long board to the wheeled stretcher?

After the patient is properly secured to the long board, the head immobilizer is positioned, applied, and secured. You continue to talk to the patient to make sure her level of responsiveness has not changed and no breathing difficulty has developed. You perform another quick neuro exam, with the patient having pulses, movement, and sensation in all four extremities.

The long board needs to be carried about 30 feet to the stretcher, so you and your partner decide to have someone on each corner of the long board. This will provide stability and all EMS personnel can be facing forward. The move is uneventful, and after placing the stretcher in the ambulance, you recheck the stretcher locking device. During transport to the hospital, you take the patient's vital signs and obtain a patient history. At the hospital, the crew moves the stretcher from the ambulance and raises it onto its wheels. You take the patient to an examination room in the emergency department and, with assistance, move the long board to the hospital gurney.

After the call, you return to the station. The folks are still in the ready room having the same discussion about the role of an EMT. You pipe in and say, "You know, after this last call, I have to agree with Kim. EMS has a lot to do with knowing how to properly, effectively, and safely move patients."

4

Medical, Legal, and Ethical Issues

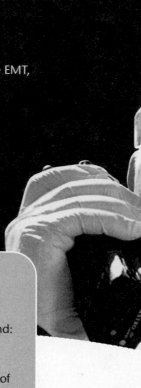

○ **STANDARD**
Preparatory (Medical/Legal and Ethics)

○ **COMPETENCY**
Applies fundamental knowledge of the EMS system, safety/well-being of the EMT, medical/legal and ethical issues to the provision of emergency care.

○ **CORE CONCEPTS**
— The scope of practice of an EMT

— How a patient may consent to or refuse emergency care

— The legal concepts of negligence, torts, and abandonment

— What it means to have a duty to act

— The responsibilities of an EMT at a crime scene

EXPLORE Resource**C**entral

To access Resource Central, follow directions on the Student Access Card provided with this text. If there is no card, go to **www.bradybooks.com** and follow the Resource Central link to Buy Access from there. Under Media Resources, you will find:

▶ **Legal Issues in Healthcare**
Learn how to protect your patient, as well as yourself! As an EMT, you should have a basic understanding of legal issues in health care. Read about the types of communication protected by HIPAA and the importance of obtaining a consent form from your patient. Knowledge is power!

▶ **Organ Donation**
Explore the topic of organ donation and how you can continue to save lives even after you're gone! But in the meantime . . . discuss your role as a living, breathing EMT in this important process.

▶ **Reporting Child Abuse**
Read about what defines sexual abuse, why it is necessary for an EMT to report suspected abuse and neglect, and what information can be found on the Child Welfare Information Gateway.

OBJECTIVES

After reading this chapter you should be able to:

4.1 Define key terms introduced in this chapter.

4.2 Describe your scope of practice as an EMT. (pp. 75–76)

4.3 Differentiate between scope of practice and standard of care. (p. 76)

4.4 Given a variety of scenarios, determine which type of patient consent applies. (pp. 76–77)

4.5 Given a variety of ethical dilemmas, discuss the issues that must be considered in each situation. (pp. 76, 83)

4.6 Explain legal and ethical considerations in situations where patients refuse care. (pp. 77–80)

4.7 Discuss the EMT's obligations with respect to advance directives, including do not resuscitate orders. (pp. 80–81)

(continued)

KEY TERMS

E very time you respond to a call, you will be faced with some aspect of medical/legal or medical/ethical issues. The issue may be as simple as making sure that the patient will accept help or as complex as a terminally ill patient who refuses all care. You may also be faced with decisions such as, "Should I stop and help even though I am off duty?" or "Can I get sued if I stop to help outside of my ambulance district?" Understanding of medical, legal, and ethical issues is an essential foundation for all emergency care. This knowledge may also reduce or prevent the legal liability that you may face as a result of calls.

SCOPE OF PRACTICE

The EMT is governed by many medical, legal, and ethical guidelines. This collective set of regulations and ethical considerations may be referred to as a *scope of practice*, which defines the scope, or extent and limits, of an EMT's job. The skills and medical interventions the EMT may perform (what you do to help the patient) are defined by legislation, which varies from state to state. Sometimes different regions within the same state may have different rules and guidelines for their EMTs.

For example, an EMT in one area may be able to perform certain basic procedures and levels of care. In the adjoining region, EMTs may provide that care and in addition perform special advanced procedures. Your duty is to provide for the well-being of the patient by rendering necessary and legally allowed care as defined under the scope of practice in your area.

Falling within your scope of practice are certain ethical responsibilities. The primary ethical consideration is to make patient care and well-being a priority, even if this requires some personal sacrifice. For example, there may be times when a patient feels cold, even in a hot climate. You may want to turn on the air conditioner in the ambulance, but you refrain out of consideration for your patient. Actions such as this may seem small but mean a lot to the patient.

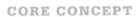

CORE CONCEPT
The scope of practice of an EMT

scope of practice
a set of regulations and ethical considerations that define the scope, or extent and limits, of the EMT's job.

standard of care
for an EMT providing care for a specific patient in a specific situation, the care that would be expected to be provided by an EMT with similar training when caring for a patient in a similar situation.

The scope of practice, as the name indicates, describes the scope of the EMT's job but does not define the ***standard of care***, which is usually defined as the care that would be expected to be provided by an EMT with similar training when caring for a patient in a similar situation. Standard of care will be discussed again later in this chapter with regard to the concept of negligence. In general, scope of practice refers to what you should do, while standard of care refers to how you should do it.

To be an effective EMT, you must maintain your skills and knowledge. This includes practicing until you have obtained confidence and mastery of the skills. After that, continuing education and recertification are necessary to maintain mastery. Every patient deserves the best care.

Emergency care can be improved on a crew and agency level as well as on an individual level. After a call, constructively critique both yourself and the crew. Accept suggestions from others to improve your skills, communication, and patient outcome. Participation in this kind of mutual critique is part of the process known as *quality improvement*. It should be practiced with the aim of maintaining the standards you would wish to have provided for yourself or someone in your family.

During the rest of this chapter, you will learn about some specific aspects of the scope of practice.

PATIENT CONSENT AND REFUSAL

Consent

CORE CONCEPT

How a patient may consent to or refuse emergency care

consent
permission from the patient for care or other action by the EMT.

Consent, or permission from the patient, is required for any treatment or action taken by the EMT. Most patients or their families will have called for your assistance and will readily accept it. A simple statement, such as, "I'm Karla Maguire, an EMT from the ambulance. I'd like to help you, okay?" is enough to request consent. Most patients will respond positively. Expressed consent must be obtained from every conscious, mentally competent adult before providing care and transportation.

The principle of consent may seem simple, but it often brings up complex issues in patient care. There are three types of consent: expressed, implied, and consent to treat minors or incompetent patients.

Expressed Consent

expressed consent
consent given by adults who are of legal age and mentally competent to make a rational decision in regard to their medical well-being.

Expressed consent, the consent given by adults who are of legal age and mentally competent to make a rational decision in regard to their medical well-being, must be obtained from all patients who are physically and mentally able to give it. Expressed consent must be *informed consent*.

CRITICAL DECISION MAKING

Ethical Dilemmas

Not all critical or difficult decisions you make will be clinical in nature. You may be faced with an ethical dilemma that will test your decision-making skills. For each of the following situations, describe how you would handle the situation. It may be helpful to list the options available to you in each case and then choose the course you think best.

1. You are driving the ambulance to the hospital and listening to the conversation in the back between a paramedic and an EMT. You hear the paramedic say, "Oh, no! I can't believe I just did that. I gave her 10 times the dose I was supposed to." You hear the paramedic ask the EMT not to tell anyone. What do you do?

2. You are on the way home from a sporting event. While there you had two drinks. You come across a crash with injury. What do you do?

3. A patient tells you that he received the injury you are treating while climbing a fence after being involved in a break-in at a local business. The patient swears he was just the lookout, and if anyone knows he told he may be killed. What do you do?

That is, patients must understand the risks associated with the care they will receive. It is not only a legal requirement but also sound emotional care to explain all procedures to the patient.

Implied Consent

In the case of an unconscious patient (or one who may be physically or mentally incapacitated but in need of emergency care), consent may be assumed. The law states that rational patients would consent to treatment if they were conscious. This is known as *implied consent*. In this situation, the law allows EMTs and other health care providers to provide treatment, at least until the patient becomes conscious and able to make rational decisions.

Children and Mentally Incompetent Adults

Children and mentally incompetent adults are not legally allowed to provide consent or refuse medical care and transportation. The parents and guardians of these patients have the legal authority to give consent, so it must be obtained before care can be given. There are times, however, when care may be given without this direct consent from a parent or guardian.

One situation where care may be given without direct consent from a parent or guardian is a child care provider or school authority who may act *in loco parentis* (in place of the parents) when the parents are not physically present. Parents may provide written documentation to these individuals allowing them to act in their absence.

In cases of life-threatening illness or injury when a parent or guardian is not present, care may be given based on implied consent. The law provides that it is reasonable to believe that a responsible parent or guardian would consent to care if he were present. In some states, statutes allow emancipated minors—those who are married or of a certain age—to provide consent. Finally, minors who themselves have children and those who serve in the armed forces may also be able to provide consent for their own care. Find out the laws where you will practice as an EMT in reference to consent of minors.

Involuntary Transportation

There will be times when the patient is going to the hospital involuntarily (against his will). This is frequently the result of a decision made by police officers or mental health workers when they believe a patient poses a threat of harm to himself or others. A patient may also be transported against his will as a result of a court order.

In some of these cases you will be transporting a patient who is physically restrained. This is a significant legal responsibility. Many lawsuits alleging negligence are brought against EMS providers for improper restraint or for harm caused to patients during restraint or transport. Because the patient has been denied the ability to move freely, it is a great responsibility for the EMT to ensure the patient's health and well-being during this time. It is essential to frequently and thoroughly monitor the patient's mental status and vital signs while the patient is in your care.

Restraint is discussed in two other places in this text: Chapter 3, "Lifting and Moving Patients," and Chapter 25, "Behavioral and Psychiatric Emergencies and Suicide."

When a Patient Refuses Care

You may think that all patients who need medical care will accept it. Most do. However, you will find that some patients who require treatment and transportation to the hospital will refuse care. Many reasons exist for this, including denial, fear, failing to understand the seriousness of the situation, intoxication, and others.

Although patients generally have the right to refuse care, it is your responsibility as an EMT to be sure that the patient is fully informed about his situation and the implications of refusing care.

In order for a patient to refuse care or transport, several conditions must be fulfilled:

- **Patient must be legally able to consent.** He must be of legal age or an emancipated minor.
- **Patient must be mentally competent and oriented.** He must not be affected by any disease or condition that would impair judgment. These conditions include unstable vital signs, alcohol intoxication or being under the influence of drugs, and altered mental status.

implied consent
the consent it is presumed a patient or patient's parent or guardian would give if they could, such as for an unconscious patient or a parent who cannot be contacted when care is needed.

in loco parentis
in place of the parents, indicating a person who may give consent for care of a child when the parents are not present or able to give consent.

- **Patient must be fully informed.** He must understand the risks associated with refusing treatment and/or transport.

- **Patient will be asked to sign a "release" form.** Such a form is designed to release the ambulance agency and individuals from *liability* (legal responsibility) arising from the patient's informed refusal.

Even carefully following these steps will not guarantee that you will be free from liability if a patient refuses care or transport. Leaving a patient who will not accept care or transport is a leading cause of lawsuits against EMS agencies and providers, even though it was the patient who refused. Occasionally, the patient's condition deteriorates to the point of unconsciousness, which leaves the patient unable to summon help, leading to a severely worsened condition or even death.

In addition to the liability factor, there is also an ethical issue. You would undoubtedly feel guilty if a patient was found unconscious or deceased after refusing care and you felt that transportation would have prevented the circumstance.

If in doubt, do everything possible to persuade the patient to accept care and transport. Take all possible actions to persuade a patient who you feel should go to the hospital but refuses. These actions may include:

- **Spend time speaking with the patient.** Use principles of effective communication. It may take reasoning, persistence, "dealing" ("We'll call a neighbor to take care of your cat, but then you go to the hospital"), or other strategies.

- **Inform the patient of the consequences of not going to the hospital,** even if they are not pleasant.

- **Consult medical direction.** If you are in a residence, use the patient's phone to contact medical direction. If the on-line doctor is willing, let him speak to the patient when all else fails. Many services require physician contact before accepting a refusal.

- **Ask the patient if it is all right if you call a family member—or advise the patient that you would like to call a family member.** Often family members can provide the patient with reasons to go to the hospital. An offer from a loved one to meet the patient at the hospital may be very helpful. *Note, however, that notifying others and sharing protected information against a patient's wishes may constitute a HIPAA violation.* If you ask for permission or if you advise the patient of your intention to call a family member and the patient either agrees or does not object, this constitutes consent. Be sure you understand your agency's policy on how to handle this issue.

- **Call law enforcement personnel if necessary.** Police may be able to order or "arrest" the patient who refuses care to force him to go to the hospital. This is done under the premise that the patient is temporarily mentally incompetent as demonstrated by refusing care that might save his life. Be very sure that there is evidence of incompetence, because you are assuming possible legal liability if you are wrong. Remember that a patient is not mentally incompetent just because he refuses lifesaving care. Again, be sure you understand your agency's policies on this issue.

- **Listen carefully to try to determine why the patient is refusing care.** Often the patient has a fear of the hospital, procedures, prolonged hospitalization, or even death. Refusal to go to the hospital may be a form of denial or unwillingness to accept the idea of being ill. If you identify the cause of the refusal, you may be able to develop a strategy to persuade the patient to accept your care and transportation to the hospital. Listening to the patient is the key to determining why he is refusing.

Always bear in mind that you do not have the right in most cases to force a competent patient to go to the hospital against his will. Subjecting the patient to unwanted care and transport has actually been viewed in court as *assault* (placing a person in fear of bodily harm) or *battery* (causing said harm or restraining).

If all efforts fail and the patient does not accept your care or transportation, it becomes vital to document the attempts you made—to make your efforts a part of the official record—in order to prevent liability. Write into your records every step you took to persuade the patient to accept care or to go to the hospital. Include the names of any witnesses to your attempts and the patient's refusal. (A sample EMS patient refusal procedures checklist is shown in Figure 4-1.)

FIGURE 4-1 Certain procedures should be followed when a patient refuses care or transport. The checklist is from Spokane County Emergency Medical Services, Washington State.

EMS PATIENT REFUSAL CHECKLIST

PATIENT'S NAME:_____ AGE:_____

LOCATION OF CALL: _____ DATE:_____

AGENCY INCIDENT #:_____ AGENCY CODE:_____

NAME OF PERSON FILLING OUT FORM: _____

I. ASSESSMENT OF PATIENT (Check appropriate response for each item)

1. Oriented to: Person? ☐ Yes ☐ No
    Place? ☐ Yes ☐ No
    Time? ☐ Yes ☐ No
    Situation? ☐ Yes ☐ No

2. Altered level of consciousness? ☐ Yes ☐ No

3. Head injury? ☐ Yes ☐ No

4. Alcohol or drug ingestion by exam or history? ☐ Yes ☐ No

II. PATIENT INFORMED (Check appropriate response for each item)

☐ Yes ☐ No Medical treatment/evaluation needed

☐ Yes ☐ No Ambulance transport needed

☐ Yes ☐ No Further harm could result without medical treatment/evaluation

☐ Yes ☐ No Transport by means other than ambulance could be hazardous in light of patient's illness/injury

☐ Yes ☐ No Patient provided with Refusal Information Sheet

☐ Yes ☐ No Patient accepted Refusal Information Sheet

III. DISPOSITION

☐ Refused all EMS assistance

☐ Refused field treatment, but accepted transport

☐ Refused transport, but accepted field treatment

☐ Refused transport to recommended facility

☐ Patient transported by private vehicle to_____

☐ Released in care or custody of self

☐ Released in care or custody of relative or friend

   Name:_____ Relationship:_____

☐ Released in custody of law enforcement agency

   Agency:_____ Officer:_____

☐ Released in custody of other agency

   Agency:_____ Officer:_____

IV. COMMENTS: _____

_____

_____

_____

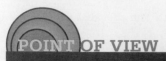
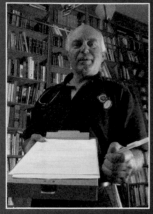

"My wife said I passed out. I don't remember passing out. To be honest, I don't remember much about it at all. I woke up and the ambulance was there. They said they'd take me to the hospital if I wanted. Who wants to go to the hospital? Not me, that's for sure. My parents died in the hospital. My brother died at the hospital. The best thing I could do was stay out of the hospital.

"My wife looked so nervous. She almost convinced me to go. And the boys on the ambulance. No, one was a girl. Nice kids. But I said no, I didn't want to go. They put a clipboard in front of me. Wanted me to sign something. Not sure what. I can't hear much anymore anyway. They were telling me all kinds of things in big medical words. At my age what difference does it make anyway?

"So I signed it."

In all cases of refusal, you should advise the patient that he should call back at any time if he has a problem or wishes to be cared for or transported. It is advisable to call a relative or neighbor who can stay with the patient in case problems develop. Leave phone stickers with emergency numbers so the patient will be able to call for help if necessary. You should also recommend that the patient or a relative call the family physician to report the incident and arrange for follow-up care. Document all actions you have taken for the patient.

Although there may be patients who legitimately refuse care (for minor wounds, unfounded calls, and the like), a patient with any significant medical condition should be transported and seen at a hospital.

Do Not Resuscitate Orders

do not resuscitate (DNR) order
a legal document, usually signed by the patient and his physician, which states that the patient has a terminal illness and does not wish to prolong life through resuscitative efforts.

advance directive
a DNR order; instructions written in advance of an event.

It will only be a matter of time before you come upon a patient who has a ***do not resuscitate (DNR) order*** (Figure 4-2). This is a legal document, usually signed by the patient and his physician, which states that the patient has a terminal illness and does not wish to prolong life through resuscitative efforts. A DNR order is called an ***advance directive***, because it is written and signed in advance of any event where resuscitation might be undertaken. It is more than the expressed wishes of the patient or family. It is an actual legal document.

There are varying degrees of DNR orders, expressed through a variety of detailed instructions that may be part of the order. Such an instruction might stipulate, for example, that resuscitation be attempted only if cardiac or respiratory arrest is observed, but not attempted if the patient is found already in arrest (to avoid the possibility of resuscitating a patient who may already have sustained brain damage).

Many states also have laws governing living wills, which are statements signed by the patient, usually regarding use of long-term life support and comfort measures such as respirators, intravenous feedings, and pain medications. Other states require naming a *proxy*—a person whom the signer of the document names to make health care decisions in case he is unable to make such decisions for himself. Living wills and health care proxies usually pertain to situations that will occur in the hospital rather than in the prehospital situation.

Become familiar with the laws regarding DNR orders, living wills, and health care proxies for your region or state and the laws and rules governing their implementation. It is important to know the forms and policies before you go to the call, since often the patient is in cardiac arrest (heart and breathing have stopped) or near death. These are stressful times for the family and for you, occasions when the window of time for making a resuscitation decision may be only a few moments.

A legal DNR order prevents unwanted resuscitation and awkward situations. In most cases, the oral requests of a family member are not reason to withhold care. If the family requests you to not resuscitate the patient, and if there are no legal DNR orders available, it

FIGURE 4-2 Example of a do not resuscitate (DNR) order.

PREHOSPITAL DO NOT RESUSCITATE ORDERS

ATTENDING PHYSICIAN

In completing this prehospital DNR form, please check part A if no intervention by prehospital personnel is indicated. Please check Part A and options from Part B if specific interventions by prehospital personnel are indicated. To give a valid prehospital DNR order, this form must be completed by the patient's attending physician and must be provided to prehospital personnel.

A) _____**Do Not Resuscitate (DNR):**
No Cardiopulmonary Resuscitation or Advanced Cardiac Life Support be performed by prehospital personnel

B) _____**Modified Support:**
Prehospital personnel administer the following checked options:
_____Oxygen administration
_____Full airway support: intubation, airways, bag/valve/mask
_____Venipuncture: IV crystalloids and/or blood draw
_____External cardiac pacing
_____Cardiopulmonary resuscitation
_____Cardiac defibrillator
_____Pneumatic anti-shock garment
_____Ventilator
_____ACLS meds
_____Other interventions/medications (physician specify)
_____

Prehospital personnel are informed that (print patient name)_____
should receive no resuscitation (DNR) or should receive Modified Support as indicated. This directive is medically appropriate and is further documented by a physician's order and a progress note on the patient's permanent medical record. Informed consent from the capacitated patient or the incapacitated patient's legitimate surrogate is documented on the patient's permanent medical record. The DNR order is in full force and effect as of the date indicated below.

_____   _____

Attending Physician's Signature   _____

_____   _____
Print Attending Physician's Name   Print Patient's Name and Location
                                             (Home Address or Health Care Facility)

_____
Attending Physician's Telephone

_____   _____
Date   Expiration Date (6 Mos from Signature)

is a legal and ethical dilemma that is usually best resolved by providing care. It is better to be criticized or sued for attempting to save a life than for letting a patient die. At times, a family under duress may ask that a DNR order be ignored and resuscitation be initiated despite the DNR. In such a situation, contact medical direction for advice and, if necessary, ask the medical direction physician to speak to the family.

OTHER LEGAL ISSUES

Negligence

To the layperson, *negligence* means that something that should have been done was not done or was done incorrectly. The legal concept of negligence in emergency care is not that

CORE CONCEPT

The legal concepts of negligence, torts, and abandonment

negligence
a finding of failure to act properly in a situation in which there was a duty to act, that needed care as would reasonably be expected of the EMT was not provided, and that harm was caused to the patient as a result.

simple. A finding of negligence, or failure to act properly, requires that *all* of the following circumstances be proved:

- The EMT had a duty to the patient (duty to act—see the next section).

- The EMT did not provide the standard of care (committed a breach of duty). This may include the failure to act; that is, he did not provide needed care as would be expected of an EMT in your locality. Failure to act is a major cause of legal actions against EMS systems or EMTs.

- There was *proximate causation* (the concept that the damages to the patient were the result of action or inaction of the EMT). This means that by not providing the standard of care, the EMT caused harm to the patient. The harm can be physical or psychological. An example of proximate causation would be injuries caused when EMTs dropped the stretcher carrying a patient.

    This concept cannot be applied to patients who are seriously injured and cannot be saved. If you perform CPR according to guidelines and the patient dies, there is no proximate causation between your actions and the patient's death.

Negligence is the basis for a large number of lawsuits involving prehospital emergency care. If the previously listed circumstances are proved, the EMT may be required to pay damages if the court considers the harm to the patient to be a loss that requires reimbursement (compensable). The negligent EMT may be required to pay for medical expenses, lost wages (possibly including future earnings), pain and suffering, and various other factors as determined by the court.

The proceedings or lawsuits against EMTs are usually classified as torts. A ***tort*** is a civil offense (as opposed to a criminal offense resulting in arrest). A tort may be defined as an action or injury caused by negligence from which a lawsuit may arise.

A concept used in tort law is ***res ipsa loquitur***, a Latin term meaning "the thing speaks for itself." This is a foundational concept in negligence, because it allows a finding of negligence even when there is no specific evidence of a negligent act. Looking back at the stretcher-drop example in which the patient was injured, the plaintiff would not have to prove specific intent or negligence on the part of the EMTs or even that the EMTs were the ones who caused the stretcher to drop. Because the EMTs had exclusive control over the stretcher when it was dropped, there is a reasonable assumption that the EMTs caused the accident and that without negligence of some sort the accident would not have happened.

Two of the most common and significant causes of lawsuits against EMTs are patient refusal and ambulance collisions (Figure 4-3). In patient refusal situations, EMTs are sued be-

tort
a civil, not a criminal, offense; an action or injury caused by negligence from which a lawsuit may arise.

res ipsa loquitur
a Latin term meaning "the thing speaks for itself."

FIGURE 4-3 Ambulance collisions cause injuries and may prompt lawsuits. (© *Canandaigua Emergency Squad*)

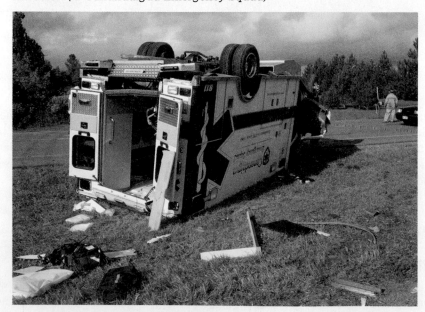

cause the patient's condition deteriorated after the ambulance left the scene. This makes it critical to follow your agency's guidelines when a patient refuses care.

Collisions are dangerous in any vehicle. When an ambulance is involved, collisions become serious because of the size and weight of the vehicle, the number of occupants (including the patient), and the nature of emergency driving. It is important to remember that most collisions are preventable. (This is why they are no longer referred to as "accidents.") Emergency driving must be done responsibly.

Lawsuits against EMTs are uncommon, especially when compared to the number of calls that are dispatched each day in this country. Although liability and negligence should be important considerations, you should not live or work in fear of a lawsuit. When you perform proper care that is within your scope of practice and is properly documented, you will prevent most, if not all, legal problems.

Duty to Act

An EMT in certain situations has a ***duty to act***, or an obligation to provide emergency care to a patient. An EMT who is on an ambulance and is dispatched to a call clearly has a duty to act. If there is no threat to safety, the EMT must provide care. This duty to act continues throughout the call.

If an EMT has initiated care, then leaves a patient without ensuring that the patient has been turned over to someone with equal or greater medical training, ***abandonment*** exists. Similarly, if a paramedic has begun advanced care, then turns the patient over to an EMT for transport, abandonment (on the part of the paramedic) may exist.

The duty to act is not always clear. It depends on your state and local laws. In many states, an off-duty EMT has no legal obligation to provide care. However, you may feel a ***moral*** or ***ethical*** obligation to act; for example, if you observe a motor-vehicle collision while off duty, you may feel morally bound to provide care, even if no legal obligation exists. If you are off duty, begin care, and then leave before other trained personnel arrive, you may still be considered to have abandoned the patient.

Other situations are even more confusing. If you are an EMT in an ambulance, but you are out of your jurisdiction, the laws are again often unclear. In general, if you follow your conscience and provide care, you will incur less liability than if you do not act. Always follow your local protocols and laws. Your instructor will provide information about local issues.

Good Samaritan Laws

Good Samaritan laws have been developed in all states to provide immunity to individuals trying to help people in emergencies. Most of these laws will grant immunity from liability if the rescuer acts in good faith to provide care to the level of his training and to the best of his ability. These laws do not prevent someone from initiating a lawsuit, nor will they protect the rescuer from being found liable for acts of gross negligence and other violations of the law.

You must familiarize yourself with the laws that govern your state. Good Samaritan laws may not apply to EMTs in your locality. In some states, the Good Samaritan laws apply only to volunteers. If you are a paid EMT, different laws and regulations may apply.

Some states have specific statutes that authorize, regulate, and protect EMS personnel. Typically, to be protected by such laws, you must be recognized as an EMT in the state where care was provided. Some states have specific licensing and certification requirements that must be met for recognition under Good Samaritan laws.

Confidentiality

When you act as an EMT, you obtain a considerable amount of information about a patient. You also are allowed into homes and other personal areas that are private and contain much information about people.

Any information you obtain about a patient's history, condition, or treatment is considered confidential and must not be shared with anyone else. This principle is known as ***confidentiality***. Such information may be disclosed only when a written release is signed by the patient. Your organization will have a policy on this. Patient information should not be disclosed based on verbal permission, nor should information be disclosed over the telephone.

"Follow your protocols. Treat people well. Ask for help when you need it. That is how to stay legally safe."

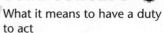
CORE CONCEPT
What it means to have a duty to act

duty to act
an obligation to provide care to a patient.

abandonment
leaving a patient after care has been initiated and before the patient has been transferred to someone with equal or greater medical training.

moral
regarding personal standards or principles of right and wrong.

ethical
regarding a social system or social or professional expectations for applying principles of right and wrong.

Good Samaritan laws
a series of laws, varying in each state, designed to provide limited legal protection for citizens and some health care personnel when they are administering emergency care.

confidentiality
the obligation not to reveal information obtained about a patient except to other health care professionals involved in the patient's care, or under subpoena, or in a court of law, or when the patient has signed a release of confidentiality.

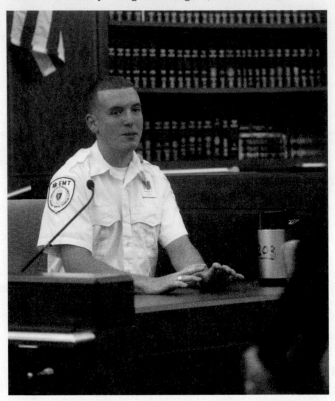

FIGURE 4-4 An EMT may be required to testify in court in a variety of legal settings. *(© Mark C. Ide)*

However, you may be subpoenaed, or ordered into court by a legal authority, where you may legally disclose patient information (Figure 4-4). If you have a question about the validity of a legal document, contact a supervisor or your agency's attorney for advice.

Patient information also may be shared with other health care professionals who will have a role in the patient's care or in quality improvement. It is appropriate to turn over information about the patient to the nurse and physician at the receiving hospital. This is necessary for continuity in patient care. It may also be necessary and permissible to supply certain patient-care information for insurance billing forms.

HIPAA

the Health Insurance Portability and Accountability Act, a federal law protecting the privacy of patient-specific health care information and providing the patient with control over how this information is used and distributed

Although confidentiality has always been a part of health care, newer regulations have given it even greater emphasis. The Health Insurance Portability and Accountability Act (**HIPAA**) has brought significant changes to the record-keeping, storage, access, and discussion of patient-specific medical information. Ambulance services that bill for services (electronically or by employing a service that does this work) are mandated to have policies, procedures, and training in place to deal with these privacy issues. Table 4-1 summarizes key points about HIPAA and how it will impact your work as an EMT.

Table 4-1   Health Insurance Portability and Accountability Act (HIPAA)

When you go through ambulance orientation, or when you begin to work or volunteer, you will likely hear much about HIPAA regulations. These federal regulations are designed to limit access to records by unnecessary personnel as well as to provide the patient the right to review his or her information and have a greater say in its use and distribution. How will this affect you as an EMT?

- You will discuss patient-specific information only with those with whom it is medically necessary to do so.
- Your EMS agency will have specific privacy policies and procedures in place.
- You will get a printed copy of these policies and procedures as will the patients in your care. You will ask your patients to sign a form indicating they have received this information. This form may be combined with your insurance-release form.
- Your EMS agency will have a Privacy Officer to oversee HIPAA issues and deal with the documentation required by law.

Remember that you will be provided information about your agency's specific privacy policies and procedures.

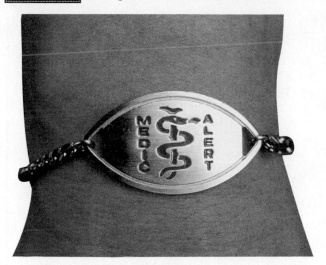
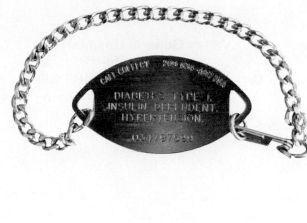

Libel and slander are two legal terms that may apply when information is shared inappropriately or falsely. *Libel* is when information that is false or injurious to another is spread in written form. *Slander* is when the information is shared verbally. Note that libel or slander can occur even if the shared information is true.

libel
false or injurious information in written form.

slander
false or injurious information stated verbally.

Special Situations
Medical Identification Devices

A patient may wear a medical identification device (Figure 4-5) to alert EMTs and other health care professionals that he has a particular medical condition. If the patient is found unconscious, the device provides important medical information. The device may be a necklace, bracelet, or card and may indicate a number of conditions including:

- Heart conditions
- Allergies
- Diabetes
- Epilepsy

Organ Donors

You may respond to calls where a patient is critically injured, perhaps near death, and is an *organ donor*. An organ donor is a patient who has completed a legal document that allows for donation of organs and tissues in the event of his death. Many people have benefited from the donation of organs by persons who have completed this paperwork (Figure 4-6).

You may find that the patient is an organ donor when told so by a family member. Often a patient may have an organ donor card on him. The back of the patient's driver's license may also contain an indication that the patient wishes to donate organs upon his death.

The emergency care of a patient who is an organ donor must not differ from the care of a patient who is not a donor. All emergency care measures must be taken. If a patient is recognized as an organ donor, contact medical direction. The on-line physician may order you to perform CPR on a patient when you might normally not resuscitate due to fatal injuries. The oxygen delivered to body cells by CPR will help preserve the organs until they can be harvested for implantation in another person.

organ donor
a person who has completed a legal document that allows for donation of organs and tissues in the event of death.

Safe Haven Laws

Most states have implemented some sort of *safe haven law*. Under such a law, a person may drop off an infant or child at any police, fire, or EMS station or deliver the infant or child to any available public safety personnel. Each state has different guidelines for the ages of children that are included under the act—usually infants to young children.

safe haven law
a law that permits a person to drop off an infant or child at a police, fire, or EMS station or to deliver the infant or child to any available public safety personnel. The intent of the law is to protect children who may otherwise be abandoned or harmed.

FIGURE 4-6 Example of an organ donor form.

Valley General Hospital
Permission for
Organ Donation/Anatomical Gift
by an Individual Prior to Death

PATIENT IDENTIFICATION PLATE

I, _____ , currently residing at _____

_____ , being eighteen (18) years of age or older, do hereby make the

following organ donation/anatomical gift to take effect upon my death:

1.   I give, if medically acceptable:

☐ My body
☐ Any needed organs or parts
☐ The following organs or parts: _____

_____

_____

2.   I make this gift to Valley General Hospital or to physicians or institutions designated by them for
the following purposes:

☐ Any purpose authorized by law
☐ Transplantation
☐ Therapy
☐ Medical Research and/or Education

3.   I acknowledge that I have read this document in its entirety and that I fully understand it and that
all blank spaces have either been completed or crossed off prior to my signing.

4.   I understand that Valley General Hospital and its authorized designees will rely upon this consent.

_____   _____   _____   _____
SIGNATURE   DATE   WITNESS TO SIGNATURE   DATE
                                                    (PRINT NAME and ADDRESS BELOW)

_____   _____
PRINT NAME

_____   _____
ADDRESS

_____
TELEPHONE NUMBER   _____   _____
                                                    WITNESS TO SIGNATURE   DATE
                                                    (PRINT NAME and ADDRESS BELOW)

                                                    _____

                                                    _____

A safe haven law is designed to protect children who may otherwise be abandoned or harmed by parents who are unable or unwilling to care for them.

Crime Scenes

A *crime scene* is defined as the location where a crime has been committed or any place that evidence relating to a crime may be found. Many crime scenes involve crimes against people. These crimes cause injuries that are often serious. Once police have made the scene safe, the EMT's priority at a crime scene is to provide patient care.

While you are providing care at the crime scene, there are actions that you can take to help preserve evidence. To preserve evidence, you must first know what evidence is, as described in the following list:

- **Condition of the scene.** The way you find the scene is important evidence to the police. Should you arrive first, make a mental note of the exterior of the scene. Remember how you gained access. Doors found ajar, pry marks, and broken windows are signs of danger for you and important evidence for the police. Make a note of whether the lights were on or off and the condition of the TV and radio.

- **The patient.** The patient himself provides valuable information. The position the patient is found in, condition of clothing, and injuries are all valuable pieces of evidence.

- **Fingerprints and footprints.** Fingerprints are perhaps the most familiar kind of evidence. They may be obtained from almost any surface. It is important for you to avoid unnecessarily touching anything at the scene in order to preserve prints. Since you will be wearing gloves at most scenes, you will not leave your fingerprints on objects. If you touch these objects, however, even while wearing gloves, you may smudge fingerprints that were left by someone else.

- **Microscopic evidence.** Microscopic evidence is a wide range of evidence that is usually invisible to the naked eye. It consists of small pieces of evidence such as dirt and carpet fibers. To the eye, there may be no way to distinguish one from another. Under the microscope, scientists can develop valuable information. From just a few fibers, the materials and sometimes the brand name of carpets or clothes can be determined. Traces of blood may be enough to determine blood type or to be used for DNA comparison.

To preserve evidence at the crime scene (Figure 4-7), the following actions will be helpful to the police. Remember that your first priority is always patient care.

- **Remember what you touch.** It may be necessary to move the patient or furniture to begin CPR or other patient care. Although this cannot be avoided, it is helpful to tell the police what you have touched or moved. Once you leave, if they find furniture moved or blood stains in two locations, they may think that a scuffle took place when in fact it did not. If you are forced to break a window to get to the patient and do not tell the police, they will think that a breaking-and-entering has occurred.

- **Minimize your impact on the scene.** If you are forced to move the patient or furniture to begin care, move as little as possible. Do not wander through the house or go to areas where it is not necessary to go. Avoid using the phone, as this will prevent the police from using the "redial" button to determine who the victim called last. Do not use the bathroom since this may also destroy evidence. Do not cut through holes left in clothing by bullets or knives, which will also destroy evidence. Cut at least 6 inches from these holes.

- **Work with the police.** The police may require you to provide a statement about your actions or observations at the scene. Although it may not be possible to make notes while patient care is going on, after you arrive at the hospital make notes about your observations and actions at the scene.

You may also wish to critique the scene—both with your crew and, if possible, with the police. Invite a member of your local or state police department to your agency for an in-service drill on crime scenes. Evidence recovery methods and procedures vary from area to area. The police officer who comes to your station will brief you on local procedures.

crime scene
the location where a crime has been committed or any place that evidence relating to a crime may be found.

FIGURE 4-7 A crime scene. *(© Kevin Link)*

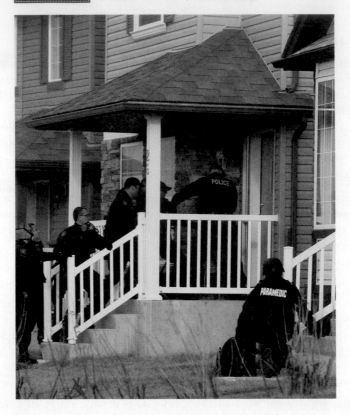

Interestingly enough, police are often as unfamiliar with EMS procedures as you are with police evidence procedures. The police may ask you to delay your work at the scene so they can take photographs or interview the patient. They may do this because they do not understand—as you will learn in later chapters—that in the case of serious injury, the time that elapses before on-scene care and transport to the hospital must be kept to a minimum for the patient to have the best chance of survival. Education and critiques can be beneficial to both EMTs and police officers.

Special Reporting Requirements

Many states require EMTs and other health care professionals to report certain types of incidents. Many areas have hotlines for reporting crimes such as child, elder, or domestic abuse. This may be mandatory in your area. Failure to report certain incidents may actually be a crime. There is also a strong moral obligation to report these crimes. Many states offer immunity from liability for people who report incidents such as these in good faith.

Other crimes may also require reports. Violence (such as gunshot wounds or stabbings) and sexual assaults often fall into this category. If you are required by law to report such incidents, you are usually exempt from confidentiality requirements in making these reports.

You may also be required to notify police of other situations, such as cases where restraint may be necessary, intoxicated persons found with injuries, or mentally incompetent people who have been injured.

CHAPTER REVIEW

Key Facts and Concepts

- Medical, legal, and ethical issues are a part of every EMS call.

- Morals are how a person expresses his belief of right and wrong.

- Consent may be expressed or implied. If a competent patient refuses care or transport, you should make every effort to persuade him, but you cannot force him to accept care or go to the hospital.

- Negligence is failing to act properly when you have a duty to act. As an EMT, you have a duty to act whenever you are dispatched on a call. You may have a legal or moral duty to act even when off duty or outside your jurisdiction.

- Abandonment is leaving a patient after you have initiated care and before you have transferred the patient to a person with equal or higher training.

- Confidentiality is the obligation not to reveal personal information you obtain about a patient except to other health care professionals involved in the patient's care, under court order, or when the patient signs a release.

- As an EMT, you may be sued or held legally liable on any of these issues. However, EMTs are rarely held liable when they have acted within their scope of practice and according to the standard of care and have carefully documented the details of the call.

- At a crime scene, care of the patient takes precedence over preservation of evidence; however, you should make every effort not to disturb the scene unnecessarily and to report your actions and observations to the police.

Key Decisions

- Does the care I wish to give fall into my scope of practice?

- Does this patient consent to my care? Can this patient consent to my care?

- Does this patient need to go to the hospital? How can I convince him to go if he doesn't want to?

- Is the DNR order valid? Does it apply to this patient?

- How should I act on each call and what can I do to prevent lawsuits?

- Do I have a duty to act in this situation?

- Is this confidential information? Can I tell anyone or share the information?

- Is this a crime scene? If so, how do I preserve evidence while taking care of the patient?

- Is this a crime that I am required to report?

Chapter Glossary

abandonment leaving a patient after care has been initiated and before the patient has been transferred to someone with equal or greater medical training.

advance directive a DNR order; instructions written in advance of an event.

assault placing a person in fear of bodily harm.

battery causing bodily harm to or restraining a person.

confidentiality the obligation not to reveal information obtained about a patient except to other health care professionals involved in the patient's care, or under subpoena, or in a court of law, or when the patient has signed a release of confidentiality.

consent permission from the patient for care or other action by the EMT.

crime scene the location where a crime has been committed or any place that evidence relating to a crime may be found.

do not resuscitate (DNR) order a legal document, usually signed by the patient and his physician, which states that the pa-

tient has a terminal illness and does not wish to prolong life through resuscitative efforts.

duty to act an obligation to provide care to a patient.

ethical regarding a social system or social or professional expectations for applying principles of right and wrong.

expressed consent consent given by adults who are of legal age and mentally competent to make a rational decision in regard to their medical well-being.

Good Samaritan laws a series of laws, varying in each state, designed to provide limited legal protection for citizens and some health care personnel when they are administering emergency care.

HIPAA the Health Insurance Portability and Accountability Act, a federal law protecting the privacy of patient-specific health care information and providing the patient with control over how this information is used and distributed.

implied consent the consent it is presumed a patient or patient's parent or guardian would give if they could, such as for an unconscious patient or a parent who cannot be contacted when care is needed.

in loco parentis in place of the parents, indicating a person who may give consent for care of a child when the parents are not present or able to give consent.

liability being held legally responsible.

libel false or injurious information in written form.

moral regarding personal standards or principles of right and wrong.

negligence a finding of failure to act properly in a situation in which there was a duty to act, that needed care as would reasonably be expected of the EMT was not provided, and that harm was caused to the patient as a result.

organ donor a person who has completed a legal document that allows for donation of organs and tissues in the event of death.

res ipsa loquitur a Latin term meaning "the thing speaks for itself."

safe haven law a law that permits a person to drop off an infant or child at a police, fire, or EMS station or to deliver the infant or child to any available public safety personnel. The intent of the law is to protect children who may otherwise be abandoned or harmed.

scope of practice a set of regulations and ethical considerations that define the scope, or extent and limits, of the EMT's job.

slander false or injurious information stated verbally.

standard of care for an EMT providing care for a specific patient in a specific situation, the care that would be expected to be provided by an EMT with similar training when caring for a patient in a similar situation.

tort a civil, not a criminal, offense; an action or injury caused by negligence from which a lawsuit may arise.

Preparation for Your Examination and Practice

Short Answer

1. Explain the difference between expressed and implied consent.

2. What are the components required to prove negligence?

3. What is your first priority at a crime scene: preserving evidence or patient care? Why?

4. You bring a patient to the hospital and the nurse tells you, "Put the patient in bed 5—I'll be right there." The nurse doesn't come over, and you leave. Is this abandonment? Why or why not?

5. You have a patient who weighs 400 pounds. You want other EMTs at your squad to know this so they can be prepared. Can you leave a copy of your run report on the bulletin board at the station to notify the others?

Thinking and Linking

As you work on this exercise, think back to what you have learned in Chapter 1, "Introduction to Emergency Medical Services and the Health Care System," Chapter 2, "The Well-Being of the EMT," and Chapter 3, "Lifting and Moving Patients" and combine those concepts with concepts explained in this chapter.

1. What roles and responsibilities of an EMT are important in preventing lawsuits?

2. What can I do when lifting and moving patients to help prevent injury to patients and the lawsuits that may result?

Critical Thinking Exercises

Many aspects of EMS require moral or ethical decisions. The purpose of this exercise will be to apply these considerations to several situations you might encounter.

1. You and your partner are in your ambulance on the way back from a call when you come upon a motor-vehicle crash. It is in an adjoining ambulance district. Do you have a duty to act? Do you have a moral or ethical obligation?

2. You are transporting a patient who was seriously injured when he was ejected from his vehicle in a high-speed colli-sion. You talk to another member of your crew who tells you the patient died the next day. That crew member is worried about getting sued over the death. Do you think that a lawsuit against you is likely? Why or why not?

3. You respond to a motor-vehicle crash and find a seriously injured patient. You find he has no pulse and are about to begin CPR when someone tells you, "He's got cancer and a DNR. Don't do that, man!" No one has the DNR order at the scene. Do you do CPR and transport the patient?

On a hot summer day you receive a call for a 37-year-old woman with general body weakness. After your primary assessment, you ask the patient about her medical history. She informs you that she has AIDS. You continue to take vital signs, find it appropriate to provide oxygen, and package her for transport. Your partner makes the radio report to the hospital, and you notice that he makes no reference to AIDS. When you arrive at the hospital, your partner gives the patient report in the hallway leading to the examination room. He provides all the patient information but does not tell the doctor the patient reported she has AIDS until he can do it discreetly in the room. He asks the patient to sign a form that allows release of information for insurance billing and acknowledges receipt of the Notice of Privacy Practices in place at your agency.

Street Scene Questions

1. Was it appropriate not to include the information that the patient has AIDS during the radio report to the hospital?
2. What is the obligation of these EMTs concerning the confidentiality of patient information?
3. Would you have handled the transfer of information differently?

After the call is over, you discuss with your partner issues of confidentiality. He tells you that he felt the fact the patient had AIDS did not need to be part of the radio report. He was concerned that it might breach the patient's confidentiality if it was said over the radio. But your partner was quick to add that AIDS was definitely a pertinent part of the medical history and he made sure it was conveyed in a discreet manner at the hospital.

Street Scene Question

4. Would it be appropriate to tell all the hospital staff about the patient's AIDS so they would know to take infection control precautions?

As you and your partner further discuss the issue, you tell him that alerting the hospital staff so they would know to use infection control precautions would be appropriate. He responds by telling you that all emergency medical personnel, whether EMS or in-hospital, should be taking infection control precautions. However, this should not be a reason for being careless with patient information and possibly breaching a patient's confidentiality.

Street Scene Questions

5. Should the information that this patient has AIDS be shared with other EMS providers in case they get a call for this patient?
6. What are the principles for confidentiality that EMTs should always maintain?

As you pull into the garage, you suggest to your partner that you should alert the other crews about this patient having AIDS. Your partner tells you that this would be a breach of the patient's confidentiality. It would be very inappropriate to do this. He reminds you that patient information is always to be kept confidential unless it needs to be shared for the purpose of giving care. "For example," he says, "the patient's information on the report to the hospital included the fact that she told us she had AIDS. Also, the physician needed to know because it was part of the medical history that we obtained. Unless there is another reason to share this information that I haven't thought of, no one else needs to hear from us that this patient has AIDS. Confidentiality is an EMS standard that pertains to the history, condition, and treatment of all the patients we see." As he gets out of the ambulance at the station, he adds: "Remember, confidentiality is a professional responsibility."

5

Medical Terminology and Anatomy and Physiology

EXPLORE ResourceCentral

To access Resource Central, follow directions on the Student Access Card provided with this text. If there is no card, go to **www.bradybooks.com** and follow the Resource Central link to Buy Access from there. Under Media Resources, you will find:

▸ **Medical Term Components**
Learn to use proper medical terms when communicating with other medical professionals. But keep the complicated medical language to yourself when talking with patients. They are probably scared enough already!

▸ **Online Human Anatomy**
Read all about the body systems and the organs that make up each system. And you thought our personalities were complicated!

▸ **Heart and Major Vessels**
Observe the heart at work in this animation and identify its main structures.

OBJECTIVES

After reading this chapter you should be able to:

5.1 Define key terms introduced in this chapter.

5.2 Describe the importance of the proper use of medical terminology. (p. 93)

5.3 Apply definitions of common prefixes, suffixes, and roots to determine the meaning of medical terms. (pp. 93–95)

5.4 Recognize the meaning of acronyms and abbreviations commonly used in EMS. (p. 95)

5.5 Give examples of when it is better to use a common or lay term to describe something than it is to use a medical term. (p. 95)

5.6 Use anatomical terms of position and direction to describe the location of body structures and position of the body. (pp. 96–100)

5.7 Utilize topographical anatomical landmarks as points of reference. (p. 100)

5.8 Describe the structures and functions of each of the following body systems:

a. Musculoskeletal (pp. 100–102, 105–109)
b. Respiratory (pp. 102, 109–111)
c. Cardiovascular (pp. 102–103, 112–120)
d. Nervous (pp. 103, 120–122)
e. Digestive (pp. 103, 122–123)
f. Integumentary (pp. 104, 123–124)
g. Endocrine (pp. 104, 124–125)
h. Renal (pp. 104, 124, 126–127)
i. Male and female reproductive (pp. 105, 127–129)

5.9 Given a series of models or diagrams, label the anatomical structures of each of the following body systems:

a. Skeletal (p. 101)
b. Respiratory (p. 110)
c. Cardiovascular (pp. 112–114, 118–119)
d. Nervous (p. 126)
e. Skin (p. 123)
f. Endocrine (p. 125)
g. Renal/urinary (p. 126)
h. Male and female reproductive (pp. 128–129)

5.10 Describe the differences in the respiratory anatomy of children as compared to adults (p. 111)

5.11 Apply understanding of anatomy and physiology to explain the function of the life support chain. (p. 120)

KEY TERMS

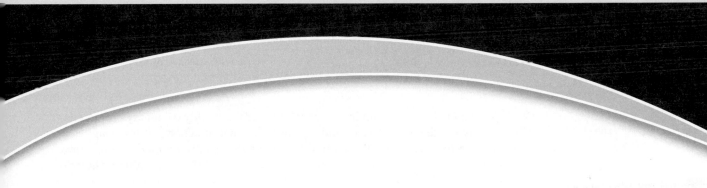

MEDICAL TERMINOLOGY

<<<<<<<

CORE CONCEPT ●- - - - - - - - -
Medical terminology and how terms are constructed

Although you are only a few chapters into the book, you have already seen some sizeable words and probably heard a few more from your instructors. You will encounter more as you begin the patient assessment and care sections of this text. Some say medicine has a language of its own. As with any language, understanding some of the basics will make it easier to understand and use correctly in communicating with other medical professionals.

The Components of Medical Terms

Medical terms are composed of words, and medical words may be composed of roots, prefixes, and/or suffixes—each with its own definition. (See the examples in Table 5-1.)

Sometimes medical words are **compounds**, made up of two or more whole words. For example, the word *small* is joined with the word *pox* to form the medical term *smallpox*, the name of a disease.

Roots are the foundations of words and are not used by themselves. *Therm* is a root that means "heat." Used alone, it would make no sense. But when a vowel is added to the end of the root (in this case, the added vowel is *o*) it becomes a **combining form**, *therm/o*, which can be joined with other words, roots, or suffixes. For example, *therm/o* and *meter* combine to form *thermometer*, an instrument for measuring heat or temperature.

Some medical terms combine more than one root or combining form. *Electrocardiogram* is a good example. The combining forms *electr/o* (electric) and *cardi/o* (heart) are joined to *gram* (a written record) to form the term. An electrocardiogram is a written record of the heart's electrical activity.

compound
a word formed from two or more whole words.

root
foundation of a word that is not a word that can stand on its own.

combining form
a word root with an added vowel that can be joined with other words, roots, or suffixes to form a new word.

Table 5-1 Common Roots, Prefixes, and Suffixes

EXAMPLE	WORD PART	MEANING
Cardi	Root	Heart
Neur	Root	Nerve
Nas	Root	Nose/nasal
Or	Root	Mouth/oral
Hyper-	Prefix	Above normal, high
Hypo-	Prefix	Below normal, low
Tachy-	Prefix	Above normal, rapid
Brady-	Prefix	Below normal, slow
-ac	Suffix	Pertaining to
-ology	Suffix	Study of
-al	Suffix	Pertaining to
-ist	Suffix	One who specializes in

prefix
word part added to the beginning of a root or word to modify or qualify its meaning.

suffix
word part added to the end of a root or word to complete its meaning.

Prefixes are added to the beginnings of roots or words to modify or qualify their meaning. They usually tell the reader what kind of, where, in what direction, or how many. The root *pnea* relates to breathing but says nothing about the quality or kind of breathing. Adding the prefix *dys-* (painful; difficult) makes it *dyspnea*, or difficult breathing. The prefix *tachy-* (rapid; fast) when combined with *pnea* creates *tachypnea*, or rapid breathing.

Abdominal pain is a broad term. Adding the prefix *intra-* (within; inside) narrows the meaning. *Intraabdominal pain* is pain within the abdomen.

Plegia refers to paralysis of the limbs. The prefix *quadri-* (four) tells the reader how many limbs are paralyzed. *Quadraplegia* is paralysis of all four limbs.

Suffixes are word parts added to the ends of roots or words to complete their meaning. A number of suffixes have specialized meanings. The suffix *-itis* means inflammation and the root *arthr* refers to a joint; thus, *arthritis* is inflammation of a joint. The suffix *-iac* forms a noun indicating a person afflicted with a certain disease; for example, *hemophiliac*, a patient suffering from the bleeding disorder hemophilia.

Some suffixes are joined to roots to form terms that indicate a state, quantity, condition, procedure, or process. *Pneumonia* and *psoriasis* are examples of medical conditions, whereas *appendectomy* and *arthroscopy* are examples of medical procedures. The suffixes in each case are underlined.

Some suffixes combine with roots to form adjectives, words that modify nouns by indicating quality or quantity or by distinguishing one thing from another. *Gastric*, *cardiac*, *fibrous*, *arthritic*, and *diaphoretic* are all examples of adjectives formed by adding suffixes (underlined) to roots.

Some suffixes are added to roots to express reduction in size, such as *-iole* and *-ule*. An *arteriole* is smaller than an artery, and a *venule* is smaller than a vein.

When added to roots, *-e* and *-ize* form verbs. *Excise* and *catheterize* are examples. Given the definitions of its root and suffixes, a *cardiologist* is one who specializes in the study of the heart, as shown in Figure 5-1.

This textbook will help you understand medical terminology by providing definitions in the margins and in a glossary. Online you will find a medical terminology guide as well as an audio glossary, which will allow you to hear the proper pronunciation of a term.

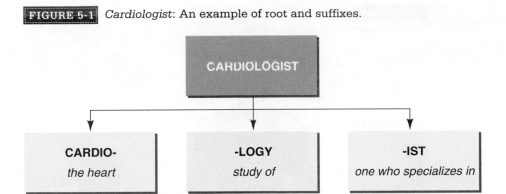

FIGURE 5-1 *Cardiologist:* An example of root and suffixes.

CARDIOLOGIST

CARDIO-	-LOGY	-IST
the heart	study of	one who specializes in

Abbreviations and Acronyms

Abbreviations and acronyms also abound in the world of EMS. (An acronym is an abbreviation made up of initials that can be pronounced as a word, such as *CPAP*, pronounced "SEE-pap," for continuous positive airway pressure—which will be discussed in Chapter 19, "Respiratory Emergencies.") You will encounter many abbreviations and acronyms in your class and in the field.

Abbreviations and acronyms can be helpful when completing documentation on a run. For example, you may write that a patient had *CHF*, which is an abbreviation for congestive heart failure. You will learn that the first care you give a patient is the *ABCs*, standing for airway, breathing, and circulation. This will help you remember your priorities during the primary assessment.

There are downsides to using initials instead of words. You must be sure that the acronym or abbreviation you are using is standard and accepted. Many services and regions have policies regarding acceptable use of these terms.

When and When Not to Use Medical Terms

You should avoid using any type of obscure medical terminology, jargon, abbreviations, or acronyms when you are talking to patients and families. For example, if you ask a patient if he has ever had "an MI" (for myocardial infarction—a heart attack), the patient will not be able to provide the correct answer if he is not familiar with the term you used.

Finally, resist the urge to use complex medical terminology—even correctly—when a simple, accurate term will do. The language of medicine, like any other language, must be applied appropriately and practically in any given situation.

ANATOMY AND PHYSIOLOGY

Think of anatomy and physiology as the owner's manual to the body. When a mechanic works on your car, he often refers to the manual to help him better understand where the specific parts are placed and what those parts do. As an EMT, you will use a knowledge of the body's anatomy and physiology to better understand where vital structures are located and how injuries and illnesses will affect the body in general.

Anatomy is the study of body structure. A working knowledge of anatomy will help you understand where organs and organ systems are located and also how external injuries may impact internal systems. *Physiology*, the study of body function, will give you a baseline idea of how the body should work normally. Understanding this will help you identify abnormal function and predict the impact of challenges to normal function.

Anatomy and physiology will be helpful guides to decision making throughout your experience as an EMT. You should use basic understanding to help you assess and treat ill or injured patients. As you assess, ask yourself, "What organs and organ systems could be affected, and what does affecting these organs do to normal body function?" Think of it as referring to the owner's manual.

anatomy
the study of body structure.

physiology
the study of body function.

FIGURE 5-2 Body regions and anatomical position.

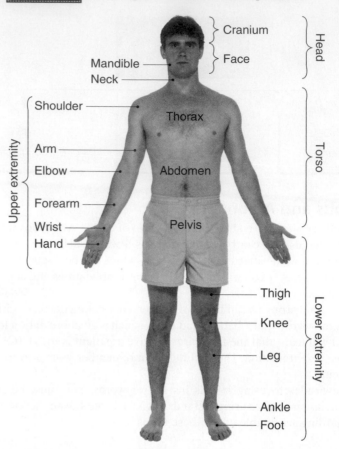

ANATOMICAL TERMS

In anatomy and physiology, being precise is important. We use specific terms to refer to exact locations. Learning these terms will be similar to learning a new language. In this case, you will be learning the language of health care. Using this new language will keep you on a par with your peers in the hospital and other health care fields, and will allow you to describe the body in a far more exact and objective manner.

Directional Terms

CORE CONCEPT
Directional terms

anatomical position
the standard reference position for the body in the study of anatomy. In this position, the body is standing erect, facing the observer, with arms down at the sides and the palms of the hands forward.

plane
a flat surface formed when slicing through a solid object.

For clear communication among health care professionals, there must be a standardized way of referring to places on the body when describing illness or injury. For this purpose, the body is divided into regions (Figure 5-2), and standardized anatomical directional terms are used (Figure 5-3). For example, the directions *left* and *right* always refer to the patient's left and right.

A universal reference when discussing human anatomy is called **anatomical position**. All descriptions of the body use anatomical position as their starting point. Anatomical position is a person standing, facing forward, with palms forward (review Figure 5-2). When describing locations on the body, you will use anatomical position as a reference even if your patient is not in this position himself. For example, your patient's face would be referred to as anterior (at the front) because the face is anterior in anatomical position, even if the patient you are describing is lying face down. The importance of always referring to this standardized position is that all health care providers, everywhere, will use the same anatomical starting point when describing the body and will understand each other's references.

For direction and spatial relationships, we divide the body into planes. A **plane** is a flat surface, the kind that would be formed if you sliced straight through a department store dummy or an imaginary human body. Cutting through from top to bottom, you could slice the body either into right and left halves or into front and back halves. Slicing the body down the middle to create two side-by-side halves would create *sagittal* or *median planes*. Slicing

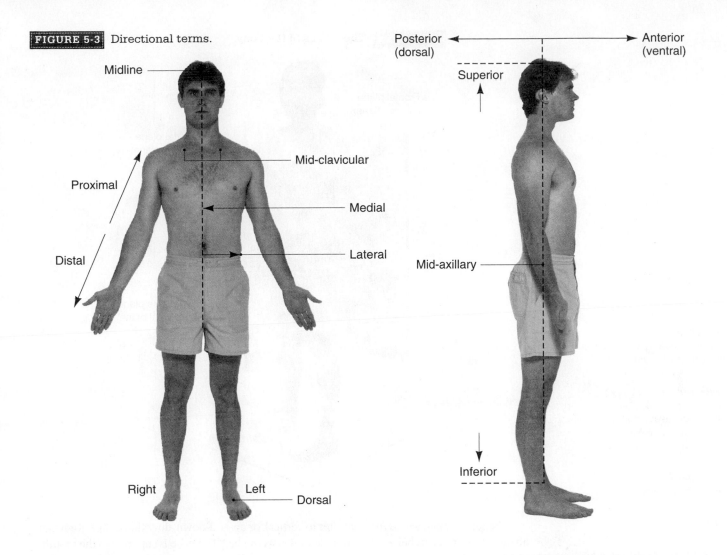

FIGURE 5-3 Directional terms.

the body into two halves, front and back, would create *frontal* or *coronal planes*. Finally, slicing the body into two halves, top and bottom, would create *transverse* or *horizontal planes* (Figure 5-4). Note that, although it is good to understand the meaning of terms referring to planes of the body, terms referring to planes are not usually used in communications among health care providers.

The *midline* of the body is created by drawing an imaginary line down the center of the body; passing between the eyes and extending down through the umbilicus (navel) (refer again to Figure 5-3). Slicing through the imaginary body at the midline divides the body into right and left halves.

The term *medial* refers to a position closer to the midline (with regard to anatomical position). The term *lateral* refers to a position farther away from the midline. For example, you would say, "The bridge of the nose is medial to the eyes." You also can say that an arm has a medial side (close to the body) and a lateral side (the outer arm, away from the body).

The term *bilateral* refers to "both sides" of anything. Patients may have diminished lung sounds on both sides when you listen with a stethoscope. This would be reported as, "The patient has diminished lung sounds bilaterally."

The *mid-axillary line* extends vertically from the mid-armpit to the ankle. (The anatomical term for the armpit is axilla, so mid-axillary means "middle of the armpit.") This line divides the body into front and back halves. The term for the front is *anterior*. The term for the back is *posterior*. For example, you would say: "The patient has wounds to the posterior arm and the anterior thigh." A synonym for anterior is *ventral* (referring to the front of the body). A synonym for posterior is *dorsal* (referring to the back of the body or back of the hand or foot). Remember that these terms always reference anatomical position regardless of the current position of the patient.

midline
an imaginary line drawn down the center of the body, dividing it into right and left halves.

medial
toward the midline of the body.

lateral
to the side, away from the midline of the body.

bilateral
on both sides.

mid-axillary (mid-AX-ııh-lair-e)
line
a line drawn vertically from the middle of the armpit to the ankle.

anterior
the front of the body or body part.

posterior
the back of the body or body part.

ventral
referring to the front of the body. A synonym for anterior.

dorsal
referring to the back of the body or the back of the hand or foot. A synonym for posterior.

FIGURE 5-4 The planes of the body.

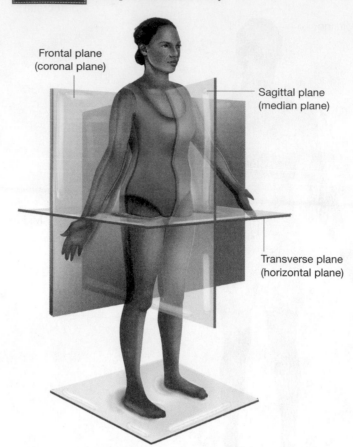

Frontal plane
(coronal plane)

Sagittal plane
(median plane)

Transverse plane
(horizontal plane)

superior
toward the head (e.g., the chest is
superior to the abdomen).

inferior
away from the head; usually compared
with another structure that is closer to
the head (e.g., the lips are inferior to
the nose).

proximal
closer to the torso.

distal
farther away from the torso.

torso
the trunk of the body; the body
without the head and the extremities.

palmar
referring to the palm of the hand.

plantar
referring to the sole of the foot.

mid-clavicular
(mid-clah-VIK-yuh-ler) **line**
the line through the center of each
clavicle.

abdominal quadrants
four divisions of the abdomen used to
pinpoint the location of a pain or
injury: the right upper quadrant
(RUQ), the left upper quadrant (LUQ),
the right lower quadrant (RLQ), and
the left lower quadrant (LLQ).

The terms *superior* and *inferior* refer to vertical, or up-and-down, directions. Superior means above; inferior means below. An example of this would be, "The nose is superior to the mouth."

The terms *proximal* and *distal* are relative terms. Proximal means closer to the *torso* (the trunk of the body, or the body without the head and the extremities). Distal means farther away from the torso. For example, think of an elbow. It is proximal to the hand, because it is closer to the torso than the hand. The elbow also is distal to the shoulder, since the elbow is farther away from the torso than the shoulder. The terms are usually used when describing locations on extremities. For example, to be sure circulation has not been cut off after splinting an arm or leg, you must feel for a distal pulse. This is a pulse found in an extremity, a pulse point that is farther away from the torso than the splint. When using relative terms like *proximal* and *distal*, it is helpful to give a point of reference. For example, you might say a laceration is proximal to the elbow. In this case, the elbow is your point of reference.

Two other terms you may sometimes hear are *palmar* (referring to the palm of the hand) and *plantar* (referring to the sole of the foot).

The *mid-clavicular line* divides the chest into regions. It runs through the center of a clavicle (collarbone) and extends inferiorly. Since there are two clavicles, there are two mid-clavicular lines. When you use a stethoscope to listen for breath sounds, you will place the stethoscope at the mid-clavicular lines to listen to each side of the chest and assess the function of both lungs.

The abdomen is divided into four parts, or quadrants, by drawing horizontal and vertical lines through the navel. The *abdominal quadrants* are described as the right upper quadrant, the left upper quadrant, the right lower quadrant, and the left lower quadrant (Figure 5-5). These are often abbreviated as, respectively, RUQ, LUQ, RLQ, and LLQ.

Positional Terms

There are five terms that describe specific patient positions: supine, prone, recovery, Fowler, and Trendelenburg.

● **CORE CONCEPT**
Positional terms

 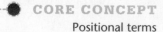

FIGURE 5-5 Abdominal quadrants.

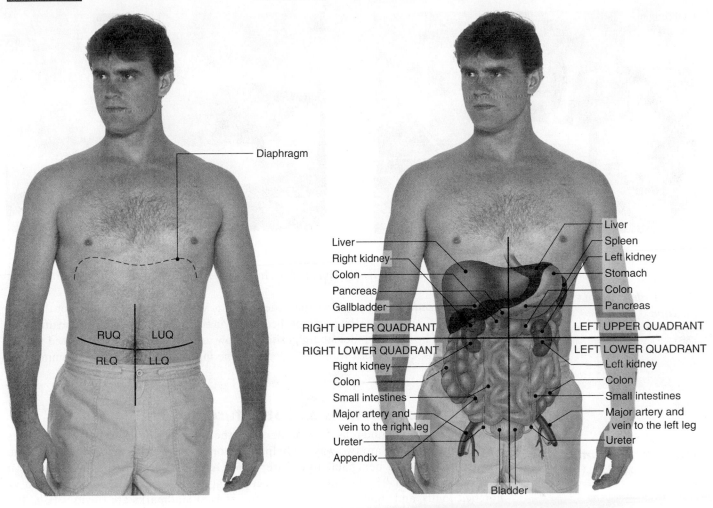

Diaphragm

Liver
Right kidney
Colon
Pancreas
Gallbladder

Liver
Spleen
Left kidney
Stomach
Colon
Pancreas

RUQ   LUQ
RLQ   LLQ

RIGHT UPPER QUADRANT   LEFT UPPER QUADRANT
RIGHT LOWER QUADRANT   LEFT LOWER QUADRANT

Right kidney
Colon
Small intestines
Major artery and
  vein to the right leg
Ureter
Appendix

Left kidney
Colon
Small intestines
Major artery and
  vein to the left leg
Ureter

Bladder

A *supine* patient is lying on his back. A *prone* patient is lying on his abdomen. A person may also be lying on his side, a position traditionally called the ***recovery position***. It is the preferred position for any unconscious nontrauma patient, because it is a position in which fluids or vomitus can drain from the mouth and be less likely to be aspirated (inhaled) into the lungs. Because the patient is lying on his side, this position is also called the *lateral recumbent position* (Figure 5-6).

When patients are transported on a stretcher, there are several positions that they may be placed in. In the ***Fowler position***, the patient is seated. This is usually accomplished by raising the head end of the stretcher so the body is at a 45° to 60° angle. The patient may be sitting straight up or leaning slightly back. If leaning back in a semi-sitting position, this is

supine
lying on the back.

prone
lying face down.

recovery position
lying on the side. Also called *lateral recumbent position*.

Fowler position
a sitting position.

FIGURE 5-6 Anatomical positions.

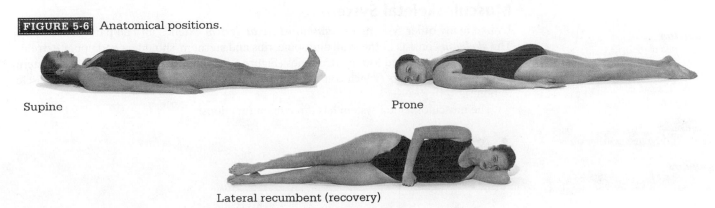

Supine

Prone

Lateral recumbent (recovery)

FIGURE 5-7 Semi-Fowler position.

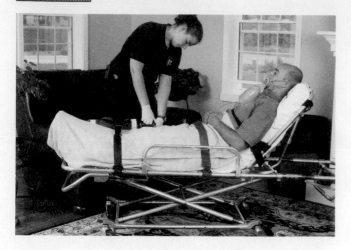

FIGURE 5-8 Trendelenburg position.

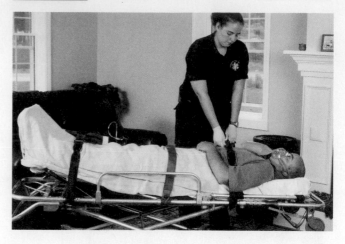

Trendelenburg (trend-EL-un-berg) *position*
a position in which the patient's feet and legs are higher than the head.

thyroid (THI-roid) *cartilage*
the wing-shaped plate of cartilage that sits anterior to the larynx and forms the Adam's apple.

musculoskeletal
(MUS-kyu-lo-SKEL-e-tal) *system*
the system of bones and skeletal muscles that support and protect the body and permit movement.

sometimes called *semi-Fowler* (Figure 5-7). In a Fowler position, the legs may be straight out or bent.

In the ***Trendelenburg position***, the patient is lying with the head slightly lower than the feet (Figure 5-8). This may be accomplished by having the patient lie flat and elevating the legs a few inches. The Trendelenburg position is now seldom used. It was once used for patients with suspected shock without suspected spine injury but is no longer recommended for shock.

Locating Body Organs and Structures

As an EMT, you will find it useful to understand the positions of the body's major organs and structures. There are two ways to help locate organs and structures of the body. The first is visualizing, or being able to picture, organs and structures inside the body as you look at the external body. The second is topography, or external landmarks, such as notches, joints, and "bumps" on bones. Some external landmarks are obvious (e.g., the navel, the nipples), some you know by other names but will have to learn the medical terms (e.g., the "Adam's apple," which is properly called the ***thyroid cartilage***), and some will probably be new to you (e.g., the xiphoid process). It is important to learn where internal organs and structures are in relation to these landmarks, which you can easily see or feel from outside the body

 CORE CONCEPT
The structure and function of major body systems

BODY SYSTEMS

Refer to Table 5-2 as you read the following sections about the various body systems.

Musculoskeletal System

skeleton
the bones of the body.

muscle
tissue that can contract to allow movement of a body part.

ligament
tissue that connects bone to bone.

tendon
tissue that connects muscle to bone.

Unlike many other systems, the ***musculoskeletal system*** extends into all parts of the body. The ***skeleton*** consists of the skull and spine, ribs and sternum, shoulders and upper extremities, and the pelvis and lower extremities (Figure 5-9). Interacting with the skeletal system are ***muscles***, ***ligaments*** (which connect bone to bone), and ***tendons*** (which connect muscle to bone).

The musculoskeletal system has three main functions:

- To give the body shape
- To protect vital internal organs
- To provide for body movement

FIGURE 5-9 The skeleton.

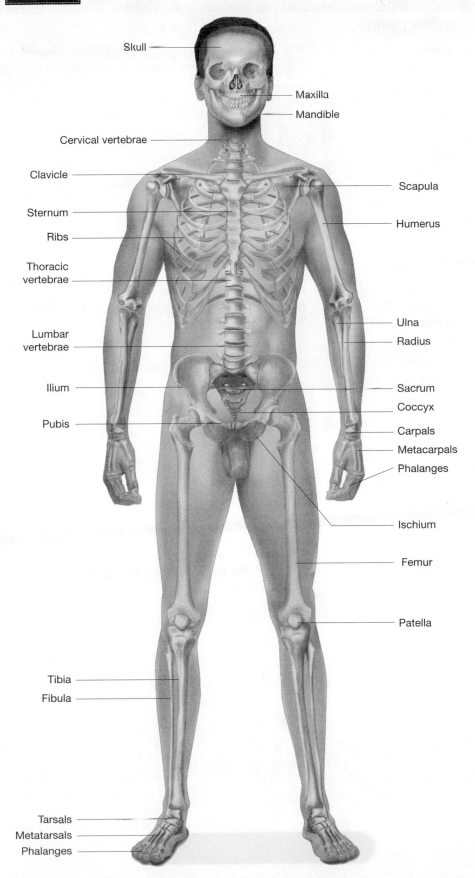

Skull

Maxilla

Mandible

Cervical vertebrae

Clavicle

Scapula

Sternum

Humerus

Ribs

Thoracic
vertebrae

Lumbar
vertebrae

Ulna

Radius

Ilium

Sacrum

Coccyx

Pubis

Carpals

Metacarpals

Phalanges

Ischium

Femur

Patella

Tibia

Fibula

Tarsals

Metatarsals

Phalanges

Table 5-2 Systems and Structures of the Human Body

SYSTEM	STRUCTURES		FUNCTIONS
Musculoskeletal	• Bones • Joints • Muscles		Skeleton supports and protects the body, forms blood cells, and stores minerals. Muscles produce movement.
Respiratory	• Nasal cavity • Pharynx • Larynx • Trachea • Bronchial tubes • Lungs		Obtains oxygen and removes carbon dioxide from the body.
Cardiovascular	• Heart • Arteries • Veins		Pumps blood throughout the entire body to transport nutrients, oxygen, and wastes.

Table 5-2 Systems and Structures of the Human Body (continued)

SYSTEM	STRUCTURES		FUNCTIONS
Blood	• Plasma • Red blood cells • White blood cells • Platelets		Transports oxygen, protects against pathogens, and promotes clotting to control bleeding.
Nervous	• Brain • Spinal cord • Nerves		Receives sensory information and coordinates the body's response.
Digestive	• Oral cavity • Pharynx • Esophagus • Stomach • Small intestine • Large intestine (colon) • Liver • Gallbladder • Pancreas		Ingests, digests, and absorbs nutrients for the body.

(continued)

Table 5-2 **Systems and Structures of the Human Body** (continued)

SYSTEM	STRUCTURES	FUNCTIONS
Integumentary	• Skin • Hair • Nails • Sweat glands	Forms protective barrier and aids in temperature regulation.
Endocrine	• Pituitary gland • Pineal gland • Thyroid gland • Parathyroid glands • Thymus gland • Adrenal glands • Pancreas • Testes • Ovaries	Regulates metabolic/hormonal activities of the body
Renal/Urinary	• Kidneys • Ureters • Urinary bladder • Urethra	Filters waste products out of the blood and removes them from the body.

Table 5-2   Systems and Structures of the Human Body (continued)

SYSTEM	STRUCTURES	FUNCTIONS
Male Reproductive	• Testes • Epididymis • Vas deferens • Penis • Seminal vesicles • Prostate gland	Produces sperm for reproduction.
Female Reproductive	• Ovaries • Fallopian tubes (oviducts) • Uterus • Vagina • Vulva • Breasts	Produces eggs for reproduction and provides place for growing baby.

Skull

To list the parts of the skeleton from top to bottom, you would begin with the skull (Figure 5-10). The *skull* is the bony structure of the head. A main function of the skull is to enclose and protect the brain. The *cranium* consists of the top, back, and sides of the skull. The face is the front of the skull.

The bones of the anterior cranium connect to facial bones, including the *mandible* (lower jaw), *maxillae* (fused bones of the upper jaw), and the *nasal bones* (which provide some of the structure of the nose). These bones form the facial structures. Some of these structures consist of multiple bones, such as the *orbits*, which surround the eyes, and the *zygomatic arches*, which form the structures of the cheeks.

Spinal Column

The spinal column provides structure and support for the body and houses and protects the spinal cord.

The spinal column (also referred to simply as the spine) consists of 33 *vertebrae*, the separate bones of the spine. Like building blocks, vertebrae are stacked one upon the other to form the spinal column. Vertebrae are open in the middle, somewhat like donuts, creating a hollow center for the spinal cord. Since the spinal cord is essential for movement, sensation, and vital functions, injuries to the spine have the potential to damage the cord, possibly resulting in paralysis or death. For this reason, you will see references throughout this text to "taking spinal precautions" for some patients.

skull
the bony structure of the head.

cranium
the top, back, and sides of the skull.

mandible (MAN-di-bul)
the lower jaw bone.

maxillae (mak-SIL-e)
the two fused bones forming the upper jaw.

nasal (NAY-zul) *bones*
the nose bones.

orbits
the bony structures around the eyes; the eye sockets.

zygomatic (ZI-go-MAT-ik) *arches*
bones that form the structure of the cheeks.

vertebrae (VER-te-bray)
the 33 bones of the spinal column.

FIGURE 5-10 The skull consists of the cranium and face.

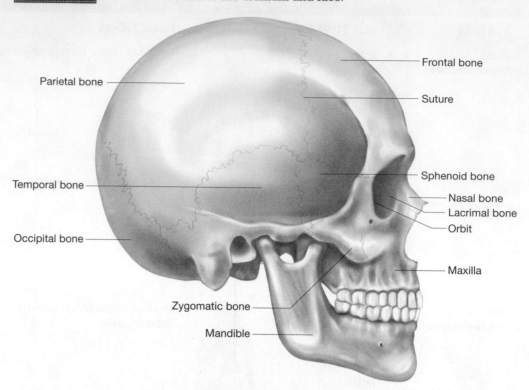

Parietal bone

Frontal bone

Suture

Temporal bone

Sphenoid bone

Nasal bone

Lacrimal bone

Orbit

Occipital bone

Maxilla

Zygomatic bone

Mandible

The five divisions of the spine are listed in Table 5-3 and shown in Figure 5-11.

The anatomy of the body allows some vertebrae to be injured more easily than others. Since the head is large and heavy, resting on the slender neck, incidents such as car crashes may cause the head to whip back and forth or strike an object such as the windshield. This frequently causes injuries to the cervical spine. An injury to the spinal cord at this level may be fatal because control of the muscles of breathing, such as the diaphragm and the muscles between the ribs, arise from the spinal cord in the cervical region. The lumbar region is also subject to injury because it is not supported by other parts of the skeleton. The thoracic spine, to which the ribs are attached, and the sacral spine and coccyx, which are supported by the pelvis, are less easily injured.

thorax (THOR-ax)
the chest.

Thorax

sternum (STER-num)
the breastbone.

The **thorax** is the chest. The bones of the thorax form an internal space called the thoracic cavity. This cavity contains the heart, lungs, and major blood vessels. An important function of the thorax is to protect these vital organs. This is accomplished by the 12 pairs of ribs that attach to the 12 thoracic vertebrae of the spine. In the front, 10 of these pairs of ribs are attached to the **sternum** (breastbone) and two are called "floating ribs" since they have no anterior attachment. You will remember the sternum from your CPR training. This flat bone is divided into three sections: the **manubrium** (superior portion), the body (center portion), and the **xiphoid process** (inferior tip).

manubrium (man-OO-bre-um)
the superior portion of the sternum.

xiphoid (ZI-foid) **process**
the inferior portion of the sternum.

Table 5-3	The Divisions of the Spine	
DIVISION	**CORRESPONDING ANATOMY**	**NUMBER OF VERTEBRAE**
Cervical	Neck	7
Thoracic	Thorax, ribs, upper back	12
Lumbar	Lower back	5
Sacral	Back wall of pelvis	5
Coccyx	Tailbone	4

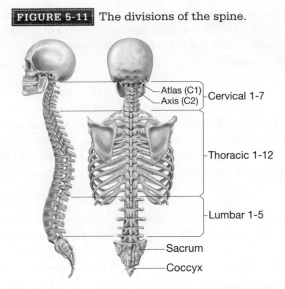

FIGURE 5-11 The divisions of the spine.

Atlas (C1)
Axis (C2)
Cervical 1-7

Thoracic 1-12

Lumbar 1-5

Sacrum

Coccyx

Pelvis

The *pelvis* is sometimes referred to by laypeople as the hip, although the hip is actually the joint where the femur (thigh bone) and pelvis join. The pelvis contains bones that are fused together. The *ilium* is the superior bone that contains the iliac crest, which is the wide bony wing that can be felt near the waist. The *ischium* is the inferior, posterior portion of the pelvis. The *pubis* is formed by the joining of the bones of the anterior pubis. The pelvis is joined posteriorly to the sacral spine.

The hip joint consists of the *acetabulum* (the socket of the hip joint) and the ball at the proximal end of the femur.

Lower Extremities

The pelvis and hip joint, described previously, may be considered part of the lower extremities. Moving downward from the hip, the large thigh bone is the *femur*. The femur, the largest long bone in the body, has a slight bend at its proximal end where it attaches to the pelvis. This bend is a frequent site of fractures and is commonly what breaks when a patient "breaks a hip." Progressing down the leg, the *patella*, or kneecap, sits anterior to the knee joint. The knee connects with the femur superiorly and with the bones of the lower leg, the tibia and fibula, inferiorly. The *tibia* is the medial and larger bone of the lower leg, also referred to as the shin bone. The *fibula* is the lateral and smaller bone of the lower leg.

The ankle connects the tibia and fibula with the foot. Two distinct landmarks are the *malleolus* at each side of the ankle: the *lateral malleolus* (at the lower end of the fibula) and the *medial malleolus* (at the lower end of the tibia). These are the protrusions that you see on the lateral and medial aspects of your ankles. The ankle consists of bones called *tarsals*. The foot bones are called *metatarsals*. The heel bone is called the *calcaneus*. The toe bones are the *phalanges*.

Upper Extremities

Each shoulder consists of several bones: the clavicle, the scapula, and the proximal humerus. The *clavicle*, or collarbone, is located anteriorly. The *scapula*, or shoulder blade, is located posteriorly. The *acromion process* of the scapula is the highest portion of the shoulder. It forms the *acromioclavicular joint* with the clavicle and is a frequent area of shoulder injury.

The upper arm and forearm consist of three bones connected at the elbow. The bone between the shoulder and the elbow is the *humerus*. The *radius* and *ulna* are the two bones between the elbow and the hand. The radius is the lateral bone of the forearm. It is always aligned with the thumb. (The radial pulse is taken over the radius.) The ulna is the medial forearm bone.

The wrist consists of several bones called *carpals*. The bones of the hand are the *metacarpals*. The finger bones, like the toe bones, are called *phalanges*.

pelvis
the basin-shaped bony structure that supports the spine and is the point of proximal attachment for the lower extremities.

ilium (IL-e-um)
the superior and widest portion of the pelvis.

ischium (ISH-e-um)
the lower, posterior portions of the pelvis.

pubis (PYOO-bis)
the medial anterior portion of the pelvis.

acetabulum (AS-uh-TAB-yuh-lum)
the pelvic socket into which the ball at the proximal end of the femur fits to form the hip joint.

femur (FEE-mer)
the large bone of the thigh.

patella (pah-TEL-uh)
the kneecap.

tibia (TIB-e-uh)
the medial and larger bone of the lower leg.

fibula (FIB-yuh-luh)
the lateral and smaller bone of the lower leg.

malleolus (mal-E-o-lus)
protrusion on the side of the ankle. The *lateral malleolus*, at the lower end of the fibula, is seen on the outer ankle; the *medial malleolus*, at the lower end of the tibia, is seen on the inner ankle.

tarsals (TAR-sulz)
the ankle bones.

metatarsals (MET-uh-TAR-sulz)
the foot bones.

calcaneus (kal-KAY-ne-us)
the heel bone.

phalanges (fuh-LAN-jiz)
the toe bones and finger bones.

clavicle (KLAV-i-kul)
the collarbone.

scapula (SKAP-yuh-luh)
the shoulder blade.

acromion (ah-KRO-me-on) **process**
the highest portion of the shoulder.

acromioclavicular (ah-KRO-me-o-klav-IK-yuh-ler) **joint**
the joint where the acromion and the clavicle meet.

humerus (HYU-mer-us)
the bone of the upper arm, between the shoulder and the elbow.

radius (RAY-de-us)
the lateral bone of the forearm.

ulna (UL-nah)
the medial bone of the forearm.

carpals (KAR-pulz)
the wrist bones.

metacarpals (MET-uh-KAR-pulz)
the hand bones.

By this point in the chapter, you are realizing the importance of anatomical terms such as *superior*, *inferior*, *medial*, *lateral*, *anterior*, and *posterior*. These terms will be used throughout the text, and you will need to use them correctly to properly document and report your patient's injuries and complaints.

Joints

joint
the point where two bones come together.

Joints are formed when bones connect to other bones. There are several types of joints, including ball-and-socket joints and hinge joints. The hip is an example of a ball-and-socket joint, in which the ball of the femur rotates in a round socket in the pelvis. The elbow is an example of a hinge joint in which the angle between the humerus and ulna—which are connected by ligaments—bends and straightens, as the name suggests, like a hinge.

Muscles

Like the skeleton, the muscles protect the body, give it shape, and allow for movement. There are three types of muscle (Figure 5-12): voluntary muscle, involuntary muscle, and cardiac muscle.

voluntary muscle
muscle that can be consciously controlled.

Voluntary muscle, or skeletal muscle, is under conscious control of the brain via the nervous system. Attached to the bones, the voluntary muscles form the major muscle mass of the body. They are responsible for movement. Voluntary muscle can contract upon voluntary command of the individual. For example, if you want to, you can reach to pick up an item or walk away. These are examples of voluntary muscle use.

involuntary muscle
muscle that responds automatically to brain signals but cannot be consciously controlled.

Involuntary muscle, or smooth muscle, is found in the gastrointestinal system, lungs, blood vessels, and urinary system and controls the flow of materials through these structures. Involuntary muscles respond automatically to orders from the brain. You do not have to

FIGURE 5-12 Three types of muscle.

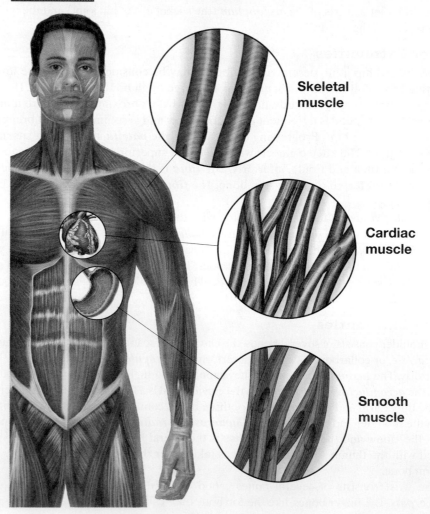

Skeletal muscle

Cardiac muscle

Smooth muscle

consciously think about using them to breathe, digest food, or perform other functions that occur under their control. In fact, we have no direct control over involuntary muscles. Involuntary muscles do respond to stimuli such as stretching, heat, and cold.

Cardiac muscle, a specialized form of involuntary muscle, is found only in the heart. Cardiac muscle is extremely sensitive to decreased oxygen supply and can tolerate an interruption of its blood supply only for very short periods. The heart muscle has its own blood supply through the coronary artery system.

The heart also has a property called *automaticity*. This means that the heart has the ability to generate and conduct electrical impulses on its own. The heartbeat (contraction) is controlled by these electrical impulses.

Respiratory System

The purposes of the *respiratory system* are ventilation and oxygenation. Oxygen (O_2) is moved into the bloodstream through inhalation, and carbon dioxide (CO_2) is picked up by the blood and excreted through exhalation.

Respiratory Anatomy

A number of structures make up the respiratory system (Figure 5-13). Air enters the body through the mouth and nose. It moves through the *oropharynx* (the area directly posterior to the mouth) and the *nasopharynx* (the area directly posterior to the nose). The *pharynx* is the area that includes both the oropharynx and the nasopharynx.

From the pharynx, air moves on a path toward the lungs. A leaf-shaped structure called the *epiglottis* closes over the *glottis*, the opening to the trachea, to prevent foods and foreign objects from entering the trachea during swallowing. The *larynx*, or voice box, contains the vocal cords. The *cricoid cartilage*, a ring-shaped structure, forms the lower portion of the larynx.

The *trachea*, or windpipe, is the tube that carries inhaled air from the larynx down toward the *lungs*. It is formed and protected by 16 C-shaped (incomplete) rings of cartilage. At the level of the lungs, the trachea splits (bifurcates) into two branches called the *bronchi*. One "mainstem" bronchus goes to each lung. Inside each lung, the bronchi continue to branch and split (the branches are called *bronchioles*), like the branches of a tree, and the air passages get smaller and smaller. Eventually, each branch ends at a group of alveoli. The *alveoli* are the small sacs within the lungs where gas exchange—the exchange of oxygen and carbon dioxide—takes place with the bloodstream.

The *diaphragm* is a structure that divides the chest cavity from the abdominal cavity. It is a large muscle that is primarily controlled by the *phrenic nerve*. During a normal respiratory cycle, the diaphragm and other parts of the body work together to allow the body to inhale and exhale. The role of the diaphragm and other muscles in the respiratory cycle is described next.

Respiratory Physiology

Inhalation is an active process. The muscles of the rib cage (*intercostal muscles*) and the diaphragm contract. The diaphragm lowers, and the ribs move upward and outward. This expands the size of the chest and thereby creates a negative pressure inside the chest cavity. This negative pressure pulls air into the lungs.

Exhalation is a passive process during which the intercostal muscles and the diaphragm relax. The ribs move downward and inward, while the diaphragm rises. This movement causes the chest to decrease in size and positive pressure to build inside the chest cavity. This positive pressure pushes air out of the lungs.

During inhalation, air is moved through the airway and into the alveoli. These tiny sacs in the lungs are the site of gas exchange between air and blood. Each single alveolus is surrounded by pulmonary capillaries. The pulmonary capillaries bring circulating blood to the outside of the alveoli. Through the very thin walls of the alveoli and the capillaries, oxygen is transferred from the air inside the alveoli to the bloodstream and carbon dioxide is moved from the bloodstream into the air within the alveoli. This movement of gases to and from the alveoli is called *ventilation*.

Oxygenated blood is carried from the lungs to the heart so it can be pumped into the body's circulatory system. As the blood leaves the heart, it travels through a branching series of arteries that gradually become smaller and finally connect to capillaries. Just as happened

cardiac muscle
specialized involuntary muscle found only in the heart.

automaticity (AW-to-muh-TISS-it-e)
the ability of the heart to generate and conduct electrical impulses on its own.

respiratory (RES-pir-ah-tor-e) **system**
the system of nose, mouth, throat, lungs, and muscles that brings oxygen into the body and expels carbon dioxide.

oropharynx (OR-o-FAIR-inks)
the area directly posterior to the mouth.

nasopharynx (NAY-zo-FAIR-inks)
the area directly posterior to the nose.

pharynx (FAIR-inks)
the area directly posterior to the mouth and nose. It is made up of the oropharynx and the nasopharynx.

epiglottis (EP-i-GLOT-is)
a leaf-shaped structure that prevents food and foreign matter from entering the trachea.

larynx (LAIR-inks)
the voice box.

cricoid (KRIK-oid) **cartilage**
the ring-shaped structure that forms the lower portion of the larynx.

trachea (TRAY-ke-uh)
the "windpipe"; the structure that connects the pharynx to the lungs.

lungs
the organs where exchange of atmospheric oxygen and waste carbon dioxide take place.

bronchi (BRONG-ki)
the two large sets of branches that come off the trachea and enter the lungs. There are right and left bronchi. *Singular* bronchus.

alveoli (al-VE-o-li)
the microscopic sacs of the lungs where gas exchange with the bloodstream takes place.

diaphragm (DI-uh-fram)
the muscular structure that divides the chest cavity from the abdominal cavity. A major muscle of respiration.

inhalation (IN-huh-LAY-shun)
an active process in which the intercostal (rib) muscles and the diaphragm contract, expanding the size of the chest cavity and causing air to flow into the lungs.

exhalation (EX-huh-LAY-shun)
a passive process in which the intercostal (rib) muscles and the diaphragm relax, causing the chest cavity to decrease in size and air to flow out of the lungs.

ventilation
the process of moving gases (oxygen and carbon dioxide) between inhaled air and the pulmonary circulation of blood.

FIGURE 5-13 The respiratory system.

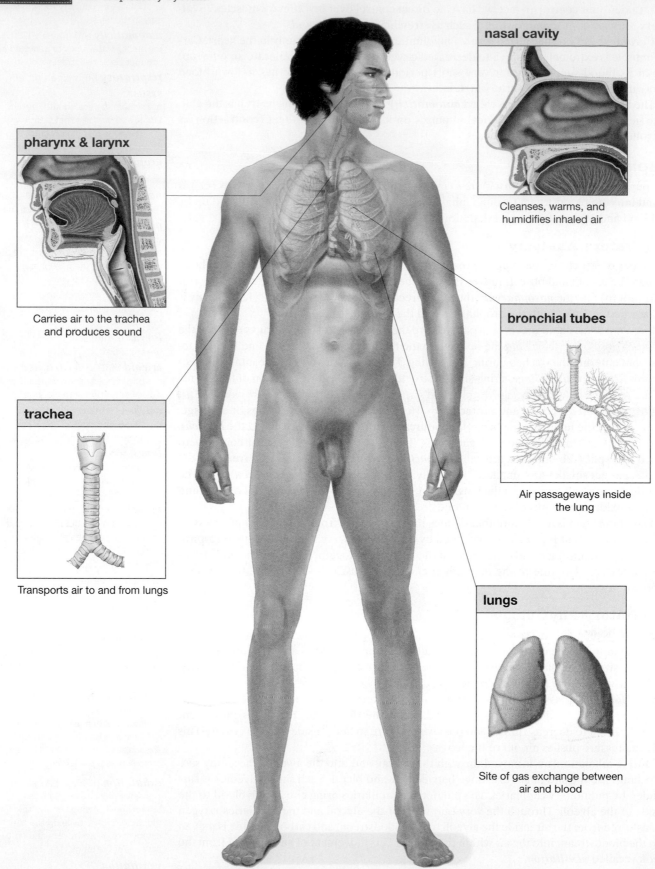

nasal cavity

Cleanses, warms, and humidifies inhaled air

pharynx & larynx

Carries air to the trachea and produces sound

bronchial tubes

Air passageways inside the lung

trachea

Transports air to and from lungs

lungs

Site of gas exchange between air and blood

with the capillaries that pass by the alveoli of the lungs, the capillaries that pass by the cells throughout the body's tissues conduct a gas exchange. At a cellular level, oxygen that was picked up from the lungs and carried by the blood is now transferred through the capillary walls and across cell membranes into the cells. Waste carbon dioxide from the cells moves in the opposite direction, out of the cells and into the capillaries. Capillaries then connect to veins and veins return blood to the heart where it can be pumped to the lungs to get rid of the waste carbon dioxide and pick up oxygen, completing the cycle of gas exchange. The process of moving gases (and other nutrients) between the cells and the blood is called *respiration*.

The exchange of gases, both in the lungs and at the body's cells, is critical to support life. Oxygen is essential to sustain normal cellular function, and the removal of carbon dioxide helps regulate the body's pH, or relative acidity. In general, the body regulates its pH through the *buffer system*, and the removal of carbon dioxide is an extremely important element of this system.

respiration (cellular)
the process of moving oxygen and carbon dioxide between circulating blood and the cells.

PEDIATRIC NOTE

There are a number of special aspects of the respiratory anatomy of infants and children (Figure 5-14). In general, all structures in a child are smaller than in an adult. A child's tongue takes up proportionally more space in the pharynx than does an adult's. The trachea is relatively narrower than in adults and, therefore, more easily obstructed by swelling or foreign matter. The trachea is also softer and more flexible in infants and children, so more care must be taken during any procedure when pressure might be placed on the neck, such as in applying a cervical collar. The cricoid cartilage is also less developed and less rigid in infants and children. Because the chest wall is softer, infants and children tend to rely more on the diaphragm when they are having breathing difficulty. This causes a visible "seesaw" breathing pattern in which the chest and abdomen alternate movement.

Special procedures that take into account the respiratory anatomy of infants and children will be discussed in later chapters on the airway and the respiratory system.

Breathing (the process of inhaling and exhaling air) may be classified as adequate or inadequate. Simply stated, adequate breathing is sufficient to support life. Inadequate breathing is not. Adequate and inadequate breathing, and how you as an EMT should assess and care for breathing problems, will be discussed in detail in Chapter 19, "Respiratory Emergencies."

FIGURE 5-14 Comparison of child and adult respiratory anatomy.

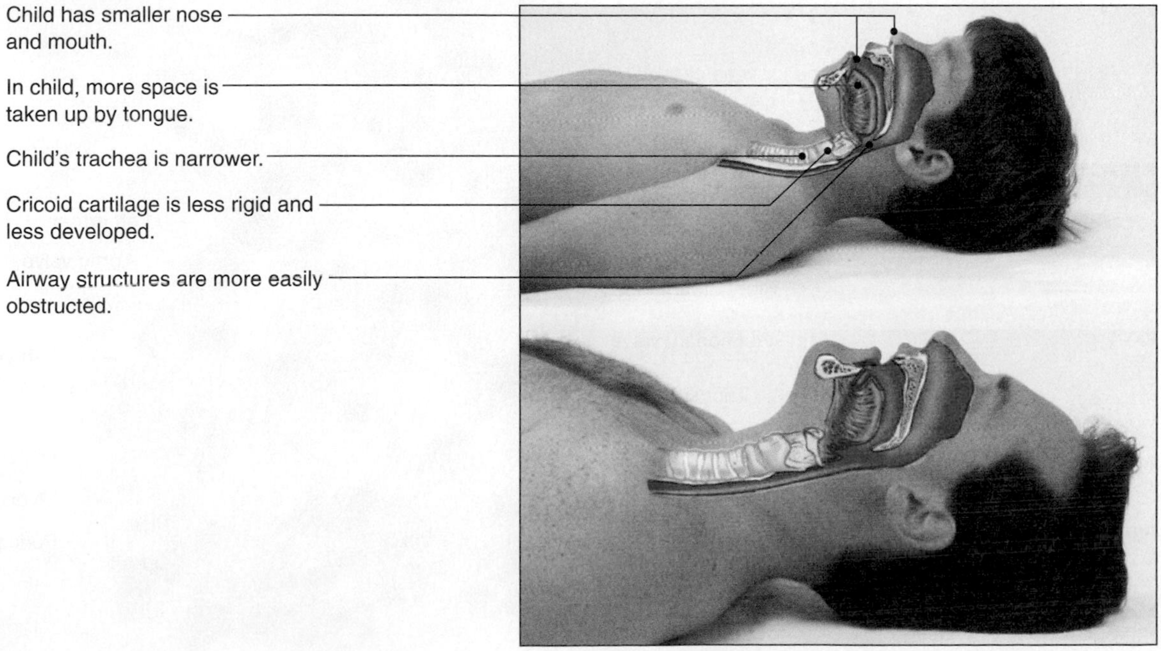

Child has smaller nose and mouth.

In child, more space is taken up by tongue.

Child's trachea is narrower.

Cricoid cartilage is less rigid and less developed.

Airway structures are more easily obstructed.

Cardiovascular System

The **cardiovascular system** consists of the heart, the blood, and the blood vessels. It is also called the *circulatory system.*

cardiovascular (KAR-de-o-VAS-kyu-ler) **system**
the system made up of the heart (cardio) and the blood vessels (vascular); the *circulatory system.*

atria (AY-tree-ah)
the two upper chambers of the heart. There is a right atrium (which receives unoxygenated blood returning from the body) and a left atrium (which receives oxygenated blood returning from the lungs).

ventricles (VEN-tri-kulz)
the two lower chambers of the heart. There is a right ventricle (which sends oxygen-poor blood to the lungs) and a left ventricle (which sends oxygen-rich blood to the body).

venae cavae (VE-ne KA-ve)
the superior vena cava and the inferior vena cava. These two major veins return blood from the body to the right atrium. (Venae cavae is plural, vena cava singular.)

Anatomy of the Heart

The human heart is a muscular organ about the size of your fist, located in the center of the thoracic cavity. The heart has four chambers: two upper chambers called **atria** and two lower chambers called **ventricles** (Figure 5-15A).

Blood is circulated through the heart and out to the body via a very specific pathway (Figure 5-15B). This pathway is governed by the chambers of the heart, as follows:

- **Right atrium.** The **venae cavae** (the superior vena cava and the inferior vena cava) are the two large veins that return blood to the heart. The right atrium receives this blood and, upon contraction, sends it to the right ventricle.

- **Right ventricle.** The right ventricle receives blood from the chamber above it, the right atrium. When the right ventricle contracts, it pumps this blood out to the lungs via the pulmonary arteries. Remember, this blood is very low in oxygen and is carrying waste carbon dioxide that was picked up as the blood circulated through the body. While this blood is in the lungs, the carbon dioxide is excreted (taken out of the blood and, when the person exhales, carried out of the body), and oxygen is obtained (taken into the blood from air the person has inhaled). The oxygen-rich blood is now returned to the left atrium via the pulmonary veins.

- **Left atrium.** The left atrium receives the oxygen-rich blood from the lungs. When it contracts, it sends this blood to the left ventricle.

- **Left ventricle.** The left ventricle receives oxygen-rich blood from the chamber above it, the left atrium. When it contracts, it pumps this blood into the aorta, the body's largest artery, for distribution to the entire body. Since the blood must reach all parts of the body, the left ventricle is the most muscular and strongest part of the heart.

FIGURE 5-15 (A) Cross-section of the heart showing chambers, layers, valves, and major associated blood vessels.

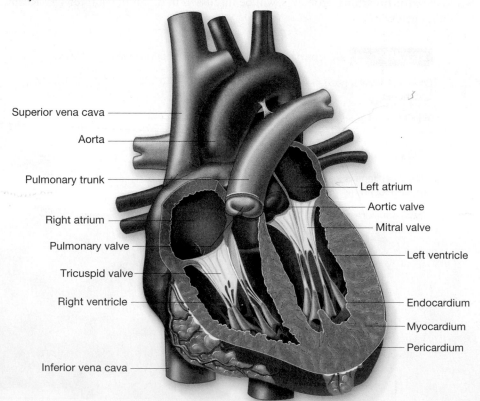

Superior vena cava

Aorta

Pulmonary trunk

Right atrium

Pulmonary valve

Tricuspid valve

Right ventricle

Inferior vena cava

Left atrium

Aortic valve

Mitral valve

Left ventricle

Endocardium

Myocardium

Pericardium

Know this

FIGURE 5-15 (B) The path of blood flow through the heart.

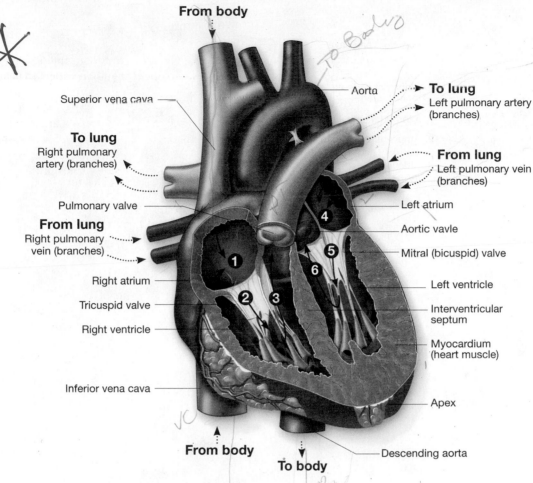

From body

Superior vena cava

Aorta — To Body

To lung

Right pulmonary artery (branches)

To lung
Left pulmonary artery (branches)

Pulmonary valve

From lung
Right pulmonary vein (branches)

From lung
Left pulmonary vein (branches)

Left atrium

Aortic valve

Mitral (bicuspid) valve

Right atrium

Tricuspid valve

Right ventricle

Left ventricle

Interventricular septum

Myocardium (heart muscle)

Inferior vena cava

Apex

From body

To body

Descending aorta

Between each atrium and ventricle is a one-way *valve* that prevents blood in the ventricle from being forced back up into the atrium when the ventricle contracts. The pulmonary artery has a one-way valve so that blood in the artery does not return to the right ventricle. The aorta also has a one-way valve to prevent backflow to the left ventricle. This system of one-way valves keeps the blood moving in the correct direction along the path of circulation.

The contraction, or beating, of the heart is an automatic, involuntary process. The heart has its own natural "pacemaker" and a system of specialized muscle tissues that conduct electrical impulses that stimulate the heart to beat. This network is called the *cardiac conduction system* (Figure 5-16). Regulation of rate, rhythm, and force of heartbeat comes, in part, from the cardiac control centers of the brain. Nerve impulses from these centers are sent to the pacemaker and conduction system of the heart. These nerve impulses and chemicals (epinephrine, for example) released into the blood control the heart's rate and strength of contractions.

Circulation of the Blood

When the blood leaves the heart, it travels throughout the body through several types of blood vessels. Blood vessels are described by their function, location, and whether they carry blood away from or to the heart.

The kind of vessel that carries blood away from the heart is called an *artery*. There are several arteries that are important to know:

- **Coronary arteries.** The *coronary arteries* (Figure 5-17) branch off from the aorta and supply the heart muscle with blood. Although the heart has blood constantly moving through it, it receives its own blood supply from the coronary arteries. Damage, severe narrowing, or blockage to these arteries usually results in chest pain.

valve
a structure that opens and closes to permit the flow of a fluid in only one direction.

cardiac conduction system
a system of specialized muscle tissues that conducts electrical impulses that stimulate the heart to beat.

artery
any blood vessel carrying blood away from the heart.

coronary (KOR-o-nar-e) *arteries*
blood vessels that supply the muscle of the heart (myocardium).

FIGURE 5-16 The cardiac conduction system.

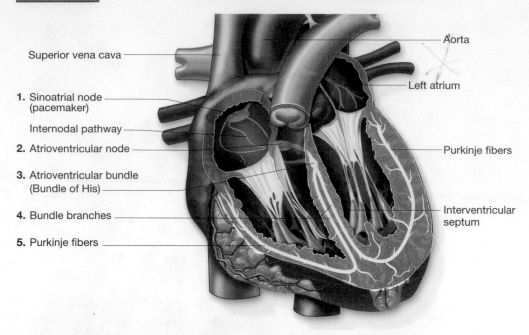

- Superior vena cava
- Aorta
- Left atrium
- **1.** Sinoatrial node (pacemaker)
- Internodal pathway
- **2.** Atrioventricular node
- **3.** Atrioventricular bundle (Bundle of His)
- **4.** Bundle branches
- **5.** Purkinje fibers
- Purkinje fibers
- Interventricular septum

FIGURE 5-17 The coronary arteries.

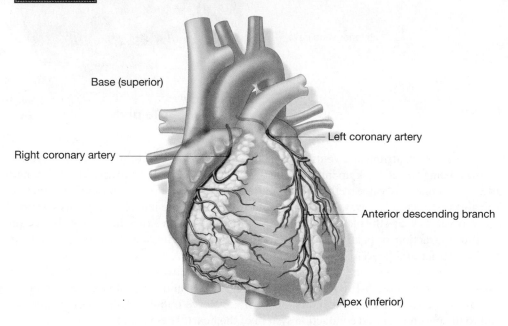

- Base (superior)
- Left coronary artery
- Right coronary artery
- Anterior descending branch
- Apex (inferior)

aorta (ay-OR-tah)
the largest artery in the body. It transports blood from the left ventricle to begin systemic circulation.

pulmonary (PUL-mo-nar-e) ***arteries***
the vessels that carry deoxygenated blood from the right ventricle of the heart to the lungs.

carotid (kah-ROT-id) ***arteries***
the large neck arteries, one on each side of the neck, that carry blood from the heart to the head.

- **Aorta.** The *aorta* is the largest artery in the body. It begins at its attachment to the left ventricle, travels superiorly, then arches inferiorly in front of the spine through the thoracic and abdominal cavities. At the level of the navel, it splits into the iliac arteries.

- **Pulmonary artery.** The *pulmonary artery* begins at the right ventricle. It carries oxygen-poor blood to the lungs. You may notice that this is an exception to the rule that arteries carry oxygen-rich blood and veins carry oxygen-poor blood. It does, however, follow the rule that arteries carry blood away from the heart while veins carry blood to the heart.

- **Carotid artery.** The *carotid artery* is the major artery of the neck. You will be familiar with this vessel from your CPR class. It is the artery that is palpated during CPR pulse checks for adults and children. It carries the main supply of blood for the head. There is a carotid artery on each side of the neck. Never palpate both at the same time because of the danger of interrupting the supply of blood to the brain.

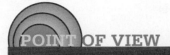
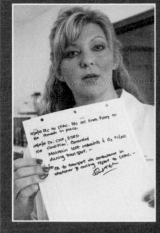
- **Femoral artery.** The *femoral artery* is the major artery of the thigh. You can relate the name *femoral* to the bone in the thigh, the femur. Pulsations for this artery can be felt in the crease between the abdomen and the groin. This artery is the major source of blood supply to the thigh and leg.

- **Brachial artery.** The *brachial artery* in the upper arm is the pulse checked during infant CPR. Its pulse can be felt anteriorly in the crease over the elbow and along the medial aspect of the upper arm. It is also the artery that is used when determining blood pressure with a blood pressure cuff and a stethoscope.

- **Radial artery.** This artery travels through, and supplies, the lower arm. The *radial artery* is the artery felt when taking a pulse at the thumb side of the wrist. Again, you can relate the name *radial* to the radius, a bone in the forearm which the radial artery is near.

- **Posterior tibial artery.** This artery is often used when determining the circulatory status of the lower extremity. The *posterior tibial artery* may be palpated on the posterior aspect of the medial malleolus.

- **Dorsalis pedis artery.** The *dorsalis pedis artery* lies on the top (dorsal portion) of the foot, lateral to the large tendon of the big toe.

Arteries begin with large vessels, like the aorta. They gradually branch into smaller and smaller vessels. The smallest branch of an artery is called an *arteriole*. These small vessels lead to the capillaries. *Capillaries* are tiny blood vessels found throughout the body. As explained earlier, the capillaries are where gases, nutrients, and waste products are exchanged between the body's cells and the bloodstream. From the capillaries the blood begins its return journey to the heart by entering the smallest veins. One of these small veins is called a *venule* (Figure 5-18).

The kind of vessel that carries the blood from the capillaries back to the heart is called a *vein*. Remember that the blood flow from the heart started in the largest arteries and moved into smaller and smaller arteries until it reached the capillaries. The blood takes an opposite course through the veins. The blood travels from the smaller to the larger vessels on its return trip to the heart. Immediately after leaving the capillaries, the blood enters venules, the smallest veins. From the venules, the veins get gradually larger, eventually reaching the venae cavae.

There are two *venae cavae*. The superior vena cava collects blood that is returned from the head and upper body. The inferior vena cava collects blood from the portions of the body below the heart. The superior and inferior venae cavae meet to return blood to the right atrium, where the process of circulation begins again.

The *pulmonary vein* carries oxygenated blood from the lungs to the left atrium of the heart. This is an exception to the rule that veins carry oxygen-poor blood. However, it does follow the rule that arteries carry blood away from the heart while veins return blood to the heart.

---

femoral (FEM-o-ral) *artery*
the major artery supplying the leg.

brachial artery
artery of the upper arm, the site of the pulse checked during infant CPR.

radial artery
artery of the lower arm. It is felt when taking the pulse at the wrist.

posterior tibial (TIB-ee-ul) *artery*
artery supplying the foot, behind the medial ankle.

dorsalis pedis (dor-SAL-is PEED-is) *artery*
artery supplying the foot, lateral to the large tendon of the big toe.

arteriole (ar-TE-re-ol)
the smallest kind of artery.

capillary (KAP-i-lair-e)
a thin-walled, microscopic blood vessel where the oxygen/carbon dioxide and nutrient/waste exchange with the body's cells takes place.

venule (VEN-yul)
the smallest kind of vein.

vein
any blood vessel returning blood to the heart.

pulmonary veins
the vessels that carry oxygenated blood from the lungs to the left atrium of the heart.

FIGURE 5-18 Arteries, capillaries, and veins.

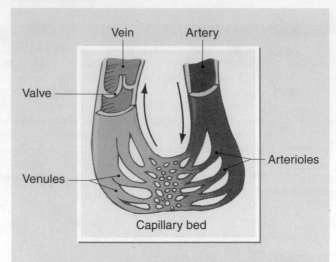

From the heart, oxygen-rich blood is carried out into the body by arteries. The arteries gradually branch into smaller arteries called arterioles. The arterioles gradually branch into tiny vessels called capillaries.

In the capillaries, the blood gives up oxygen and nutrients, which move through the thin walls of the capillaries into the body's cells. At the same time, carbon dioxide and other wastes move in the opposite direction, from the cells and through the capillary walls, to be picked up by the blood.

On its return journey to the heart, the oxygen-poor blood, now carrying carbon dioxide and other wastes, flows from the capillaries into small veins called venules which gradually merge into larger veins.

Composition of the Blood

The blood is made up of several components: plasma, red and white blood cells, and platelets (Figure 5-19).

plasma (PLAZ-mah)
the fluid portion of the blood.

- **Plasma.** *Plasma* is a watery, salty fluid that makes up over half the volume of the blood. The red and white blood cells and platelets are carried in the plasma.

red blood cells
components of the blood. They carry oxygen to, and carbon dioxide away from, the cells.

- **Red blood cells.** *Red blood cells* are also called *RBCs, erythrocytes*, or *red corpuscles*. Their primary function is to carry oxygen to the tissues and carbon dioxide away from the tissues. These cells also provide the red color to the blood.

white blood cells
components of the blood. They produce substances that help the body fight infection.

- **White blood cells.** *White blood cells* are also called *WBCs, leukocytes*, or *white corpuscles*. They are involved in destroying microorganisms (germs) and producing substances called antibodies, which help the body resist infection.

platelets
components of the blood; membrane-enclosed fragments of specialized cells.

- **Platelets.** *Platelets* are membrane-enclosed fragments of specialized cells. When these fragments are activated, they release chemical *clotting factors* needed to form blood clots.

As you can see, the blood has a variety of functions. It is used to transport gases like oxygen and carbon dioxide and also can serve as a reservoir for oxygen dissolved in its plasma. Blood also plays a role in fighting infection and the production of clotting factors. Other functions include the regulation of body pH through chemicals transported in the blood (otherwise known as the *blood buffer*).

Pulse

pulse
the rhythmic beats caused as waves of blood move through and expand the arteries.

A *pulse* is formed when the left ventricle contracts, sending a wave of blood through the arteries. The pulse is felt by compressing an artery over a bone. This allows you to feel the wave of blood, or pulse, as it comes through the artery.

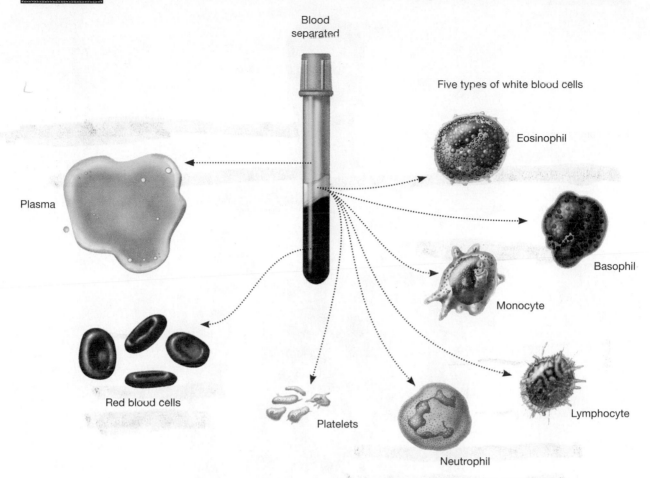

Earlier in this chapter, several arteries were named. Among them were the primary arteries where a pulse is taken for vital signs or CPR: the carotid, brachial, and radial arteries. You will also use the pulses at the ankles and feet (posterior tibial and dorsalis pedis) to check for adequate circulation to the lower extremities.

The radial, brachial, posterior tibial, and dorsalis pedis pulses are called *peripheral pulses* because they can be felt on the periphery, or outer reaches, of the body. The carotid and femoral pulses are called *central pulses* because they can be felt in the central part of the body. Because they are larger vessels closer to the heart, the carotid and femoral pulses can be felt even when peripheral pulses are too weak to be felt.

Blood Pressure

The force blood exerts against the walls of blood vessels is known as *blood pressure*. Usually, arterial blood pressure (pressure in an artery) is measured.

Each time the left ventricle of the heart contracts, it forces blood out into circulation. The pressure created in the arteries by this blood is called the *systolic blood pressure*. When the left ventricle of the heart is relaxed and refilling, the pressure remaining in the arteries is called the *diastolic blood pressure*. The systolic pressure is reported first, the diastolic second, as in "120 over 80," which is written as "120/80."

Perfusion

The movement of blood through the heart and blood vessels is called circulation. In healthy individuals, circulation is adequate. That is, there is enough blood within the system and there is a means to pump and deliver it to all parts of the body efficiently (Figure 5-20). The adequate supply of oxygen and nutrients to the organs and tissues of the body, with the removal of waste products, is called *perfusion*.

peripheral pulses
the radial, brachial, posterior tibial, and dorsalis pedis pulses, which can be felt at peripheral (outlying) points of the body.

central pulses
the carotid and femoral pulses, which can be felt in the central part of the body.

blood pressure
the pressure caused by blood exerting force against the walls of blood vessels. Usually arterial blood pressure (the pressure in an artery) is measured. There are two parts: *diastolic blood pressure* and *systolic blood pressure*.

systolic (sis-TOL-ik) *blood pressure*
the pressure created in the arteries when the left ventricle contracts and forces blood out into circulation.

diastolic (di-as-TOL-ik) *blood pressure*
the pressure in the arteries when the left ventricle is refilling.

perfusion
the supply of oxygen to, and removal of wastes from, the cells and tissues of the body as a result of the flow of blood through the capillaries.

FIGURE 5-20 (A) The major arteries of the body.

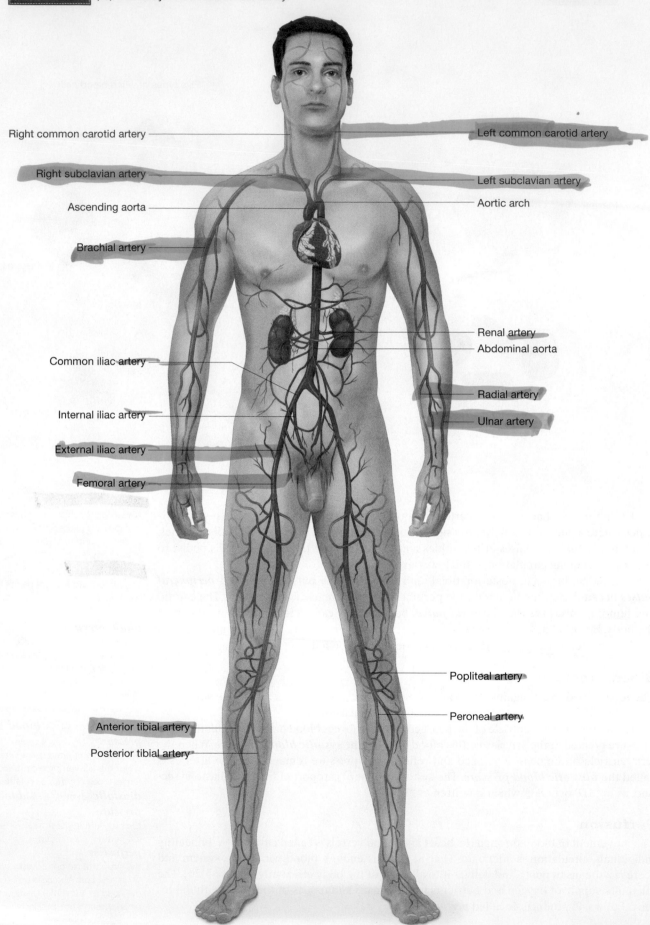

Right common carotid artery

Left common carotid artery

Right subclavian artery

Left subclavian artery

Ascending aorta

Aortic arch

Brachial artery

Renal artery

Abdominal aorta

Common iliac artery

Radial artery

Internal iliac artery

Ulnar artery

External iliac artery

Femoral artery

Popliteal artery

Peroneal artery

Anterior tibial artery

Posterior tibial artery

FIGURE 5-20 (B) The major veins of the body.

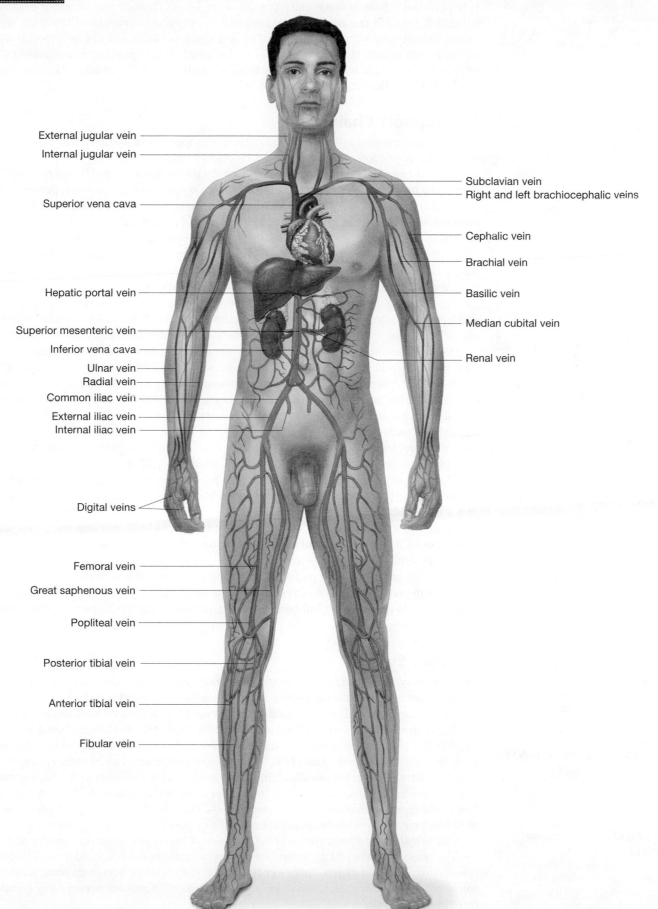

External jugular vein

Internal jugular vein

Superior vena cava

Hepatic portal vein

Superior mesenteric vein

Inferior vena cava

Ulnar vein

Radial vein

Common iliac vein

External iliac vein

Internal iliac vein

Digital veins

Femoral vein

Great saphenous vein

Popliteal vein

Posterior tibial vein

Anterior tibial vein

Fibular vein

Subclavian vein

Right and left brachiocephalic veins

Cephalic vein

Brachial vein

Basilic vein

Median cubital vein

Renal vein

Hypoperfusion (inadequate perfusion), also known as *shock*, is a serious condition. With hypoperfusion, there is inadequate circulation of blood through one or more organs or structures. Blood is not reaching and filling all the capillary networks of the body, which means that oxygen will not be delivered to, and waste products will not be removed from, all the body's tissues. Hypoperfusion can lead to death. It is important to understand what hypoperfusion is, how it occurs, and how to recognize it. This will be discussed in more depth in Chapter 27, "Bleeding and Shock."

Life Support Chain

The respiratory system and the cardiovascular system together make up the *cardiopulmonary system*. The interaction of these two systems is essential to life.

Oxygen and glucose are necessary to the cells. Glucose is converted by the cells into energy in the form of adenosine triphosphate (ATP). Oxygen is a necessary component of this conversion process. When oxygen is present, glucose is converted in a process called *aerobic metabolism*. This process produces efficient amounts of energy and minimal waste products, such as carbon dioxide and water. If oxygen is not present in sufficient supply, the process will shift to *anaerobic metabolism*. This process produces less energy and more waste products, such as *lactic acid*. Waste products, in turn, make the body more acidotic. Acidosis injures the body's cells and limits the blood's ability to carry oxygen.

The movement of oxygen from the blood into the cells, coupled with the removal of waste products, is referred to as perfusion. As stated previously, perfusion is essential to normal cell function. Perfusion depends on the cardiopulmonary system, as described next.

In order for cells to be oxygenated and carbon dioxide to be removed, a variety of factors must be working properly. First and foremost, air must be reaching the alveoli of the lungs and, once there, must be matched up with a sufficient supply of blood in the pulmonary capillaries. If, for example, air is obstructed from getting to the alveoli, as in a foreign body obstruction, gas exchange cannot occur. Similarly, if there is not enough blood passing through the pulmonary capillaries, as in the case of severe external bleeding, gas exchange cannot occur. This coupling of a sufficient amount of air with a sufficient amount of blood is called a ventilation perfusion match and abbreviated as a V/Q match.

There are other critical elements to normal perfusion as well. The heart must pump effectively. If the pump fails, blood will not move. There must be sufficient oxygen in the air that is breathed. There must be an effective capability to carry oxygen in the blood (anemia is a condition that in some cases reduces the number of oxygen-carrying red blood cells). Furthermore, if the mechanics of respiration are disrupted, air will not move. All of these elements are critical components to perfusion.

There are other potential perfusion problems; to simplify things, consider anything that threatens the normal function of the cardiopulmonary system to be a threat to quality perfusion. Threats to perfusion will be discussed in greater detail in Chapter 6, "Principles of Pathophysiology."

Nervous System

The *nervous system* (Figure 5-21) consists of the brain, spinal cord, and nerve tissue. It transmits impulses that govern sensation, movement, and thought. It also controls the body's voluntary and involuntary activity. It is subdivided into the central and peripheral nervous systems.

The *central nervous system (CNS)* is composed of the brain and the spinal cord. The brain could be likened to a powerful computer that receives information from the body and, in turn, sends impulses to different areas of the body to respond to internal and external changes. The spinal cord rests within the spinal column and stretches from the brain to the lumbar vertebrae. Nerves branch from each part of the cord and reach throughout the body. A key function of the central nervous system is consciousness. The reticular activating system is a series of nervous pathways in the brain and is essentially responsible for keeping you awake.

The *peripheral nervous system (PNS)* consists of two types of nerves: sensory and motor. The sensory nerves pick up information from throughout the body and transmit it to the spinal cord and brain. If you touch something hot, your sensory nerves transmit this to the spinal cord and brain so immediate action may be taken. The motor nerves carry messages from the brain to the body.

FIGURE 5-21 The nervous system.

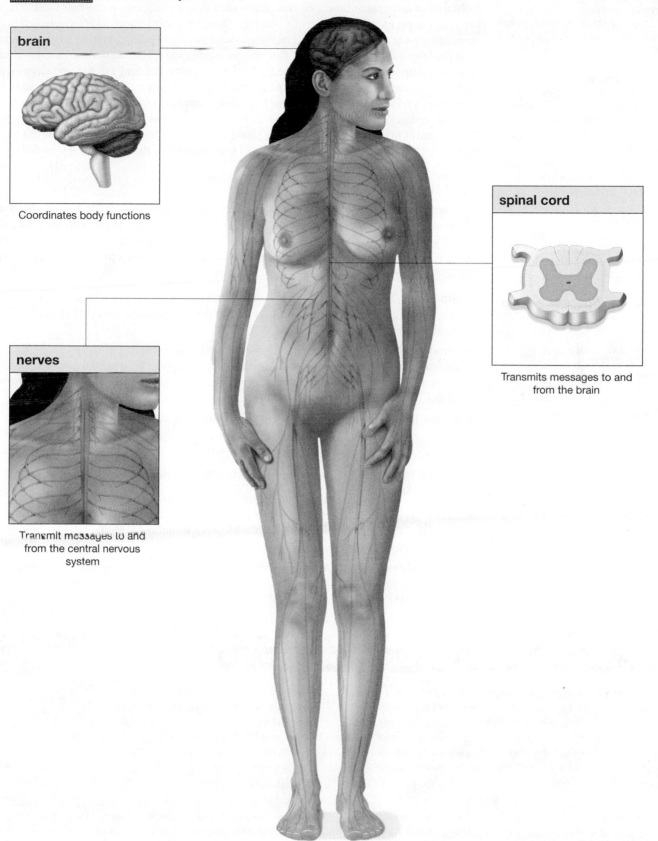

brain

Coordinates body functions

spinal cord

Transmits messages to and from the brain

nerves

Transmit messages to and from the central nervous system

autonomic (AW-to-NOM-ik)
nervous system
the division of the peripheral nervous system that controls involuntary motor functions.

digestive system
system by which food travels through the body and is digested, or broken down into absorbable forms.

stomach
muscular sac between the esophagus and the small intestine where digestion of food begins.

small intestine
the muscular tube between the stomach and the large intestine, divided into the duodenum, the jejunum, and the ileum, which receives partially digested food from the stomach and continues digestion. Nutrients are absorbed by the body through its walls.

large intestine
the muscular tube that removes water from waste products received from the small intestine and moves anything not absorbed by the body toward excretion from the body.

liver
the largest organ of the body, which produces bile to assist in breakdown of fats and assists in the metabolism of various substances in the body.

gallbladder
a sac on the underside of the liver that stores bile produced by the liver.

The *autonomic nervous system* is the division of the peripheral nervous system that controls involuntary motor functions and affects such things as digestion and heart rate. The autonomic nervous system can be further broken down into the *sympathetic and parasympathetic nervous systems*. The sympathetic nervous system function is often referred to as the "fight-or-flight" response. This system is engaged when the body is in crisis. Stimulation of sympathetic tone causes the heart to beat faster, the lungs to breathe deeper, and the blood vessels to constrict. Imagine all the responses you might need if you had to run away from a potential threat. The *parasympathetic nervous system* asserts an opposite effect. It is engaged in times of relaxation and is often referred to as the "feed-or-breed" response. Parasympathetic tone causes increased blood flow to the digestive tract and to the reproductive organs. It also can cause the heart to slow down and the blood vessels to dilate.

Digestive System

The *digestive system* provides the mechanisms by which food travels through the body and is digested, or broken down into absorbable forms. Food enters the mouth and is broken down by both saliva and chewing. The food passes from the mouth through the oropharynx and into the esophagus, where it is transported to the stomach. Except for the mouth and the esophagus, all of the organs of digestion are contained in the abdominal cavity.

- **Stomach.** The *stomach* is a hollow organ that expands as it fills with food. In the stomach, acidic gastric juices begin to break food down into components that the body will be able to convert into energy.

- **Small intestine.** The *small intestine* is divided into three parts: the *duodenum*, the *jejunum*, and the *ileum*. This organ receives food from the stomach and continues to break it down for absorption. These nutrients are absorbed by the body through the wall of the small intestine.

- **Large intestine (colon).** The *large intestine* removes water from waste products as they move toward elimination from the body. Anything not absorbed from this point is moved through the colon and excreted as feces.

Several organs located outside of the stomach–intestines continuum assist in the food breakdown process.

- **Liver.** The *liver* produces bile, which is excreted into the small intestine to assist in the breakdown of fats. The liver has many additional functions, including detoxifying harmful substances, storing sugar, and assisting in production of blood products.

- **Gallbladder.** The *gallbladder* serves as a storage system for bile from the liver.

Inside/Outside

RECOGNIZING SYMPATHETIC NERVOUS SYSTEM RESPONSE

Recognizing a sympathetic nervous system response can be an important part of a patient assessment. Often a patient's sympathetic nervous system will be engaged as the result of injury or illness, and recognizing its signs can help alert you to a problem even when the immediate cause is unknown. Let's use the example of a 62-year-old male having an acute myocardial infarction:

■ Inside

In this patient something very wrong is happening. A coronary artery is blocked, and his heart is not getting the oxygen supply it desperately needs. In most people this will cause chest pain, but in this case the patient is diabetic and, for an unknown reason, no chest pain is present. He does, however, feel weak and nauseated. Despite his obscure symptoms, his body is reacting. His brain engages the sympathetic nervous system to respond to the challenge. His heart beats a bit faster, he breathes a bit quicker. His blood vessels constrict and divert blood away from the skin.

■ Outside

Although he is presenting atypically, that is, in an unusual fashion, your assessment reveals a few red flags. You notice he is pale and sweaty (a result of constricted blood vessels). You also observe the elevated heart rate and respiratory rate. By noticing these signs you recognize a "sympathetic discharge" and know that the body is responding to a serious problem. *This may be more than an upset stomach.*

- **Pancreas.** Perhaps best known for production of the hormone insulin, which is involved in the regulation of sugar in the bloodstream, the **pancreas** also secretes juices that assist in breaking down proteins, carbohydrates, and fat.
- **Spleen.** Acting as a blood filtration system, the **spleen** filters out older blood cells. It has many blood vessels and at any given time holds significant quantities of blood, reserves the body can use in case of significant blood loss.
- **Appendix.** Located near the junction of the small and large intestines, the **appendix** is made up of lymphatic tissue. Its exact function is not well understood, but it is often considered with the digestive system because an infected appendix (appendicitis) is a common cause of abdominal pain.

Integumentary System

The integumentary system consists primarily of the skin. The **skin** performs a variety of functions, such as protection, water balance, temperature regulation, excretion, and shock absorption.

- **Protection.** The skin serves as a barrier to keep out microorganisms, debris, and unwanted chemicals. Underlying tissues and organs are protected from environmental contact. This helps preserve the chemical balance of body fluids and tissues.
- **Water balance.** The skin helps prevent water loss and stops environmental water from entering the body.
- **Temperature regulation.** Blood vessels in the skin can dilate (increase in diameter) to carry more blood to the skin, allowing heat to radiate from the body. When the body needs to conserve heat, these vessels constrict (decrease in diameter) to prevent heat loss. The sweat glands found in the skin produce perspiration, which will evaporate and help cool the body. The fat layer beneath the skin also serves as a thermal insulator.
- **Excretion.** Salts and excess water can be released through the skin.
- **Shock (impact) absorption.** The skin and its layers of fat help protect the underlying organs from minor impacts and pressures.

The skin has three major layers: the epidermis, dermis, and subcutaneous layers (Figure 5-22). The outer layer of the skin is called the **epidermis**. It is composed of four layers (strata) everywhere except at the palms of the hands and soles of the feet. These two regions have five skin layers. The

pancreas
a gland located behind the stomach that produces insulin and juices that assist in digestion of food in the duodenum of the small intestine.

spleen
an organ located in the left upper quadrant of the abdomen that acts as a blood filtration system and a reservoir for reserves of blood.

appendix
a small tube located near the junction of the small and large intestines in the right lower quadrant of the abdomen, the function of which is not well understood. Its inflammation, called appendicitis, is a common cause of abdominal pain.

skin
the layer of tissue between the body and the external environment.

epidermis (ep-i-DER-mis)
the outer layer of skin.

FIGURE 5-22 The layers of the skin.

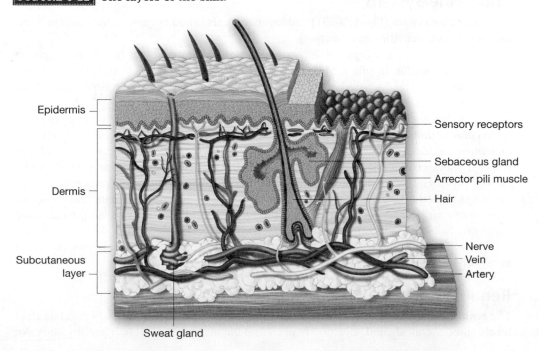

Epidermis

Dermis

Subcutaneous layer

Sensory receptors

Sebaceous gland

Arrector pili muscle

Hair

Nerve

Vein

Artery

Sweat gland

outermost layers of the epidermis are composed of dead cells, which are rubbed off or sloughed off and replaced. The pigment granules of the skin and living cells are found in the deeper layers. The cells of the innermost layer actively divide, replacing the dead cells of the outer layers. Note that the epidermis contains no blood vessels or nerves. Except for certain types of burns and injuries due to cold, injuries of the epidermis present few problems in EMT-level care.

The layer of skin below the epidermis is the ***dermis***, which is rich with blood vessels, nerves, and specialized structures such as sweat glands, sebaceous (oil) glands, and hair follicles. Specialized nerve endings are also found in the dermis. They are involved with the senses of touch, cold, heat, and pain. Once the dermis is opened to the outside world, contamination and infection become major problems. These wounds can be serious, accompanied by profuse bleeding and intense pain.

The layers of fat and soft tissue below the dermis makes up the ***subcutaneous layers***. Shock absorption and insulation are major functions of this layer. Again, there are the problems of tissue and bloodstream contamination, bleeding, and pain when these layers are injured or exposed.

dermis (DER-mis)
the inner (second) layer of skin, rich in blood vessels and nerves, found beneath the epidermis.

subcutaneous (SUB-ku-TAY-ne-us) ***layers***
the layers of fat and soft tissues found below the dermis.

CRITICAL DECISION MAKING

Identifying Possible Areas of Injury

Your knowledge of anatomy is a critical foundation for making solid clinical decisions in the field. For each of the patients in the following list, identify what organ or body system may be involved in that patient's complaint. This exercise requires no knowledge of diseases or conditions—just the anatomy of the body.

1. Your patient falls in an icy parking lot. She tries to catch herself and breaks the bones of the arm just above the wrist. What are these bones called?

2. Your patient was the driver of a car that was hit in a "T-bone," or side impact, crash. He was the driver. He complains of pain in the left upper abdominal quadrant. What organ is located in this area that can cause severe internal bleeding?

3. Your patient was riding a motorcycle and was thrown over the handlebars in a crash. She has broken the large bone in her right thigh. What bone is this, and would you expect blood loss from the fracture?

Endocrine System

endocrine (EN-do-krin) ***system***
system of glands that produce chemicals called hormones that help to regulate many body activities and functions

insulin (IN-suh-lin)
a hormone produced by the pancreas or taken as a medication by many diabetics.

epinephrine (EP-uh-NEF-rin)
a hormone produced by the body. As a medication, it dilates respiratory passages and is used to relieve severe allergic reactions.

The ***endocrine system*** (Figure 5-23) produces chemicals called hormones that help to regulate many body activities and functions.

The pancreas is a key organ of the endocrine system. Among other functions, it secretes the hormone ***insulin***. Insulin is critical to the body's use of glucose, a sugar that fuels the body. (Insulin will be discussed in greater detail in Chapter 21, "Diabetic Emergencies and Altered Mental Status.")

The adrenal glands are also an essential component of the endocrine system. They secrete ***epinephrine*** (also known as adrenaline) and norepinephrine. These chemicals serve as neurotransmitters (chemical messengers) and engage the sympathetic nervous system through a series of chemical receptors located in specific organ systems. For example, when the fight-or-flight response is engaged, norepinephrine is released. It activates receptors in the lungs (called *beta 2 receptors*) which stimulate the bronchioles to dilate and therefore move more air. Receptors in the heart (called *beta 1 receptors*) are activated to increase heart rate and increase the force of contraction.

The endocrine system is a complex system of chemical messaging that also interacts with many other body systems.

Renal System

renal system
the body system that regulates fluid balance and the filtration of blood. Also called the *urinary system*.

The ***renal system***, also called the *urinary system* (Figure 5-24), helps the body regulate fluid levels, filter chemicals, and adjust body pH. Fluid balance is essential to a healthy body. An

FIGURE 5-23 The endocrine system.

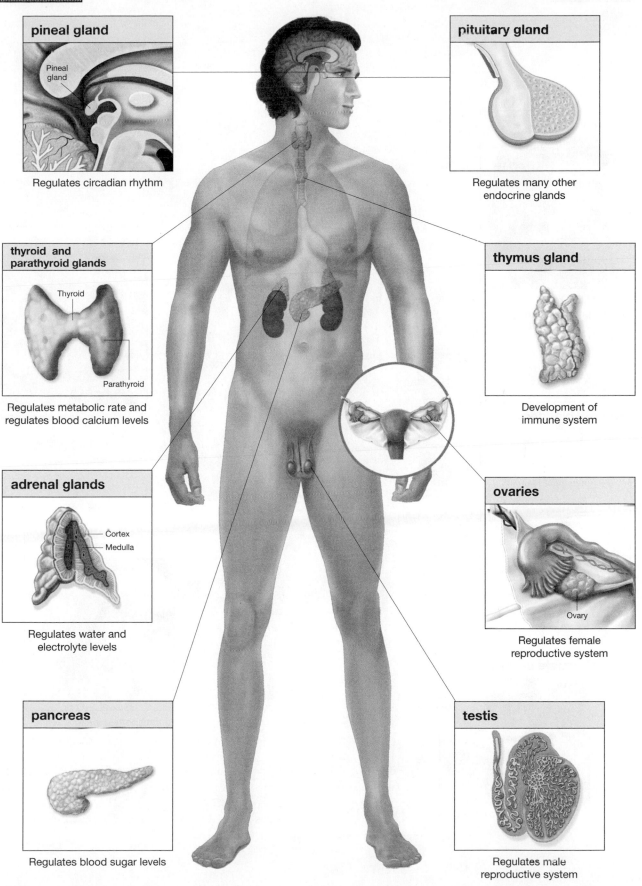

pineal gland

Pineal gland

Regulates circadian rhythm

pituitary gland

Regulates many other endocrine glands

thyroid and parathyroid glands

Thyroid

Parathyroid

Regulates metabolic rate and regulates blood calcium levels

thymus gland

Development of immune system

adrenal glands

Cortex

Medulla

Regulates water and electrolyte levels

ovaries

Ovary

Regulates female reproductive system

pancreas

Regulates blood sugar levels

testis

Regulates male reproductive system

FIGURE 5-24 The renal/urinary system.

kidney

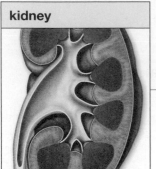

Filters blood and
produces urine

urinary bladder

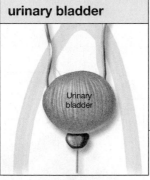

Stores urine

female urethra

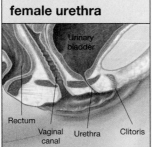

Transports urine to exterior

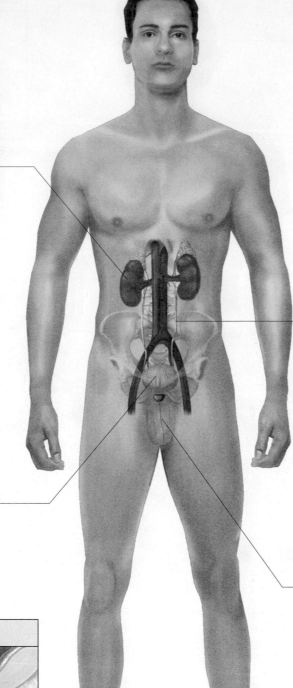

ureter

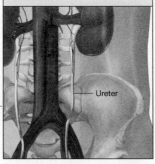

Transports urine to the bladder

male urethra

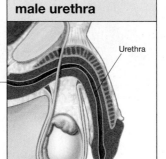

Transports urine to exterior

average adult excretes roughly a liter and a half of urine per day. The renal system can adjust this fluid movement to account for changes in fluid intake or fluid loss such as bleeding.

The **kidneys** are the principal organs of the renal system. They help filter a waste product called urea from the blood and provide fluid balance by regulating the uptake of sodium and the excretion of urine. The kidneys also assist the buffer system with the production of bicarbonate for the blood. Bicarbonate is an essential substance used to help regulate acidity or pH in the body.

The renal system also includes the **bladder** and its connecting passages. The bladder is a round, hollow sac that serves as a fluid reservoir for urine. It receives urine from the kidneys via small tubes called **ureters**. Urine is excreted from the bladder to the outside world through a tube called the **urethra**. In males, the urethra passes through the penis. In females, the urethra is shorter and emerges from the body just above the vaginal opening.

Reproductive System

The **reproductive system** is a group of organs and glands designed for the specific purpose of reproduction. It is important to note here, and as you probably already know, the reproductive systems of men and women vary greatly and contain different organs. The female reproductive system will be discussed in more detail in Chapter 34, "Obstetric and Gynecologic Emergencies."

Male Reproductive System

The primary organs of the male reproductive system (Figure 5-25A) are the testes and the penis. The **testes** produce sperm, the male component of reproduction, and are housed outside the body in the *scrotum*. The testes are connected to the penis through a small tube called the *epididymis*. The **penis** is the external reproductive organ of the male and is used for both sexual intercourse and urination.

Female Reproductive System

The primary organs of the female reproductive system (Figure 5-25B) are the ovaries, the uterus, and the vagina. The **ovaries** are located bilaterally in the lower quadrants of a female's abdomen and serve to produce ova or (eggs) for reproduction. The ovaries are connected to the uterus via the *fallopian tubes*, also called the *oviducts*. The fallopian tubes, or oviducts, are the site where sperm fertilizes the descending ovum. The **uterus** is a muscular organ located along the midline in the lower quadrants of a female abdomen. The uterus is designed to contain the developing fetus through the 40 weeks of pregnancy. Although it is a small organ, it has a huge potential to grow as pregnancy develops. It is also highly vascular and at times of pregnancy can be prone to serious bleeding. The uterus connects to the **vagina**, or birth canal. The vagina serves not only as the exit route for the fetus, but also as the female reproductive organ and site of sexual intercourse.

kidneys
organs of the renal system used to filter blood and regulate fluid levels in the body.

bladder
the round sac-like organ of the renal system used as a reservoir for urine.

ureters (YER-uh-terz)
the tubes connecting the kidneys to the bladder.

urethra (you-RE-thra)
tube connecting the bladder to the vagina or penis for excretion of urine.

reproductive system
the body system that is responsible for human reproduction.

testes (TES-tees)
the male organ of reproduction used for the production of sperm.

penis
the organ of male reproduction responsible for sexual intercourse and the transfer of sperm.

ovaries
egg-producing organs within the female reproductive system.

uterus (YOU-ter-us)
female organ of reproduction used to house the developing fetus.

vagina (vuh-JI-na)
the female organ of reproduction used for both sexual intercourse and as an exit from the uterus for the fetus.

FIGURE 5-25 (A) The male reproductive system.

testes

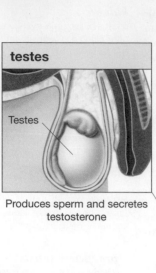

Testes

Produces sperm and secretes testosterone

epididymis

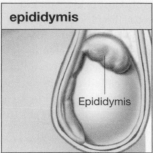

Epididymis

Stores sperm

vas deferens

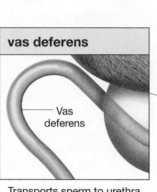

Vas deferens

Transports sperm to urethra

seminal vesicles

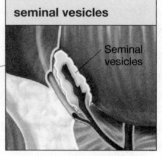

Seminal vesicles

Secretes fluid for semen

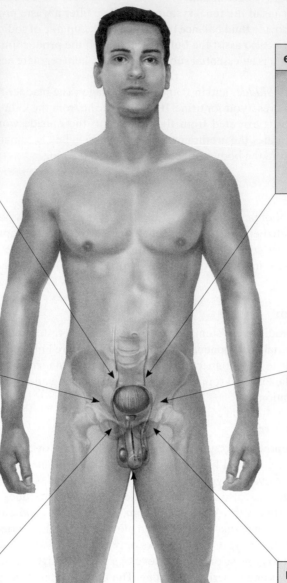

prostate gland

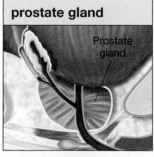

Prostate gland

Secretes fluid for semen

penis

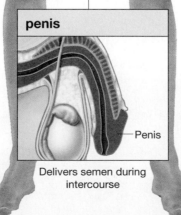

Penis

Delivers semen during intercourse

bulbourethral gland

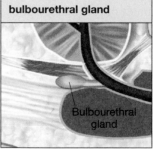

Bulbourethral gland

Secretes fluid for semen

FIGURE 5-25 (B) The female reproductive system.

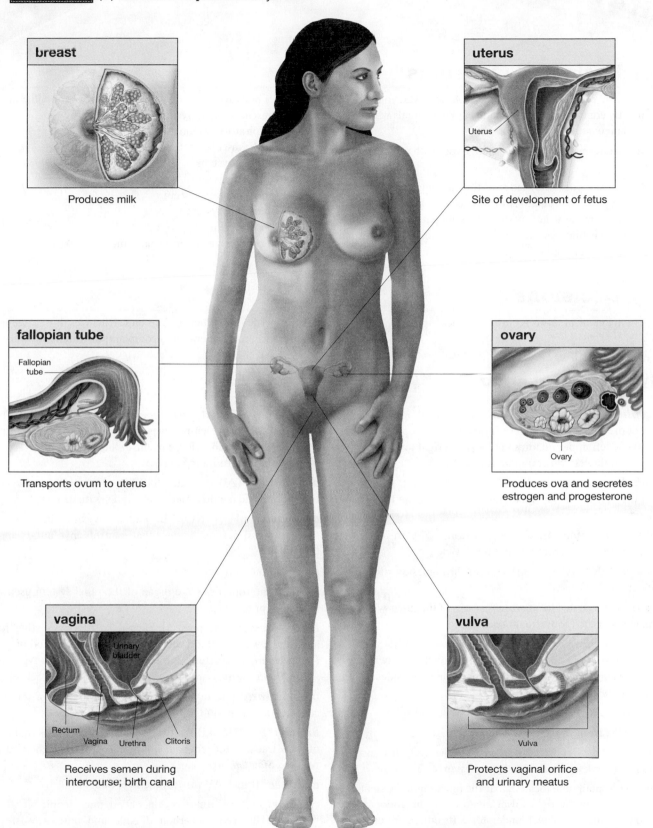

breast

Produces milk

uterus

Uterus

Site of development of fetus

fallopian tube

Fallopian tube

Transports ovum to uterus

ovary

Ovary

Produces ova and secretes estrogen and progesterone

vagina

Urinary bladder

Rectum   Vagina   Urethra   Clitoris

Receives semen during intercourse; birth canal

vulva

Vulva

Protects vaginal orifice and urinary meatus

Key Facts and Concepts

- Medicine has a language of its own. As an EMT, you will frequently communicate with medical professionals who speak this language.

- Medical terms generally consist of a root with a prefix and/or suffix.

- As an EMT, your knowledge of the anatomy, or structure, of the body and the functions, or physiology, of the body will be important in allowing you to assess your patient and communicate your findings with other EMS personnel and hospital staff accurately and efficiently.

- Major body systems with which you should be familiar are the
  - Musculoskeletal system
  - Respiratory system
  - Cardiovascular system
  - Nervous system
  - Digestive system
  - Integumentary system
  - Endocrine system
  - Renal system
  - Reproductive systems (male and female)

Key Decisions

- Are my medical terms accurate and descriptive?

- Can I identify critical organs and structures that reside in an area where a patient has a complaint or traumatic injury?

Chapter Glossary

abdominal quadrants four divisions of the abdomen used to pinpoint the location of a pain or injury: the right upper quadrant (RUQ), the left upper quadrant (LUQ), the right lower quadrant (RLQ), and the left lower quadrant (LLQ).

acetabulum (AS-uh-TAB-yuh-lum) the pelvic socket into which the ball at the proximal end of the femur fits to form the hip joint.

acromioclavicular (ah-KRO-me-o-klav-IK-yuh-ler) ***joint*** the joint where the acromion and the clavicle meet.

acromion (ah-KRO-me-on) ***process*** the highest portion of the shoulder.

alveoli (al-VE-o-li) the microscopic sacs of the lungs where gas exchange with the bloodstream takes place.

anatomical position the standard reference position for the body in the study of anatomy. In this position, the body is standing erect, facing the observer, with arms down at the sides and the palms of the hands forward.

anatomy the study of body structure.

anterior the front of the body or body part.

aorta (ay-OR-tah) the largest artery in the body. It transports blood from the left ventricle to begin systemic circulation.

appendix a small tube located near the junction of the small and large intestines in the right lower quadrant of the abdomen, the function of which is not well understood. Its inflammation, called appendicitis, is a common cause of abdominal pain.

arteriole (ar-TE-re-ol) the smallest kind of artery.

artery any blood vessel carrying blood away from the heart.

atria (AY-tree-ah) the two upper chambers of the heart. There is a right atrium (which receives unoxygenated blood returning from the body) and a left atrium (which receives oxygenated blood returning from the lungs).

automaticity (AW-to-muh-TISS-it-e) the ability of the heart to generate and conduct electrical impulses on its own.

autonomic (AW-to-NOM-ik) ***nervous system*** the division of the peripheral nervous system that controls involuntary motor functions.

bilateral on both sides.

bladder the round sac-like organ of the renal system used as a reservoir for urine.

blood pressure the pressure caused by blood exerting force against the walls of blood vessels. Usually arterial blood pressure (the pressure in an artery) is measured. There are two types: ***diastolic blood pressure*** and ***systolic blood pressure.***

brachial artery artery of the upper arm; the site of the pulse checked during infant CPR.

bronchi (BRONG-ki) the two large sets of branches that come off the trachea and enter the lungs. There are right and left bronchi. *Singular* bronchus.

calcaneus (kal-KAY-ne-us) the heel bone.

capillary (KAP-i-lair-e) a thin-walled, microscopic blood vessel where the oxygen/carbon dioxide and nutrient/waste exchange with the body's cells takes place.

cardiac conduction system a system of specialized muscle tissues that conducts electrical impulses that stimulate the heart to beat.

cardiac muscle specialized involuntary muscle found only in the heart.

cardiovascular (KAR-de-o-VAS-kyu-ler) *system* the system made up of the heart (cardio) and the blood vessels (vascular); the circulatory system. Sometimes called the circulatory system.

carotid (kah-ROT-id) *arteries* the large neck arteries, one on each side of the neck, that carry blood from the heart to the head.

carpals (KAR-pulz) the wrist bones.

central nervous system (CNS) the brain and spinal cord.

central pulses the carotid and femoral pulses, which can be felt in the central part of the body.

clavicle (KLAV-i-kul) the collarbone.

combining form a word root with an added vowel that can be joined with other words, roots, or suffixes to form a new word; for example, the combining form *therm/o*, which added to *meter* makes the new word *thermometer*.

compound a word formed from two or more whole words; for example, the compound *smallpox* formed from *small* and *pox*.

coronary (KOR-o-nar-e) *arteries* blood vessels that supply the muscle of the heart (myocardium).

cranium the top, back, and sides of the skull.

cricoid (KRIK-oid) *cartilage* the ring-shaped structure that forms the lower portion of the larynx.

dermis (DER-mis) the inner (second) layer of skin, rich in blood vessels and nerves, found beneath the epidermis.

diaphragm (DI-uh-fram) the muscular structure that divides the chest cavity from the abdominal cavity. A major muscle of respiration.

diastolic (di-as-TOL-ik) *blood pressure* the pressure in the arteries when the left ventricle is refilling.

digestive system system by which food travels through the body and is digested, or broken down into absorbable forms.

distal farther away from the torso. *See also* proximal.

dorsal referring to the back of the body or the back of the hand or foot. A synonym for posterior.

dorsalis pedis (dor-SAL-is PEED-is) *artery* artery supplying the foot, lateral to the large tendon of the big toe.

endocrine (EN-do-krin) *system* system of glands that produce chemicals called hormones that help to regulate many body activities and functions.

epidermis (ep-i-DER-mis) the outer layer of skin.

epiglottis (EP-i-GLOT-is) a leaf-shaped structure that prevents food and foreign matter from entering the trachea.

epinephrine (EP-uh-NEF-rin) a hormone produced by the body. As a medication, it dilates respiratory passages and is used to relieve severe allergic reactions.

exhalation (EX-huh-LAY-shun) a passive process in which the intercostal (rib) muscles and the diaphragm relax, causing the chest cavity to decrease in size and air to flow out of the lungs.

femoral (FEM-o-ral) *artery* the major artery supplying the leg.

femur (FEE-mer) the large bone of the thigh.

fibula (FIB-yuh-luh) the lateral and smaller bone of the lower leg.

Fowler position a sitting position.

gallbladder a sac on the underside of the liver that stores bile produced by the liver.

humerus (HYU-mer-us) the bone of the upper arm, between the shoulder and the elbow.

hypoperfusion inadequate perfusion of the cells and tissues of the body caused by insufficient flow of blood through the capillaries. Also called *shock*. *See also* perfusion.

ilium (IL-e-um) the superior and widest portion of the pelvis.

inferior away from the head; usually compared with another structure that is closer to the head (e.g., the lips are inferior to the nose).

inhalation (IN-huh-LAY-shun) an active process in which the intercostal (rib) muscles and the diaphragm contract, expanding the size of the chest cavity and causing air to flow into the lungs.

insulin (IN-suh-lin) a hormone produced by the pancreas or taken as a medication by many diabetics.

involuntary muscle muscle that responds automatically to brain signals but cannot be consciously controlled.

ischium (ISH-e-um) the lower, posterior portions of the pelvis.

joint the point where two bones come together.

kidneys organs of the renal system used to filter blood and regulate fluid levels in the body.

large intestine the muscular tube that removes water from waste products received from the small intestine and moves anything not absorbed by the body toward excretion from the body.

larynx (LAIR-inks) the voice box.

lateral to the side, away from the midline of the body.

ligament tissue that connects bone to bone.

liver the largest organ of the body, which produces bile to assist in breakdown of fats and assists in the metabolism of various substances in the body.

lungs the organs where exchange of atmospheric oxygen and waste carbon dioxide take place.

malleolus (mal-E-o-lus) protrusion on the side of the ankle. The *lateral malleolus*, at the lower end of the fibula, is seen on the outer ankle; the *medial malleolus*, at the lower end of the tibia, is seen on the inner ankle.

mandible (MAN-di-bul) the lower jaw bone.

manubrium (man-OO-bre-um) the superior portion of the sternum.

maxillae (mak-SIL-e) the two fused bones forming the upper jaw.

medial toward the midline of the body.

metacarpals (MET-uh-KAR-pulz) the hand bones.

metatarsals (MET-uh-TAR-sulz) the foot bones.

mid-axillary (mid-AX-uh-lair-e) *line* a line drawn vertically from the middle of the armpit to the ankle.

mid-clavicular (mid-clah-VIK-yuh-ler) *line* the line through the center of each clavicle.

midline an imaginary line drawn down the center of the body, dividing it into right and left halves.

muscle tissue that can contract to allow movement of a body part.

musculoskeletal (MUS-kyu-lo-SKEL-e-tal) **system** the system of bones and skeletal muscles that support and protect the body and permit movement.

nasal (NAY-zul) **bones** the nose bones.

nasopharynx (NAY-zo-FAIR-inks) the area directly posterior to the nose.

nervous system the system of brain, spinal cord, and nerves that govern sensation, movement, and thought.

orbits the bony structures around the eyes; the eye sockets.

oropharynx (OR-o-FAIR-inks) the area directly posterior to the mouth.

ovaries egg-producing organs within the female reproductive system.

palmar referring to the palm of the hand.

pancreas a gland located behind the stomach that produces insulin and juices that assist in digestion of food in the duodenum of the small intestine.

patella (pah-TEL-uh) the kneecap.

pelvis the basin-shaped bony structure that supports the spine and is the point of proximal attachment for the lower extremities.

penis the organ of male reproduction responsible for sexual intercourse and the transfer of sperm.

perfusion the supply of oxygen to, and removal of wastes from, the cells and tissues of the body as a result of the flow of blood through the capillaries.

peripheral nervous system (PNS) the nerves that enter and leave the spinal cord and travel between the brain and organs without passing through the spinal cord.

peripheral pulses the radial, brachial, posterior tibial, and dorsalis pedis pulses, which can be felt at peripheral (outlying) points of the body.

phalanges (fuh-LAN-jiz) the toe bones and finger bones.

pharynx (FAIR-inks) the area directly posterior to the mouth and nose. It is made up of the oropharynx and the nasopharynx.

physiology the study of body function.

plane a flat surface formed when slicing through a solid object.

plantar referring to the sole of the foot.

plasma (PLAZ-mah) the fluid portion of the blood.

platelets components of the blood; membrane-enclosed fragments of specialized cells.

posterior the back of the body or body part.

posterior tibial (TIB-ee-ul) **artery** artery supplying the foot, behind the medial ankle.

prefix word part added to the beginning of a root or word to modify or qualify its meaning; for example, the prefix *bi-* added to the word *lateral* to form the word *bilateral*.

prone lying face down.

proximal closer to the torso. *See also* distal.

pubis (PYOO-bis) the medial anterior portion of the pelvis.

pulmonary (PUL-mo-nar-e) **arteries** the vessels that carry deoxygenated blood from the right ventricle of the heart to the lungs.

pulmonary veins the vessels that carry oxygenated blood from the lungs to the left atrium of the heart.

pulse the rhythmic beats caused as waves of blood move through and expand the arteries.

radial artery artery of the lower arm. It is felt when taking the pulse at the wrist.

radius (RAY-de-us) the lateral bone of the forearm.

recovery position lying on the side. Also called *lateral recumbent position*.

red blood cells components of the blood. They carry oxygen to, and carbon dioxide away from, the cells.

renal system the body system that regulates fluid balance and the filtration of blood. Also called the *urinary system*.

reproductive system the body system that is responsible for human reproduction.

respiration (cellular) the process of moving oxygen and carbon dioxide between circulating blood and the cells.

respiratory (RES-pir-ah-tor-e) **system** the system of nose, mouth, throat, lungs, and muscles that brings oxygen into the body and expels carbon dioxide.

root foundation of a word that is not a word that can stand on its own; for example, the root *cardi*, meaning "heart," in words such as *cardiac* and *cardiology*.

scapula (SKAP-yuh-luh) the shoulder blade.

shock *See* hypoperfusion.

skeleton the bones of the body.

skin the layer of tissue between the body and the external environment.

skull the bony structure of the head.

small intestine the muscular tube between the stomach and the large intestine, divided into the duodenum, the jejunum, and the ileum, which receives partially digested food from the stomach and continues digestion. Nutrients are absorbed by the body through its walls.

spleen an organ located in the left upper quadrant of the abdomen that acts as a blood filtration system and a reservoir for reserves of blood.

sternum (STER-num) the breastbone.

stomach muscular sac between the esophagus and the small intestine where digestion of food begins.

subcutaneous (SUB-ku-TAY-ne-us) **layers** the layers of fat and soft tissues found below the dermis.

suffix word part added to the end of a root or word to complete its meaning; for example, the suffix *–itis* added to the root *laryng* to form the word *laryngitis*.

superior toward the head (e.g., the chest is superior to the abdomen).

supine lying on the back.

systolic (sis-TOL-ik) *blood pressure* the pressure created in the arteries when the left ventricle contracts and forces blood out into circulation.

tarsals (TAR-sulz) the ankle bones.

tendon tissue that connects muscle to bone.

testes (TES-tees) the male organs of reproduction used for the production of sperm.

thorax (THOR-ax) the chest.

thyroid (THI-roid) *cartilage* the wing-shaped plate of cartilage that sits anterior to the larynx and forms the Adam's apple.

tibia (TIB-e-uh) the medial and larger bone of the lower leg.

torso the trunk of the body; the body without the head and the extremities.

trachea (TRAY-ke-uh) the "windpipe"; the structure that connects the pharynx to the lungs.

Trendelenburg (trend-EL-un-berg) *position* a position in which the patient's feet and legs are higher than the head.

ulna (UL-nah) the medial bone of the forearm.

ureters (YER-uh-terz) the tubes connecting the kidneys to the bladder.

urethra (you-RE-thra) tube connecting the bladder to the vagina or penis for excretion of urine.

uterus (YOU-ter-us) female organ of reproduction used to house the developing fetus.

vagina (vu-JI-na) the female organ of reproduction used for both sexual intercourse and as an exit from the uterus for the fetus.

valve a structure that opens and closes to permit the flow of a fluid in only one direction.

vein any blood vessel returning blood to the heart.

venae cavae (VE-ne KA-ve) the superior vena cava and the inferior vena cava. These two major veins return blood from the body to the right atrium. (Venae cavae is plural, vena cava singular.)

ventilation the process of moving gases (oxygen and carbon dioxide) between inhaled air and the pulmonary circulation of blood.

ventral referring to the front of the body. A synonym for anterior.

ventricles (VEN-tri-kulz) the two lower chambers of the heart. There is a right ventricle (which sends oxygen-poor blood to the lungs) and a left ventricle (which sends oxygen-rich blood to the body).

venule (VEN-yul) the smallest kind of vein.

vertebrae (VER-te-bray) the 33 bones of the spinal column.

voluntary muscle muscle that can be consciously controlled.

white blood cells components of the blood. They produce substances that help the body fight infection.

xiphoid (ZI-foid) *process* the inferior portion of the sternum.

zygomatic (ZI-go-MAT-ik) *arches* bones that form the structure of the cheeks.

Preparation for Your Examination and Practice

Short Answer

1. Define the following pairs of anatomical terms:
   medial   lateral
   anterior   posterior
   proximal   distal

2. List the three functions of the musculoskeletal system.

3. Name the five divisions of the spine and describe the location of each.

4. Describe the physical processes of inhalation and exhalation.

5. List four places a peripheral pulse may be felt.

6. Describe the central nervous system and peripheral nervous system.

7. List three functions of the skin.

Thinking and Linking

Linking your knowledge of medical terminology and anatomy with common diseases will help you to understand the diseases and communicate about them. For each of the following diseases, use word parts (root, prefix, suffix—as appropriate) to determine what organs the disease affects. (The on-line medical terminology reference included in Resource Central will assist you.)

Hepatitis

Appendicitis

Splenomegaly

Cholecystitis

Polynephritis

Hydrocephalus

Pneumothorax

Critical Thinking Exercises

Understanding medical terminology and knowing how to use it is important in your practice as an EMT. The purpose of this exercise will be to consider how you might appropriately use medical terminology in your radio report about a patient's injuries.

- As an EMT, you are called to respond to a teenage boy who has taken a hard fall from his dirt bike. He has a deep gash on the outside of his left arm about halfway between the shoulder and the elbow and another on the inside of his right arm just above the wrist. His left leg is bent at a funny angle about halfway between hip and knee, and when you cut away his pants leg, you see a bone sticking out of a wound on the front side. You take the necessary on-scene assessment and care steps and are on the way to the hospital in the ambulance. How do you describe your patient's injuries over the radio to the hospital staff?

Street Scenes

"Respond to Elm Street near the intersection on Central Avenue for a report of a motor-vehicle crash. Third-party call from a passerby on a cell phone. The time is now 1505 hours." Your response time is relatively fast, and you arrive before the dispatcher can provide any additional information. As you approach the scene, you see that two vehicles are involved in the crash. It appears the truck rear-ended the four-door sedan. A police officer on-scene has already taken charge of traffic control. You ask him, "How many patients?" He replies, "Three." You find an open area to place the ambulance. Once assured that the scene is safe, you begin your assessment.

The driver of the truck is walking around the scene. The other vehicle had two occupants—a mother and her son, who was belted in the back seat. The mother is tending to the child, who appears to be unresponsive. It doesn't look as if the impact speed was great, but the child hit his head fairly hard on the arm rest and you can still see the dent. An Emergency Medical Response unit is also on-scene and they tell you they will check on the driver of the truck. You turn your attention to the child.

The mother tells you she is fine. "Just take care of Peter. He's only 6 years old." You get into the vehicle next to the child and hear that he has snoring respirations. You remember that the tongue is the most likely cause, so you manually stabilize the head and neck to prevent any further injury to his head and cervical spine. As you do so, you push Peter's jaw forward to move the tongue in the direction of the mandible. It works, and the snoring sound stops. Your partner prepares for extrication to the backboard.

Street Scene Questions

1. As you assess your young patient, how does his anatomy impact on the process?
2. What should you be alert to when examining the child's abdomen?

Before rotating Peter onto the backboard, you apply a cervical collar. Then you rotate him onto the board. Remembering that a child's head is larger in proportion to the rest of the body than an adult's, you place a folded towel under Peter's shoulders in order to keep his head in a neutral position with the airway open. Your partner calls out to Peter to see if his mental status has changed. Peter responds to painful stimuli only.

Once Peter has been moved into the ambulance, you perform a head-to-toe exam. When you get to the abdomen, you palpate all four quadrants and observe a bruise, probably caused by the lap portion of the seat belt. Peter reacts as if in pain when you touch the left upper quadrant, and you think that his spleen may have been injured.

En route to the hospital, you find the patient is breathing at a rate of 32 and has a pulse of 150. You call out to Peter, and this time he responds to your voice.

Street Scene Questions

3. What are the significant findings based on the assessment and your knowledge of the human body?
4. Do you have any concerns about additional injuries to this patient? If so, what are they?

You take another set of vital signs and find that Peter has an increase in pulse and respiration rates. You perform a reassessment and find there is still pain in the upper left quadrant of the abdomen. As you run your hands over the patient's back, you are concerned by his apparent pain in the lumbar region of the spine, which may have been caused by the force of the crash.

Your partner tells you the ETA to the hospital is 10 minutes and notifies emergency department personnel by radio. The transmission gives an overview of the injuries and the vital signs, noting the change in the last 10 minutes. He mentions how the patient's mental status has changed and describes the abdominal and lumbar pain and location.

When the patient is being wheeled into the trauma room, the staff do a quick assessment and check the abdomen. The emergency department physician tells you that because of assessment findings given in the radio report, she has a surgeon on the way to check Peter.

"Good job!" she adds.

Principles of Pathophysiology

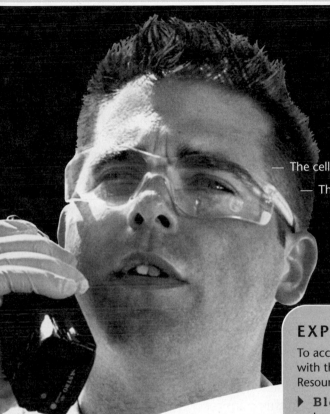

STANDARD ⊙------
Pathophysiology

COMPETENCY ⊙------
Uses fundamental knowledge of the pathophysiology of respiration
and perfusion to patient assessment and management.

CORE CONCEPTS ⊙------
— The cell, cellular metabolism, and results of the alteration of cellular metabolism
— The respiratory system and the importance of oxygenation and ventilation
— The cardiovascular system and the movement of blood
— The principles of perfusion, hypoperfusion, and shock
— Disrupted physiology of major body systems

EXPLORE Resource**Central**

To access Resource Central, follow directions on the Student Access Card provided
with this text. If there is no card, go to **www.bradybooks.com** and follow the
Resource Central link to Buy Access from there. Under Media Resources, you will find:

▶ **Blood Composition**
Learn about the blood's components, the functions of each component and
identify some disorders associated with the blood. It'll have you seeing red!

▶ **Cellular Structures and Respiration**
View an animation of the cell and learn about its main components and the
purpose of the cell membrane.

▶ **Frank Starling's Law and Heart Failure**
Read about and watch an animation on Starling's Law. Discuss the body's
response when the heart is unable to meet the demands of the body.

OBJECTIVES

After reading this chapter you should be able to:

6.1 Define key terms introduced in this chapter.

6.2 Describe the basic roles and structures of body
cells. (pp. 136–137)

6.3 Describe the roles of water, glucose, and oxygen in
the cell. (pp. 137–138)

6.4 Describe conditions that can threaten
cardiopulmonary function. (pp. 142–147)

6.5 Explain how impaired cardiopulmonary function
affects the body. (pp. 147–148)

6.6 Discuss the mechanisms the body uses to
compensate for impaired cardiopulmonary
function. (pp. 148–149)

6.7 Explain the pathophysiology of shock. (p. 148)

6.8 Identify signs and symptoms that indicate the
body is attempting to compensate for impaired
cardiopulmonary function. (pp. 148–149)

6.9 Describe ways in which the body's fluid balance
can become disrupted. (pp. 149–150)

(continued)

6.10 Recognize indications that the body's fluid balance has been disrupted. (pp. 149–150)

6.11 Describe ways in which the nervous system may be impaired. (p. 151)

6.12 Recognize indications that the nervous system may be impaired. (p. 151)

6.13 Describe the effects on the body of:
  a. Endocrine dysfunction (pp. 151–152)
  b. Digestive system dysfunction (p. 152)
  c. Immune system dysfunction (p. 153)

KEY TERMS

aerobic metabolism, *p. 137*
anaerobic metabolism, *p. 138*
cardiac output, *p. 147*
chemoreceptors, *p. 143*
dead air space, *p. 142*
dehydration, *p. 149*

edema, *p. 150*
electrolyte, *p. 137*
FiO₂, *p. 138*
hydrostatic pressure, *p. 143*
hypersensitivity, *p. 153*
hypoperfusion, *p. 148*

minute volume, *p. 142*
pathophysiology, *p. 137*
perfusion, *p. 148*
plasma oncotic pressure, *p. 143*
shock, *p. 148*

stretch receptors, *p. 145*
stroke volume, *p. 146*
systemic vascular resistance (SVR), *p. 146*
tidal volume, *p. 142*
V/Q match, *p. 148*

The body is an amazing system. Its capacity to adapt to and overcome challenges seems limitless. As an EMT, it is very useful to understand how common illnesses and injury affect the body and, more important, how the body will react to and compensate for these insults.

Pathophysiology is the study of how disease processes affect the function of the body. In Chapter 5, "Medical Terminology and Anatomy and Physiology," you learned about how the body systems work under normal circumstances. In this chapter, we will discuss what happens to those systems when disease and outside forces interfere with normal function. Understanding pathophysiology will help you recognize the changes your patient is going through as a result of illness or injury. It will also help you understand how to best counteract those changes to improve the outcome of your patient.

> **NOTE:** *Throughout this chapter, we attempt to simplify topics that are just not simple. Also, we don't attempt to cover every aspect of human pathophysiology. It would be impossible and beyond the scope of the EMT to cover all the topics pertaining to pathophysiology in this short chapter. Instead, we focus narrowly on the cardiopulmonary system.*

Maintaining professionalism requires the EMT to undergo constant self-improvement. There are many available informative resources and courses on pathophysiology. Learning more will only make you a better provider.

THE CELL

CORE CONCEPT

The cell, cellular metabolism, and results of the alteration of cellular metabolism

A normal cell incorporates a series of structures that are designed to accomplish specific functions. Common cell structures include the *nucleus*, the *endoplasmic reticulum*, and the *mitochondria*. The cell nucleus, for example, contains DNA, the genetic blueprint for reproduction. The structures within a cell are covered by a *cell membrane* that protects and selectively allows water and other substances into and out of the cell (Figure 6-1).

Although some types of cells, like cardiac muscle cells, are specialized to serve specific purposes, some important components and functions are common to most cells. The endoplasmic reticulum, for example, plays a key role in synthesizing proteins. The mitochondria

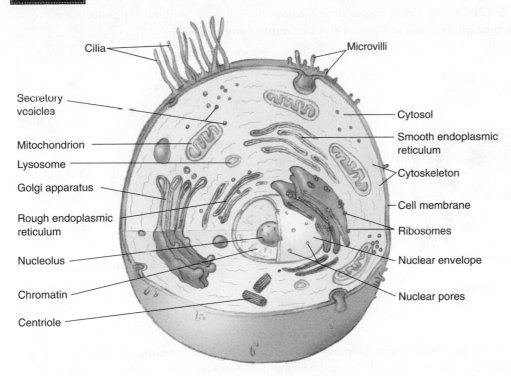

FIGURE 6-1 The cell.

Cilia
Microvilli
Secretory vesicles
Cytosol
Mitochondrion
Smooth endoplasmic reticulum
Lysosome
Cytoskeleton
Golgi apparatus
Cell membrane
Rough endoplasmic reticulum
Ribosomes
Nucleolus
Nuclear envelope
Chromatin
Nuclear pores
Centriole

are responsible for converting glucose and other nutrients into energy in the form of *adenosine triphosphate (ATP)*. This is one of the processes known as ***metabolism***. ATP is essentially the cell's internally created fuel and is responsible for powering all the other cellular functions. Without ATP, many of the cell's specialized structures cannot function. For example, without ATP, a specialized mechanism called the *sodium potassium pump* cannot actively move ions back and forth across the cell membrane. This movement of ions is responsible for generating an electrical charge to cause depolarization, which is the stimulus for muscle contraction, including contractions of the heart.

To accomplish these very important functions, cells have some basic requirements, principally water, glucose, and oxygen.

Water and the Cell

A cell needs the correct balance of water between its inside and outside. Without enough water, the cell will dehydrate and die. In contrast, with too much water, basic cellular function will be interrupted. Water also influences the concentrations of important chemicals called ***electrolytes***. Electrolytes are substances that, when dissolved in water, separate into charged particles. The movement of these charged particles enables the electrical functions of cells such as nerve transmission and cardiac muscle depolarization. Levels of water in the body are controlled by the circulatory and renal systems.

Glucose and the Cell

Glucose, a simple sugar converted from the foods we eat, is the basic nutrient of the cell. It is also the building block for energy in the form of ATP. Without glucose, energy is not created and cell function ceases.

Oxygen and the Cell

Healthy metabolism requires oxygen. Oxygen is used by the cell to metabolize glucose into energy. One of the waste products of this metabolism is carbon dioxide. When oxygen enters the cell in the correct quantity, energy is produced in an efficient manner with minimal waste products. When this process (metabolism) takes place in the presence of oxygen, it is called ***aerobic metabolism*** (Figure 6-2A).

pathophysiology
(path-o-fiz-e-OL-o-je)
the study of how disease processes affect the function of the body.

metabolism (meh-TAB-o-lizm)
the cellular function of converting nutrients into energy.

electrolyte (e-LEK-tro-lite)
a substance that, when dissolved in water, separates into charged particles.

aerobic (air-O-bik) ***metabolism***
the cellular process in which oxygen is used to metabolize glucose. Energy is produced in an efficient manner with minimal waste products.

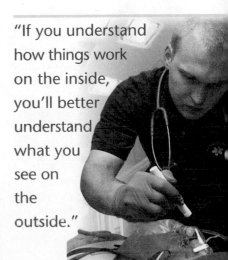

"If you understand how things work on the inside, you'll better understand what you see on the outside."

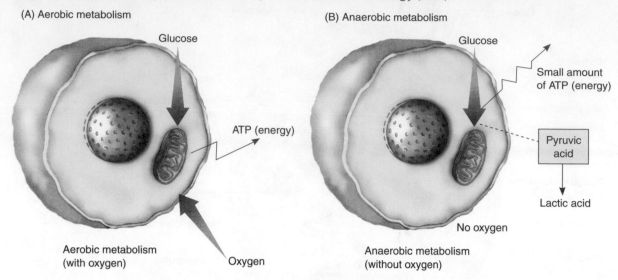

FIGURE 6-2 (A) Aerobic metabolism. Glucose broken down in the presence of oxygen produces a large amount of energy (ATP). (B) Anaerobic metabolism. Glucose broken down without the presence of oxygen produces acidic by-products and only a small amount of energy (ATP).

When glucose is metabolized without oxygen, or without enough oxygen, energy is produced inefficiently and with a great deal more waste. In addition to carbon dioxide, lactic acid is produced. When this process (metabolism) takes place without oxygen, it is called ***anaerobic metabolism***, a form of energy conversion that is not healthy for the body (Figure 6-2B). The waste products of anaerobic metabolism make the body more acidic than normal, and this acidity impacts many systems negatively.

Oxygenation of the cells and the removal of the waste products of metabolism are among the responsibilities of the respiratory system.

The cell membrane is also a vulnerable element of the cell. Many disease processes alter its *permeability*, or its ability to effectively transfer fluids, electrolytes, and other substances in and out. An ineffective cell membrane can allow substances into the cell that should not be there (like toxins) and interfere with the regulation of water.

Thus far we have been discussing the structure and function of one cell. Remember, however, that many cells working together to form organ systems, and just as a single cell's function can be disturbed by illness or injury, so can the function of an entire organ system.

THE CARDIOPULMONARY SYSTEM

Air goes in, air goes out, and blood goes round and round. This is an old saying in EMS, referring to the proper function of the lungs and heart. It is an oversimplification of a complicated process, but it sums up the importance of some of the body's most basic functions.

We previously noted that cells need oxygen for the efficient production of energy. As humans, we obtain oxygen from the air we breathe. Typically, inhaled air contains mostly nitrogen (79 percent) but also oxygen (21 percent). The concentration of oxygen in the air we breathe in is referred to as the fraction of inspired oxygen, or ***FiO_2***. We use our lungs to bring that oxygen into our bodies and our blood to distribute it to the cells. Our blood also picks up waste carbon dioxide from the cells and transports it back to the lungs, where it can be breathed out.

The term *cardiopulmonary system* refers to the combination of the respiratory and cardiovascular systems. (See *Visual Guide: Ventilation, Respiration, and Perfusion.*) The lungs (pulmonary system), heart, blood vessels, and the blood itself (cardiovascular system) work in concert to perform cardiopulmonary functions. The primary function of the cardiopulmonary system is to deliver oxygen and nutrients to the cells and to remove waste products from the cells. These basic operations rely on the coordinated movements of blood and air. Interruption of any part of this balance results in a compromise to, or even a failure of, the system.

FIGURE 6-3 The bronchial tree. Each mainstem bronchus enters a lung and then branches into smaller and smaller bronchi, ending in the smallest bronchioles.

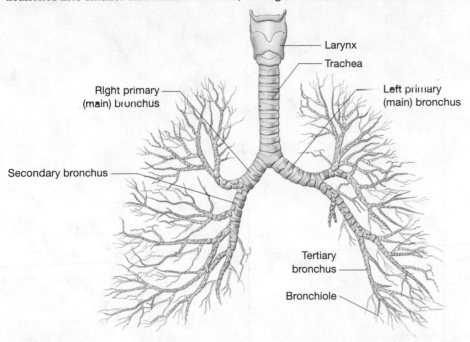

Larynx

Trachea

Right primary (main) bronchus

Left primary (main) bronchus

Secondary bronchus

Tertiary bronchus

Bronchiole

The Airway

The respiratory system begins at the airway. The airway is made up of the structures from the mouth and nose to the alveoli of the lungs. Air follows a path from the openings of the mouth and nose into the pharynx and/or nasopharynx, travels to the rear of the throat (or hypopharynx), then enters the larynx, below which the trachea begins. Air travels down the trachea to the point where it branches into two large tubes called the mainstem bronchi, one leading to each lung. Air follows the paths of the bronchi as they subdivide and subdivide again (like branches of a tree) (Figure 6-3) until they reach their endpoints at the multitude of tiny air pockets in the lungs called alveoli (Figure 6-4A). The alveoli are where the exchange of oxygen and carbon dioxide with the blood takes place (Figure 6-4B).

FIGURE 6-4 (A) Each bronchiole terminates in a tiny air pocket called an alveolar sac. (B) The alveoli are encased by networks of capillaries; oxygen and carbon dioxide are exchanged between the air in the alveoli and the blood in the capillaries.

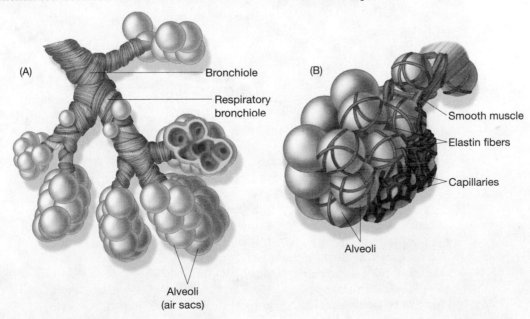

(A)

Bronchiole

Respiratory bronchiole

(B)

Smooth muscle

Elastin fibers

Capillaries

Alveoli

Alveoli (air sacs)

CHAPTER 6
Ventilation, Respiration, and Perfusion

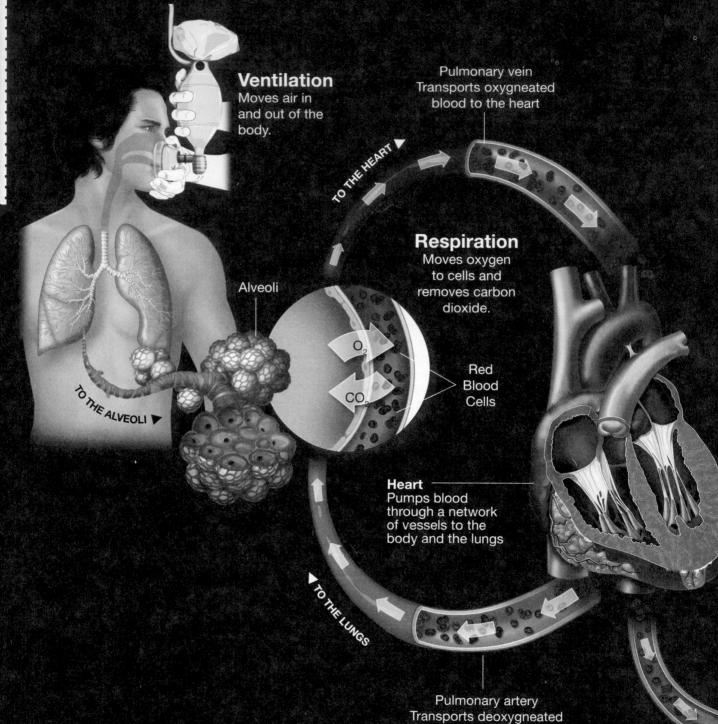

Ventilation
Moves air in and out of the body.

Pulmonary vein
Transports oxygneated blood to the heart

TO THE HEART ▶

Alveoli

Respiration
Moves oxygen to cells and removes carbon dioxide.

O_2

CO_2

Red Blood Cells

TO THE ALVEOLI ▶

Heart
Pumps blood through a network of vessels to the body and the lungs

▶ TO THE LUNGS

Pulmonary artery
Transports deoxygneated blood to the lungs

The ultimate goal of emergency care is to move air into the body so that all cells are perfused with oxygen.

Cells die when they don't receive oxygen. People die when too many cells die.

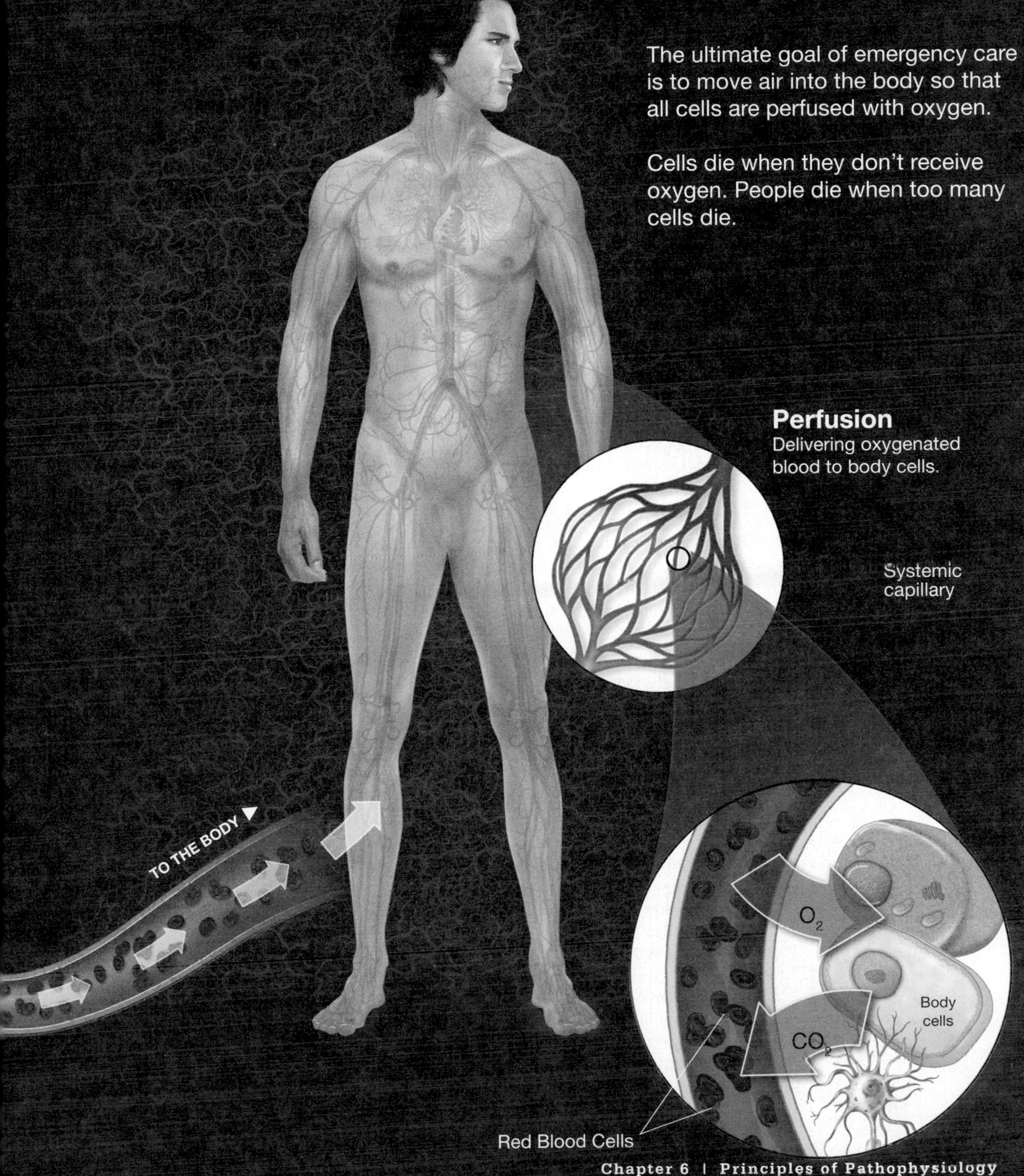

Perfusion
Delivering oxygenated blood to body cells.

Systemic capillary

TO THE BODY ▶

O_2

CO_2

Body cells

Red Blood Cells

Moving air in and out of the chest requires an open pathway. In EMS, we refer to this open pathway as a **patent** airway. Although a healthy person with a normal mental status should have no problem keeping his airway open, there are a number of potential airway challenges that occur with disease and trauma.

Upper airway (above the trachea) obstructions are common. These obstructions can be caused by foreign bodies (as in a person choking), by infection (such as a child with croup), or even by trauma or burns causing the soft tissue of the larynx to swell. Any of these obstructions can seriously and significantly inhibit the flow of air and interrupt the process of moving oxygen in and carbon dioxide out.

The Lungs

The lungs are part of the lower airway (below the opening of the trachea). The lungs, together with the diaphragm and the muscles of the chest wall, change their internal pressures to pull air in or push air out. The volume of air moved in one in-and-out cycle of breathing is called the **tidal volume**. We multiply tidal volume by the respiratory rate to obtain **minute volume**, the amount of air that gets into and out of the lungs in 1 minute. Obviously, minute volume can be affected by changes in either tidal volume or rate (or both). Here are two examples of how minute volume can be impacted by very different mechanisms:

- A 25-year-old male has a normal minute volume of 5,000 mL. (Tidal volume of 500 mL × 10 breaths per minute). He overdoses on heroin. Because heroin is a narcotic, it interferes with the respiratory center in his brain, and his breathing rate slows to 4 breaths per minute. He is breathing the same tidal volume as he was before, but because his rate has become so slow, his minute volume has significantly decreased. (Tidal volume of 500 mL × 4 breaths per minute = 2,000 mL minute volume.)

- A 30-year-old woman has a normal minute volume of 6,000 mL (tidal volume of 500 mL × 12 breaths per minute). She has an asthma attack and, as the attack grows more severe, her tidal volume decreases to 250 mL. Even though her breathing rate has not changed, she is taking in less air with each breath, so her minute volume has significantly decreased. (Tidal volume of 250 mL × 12 breaths per minute = 3,000 mL minute volume.)

Remember also that not all of the minute volume of air reaches the alveoli. About 150 mL of a normal tidal volume occupies the space between the mouth and alveoli but does not actually reach the area of gas exchange. We refer to this as **dead air space**. *Alveolar ventilation* occurs only with the air that reaches the alveoli.

Respiratory Dysfunction

Specific lung diseases and dysfunctions will be discussed later, in Chapter 19, "Respiratory Emergencies." However, in general, a respiratory dysfunction occurs any time minute volume is interfered with.

Disruption of Respiratory Control   A section of the brain called the medulla oblongata is the seat of respiratory control. From time to time, disorders that affect this portion of the brain can interfere with respiratory function. Medical events like stroke and infection can disrupt the medulla's function and alter the control of effective breathing. Toxins and drugs like narcotics can also affect the medulla's capabilities and adversely impact minute volume. Brain trauma and intracranial pressure can physically harm the medulla and disrupt its function. Even with an intact brain, messages must make their way to the muscles of respiration. Spinal cord injuries and other neurologic disorders can interrupt these transmissions.

Disruption of Pressure   The thorax is essentially a vault. The large muscle called the diaphragm forms its lower boundary just below the rib cage. The lungs are encased by the chest walls, where ribs are separated by intercostal muscles that contract and relax to create the motion of breathing. The lungs are in direct contact with the inner walls of the chest. Although they are in contact, there is a slight space between the lung tissue and chest wall called the pleural space. There is typically a small amount of fluid in this space between the lung and chest wall. This fluid both lubricates the space to reduce the friction of movement and helps the lung to adhere to the inside of the chest wall. However, this area between the lung and the chest wall is also a potential space where blood and air may accumulate.

Ventilation is activated by changing pressures within this vault. Inhalation is an *active* process. To inhale, the diaphragm contracts, the muscles of the chest expand, and a negative pressure is created in the lungs. This negative pressure pulls air in through the trachea. By contrast, exhalation is a *passive* process. To exhale, those same muscles relax to make the chest contract, creating a positive pressure that pushes air out. These changing pressures rely on an intact chest compartment. If a hole is created in the chest wall and air is allowed to escape or be drawn in, the pressures necessary for breathing can be disrupted and minute volume impaired. Furthermore, if bleeding develops within the chest, blood can accumulate in the pleural space and force the lung to collapse away from the chest wall. This can also occur if a hole in either the lung or the chest wall (or both) allows air to accumulate between the lung and the chest wall.

Disruption of Lung Tissue Besides changing the actual amount of air moved per minute, lung function can also be interfered with by disrupting the lung tissue itself. Obviously, trauma is the chief culprit. When lung tissue is displaced or destroyed by mechanical force, it cannot exchange gas. Keep in mind, however, that medical problems can also disrupt lung tissue. For example, medical problems such as congestive heart failure and sepsis change the ability of the alveoli to transfer gases across their membranes. Diffusion of gas is altered, and when this happens, the blood in the alveolar capillaries can neither receive oxygen nor off-load carbon dioxide normally or at all.

The net result of any of these challenges is low oxygen (hypoxia) and high carbon dioxide (hypercapnia) within the body. The more the challenge interferes with the movement of air, the more significant the disruption in oxygenation and ventilation.

Respiratory Compensation

When the respiratory system is affected by any of the challenges we have already discussed, the body attempts to compensate for the gas exchange deficits. Specific sensors in the brain and vascular system register low oxygen levels and high carbon dioxide levels. These ***chemoreceptors*** send messages to the brain that assistance is required. Normally, respiration or the need to breathe is triggered in the brain by changing carbon dioxide levels. When carbon dioxide levels are increased, the brain stimulates the respiratory system to take a breath. In a similar fashion, when the respiratory system is challenged, chemoreceptors sense changing gas levels and send messages to the brain. The brain then stimulates the respiratory system to increase rate and/or tidal volume. From a patient assessment standpoint, the most obvious sign of these changes is an evident increase in respiratory rate.

The respiratory system moves air in and out, but to *perfuse* cells the air that is breathed in must be matched up with blood. The cardiovascular system moves blood that has been oxygenated as it passes by the alveoli to the cells to provide the second half of the cardiopulmonary equation.

chemoreceptors
(ke-mo-re-cept-erz)
chemical sensors in the brain and blood vessels that identify changing levels of oxygen and carbon dioxide.

The Blood

Blood is the vehicle by which oxygen and carbon dioxide are transported. The liquid portion of blood is called plasma. Other components include red blood cells that contain oxygen-carrying hemoglobin, white blood cells that fight infection, and platelets that form clots (Figure 6-5). Blood transports oxygen by binding it to the hemoglobin in red blood cells and, to a lesser extent, by dissolving it into the *plasma*. Carbon dioxide is also dissolved into the plasma.

Blood plasma contains large proteins, which tend to attract water away from the area around body cells and pull it into the bloodstream. This force is called ***plasma oncotic pressure***. It is counterbalanced by the pressure created inside the vessels when the heart beats. This pressure tends to push fluid back out of the blood vessels toward the cells and is called ***hydrostatic pressure***.

The balance between the pulling-in force of plasma oncotic pressure and the pushing-out force of hydrostatic pressure is critical to regulating both blood pressure and cell hydration. A loss or disruption of either of these pressures can be devastating. For example, albumin, one of the large proteins in plasma, is created in the liver. Liver-failure patients often do not produce enough albumin. Without the pulling-in force of albumin, water freely leaves the bloodstream and accumulates around the body cells, leading to dehydration of the blood and massive edema (swelling) in the patient.

CORE CONCEPT ●--------

The cardiovascular system and the movement of blood

plasma oncotic (PLAZ-ma on-KOT-ik) *pressure*
the pull exerted by large proteins in the plasma portion of blood that tends to pull water from the body into the bloodstream.

hydrostatic (HI-dro-STAT ik) *pressure*
the pressure within a blood vessel that tends to push water out of the vessel.

FIGURE 6-5 Blood components.

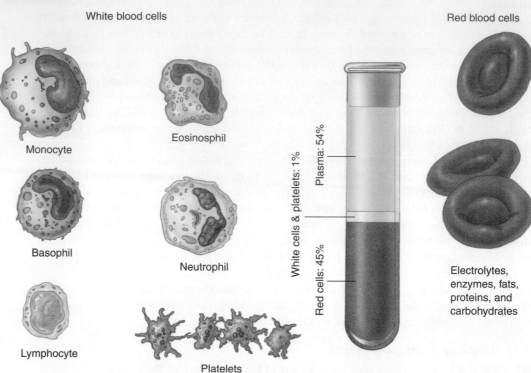

White blood cells

Monocyte

Eosinosphil

Basophil

Neutrophil

Lymphocyte

Platelets

Plasma: 54%

White cells & platelets: 1%

Red cells: 45%

Red blood cells

Electrolytes, enzymes, fats, proteins, and carbohydrates

Blood Dysfunction

The most common blood dysfunctions relate to volume. You simply have to have enough blood to accomplish the goals of moving oxygen and carbon dioxide. Bleeding obviously defeats this goal, as does dehydration.

Other blood dysfunctions are caused by conditions that affect the components of the blood. Certain types of anemia decrease the number of red blood cells, which decreases the blood's ability to carry oxygen. Other conditions (like liver failure) affect water-retaining proteins in the blood (such as albumin), causing a decrease in volume.

The Blood Vessels

Blood is distributed throughout the body, then returned to the heart, by a network of blood vessels. Arteries, veins, and capillaries form this network (Figure 6-6). Arteries carry blood away from the heart. Artery walls are composed of layers, and arteries can change diameter by contracting their middle layer of smooth muscle. Veins carry blood back to the heart and also can change diameter with a layer of smooth muscle. Arteries carry oxygenated blood while veins carry deoxygenated blood. The only exceptions to this rule are the pulmonary arteries (they carry deoxygenated blood from the heart to the lungs) and the pulmonary veins (they carry oxygenated blood from the lungs to the heart).

As blood leaves the heart, it travels through arteries, whose diameter decreases as they approach the cellular level, eventually reaching the smallest arteries, known as arterioles. Arterioles then feed the *oxygenated* blood into tiny vessels called capillaries. Capillaries have thin walls, like cell membranes, that allow for movement of substances into and out of the bloodstream. Through these thin capillary walls oxygen is off-loaded and carbon dioxide is picked up from the cells of the body. Capillaries then connect to the smallest veins, called venules. Venules turn into veins as they grow larger, and veins transport blood back to the heart.

A similar process takes place in the lungs, but it is reversed from the process that happened at the level of the body cells. *Deoxygenated* blood that has been returned to the right side of the heart is pumped to the lungs via the pulmonary arteries and arterioles. The pulmonary arterioles connect with pulmonary capillaries that surround the alveoli, the tiny air pockets in the lungs. Carbon dioxide is off-loaded from the capillaries across the alveolar

FIGURE 6-6 The network of arteries, veins, and capillaries.

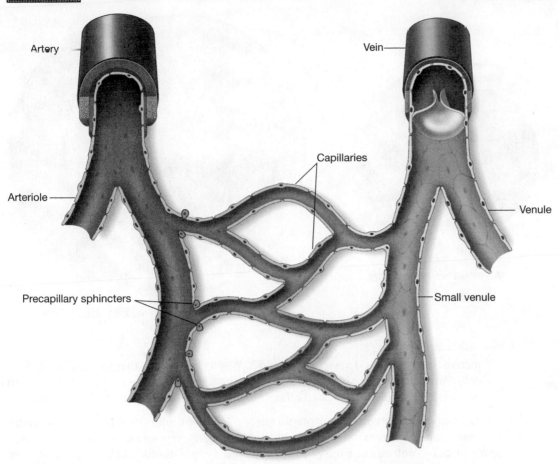

Artery

Vein

Capillaries

Arteriole

Venule

Precapillary sphincters

Small venule

membrane to the alveoli to be exhaled from the lungs. Oxygen is transferred from the air in the alveoli across the alveolar membrane and into the surrounding capillaries. The newly oxygenated blood then continues on its way from the pulmonary capillaries to the pulmonary venules and into the pulmonary veins. The pulmonary veins return the oxygenated blood to the left side of the heart, which pumps it out to the body.

The movement of blood through the blood vessels depends on pressure in the system. For the leading blood molecule to get where it is going, it must have other molecules behind it, pushing it along (normal pressure). If the molecules are too spread out, there is no push on that leading molecule, and it does not move (low pressure). We will discuss the heart's role in creating the needed pressure later in the chapter, but one factor besides the heart that helps determine pressure within a blood vessel is its size or, more specifically, the vessel's diameter.

We noted earlier that most vessels can change their diameter by using a layer of smooth muscle in the vessel wall. Depending on the circumstances, vessels will frequently change size to adjust for changes in pressure. In fact, certain blood vessels contain specialized sensors called ***stretch receptors*** that detect the level of internal pressure and transmit messages to the nervous system, which then triggers the smooth muscle in the vessel walls to make any needed size adjustments. Pressure may need to be adjusted for a variety of reasons, including loss of volume (blood) in the system or too much volume in the system. For example:

stretch receptors
sensors in blood vessels that identify internal pressure.

- An 18-year-old patient lacerates his femoral artery and is bleeding severely. The volume of blood in his blood vessels is significantly decreased. As a result, the pressure in the system decreases and the existing blood has a difficult time moving. Stretch receptors in his aorta sense the falling pressures. Messages are transmitted to the central nervous system and the blood vessels are stimulated to contract. Because this decreases the container size, the pressure within the system normalizes (for now).

- A 30-year-old woman experiences a spike in blood pressure after a frightening near-collision on the highway as her sympathetic nervous system causes her heart rate to

FIGURE 6-7 Dilated blood vessel.

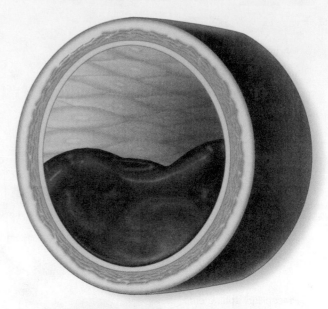

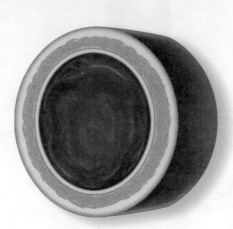

(A) Normal vessel

(B) Dilated vessel with reduced blood volume

FIGURE 6-8 Increased permeability allows too much fluid to escape through capillary walls.

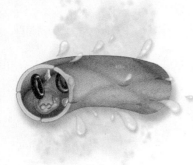

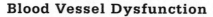

Permeable capillaries

systemic vascular resistance (SVR)

the pressure in the peripheral blood vessels that the heart must overcome in order to pump blood into the system.

increase and her blood vessels to constrict. When she realizes that she has averted the collision and everything is all right, her parasympathetic nervous system causes her heart rate to slow and blood vessels to relax, bringing her blood pressure back to normal.

The autonomic nervous system plays a major role in controlling vessel diameter. In particular, the sympathetic nervous system in its "fight-or-flight" response stimulates blood vessels to constrict. By contrast, the parasympathetic nervous system stimulates blood vessels to relax.

Blood Vessel Dysfunction

Loss of Tone   A major problem with blood vessels occurs with their inability to control their diameter. If blood vessels are unable to constrict when necessary or, worse, if they are forced into an uncontrolled dilatation, internal pressure can seriously drop (Figure 6-7). Many conditions can cause this loss of tone. Injuries to the brain and spinal cord can cause uncontrolled dilation of the blood vessels (vasodilation). Systemic infections (sepsis) can also cause vessel dilation. Severe allergic reactions also can cause similar problems.

Permeability   Certain conditions cause capillaries to become overly permeable, or "leaky," allowing too much fluid to flow out through their walls (Figure 6-8). Sepsis and certain diseases can frequently cause increases in capillary permeability.

Hypertension   The pressure inside the vessels that the heart has to pump against is called ***systemic vascular resistance (SVR)***. Normally, this pressure is an important factor in moving blood. However, in some patients, the pressure is abnormally increased. Chronic smoking, certain drugs, and even genetics can cause an abnormal constriction of the peripheral blood vessels and, therefore, an unhealthy high pressure level. This increased pressure can be a major risk factor in heart disease and stroke.

The Heart

The heart is the key to cardiovascular function. The movement of blood and the resulting transportation of oxygen and carbon dioxide depend on the heart working properly.

At its most basic level, the heart is a pump. Its job is very straightforward: to move blood. To do this, it mechanically contracts and ejects blood. The volume of blood ejected in one squeeze is known as the ***stroke volume***. An average person ejects roughly 60 mL of blood per contraction. Stroke volume depends on a series of factors:

stroke volume

the amount of blood ejected from the heart in one contraction.

- *Preload* is how much blood is returned to the heart prior to the contraction; in other words, how much it is filled. The greater the filling of the heart, the greater the stroke volume.

- *Contractility* is the force of contraction; that is, how hard the heart squeezes. The more forceful the muscle squeezes, the greater the stroke volume.
- *Afterload* is a function of systemic vascular resistance. It is how much pressure the heart has to pump against in order to force blood out into the system. The greater the pressure in the system, the lower the stroke volume.

When we discussed the lungs we determined the *minute volume* by multiplying the tidal volume (amount of air breathed in per respiration) by the respiratory rate (number of respirations in 1 minute). *Cardiac output*, like minute volume, is a per-minute measurement and is calculated in a similar fashion. Cardiac output is determined by examining the stroke volume (amount of blood ejected in one beat) and the heart rate (number of beats in 1 minute). In other words, to calculate cardiac output, you would multiply the stroke volume by the heart rate.

cardiac output
the amount of blood ejected from the heart in 1 minute (heart rate × stroke volume).

Just like minute volume, cardiac output can be affected by changes to either part of the equation. Either slowing the heart rate or decreasing the stroke volume will decrease cardiac output. Cardiac output can also be impacted by heart rates that are too fast. Although increasing heart rate would normally increase cardiac output, very fast rates (usually >180 in adults) limit the filling of the heart and in fact *decrease* stroke volume. Some examples of impaired cardiac output include:

- A 46-year-old woman has a tachycardia (rapid heartbeat) at a rate of 220. Her cardiac output has dropped, even though she has increased her rate. As a result of the tachycardia, her ventricles have little time to fill and her stroke volume has decreased.
- An 82-year-old woman has a bradycardia (slow heartbeat) at a rate of 38. Her heart rate has decreased and, because of this, so has her cardiac output.
- A 25-year-old male has been stabbed in the abdomen. Because he has severe internal bleeding, not as much blood is returning to the heart, and therefore stroke volume is decreased. Cardiac output has decreased as a result.
- A 90-year-old male is having his fourth heart attack. In this case, the muscle wall of the left ventricle is no longer working. Because his heart is having difficulty squeezing out blood, his cardiac output has dropped.

The autonomic nervous system also plays a large role in adjusting cardiac output. The sympathetic nervous system's "fight-or-flight" response increases heart rate and the strength of heart muscle contraction. The parasympathetic nervous system slows the heart down and decreases contractility.

On an ongoing basis, it is the heart that creates the pressure in the cardiovascular system. Without its pumping force, blood does not move.

Heart Dysfunction

Heart dysfunctions can be either mechanical or electrical. That is, they can be a result of a structural/muscle problem or the result of a problem with the electrical stimulation of that muscle.

Mechanical problems include physical trauma (like bullet holes and stab wounds), squeezing forces (like when the heart is compressed by bleeding inside its protective pericardial sac), or loss of cardiac muscle function from cell death (as in a heart attack).

Electrical problems typically occur from diseases such as heart attacks or heart failure that damage the electrical system of the heart. These cardiac electrical problems include unorganized rhythms, such as ventricular fibrillation, and rate problems, such as bradycardias and tachycardias. In infants and children, bradycardia is often the result of acute hypoxia from inadequate ventilation rather than from a primary cardiac cause.

(For more information on cardiac dysfunctions see Chapter 20, "Cardiac Emergencies.")

The Cardiopulmonary System: Putting It All Together

Air goes in, air goes out, and blood goes round and round. Now that you have had an opportunity to explore what really happens in the cardiopulmonary system, you may see just how important that old saying is to understanding the big picture. (Review *Visual Guide: Ventilation, Respiration, and Perfusion.*) See the following discussion of the term *perfusion* and the discussion in the following section on shock.

V/Q match

ventilation/perfusion match. This implies that the alveoli are supplied with enough air and that the air in the aveoli is matched with sufficient blood in the pulmonary capillaries to permit optimum exchange of oxygen and carbon dioxide.

perfusion (pur-FEW-zhun)

the supply of oxygen to, and removal of wastes from, the cells and tissues of the body as a result of the flow of blood through the capillaries.

hypoperfusion

(HI-po-per-FEW-zhun) inability of the body to adequately circulate blood to the body's cells to supply them with oxygen and nutrients. Also called *shock*.

shock

the inability of the body to adequately circulate blood to the body's cells to supply them with oxygen and nutrients. Also called *hypoperfusion*. A life-threatening condition.

● CORE CONCEPT

The principles of perfusion, hypoperfusion, and shock

For the system to do its job, all of the components must be doing theirs. In the respiratory system, air movement must bring oxygen all the way to the alveoli and move carbon dioxide back all the way out; there must be a significant quantity of air moving, and the alveoli must be capable of exchanging gas. In the cardiovascular system, there must be enough blood; the heart must adequately pump the blood, and there must be enough pressure in the system to provide perfusion throughout the body—that is, to move the blood between the alveoli and the body cells and between the body cells and the alveoli. Furthermore, the blood must be capable of carrying oxygen and carbon dioxide.

When all these functions are in place we have what is called a ventilation/perfusion match, otherwise known as a *V/Q match*. What this implies is that the alveoli have sufficient air and that air is matched up with sufficient blood in the pulmonary capillaries. V/Q matching is rarely perfect. In fact, even in healthy lungs a force as simple as gravity can mean that alveoli in the upper areas of the lungs may not be matched with as much blood as alveoli in the lower areas. As a result, we often express the V/Q match as a ratio rather than a true match.

The V/Q ratio can be disrupted by any challenge that interferes with any element of the cardiopulmonary system. Minute volume problems, cardiac output problems, and structural damage to the lungs all can disrupt the match between air and blood.

Shock

Shock will be discussed in greater detail in Chapter 27, "Bleeding and Shock," but it is worth noting that shock occurs when a V/Q mismatch happens. As we noted previously, all cells require regular delivery of oxygen and nutrients and removal of waste products. This is a function of a regular supply of blood and is referred to as *perfusion*. Shock occurs when perfusion is inadequate. Inadequate perfusion is referred to as *hypoperfusion*, which is considered to be a synonym for *shock*. In other words, shock occurs when the regular delivery of oxygen and nutrients to cells and the removal of their waste products is interrupted. Without a regular supply of oxygen, cells become hypoxic and must rely on anaerobic metabolism. When this type of metabolism occurs, lactic acid and other waste products accumulate and harm the cells. Without the removal of carbon dioxide, the buildup of harmful waste products is accelerated. Unless it is reversed, shock will kill cells, organs, and eventually the patient.

PATHOPHYSIOLOGY OF OTHER SYSTEMS

Fluid Balance

● CORE CONCEPT

Disrupted physiology of major body systems

About 60 percent of the body is made up of water, and without this fluid the functions of the cells would cease. Water is distributed throughout the body, both inside and outside the cells, and balancing this distribution is an important part of maintaining normal cellular function.

Inside/Outside

RECOGNIZING COMPENSATION

When a V/Q mismatch occurs, the body compensates in predictable ways. Commonly, the autonomic nervous system engages the "fight-or-flight" mechanism of its sympathetic arm. This causes blood vessels to constrict and the heart to beat faster and stronger. The sympathetic nervous response also causes pupils to dilate and the skin to sweat. Chemoreceptors in the brain and blood vessels sense increasing carbon dioxide and hypoxia and stimulate the respiratory system to breathe faster and deeper.

The signs and symptoms of these changes are often readily apparent. Look for increased pulse and respirations. You may note delayed capillary refill and pale skin. Pupils may be dilated and the patient may be sweaty even in cool environments.

Although you may not know exactly what the nature of the V/Q mismatch is, recognizing these common signs of compensation will help you identify that the mismatch exists. Each of these signs should serve as a red flag when you assess your patient. Learn to recognize the signs of compensation as a warning that the body is dealing with a challenge. Consider that these findings point out that something important and dangerous may be taking place.

CRITICAL DECISION MAKING

Why Is Her Heart Beating Rapidly?

You and your partner respond to a 10-year-old female who has crashed her bicycle. When you arrive, her mother is with the child and says, "Everything is fine. She's just a little upset." The child is crying but is able to tell you she fell off her bike and "hurt her belly on the handle bars." Mom allows you to examine the child. She is awake and alert. She is crying, so she seems to be moving air and breathing without any problems. Her radial pulse is present, but you note it to be 128. You double check your pediatric vital sign chart and find that the rate is faster than it should be for her age group.

In your head, you are facing an important question. Why is her heart beating rapidly? The easy answer is that the rate is caused by her crying and emotional response to the situation. This may very well be the correct answer. However, you also must consider that she has a mechanism of injury—that is, a force that you would expect to cause injury (striking the handlebars)—and she has pain as a result of that force. You recall that a rapid heart rate can be a sign of compensation.

You say to yourself, *"This is a red flag. Could her heart be beating fast because she is bleeding into her belly and going into shock? Maybe I need to err on the side of caution and assume this is the case. After all, if it turns out that she just is upset and I've taken this call too seriously, then the little girl is still OK and no harm has been done. On the other hand, if I treat it like it's nothing and the girl really has internal bleeding. . . ."*

Clues to your assessment come in many forms. Learn to recognize the important ones.

PEDIATRIC NOTE

You will learn in Chapter 35, "Pediatric Emergencies," that children compensate a bit differently than adults. For example, a child will rely more on heart rate and less on increases in contractility to overcome a deficit in cardiac output. Pediatric differences in compensation must be incorporated into your assessment. Always be sure to look out for more subtle signs of shock and compensation in children. For more information on assessing children, see Chapter 35.

Normally, water is divided among three spaces in the body, with the following percentages representing averages (Figure 6-9):

- Intracellular (70 percent)—This is water that is inside the cells.
- Intravascular (5 percent)—This is water that is in the bloodstream.
- Interstitial (25 percent)—This water can be found between cells and blood vessels.

We regulate the levels of water in our body by drinking fluids and making/excreting urine. This allows us to constantly adjust our hydration based on our levels of activity. Inside our bodies, fluid is distributed appropriately through a number of factors:

- The brain and kidneys regulate thirst and elimination of excess fluid.
- The large proteins in our blood plasma pull fluid into the bloodstream.
- The permeability of both cell membranes and the walls of capillaries help determine how much water can be held in and pushed out of cells and blood vessels.

Each of these factors helps us regulate the amount and distribution of fluid. If these factors were to be interfered with, fluid levels and distribution can become problematic.

Disruptions of Fluid Balance

Fluid Loss **Dehydration** is an abnormal decrease in the total amount of water in the body. This may be caused by a decreased fluid intake or a significant loss of fluid from the body by one or more of a variety of means. Remember, however, that maintaining a balance

dehydration (de-hi-DRAY-shun) an abnormally low amount of water in the body.

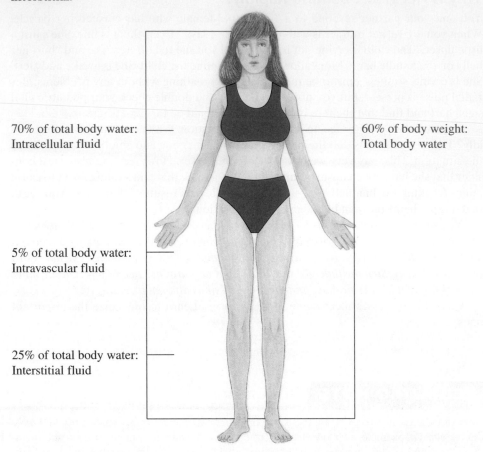

FIGURE 6-9 Water comprises approximately 60 percent of body weight. The water is distributed into three spaces: intracellular, intravascular, and interstitial.

70% of total body water:
Intracellular fluid

60% of body weight:
Total body water

5% of total body water:
Intravascular fluid

25% of total body water:
Interstitial fluid

of water relies on a healthy gastrointestinal system. Severe vomiting or diarrhea can also significantly alter the amount of water in the body. Fluid can be lost, as well, through rapid breathing (as in a respiratory distress patient) and profuse sweating. The plasma portion of blood can be lost with injuries such as burns.

Fluid Distribution   Sometimes the body has enough water but cannot get it to where it needs to go. Certain disease processes interfere with the body's mechanisms of moving fluid. We discussed previously the loss of proteins in blood from liver failure and the changes in capillary membrane permeability that occur with severe infections. In these cases, water migrates out of the bloodstream and cells and into the interstitial space (where it is much less useful). Often this can be seen in the form of edema.

Edema is swelling associated with the movement of water. Edema can be seen best in *dependent* parts of the body; that is, those parts most subject to gravity such as the hands, feet, and legs. Edema can also occur because of an injury (for example, when your thumb swells up after hitting it with a hammer). In this case, the injury has altered the permeability of local capillaries and fluid has shifted. The larger the injury, the more the fluid shifts. Occasionally, fluid can be shifted by changing pressures inside the blood vessels. When pressure is high, the tendency will be to move the fluid portion of the blood out. This can be seen in disorders like acute pulmonary edema.

edema (eh-DEE-muh)
swelling associated with the movement of water into the interstitial space.

The Nervous System

The brain and spinal cord will be discussed in greater detail in Chapter 31, "Trauma to the Head, Neck, and Spine." However, it is important to note here that almost all body functions are regulated by the brain and the spinal cord. The brain is the control center and the spinal cord is the messenger. Trauma or disease to either of these organs can be devastating to body functions.

The brain and spinal cord are well-protected by bone and muscle. Additionally, they are covered by protective layers called meninges. They are further defended by a layer of shock absorbing fluid called cerebrospinal fluid.

Although they are well protected, brain and spinal cord function can be damaged by trauma or disease.

Nervous System Dysfunction

Trauma Despite all their defenses, occasionally the brain and spinal cord are subjected to forces that injure them. Motor-vehicle crashes, falls, and diving accidents all can cause injury to these systems. In the brain, mechanical damage will interrupt the function of the area that has been harmed. For example, injuries to the area that controls speech will result in an inability to speak or to speak normally.

Because the brain is enclosed in the cranial vault, bleeding and swelling also are a concern. Since the skull is a closed container, blood or edema takes up space where brain tissue would otherwise be and presses on the brain. Blood pressure inside the vault (intracranial pressure) can also be increased, and this pressure can damage additional structures and alter functions as well.

Mechanical damage to the spine and other nervous pathways results in disruption of nervous system communication. When we think of severing the spinal cord, paralysis comes to mind. However, remember that, beyond motor function, the patient also loses sensory and autonomic messaging. That means when a nervous pathway is destroyed, movement, sensation, and even automatic functions like breathing and blood vessel dilation may be altered. As in the brain, bleeding and edema are also threats in the closed container of the spinal column.

Medical Dysfunction Medical problems, both acute and chronic, can alter nervous system function. Strokes result from clots and bleeding in the arteries that perfuse the brain. In these cases, brain cells are deprived of oxygen and die. As with trauma, the net result of the damage will depend on the affected area's function. Diseases can also affect the brain and spinal cord. Meningitis, an infection of the protective layers of the brain and spinal cord; encephalitis, an infection of the brain itself; and a variety of diseases that affect the nerves, such as Lou Gehrig's disease and multiple sclerosis, all can impair the transmission of messages in the nervous system. General medical problems can also affect normal brain function; for example, a diabetic with low blood sugar (hypoglycemia) who becomes confused and eventually unresponsive when his brain is deprived of the glucose it needs for proper functioning.

Signs of neurologic impairment include:

- Altered mental status
- Inability to speak or difficulty speaking
- Visual or hearing disturbance
- Inability to walk or difficulty walking
- Paralysis (sometimes limited to one side)
- Weakness (sometimes limited to one side)
- Loss of sensation (sometimes limited to one side or area of the body)
- Pupil changes

The Endocrine System

The endocrine system is made up of a variety of glands that secrete chemical messages in the form of hormones. These hormones dictate and control a variety of body functions, such as glucose transfer and water absorption in the kidneys among many others. The major organs of this system include the kidneys and the brain. The endocrine system also includes several glands, such as the pancreas and the pituitary, thyroid, and adrenal glands.

Endocrine System Dysfunction

Dysfunctions of the endocrine system are primarily the result of organ or gland problems. Although trauma can cause injury to organs, typically endocrine dysfunctions are either present at birth or the result of illness. Endocrine disorders generally fall into one of two categories: too many hormones or not enough hormones.

Too Many Hormones In some disease states, glands produce an excessive amount of hormones. Graves' disease, for example, is a condition in which the thyroid gland overproduces its hormone. Patients with this condition can suffer from difficulties like regulating temperature and fast heart rates.

Not Enough Hormones More common are endocrine disorders where glands produce too few hormones. In diabetes, the pancreas does not secrete enough of the hormone insulin. Insulin helps move glucose from our bloodstream into our body cells. Without enough insulin, our cells starve.

For more information on endocrine disorders, see Chapter 21, "Diabetic Emergencies and Altered Mental Status."

The Digestive System

The digestive system consists of the esophagus, stomach, intestines, and a few additional associated organs. The digestive system allows food, water, and other nutrients to enter the body. It also controls the absorption of those substances into our bloodstream.

Digestive Dysfunction

Digestive disorders can seriously impact both hydration levels and nutrient transfer.

Gastrointestinal Bleeding The digestive system is supported by a rich blood supply, which enables absorption of nutrients from the digestive tract into the bloodstream. Gastrointestinal (GI) bleeding can occur anywhere in the digestive tract from the esophagus to the anus. Digestive system bleeding can be slow and chronic or can present with shock from acute massive bleeding in the form of rectal bleeding or vomiting blood.

Vomiting and Diarrhea Probably the most common digestive disorders are vomiting and diarrhea. Vomiting and diarrhea are not diseases themselves, but rather are symptoms of other disorders. There are literally hundreds of potential causes, but you should be aware that both can be related to serious problems. Aside from digestive complications, vomiting is often a sign of acute myocardial infarction (heart attack) and stroke. More commonly, however, vomiting and diarrhea are caused by viral or bacterial infection. When isolated, the serious complications of nausea and vomiting include dehydration and malnutrition.

The Immune System

The immune system is responsible for fighting infection. It responds to specific body invaders by identifying them, marking them, and destroying them. The blood plays a major role in the immune system. Once a foreign body is identified, the body dispatches specialized cells and chemicals. White blood cells and antibodies are transported in the

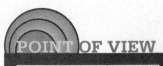

POINT OF VIEW

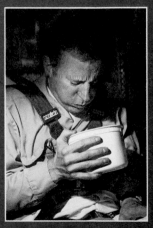

"So this patient told me he woke up at 3 a.m. with a terrible stomachache and immediately threw up. At first he thought it might have been the fish tacos he ate for dinner. When he walked back into the bedroom he felt a little out of breath. So he figured maybe it was a stomach virus. He hated to call 911—you know, wake up the poor EMTs in the middle of the night and make a big deal over nothing. But he felt pretty awful, so he made the call.

"When we arrived, we assured him it was OK that he called. He didn't want to go to the hospital. He said he was sure he wasn't having a heart attack because he didn't have any chest pain. But one thing I know: What's happening on the inside can produce a lot of different symptoms on the outside. In my EMT courses, they called those inside/outside relationships 'pathophysiology.' I realized that nausea plus shortness of breath could be indications of a cardiac problem, with or without chest pain.

"So I told him better safe than sorry. Sure, maybe it was the fish tacos, but it could be something more severe. Best to go to the ED and get it checked out. He agreed. My instinct was to not linger at the scene but to get him transported right away.

"It turned out he was having a heart attack. To make a long story short, he recovered and has made some lifestyle changes to help prevent another one. The ED doc told me this patient might not have made it if we hadn't got him to the hospital so quickly.

"Boy was I glad I took my pathophysiology studies seriously and realized that something critical could be causing the man's symptoms. It meant saving a life!"

bloodstream to attack the invaders. (More information on this process can be found in Chapter 22, "Allergic Reaction.")

This is a normal body response to infection or invasion by a foreign substance. An allergic reaction or anaphylactic reaction is an abnormally exaggerated version of this response that occurs as a result of a flaw in the immune system.

Hypersensitivity (Allergic Reaction)

An exaggerated immune response is referred to as **hypersensitivity** (also known as an allergic reaction). Hypersensitivity can occur in a response to certain foods, drugs, animals, or a variety of substances. In a hypersensitivity reaction, the immune system, in responding to these specific substances, releases chemical toxins that cause more of a reaction than necessary. The allergic reaction occurs when these chemicals affect more than just the designated invader.

hypersensitivity
an exaggerated response by the immune system to a particular substance.

One of the chemicals released, called histamine, produces edema and, in some cases, a narrowing of the airways. Other chemicals can cause dilation of the smooth muscles of blood vessels, resulting in a rapid drop in blood pressure. Hypersensitivity reactions range from minor and localized reactions to severe and life-threatening ones. Rapid identification and treatment is often lifesaving.

For more information on allergies and anaphylaxis, see Chapter 22, "Allergic Reaction."

CHAPTER REVIEW

Key Facts and Concepts

- Pathophysiology allows us to understand how negative forces impact the normal function of the body.

- Pathophysiology helps us understand how common disorders cause changes in the body.

- Understanding how the body compensates for insults sheds light on the signs and symptoms we may see during assessment.

- Understanding what compensation looks like helps us rapidly identify potentially life-threatening problems.

Key Decisions

- Is the airway obstructed? Is it open? Will it stay open?

- Is air reaching the alveoli? Is breathing adequate?

- Is perfusion adequate in my patient? Is he in shock?

- Is anything interrupting the ventilation/perfusion match of this patient?

Chapter Glossary

aerobic (air-O-bik) **metabolism** the cellular process in which oxygen is used to metabolize glucose. Energy is produced in an efficient manner with minimal waste products.

anaerobic (AN-air-o-bik) **metabolism** the cellular process in which glucose is metabolized into energy without oxygen. Energy is produced in an inefficient manner with many waste products.

cardiac output the amount of blood ejected from the heart in 1 minute (heart rate × stroke volume).

chemoreceptors (ke-mo-re-cept-erz) chemical sensors in the brain and blood vessels that identify changing levels of oxygen and carbon dioxide.

dead air space air that occupies the space between the mouth and alveoli but that does not actually reach the area of gas exchange.

dehydration(de-hi-DRAY-shun) an abnormally low amount of water in the body.

edema (eh-DEE-muh) swelling associated with the movement of water into the interstitial space.

electrolyte (e-LEK-tro-lite) a substance that, when dissolved in water, separates into charged particles.

FiO₂ fraction of inspired oxygen; the concentration of oxygen in the air we breathe.

hydrostatic (HI-dro-STAT-ik) *pressure* the pressure within a blood vessel that tends to push water out of the vessel.

hypersensitivity an exaggerated response by the immune system to a particular substance.

hypoperfusion (HI-po-per-FEW-zhun) inability of the body to adequately circulate blood to the body's cells to supply them with oxygen and nutrients. Also called *shock*.

metabolism (meh-TAB-o-lizm) the cellular function of converting nutrients into energy.

minute volume the amount of air breathed in during each respiration multiplied by the number of breaths per minute.

patent (PAY-tent) open and clear; free from obstruction.

pathophysiology (path-o-fiz-e-OL-o-je) the study of how disease processes affect the function of the body.

perfusion (pur-FEW-zhun) the supply of oxygen to, and removal of wastes from, the cells and tissues of the body as a result of the flow of blood through the capillaries.

plasma oncotic (PLAZ-ma on-KOT-ik) *pressure* the pull exerted by large proteins in the plasma portion of blood that tends to pull water from the body into the bloodstream.

shock the inability of the body to adequately circulate blood to the body's cells to supply them with oxygen and nutrients. Also called *hypoperfusion*. A life-threatening condition.

stretch receptors sensors in blood vessels that identify internal pressure.

stroke volume the amount of blood ejected from the heart in one contraction.

systemic vascular resistance (SVR) the pressure in the peripheral blood vessels that the heart must overcome in order to pump blood into the system.

tidal volume the volume of air moved in one cycle of breathing.

V/Q match ventilation/perfusion match. This implies that the alveoli are supplied with enough air and that the air in the alveoli is matched with sufficient blood in the pulmonary capillaries to permit optimum exchange of oxygen and carbon dioxide.

Preparation for Your Examination and Practice

Short Answer

1. Define metabolism. Explain the necessary components of efficient metabolism.
2. Describe three types of respiratory dysfunction and how those dysfunctions affect the body.
3. Describe why it is important that blood vessels have the capability to dilate and constrict. How do these impact the cardiovascular system as a whole?
4. Define cardiac output. What are the key components of cardiac output?
5. Describe how the body might compensate for a challenge to the cardiopulmonary system. How might these compensations be seen in a patient?

Thinking and Linking

Pathophysiology, or the dysfunction of a particular system, can typically be identified through signs and symptoms. For the following situations, link each listed pathophysiology with its likely external manifestations to describe probable signs/symptoms, including changes in vital signs, that may result from the dysfunction.

PATHOPHYSIOLOGY	SIGN/SYMPTOM
Obstructed airway	
Bronchospasm (narrowed air passages)	
Massive external hemorrhage	
Heart rate too slow to maintain perfusion	

Critical Thinking Exercises

An understanding of cellular metabolism pathophysiology is important. The purpose of this exercise will be to consider some aspects of cellular metabolism.

1. What are the requirements for normal cellular metabolism? What changes occur when those requirements are not available?

2. Considering the requirements of normal cellular metabolism, discuss how each of the following systems and/or organs contributes to the delivery of those requirements

   - Respiratory
   - Circulatory
   - Blood vessels
   - Blood

Pathophysiology to Practice

The following questions are designed to assist you in gathering relevant clinical information and making accurate decisions in the field.

1. We discussed that the heart plays a major role in compensation. Consider a patient with a traumatic injury to the heart. What impact on the patient's ability to compensate might an injury like this have?

2. We discussed that the blood vessels play a major role in compensation. Consider a patient with an inability to control the diameter of the blood vessels (as in sepsis). What impact might an illness like this have on the patient's ability to compensate?

3. Certain types of anemia decrease the amount of red blood cells in a patient's blood. What might be the impact of not having enough red blood cells? How might this condition affect that patient's ability to compensate for an illness or injury?

Street Scenes -----------------------------------

It is 2000 hours. Your unit is dispatched to a run-down home for a man complaining of diarrhea. When you arrive you notice a foul, fecal smell. You meet the patient in the living room. He is a 68-year-old man. He complains of nausea and diarrhea over the last 3 days. He notes his bowel movements have been "very dark, almost black." He is awake, alert, and breathing at a rate of 24/min. His skin is slightly pale. You have a difficult time finding a radial pulse, but feel a carotid pulse at 124.

Street Scene Questions

1. What additional patient history should you obtain?
2. What does your primary assessment reveal about this patient's condition? How sick is he and why?
3. Why might this patient not have a palpable radial pulse? How is this related to his heart and respiratory rates?

You place the patient on high-concentration oxygen and continue your assessment while your partner readies the stretcher for transport. You locate a very weak radial pulse and obtain a blood pressure of 82/62. You notice no injuries but find his abdomen to be slightly tender in the left quadrants. You load the patient on the stretcher and prepare to transfer him to the ambulance.

Street Scene Questions

4. Was a low blood pressure predictable based on your primary assessment?
5. What is the cause of this patient's low blood pressure?
6. Should you contact ALS for this call or simply transport him to the hospital yourself?

When the patient stands to transfer from the chair to the stretcher he becomes very dizzy and "feels like he is going to pass out." Once he lies down on the stretcher he feels better.

En route to the hospital, you obtain a SAMPLE history. He states that his biggest problem tonight is the diarrhea, but his stomach hurts, too. He has no allergies. He tells you he has a history of "drinking too much" and that he has had some "stomach problems because of it." He can't tell you what those problems are, but he "takes a pill for them." He hasn't been able to eat much over the last couple days. In fact, he tells you he has been feeling weak for a few days and now the diarrhea has really made him feel bad.

You continue to transport him to the hospital. There he is diagnosed with a severe gastrointestinal bleed and prepared for surgery.

7
Life Span Development

COMPETENCY
Applies fundamental knowledge of life span development to patient assessment and management.

CORE CONCEPTS
— The physiological (physical) characteristics of different age groups from infancy through late adulthood

— The psychosocial (mental and social) characteristics of different age groups from infancy through late adulthood

EXPLORE Resource**C**entral

To access Resource Central, follow directions on the Student Access Card provided with this text. If there is no card, go to **www.bradybooks.com** and follow the Resource Central link to Buy Access from there. Under Media Resources, you will find:

▶ **Life Span Development**
Watch this video to learn how to deal with different types of patients at all stages of life and why you should understand a patient's developmental stage.

▶ **American Academy of Pediatrics Stages of Development**
Learn about the milestones children reach at different ages and what bodily changes occur at different stages. They grow up so fast!

▶ **APA Website on Aging**
Read about the normal process of aging, why good nutrition and fitness is important after age 50, and learn about what challenges individuals may face in late adulthood. At least until someone finds that elusive fountain of youth!

OBJECTIVES

After reading this chapter you should be able to:

7.1 Define key terms introduced in this chapter.

7.2 Describe the physical and physiological characteristics, including normal vital signs, for individuals in each of the following age groups:
  a. Infant (pp. 157–160)
  b. Toddler (pp. 160–161)
  c. Preschool age (pp. 161–162)
  d. School age (pp. 162–163)
  e. Adolescent (pp. 163–164)
  f. Early adult (pp. 164–165)
  g. Middle adult (pp. 165–166)
  h. Late adult (pp. 166–167)

7.3 Describe the typical psychosocial characteristics and concerns of individuals at each stage during the life span. (pp. 157–167)

7.4 Use knowledge of physical, physiological, and psychosocial development to anticipate the needs and concerns of patients of all ages. (pp. 157–167)

L ife span development looks at the physiological (physical) and psychosocial (mental and social) changes that occur from birth to death. You will learn more about the pediatric patient in Chapter 35, "Pediatric Emergencies," and about the geriatric patient in Chapter 36, "Geriatric Emergencies."

In this chapter, we will follow Jamie as she develops through the following stages of life:

- Infancy
- Toddler phase
- Preschool age
- School age
- Adolescence
- Early adulthood
- Middle adulthood
- Late adulthood

INFANCY (BIRTH TO 1 YEAR)

If you have ever spent time around infants, you can attest to the phenomenal changes that occur during this first year of life. This is the period referred to as *infancy*. The infant is a small bundle of joy, totally dependent upon others, and grows to begin walking and developing a unique personality (Figures 7-1 and 7-2).

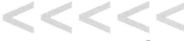

CORE CONCEPT

The physiological (physical) characteristics of different age groups from infancy through late adulthood

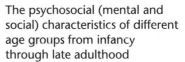

CORE CONCEPT

The psychosocial (mental and social) characteristics of different age groups from infancy through late adulthood

infancy
stage of life from birth to 1 year of age.

FIGURE 7-1 A newborn infant.

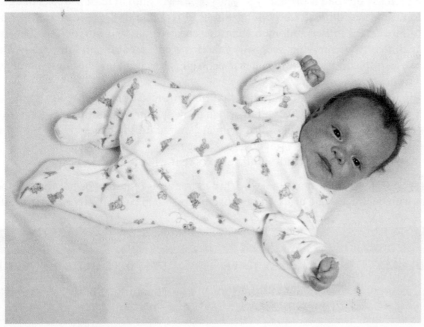

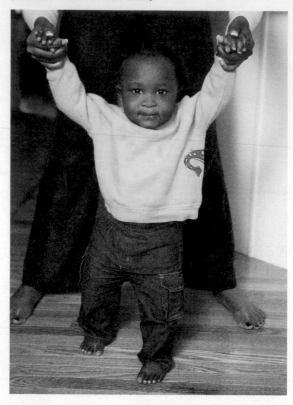

FIGURE 7-2 A year-old infant.

(© Chad Johnson/Masterfile)

Physiological

As Jamie ages, her normal pulse rate and respiratory rate will decrease and her blood pressure will increase. Her vital signs are listed in Table 7-1. At birth, Jamie will weigh 3.0–3.5 kg (6.6–7.7 lbs). Her weight will likely double by 6 months and triple by 12 months. Her head will be equal to 25 percent of her total body weight.

While in her mother's uterus, Jamie's lungs did not function, and she had a different pattern of circulation before birth than after. The transition from fetal circulation to pulmonary circulation occurs quickly—usually within the first minutes or hours after birth.

Jamie's airway is shorter, narrower, less stable, and more easily obstructed than at any other stage in her life. She is primarily a "nose breather" until at least 4 weeks of age. Nasal congestion can cause difficulty breathing. She is also a diaphragm breather; thus, you may see more movement in her abdomen than the chest. Jamie will fatigue more easily with breathing difficulty, because her accessory muscles are less mature and tire easily. She may be more susceptible to trauma, since her chest wall is less rigid and her lung tissue is more prone to trauma from pressure.

During pregnancy, certain antibodies that help protect from disease are passed to her from her mother. Jamie is also breast fed, which provides her with antibodies to many of the diseases her mother has had. This helps protect Jamie until she can produce her own antibodies, either from vaccination or exposure to diseases.

Jamie's nervous system includes four reflexes that will diminish over time:

- **Moro reflex.** When you startle her, she throws her arms out, spreads her fingers, and then grabs with her fingers and arms. These movements should be relatively equal on both sides.

Moro reflex
when startled, an infant throws his arms out, spreads his fingers, then grabs with his fingers and arms.

Table 7-1 Vital Signs: Infant			
HEART RATE	**RESPIRATORY VOLUME**	**RESPIRATORY RATE**	**SYSTOLIC BLOOD PRESSURE**
140–160/minute	7–8 mL/kg at birth increasing to 10–15 mL/kg at 1 year	40–60/minute (Drops to 30–40 soon after birth)	70 mmHg at birth to 90 mmHg at 1 year

- *Palmar reflex.* When you place your finger in her palm, she grasps it. Within a couple of months, this merges with the ability to release an object from the hand.
- *Rooting reflex.* When you touch Jamie's cheek when she is hungry, she turns her head toward the side touched.
- *Sucking reflex.* When you stroke Jamie's lips, she starts sucking. This reflex works in conjunction with the rooting reflex.

Initially, Jamie will sleep from 16 to 18 hours in total throughout the day and night. This will soon change to about 4 to 6 hours during the day and 9 to 10 hours during the night. Although each infant varies, usually in 2 to 4 months the infant will sleep through the night. Even though infants do sleep a lot, they are easy to awaken.

Jamie's extremities grow in length from a combination of growth plates that are located at the ends of the long bones (humerus and femur), and the epiphyseal plates located near the ends of the long bones. As mentioned in Chapter 5, "Medical Terminology and Anatomy and Physiology," the bones at the top of the skull are not fused at birth. The "soft spot" where these bones meet is called a fontanelle. The posterior fontanelle usually closes in 2 or 3 months, and the anterior one closes between 9 and 18 months. Looking at the anterior fontanelle, you can get a good idea of Jamie's state of hydration. Normally, the fontanelle is level with, or slightly below, the surface of the skull. If the fontanelle is sunken, this indicates dehydration. If the fontanelle is bulging, you should suspect increased pressure inside the skull.

There are certain milestones during Jamie's first year. Some of these are listed in Table 7-2.

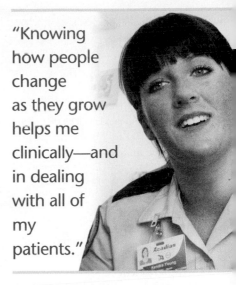

"Knowing how people change as they grow helps me clinically—and in dealing with all of my patients."

palmar reflex
when you place your finger in an infant's palm, he will grasp it.

rooting reflex
when you touch a hungry infant's cheek, he will turn his head toward the side touched.

sucking reflex
when you stroke a hungry infant's lips, he will start sucking.

Table 7-2	Developmental Changes: Infant
AGE	**CHARACTERISTICS**
2 months	• Tracks objects with eyes • Recognizes familiar faces
3 months	• Moves objects to mouth with hands • Distinct facial expressions (smile, frown)
4 months	• Drools without swallowing • Begins to reach out to people
5 months	• Sleeps through the night without waking for feeding • Discriminates between family and strangers
5–7 months	• Teeth begin to appear
6 months	• Sits upright in high chair • Begins making one-syllable sounds
7 months	• Fear of strangers • Moods shift quickly (crying to laughing to crying)
8 months	• Begins responding to word no • Can sit alone • Can play "peek-a-boo"
9 months	• Responds to adult anger • Pulls himself up to standing position • Explores objects by mouthing, sucking, chewing, and biting
10 months	• Pays attention to his name • Crawls well
11 months	• Attempts to walk without assistance • Begins to show frustration about restrictions
12 months	• Walks with help • Knows own name

Psychosocial

Jamie's primary means of communication is crying. Those close to Jamie will soon learn if she is crying because she is hungry, is tired, needs to be changed, or for some other reason.

Within the first 6 months, Jamie will bond with her caregivers and start displaying the following characteristics:

- *Bonding.* This is her sense that her needs will be met. When she is hungry, she is fed. When she needs to be held, she is.
- *Trust vs. mistrust.* Jamie likes an orderly, predictable environment. When her environment is disorderly and irregular, she develops anxiety and insecurity.
- *Scaffolding.* She learns by building on what she already knows.
- *Temperament.* This is her reaction to her environment.

TODDLER PHASE (12–36 MONTHS)

During the *toddler phase*, physical, mental, and social development continues. Body systems continue to grow and refine themselves, and the toddler develops more individuality. This age group's curiosity has led to such affectionate terms as *curtain climbers* or *rug rats*. Their developing personality is sometimes referred to as the "terrible twos." Like all phases of childhood, these years can be a very rewarding time for both toddler and caregivers (Figure 7-3).

Physiological

Jamie's body temperature now ranges from 96.8°F–99.6°F (36.3°C–37.9°C). She will gain approximately 2.0 kg (4.4 lb) per year. Her vital signs are listed in Table 7-3.

All of Jamie's body systems will continue to develop and improve in efficiency.

- **Pulmonary system.** Terminal airways branch and grow. Alveoli increase in number.
- **Nervous system.** Jamie's brain is now 90 percent of adult brain weight. Fine motor skills develop.

FIGURE 7-3 A toddler. (© Rommel/Masterfile)

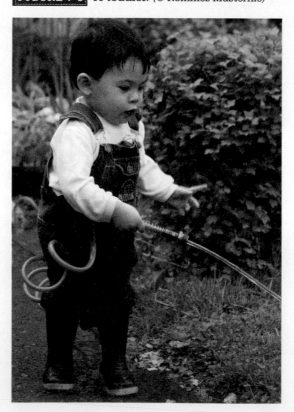

Table 7-3 Vital Signs: Toddler

HEART RATE	RESPIRATORY RATE	SYSTOLIC BLOOD PRESSURE
80–130/minute	20–30/minute	70–100 mmHg

Table 7-4 Cognitive Developmental Changes: Toddler

AGE	CHARACTERISTICS
12 months	Begins to grasp that words "mean" something
18–24 months	Begins to understand cause and effect Develops separation anxiety, shown by clinging and crying when a parent leaves
24–36 months	Begins developing "magical thinking" and engages in play-acting, such as playing house
3–4 years	Masters the basics of language that will continue to be refined throughout childhood

- **Musculoskeletal system.** Muscle mass and bone density increase.
- **Immune system.** The toddler is more susceptible to illness. She develops immunity to pathogens as exposure occurs and through vaccination.
- **Teeth.** By 36 months of age, Jamie has all her primary teeth.

Although Jamie is physiologically capable of being toilet trained by 12 to 15 months of age, she is not psychologically ready until 18 to 30 months. It is important not to rush toilet training. She will let her parents know when she is ready. The average age for completion of toilet training is 28 months.

Psychosocial

Cognitive development deals with the development of knowledge and thinking. Table 7-4 shows some of the cognitive development Jamie will experience.

PRESCHOOL AGE (3–5 YEARS)

Preschool age is a time of continued physiological and psychosocial development. This is often a time when preschoolers are put into social interaction situations such as day care or preschools (Figure 7-4).

preschool age
stage of life from 3 to 5 years.

Physiological

Jamie's body systems continue to develop and refine their various processes. Her vital signs are listed in Table 7-5.

Psychosocial

Jamie attends a preschool where she is involved with peer groups. Peer groups provide a source of information about other families and the outside world. Interaction with peers offers opportunities for learning skills, comparing herself to others, and feeling part of a group.

Table 7-5 Vital Signs: Preschool Age

HEART RATE	RESPIRATORY RATE	SYSTOLIC BLOOD PRESSURE
80–120/minute	20–30/minute	80–110 mmHg

FIGURE 7-4 A preschooler. (© Daniel Limmer)

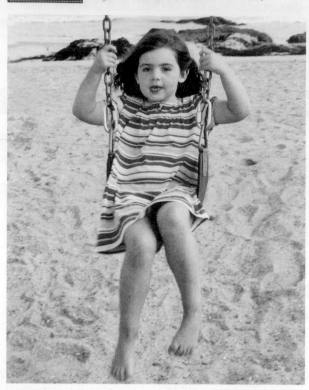

SCHOOL AGE (6–12 YEARS)

Whether attending a public or private school, or being home-schooled, the stage of development referred to as **school age** opens vast opportunities for the child.

school age
stage of life from 6 to 12 years.

Physiological

Jamie's body temperature is approximately 98.6°F (37°C), and she will gain 3 kg (6.6 lb) and grow 6 cm (2.4 in.) per year (Figure 7-5). Her vital signs are listed in Table 7-6.

One of the most obvious changes in Jamie during this time is the loss of her primary teeth. Replacement with permanent teeth begins.

FIGURE 7-5 School-age children. (© Roy Ooms/Masterfile)

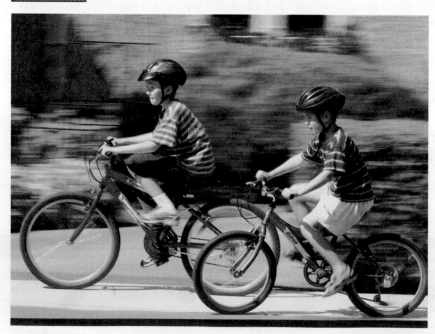

Table 7-6 Vital Signs: School Age		
HEART RATE	**RESPIRATORY RATE**	**SYSTOLIC BLOOD PRESSURE**
70–110/minute	20–30/minute	80–120 mmHg

Psychosocial

This is a transition time for both Jamie and her parents. Her parents spend less time with her than they did at earlier ages and provide more general supervision. Jamie develops better decision-making skills and is allowed to make more decisions on her own.

Self-esteem develops and may be affected by popularity with peers, rejection, emotional support, and neglect. Negative self-esteem can be very damaging to further development.

As Jamie matures, moral development begins when she is rewarded for what her parents believe to be right and punished for what her parents believe to be wrong. With cognitive growth, moral reasoning appears and the control of her behavior gradually shifts from external sources to internal self-control.

ADOLESCENCE (13–18 YEARS)

Although life span development is a continual process, dynamic physiological and psychosocial changes occur during three major developmental ages: infancy, with the transition from fetal life to life in the world; *adolescence*, with the transition from childhood to adulthood (Figure 7-6); and late adulthood, with its deterioration of systems.

adolescence
stage of life from 13 to 18 years.

Physiological

During this stage, Jamie will usually experience a rapid 2- to 3-year growth spurt, beginning distally with enlargement of her feet and hands followed by enlargement of her arms and legs. Her chest and trunk enlarge in the final stage of growth. Girls are usually finished growing by

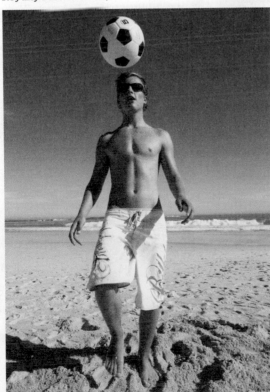

FIGURE 7-6 An adolescent. *(Masterfile Royalty Free Division)*

Table 7-7 Vital Signs: Adolescence		
HEART RATE	**RESPIRATORY RATE**	**SYSTOLIC BLOOD PRESSURE**
55–105/minute	12–20/minute	80–120 mmHg

the age of 16 and boys by the age of 18. In late adolescence, the average male is taller and stronger than the average female. Jamie's vital signs are listed in Table 7-7.

At this age, both males and females reach reproductive maturity. Secondary sexual development occurs, with noticeable development of the external sexual organs. In females, menstruation begins and breasts develop.

Psychosocial

Adolescence can be a time of serious family conflicts as the adolescent strives for independence and parents strive for continued control.

At this age, Jamie is trying to achieve more independence and develop her own identity. She becomes interested in the opposite sex, and finds this somewhat embarrassing. She not only wants to be treated like an adult but also enjoys the comforts of childhood.

Body image is a great concern at this point in life. This is a time when eating disorders are common. It also is a time when self-destructive behaviors begin, such as use of tobacco, alcohol, illicit drugs, and unsafe driving. Depression and suicide are alarmingly common in this age group.

As adolescents develop their capacity for logical, analytical, and abstract thinking, they begin to develop a personal code of ethics.

EARLY ADULTHOOD (19–40 YEARS)

early adulthood
stage of life from 19 to 40 years.

With great pomp and circumstance, the adolescent graduates from childhood to adulthood (Figure 7-7). Some say the best years are behind; some say the best years are ahead. But life is what you make of it, and *early adulthood* opens up great opportunities.

FIGURE 7-7 A young adult. *(© Mark Leibowitz/Masterfile)*

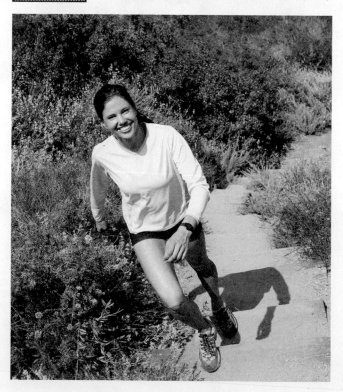

Table 7-8 Vital Signs: Early Adulthood		
HEART RATE	**RESPIRATORY RATE**	**BLOOD PRESSURE**
Average 70/minute	16–20/minute	120/80 mmHg

Physiological

This is the period of life when Jamie will develop lifelong habits and routines. Her vital signs are listed in Table 7-8.

Peak physical condition occurs between 19 and 26 years of age, when all body systems are at optimal performance levels. At the end of this period, the body begins its slowing process.

Psychosocial

The highest levels of job stress occur at this point in life, when Jamie is trying to establish her identity. Love develops, both romantic and affectionate. Childbirth is most common in this age group, with new families providing new challenges and stresses. Accidents are a leading cause of death in this age group.

MIDDLE ADULTHOOD (41–60 YEARS)

For most, **middle adulthood** is a time of reflecting on how far they have come and where they want to go. This internal conflict is often called "midlife crisis."

middle adulthood
stage of life from 41 to 60 years.

Physiological

During this stage of development, Jamie has no significant changes in vital signs from her early adulthood. She is starting to have some vision problems and is now wearing prescription glasses. Her cholesterol is a little high, and she is concerned about health problems. Cancer often develops in this age group, weight control becomes more difficult, and for women in the late 40s to early 50s, menopause commences. Heart disease is the major killer after the age of 40 in all age, sex, and racial groups (Figure 7-8).

FIGURE 7-8 A middle-aged adult. (© Blend Images/Masterfile)

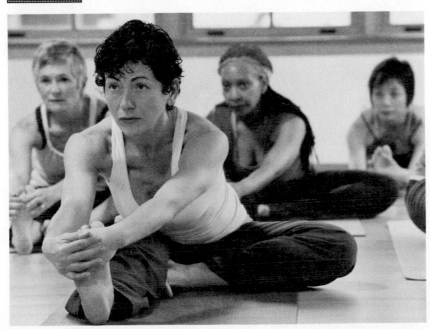

Psychosocial

Jamie is becoming more task oriented as she sees the time for accomplishing her lifetime goals diminish. Still, she tends to approach problems more as challenges than as threats. With her children starting lives of their own, she is experiencing "empty-nest syndrome," the time after the last offspring has left home. This may also be a time of increased freedom and opportunity for self-fulfillment.

Jamie is concerned about her children as they start their new lives, and she is also concerned about caring for aging parents.

LATE ADULTHOOD (61 YEARS AND OLDER)

late adulthood
stage of life from 61 years and older.

Late adulthood is often referred to as the "twilight years." This stage of development brings about several physiological and psychosocial changes, second only to those seen during infancy or adolescence (Figure 7-9).

Physiological

Jamie's vital signs will depend on her physical and health condition. Her cardiovascular system becomes less efficient, and the volume of blood decreases. She is less tolerant of tachycardia (fast heart rate). Her respiratory system deteriorates and makes her more likely to develop respiratory disorders. Changes in the endocrine system result in decreased metabolism. Her sleep-wake cycle also is disrupted, causing her to have sleep problems. All other body systems are deteriorating as time progresses.

Psychosocial

As Jamie ages she will face many challenges. Motivation, personal interests, and the level of activities will enhance this later time of life. She faces the following challenges:

- **Living environment.** How long can she live at home? Does she need to be in an assisted living facility, or perhaps a nursing home?

FIGURE 7-9 An older adult. *(© Norbert Schafer/Masterfile)*

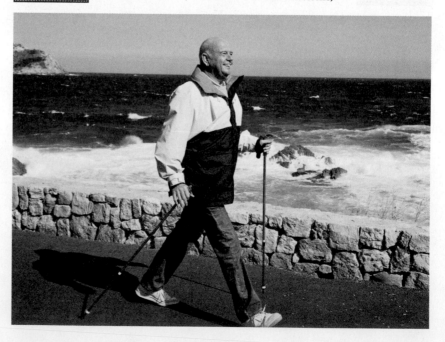

- **Self-worth.** Though she has slowed down a bit, she is concerned with producing quality work that benefits herself and others.

- **Financial burdens.** With limited income and increasing expenses, financial concerns weigh heavily on her decisions.

- **Death and dying.** She sees friends and relatives become ill and die. Concerns of her own health condition and mortality often come to mind.

CRITICAL DECISION MAKING

Determining If Vital Signs Are Normal

Although you don't have to memorize vital signs (you can use a reference chart much of the time) you should have a general idea of whether vital signs are normal or abnormal for different age groups. For each of the vital signs in the following list, indicate whether you believe they are normal or abnormal. Note what the normal rate for each patient should be.

A 3-year-old boy who seems groggy and has a pulse of 60/minute

A 65-year-old man who feels like his heart is skipping beats and has a pulse of 130/minute

A 42-year-old man with a respiratory rate of 16 who fell off a curb and hurt his ankle

A 77-year-old woman with dizziness and a pulse of 56

A 3-month-old baby with a respiratory rate of 30

POINT OF VIEW

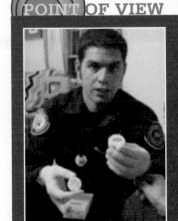

"It is hard to believe I've been alive this long. Life has been good to me. It is my 89th birthday today. Things have changed a lot since I was born. I lost a sister when she was little. People died right and left from the flu and pneumonia. Doctors then couldn't do anything like they do now. Somehow they keep me going."

CHAPTER REVIEW

Key Facts and Concepts

- Understanding the basic physiological and psychosocial development for each age group will assist you in communicating with and assessing patients of various ages.

- Physiological differences between the ages will also affect your care. Examples include differences in the respiratory systems of younger patients and the effect of preexisting medical conditions of older patients.

- Infants and young children have less developed and smaller respiratory structures which can make respiratory conditions worse.

- Your ability to communicate with younger patients will depend on their stage of development. This can range from fear of strangers to separation anxiety from parents and embarrassment during adolescence. Older patients may have issues with denial or depression over medical conditions.

Key Decisions

- How do I approach this patient most effectively based on his developmental characteristics?

- Does the age of my patient pose any assessment or care challenges based on the physiologic development?

Chapter Glossary

adolescence stage of life from 13 to 18 years.

bonding the sense that needs will be met.

early adulthood stage of life from 19 to 40 years.

infancy stage of life from birth to 1 year of age.

late adulthood stage of life from 61 years and older.

middle adulthood stage of life from 41 to 60 years.

Moro reflex when startled, an infant throws his arms out, spreads his fingers, then grabs with his fingers and arms.

palmar reflex when you place your finger in an infant's palm, he will grasp it.

preschool age stage of life from 3 to 5 years.

rooting reflex when you touch a hungry infant's cheek, he will turn his head toward the side touched.

scaffolding building on what one already knows.

school age stage of life from 6 to 12 years.

sucking reflex when you stroke a hungry infant's lips, he will start sucking.

temperament the infant's reaction to his environment.

toddler phase stage of life from 12 to 36 months.

trust vs. mistrust concept developed from an orderly, predictable environment versus a disorderly, irregular environment.

Preparation for Your Examination and Practice

Short Answer

1. For each of the following, decide which age group would most likely fit the description given:
   Decreased metabolism
   Toilet trained
   "Empty nest" syndrome
   Noticeable development of external sex organs
   Rooting reflex
   Self-destructive behaviors common
   Peak physical condition
   "Twilight years"

2. How would a child's response to EMS change from birth through adolescence?

Thinking and Linking

Thinking back to the anatomy, physiology, and pathophysiology chapters, link information from those chapters to information in this chapter to answer the following questions:

- What is the difference between pediatric and geriatric bones? How would fractures be different between the two age groups?

- How does heart rate change from birth through adulthood? Does the heart get stronger or weaker as a person enters late adulthood?

- Does the respiratory system improve or decrease with age? Who is more likely to get a chronic respiratory condition, a child or geriatric patient?

Critical Thinking Exercises

Adolescent patients can offer special challenges to the EMT. The purpose of this exercise will be to consider how you might handle the challenge described here.

- You are called for a 16-year-old girl with abdominal pain. She is with friends at the park. She seems hesitant to answer any of your questions. What characteristic of adolescent development is most likely the cause of this? How could you overcome it?

Pathophysiology to Practice

The following questions are designed to assist you in gathering relevant clinical information and making accurate decisions in the field.

1. Your patient is a young child who has been thrown from her bicycle, possibly striking her abdomen on the handlebars. Her vital signs seem mostly OK, but her heart rate is faster than normal. What does this cause you to suspect regarding her condition?

2. Elderly patients often take many medications. How will knowing what medications a patient takes help in your assessment and care of that patient?

Street Scenes

Your ambulance is called to an auto vs. pedestrian collision. You arrive to find a child lying on the ground near the front of a mid-sized car. The child is crying and being held by his mother.

The driver meets you as you approach. She is crying and tells you she didn't see the child run out of the driveway into the path of her car until it was too late. She tells you she was fortunately going slowly—about 20–25 miles per hour.

You approach the scene and introduce yourself. The child appears to be 3 or 4 years old. He clings fiercely to his mother as you begin to talk. You see an abrasion on his right arm and another on the right side of his forehead.

Because of the mechanism of injury and abrasions on the patient's forehead, you decide you should immobilize the patient's spine.

Street Scene Questions

1. How would you interpret the child's behavior of clinging to his mother? Do you believe it is a normal/good sign or a sign of serious injury?
2. Immobilizing the patient's spine will mean restricting his movement. How do you anticipate the patient will respond to this?
3. Would involving the mother be helpful? How?

You continue to assess the child. You find his vital signs are: pulse 102 strong and regular, respirations 28 and adequate, blood pressure 96/58, and capillary refill time is less than 2 seconds. The boy's pupils react to light and appear to be of a normal size.

Street Scene Questions

4. Are these vital signs normal for this patient?
5. Do you need to memorize a list of vital sign ranges for various ages? If not, how would you know what is normal when on a call?
6. How should you explain your assessment and care to this child?

With the help of his mother and a stuffed animal from the ambulance, you are able to calm the child and immobilize him on a backboard. You splint his right arm. The child remains alert and is transported to the hospital uneventfully.

You later find that the child was very lucky and escaped serious injury. His only significant injury was a fracture of his arm—for which he was able to choose the color of his cast.

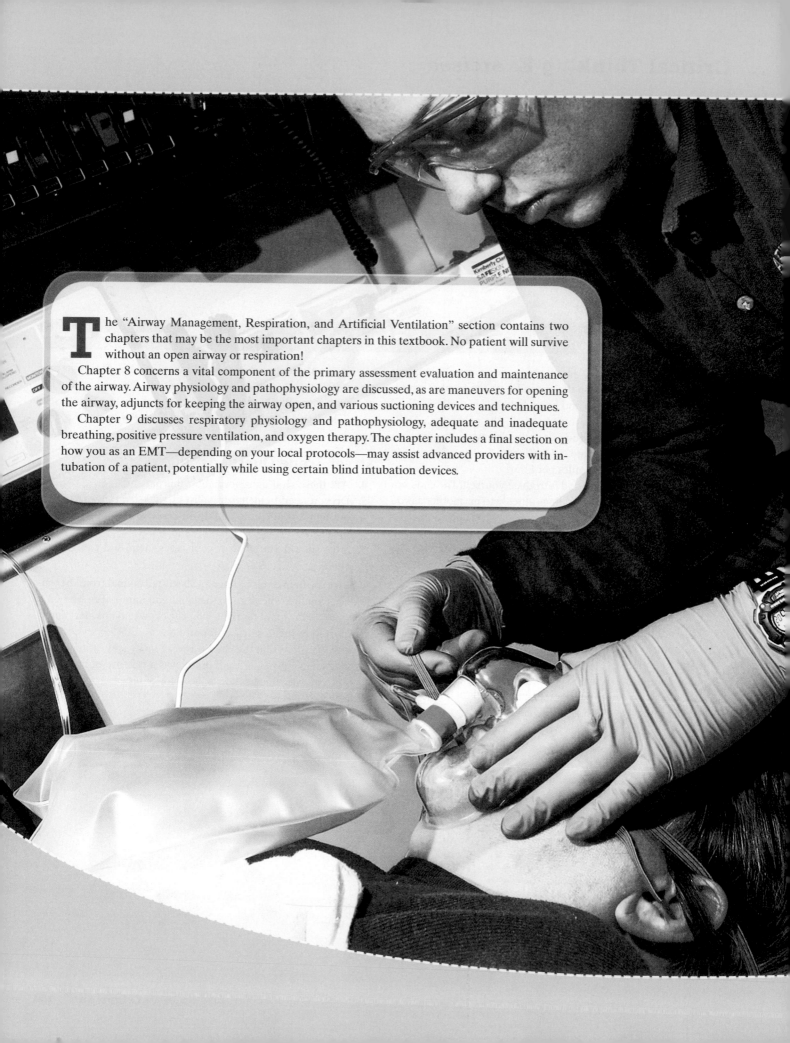

The "Airway Management, Respiration, and Artificial Ventilation" section contains two chapters that may be the most important chapters in this textbook. No patient will survive without an open airway or respiration!

Chapter 8 concerns a vital component of the primary assessment evaluation and maintenance of the airway. Airway physiology and pathophysiology are discussed, as are maneuvers for opening the airway, adjuncts for keeping the airway open, and various suctioning devices and techniques.

Chapter 9 discusses respiratory physiology and pathophysiology, adequate and inadequate breathing, positive pressure ventilation, and oxygen therapy. The chapter includes a final section on how you as an EMT—depending on your local protocols—may assist advanced providers with intubation of a patient, potentially while using certain blind intubation devices.

Airway Management, Respiration, and Artificial Ventilation

8

Airway Management

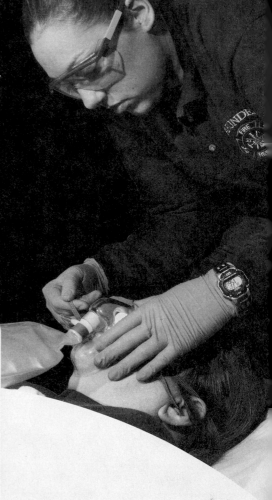

-------○ **STANDARD**
Airway Management, Respiration, and Artificial Ventilation (Airway Management)

-------○ **COMPETENCY**
Applies knowledge (fundamental depth, foundational breadth) of general anatomy and physiology to patient assessment and management in order to assure a patent airway, adequate mechanical ventilation, and respiration for patients of all ages.

-----○ **CORE CONCEPTS**

— Physiology of the airway

— Pathophysiology of the airway

— How to recognize an adequate or an inadequate airway

— How to open an airway

— How to use airway adjuncts

— Principles and techniques of suctioning

EXPLORE Resource Central

To access Resource Central, follow directions on the Student Access Card provided with this text. If there is no card, go to **www.bradybooks.com** and follow the Resource Central link to Buy Access from there. Under Media Resources, you will find:

▶ **Adult Foreign Body Airway Obstruction**
Watch a video on how to provide emergency care for an adult with a foreign body airway obstruction and don't get all choked up when you encounter this emergency!

▶ **Airway Maintenance for Trauma Patients**
Take a deep breath and read about the categories of patients with traumatic injuries that require a secured airway, types of advanced airway devices that can be used to secure the airway of a trauma patient, and so much more!

▶ **OPA, NPA, Suction Techniques**
See an animation on using an OPA and NPA and how to properly suction a patient.

OBJECTIVES

After reading this chapter you should be able to:

8.1 Define key terms introduced in this chapter.

8.2 Describe the anatomy and physiology of the upper and lower airways. (pp. 173–176)

8.3 Given a diagram or model, identify the structures of the upper and lower airways. (pp. 173–176)

8.4 Describe common pathophysiologic problems leading to airway obstruction. (pp. 176–180)

8.5 Demonstrate assessment of the airway in a variety of patient scenarios. (pp. 177–179)

8.6 Associate abnormal airway sounds with likely pathophysiologic causes. (pp. 177–179)

8.7 Identify patients who have an open airway but who are at risk for airway compromise. (pp. 178–179)

8.8 Recognize patients who have an inadequate airway. (pp. 177–179)

8.9 Demonstrate manually opening the airway in pediatric and adult medical and trauma patients.
  a. Head-tilt, chin-lift maneuver (pp. 181–182)
  b. Jaw-thrust maneuver (pp. 182–183)

(continued)

8.10 Describe the indications, contraindications, use, and potential complications of airway adjuncts, including:
   a. Oropharyngeal airway (pp. 184–186)
   b. Nasopharyngeal airway (pp. 186–188)

8.11 Recognize the indications for suctioning of the mouth and oropharynx. (pp. 188–192)

8.12 Describe risks and limitations associated with suctioning the mouth and oropharynx. (pp. 190–192)

8.13 Demonstrate the following airway management skills:
   a. Inserting an oropharyngeal airway (pp. 185–186)
   b. Inserting a nasopharyngeal airway (p. 187)
   c. Suctioning the mouth and oropharynx (p. 191)

8.14 Describe modifications in airway management for pediatric patients, patients with facial trauma, and patients with airway obstruction. (pp. 192–193)

KEY TERMS

airway, p. 173
bronchoconstriction, p. 177
gag reflex, p. 184

head-tilt, chin-lift maneuver, p. 181
jaw-thrust maneuver, p. 182

nasopharyngeal airway, p. 183
oropharyngeal airway, p. 183
patent airway, p. 174

stridor, p. 177
suctioning, p. 188

The cells of the human body must have oxygen to survive. The reason the ABCs—airway, breathing, and circulation—are so important is they are the means by which oxygen is brought into the body and transported to the cells. In this chapter we will discuss the airway, the "A" of the ABCs, and its role in delivering oxygen to the cells. You will learn that much of our primary assessment and treatment will focus on the *airway*. The reason for this is simple: When the airway fails, air cannot reach the lungs. When air cannot reach the lungs, oxygen cannot be delivered to the cells. In essence, without an airway, the patient will die. As you proceed through this chapter, keep in mind how important this statement really is.

In Chapter 5, "Medical Terminology and Anatomy and Physiology," you reviewed the anatomy and physiology of the respiratory system. In preparation for this chapter, you should review the following structures of the respiratory system and be able to label them on a blank diagram of the respiratory system (Figures 8-1, 8-2, and 8-3):

- Nose
- Mouth
- Tongue
- Nasopharynx
- Oropharynx
- Laryngopharynx
- Epiglottis
- Trachea
- Larynx

- Cricoid cartilage
- Carina
- Bronchi (right mainstem bronchus, left mainstem bronchus)
- Bronchioles
- Lungs
- Alveoli (alveolar sacs)
- Diaphragm

This chapter will also discuss a variety of topics you have previously covered in the CPR course you took as a prerequisite to your EMT course. This information included providing rescue breathing, performing cardiopulmonary resuscitation (CPR), and treating airway obstructions in infants, children, and adults. We will discuss each of these topics, but for more detail you should review Appendix A, "Basic Cardiac Life Support Review," in the back of this book.

airway

the passageway by which air enters or leaves the body. The structures of the airway are the nose, mouth, pharynx, larynx, trachea, bronchi, and lungs. *See also* patent airway.

FIGURE 8-1 The respiratory system.

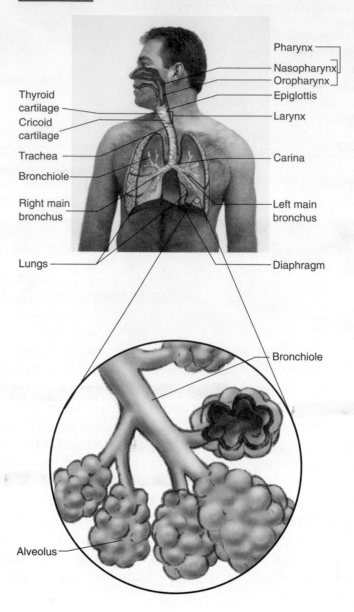

- Pharynx
- Nasopharynx
- Oropharynx
- Epiglottis
- Thyroid cartilage
- Larynx
- Cricoid cartilage
- Trachea
- Carina
- Bronchiole
- Right main bronchus
- Left main bronchus
- Lungs
- Diaphragm
- Bronchiole
- Alveolus

AIRWAY PHYSIOLOGY

CORE CONCEPT

Physiology of the airway

patent airway

an airway (passage from nose or mouth to lungs) that is open and clear and will remain open and clear, without interference to the passage of air into and out of the body.

The movement of air into and out of the lungs requires an intact and open airway, or *patent airway*. That means that air flow is unobstructed and capable of moving freely along its path.

In the upper airway (Figure 8-2), air enters the body through the mouth and nose. The nose is specifically designed to accept air and, through a series of turns and curves, air is warmed and humidified as it proceeds through the nasal passages. The mouth is primarily designed to be the entrance to the digestive system, but it also is an entryway for air (especially in an emergency). Distal to the mouth and nasal passages, air enters the throat or *pharynx*. The pharynx is divided into three regions: the *oropharynx*—where the oral cavity joins the pharynx; the *nasopharynx*—where the nasal passages empty into the pharynx, and finally the *laryngopharynx*—the structures surrounding the entrance to the trachea.

The laryngopharynx, also known as the hypopharynx, is designed to provide structure to, and protect, the opening to the trachea. It also is the point of division between the upper airway and the lower airway. The entry point into the larynx, called the *glottic opening*, is protected by a large leaflike structure called the *epiglottis*. This protective flap that sits above the glottic opening is designed to seal off the trachea during swallowing or in response to the gag reflex. The glottic opening is also protected by the vocal cords. These curtainlike fibers

FIGURE 8-2 The upper airway.

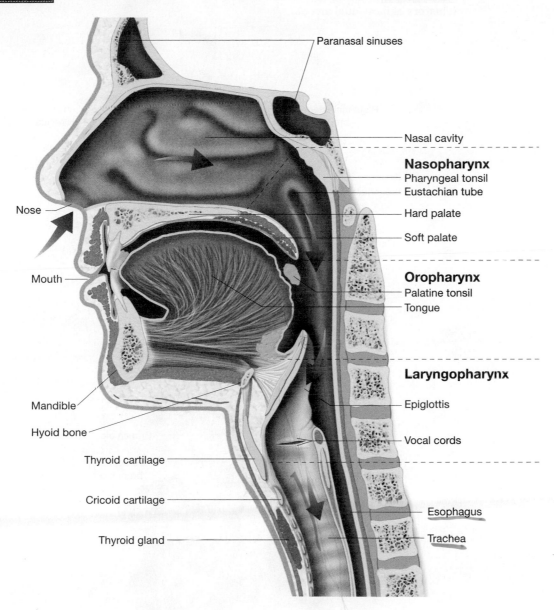

Paranasal sinuses

Nasal cavity

Nasopharynx
Pharyngeal tonsil
Eustachian tube

Nose

Hard palate

Soft palate

Oropharynx
Palatine tonsil
Tongue

Mouth

Laryngopharynx

Mandible

Epiglottis

Hyoid bone

Vocal cords

Thyroid cartilage

Cricoid cartilage

Esophagus

Thyroid gland

Trachea

that line either side of the tracheal opening not only can close shut for protection, but also vibrate with the passage of air to create the voice.

The larynx itself is framed and protected by cartilage. The shieldlike thyroid cartilage protects the front of the larynx and forms the Adam's apple. The cricoid ring, a complete circle of cartilage, forms the lower aspect of the larynx and provides structure to the proximal trachea.

The lower airway (Figure 8-3) begins below the larynx and is comprised of the trachea, bronchial passages, and the alveoli. From the glottic opening, air enters the trachea. The trachea is a tube protected by 16 rings of cartilage. These rings provide structure and prevent the trachea from collapsing. The top ring is the cricoid ring, which extends fully 360 degrees around. In the other rings, the cartilage extends only about three-fourths of the way around and is connected posteriorly by smooth muscle. The trachea branches at the *carina* and forms two mainstem bronchi. These large branches then further subdivide to form smaller and smaller air passages called bronchioles. All the air passages are supported by cartilage and are lined with smooth muscle. This smooth muscle allows the bronchioles to change their internal diameter in response to specific stimulation. The bronchioles end at the alveoli. Alveoli are tiny sacs that occur in grapelike bunches at the end of the airway. These alveoli are surrounded by pulmonary capillaries and it is through their thin membranes that oxygen and

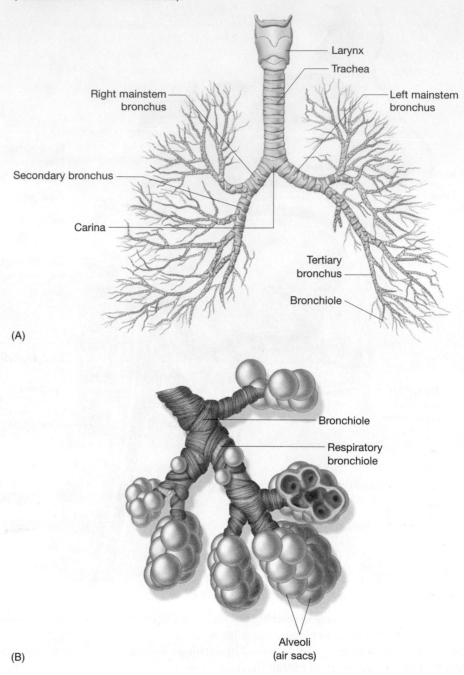

FIGURE 8-3 The lower airway. (A) The bronchial tree. (B) The alveolar sacs (clusters of individual alveoli).

Larynx

Trachea

Right mainstem bronchus

Left mainstem bronchus

Secondary bronchus

Carina

Tertiary bronchus

Bronchiole

(A)

Bronchiole

Respiratory bronchiole

Alveoli (air sacs)

(B)

carbon dioxide are diffused. Gas exchange will be discussed in greater detail in the following chapter.) It is important to remember that the bronchioles divide and travel in every direction. As a result, tiny bronchioles and the millions of alveoli they connect to cover most anatomic regions of the chest from the collarbones to the diaphragm.

AIRWAY PATHOPHYSIOLOGY

CORE CONCEPT

Pathophysiology of the airway

In order for air to make the journey from the nose and mouth to the lungs, the pathway must be relatively unobstructed. A variety of obstructions can interfere with air flow. Foreign bodies like food and small toys are common obstructions, as are fluids including blood and vomit. The airway can also be obstructed by the patient himself. A patent airway requires control of the muscles that form the airway. This is referred to as intact muscle tone. Conditions like altered mental status and neurologic disorders can result in a loss of this muscle tone and lead to collapse of the airway. A common obstruction in a person with a decreased mental status is the tongue—or, more precisely, the epiglottis connected to the tongue. This obstruction occurs when a lack of tone causes the tongue to relax and fall back. When it does, the epiglottis falls back and covers the entrance to the trachea. Often people consider this as the tongue obstructing the airway but, in reality, the epiglottis actually causes the obstruction.

Airway obstruction can occur acutely, as in choking on a foreign body, or it can occur over time. Burns, blunt force trauma, and certain infections can cause swelling of the tissues in and around the glottic opening. This can also impede the movement of air. As such, it is always important to evaluate the patency of an airway not just in the immediate sense but also in an ongoing sense. "Yes, the airway is open now, but will it stay open?"

In the lower airway, smooth muscle can constrict and decrease the internal diameter of the airway. Changing the internal diameter even slightly causes a significant increase in the resistance to air flow and can seriously impact the patient's ability to move air. This is commonly referred to as **bronchoconstriction** or bronchospasm and is common in diseases like asthma.

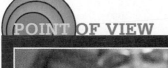

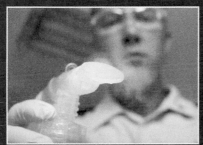

POINT OF VIEW

"It was hissin' and spittin' and smokin' but I know that darn thing saves my life once or twice a month. I have asthma real bad and as hard as I try to take my meds and do the right things it gets away from me. Sometimes it is when I have to run and catch the bus. Other times it is allergy season. Other times I don't know—but I end up in the ambulance and I need my nebs.

"Until recently the EMTs on the ambulance didn't have them. Now they do. Some new law or rule in my state means I can get them from the EMTs instead of waiting until the hospital. That is a good thing."

PATIENT ASSESSMENT

The Airway

There are really two questions you must consider when assessing a patient's airway: "Is the airway open?" and "Will the airway stay open?" (See Table 8-1.)

Is the Airway Open?

You can determine the presence of an airway in most patients by simply saying hello. The patient's ability to speak is an immediate indicator that he is capable of moving air. At the same time, a person who is unable to speak, or one that speaks in an unusually raspy or hoarse voice, may be indicating to you a difficulty moving air. **Stridor** is a high-pitched sound generated from partially obstructed air flow in the upper airway. This sound can be present on inhalation or exhalation (or both) and is an ominous sign of poor air movement. The sounds of breathing from the mouth and nose should be typically free of gurgling, gasping, crowing, wheezing, snoring, and stridor. You may also see patients use position to keep an airway open. When swelling obstructs air flow through the upper airway (typically due to infection), patients may present in the "sniffing position." You will notice a bolt upright position with their head pitched forward as if they were attempting to smell something. In a person with a partially obstructed airway, this position can be critical to keeping air moving.

Often it is not immediately apparent if an airway is present. In your CPR class you learned about the "Look-Listen-Feel" method. If a person is unconscious, you may need to employ this method to ensure an airway is present. In this case, look at the chest to see if it is rising and falling. The airway should also be visually inspected for foreign bodies including objects and fluid. You should listen at the mouth for sounds of breathing while placing your hand on the chest to feel for movement. You may also need to place your hand near the patient's mouth to feel for air flow. In these cases you may detect subtle air movement that might not be apparent with just visual observation.

Remember that you assess the airway as part of the primary assessment and when you find a problem in the primary assessment, you must stop and fix that problem. In this case,

↓ Internal diameter

↑ resistance

bronchoconstriction
(BRON-ko-kun-STRIK-shun)
the contraction of smooth muscle that lines the bronchial passages that results in a decreased internal diameter of the airway and increased resistance to air flow.

CORE CONCEPT
How to recognize an adequate or an inadequate airway

stridor (STRI-dor)
a high pitched sound generated from partially obstructed air flow in the upper airway.

Table 8-1   The Airway in the Primary Assessment – ABC

- Is the airway open?
- Are they able to speak?
- Look
  - Visually inspect the airway to ensure it is free from foreign bodies and obvious trauma
  - Look for visual signs of breathing such as chest rise
- Listen
  - Listen for the sound of breathing
  - Listen for sounds of obstructed air movement such as stridor, snoring, gurgling, and gasping
- Feel
  - Feel for air movement at the mouth
  - Feel the chest for rise and fall
- Will the airway stay open?
  - Are there immediate correctable threats?
  - If no airway, then open it
  - Consider how you might keep open an unstable airway
  - Consider ALS for more definitive airway care
- Are there potential threats that may develop later?
  - Reassess, reassess, reassess
  - Assess for signs of impending collapse such as stridor or voice changes
  - Consider conditions that may later threaten the airway (such as anaphylaxis)

if there is no airway present, stop and provide one. We will discuss airway treatment later in this chapter.)

Will the Airway Stay Open?

The first part of this chapter discussed ensuring an open airway. That is certainly important, but of equal importance now will be ensuring that the airway stays open. Airway assessment is not just a moment in time, but rather a constant consideration, especially in a critical patient. In some cases you may need to immediately consider how to keep an airway open after initially establishing it. In a person with no ability to keep an airway open, you may manually open it with a head-tilt, chin lift. However, the moment you take your hands away, that airway will be lost. At this point you must consider additional steps. Similarly, if you identify a partially obstructed airway, you must ask yourself, "How long will it be until this airway is completely obstructed?" and "What are the necessary steps to take to prevent or resolve this problem?" Consider the following examples:

- You assess the airway of an unconscious victim of a fall off a ladder. He has no airway so you apply the jaw thrust. The airway opens and he begins to breathe. However, when you take your hands away, the airway closes and he stops breathing. In this case the airway is open, but it will not stay open.

- You assess a child after multiple bee stings. He speaks to you with a hoarse voice but is breathing. You note stridor on inspiration. He has an airway, but his voice changes indicate that his airway is swelling and partially obstructing air movement. How long will he be able to move air? What steps must you take immediately to keep air moving?

Remember also that the ability to maintain an airway can change over time. As mental status decreases, so might the ability to protect an airway. Always reassess this capability and remember that just because your patient has an open airway now, there is no guarantee he will continue to have an open airway later.

Signs of an Inadequate Airway

Signs that would indicate no airway or a potentially inadequate airway include the following:

- There are no signs of breathing or air movement.
- There is evidence of foreign bodies in the airway including blood, vomit, or objects like broken teeth.

- No air can be felt or heard at the nose or mouth, or the amount of air exchanged is below normal.
- The patient is unable to speak, or has difficulty speaking.
- The patient has an unusual hoarse or raspy quality to his voice.
- Chest movements are absent, minimal, or uneven.
- Movement associated with breathing is limited to the abdomen (abdominal breathing).
- Breath sounds are diminished or absent.
- Noises such as wheezing, crowing, stridor, snoring, gurgling, or gasping are heard during breathing.
- In children, there may be retractions (a pulling in of the muscles) above the clavicles and between and below the ribs.
- Nasal flaring (widening of the nostrils of the nose with respirations) may be present, especially in infants and children.

CRITICAL DECISION MAKING

Will the Airway Stay Open?

You have learned about the signs of an unstable airway. Use this information to consider whether the following patients have an airway that will "stay open."

1. A 16-year-old asthma patient who tells you he is tired and seems to be nodding off to sleep.

2. A 72-year-old female who was recently diagnosed with pneumonia. Today she has called you because her breathing is much worse. She is breathing rapidly and has diminished lung sounds on the left side.

3. A 35-year-old male who tells you he is having trouble breathing. You notice he is drooling and is sitting bolt upright. When you attempt to lean him back on the stretcher he coughs, gags, and repositions himself in a "sniffing position."

4. A 16-month-old whose mother tells you the child has had a cold for two days and woke up with a cough tonight. The child is awake and alert but barking like a seal when she coughs.

Inside/Outside

THE SOUNDS OF A PARTIALLY OBSTRUCTED AIRWAY

A partially obstructed airway can often be identified by the sounds of limited air movement. Understanding these sounds can help you better understand the pathophysiology of the obstruction.

- **Stridor.** Stridor is typically caused by severely restricted air movement in the upper airway. As air is forced by pressure through a partial obstruction, a high pitched, sometimes almost whistling sound can be heard. Typically stridor indicates a severely narrowed passage of air and suggests near obstruction. In stridor, the obstruction can be a foreign body, such as a toy, or it can be caused by swelling of the upper airway tissues, as in an infection.

- **Hoarseness.** Voice changes, like stridor, often reflect a narrowing of the upper airway passages. Voice changes are often useful in assessing an ongoing airway issue. For example, in a person whose airway is swelling after a burn, you may note a normal voice to begin with, but a raspy voice as the swelling builds up around the vocal cords. The development of hoarseness is often an ominous sign.

- **Snoring.** Snoring is the sound of the soft tissue of the upper airway creating impedance (or partial obstruction) to the flow of air. Many persons normally snore while asleep, but snoring in the case of injury or illness can often indicate a decrease in mental status such that airway muscle tone is diminished. It is also an indication that the airway needs assistance to stay open.

- **Gurgling.** Gurgling is the sound of fluid obstructing the airway. As air is forced through the liquid, the gurgling sound is made. Common liquid obstructions include vomit, blood, and other airway secretions. Gurgling is a sign that immediate suctioning is necessary.

The Airway

When the patient's signs indicate an inadequate airway, a life-threatening condition exists and prompt action must be taken to open and maintain the airway. The following text explains the procedures for opening the airway.

OPENING THE AIRWAY

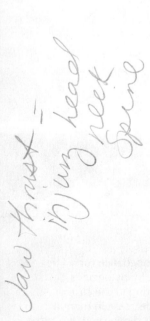

● CORE CONCEPT

How to open an airway

Assessing the airway will be one of the highest priorities of your assessment. When an airway problem is detected, it must be dealt with immediately.

For most patients, the airway can be assessed by simply assessing their speech. In a person with a diminished mental status, other steps may be necessary. In the latter case, the procedures for airway evaluation, opening the airway, and artificial ventilation are best carried out with the patient lying supine (flat on his back). Scan 8-1 illustrates the technique for positioning a patient found lying on the floor or ground. Patients who are found in positions other than supine or on the ground should be moved to a supine position on the floor or stretcher for evaluation and treatment.

Any movement of a trauma (injured) patient before immobilization of the head and spine can produce serious injury to the spinal cord. If injury is suspected, protect the head and neck as you position the patient. Airway and breathing, however, have priority over protection of the spine and must be ensured as quickly as possible. If the trauma patient must be moved in order to open the airway or to provide ventilations, you will probably not have time to provide immobilization with a cervical collar or head immobilization device on a stretcher but, instead, will provide as much manual stabilization as possible.

Use the following as indications that head, neck, or spinal injury may have occurred, especially when the patient is unconscious and cannot tell you what happened:

- Mechanism of injury is one that can cause head, neck, or spine injury. For example, a patient who is found on the ground near a ladder or stairs may have such injuries. Motor-vehicle collisions are another common cause of head, neck, and spine injuries.

- Any injury at or above the level of the shoulders indicates that head, neck, or spine injuries may also be present.

- Family or bystanders may tell you that an injury to the head, neck, or spine has occurred, or they may give you information that leads you to suspect it.

You must open and maintain the airway in any patient who cannot do so for himself. This includes patients who have an altered mental status (including unconsciousness) or who are in respiratory or cardiac arrest. Insertion of an oral or nasal airway and suctioning may be required to maintain a patent airway.

As stated previously, most airway problems are caused by lack of tone in the muscles that keep the airway open. As control over these muscles diminishes, muscles such as the tongue relax and allow the airway to be obstructed. Often position contributes to this problem. As the head flexes forward, the tongue may slide into the airway, causing the epiglottis to obstruct the airway. If the patient is unconscious, the tongue loses muscle tone and muscles of the lower jaw relax. Since the tongue is attached to the lower jaw, the risk of airway obstruction is even greater during unconsciousness. The basic procedures for opening the airway help to correct the position of the tongue and therefore move laryngeal tissues like the epiglottis out of the way of the glottic opening.

Two procedures are commonly recommended for opening the airway: the head-tilt, chin-lift maneuver and the jaw-thrust maneuver, the latter being recommended when head, neck, or spine injury is suspected.

NOTE: *If any indication of head, neck, or spine injury is present, do not use the head-tilt, chin-lift maneuver. (Use the jaw-thrust maneuver instead.) Remember that any unconscious, and many conscious, trauma patients should be suspected of having an injury to the head, neck, or spine.*

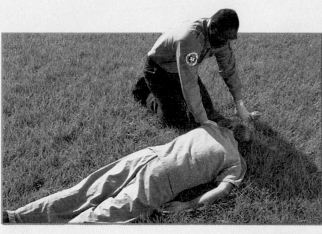

1 Straighten the legs and position the closer arm above the patient's head.

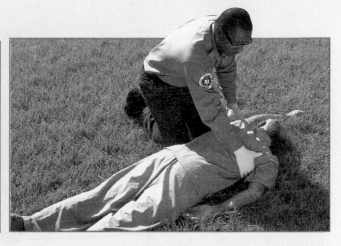

2 Grasp under the distant armpit.

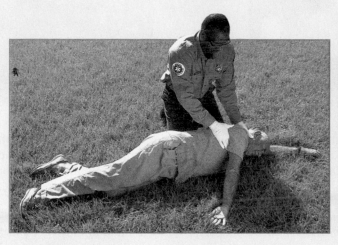

3 Cradle the head and neck, and move the patient as a unit onto his side.

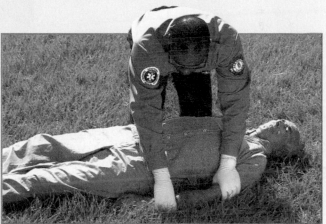

4 Move the patient onto his back and reposition the extended arm.

NOTE: *This maneuver is used when the rescuer must act alone.*

Head-Tilt, Chin-Lift Maneuver

The *head-tilt, chin-lift maneuver* (Figure 8-4) uses head position to align the structures of the airway and provide for the free passage of air. By moving the jaw in an anterior fashion, the tongue is drawn forward, clearing the airway, and with it the tissues of the larynx are moved off the glottic opening.

To perform the head-tilt, chin-lift maneuver, follow these steps:

1. Once the patient is supine, place one hand on the forehead and place the fingertips of the other hand under the bony area at the center of the patient's lower jaw.

2. Tilt the head by applying gentle pressure to the patient's forehead.

3. Use your fingertips to lift the chin and to support the lower jaw. Move the jaw forward to a point where the lower teeth are almost touching the upper teeth. Do not compress the soft tissues under the lower jaw, which can obstruct the airway.

head-tilt, chin-lift maneuver
a means of correcting blockage of the airway by the tongue by tilting the head back and lifting the chin. Used when no trauma, or injury, is suspected.

FIGURE 8-4 Head-tilt, chin-lift maneuver, side view. Inset shows EMT's fingertips under the bony area at the center of the patient's lower jaw.

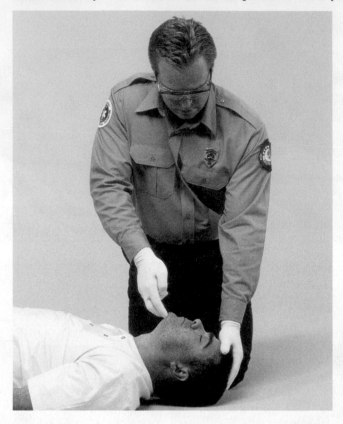
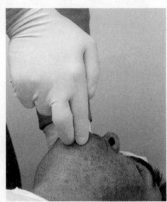

4. Do not allow the patient's mouth to be closed. To provide an adequate opening at the mouth, you may need to use the thumb of the hand supporting the chin to pull back the patient's lower lip. Do not insert your thumb into the patient's mouth (to avoid being bitten).

NOTE: *The jaw-thrust maneuver is the only recommended airway procedure for unconscious patients with possible head, neck, or spine injury or unknown mechanism of injury.*

Jaw-Thrust Maneuver

jaw-thrust maneuver
a means of correcting blockage of the airway by moving the jaw forward without tilting the head or neck. Used when trauma, or injury, is suspected to open the airway without causing further injury to the spinal cord in the neck.

The ***jaw-thrust maneuver*** (Figure 8-5) is most commonly used to open the airway of an unconscious patient with suspected head, neck, or spine injury or unknown mechanism of injury.

NOTE: *The purpose of the jaw-thrust maneuver is to open the airway without moving the head or neck.*

Follow these steps:

1. Carefully keep the patient's head, neck, and spine aligned, moving him as a unit as you place him in the supine position.
2. Kneel at the top of the patient's head. For long-term comfort it may be helpful to rest your elbows on the same surface as the patient's head.
3. Carefully reach forward and gently place one hand on each side of the patient's lower jaw, at the angles of the jaw below the ears.
4. Stabilize the patient's head with your forearms.
5. Using your index fingers, push the angles of the patient's lower jaw forward.
6. You may need to retract the patient's lower lip with your thumb to keep the mouth open.
7. Do not tilt or rotate the patient's head.

FIGURE 8-5 Jaw-thrust maneuver, side view. Inset shows EMT's finger position at angle of the jaw just below the ears.

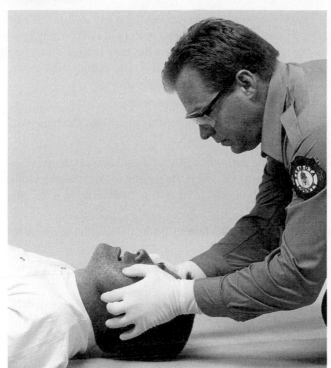
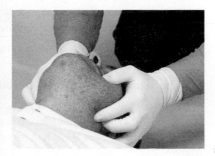

In addition to physically opening the airway with the head-tilt, chin-lift or the jaw-thrust maneuver, it is imperative that the airway also be cleared of any secretions, blood, or vomitus. The most effective way to clear the patient's airway is with a wide-bore, rigid-tip Yankauer suction device. *It is crucial that a suction unit be ready for immediate use when opening and maintaining the airway.* The equipment and techniques used for suctioning will be discussed later in this chapter.

AIRWAY ADJUNCTS

If you determine that your patient does not have a patent airway, you must take action to secure it. The airway must be maintained throughout all care procedures.

The most common impediment to an open airway is a lack of airway muscle tone. When a patient becomes unconscious, the muscles relax. The tongue and tissues of the larynx will slide back into the pharynx and obstruct the airway. Even though a head-tilt, chin-lift or jaw-thrust maneuver will help open a patient's airway, the obstruction may resume once the maneuver is released. Sometimes even when the head-tilt, chin-lift or jaw-thrust is maintained, soft tissues and the tongue may continue to partially obstruct the airway.

Airway adjuncts, devices that aid in maintaining an open airway, may be used to initially assist in the opening of an airway and continually used to help keep an airway open. There are several types of airway adjuncts.

The two most common airway adjuncts, whose main function is to keep the tongue from blocking the airway, are the ***oropharyngeal airway*** (also known as the oral airway or OPA) and the ***nasopharyngeal airway*** (also known as the nasal airway or NPA). The structure and use of these airways can be understood by analyzing their names. *Oro* refers to the mouth, *naso* the nose, and *pharyngeal* the pharynx. Oropharyngeal airways are inserted into the mouth and help properly position the tongue. Nasopharyngeal airways are inserted through the nose and rest in the pharynx, also to help properly position the tongue.

CORE CONCEPT ●
How to use airway adjuncts

oropharyngeal (OR-o-fah-RIN-jul)
airway
a curved device inserted through the patient's mouth into the pharynx to help maintain an open airway.

nasopharyngeal
(NAY-zo-fah-RIN-jul) ***airway***
a flexible breathing tube inserted through the patient's nose into the pharynx to help maintain an open airway.

Rules for Using Airway Adjuncts

Some general rules apply to the use of oropharyngeal and nasopharyngeal airways:

gag reflex
vomiting or retching that results when
something is placed in the back of the
pharynx. This is tied to the swallow
reflex.

- Only use an oropharyngeal airway on patients who do not exhibit a ***gag reflex***. The gag reflex causes vomiting or retching when something is placed in the pharynx. When a patient is deeply unconscious, the gag reflex usually disappears but may reappear as a patient begins to regain consciousness. A patient with a gag reflex who cannot tolerate an oropharyngeal airway may be able to tolerate a nasopharyngeal airway.

- Open the patient's airway manually before using an adjunct device.

- When inserting the airway, take care not to push the patient's tongue into the pharynx.

- Have suction ready prior to inserting any airway.

- Do not continue inserting the airway if the patient begins to gag. Continue to maintain the airway manually and do not use an adjunct device. If the patient remains unconscious for a prolonged time, you may later attempt to insert an airway to determine if the gag reflex is still present.

- When an airway adjunct is in place, you must maintain the head-tilt, chin-lift or jaw-thrust maneuver and monitor the airway.

- After an airway adjunct is in place, continue to be ready to provide suction if the gag reflex returns.

- If the patient regains consciousness or develops a gag reflex, remove the airway immediately.

- Use infection control practices while maintaining the airway. Wear disposable gloves. In airway maintenance, there is a chance of a patient's body fluids coming in contact with your face and eyes. Wear a mask and goggles or other protective eyewear to prevent this contact.

Oropharyngeal Airway

Once a patient's airway is opened, an oropharyngeal airway can be inserted to help keep it open. An oropharyngeal airway is a curved device, usually made of plastic, that can be inserted into the patient's mouth. The oropharyngeal airway has a flange that will rest against the patient's lips. The rest of the device moves the tongue forward as it curves back to the pharynx.

There are standard sizes of oropharyngeal airways (Figure 8-6). Many manufacturers make a complete line, ranging from airways for infants to large adult sizes. An entire set should be carried to allow for quick, proper selection.

The airway adjunct cannot be used effectively unless you select the correct airway size for the patient. To determine the appropriate size oral airway, measure the device from the corner of the patient's mouth to the tip of the earlobe on the same side of the patient's face. An alternative method is to measure from the center of the patient's mouth to the angle of the lower jaw bone. Do not use an airway device unless you have measured it against the patient and verified it as being the proper size. Remember that if an airway is too big, its distal tip will rest close to the esophagus and direct air into the stomach. If it is too small, it will not properly displace the tongue forward to open the airway. If the airway is not the correct size, do not use it on the patient.

FIGURE 8-6 Oropharyngeal airways.

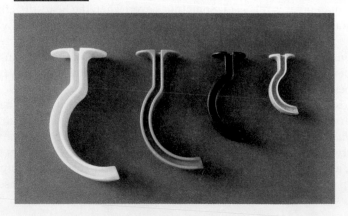

To insert an oropharyngeal airway, follow these steps (Scan 8-2):

1. Place the patient on his back and use an appropriate manual method to open the airway. If no spinal injuries are suspected, use a head-tilt, chin-lift maneuver. If there are possible spinal injuries, use the jaw-thrust maneuver, moving the patient no more than necessary to ensure an open airway (the airway takes priority over the spine).

2. Perform a crossed-finger technique to open the mouth. That is, cross the thumb and forefinger of one hand and place them on the upper and lower teeth at the corner of the patient's mouth. Spread your fingers apart to open the patient's jaws.

3. Position the airway device so that its tip is pointing toward the roof of the patient's mouth.

4. Insert the device and slide it along the roof of the patient's mouth, past the soft tissue hanging down from the back (the uvula), or until you meet resistance against the soft

SCAN 8-2 Inserting an Oropharyngeal Airway

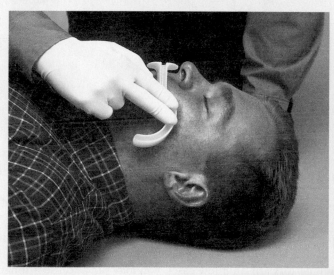

❶ Ensure the oropharyngeal airway is the correct size by checking to make sure it either extends from the center of the mouth to the angle of the jaw or . . .

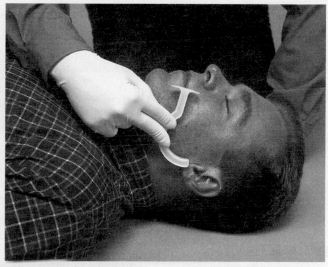

❷ Measure from the corner of the patient's mouth to the tip of the earlobe.

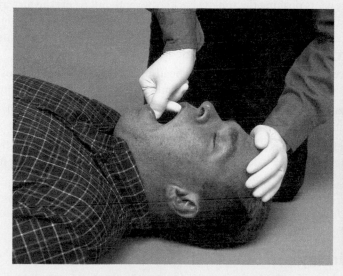

❸ Use the crossed-fingers technique to open the patient's mouth.

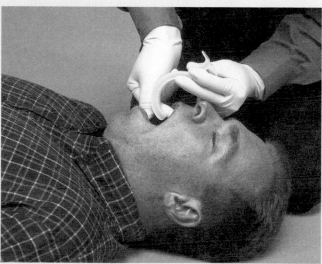

❹ Insert the airway with the tip pointing to the roof of the patient's mouth.

(continued)

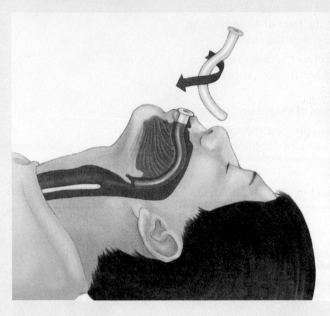
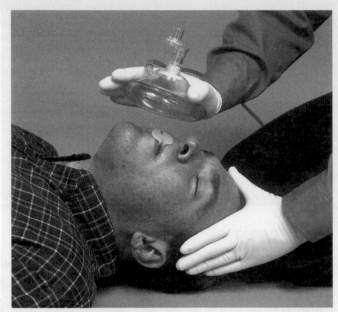

5 Rotate it 180 degrees into position. When the airway is properly positioned, the flange rests against the patient's mouth.

NOTE: *Monitor the patient closely. If there is a gag reflex, remove the airway adjunct at once by following the anatomical curvature. You do not need to rotate the device when removing it.*

palate. Be certain not to push the patient's tongue back into the pharynx. Any airway insertion is made easier by using a tongue blade (tongue depressor) or a rigid suction tip to assist in moving the tongue forward. In a few cases, you may have to use a tongue blade to hold the tongue in place. Watch what you are doing when inserting the airway. This procedure should not be performed by "feel" only.

5. Gently rotate the airway 180 degrees so that the tip is pointing down into the patient's pharynx. This method prevents pushing the tongue back. Alternatively, insert the airway with the tip already pointing "down" toward the patient's pharynx, using a tongue depressor or rigid suction tip to press the tongue down and forward to avoid obstructing the airway. *This is the preferred method for airway insertion in an infant or child.*

6. Position the patient. Place the nontrauma patient in a head-tilt position. If there are possible spine injuries, maintain cervical stabilization at all times during airway management.

7. Check to see that the flange of the airway is against the patient's lips. If the airway device is too long or too short, remove it and replace it with the correct size.

8. Monitor the patient closely. If there is a gag reflex, remove the airway adjunct at once by following the anatomical curvature. You do not need to rotate the device when removing it.

NOTE: *Some EMS systems allow an oropharyngeal airway to be inserted with the tip pointing to the side of the patient's mouth. The device is then rotated 90 degrees so that its tip is pointing down the patient's pharynx. Use this approach only if it is part of the protocol of your EMS system.*

Nasopharyngeal Airway

The nasopharyngeal airway has gained popularity because it often does not stimulate the gag reflex. This allows the nasopharyngeal airway to be used in patients who have a reduced level of responsiveness but still have an intact gag reflex. Other benefits include the fact that it can be used when the teeth are clenched and when there are oral injuries.

Use the soft flexible nasal airway and not the rigid clear plastic airway in the field. The soft ones are less likely to cause soft-tissue damage or bleeding. The typical sizes for adults are 34, 32, 30, and 28 French.

To insert a nasopharyngeal airway, follow these steps (Scan 8-3):

1. Measure the nasopharyngeal airway from the patient's nostril to the tip of the earlobe or to the angle of the jaw. Choosing the correct length will ensure an appropriate diameter.

2. Lubricate the outside of the tube with a water-based lubricant before insertion. Do not use a petroleum jelly or any other type of non-water-based lubricant. Such substances can damage the tissue lining of the nasal cavity and the pharynx and increase the risk of infection.

3. Gently push the tip of the nose upward. Keep the patient's head in a neutral position. Most nasopharyngeal airways are designed to be placed in the right nostril. The bevel

SCAN 8-3 Inserting a Nasopharyngeal Airway

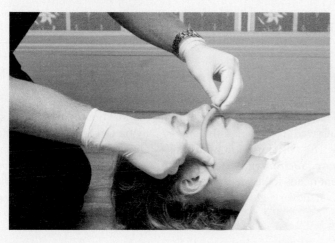

① Measure the nasopharyngeal airway from the patient's nostril to the tip of the earlobe or to the angle of the jaw.

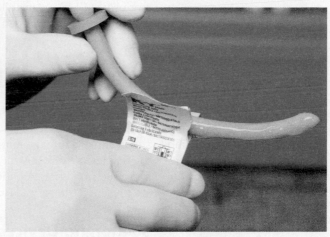

② Apply a water-based lubricant before insertion.

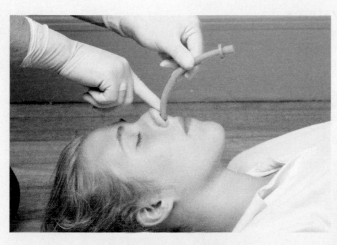

③ Gently push the tip of the nose upward, and insert the airway with the beveled side toward the base of the nostril or toward the septum (wall that separates the nostrils). Insert the airway, advancing it until the flange rests against the nostril.

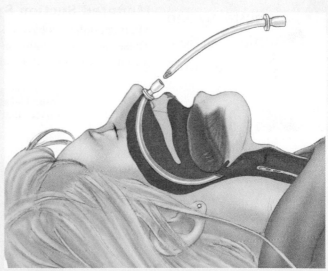

④ Never force a nasopharyngeal airway. If you experience difficulty advancing the airway, pull the tube out and try the other nostril.

(angled portion at the tip) should point toward the base of the nostril or toward the septum (wall that separates the nostrils).

4. Insert the airway into the nostril. Gently advance the airway until the flange rests firmly against the patient's nostril. Never force a nasopharyngeal airway. If you experience difficulty advancing the airway, pull the tube out and try the other nostril.

Oropharyngeal and nasopharyngeal airways can be a tremendous asset to the EMT when used properly. However, no device can replace the EMT. The proper use of these airways or any other device depends on the appropriate use, good judgment, and adequate monitoring of the patient by the EMT.

NOTE: *Do not use a nasopharyngeal airway if clear (cerebrospinal) fluid is coming from the nose or ears. This may indicate a skull fracture where the airway would pass.*

Oropharyngeal and nasopharyngeal airways help move soft tissue of the upper airway to provide clear passage for air. To ensure an open airway to the level of the lungs, it is sometimes necessary to insert an endotracheal (through-the-trachea) tube. Endotracheal intubation is an advanced-life-support procedure in which EMTs may assist advanced-level providers. Furthermore, some EMS systems allow for the use of blind insertion airway devices. These devices and procedures will be discussed in Chapter 9, "Respiration and Artificial Ventilation."

SUCTIONING

suctioning (SUK-shun-ing) use of a vacuum device to remove blood, vomitus, and other secretions or foreign materials from the airway.

"Aspiration kills. Watch that airway constantly and suction, suction, suction."

The patient's airway must be kept clear of foreign materials, blood, vomitus, and other secretions. Materials that are allowed to remain in the airway may be forced into the trachea and eventually into the lungs. This will cause complications ranging from severe pneumonia to complete airway obstruction. *Suctioning* is the method of using a vacuum device to remove such materials. A patient needs to be suctioned immediately when fluids or secretions are present in the airway or whenever a gurgling sound is heard.

Suctioning Devices

Each suction unit consists of a suction source, a collection container for materials you suction, tubing, and suction tips or catheters. Systems are either mounted in the ambulance or are portable and may be brought to the scene.

Mounted Suction Systems

Many ambulances have a suction unit mounted in the patient compartment (Figure 8-7). These units are usually installed near the head of the stretcher so they are easily used. Mounted systems, often called "on-board" units, create a suctioning vacuum produced by

FIGURE 8-7 A mounted suction unit installed in the ambulance's patient compartment.

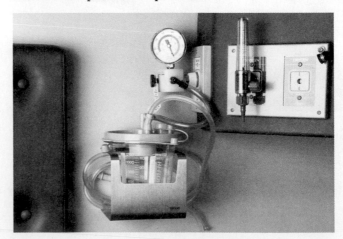

FIGURE 8-8 (A) Oxygen-powered portable suction unit, (B) battery-powered portable unit, and (C) manually operated unit.

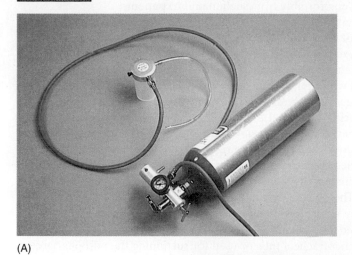

(A)

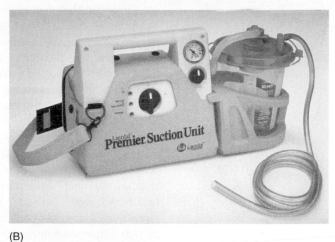

(B)

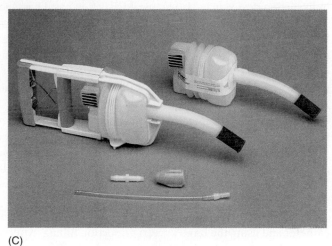

(C)

the engine's manifold or an electrical power source. To be effective, suction devices must furnish an air intake of at least 30 liters per minute at the open end of a collection tube. This will occur if the system can generate a vacuum of no less than 300 mmHg (millimeters of mercury) when the collecting tube is clamped.

Portable Suction Units

There are many different types of portable suction units (Figure 8-8). They may be oxygen- or air-powered, electrically powered (by batteries or household current), or manually operated. The requirement for the amount of suction a portable unit must provide is identical to that of the fixed unit (30 liters per minute, 300 mmHg). It is important to have the ability to suction anywhere. Portable suction devices provide that ability.

Tubing, Tips, and Catheters

For suctioning to be effective, the proper equipment must be used. Although a suction unit might be the most powerful available, it will do no good unless used with the proper attachments. Before operating a suction unit, you must have:

- Tubing
- Suction tips
- Suction catheters
- Collection container
- Container of clean or sterile water

The *tubing* attached to a suction unit must be thick-walled, nonkinking, wide-bore tubing. This is because the tubing must not collapse due to the suction, must allow "chunks" of suctioned material to pass, and must not kink, which would reduce the suction. The tubing must be long enough to reach comfortably from suction unit to patient.

Currently, the most popular type of *suction tip* is the rigid pharyngeal tip, also called "Yankauer," "tonsil sucker," or "tonsil-tip" suction. This rigid device allows you to suction the mouth and pharynx with excellent control over the distal end of the device. It also has a larger bore than flexible catheters. Most successfully used with an unresponsive patient, rigid-tip suction must be used with caution, especially if the patient is not completely unresponsive or may be regaining consciousness. When the tip is placed into the pharynx, the gag reflex may be activated, producing additional vomiting. It is also possible to stimulate the vagus nerve in the back of the pharynx, which can slow the heart rate. Therefore, be careful not to suction more than a few seconds at a time with a rigid tip and never lose sight of the tip.

Suction catheters are flexible plastic tubes. They come in various sizes identified by a number "French." The larger the number, the larger the catheter. A "14 French" catheter is larger than an "8 French" catheter. These catheters are usually not large enough to suction vomitus or thick secretions and may kink. Flexible catheters are designed to be used in situations when a rigid tip cannot be used. For example, a soft catheter can be passed through a tube such as a nasopharyngeal or endotracheal tube or used for suctioning the nasopharynx. (A bulb suction device may also be used to suction nasal passages.)

Another important part of a suction device is the *collection container*. All units should have a nonbreakable container to collect the suctioned materials. These containers must be easily removed for disposal or decontamination. Remember to wear gloves, protective eyewear, and a mask not only while suctioning but also while cleaning the equipment. Most modern suction devices have disposable containers to eliminate the time and risks involved in decontamination.

Suction units also must have a *container of clean (preferably sterile) water* nearby. This water is used to clear matter that is partially blocking the tubing. When this partial blockage of the tube occurs, place the suction tip or catheter in the container of water. This will cause a stream of water to flow through the tip and tubing, usually forcing the clog to dislodge. When the tip or tubing becomes clogged with an item that will not dislodge, replace it with a new tip or tubing.

In the event of copious, thick secretions or vomiting, consider removing the rigid tip or catheter and using the large bore, rigid suction tubing. After you are finished, place the standard tip back on for further suctioning.

Techniques of Suctioning

Although there may be some variations in suction technique (a suggested technique is shown in Scan 8-4), a few rules always apply. *The first rule is always use appropriate infection control practices while suctioning.* These practices include the use of protective eyewear, mask, and disposable gloves. Proper suctioning requires you to have your fingers around and sometimes inside the patient's mouth. Disposable gloves prevent contact between the EMT and the patient's bodily fluids. Protective eyewear and mask are also recommended since these fluids might splatter, or the patient may gag or cough, sending droplets to your face, eyes, and mouth.

The second rule is to try limiting suctioning to no longer than 10 seconds at a time. This is because prolonged suctioning will cause hypoxia and, potentially, death. If the patient continues to vomit longer than 10 seconds, however, you must still continue to suction. Ventilating foreign matter into the lungs will also cause hypoxia and possible death. In short, suction quickly and efficiently for as short a time as possible.

Patients who need airway control and suctioning are often unconscious and may be in cardiac or respiratory arrest. Oxygen delivery to this patient is very important. During suctioning, the ventilations or other methods of oxygen delivery are discontinued to allow for the passage of the suction catheter. To prevent critical delays in oxygen delivery, limit suctioning to a few seconds, then resume ventilations or oxygen delivery.

In a few cases you will preoxygenate a patient before suctioning. This means that you will adequately ventilate the patient with supplemental oxygen before suctioning, because oxygen levels will drop during suctioning; for example, during routine suctioning of an endotracheal tube. If you come upon a patient with vomitus or other materials in his airway, or if a patient

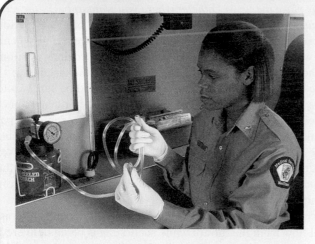

1 Turn the unit on, attach a catheter, and test for suction at the beginning of your shift.

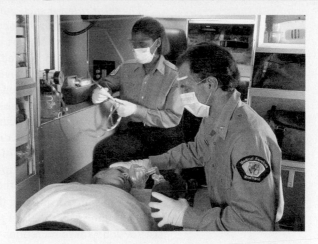

2 Position yourself at the patient's head and turn the patient's head or entire body to the side.

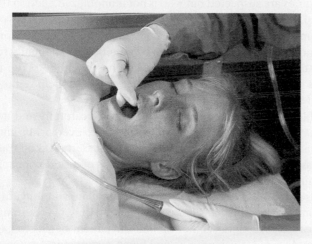

3 Open and clear the patient's mouth.

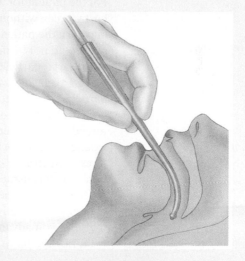

4 Place the convex side of the rigid tip against the roof of the mouth. Insert just to the base of the tongue.

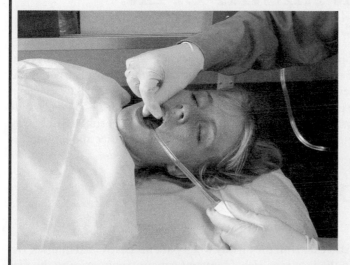

5 Apply suction only after the rigid tip is in place. Do not lose sight of the tip while suctioning. Suction while withdrawing the tip.

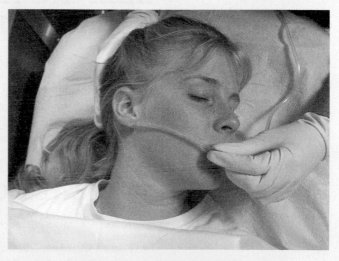

If you are using a flexible catheter, measure it from the patient's earlobe to the corner of the mouth or from the center of the mouth to the angle of the jaw.

vomits suddenly and unexpectedly, you should suction immediately, *without* preoxygenation. In these cases, preoxygenation would force foreign substances into the lungs, which can be fatal.

The third rule for suctioning is place the tip or catheter where you want to begin the suctioning and suction on the way out. Most suction tips and catheters do not produce suction at all times. You have to start the suctioning. The tip or catheter will have an open distal end where the suction is delivered. It will also have an opening, or port, in the proximal portion. When you put your finger over the proximal port, suctioning begins from the distal end.

It is not necessary to measure when using a rigid tip. Rather, you should be sure not to lose sight of the tip when inserting it. However, do measure the suction catheter in a manner similar to an oropharyngeal airway. The length of catheter that should be inserted into the patient's mouth is equal to the distance between the corner of the patient's mouth and earlobe.

Carefully bring the tip of the catheter to the area where suctioning is needed. Never "jab" or force the suction tip into the mouth or pharynx. Then place your finger over the proximal opening to begin the suctioning, and suction as you slowly withdraw the tip from the patient's mouth, moving the tip from side to side.

Suctioning is best delivered with the patient turned on his side. This allows gravity to assist suction as free secretions will flow from the mouth while suctioning is being delivered. Caution must be used in patients with suspected neck or spine injuries. If the patient is fully and securely immobilized, the entire backboard may be tilted to place the patient on his side. For the patient for whom such injuries are suspected but who is not immobilized, suction the best you can without turning the patient. If all other methods have failed, as a last resort you may turn the patient's body as a unit, attempting to keep the neck and spine in line. Suctioning should not be delayed to immobilize a patient. It may also be beneficial to manually remove large particles prior to or during suctioning. As always, caution should be taken in placing your fingers in a patient's mouth. However, a shallow sweep will often help remove particles not able to be suctioned through the lumen of the suction device.

The rigid suction tip or flexible catheter should be moved into place carefully and not forced. Rigid suction devices may cause tissue damage and bleeding. Never probe into wounds or attempt to suction away attached tissue with a suction device. Certain skull fractures may actually cause brain tissue to be visible in the pharynx. If this occurs, do not suction near this tissue; limit suctioning to the mouth.

Suction devices may also cause activation of the gag reflex and stimulate vomiting. In a patient who already has secretions that need to be suctioned, vomiting only makes things worse. If you advance a suction catheter or rigid suction tip and the patient begins to gag, withdraw the tip to a position that does not cause gagging and begin suctioning.

KEEPING AN AIRWAY OPEN: DEFINITIVE CARE

At times keeping an airway open will exceed the capabilities of the basic EMT. Medications and/or surgical procedures may be necessary to resolve the cause of airway obstruction. As an EMT you should rapidly evaluate and treat airway problems, but also quickly recognize the need for more definitive care. In some systems definitive care may be an advanced life support intercept. In other systems, definitive care might be the closest hospital. Either way, you must know your local system resources and recognize your capabilities and limitations.

SPECIAL CONSIDERATIONS

There are a number of special considerations in airway management:

- **Facial injuries.** Take extra care with the airway when patients have facial injuries. Because the blood supply to the face is so rich, blunt and penetrating injuries to the face frequently result in severe swelling or bleeding that may block or partially block the airway. Frequent suctioning may be required. Insertion of an airway adjunct or endotracheal tube may be necessary.

- **Obstructions.** Many suction units are not adequate for removing solid objects like teeth and large particles of food or other foreign objects. These must be removed using manual techniques for clearing airway obstructions, such as abdominal thrusts, chest thrusts, or finger sweeps, which you learned in your basic life support course and which are reviewed in Appendix A, "Basic Cardiac Life Support Review," at the back of this book. You may need to log roll the patient into a supine position to clear the oropharynx manually.

- **Dental appliances.** Dentures should ordinarily be left in place during airway procedures. Partial dentures may become dislodged during an emergency. Leave a partial denture in place if possible, but be prepared to remove it if it endangers the airway.

PEDIATRIC NOTE

There are several special considerations that you must take into account when managing the airway of an infant or child (Figure 8-9):

Anatomic Considerations

- The mouth and nose of infants and children are smaller and more easily obstructed than those of adults.
- In infants and children, the tongue takes up more space proportionately in the mouth than in adults.
- The trachea (windpipe) is softer and more flexible in infants and children.
- The trachea is narrower and is easily obstructed by swelling.
- The chest wall is softer, and infants and children tend to depend more on their diaphragm for breathing.

Management Considerations

- Open the airway gently. Infants can be placed in a neutral neck position and children only require slight extension of the neck. Do not hyperextend the neck, because it may collapse the trachea.
- An oral or nasal airway may be considered when other measures fail to keep the airway open.
- In suctioning infants and children, use a rigid tip but be careful not to touch the back of the airway.

FIGURE 8-9 Comparison of child and adult respiratory passages.

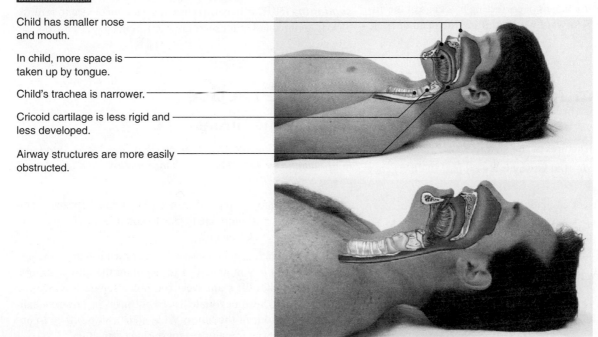

Child has smaller nose and mouth.

In child, more space is taken up by tongue.

Child's trachea is narrower.

Cricoid cartilage is less rigid and less developed.

Airway structures are more easily obstructed.

Key Facts and Concepts

- The airway is the passageway by which air enters the body during respiration, or breathing.
- A patient cannot survive without an open airway.
- Airway adjuncts—the oropharyngeal and nasopharyngeal airway—can help keep the airway open.

- It may be necessary to suction the airway or to use manual techniques to remove fluids and solids from the airway before, during, or after artificial ventilation

Key Decisions

- Is the airway open?
- Will the airway stay open?

- Do I need to suction the airway?
- Do I need an adjunct to keep the airway open?

Chapter Glossary

airway the passageway by which air enters or leaves the body. The structures of the airway are the nose, mouth, pharynx, larynx, trachea, bronchi, and lungs. *See also* patent airway.

bronchoconstriction (BRON-ko-kun-STRIK-shun) the contraction of smooth muscle that lines the bronchial passages that results in a decreased internal diameter of the airway and increased resistance to air flow.

gag reflex vomiting or retching that results when something is placed in the back of the pharynx. This is tied to the swallow reflex.

head-tilt, chin-lift maneuver a means of correcting blockage of the airway by the tongue by tilting the head back and lifting the chin. Used when no trauma, or injury, is suspected.

jaw-thrust maneuver a means of correcting blockage of the airway by moving the jaw forward without tilting the head or neck.

Used when trauma, or injury, is suspected to open the airway without causing further injury to the spinal cord in the neck.

nasopharyngeal (NAY-zo-fah-RIN-jul) *airway* a flexible breathing tube inserted through the patient's nostril into the pharynx to help maintain an open airway.

oropharyngeal (OR-o-fah-RIN-jul) *airway* a curved device inserted through the patient's mouth into the pharynx to help maintain an open airway.

patent airway an airway (passage from nose or mouth to lungs) that is open and clear and will remain open and clear, without interference to the passage of air into and out of the body.

stridor (STRI-dor) a high pitched sound generated from partially obstructed air flow in the upper airway.

suctioning (SUK-shun-ing) use of a vacuum device to remove blood, vomitus, and other secretions or foreign materials from the airway.

Preparation for Your Examination and Practice

Short Answer

1. Name the main structures of the airway.
2. Explain why care for the airway is a vital part of emergency care.
3. Describe the signs of an inadequate airway.
4. Explain when the head-tilt, chin-lift maneuver should be used and when the jaw-thrust maneuver should be used to open the airway—and why.
5. Explain how airway adjuncts and suctioning help in airway management.

Thinking and Linking

Think back to Chapter 3, "Lifting and Moving Patients," and link information from that chapter with information from this chapter as you consider the following questions:

1. You are treating a patient with a spine injury who is immobilized on a backboard. He begins to vomit. In addition to suctioning, what do you do?
2. You are treating an unconscious patient with an unsecure airway. Thus far, you have had to maintain the airway using a head-tilt, chin-lift maneuver. You now prepare to move the patient and must negotiate a series of turns in a narrow hallway to get out of the house. What steps can you take to ensure the airway remains patent during extrication?

Critical Thinking Exercises

Airway assessment is a critical skill. The purpose of this exercise will be to consider how you might assess and manage patients with signs of an airway problem.

1. On arrival at the emergency scene, you find an adult female patient with gurgling sounds in the throat and inadequate breathing slowing to almost nothing. How do you proceed to protect the airway?

2. When evaluating a small child you hear stridor. What does this sound tell you? What are your immediate concerns regarding this sound?

3. When assessing an unconscious patient, you note snoring respirations. Should you be concerned with this and, if so, what steps can you take to correct this situation?

Pathophysiology to Practice

The following questions are designed to assist you in gathering relevant clinical information and making accurate decisions in the field.

- Describe the signs of a partially obstructed airway
- Describe how an altered mental status might impact the airway of your patient.
- Describe why trauma to the neck might be both an immediate and an ongoing threat to the airway.

Street Scenes

"Control to unit 144," your radio blurts out. You respond, "Go ahead, control." Dispatch tells you that you have a priority-one response to a man down, age unknown, found on the corner of Salina and Jefferson Street. Dispatch also notes that prearrival questioning indicates the patient is not breathing. Brian, your partner, drives, and while en route you make sure that you have a plan. Brian will take the lead. When he pulls up to the scene, a frantic bystander is waving his arms. He points to a man lying on the ground who is not moving.

Street Scene Questions

1. What is your first priority when starting to assess this patient?
2. What type of emergency care should you be prepared to give?
3. What equipment should you proceed into the scene with?

As you approach, you observe a middle-aged man lying left lateral recumbent on the ground. The bystanders tell you they just found him and don't know how he got there. Your scene survey reveals no obvious trauma or bleeding. You address the patient in a loud voice but he does not respond.

Street Scene Questions

4. After assuring the scene is safe, what are your immediate assessment priorities?
5. Describe the steps involved in assessing the airway of this unresponsive patient.

Brian assists you in rolling the patient supine. Because you are unsure about the mechanism of injury, you maintain spinal precautions. You observe gurgling and snoring respirations. The patient has some chest rise, but there appears to be a substantial amount of vomit present in his airway.

Street Scene Questions

6. What immediate actions must be taken to clear the airway?
7. Once the airway has been cleared, describe how you might open the airway.

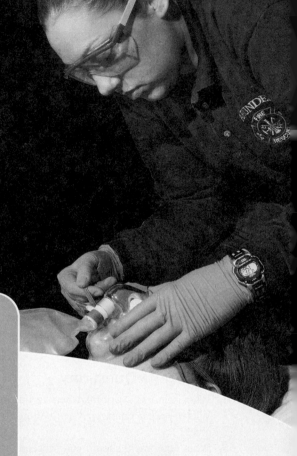

9

Respiration and Artificial Ventilation

⟳ **STANDARD**
Airway Management, Respiration, and Artificial Ventilation
(Respiration, Artificial Ventilation)

⟳ **COMPETENCY**
Applies knowledge (fundamental depth, foundational breadth) of general
anatomy and physiology to patient assessment and management in order to
assure a patent airway, adequate mechanical ventilation, and respiration for
patients of all ages.

⟳ **CORE CONCEPTS**
— Physiology and pathophysiology of the respiratory system

— How to recognize adequate and inadequate breathing

— Principles and techniques of positive pressure ventilation

— Principles and techniques of oxygen administration

EXPLORE Resource⊙entral

To access Resource Central, follow directions on the Student Access Card provided
with this text. If there is no card, go to **www.bradybooks.com** and follow the
Resource Central link to Buy Access from there. Under Media Resources, you will find:

▶ **Effective BVM Ventilations**
Learn how to give effective BVM ventilations, how to properly position a patient's
head and why it is important to have the proper mask size.

▶ **Oxygen Delivery Devices**
See a video on different types of oxygen delivery devices. Who knew there were
so many choices? Learn the flow rates and oxygen delivery amounts associated
with each device as well as the pros and cons of these devices.

▶ **King Airway Insertion**
Watch this video to learn how to insert a King airway and what you should do
directly after insertion of this device.

 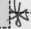

OBJECTIVES

After reading this chapter you should be able to:

9.1 Define key terms introduced in this chapter.

9.2 Explain the physiological relationship between
assessing and maintaining an open airway,
assessing and ensuring adequate ventilation,
and assessing and maintaining adequate
circulation. (pp. 198–201)

9.3 Describe the mechanics of ventilation. (pp. 198–199)

9.4 Explain mechanisms that control the depth and
rate of ventilation. (pp. 198–199)

9.5 Explain the relationships between tidal volume,
respiratory rate, minute volume, dead air space,
and alveolar ventilation. (pp. 198–199)

9.6 Describe the physiology of external and internal
respiration. (p. 199)

KEY TERMS

alveolar ventilation, *p. 199*
artificial ventilation, *p. 208*
cellular respiration, *p. 199*
cricoid pressure, *p. 215*

cyanosis, *p. 206*
diffusion, *p. 199*
hypoxia, *p. 201*
positive pressure ventilation, *p. 208*

pulmonary respiration, *p. 199*
respiration, *p. 201*
respiratory arrest, *p. 202*
respiratory distress, *p. 201*

respiratory failure, *p. 201*
stoma, *p. 215*
ventilation, *p. 198*

By securing the airway, you provide an open pathway for air to move into and out of the body, as we discussed in Chapter 8, "Airway Management." However, a patent airway does not guarantee that the air will move, and it certainly does not guarantee that air will move in adequate volumes to support life. To ensure this, the EMT must assess breathing, or the "B" of the ABCs.

Recall that breathing accomplishes two essential functions: It brings oxygen into the body and it eliminates carbon dioxide. Although your body will tolerate the buildup of carbon dioxide longer than it will tolerate a lack of oxygen, both of these functions are absolutely necessary to support life.

Proper airway management must always be paired with the assessment of adequate breathing to ensure that both of these critical functions are occurring. If you determine that the patient's breathing is not meeting the body's needs, then you must take immediate corrective action. A thorough primary assessment focuses on a rapid evaluation of both airway *and* breathing and identifies immediate life threats associated with the airway and the respiratory system.

In this chapter, you will learn the skills necessary to correct inadequate breathing. However, it is just as important to learn the decision-making process that will tell you when to employ those skills. You must learn not just "how to" but, equally important, "when to" assist a patient with breathing.

PHYSIOLOGY AND PATHOPHYSIOLOGY

Mechanics of Breathing

----------● CORE CONCEPT

Physiology and pathophysiology of the respiratory system

ventilation

breathing in and out (inhalation and exhalation), or artificial provision of breaths.

Air is moved into and out of the chest in a process called *ventilation*. To move air, the diaphragm and the muscles of the chest are contracted and relaxed to change the pressure within the chest cavity. This changing pressure inflates and deflates the lungs. *Inhalation* is an active process. The muscles of the chest, including the intercostal muscles between the ribs, expand at the same time the diaphragm contracts in a downward motion. These movements increase the size of the chest cavity and create a negative pressure. This negative pressure pulls air in through the glottic opening and inflates the lungs. Conversely, *exhalation* is a passive process. That is, it occurs when the previously discussed muscles relax. As the size of the chest decreases, it creates a positive pressure and pushes air out. Because it is passive, exhalation typically takes slightly longer than inhalation.

As we discussed in Chapter 6, "Principles of Pathophysiology," the amount of air moved in one breath (one cycle of inhalation and exhalation) is called *tidal volume*. A normal tidal volume is typically 5–7 mL per kg of body weight. The amount of air moved into and out of the lungs per minute is called *minute volume*. Minute volume is calculated by multiplying the tidal volume and the respiratory rate ($MV = TV \times RR$).

Recall that ventilation (inhalation and exhalation) is ultimately designed to move air to and from the alveoli for gas exchange. However, as noted in Chapter 6, "Principles of Pathophysiology," not all the air we breathe reaches the alveoli. For example, a 100-kg adult has an average tidal volume of roughly 500 mL. Of that 500 mL, only about 350 mL reaches the alveoli. The remainder occupies the trachea, bronchioles, and other parts of the airway, the area known as *dead air space* (Figure 9-1). The alveoli are the only place where oxygen and

FIGURE 9-1 Dead air space: areas of the airway outside the alveoli.

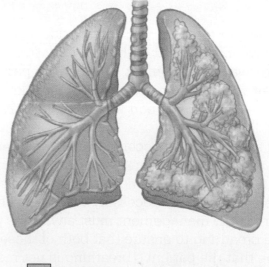

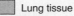 Lung tissue

Dead space (trachea and bronchi)

Alveoli/gas exchange areas

carbon dioxide are exchanged with the bloodstream; therefore, the air in the dead space contributes nothing to oxygenating the body. The term *alveolar ventilation* refers to how much air actually reaches the alveoli.

Of course, alveolar ventilation depends very much on tidal volume. Consider the following example:

An asthma patient has a normal tidal volume of 500 mL. Today, however, because his asthma attack has constricted his bronchiole tubes, he can move only 300 mL of tidal volume. If the air in the dead space remains constant at 150 mL, then only 150 mL of air reaches his alveoli per breath.

- Normal tidal volume: 500 mL $\times$ 16 breaths per minute = 8,000 mL
- Normal alveolar ventilation: 350 mL (500–150 dead space air) $\times$16 bpm = 5,600 mL
- Asthma attack tidal volume: 300 mL $\times$ 16 bpm = 4,800 mL
- Asthma attack alveolar ventilation: 150 mL (300–150 dead air space) $\times$ 16 bpm = 2,400 mL

Remember that alveolar ventilation can be altered through changes in rate as well as by changes in volume. A person breathing too slowly will have a decreased minute volume, so the amount of air reaching the alveoli per minute is decreased, just as it would be decreased by a reduction in tidal volume.

- Normal minute volume: 500 mL $\times$ 16 breaths per minute = 8,000 mL
- Slowed minute volume: 500 mL $\times$ 8 breaths per minute = 4,000 mL

Occasionally, very fast respiratory rates may decrease minute volume as well, not primarily because of rate but because the faster rate can affect the tidal volume. Fast breathing can, at times, limit the amount of time the lungs have to fill and therefore decrease tidal volume. Even though increasing the rate should increase minute volumes, exceptionally fast breathing will actually reduce minute volume and alveolar ventilation.

Physiology of Respiration

Inhaled air fills the alveoli. The pulmonary capillaries bring circulating blood to the outside of these tiny air sacs, where the thin walls of the alveoli and the thin walls of the capillaries allow oxygen from the air in the alveoli to move into the blood to circulate throughout the body. The thin walls of the capillaries and alveoli also allow carbon dioxide to move from the blood into the alveoli to be expelled during exhalation.

The movement of gases from an area of high concentration to an area of low concentration is called *diffusion*. The diffusion of oxygen and carbon dioxide that takes place between the *alveoli* and circulating blood is called *pulmonary respiration*. Carbon dioxide is off-loaded from the blood into alveoli, while oxygen from the air in the alveoli is loaded onto the hemoglobin of the blood and transported to the cells. At the cells, through a similar but reversed process of diffusion, oxygen passes from the blood, across cell membranes, and into the cells, while carbon dioxide from the cells passes into the blood. The diffusion of oxygen and carbon dioxide that takes place between the *cells* and circulating blood is called *cellular respiration* (Figure 9-2).

Remember: For this entire process to be working, the respiratory system must be appropriately matched up with a functioning cardiovascular system. The respiratory system must be moving air in and out of the alveoli and the circulatory system must be transporting adequate amounts of blood between the cells and the alveoli. These two systems working in concert are often referred to as the *cardiopulmonary system* and also referred to as a ventilation-perfusion (V/Q) match, as was discussed in Chapter 6, "Principles of Pathophysiology." When either of these systems fails, the process of respiration is defeated.

Pathophysiology of the Cardiopulmonary System

Before proceeding, take a few minutes to review the concepts of pathophysiology of the cardiopulmonary system that were discussed in detail in Chapter 6.

FIGURE 9-2 The processes of pulmonary and cellular respiration.

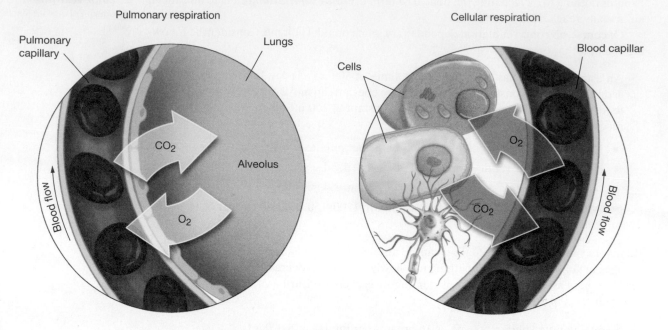

Consider the following mechanical failures of the cardiopulmonary system that may occur:

- **Mechanics of breathing disrupted.** If the chest cannot create the necessary pressure changes, air cannot be moved in and out of the lungs. Breathing can be disrupted by a variety of causes, such as:
  - *A patient stabbed in the chest.* When the diaphragm moves downward, air is pulled into the chest cavity through the stab wound in addition to the normal drawing in of air through the glottic opening. Because of the air rushing into the chest through the stab wound, a negative pressure cannot be created to efficiently pull air into the lungs through the normal airway passages.
  - *A patient loses nervous control of respiration.* A patient may lose the ability to transmit messages through nerve tissue to innervate the muscles of respiration. This can occur in diseases like muscular dystrophy and multiple sclerosis.
  - *A patient sustains painful chest wall injuries.* Pain and physical damage can both limit chest wall movement.
  - *A patient has airway problems such as bronchoconstriction.* If air cannot move, breathing cannot occur. Some diseases like asthma and chronic obstructive pulmonary disease (COPD) can cause bronchial tubes to decrease in diameter and limit the amount of air that can flow through them.

- **Gas exchange interrupted.** Sometimes the ability to diffuse oxygen and carbon dioxide is impaired. Consider the following examples:
  - *Low oxygen levels in the outside air such as in confined space rescue situations.* Here there simply is not enough oxygen in the air breathed in.
  - *Diffusion problems.* Some diseases like congestive heart failure and COPD can limit the ability of alveoli to exchange oxygen and carbon dioxide. Here oxygenated air and blood reach the alveoli, but the alveoli themselves are not working.

- **Circulation issues.** There can be problems that prevent the blood from carrying enough oxygen to the body's cells, such as:
  - *Not enough blood.* If a person has lost a significant amount of blood, not enough blood can be circulated to the alveoli. If blood is not present at the interface with the alveoli, oxygen and carbon dioxide cannot be exchanged.
  - *Hemoglobin problems.* Occasionally respiration can be impaired if there is not enough hemoglobin, the oxygen-binding protein in the blood. For example, anemia is a disease that causes low amounts of hemoglobin in the blood. In other situations,

as with a patient whose body pH becomes very acidotic, sufficient hemoglobin may be present but may have a difficulty in holding oxygen. When hemoglobin fails, oxygen cannot be transported.

RESPIRATION

respiration (RES-pir-AY-shun) the diffusion of oxygen and carbon dioxide between the alveoli and the blood (pulmonary respiration) and between the blood and the cells (cellular respiration). Also used to mean, simply, breathing.

As just discussed, *ventilation* is the term properly applied to the process of inhaling and exhaling, or breathing, whereas **respiration** refers to the exchange of gases between the alveoli and the blood (external respiration) and between the blood and the cells (internal respiration). However, in common speech, and in an overall sense, *respiration* means, simply, breathing in all its aspects.

Adequate and Inadequate Breathing

The brain and body cells need a steady supply of oxygen to accomplish the tasks of everyday living. Low levels of oxygen, or **hypoxia**, will disrupt normal function. Although it is also important for carbon dioxide to be removed, the body will tolerate high levels of carbon dioxide (*hypercapnia*) for longer periods of time than it will tolerate hypoxia. As we evaluate breathing in a patient, we will assess severity based on how well the patient's cardiopulmonary system is accomplishing the goals of oxygenation and removal of carbon dioxide.

CORE CONCEPT ●
How to recognize adequate and inadequate breathing

hypoxia (hi-POK-se-uh) an insufficiency of oxygen in the body's tissues.

When the cardiopulmonary system fails, the body makes adjustments to compensate for hypoxia and/or a buildup of carbon dioxide. These adjustments are somewhat predictable and can help us recognize the severity of the patient's problem.

In most people, the urge to breathe is caused by the buildup of carbon dioxide. Special sensors in the cardiovascular system, called chemoreceptors, detect increasing levels of carbon dioxide as well as low levels of oxygen. When these sensors detect significant changes, especially a build-up of carbon dioxide, the respiratory system is stimulated to breathe more rapidly.

When a person's cardiopulmonary system cannot keep up with the body's current demands, carbon dioxide levels increase and hypoxia occurs. The body typically responds with an increased respiratory rate to attempt to move more air. At this point, it is common for the patient to complain of the sensation of shortness of breath. The body will also typically respond by engaging the sympathetic (or "fight-or-flight") nervous system. The sympathetic nervous system will increase heart rate in an attempt to move more blood (and transport more oxygen and carbon dioxide) and will constrict blood vessels, which also aids in the movement of blood.

In some cases, the adjustments the body makes will keep up with added demands. For example, a patient will have a challenge, such as an asthma attack, and the patient's body will be compensating for that challenge. Increased respiratory rate, increased heart rate, and perhaps even position changes may be enough to meet the challenge and, at least minimally, the body's needs. The outward signs of these changes (vital signs, appearance, position) will indicate that the patient's system is working extra hard to meet his needs. If these changes are effective, there will be signs that oxygen and carbon dioxide are being adequately exchanged. These signs include normal mental status, relatively normal skin color, and a pulse oximetry reading (measurement of blood oxygen saturation) that is within normal limits. These patients are classified as having **respiratory distress**. That is, they have a challenge, but the compensatory mechanisms the body is providing are meeting their increased demands. They are, in fact, compensating.

respiratory distress increased work of breathing; a sensation of shortness of breath.

Unfortunately, some challenges are just too great for the body's compensatory mechanisms to overcome. Additionally, most of the mechanisms of compensation, such as increased respiratory muscle use, come at a cost of increased oxygen demand. If the very nature of the problem is that there was not enough oxygen to begin with, the demand for oxygen will quickly overtake the limited supply. In these cases, compensation fails and the body's metabolic needs are not met. Hypoxia becomes profound, carbon dioxide builds to dangerous levels, and the muscles used for increased respiration begin to tire. This condition represents *inadequate breathing* and is called **respiratory failure** (Figure 9-3).

respiratory failure the reduction of breathing to the point where oxygen intake is not sufficient to support life.

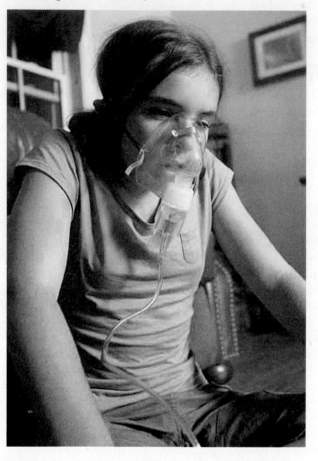

FIGURE 9-3 Respiratory distress usually involves accessory muscle use and increased work of breathing. Severe or prolonged respiratory distress can proceed to respiratory failure and inadequate ventilation when the body can no longer work so hard to breathe. In this case you will see a reduced level of responsiveness or an appearance of tiring, shallow ventilations, and other signs of inadequate breathing. *(© Dan Limmer)*

respiratory arrest
when breathing completely stops.

Respiratory failure is especially important to recognize, because it is often the precursor to the complete stoppage of breathing (***respiratory arrest***).

As an EMT, you will use your primary assessment to evaluate patients and rapidly classify their respiratory status. In essence, you will be making the decision as to whether their breathing is adequate or inadequate.

Inadequate Breathing

When you note that a patient's breathing is absent, you will provide artificial ventilation. However, there is a time before respiration completely ceases when, although the patient may show some signs of breathing, these breathing efforts are not enough to support life. That is, if the patient continues to breathe in this manner, he will eventually develop respiratory arrest and die. This is deemed inadequate breathing. In inadequate breathing, either the *rate of breathing* or the *depth of breathing* (or both) falls outside of normal ranges.

Recognizing inadequate breathing requires both keen assessment skills and prompt action (Table 9-1). Identifying this condition and providing ventilation to an inadequately breathing patient may actually keep him alive and breathing in a case where he would have stopped breathing and died without your intervention (Figure 9-4).

Table 9-1 Respiratory Conditions with Appropriate Interventions

CONDITION	SIGNS	EMT INTERVENTION	
ADEQUATE BREATHING Patient is breathing adequately but needs supplemental oxygen due to a medical or traumatic condition.	• Rate and depth of breathing are adequate. • No abnormal breath sounds. • Air moves freely in and out of the chest. • Skin color normal.	Oxygen by *nonrebreather mask* or *nasal cannula.*	
INADEQUATE BREATHING (RESPIRATORY FAILURE) Patient is moving some air in and out but it is slow or shallow and not enough to live.	• Patient has some breathing but not enough to live. • Rate and/or depth outside of normal limits. • Shallow ventilations. • Diminished or absent breath sounds. • Noises such as crowing, stridor, snoring, gurgling, or gasping. • Blue (cyanotic) or gray skin color. • Decreased minute volume.	Assisted ventilations (air forced into the lungs under pressure) with a *pocket face mask, bag-valve mask,* or *FROPVD.* See chapter text about adjusting rates for rapid or slow breathing. **NOTE:** *A nonrebreather mask requires adequate breathing to pull oxygen into the lungs. It DOES NOT provide ventilation to a patient who is not breathing or who is breathing inadequately.*	
PATIENT IS NOT BREATHING AT ALL (RESPIRATORY ARREST)	• No chest rise. • No evidence of air being moved from the mouth or nose. • No breath sounds.	Artificial ventilations with a *pocket facemask, bag-valve mask, FROPVD,* or *ATV* at 10–12/minute for an adult and 20/minute for an infant or child. **NOTE:** *DO NOT use oxygen-powered ventilation devices on infants or children.*	

FIGURE 9-4 Along the continuum from normal, adequate breathing to no breathing at all, there are milestones where an EMT should apply a nonrebreather mask or switch to positive pressure ventilation with a pocket face mask, BVM, or FROPVD for assisting the patient's own ventilations or providing artificial ventilation. It is essential to recognize the need for assisted ventilations, even before severe respiratory distress develops.

PATIENT'S CONDITION

WHEN AND HOW TO INTERVENE

Adequate breathing:
Speaks full sentences;
alert and calm

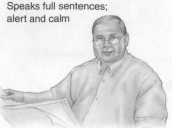

Nonrebreather mask or nasal cannula

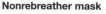

Increasing respiratory distress:
Visibly short of breath;
Speaking 3–4 word sentences;
Increasing anxiety

Nonrebreather mask

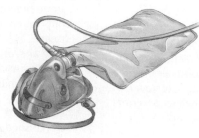

Key decision-making point:

Recognize inadequate breathing before respiratory arrest develops.

Assist ventilations before they stop altogether!

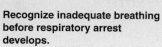

Severe respiratory distress:
Speaking only 1–2 word sentences;
Very diaphoretic (sweaty);
Severe anxiety

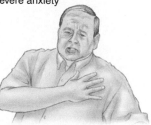

Assisted ventilations
Pocket face mask (PFM),
bag-valve mask (BVM), or
flow-restricted, oxygen-powered
ventilation device (FROPVD)

Assist the patient's own
ventilations, adjusting the
rate for rapid or slow
breathing

Continues to deteriorate:
Sleepy with head-bobbing;
Becomes unarousable

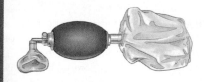

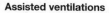

Respiratory arrest:
No breathing

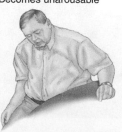

Artificial ventilation
Pocket face mask (PFM),
bag-valve mask (BVM), or
flow-restricted, oxygen-powered
ventilation device (FROPVD)

Assisted ventilations at
12/minute for an adult or
20/minute for a child or infant

Inside/Outside

Respiratory failure occurs when the mechanisms of respiratory compensation can no longer keep up with a respiratory challenge. To illustrate this process, let's review the progression of a patient having an asthma attack.

Patients with asthma have episodic attacks where their bronchiole tubes spasm and constrict. This leads to decreased air flow and decreased tidal volume. As minute volume and alveolar ventilation decrease, the body senses increased levels of carbon dioxide and slight hypoxia. The brain responds with an increased stimulus to breathe and activation of the sympathetic nervous system.

Inside the body, the respiratory system compensates. Respiratory rate and depth are increased in an attempt to increase alveolar ventilation. The heart pumps faster and harder in an attempt to move oxygen and carbon dioxide more quickly. Blood vessels constrict as the "fight-or-flight" response engages.

Outside the body, the patient may notice a sensation of shortness of breath. He may complain that he "can't catch my breath." You may notice an increased respiratory rate and an increased work of breathing. It may simply look like it is hard for the patient to breathe. You may hear wheezes, which are the sounds of the bronchoconstriction. You may also note the patient has slightly pale skin. However, since the patient's compensatory mechanisms are working, you should not see blue skin. His mental status is also normal, since adequate levels of oxygen are being supplied to the brain. At this point you would classify this patient as being in *respiratory distress*. He has a challenge, but his needs are being met by compensatory mechanisms inside the body.

Unfortunately, the asthma attack continues. Inside the body, the patient's bronchiole tubes get narrower as they begin to swell in response to the attack. Tidal volume and alveolar ventilation decrease even more, and the brain now lacks sufficient oxygen. Carbon dioxide also has been building up and is beginning to interfere with normal function. As you reassess this patient, you notice he is beginning to get anxious, maybe even a bit combative, as hypoxia increases and affects his brain. You notice it is harder to hear air moving when you listen to his chest. His wheezes have become "tighter." His fingernails are now turning blue, and you notice a similar discoloration in his lips and around his eyes. *Respiratory failure* has begun. Compensation can no longer keep up with his needs.

As the attack continues, tidal volume and alveolar ventilation decrease even further. Hypoxia is now profound. The patient's body has become acidotic from the retention of too much carbon dioxide and from anaerobic metabolism (metabolism without enough oxygen present), and he is growing tired. For a prolonged period now, the muscles in his chest have been working extra hard. These respiratory muscles demand oxygen that the patient's respiratory system cannot deliver. As a result, the respiratory muscles fatigue.

On the outside, the patient's mental status now is obviously severely impaired. He has become drowsy; in fact, he can barely stay awake. His respiratory rate has slowed, and you note he is breathing irregularly. His color is ashen with a definite bluish discoloration. He is now in profound respiratory failure. *Respiratory arrest* is imminent.

PATIENT ASSESSMENT

Assessing Breathing

As you assess breathing during the primary assessment, you should answer two important questions. The first question is, "Is the patient breathing?" You can determine this simply by their response to a simple hello. If he is unconscious, you may need to revert to BLS procedures and perform a "look-listen-feel" assessment. If he is not breathing, you must take immediate action to breathe for him. The second question you must answer is, "If he is breathing, is it adequate?" Is the effort he is putting forth enough to support his needs? If the answer is no, then you must intervene.

Signs of Adequate Breathing

To determine signs of adequate breathing, you should:

- *Look* for adequate and equal expansion of both sides of the chest when the patient inhales. If he has an obviously serious respiratory problem, expose and visually inspect the chest.
- *Listen* for air entering and leaving the nose, mouth, and chest. The breath sounds (when auscultated, or listened to with a stethoscope) should be present and equal on both sides of the chest. The sounds from the mouth and nose should be typically free of gurgling, gasping, crowing, wheezing, snoring, and stridor (harsh, high-pitched sound during inhalation).
- *Feel* for air moving out of the nose or mouth.
- Check for typical skin coloration. There should be no blue or gray colorations.
- Note the rate, rhythm, quality, and depth of breathing typical for a person at rest (Table 9–2).

Table 9-2 Adequate Breathing

NORMAL RATES	QUALITY
Adult—12–20 per minute	Breath sounds—present and equal
Child—15–30 per minute	Chest expansion—adequate and equal
Infant—25–50 per minute	Minimum effort
RHYTHM	**DEPTH**
Regular	Adequate

Signs of Inadequate Breathing

Signs of inadequate breathing include the following:

- Chest movements are absent, minimal, or uneven.
- Movement associated with breathing is limited to the abdomen (abdominal breathing).
- No air can be felt or heard at the nose or mouth, or the amount of air exchanged is below normal.
- Breath sounds are diminished or absent.
- Noises such as wheezing, crowing, stridor, snoring, gurgling, or gasping are heard during breathing.
- Rate of breathing is too rapid or too slow.
- Breathing is very shallow, very deep, or appears labored.
- The patient's skin, lips, tongue, ear lobes, or nail beds are blue or gray. This condition is called **cyanosis**, and the patient is said to be cyanotic.
- Inspirations are prolonged (indicating a possible upper airway obstruction) or expirations are prolonged (indicating a possible lower airway obstruction).
- Patient is unable to speak, or the patient cannot speak full sentences because of shortness of breath.
- In children, there may be retractions (a pulling in of the muscles) above the clavicles and between and below the ribs.
- Nasal flaring (widening of the nostrils of the nose with respirations) may be present, especially in infants and children.

cyanosis (SIGH-uh-NO-sis)
a blue or gray color resulting from lack of oxygen in the body.

Respiratory Evaluation

NORMAL BREATHING (Adequate Breathing)	RESPIRATORY DISTRESS (Adequate Breathing)	RESPIRATORY FAILURE (Inadequate Breathing)	RESPIRATORY ARREST (Inadequate Breathing)
Quiet, no unusual sounds	May have unusual sounds such as wheezing, stridor, or coughing	Same as distress; beware absent sounds	No sounds of breathing
Normal rate of breathing	Typically elevated rate of breathing; not excessively fast, though Adequate minute volume	Often too fast or too slow Sometimes irregular or slowing Inadequate minute volume	None
Normal skin color	Sometimes normal or pale due to vasoconstriction	Pale or blue; sometimes mottled (blotchy)	Pale or blue
Normal mental status	Normal, sometimes agitated or anxious	Altered mental status	Typically unconscious or rapidly becoming unconscious

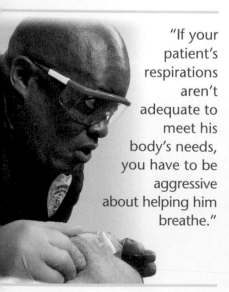

"If your patient's respirations aren't adequate to meet his body's needs, you have to be aggressive about helping him breathe."

Occasionally, respiratory arrest will be difficult to determine. Recall the steps of basic CPR. Look at the chest for rise and fall. Listen for the sounds of breathing. Feel for air movement. Although gasping breaths may occasionally be present, they should never be confused for normal breathing.

Hypoxia

As already noted, hypoxia is an insufficiency in the supply of oxygen to the body's tissues. There are several major causes of hypoxia. Consider the following scenarios:

- **A patient is trapped in a fire.** The air that the patient breathes contains smoke and reduced amounts of oxygen. Since the patient cannot breathe in enough oxygen, hypoxia develops.

- **A patient has emphysema.** This lung disease decreases the efficiency of the transfer of oxygen between the atmosphere and the body. Since the lungs cannot function properly, hypoxia develops.

- **A patient overdoses on a drug that has a depressing effect on the respiratory system.** The patient's respirations are only 5 per minute. In this case, the victim is not breathing frequently enough to support the body's oxygen needs. Hypoxia develops.

- **A patient has a heart attack.** The lungs function properly by taking atmospheric air and turning it over to the blood for distribution. The damaged heart, however, cannot pump the blood throughout the body, and hypoxia develops.

There are many causes of hypoxia in addition to the examples named, including stroke, shock, and others. The most important thing to know is how to recognize signs of hypoxia so that it may be treated. Hypoxia may be indicated by cyanosis (blue or gray color to the skin). Additionally, when the brain suffers hypoxia, the patient's mental status may deteriorate. Restlessness or confusion may result.

As an EMT, your concern will be preventing hypoxia from developing or becoming worse and, when possible, reducing the level of hypoxia. This is done with the administration of oxygen.

PATIENT CARE

Inadequate Breathing

When the patient's signs indicate inadequate breathing or no breathing (respiratory failure or respiratory arrest), a life-threatening condition exists and prompt action must be taken. In the previous chapter we discussed the procedures for opening, clearing, and securing the airway. In some patients with respiratory failure you may need to first address airway issues. Review Chapter 8, "Airway Management," for more information. The additional procedures to treat life-threatening respiratory problems are:

- Providing artificial ventilation to the nonbreathing patient and the patient with inadequate breathing
- Providing supplemental oxygen to the breathing patient

These procedures are discussed next and on the following pages.

Decision Point

When Do I Intervene?
It can sometimes be difficult to determine when a patient needs your intervention. Often patients in respiratory failure will be breathing and conscious. It is important, however, to identify not just the presence of breathing but the adequacy of breathing. Even though the patient may still be breathing, if he is displaying the signs of inadequate breathing, he absolutely needs your intervention. Keep in mind that what the patient is doing on his own is not meeting his needs. If left unchecked, his condition will progress to respiratory arrest. In general, it is better to be too aggressive than not aggressive enough. If the patient will allow you to intervene with a bag-valve mask, it generally means he needs it.

POSITIVE PRESSURE VENTILATION

artificial ventilation

forcing air or oxygen into the lungs
when a patient has stopped breathing
or has inadequate breathing. Also
called *positive pressure ventilation*.

positive pressure ventilation

See artificial ventilation.

If you determine that the patient is not breathing or that his breathing is inadequate, you will need to provide artificial ventilation. *Ventilation* is the breathing of air or oxygen. *Artificial ventilation*, also called *positive pressure ventilation*, is forcing air or oxygen into the lungs when a patient has stopped breathing or has inadequate breathing.

It is important to remember that when we use positive pressure, we use a force that is exactly the opposite of the force the body normally uses to draw air into the lungs. Under normal circumstances, the respiratory system creates a negative pressure within the chest cavity to pull in air. With artificial ventilations, we use positive pressure from outside to push air in. This change has some negative side effects you must be conscious of and will need to limit by using proper technique.

The negative side effects of positive pressure ventilation are:

- **Decreasing cardiac output/dropping blood pressure.** Normally, the heart uses the negative pressure of ventilation to assist the filling of its chambers with blood. When we use positive pressure to ventilate, we eliminate that negative pressure and filling assistance. Although the heart can typically compensate, the risk of causing a drop in blood pressure exists, especially when excessive positive pressures are used to ventilate. This risk from positive pressure can be minimized by using just enough volume to raise the chest.

- **Gastric distention.** Gastric distention is the filling of the stomach with air that occurs when air is pushed through the esophagus during positive pressure ventilation. The esophagus, which leads to the stomach, is a larger opening than the trachea, which leads to the lungs, and the esophagus does not have a protective "cap" like the epiglottis that covers the trachea. Consequently, air is frequently diverted through the esophagus when we attempt to push air through the trachea. Side effects of gastric distention include vomiting and restriction of the movement of the diaphragm. Gastric distention can be minimized by using airway adjuncts when ventilating and also by establishing proper head position and airway opening techniques. Later in this chapter we will discuss cricoid pressure, a technique that can also help minimize gastric distention.

- **Hyperventilation.** When we take over ventilations for a patient, it is important to pay attention to rate. There are any number of distractions and stressors that cause EMTs to ventilate too quickly, and you should know that there are negative consequences of this action. Hyperventilation causes too much carbon dioxide to be blown off. This causes a vasoconstriction (narrowing of the blood vessels) in the body and can limit blood flow to the brain. Always concentrate on maintaining proper ventilation rates while providing artificial ventilation.

Techniques of Artificial Ventilation

Various techniques are available to the EMT that can be used to provide artificial ventilation:

- Mouth-to-mask (preferably with high-concentration supplemental oxygen at 15 liters per minute)
- Two-rescuer bag-valve mask (BVM) (preferably with high-concentration supplemental oxygen at 15 liters per minute)
- Flow-restricted, oxygen-powered ventilation device
- One-rescuer bag-valve mask (preferably with high-concentration supplemental oxygen at 15 liters per minute)

NOTE: *Do not ventilate a patient who is vomiting or who has vomitus in his airway. Positive pressure ventilation will force the vomitus into the patient's lungs. Make sure the patient is not actively vomiting and suction any vomitus from the airway before ventilating.*

No matter what method you use to ventilate the patient, you must ensure that the patient is being adequately ventilated. To determine the signs of *adequate* artificial ventilation, you should:

- Watch the chest rise and fall with each ventilation.
- Ensure that the rate of ventilation is sufficient—approximately 10–12 per minute in adults, 20 per minute in children, and a minimum of 20 per minute in infants.

FIGURE 9-5 Examples of barrier devices.

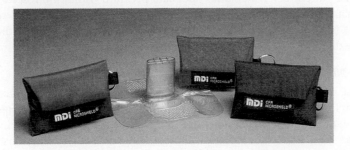

Inadequate artificial ventilation occurs when:

- The chest does not rise and fall with ventilations.
- The rate of ventilation is too fast or too slow.

Techniques used for artificial ventilation should also ensure adequate protection of the rescuer from the patient's body fluids, including saliva, blood, and vomit. For this reason, mouth-to-mouth ventilation is not recommended unless there is no alternative method of artificial ventilation available. A number of compact barrier devices are available for personal use (Figure 9-5).

NOTE: *The skill of assisting a patient's ventilations is difficult to master as it requires careful watching for the chest rise and coordinating delivery of the pocket-mask or BVM ventilation.*

As noted earlier, ventilation will also be required on a patient who is breathing but doing so inadequately. This may be due to a very rapid but shallow rate or a very slow rate. In any case, keep in mind that it may be intimidating to ventilate (use a pocket face mask or bag-valve mask on) a patient who is breathing and may even be aware of what you are doing. Follow these guidelines for ventilation of a breathing patient:

For a patient with rapid ventilations:

- Carefully assess the adequacy of respirations.
- Explain the procedure to the patient. Calm reassurance and a simple explanation such as, "I'm going to help you breathe," are essential for the awake patient.
- Place the mask (pocket face mask or BVM) over the patient's mouth and nose.
- After sealing the mask on the patient's face, squeeze the bag with the patient's inhalation. Watch as the patient's chest begins to rise and deliver the ventilation with the start of the patient's own inhalation. The goal will be to increase the volume of the breaths you deliver. Over the next several breaths, adjust the rate so you are ventilating fewer times per minute but with greater volume per breath (increasing the minute volume).

For a patient with slow ventilations:

- Carefully assess the adequacy of respirations.
- Explain the procedure to the patient. Again, calm reassurance and a simple explanation such as, "I'm going to help you breathe," are essential in the awake patient.
- Place the mask (pocket face mask or BVM) over the patient's mouth and nose.
- After sealing the mask on the patient's face, squeeze the bag every time the patient begins to inhale. If the rate is very slow, add ventilations in between the patient's own to obtain a rate of approximately 12 per minute with adequate minute volume.

CPAP/BiPAP

A new and very effective prehospital modality of therapy for treating patients with inadequate breathing and respiratory distress is *noninvasive positive pressure ventilation (NPPV)* in the form of *CPAP* (continuous positive airway pressure) and *BiPAP* (biphasic continuous positive airway pressure). NPPV assists the ventilations of a breathing patient by assuring that each breath the patient takes maintains adequate pressure within the respiratory tract, improving alveolar ventilation and gas exchange (thus preventing hypoxia and carbon dioxide accumulation). NPPV can be used only by patients who are still breathing on their own. It will be extensively discussed in Chapter 19, "Respiratory Emergencies."

Mouth-to-Mask Ventilation

pocket face mask

a device, usually with a one-way valve, to aid in artificial ventilation. A rescuer breathes through the valve when the mask is placed over the patient's face. It also acts as a barrier to prevent contact with a patient's breath or body fluids. It can be used with supplemental oxygen when fitted with an oxygen inlet.

Mouth-to-mask ventilation is performed using a **pocket face mask**. The pocket face mask is made of soft, collapsible material and can be carried in your pocket, jacket, or purse (Figure 9-6). Many EMTs purchase their own pocket face masks for workplace or auto first aid kits.

Face masks have important infection control features. Your ventilations (breaths) are delivered through a valve in the mask so that you do not have direct contact with the patient's mouth. Most pocket masks have one-way valves that allow your ventilations to enter but prevent the patient's exhaled air from coming back through the valve and into contact with you (Figure 9-7).

Some pocket masks have oxygen inlets. When high-concentration oxygen is attached to the inlet, it delivers an oxygen concentration of approximately 50 percent. This is significantly better than the 16 percent oxygen concentration (in exhaled air) delivered by mouth-to-mask ventilations without supplemental oxygen.

Most pocket face masks are made of a clear plastic. This is important because you must be able to observe the patient's mouth and nose for vomiting or secretions that need to be suctioned. You also need to observe the color of the lips, an indicator of the patient's respiratory status. Some pocket face masks have a strap that goes around the patient's head. This is helpful during one-rescuer CPR, since it will hold the mask on the patient's face while you are performing chest compressions. However, it does not replace the need for proper hand placement on the mask.

To provide mouth-to-mask ventilation (Table 9-3), follow these steps:

1. Position yourself at the patient's head and open the airway. It may be necessary to clear the airway of obstructions. If appropriate, insert an oropharyngeal airway to help keep the patient's airway open (as described later in this chapter).

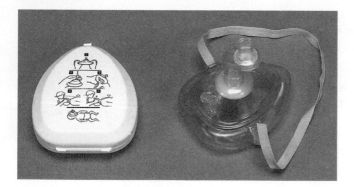

FIGURE 9-6 Pocket face mask.

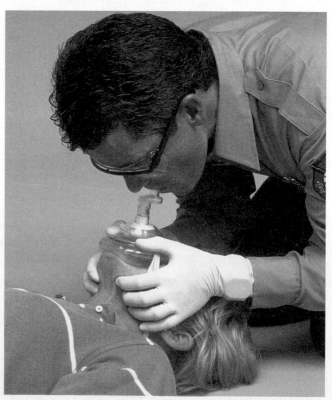

FIGURE 9-7 Use only a pocket mask with a one-way valve.

Table 9-3   Use of the Pocket Face Mask

PATIENT	USE OF THE POCKET FACE MASK
Patient *without* suspected spine injury—EMT at top of patient's head 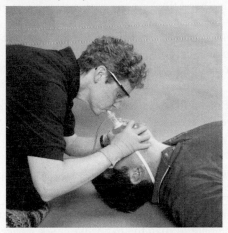	• Position yourself directly above (at the top of) the patient's head. • Apply the mask to the patient. Use the bridge of the patient's nose as a guide for correct position. • Place your thumbs over the top of the mask, your index fingers over the bottom of the mask, and the rest of your fingers under the patient's jaw. • Lift the jaw to the mask as you tilt the patient's head backward and place the remaining fingers under the angle of the jaw. • While lifting the jaw, squeeze the mask with your thumbs to achieve a seal between the mask and the patient's face. • Give breaths into the one-way valve of the mask. Watch for the chest to rise.
Patient *without* suspected spine injury—Alternative: EMT beside patient's head 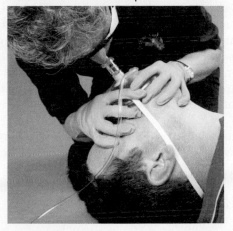	• Position yourself beside the patient's head. • Apply the mask to the patient. Use the bridge of the nose as a guide for correct position. • Seal the mask by placing your index finger and thumb of the hand closer to the top of the patient's head along the top border of the mask. • Place the thumb of the hand closer to the patient's feet on the lower margin of the mask. Place the remaining fingers of this hand along the bony margin of the jaw. • Lift the jaw while performing a head-tilt, chin-lift maneuver. • Compress the outer margins of the mask against the face to obtain a seal. • Give breaths into the one-way valve on the mask. Watch for the chest to rise.
Patient *with* suspected spine injury—EMT at top of patient's head 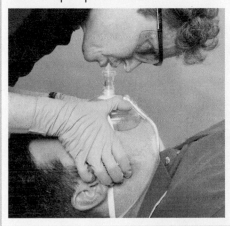	• Position yourself directly above (at the top of) the patient's head. • Apply the mask to the patient. Use the bridge of the patient's nose as a guide for correct position. • Place the thumb sides of your hands along the mask to hold it firmly on the face. • Use your remaining fingers to lift the angle of the jaw. ***Do not tilt the head backward.*** • While lifting the jaw, squeeze the mask with your thumbs and fingers to achieve a seal. • Give breaths into the one-way valve on the mask. Watch for the chest to rise. **NOTE:** *Factors such as hand size, patient size, or dentures not in place may necessitate modifications in hand position and technique to achieve the necessary tight seal.*

2. Connect oxygen to the inlet on the mask and run at 15 liters per minute. If oxygen is not immediately available, do not delay mouth-to-mask ventilations.

3. Position the mask on the patient's face so that the apex (top of the triangle) is over the bridge of the nose and the base is between the lower lip and prominence of the chin. (Center the ventilation port over the patient's mouth.)

4. Hold the mask firmly in place while maintaining head tilt. Use one of these positions or some variation—with the aim of achieving a tight seal:
   • Thumbs over the top of the mask, index fingers over the bottom of the mask, and remaining fingers under the patient's jaw (Table 9-3, top)
   • Thumbs along the side of the mask and remaining fingers under the patient's jaw (Table 9-3, bottom)

5. Take a breath and exhale into the mask port or one-way valve at the top of the mask port. Each ventilation should be delivered over 1 second in adults, infants, and children and be of just enough volume to make the chest rise. Full expansion of the chest is undesirable; the ventilation should cease as soon as you notice the chest moving.

6. Remove your mouth from the port and allow for passive exhalation. Continue as you would for mouth-to-mouth ventilations or CPR.

When properly used, and if the rescuer has an adequate expiratory capacity, the pocket face mask may deliver higher volumes of air to the patient than the bag-valve-mask device.

Bag-Valve Mask

bag-valve mask (BVM)
a handheld device with a face mask and self-refilling bag that can be squeezed to provide artificial ventilations to a patient. It can deliver air from the atmosphere or oxygen from a supplemental oxygen supply system.

The **bag-valve mask (BVM)** (also called bag mask or bag-mask device) is a handheld ventilation device. It may also be referred to as a bag-valve-mask unit, system, device, resuscitator, or simply BVM. The bag-valve-mask unit can be used to ventilate a nonbreathing patient and is also helpful to assist ventilations in the patient whose own respiratory attempts are not enough to support life, such as a patient in respiratory failure or drug overdose. The BVM also provides an infection-control barrier between you and your patient. The use of the bag-valve mask in the field is often referred to as "bagging" the patient (Table 9-4).

Bag-valve-mask units come in sizes for adults, children, and infants (Figure 9-8). Many different types of bag-valve-mask systems are available; however, all have the same basic parts. The bag must be a self-refilling shell that is easily cleaned and sterilized. (Some bag-

FIGURE 9-8 Adult, child, and infant bag-valve-mask units.

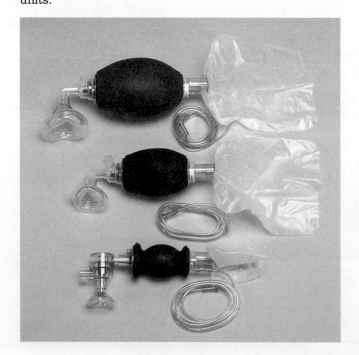

Table 9-4 Use of the Bag-Valve Mask

PATIENT	USE OF THE BAG-VALVE MASK
Patient *without* suspected spine injury 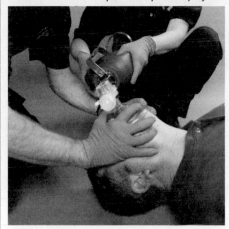	• Open the airway and insert appropriately sized oral or nasal airway (if no gag reflex). • Position your thumbs over the top of the mask, with index fingers over the bottom of the mask. • Place the mask over the patient's face. Position the mask over the patient's nose and lower to the chin. (Large, round-style masks are centered first on the mouth.) • Use your middle, ring, and little fingers to bring the jaw up to the mask. • Connect the bag to the mask and have an assistant squeeze the bag until the chest rises. • If the chest does not rise and fall, reevaluate the head position and mask seal. • If unable to ventilate, use another device (e.g., pocket face mask or FROPVD).
Patient *with* suspected spine injury 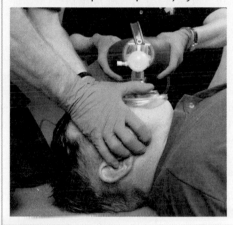	• Open the airway with a jaw thrust and insert an appropriate size airway if no gag reflex exists. • Have an assistant manually immobilize the head and neck. Immobilization of the head between your knees may be acceptable if no assistance is available. • Place the thumb sides of your hands along the mask to hold it firmly on the face. • Place the mask on the patient's face as previously described. • Use your little and ring fingers to bring the jaw up to the mask without tilting the head or neck. • Have an assistant squeeze the bag with two hands until the chest rises. • Continually evaluate ventilations.

valve-mask units are designed for single use and are then disposed of.) The system must have a non-jam valve that allows an oxygen inlet flow of 15 liters per minute. The valve should be nonrebreathing (preventing the patient from rebreathing his own exhalations) and not subject to freezing in cold temperatures. Most systems have a standard 15/22 respiratory fitting to ensure a proper fit with other respiratory equipment, face masks, and endotracheal tubes.

The mechanical workings of a bag-valve-mask device are simple. Oxygen, flowing at 15 liters per minute, is attached to the BVM and enters the reservoir. When the bag is squeezed, the air inlet to the bag is closed, and the oxygen is delivered to the patient.

When the squeeze of the bag is released, a passive expiration by the patient will occur. While the patient exhales, oxygen enters the reservoir to be delivered to the patient the next time the bag is squeezed. BVM systems without a reservoir deliver approximately 50 percent oxygen. In contrast, systems with an oxygen reservoir provide nearly 100 percent oxygen. The bag itself will hold anywhere from 1,000 to 1,600 mL of air. This means that the bag-valve-mask system must be used properly and efficiently.

The most difficult part of delivering BVM artificial ventilations is obtaining an adequate mask seal so that air does not leak out around the edges of the mask. It is difficult to maintain the seal with one hand while squeezing the bag with the other, and one-rescuer bag-valve-mask operation is often unsuccessful or inadequate for this reason. Therefore, it is strongly recommended by the American Heart Association that BVM artificial ventilation be performed by two rescuers. In two-rescuer BVM ventilation, one rescuer is assigned to squeeze the bag while the other rescuer uses two hands to maintain a mask seal.

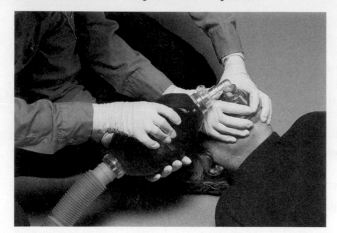

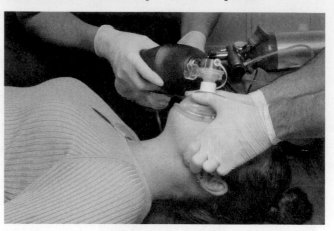

NOTE: *Many older bag-valve masks have "pop-off" valves, designed to open after certain pressures are obtained. Studies have shown that pop-off valves may prevent adequate ventilations. BVM systems with pop-off valves should be replaced. A BVM system should also have a clear face mask so that you can observe the lips for cyanosis and monitor the airway in case suctioning is needed.*

The two-rescuer technique can also be modified so that the jaw-thrust maneuver can be used during BVM ventilations. This technique is to be used when performing BVM ventilation on a patient with a suspected head, neck, or spine injury. Proficiency in this technique requires frequent mannequin practice. There are different ways to perform BVM ventilation when trauma (injury) is not suspected (Figure 9-9) and when trauma is suspected (Figure 9-10).

Two-Rescuer BVM Ventilation—No Trauma Suspected When two rescuers perform bag-valve ventilation on a patient in whom *no* trauma is suspected, follow these steps:

1. Open the patient's airway *using the head-tilt, chin-lift maneuver*. Suction and insert an airway adjunct as necessary.

2. Select the correct bag-valve mask size (adult, child, or infant).

3. Kneel at the patient's head. Position thumbs over the top half of the mask, index fingers over the bottom half.

4. Place the apex, or top, of the triangular mask over the bridge of the patient's nose. Then lower the mask over the mouth and upper chin. If the mask has a large, round cuff surrounding a ventilation port, center the port over the patient's mouth.

5. Use your middle, ring, and little fingers to bring the patient's jaw up to the mask. *Maintain the head-tilt, chin-lift maneuver*.

6. The second rescuer should connect the bag to the mask, if not already done. While you maintain the mask seal, the second rescuer should squeeze the bag with two hands until the patient's chest rises. The second rescuer should squeeze the bag *once every 5 seconds for an adult, once every 3 seconds for a child or infant*.

7. The second rescuer should release pressure on the bag and let the patient exhale passively. While this occurs, the bag is refilling from the oxygen source.

Two-Rescuer BVM Ventilation—Trauma Suspected When two rescuers perform bag-valve ventilation on a patient in whom trauma *is* suspected, follow these steps:

1. Open the patient's airway *using the jaw-thrust maneuver*. Suction and insert an airway adjunct (see later in this chapter) as necessary.

2. Select the correct bag-valve mask size (adult, child, or infant).

3. Kneel at the patient's head. Place thumb sides of your hands along the mask to hold it firmly on the face.

4. Use your remaining fingers to bring the jaw upward, toward the mask, *without tilting the head or neck*.

5. Have the second rescuer squeeze the bag to ventilate the patient as previously described for the nontrauma patient.

Cricoid Pressure Cricoid *pressure*, also known as the Sellick maneuver, is performed by applying firm backward pressure to the cricoid ring in the patient's neck. The cricoid ring surrounds the trachea, and pushing on it exerts pressure on the esophagus, which is posterior to the trachea, partially occluding the esophagus. This technique is designed to minimize air entry into the esophagus and stomach during positive pressure ventilation. The cricoid ring can be found by palpating the Adam's apple and then identifying the ring (or bump) just inferior. While one provider is providing artificial ventilation, a second provider will place two fingers on this ring and firmly press backward while ventilating. It should be noted that this technique will cause discomfort in the conscious patient and should be limited to those patients who are unconscious or have a severely impaired mental status. You should also not apply cricoid pressure if the patient is vomiting or begins to vomit.

One-Rescuer BVM Ventilation As noted, use of a bag-valve mask by a single rescuer is the last choice of artificial ventilation procedure—behind use of a pocket face mask with supplemental oxygen, a two-rescuer bag-valve-mask procedure, and use of a flow-restricted, oxygen-powered ventilation device. You should provide ventilations with a one-rescuer bag-valve-mask procedure only when no other options are available.

When you perform bag-valve ventilation alone, without assistance from a second rescuer, follow these steps:

1. Position yourself at the patient's head and establish an open airway. Suction and insert an airway adjunct as necessary.

2. Select the correct size mask for the patient. Position the mask on the patient's face as described previously for the two-rescuer BVM technique.

3. Form a "C" around the ventilation port with thumb and index finger. Use your middle, ring, and little fingers under the patient's jaw to hold the jaw to the mask.

4. With your other hand, *squeeze the bag once every 5 seconds. For infants and children, squeeze the bag once every 3 seconds.* The squeeze should be a full one, causing the patient's chest to rise.

5. Release pressure on the bag and let the patient exhale passively. While this occurs, the bag is refilling from the oxygen source.

If the chest does not rise and fall during BVM ventilation, you should:

1. Reposition the head.

2. Check for escape of air around the mask and reposition your fingers and the mask.

3. Check for airway obstruction or obstruction in the BVM system. Re-suction the patient if necessary. Consider insertion of an airway adjunct if not already done.

4. If none of these methods work, use an alternative method of artificial ventilation, such as a pocket mask or a flow-restricted, oxygen-powered ventilation device.

The BVM may also be used during CPR. In this situation, the bag is squeezed once each time a ventilation is to be delivered. In one-rescuer CPR, it is preferable to use a pocket mask with supplemental oxygen (Figure 9-11) rather than a BVM system. A single rescuer would take too much time picking up the BVM and obtaining a face seal each time a ventilation is to be delivered, in addition to the normal difficulty in maintaining a seal with the one-rescuer BVM technique.

NOTE: *Bag-valve-mask devices should be completely disassembled and disinfected after each use. Because proper decontamination is often costly and time-consuming, many hospitals and EMS agencies use single-use disposable BVMs.*

Artificial Ventilation of a Stoma Breather The BVM can be used to artificially ventilate a patient with a ***stoma***, a surgical opening in the neck through which the patient breathes. Patients with stomas who are found to be in severe respiratory distress or respiratory arrest frequently have thick secretions blocking the stoma. It is recommended that you suction the stoma frequently in conjunction with BVM-to-stoma ventilations.

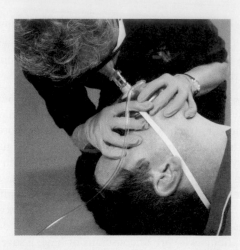

FIGURE 9-11 One-rescuer CPR using a pocket face mask with supplemental oxygen. The EMT is beside the patient, from which position chest compressions can also be performed. The strap holds the pocket mask in place while the rescuer switches tasks.

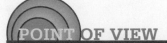

POINT OF VIEW

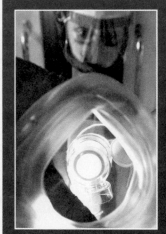

"I still can't tell you why I didn't know it was coming on. I didn't feel right for a few days. Then it hit me. I couldn't move without feeling like I would suffocate. I just couldn't breathe. Couldn't catch my breath. I could tell it was serious when the EMTs came in. It showed in their faces.

"I think I must've started getting even worse, because I remember feeling like I was losing it. I remember them trying to calm me down, but I really felt like I was going to have to be peeled off the ceiling of that ambulance.

"When they tried to put that big mask on my face I felt like it was going to kill me. To take away all my air. I fought it. The EMTs kept calming me and putting that mask on my face. Somehow I calmed down a little and they gave me air or oxygen or something. I made it to the hospital. The doctor told me that the EMTs may have saved my life.

"I appreciate that more than I can say—even if that mask felt pretty intimidating at the time."

As with other BVM uses, a two-rescuer technique is preferred over a one-rescuer technique. To provide artificial ventilation to a stoma breather using a BVM, follow these steps:

1. Clear any mucus plugs or secretions from the stoma.
2. Leave the head and neck in a neutral position, as it is unnecessary to position the airway prior to ventilations in a stoma breather.
3. Use a pediatric-sized mask to establish a seal around the stoma.
4. Ventilate at the appropriate rate for the patient's age.
5. If unable to artificially ventilate through the stoma, consider sealing the stoma and attempting artificial ventilation through the mouth and nose. (This may work if the trachea is still connected to the passageways of the mouth, nose, and pharynx. In some cases, however, the trachea has been permanently connected to the neck opening with no remaining connection to the mouth, nose, or pharynx).

Flow-Restricted, Oxygen-Powered Ventilation Device

A ***flow-restricted, oxygen-powered ventilation device (FROPVD),*** also called a *manually triggered ventilation device*, uses oxygen under pressure to deliver artificial ventilations through a mask placed over the patient's face. This device is similar to the traditional demand-valve resuscitator but includes newer features designed to optimize ventilations and safeguard the patient (Figure 9-12). Recommended features include:

- A peak flow rate of 100 percent oxygen at up to 40 liters per minute
- An inspiratory pressure relief valve that opens at approximately 60 cm of water pressure
- An audible alarm when the relief valve is activated
- A rugged design and construction

flow-restricted, oxygen-powered ventilation device (FROPVD)
a device that uses oxygen under pressure to deliver artificial ventilations. Its trigger is placed so that the rescuer can operate it while still using both hands to maintain a seal on the face mask. It has automatic flow restriction to prevent overdelivery of oxygen to the patient.

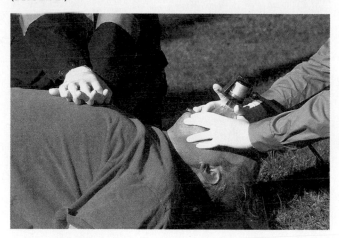

FIGURE 9-12 Providing ventilations with a flow-restricted, oxygen-powered ventilation device (FROPVD).

- A trigger that enables the rescuer to use both hands to maintain a mask seal while triggering the device
- Satisfactory operation in both ordinary and extreme environmental conditions

Follow the same procedures for mask seal as recommended for the BVM (Table 9-5). Trigger the device until the chest rises *and repeat every 5 seconds*. If the chest does not rise,

Table 9-5 Use of the Flow-Restricted, Oxygen-Powered Ventilation Device (FROPVD; Manually Triggered Ventilator)	
PATIENT	**USE OF THE FROPVD**
Patient *without* suspected spine injury 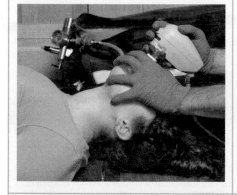	• Open the airway and insert an appropriately sized oral or nasal airway. • Position the thumbs over the top of the mask, with your index fingers over the bottom half. • Place the mask over the face and use the middle, ring, and little fingers to bring the patient's jaw up to the mask. • Trigger the ventilation device until the chest rises. Do not overinflate. • Reevaluate ventilations frequently.
Patient *with* suspected spine injury 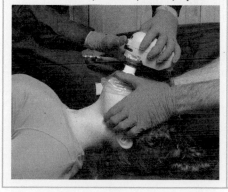	• Open the airway with a jaw thrust and insert an appropriate size airway if no gag reflex exists. • Have an assistant manually immobilize the head and neck. Immobilization of the head between your knees may be acceptable if no assistance is available. • Place the thumb side of your hands along the mask to hold it firmly on the face. • Place the mask on the patient's face as previously described. • Use your remaining fingers to bring the jaw up to the mask without tilting the head or neck. • Trigger the ventilation device until the chest rises. Do not overinflate. • Monitor ventilations.

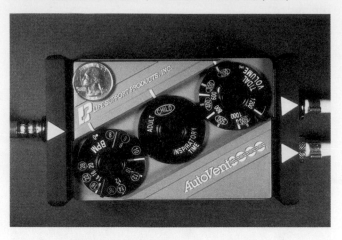

FIGURE 9-13 An automatic transport ventilator. The coin is shown for scale. (© Edward T. Dickinson, MD)

reposition the head, check the mask seal, check for obstructions, and consider the use of an alternative artificial ventilation procedure.

When using the FROPVD on a patient with chest trauma, be especially careful not to overinflate, as you may actually make the chest injury worse. Also, always make sure the airway is fully opened, and watch for chest rise. Make sure you are not forcing excess air to enter the stomach instead of the lungs, causing gastric distention, which could cause the patient to regurgitate and possibly compromise the airway with stomach contents.

If neck injury is suspected, have an assistant hold the patient's head manually or put a rigid collar or head blocks on the patient to prevent movement. (Using your knees to prevent head movement is sometimes recommended but places you too close to the patient, making it difficult to open the airway and assess chest rise properly.) Bring the jaw up to the mask without tilting the head or neck.

The flow-restricted, oxygen-powered ventilation device should be used only on adults unless you have a child unit and have been given special training in its use by your Medical Director.

Automatic Transport Ventilator

automatic transport ventilator (ATV)
a device that provides positive pressure ventilations. It includes settings designed to adjust ventilation rate and volume, is portable, and is easily carried on an ambulance.

The *automatic transport ventilator (ATV)* (Figure 9-13) may be used in EMS to provide positive pressure ventilations to a patient in respiratory arrest. The ATV has settings to adjust ventilation rate and volume. These ventilators are very portable and easily carried on

CRITICAL DECISION MAKING

Oxygen or Ventilation?

You have learned several methods to administer supplemental oxygen and to provide ventilations to a patient. It has been said that the decision on when to provide supplemental oxygen (e.g., nonrebreather mask or cannula) or to ventilate (e.g., BVM, FROPVD) is one of the most important decisions you will make.

For each of the following patients, decide whether you would administer oxygen or ventilate the patient.

1. A patient who was found on the floor by a relative. He has no pulse or respirations.

2. A 14-year-old patient who has a broken femur. She is alert; pulse 110, strong and regular; respirations 28, rapid and deep.

3. A 64-year-old male with chest pain. He is alert; pulse 56; respirations 18 and normal.

4. A 78-year-old patient with COPD. He has had increasing difficulty breathing over the past few days. He responds verbally but is not oriented. His pulse is 124; respirations 36 and shallow.

ambulances. When prolonged ventilation is necessary, and when only one rescuer is available to ventilate a patient, the ATV may be beneficial. Caution must be used to be sure the respiratory rate is appropriate for the patient's size and condition. A proper mask seal is required for these devices to effectively deliver ventilation.

OXYGEN THERAPY

Importance of Supplemental Oxygen

Oxygen administration is often one of the most important and beneficial treatments an EMT can provide. The atmosphere provides approximately 21 percent oxygen. If a person does not have an illness or injury, that 21 percent is enough to support normal functioning. However, patients EMTs come in contact with are sick or injured and often require supplemental oxygen.

CORE CONCEPT ●
Principles and techniques of oxygen administration

Conditions Requiring Oxygen

Patients with the following conditions may require supplemental oxygen:

- **Respiratory or cardiac arrest.** CPR is only 25 to 33 percent as effective as normal circulation. High-concentration oxygen administration is currently recommended when providing artificial ventilations to a patient in respiratory or cardiac arrest.

- **Heart attacks and strokes.** These emergencies result from an interruption of blood to the heart or brain. When this occurs, tissues are deprived of oxygen. Providing extra oxygen is extremely important.

- **Shock.** Since shock is the failure of the cardiovascular system to provide sufficient blood to all the vital tissues, all cases of shock reduce the amount of oxygenated blood reaching the tissues. Administration of oxygen helps the blood that does reach the tissues deliver the maximum amount of oxygen.

- **Blood loss.** Whether bleeding is internal or external, there is a reduced amount of circulating blood and red blood cells, so the blood that is circulating needs to be saturated with oxygen.

- **Respiratory distress and lung diseases.** The lungs are responsible for turning oxygen over to the blood cells to be delivered to the tissues. When the lungs are not functioning properly, supplemental oxygen helps ensure that the body's tissues receive adequate oxygen.

- **Head injuries, other serious injuries, and more.** There are very few emergencies where oxygen administration would not be appropriate. All our body's systems work together. An injury in one part may cause shock that affects the rest of the body.

Oxygen Therapy Equipment

In the field, oxygen equipment must be safe, lightweight, portable, and dependable. Some field oxygen systems are very portable and can be brought almost anywhere. Other systems are installed inside the ambulance so that oxygen can be delivered during transportation to the hospital.

Most oxygen delivery systems (Figure 9-14) contain several items: oxygen cylinders, pressure regulators, and a delivery device (nonrebreather mask or cannula). When the patient is not breathing or is breathing inadequately, additional devices (such as a pocket mask, bag-valve mask, or FROPVD) can be used to force oxygen into the patient's lungs.

Oxygen Cylinders

Outside a medical facility, the standard source of oxygen is the *oxygen cylinder*, a seamless steel or lightweight alloy cylinder filled with oxygen under pressure, equal to 2,000 to 2,200 pounds per square inch (psi) when the cylinders are full. Cylinders come in various sizes, identified by letters (Figure 9-15). The following cylinders are in common use in emergency care:

- *D cylinder* contains about 350 liters of oxygen.
- *E cylinder* contains about 625 liters of oxygen.
- *M cylinder* contains about 3,000 liters of oxygen.

oxygen cylinder
a cylinder filled with oxygen under pressure.

FIGURE 9-14 An oxygen delivery system.

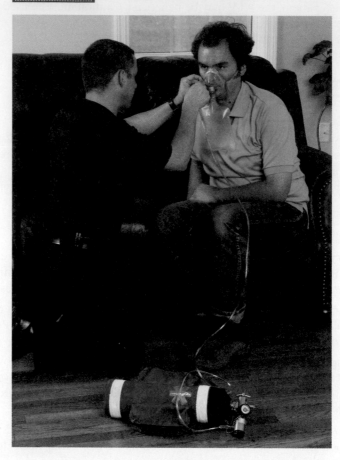

FIGURE 9-15 For safety, to prevent them from tipping over, oxygen cylinders must be placed in a horizontal position or, if upright, must be securely supported.

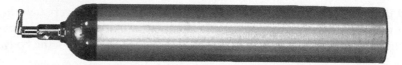

Fixed systems on ambulances (commonly called on-board oxygen) include the M cylinder and larger cylinders (Figure 9-16):

- *G cylinder* contains about 5,300 liters of oxygen.
- *H cylinder* contains about 6,900 liters of oxygen.

The *United States Pharmacopoeia* has assigned a color code to distinguish compressed gases. Green and white cylinders have been assigned to all grades of oxygen. Unpainted stainless steel and aluminum cylinders are also used for oxygen. Regardless of the color, always check the label to be certain you are using medical-grade oxygen.

Part of your duty as an EMT is to make certain that the oxygen cylinders you will use are full and ready before they are needed to provide care. The length of time you can use an oxygen cylinder depends on the pressure in the cylinder and the flow rate. You cannot tell if an oxygen cylinder is full, partially full, or empty just by lifting or moving the cylinder. The method of calculating cylinder duration is shown in Table 9-6.

Oxygen cylinders should never be allowed to empty below the safe residual or the tank may be permanently damaged. The safe residual for an oxygen cylinder is when the pressure gauge reads 200 psi or above. Below this point there is not enough oxygen in the cylinder to

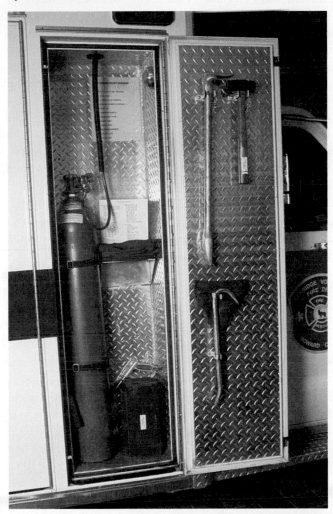

Table 9-6 Oxygen Cylinders: Duration of Flow

SIMPLE FORMULA

Gauge pressure in psi (pounds per square inch) minus the safe residual pressure (always 200 psi) times the constant (see following list) divided by the flow rate in liters per minute = duration of flow in minutes.

CYLINDER CONSTANTS

D = 0.16	G = 2.41
E = 0.28	H = 3.14
M = 1.56	K = 3.14

EXAMPLE

Determine the life of an M cylinder that has a pressure of 2,000 psi displayed on the pressure gauge and a flow rate of 10 liters per minute.

$$\frac{(2,000 - 200) \times 1.56}{10} = \frac{2,808}{10} = 280.8 \text{ minutes}$$

allow for proper delivery to the patient. Before the cylinder reaches the 200 psi reading, you must switch to a fresh cylinder.

(**NOTE:** *Some systems or services may require cylinder changes at specific psi levels. Always follow local guidelines.*)

Safety is of prime importance when working with oxygen cylinders. You should:

- *Always* use pressure gauges, regulators, and tubing that are intended for use with oxygen.
- *Always* use nonferrous (made of plastic or of metals that do not contain iron) oxygen wrenches for changing gauges and regulators or for adjusting flow rates. Other types of metal tools may produce a spark should they strike against metal objects.
- *Always* ensure that valve seat inserts and gaskets are in good condition. This prevents dangerous leaks. Disposable gaskets on oxygen cylinders should be replaced each time a cylinder change is made.
- *Always* use medical-grade oxygen. Industrial oxygen contains impurities. The cylinder should be labeled "OXYGEN U.S.P." The oxygen must not be more than 5 years old.
- *Always* open the valve of an oxygen cylinder fully, then close it half a turn to prevent someone else from thinking the valve is closed and trying to force it open. The valve does not have to be turned fully to be open for delivery.
- *Always* store reserve oxygen cylinders in a cool, ventilated room, properly secured in place.
- *Always* have oxygen cylinders hydrostatically tested every 5 years. The date a cylinder was last tested is stamped on the cylinder. Some cylinders can be tested every 10 years. These will have a star after the date (e.g., 4M86MM*).
- *Never* drop a cylinder or let it fall against any object. When transporting a patient with an oxygen cylinder, make sure the oxygen cylinder is strapped to the stretcher or otherwise secured.
- *Never* leave an oxygen cylinder standing in an upright position without being secured.
- *Never* allow smoking around oxygen equipment in use. Clearly mark the area of use with signs that read "OXYGEN–NO SMOKING."
- *Never* use oxygen equipment around an open flame.
- *Never* use grease, oil, or fat-based soaps on devices that will be attached to an oxygen supply cylinder. Take care not to handle these devices when your hands are greasy. Use greaseless tools when making connections.
- *Never* use adhesive tape to protect an oxygen tank outlet or to mark or label any oxygen cylinders or oxygen delivery apparatus. The oxygen can react with the adhesive and debris and cause a fire.
- *Never* try to move an oxygen cylinder by dragging it or rolling it on its side or bottom.

Pressure Regulators

pressure regulator
a device connected to an oxygen cylinder to reduce cylinder pressure so it is safe for delivery of oxygen to a patient.

The pressure in an oxygen cylinder (approximately 2,000 psi in a full tank—varying with surrounding temperature) is too high to be delivered to a patient. A ***pressure regulator*** must be connected to the cylinder to provide a safe working pressure of 30 to 70 psi.

On cylinders of the E size or smaller, the pressure regulator is secured to the cylinder valve assembly by a yoke assembly. The yoke is provided with pins that must mate with corresponding holes in the valve assembly. This is called a pin-index safety system. Since the pin position varies for different gases, this system prevents an oxygen delivery system from being connected to a cylinder containing another gas.

NOTE: *You must maintain the regulator inlet filter. It has to be free of damage and clean to prevent contamination of, and damage to, the regulator.*

Cylinders larger than the E size have a valve assembly with a threaded outlet. The inside and outside diameters of the threaded outlets vary according to the gas in the cylinder. This prevents an oxygen regulator from being connected to a cylinder containing another gas. In other words, a nitrogen regulator cannot be connected to an oxygen cylinder, or vice versa.

Before connecting the pressure regulator to an oxygen supply cylinder, stand to the side of the main valve opening and open (crack) the cylinder valve slightly for just a second to clear dirt and dust out of the delivery port or threaded outlet.

Flowmeters

flowmeter
a valve that indicates the flow of oxygen in liters per minute.

A ***flowmeter***, which is connected to the pressure regulator, allows control of the flow of oxygen in liters per minute. Most services keep the flowmeter permanently attached to the pressure regulator. Low-pressure and high-pressure flowmeters are available.

Low-Pressure Flowmeters Low-pressure flowmeters, specifically the pressure-compensated flowmeter and the constant flow selector valve (Figure 9-17A), are in general use in the field.

- **Pressure-compensated flowmeter.** This meter is gravity dependent and must be in an upright position to deliver an accurate reading. The unit has an upright, calibrated glass tube in which there is a ball float. The float rises and falls according to the amount of gas passing through the tube. This type of flowmeter indicates the actual flow at all times, even though there may be a partial obstruction to gas flow (e.g., from a kinked delivery tube). If the tubing collapses, the ball will drop to show the lower delivery rate. This unit is not practical for many portable delivery systems. Recommended use is for larger (M, G, and H) oxygen cylinders in the ambulance.

- **Constant flow selector valve.** This type of flowmeter, which is gaining in popularity, has no gauge and allows for the adjustment of flow in liters per minute in stepped increments (2, 4, 6, 8 . . . to 15 liters or more per minute). It can be accurately used with the nasal cannula or nonrebreather mask and with any size oxygen cylinder. It is rugged and will operate at any angle.

  When using this type of flowmeter, make certain that it is properly adjusted for the desired flow and monitor it to make certain that it stays properly adjusted. All types of meters should be tested for accuracy as recommended by the manufacturer.

High-Pressure Flowmeters The low-pressure flowmeters just listed will administer oxygen up to either 15 or 25 liters per minute. In some circumstances, however, oxygen is required at higher pressures. This may be necessary for oxygen-powered devices such as the Thumper™ CPR device or for respirators and ventilators, such as the CPAP and BiPAP devices discussed earlier in this chapter. There are several ways you will identify high-pressure connections. One is observing a threaded connection on an oxygen regulator (Figure 9-17B). You may also see thick, green hose-type tubing connected to the high-pressure regulator.

Humidifiers

A *humidifier* can be connected to the flowmeter to provide moisture to the dry oxygen coming from the supply cylinder (Figure 9-18). Oxygen without humidification can dry out the mucous membranes of the patient's airway and lungs. In most short-term use, the dryness of the oxygen is not a problem; however, the patient is usually more comfortable when given humidified oxygen. This is particularly true if the patient has COPD or is a child.

A humidifier is usually no more than a nonbreakable jar of water attached to the flowmeter. Oxygen passes (bubbles) through the water to become humidified. As with all oxygen delivery equipment, the humidifier must be kept clean. The water reservoir can become a breeding

humidifier
a device connected to the flowmeter to add moisture to the dry oxygen coming from an oxygen cylinder.

FIGURE 9-17 (A) Low-pressure flowmeters: (Left) A pressure-compensated flowmeter; (Right) A constant flow selector valve. (B) High-pressure flowmeter. High-pressure oxygen is delivered through hoses attached to a threaded connector.

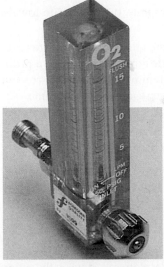
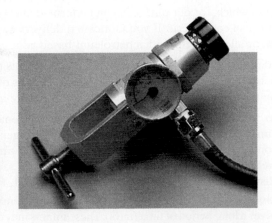
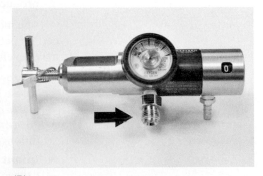

(A)

(B)

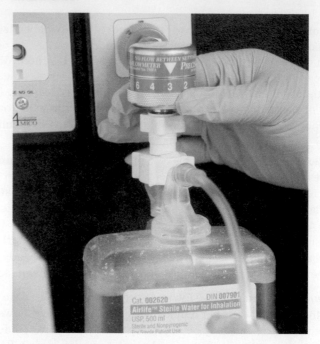

FIGURE 9-18 Humidifier in use on board an ambulance.

ground for algae, harmful bacteria, and dangerous fungal organisms. Always use fresh water in a clean reservoir for each shift. Sterile single-patient-use humidifiers are available and preferred.

In many EMS systems, humidifiers are no longer used because they are not indicated for short transports and because of the infection risk. The devices may be beneficial on long transports and on certain pediatric patients with signs of inadequate breathing.

Hazards of Oxygen Therapy

Although the benefits of oxygen are great, oxygen must be used carefully. The hazards of oxygen therapy may be grouped into two categories: nonmedical and medical.

Nonmedical hazards are extremely rare and can be avoided totally if oxygen and oxygen equipment are treated properly. Some of the most common hazards are:

- The oxygen used in emergency care is stored under pressure, usually 2,000 to 2,200 pounds per square inch (psi) or greater in a full cylinder. If the tank is punctured, or a valve breaks off, the supply tank can become a missile (damaged tanks have been able to penetrate concrete walls). Imagine what would happen in the passenger compartment of an ambulance if such an accident occurred.

- Oxygen supports combustion, causing fire to burn more rapidly. It can saturate towels, sheets, and clothing, greatly increasing the risk of fire.

- Under pressure, oxygen and oil do not mix. When they come into contact, a severe reaction occurs which, for our purposes, can be termed an explosion. This is seldom a problem, but it can easily occur if you lubricate a delivery system or gauge with petroleum products, or allow contact with a petroleum-based adhesive (e.g., adhesive tape).

The medical hazards of oxygen rarely affect the patients treated by the EMT. There are certain patients who, when exposed to high concentrations of oxygen for a prolonged time, may develop negative side effects. These situations are rare in the field:

- **Oxygen toxicity or air sac collapse.** These problems are caused in some patients whose lungs react unfavorably to the presence of oxygen and also may result from too high a concentration of oxygen for too long a period of time. The body reacts to a sensed "overload" of oxygen by reduced lung activity and air sac collapse. Like the other conditions listed here, these are extremely rare in the field.

- **Infant eye damage.** This condition may occur when premature infants are given too much oxygen over a long period of time (days). These infants may develop scar tissue on the retina of the eye. Oxygen by itself does not cause this condition but it is the result of many factors. Oxygen should never be withheld from any infant with signs of inadequate breathing.

- **Respiratory depression or respiratory arrest.** Patients in the end stage of COPD may over time lose the normal ability to use the body's blood carbon dioxide levels as a stimulus to breathe. When this occurs, the COPD patient's body may use low blood oxygen as the factor that stimulates him to breathe. Because of this so-called hypoxic drive, EMTs have for years been trained to administer only low concentrations of oxygen to these patients for fear of increasing blood oxygen levels and wiping out their "drive to breathe." It is now widely believed that more harm is done by withholding high-concentration oxygen than could be done by administering it.

As an EMT you will probably never see oxygen toxicity or any other adverse conditions that can result from oxygen administration. The time required for such conditions to develop is too long to cause any problems during emergency care in the field. The bottom line is: *Never withhold oxygen from a patient who needs it!*

Administering Oxygen

Scans 9-1 and 9-2 will take you step by step through the process of preparing the oxygen delivery system, administering oxygen, and discontinuing the administration of oxygen. Do not

---

SCAN 9-1 | Preparing the Oxygen Delivery System

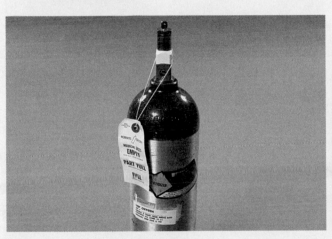

❶ Select the desired cylinder. Check for label "Oxygen U.S.P."

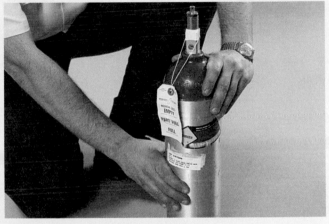

❷ Place the cylinder in an upright position and stand to one side.

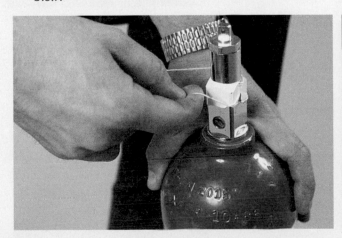

❸ Remove the plastic wrapper or cap protecting the cylinder outlet.

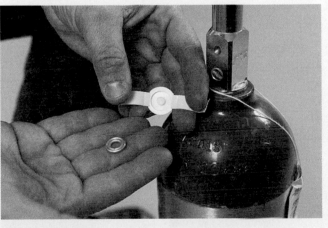

❹ Keep the plastic washer (some set-ups).

(continued)

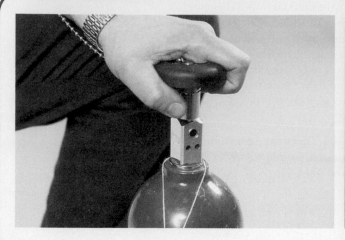

5 "Crack" the main valve for 1 second.

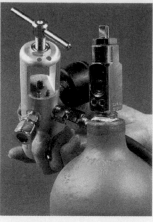 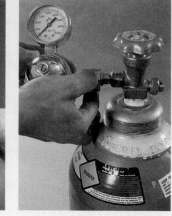

6 Select the correct pressure regulator and flowmeter. Pin yoke is shown on the left, threaded outlet on the right.

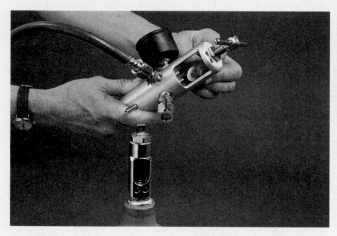

7 Place the cylinder valve gasket on the regulator oxygen port.

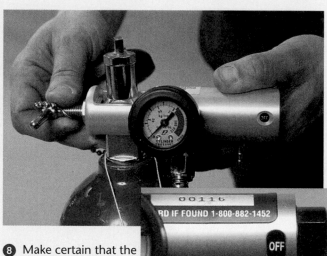

8 Make certain that the pressure regulator is closed.

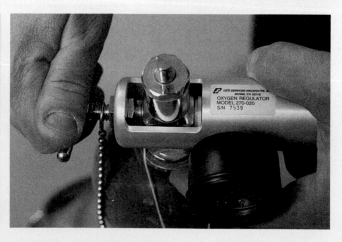

9 Align pins (left), or thread by hand (right).

10 Tighten T-screw for pin yoke or . . . Tighten a threaded outlet with a nonferrous wrench.

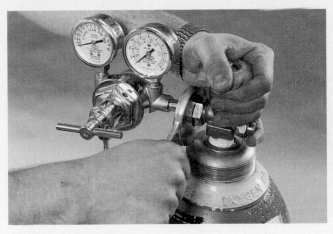

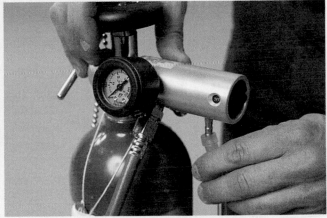

⓫ Attach tubing and delivery device.

SCAN 9-2 Administering Oxygen

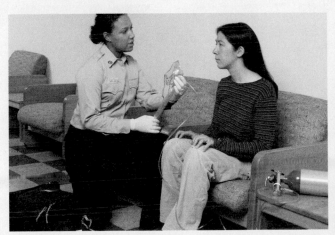

❶ Explain to the patient the need for oxygen.

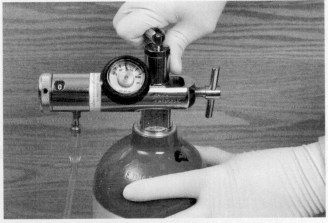

❷ Open the main valve and adjust the flowmeter.

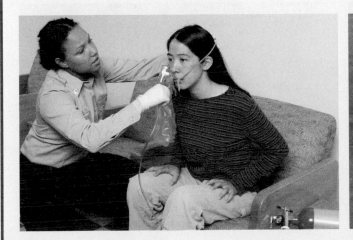

❸ Place an oxygen delivery device on the patient.

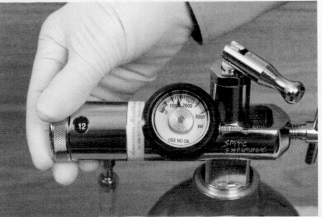

❹ Adjust the flowmeter.

(continued)

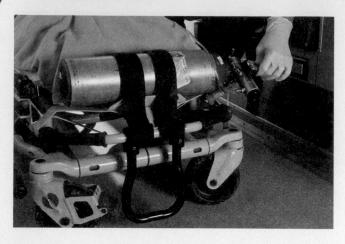

5 Secure the cylinder during transfer.

DISCONTINUING OXYGEN

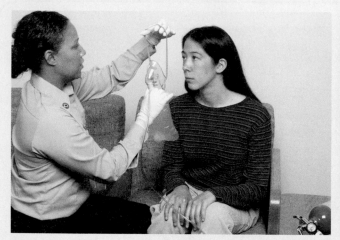

1 Remove the delivery device.

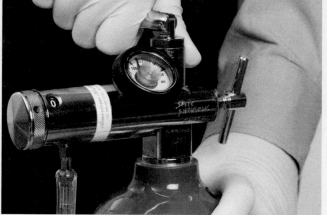

2 Close the main valve.

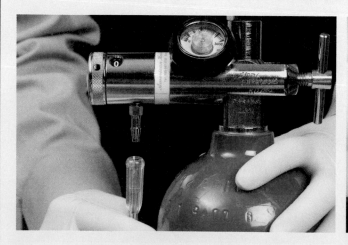

3 Remove the delivery tubing.

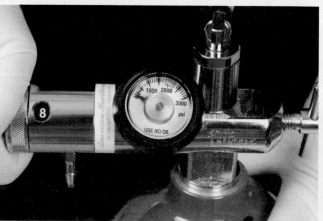

4 Bleed the flowmeter.

Table 9-7 Oxygen Delivery Devices

DEVICE	FLOW RATE	OXYGEN CONCENTRATION	APPROPRIATE USE
Nonrebreather mask	12–15 liters per minute	80–90 percent	Delivery system of choice for patients with signs of hypoxia, those short of breath, or those suffering chest pain, suffering severe injuries, or displaying an altered mental status.
Nasal cannula	1–6 liters per minute	24–44 percent	Appropriate for patients who cannot tolerate a mask.
Partial rebreather mask	9–10 liters per minute	40–60 percent	Usually not used in EMS. Some patients may use at home to keep CO levels up.
Venturi mask	Varied, depending on device; up to 15 liters per minute	24–60 percent	A device used to deliver a specific concentration of oxygen. Device delivers 24–60 percent oxygen, depending on adapter tip and oxygen flow rate.
Tracheostomy mask	8–10 liters per minute	Can be set up to deliver varying oxygen percentages as required by the patient; desired percentage of oxygen may be recommended by the home care agency	A device used to deliver ventilations/oxygen through a stoma or tracheostomy tube.

attempt to learn on your own how to use oxygen delivery systems. You should work with your instructor and follow your instructor's directions for the specific equipment you will be using.

Oxygen is administered to assist in the delivery of artificial ventilations to nonbreathing patients, as was discussed earlier in this chapter under "Techniques of Artificial Ventilation." Oxygen is also very commonly administered to breathing patients for a variety of conditions. A number of oxygen-delivery devices and systems are used. Each has benefits and drawbacks. A device that is good for one patient may not be ideal for another. The goal is to use the oxygen-delivery device that is best for each patient.

For the patient who is breathing adequately and requires supplemental oxygen due to potential hypoxia, various oxygen-delivery devices are available. In general, however, the nonrebreather mask and the nasal cannula are the two devices most commonly used by the EMT to provide supplemental oxygen (Table 9-7).

Nonrebreather Mask

The *nonrebreather (NRB) mask* (Figure 9-19) is the EMT's best way to deliver high concentrations of oxygen to a breathing patient. This device must be placed properly on the patient's face to provide the necessary seal to ensure high-concentration delivery. The reservoir bag must be inflated before the mask is placed on the patient's face.

To inflate the reservoir bag, use your finger to cover the exhaust port or the connection between the mask and the reservoir. The reservoir must always contain enough oxygen so that it does not deflate by more than one-third when the patient takes his deepest inspiration. This can be maintained by the proper flow of oxygen (15 liters per minute). Air exhaled by the patient does not return to the reservoir (is not rebreathed). Instead, it escapes through a flutter valve in the face piece.

This mask will provide concentrations of oxygen ranging from 80 to 100 percent. The optimum flow rate is 12 to 15 liters per minute. New design features allow for one emergency port in the mask so that the patient can still receive atmospheric air should the oxygen supply fail. This feature keeps the mask from being able to deliver 100 percent oxygen but is a necessary safety feature. The mask is excellent for use in patients with signs of hypoxia or who are short of breath, suffering chest pain, or displaying an altered mental status.

Nonrebreather masks come in different sizes for adults, children, and infants.

nonrebreather (NRB) mask
a face mask and reservoir bag device that delivers high concentrations of oxygen. The patient's exhaled air escapes through a valve and is not rebreathed.

FIGURE 9-19 Nonrebreather mask.

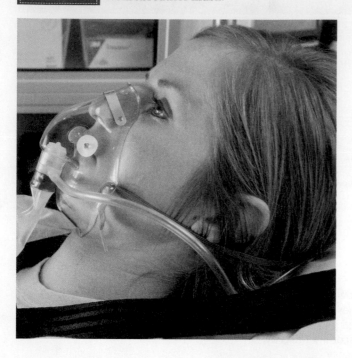

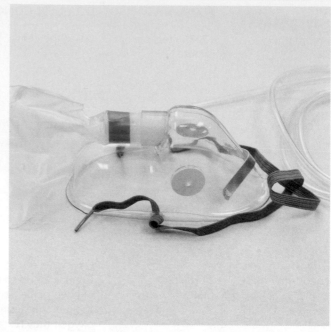

Nasal Cannula

nasal cannula

(NAY-zul KAN-yuh-luh)

a device that delivers low concentrations of oxygen through two prongs that rest in the patient's nostrils.

A *nasal cannula* (Figure 9-20) provides low concentrations of oxygen (between 24 and 44 percent). Oxygen is delivered to the patient by two prongs that rest in the patient's nostrils. The device is usually held to the patient's face by placing the tubing over the patient's ears and securing the slip-loop under the patient's chin.

Patients who have chest pain, signs of shock, hypoxia, or other more serious problems need a higher concentration than can be provided by a cannula. However, some patients will not tolerate a mask-type delivery device because they feel "suffocated" by the mask. For the patient who refuses to wear an oxygen face mask, the cannula is better than no oxygen at all. The cannula should be used only when a patient will not tolerate a nonrebreather mask.

When a cannula is used, the liters per minute delivered should be no more than 4 to 6. At higher flow rates the cannula begins to feel more uncomfortable, like a windstorm in the nose, and dries out the nasal mucous membranes.

FIGURE 9-20 Nasal cannula.

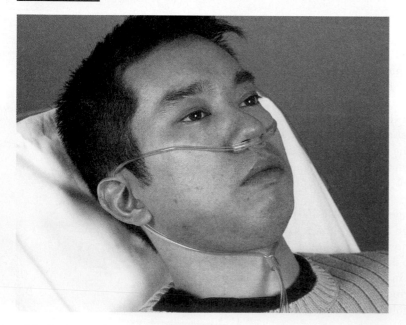

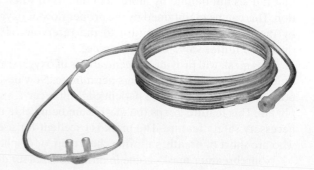

FIGURE 9-21 Partial rebreather mask.

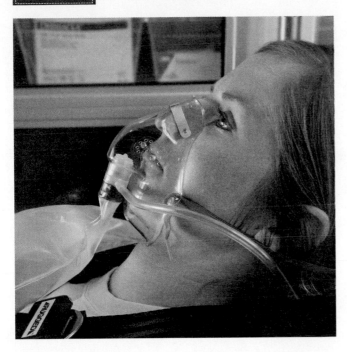 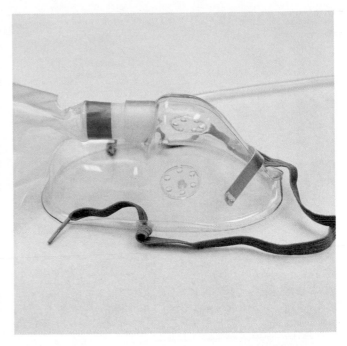

Partial Rebreather Mask

A *partial rebreather mask* (Figure 9-21) is very similar to a nonrebreather mask with the exception that there is no one-way valve in the opening to the reservoir bag. This allows the patient to rebreathe about one-third of his exhaled air. This type of mask is used for some patients to preserve the carbon dioxide levels in their blood in order to stimulate breathing. Partial rebreather masks deliver 40–60 percent oxygen at 9–10 lpm. These masks are not typically used in EMS but may be encountered when caring for a patient who uses such a mask at home.

Venturi Mask

A *Venturi mask* (Figure 9-22) delivers specific concentrations of oxygen by mixing oxygen with inhaled air. The Venturi mask package may contain several tips. Each tip will provide a

partial rebreather mask
a face mask and reservoir oxygen bag with no one-way valve to the reservoir bag so that some exhaled air mixes with the oxygen; used in some patients to help preserve carbon dioxide levels in the blood to stimulate breathing.

Venturi mask
a face mask and reservoir bag device that delivers specific concentrations of oxygen by mixing oxygen with inhaled air.

FIGURE 9-22 Venturi mask.

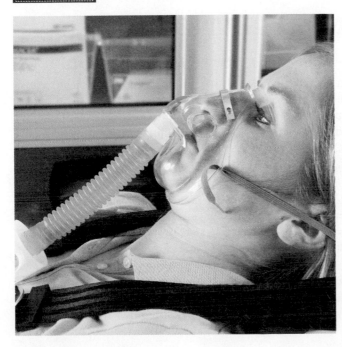 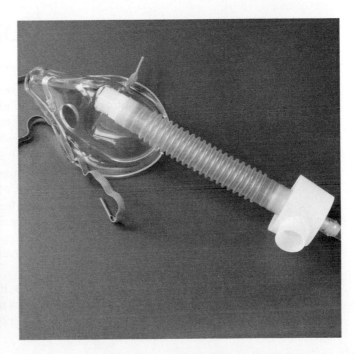

FIGURE 9-23 Tracheostomy mask.

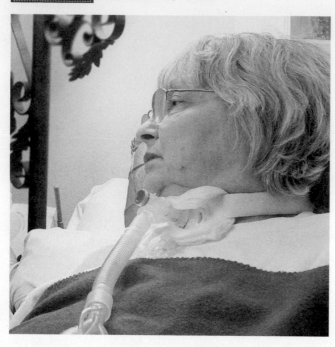 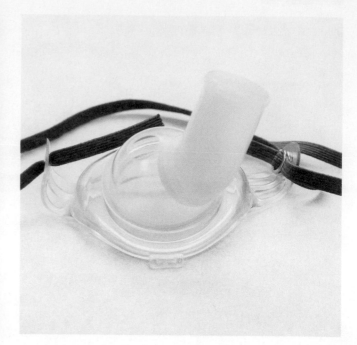

different concentration of oxygen when used at the flow rate designated on the tip. Some Venturi masks have a set percentage and flow rate whereas others have an adjustable Venturi port. These devices are most commonly used on patients with COPD.

Tracheostomy Mask

tracheostomy mask
a device designed to be placed over a stoma or tracheostomy tube to provide supplemental oxygen.

A *tracheostomy mask* (Figure 9-23) is designed to be placed over a stoma or tracheostomy tube to provide supplemental oxygen. It is typically a small cuplike mask that fits over the tracheostomy opening and is held in place by an elastic strap placed around the neck. These masks are connected to 8 to 10 lpm of oxygen via supply tubing.

SPECIAL CONSIDERATIONS

There are a number of special considerations in airway management:

- **Facial injuries.** Take extra care with a patient's airway if he has facial injuries. Because the blood supply to the face is so rich, blunt injuries to the face frequently result in severe swelling or bleeding that may block or partially block the airway. Frequent suctioning may be required. In addition, insertion of an airway adjunct or endotracheal tube may be necessary.

- **Obstructions.** Many suction units are not adequate for removing solid objects like teeth and large particles of food or other foreign objects. These must be removed using manual techniques for clearing airway obstructions, such as abdominal thrusts, chest thrusts, or finger sweeps, which you learned in your basic life support course and which are reviewed in Appendix A, "Basic Cardiac Life Support Review," at the back of this book. You may need to log roll the patient into a supine position to clear the oropharynx manually.

- **Dental appliances.** Dentures should ordinarily be left in place during airway procedures. Partial dentures may become dislodged during an emergency. Leave a partial denture in place if possible, but be prepared to remove it if it endangers the airway.

There are several special considerations that you must take into account when assessing and managing breathing in an infant or child (review Figure 8–9 in Chapter 8):

Anatomic Considerations

- In infants and children, the tongue takes up more space proportionately in the mouth than in adults. Always consider using an airway adjunct when performing artificial ventilation.
- The trachea (windpipe) is softer and more flexible in infants and children. Furthermore, small children often have a proportionally larger head, which makes it more difficult to maintain a patent airway. Often padding is necessary behind their shoulders to provide a proper airway position. Always consider this when performing artificial ventilation.
- The chest wall is softer, and infants and children tend to depend more on their diaphragm for breathing. Gastric distention can severely impair the movement of the diaphragm and therefore seriously decrease tidal volumes in children.
- Children burn oxygen at twice the rate adults do. Although they compensate well, hypoxia will often occur more rapidly and decompensation can be swift.

Management Considerations

- When ventilating, avoid excessive pressure and volume. Use only enough to make the chest rise.
- Use properly sized face masks when providing ventilations to ensure a good mask seal.
- Flow-restricted, oxygen-powered ventilation devices are contraindicated (should not be used) in infants and children, unless you have a pediatric unit and have been properly trained in its use.
- Use pediatric-sized nonrebreather masks and nasal cannulas when administering supplemental oxygen.
- Infants and children are prone to gastric distention during ventilations, which may impair adequate ventilations.

ASSISTING WITH ADVANCED AIRWAY DEVICES

You may be called to assist an advanced EMT or paramedic with an advanced airway device. There are two basic types of devices, each with different procedures for use:

- **Devices that require direct visualization of the glottic opening (endotracheal intubation).** A device called a laryngoscope is used to visualize the airway while the tube is guided into the trachea.
- **Devices that are inserted "blindly," meaning without having to look into the airway to insert the device.** These devices include the King LT™ airway, Combitube®, and laryngeal mask airway (LMA™)

In most states, the decision to use the advanced device and insertion of the device is limited to advanced level providers (always refer to your local protocol). The EMT may be called upon to assist in patient preparation for insertion of the device. The most important thing an EMT can do to further the success of the insertion and benefit to the patient is to assure a patent airway and quality ventilations prior to insertion of the device. Fortunately, this is something EMTs should be doing all the time.

NOTE: *Be especially careful not to disturb the endotracheal tube. Movement of the patient to a backboard, down stairs, and into the ambulance can easily cause displacement of the tube. If the tube comes out of the trachea, the patient receives no oxygen and will certainly die.*

Preparing the Patient for Intubation

Before the paramedic inserts the endotracheal tube, you may be asked to give the patient extra oxygen. This is referred to as hyperoxygenation, and it can easily be accomplished by

FIGURE 9-24 (A) The endotracheal tube and (B) endotracheal tube with stylet in place.

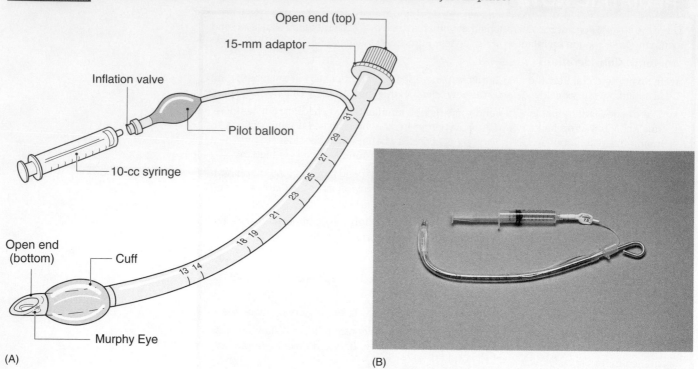

Open end (top)

15-mm adaptor

Inflation valve

Pilot balloon

10-cc syringe

Open end
(bottom)

Cuff

Murphy Eye

(A)

(B)

ventilating with a bag-valve-mask device that is connected to oxygen and includes a reservoir. To do this, ventilate at a normal to slightly increased rate. Do not administer more than 20 breaths/minute for more than 2–3 minutes nor administer breaths more forcefully during this time. Increasing the force of ventilations (bag squeeze) will force air into the stomach and cause vomiting.

The paramedic will then position the patient's head to align the mouth, pharynx, and trachea. This is sometimes referred to as a "sniffing position." The paramedic will remove the oral airway and pass the endotracheal tube (Figure 9-24) through the mouth, into the throat, past the vocal cords, and into the trachea. This procedure requires using a laryngoscope to move the tongue out of the way and provide a view of the vocal cords. The tube may also be passed through the nose. This does not require visualization of the airway.

In order to maneuver the tube past the vocal cords correctly, the paramedic will need to see them. You may be asked to help by gently pressing on the throat to push the vocal cords into the paramedic's view. You will do this by pressing your thumb and index finger just to either side of the throat over the cricoid cartilage, the ring-shaped cartilage just below the thyroid cartilage, or Adam's apple. This procedure is known as cricoid pressure (Figure 9-25).

Once the tube is properly placed, the cuff is inflated with air from a 10-cc syringe. While holding the tube, the paramedic assures proper tube placement by using at least two methods, including auscultation of both lungs and the epigastrium and using a capnometry or an end-tidal CO_2 detector device (Figure 9-26). If the tube has been correctly placed, there will be sounds of air entering the lungs but no sounds of air in the epigastrium. Air sounds in the epigastrium indicate that the tube has been incorrectly placed in the esophagus instead of the trachea so that air is entering the stomach instead of the lungs. The tube position must be corrected immediately by removing the tube, reoxygenating the patient, and repeating the process of intubation.

The correctly positioned tube is anchored in place with a commercially made tube restraint.

The entire procedure of intubation—including the last ventilation, passing the tube, and the next ventilation—should take less than 30 seconds.

You might be asked to assist the advanced providers by monitoring the lung and epigastric sounds throughout the call. Most systems now use continuous end-tidal carbon dioxide detection when an endotracheal tube is in place as one method of monitoring tube placement.

If the tube is pushed in too far, it will most likely enter the right mainstem bronchus, preventing oxygen from entering the patient's left lung. (You can identify this by noting breath sounds on the right side with no sounds over the left or the epigastrium.)

FIGURE 9-25 In cricoid pressure, press your thumb and index finger on either side of the medial throat over the cricoid cartilage.

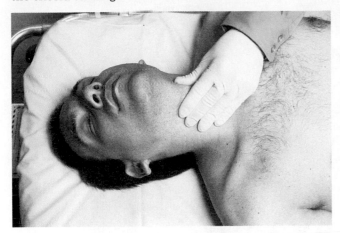

FIGURE 9-26 An end-tidal CO_2 detector can ensure proper placement of the endotracheal tube.

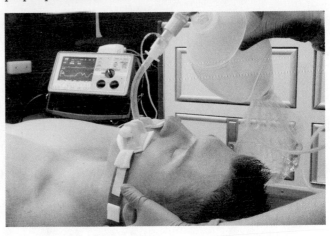

If the tube is pulled out, it can easily slip into the esophagus and send all the ventilations directly to the stomach (indicated by breath sounds over the epigastrium), denying the patient oxygen. Tube displacement is a fatal complication if it goes unnoticed.

NOTE: *Be especially careful not to disturb the endotracheal tube once it has been correctly placed and secured. Movement of the patient to a backboard, down stairs, and into the ambulance can easily cause displacement of the tube. If the tube comes out of the trachea, the patient receives no oxygen and will certainly die.*

Ventilating the Intubated Patient

When you are asked to ventilate an intubated or "tubed" patient, keep in mind that even very little movement can displace the tube. Look at the gradations on the side of the tube. In the typical adult male, for example, the 22-cm mark will be at the teeth when the tube is properly placed. If the tube moves, report this to the paramedic immediately.

Hold the tube against the patient's teeth with two fingers of one hand (Figure 9-27). Use the other hand to work the bag-valve-mask unit. (A patient with an endotracheal tube offers less resistance to ventilations, so you may not need two hands to work the bag.) If you are ventilating a breathing patient, be sure to provide ventilations that are timed with the patient's own respiratory effort as much as possible so the patient can take full breaths. It is also possible to help the patient increase his respiratory rate, if needed, by interposing extra ventilations. Remember these cautions:

- Pay close attention to what the ventilations feel like. Report any change in resistance. Increased resistance when ventilating with the bag-valve mask is one of the first signs of air escaping through a hole in the lungs and filling the space around the lungs, which is an extremely serious problem. A change in resistance can also indicate that the tube has slipped into the esophagus.

- When the patient is defibrillated, carefully remove the bag from the tube. If you do not, the weight of the unsupported bag may accidentally displace the tube.

- Watch for any change in the patient's mental status. A patient who becomes more alert may need to be restrained from pulling out the tube. In addition, an oral airway generally is used as a bite block (a device that prevents the patient from biting the endotracheal tube). If the patient's gag reflex returns along with increased consciousness, you may need to pull the bite block out a bit.

Finally, during a cardiac arrest in the absence of an IV line for administering medications, you may be asked to stop ventilating and remove the BVM. The paramedic may then inject a medication such as epinephrine down the endotracheal tube. To increase the rate at which medication enters the bloodstream through the respiratory system, you then may be asked to ventilate the patient for a few minutes. (Give ventilations at a faster-than-normal rate.)

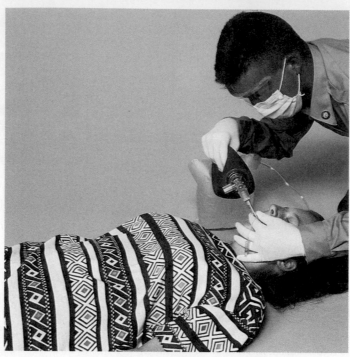

FIGURE 9-27 Make sure the endotracheal tube does not move. Hold it with two fingers against the patient's teeth.

Assisting with a Trauma Intubation

Occasionally you will be asked to assist in the endotracheal intubation of a patient with a suspected cervical spine injury. Since using the "sniffing position," which involves elevating the neck, risks worsening cervical spine injury, some modifications are necessary. Your role will change as well. You may be required to provide manual in-line stabilization during the whole procedure.

To accomplish this, the paramedic will hold manual stabilization while you apply a cervical collar. In some EMS systems, the patient may be intubated without a cervical collar in place but with attention to manual stabilization during and after intubation. Since the paramedic must stay at the patient's head, it will be necessary for you to stabilize the head and neck from the patient's side (Figure 9-28). Once you are in position, the paramedic will lean back and use the laryngoscope, which will bring the vocal cords into view. The patient can then be tubed.

FIGURE 9-28 To assist in the intubation of a patient with suspected cervical spine injury, maintain manual stabilization throughout the procedure.

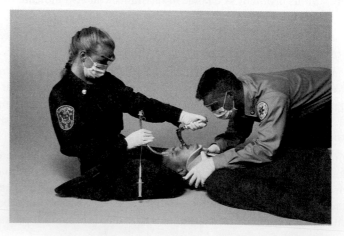

After intubation, you will hold the tube against the teeth until placement is confirmed with both an esophageal detector device and auscultation of both lungs and the epigastrium. Then the tube is anchored. At that time you can change your position to a more comfortable one. However, until the patient is immobilized on a long backboard, it will be necessary to assign another EMS worker to maintain manual stabilization while you ventilate the patient. Never assume that a collar provides adequate immobilization by itself. Manual stabilization must be used in addition to a collar until the head is taped in place on the backboard.

Blind-Insertion Airway Devices

Blind-insertion devices have increased in popularity recently because of the difficulty in inserting endotracheal tubes, a procedure that requires visualizing the glottis opening. Blind-insertion devices include the King LT ™ airway (Figure 9-29), Combitube® (Figure 9-30), and

FIGURE 9-29 The King LT-D™ airway, a disposable version of the King LT™ airway that is recommended for prehospital use. (© *Tracey Lemons/King Systems Corporation, Indianapolis, Indiana*)

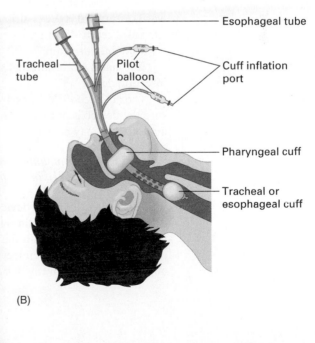

FIGURE 9-30 (A) The esophageal tracheal Combitube® and (B) the Combitube® in place.

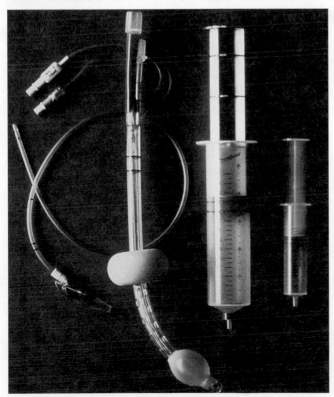

(A)

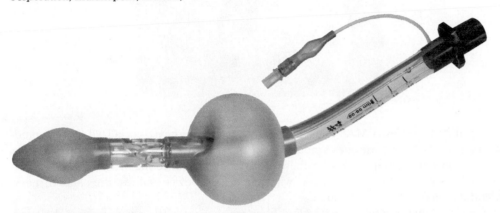

Esophageal tube

Tracheal tube

Pilot balloon

Cuff inflation port

Pharyngeal cuff

Tracheal or esophageal cuff

(B)

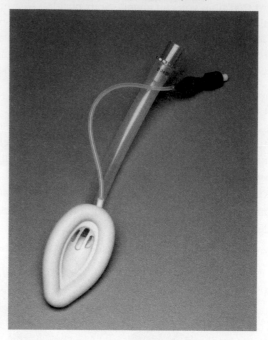

laryngeal mask airway (LMA™) (Figure 9-31). A few states have specialized training modules that allow EMTs to use one or more of these devices—always follow your local protocols.

The concepts of preparation for these airways are similar to the procedures listed earlier. The advanced EMT or paramedic will examine the device and test the balloon, mask, or cuff on the distal end of the tube.

One item that is different with blind-insertion devices is the positioning of the head. Blind-insertion devices usually do not require the head to be placed in the sniffing position. Instead, a position known as a "neutral position" where the head is not flexed either backward or forward is the position recommended by manufacturers. Depending on the device, the advanced EMT or paramedic may lubricate the device with a water-based jelly to allow for a smooth insertion.

It remains important that the patient is well-oxygenated prior to insertion of the blind-insertion device.

The advanced EMT or paramedic will listen over both lungs and the epigastrium to assure the device is properly placed. You will be asked to ventilate through the device so this auscultation may be performed. Use caution not to displace the tube during the process.

> **NOTE:** *The Combitube has two ports you can ventilate through. Begin by ventilating in the port labeled #1. Follow the instructions of the advanced provider for further ventilation.*

These blind-insertion devices do not have masks. You will ventilate directly into the tube. There are different guidelines for securing each of these devices. It is important that you follow the same rules as with the endotracheal tube: Do not let go of the BVM while it is attached to the tube. Disconnect the BVM when the patient is moved or defibrillated. Report any obvious tube movement or ventilatory changes to the advanced provider.

CHAPTER REVIEW

Key Facts and Concepts

- Respiratory failure is the result of inadequate breathing, breathing that is insufficient to support life.

- A patient in respiratory failure or respiratory arrest must receive artificial ventilations.

- Oxygen can be delivered to the nonbreathing patient as a supplement to artificial ventilation.

- Oxygen can also be administered as therapy to the breathing patient whose breathing is inadequate or who is cyanotic, cool and clammy, short of breath, suffering chest pain, suffering severe injuries, or displaying an altered mental status.

Key Decisions

- Is the patient breathing? Is the patient breathing adequately (ventilating *and* oxygenating)? Does the patient need supplemental oxygen?

- Is there a need to initiate artificial ventilation?

- Are my artificial ventilations adequate (proper rate and volume)?

Chapter Glossary

alveolar ventilation the amount of air that reaches the alveoli.

artificial ventilation forcing air or oxygen into the lungs when a patient has stopped breathing or has inadequate breathing. Also called *positive pressure ventilation*.

automatic transport ventilator (ATV) a device that provides positive pressure ventilations. It includes settings designed to adjust ventilation rate and volume, is portable, and is easily carried on an ambulance.

bag-valve mask (BVM) a handheld device with a face mask and self-refilling bag that can be squeezed to provide artificial ventilations to a patient. It can deliver air from the atmosphere or oxygen from a supplemental oxygen supply system.

cellular respiration the exchange of oxygen and carbon dioxide between cells and circulating blood.

cricoid pressure pressure applied to the cricoid ring to minimize air entry into the esophagus during positive pressure ventilation. Also called *Sellick maneuver*.

cyanosis (SIGH-uh-NO-sis) a blue or gray color resulting from lack of oxygen in the body.

diffusion a process by which molecules move from an area of high concentration to an area of low concentration.

flowmeter a valve that indicates the flow of oxygen in liters per minute.

flow-restricted, oxygen-powered ventilation device (FROPVD) a device that uses oxygen under pressure to deliver artificial ventilations. Its trigger is placed so that the rescuer can operate it while still using both hands to maintain a seal on the face mask. It has automatic flow restriction to prevent overdelivery of oxygen to the patient.

humidifier a device connected to the flowmeter to add moisture to the dry oxygen coming from an oxygen cylinder.

hypoxia (hi-POK-se-uh) an insufficiency of oxygen in the body's tissues.

nasal cannula (NAY-zul KAN-yuh-luh) a device that delivers low concentrations of oxygen through two prongs that rest in the patient's nostrils.

nonrebreather (NRB) mask a face mask and reservoir bag device that delivers high concentrations of oxygen. The patient's exhaled air escapes through a valve and is not rebreathed.

oxygen cylinder a cylinder filled with oxygen under pressure.

partial rebreather mask a face mask and reservoir oxygen bag with no one-way valve to the reservoir bag so that some exhaled air mixes with the oxygen; used in some patients to help preserve carbon dioxide levels in the blood to stimulate breathing.

pocket face mask a device, usually with a one-way valve, to aid in artificial ventilation. A rescuer breathes through the valve when the mask is placed over the patient's face. It also acts as a barrier to prevent contact with a patient's breath or body fluids. It can be used with supplemental oxygen when fitted with an oxygen inlet.

positive pressure ventilation *See* artificial ventilation.

pressure regulator a device connected to an oxygen cylinder to reduce cylinder pressure so it is safe for delivery of oxygen to a patient.

pulmonary respiration the exchange of oxygen and carbon dioxide between the alveoli and circulating blood in the pulmonary capillaries.

respiration (RES-pir-AY-shun) the diffusion of oxygen and carbon dioxide between the alveoli and the blood (pulmonary respiration) and between the blood and the cells (cellular respiration). Also used to mean, simply, breathing.

respiratory arrest when breathing completely stops.

respiratory distress increased work of breathing; a sensation of shortness of breath.

respiratory failure the reduction of breathing to the point where oxygen intake is not sufficient to support life.

stoma a permanent surgical opening in the neck through which the patient breathes.

tracheostomy mask a device designed to be placed over a stoma or tracheostomy tube to provide supplemental oxygen.

ventilation breathing in and out (inhalation and exhalation), or artificial provision of breaths.

Venturi mask a face mask and reservoir bag device that delivers specific concentrations of oxygen by mixing oxygen with inhaled air.

Preparation for Your Examination and Practice

Short Answer

1. Describe the signs of respiratory distress.
2. Describe the signs of respiratory failure.
3. Name and briefly describe the techniques of artificial ventilation (mouth-to-mask, BVM, FROPVD).
4. For BVM ventilation, describe recommended variations in technique for one or two rescuers and for a patient with trauma suspected or trauma not suspected.
5. Describe how positive pressure ventilation moves air differently from how the body normally moves air.
6. Name patient problems that would benefit from administration of oxygen and explain how to decide what oxygen delivery device (nonrebreather mask, nasal cannula, or other) should be used for a particular patient.

Thinking and Linking

Think back to Chapter 8, "Airway Management," and link information from that chapter with information from this chapter to describe how the process of moving air in and out of the chest might be interfered with by the following dysfunctions:

1. Penetrating trauma to the chest
2. A spinal injury that paralyzes the diaphragm
3. Bronchoconstriction that narrows the air passages
4. A rib fracture
5. A brain injury to the respiratory control center in the medulla

Critical Thinking Exercises

Careful assessment is needed in order to decide if a patient does or does not need artificial ventilation. The purpose of this exercise will be to apply this skill in the following situations.

1. On arrival at the emergency scene, you find an adult female patient who is semiconscious. Her respiratory rate is 7/min. She appears pale and slightly blue around her lips. What immediate actions are necessary? Is this patient in respiratory failure, and if so what signs and symptoms indicate this? Does this patient require artificial ventilations?

2. On arrival at the emergency scene, you find an adult male patient sitting bolt upright in a chair. He looks at you as you come into the room, but he is unable to speak more than two words at a time. He seems to have a prolonged expiratory phase; you hear wheezes, and his respiratory rate is 36. What immediate actions are necessary? Is this patient in respiratory failure, and if so what signs and symptoms indicate this? Does this patient require artificial ventilations?

3. On arrival at the scene of a motor-vehicle crash, you find an adult female patient pacing outside her damaged vehicle. She appears to be breathing very rapidly but acknowledges you as you approach. Her color seems normal and her respiratory rate is 48. What immediate actions are necessary? Is this patient in respiratory failure, and if so what signs and symptoms indicate this? Does this patient require artificial ventilations?

Pathophysiology to Practice

The following questions are designed to assist you in gathering relevant clinical information and making accurate decisions in the field.

1. Describe the elements you would assess to determine if a patient is breathing adequately.
2. You are assessing a breathing patient. Describe what findings might indicate the need to initiate artificial ventilations despite the fact the patient continues to breathe.
3. Describe how you would determine that you have delivered enough air (volume) when ventilating using a bag-valve mask.

"Dispatch to unit 401, respond to 244 Lisbon St. for a patient with shortness of breath." En route, you make a preliminary plan with your partners, Danielle and Jim. You discuss what equipment the team will bring in and briefly review the immediate life threats associated with shortness of breath. Going into the apartment building, you bring in the stretcher, jump kit, oxygen, portable suction, and BVM unit.

As you approach the apartment, you notice that the hall smells of cigarette smoke. The odor is worse as you enter the unit. Your patient is found sitting at the kitchen table. He is a tall, thin, 70-year-old man. He appears anxious and is obviously having trouble breathing.

Street Scene Questions

1. What is your first priority when starting to assess this patient?
2. Assuming his airway is patent, what are the essential elements in assessing this patient's breathing?
3. What type of emergency care should you be prepared to give?

As you assess the patient, you note he is breathing rapidly with an audible wheeze. He seems very tired. He can only speak one or two words at a time and you notice that his fingernails are blue. You also notice that his respiratory rate slows down and becomes slightly irregular from time to time.

Street Scene Questions

4. Is this patient's breathing adequate (why/why not)?
5. Does this patient require artificial ventilation?

The team decides that this patient is in respiratory failure, is tiring out, and needs immediate ventilation. You connect the BVM to high-concentration oxygen and begin to ventilate the patient. At first the patient is uncooperative and you find it difficult to time your ventilations with his. However, after a few breaths your timing begins to work. About every fourth patient breath you administer a breath to help increase tidal volume. The patient becomes more and more comfortable with this.

Jim continues the assessment while Danielle requests advanced life support backup and prepares for rapid transport.

You continue ventilating as the team loads the patient and initiates transport.

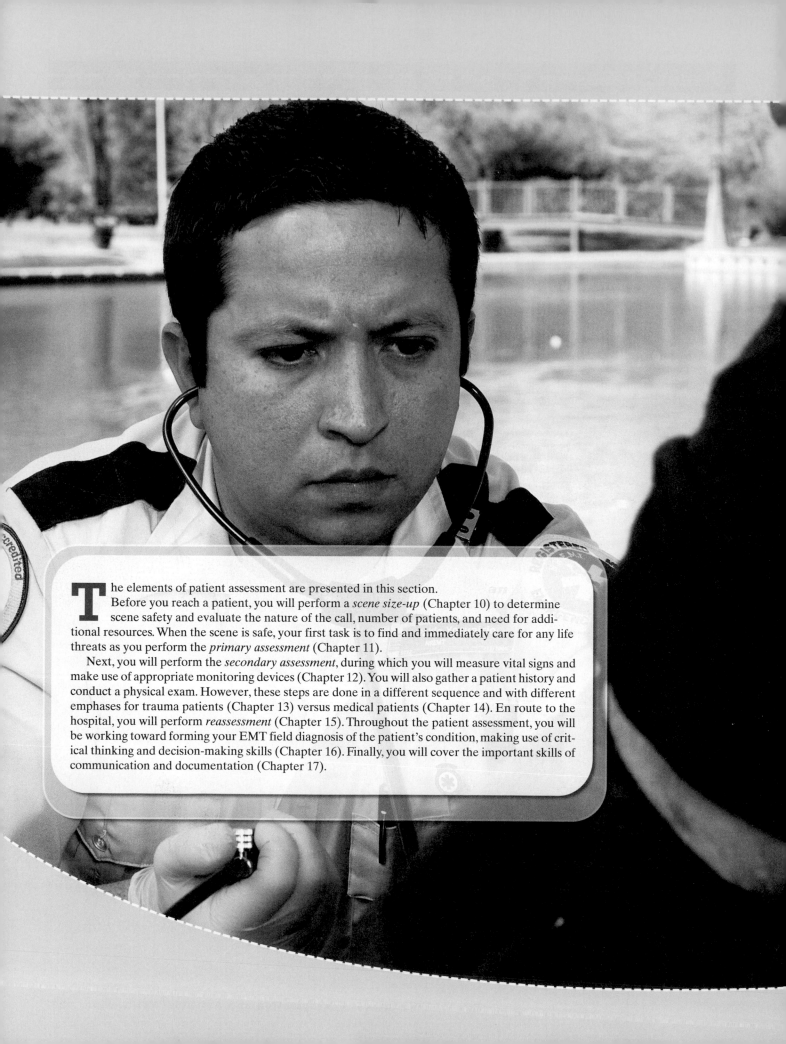

The elements of patient assessment are presented in this section.

Before you reach a patient, you will perform a *scene size-up* (Chapter 10) to determine scene safety and evaluate the nature of the call, number of patients, and need for additional resources. When the scene is safe, your first task is to find and immediately care for any life threats as you perform the *primary assessment* (Chapter 11).

Next, you will perform the *secondary assessment*, during which you will measure vital signs and make use of appropriate monitoring devices (Chapter 12). You will also gather a patient history and conduct a physical exam. However, these steps are done in a different sequence and with different emphases for trauma patients (Chapter 13) versus medical patients (Chapter 14). En route to the hospital, you will perform *reassessment* (Chapter 15). Throughout the patient assessment, you will be working toward forming your EMT field diagnosis of the patient's condition, making use of critical thinking and decision-making skills (Chapter 16). Finally, you will cover the important skills of communication and documentation (Chapter 17).

Patient Assessment

10

Scene Size-Up

EXPLORE Resource Central

To access Resource Central, follow directions on the Student Access Card provided with this text. If there is no card, go to **www.bradybooks.com** and follow the Resource Central link to Buy Access from there. Under Media Resources, you will find:

▶ **Sizing Up the Scene**
Your first priority is to protect yourself. Discover how information from dispatch impacts an EMT's ability to size up the scene and how bystander interactions could influence the scene size-up.

▶ **Mechanism of Injury (MOI)**
Watch a video on identifying mechanism of injury, how the significance of the MOI influences patient care, and what equipment might be needed when an EMT assesses a trauma patient.

▶ **Traffic Injuries and Fatalities Information**
Think getting stuck in traffic is bad? It's better than being the cause of it! Find statistics on traffic injuries and fatalities in 2009 and read about some safety concerns an EMT should have when approaching the scene of a motor vehicle collision.

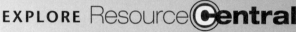

OBJECTIVES

After reading this chapter you should be able to:

10.1 Define key terms introduced in this chapter.

10.2 Explain the ongoing nature of scene size-up beyond the initial moments at the scene. (p. 245)

10.3 Given a scene-arrival scenario, list several examples of potential hazards for which the EMT should actively search. (pp. 245–248)

10.4 Describe considerations in establishing a danger zone at the scene of a vehicle collision. (pp. 248–250)

10.5 Recognize indications of possible crime scenes and the potential for violence. (pp. 250–252)

10.6 Use information from the scene size-up to make decisions about the use of Standard Precautions to protect against disease exposure. (p. 252)

10.7 Use information from the scene size-up to determine the mechanism of injury or nature of the illness. (pp. 253–260)

(continued)

10.8 Explain the importance of determining the number of patients and the need for additional resources in the scene size-up. (pp. 260–261)

10.9 Given a number of scenarios, perform a scene size-up, including:

a. Recognizing potential dangers (pp. 245–252)

b. Making decisions about body substance isolation (p. 252)

c. Determining the nature of the illness or mechanism of injury (pp. 253–260)

d. Determining the number of patients (pp. 260–261)

e. Determining the need for additional resources. (pp. 260–261)

KEY TERMS

blunt-force trauma, *p. 259*

danger zone, *p. 248*

index of suspicion, *p. 260*

mechanism of injury, *p. 253*

nature of the illness, *p. 260*

penetrating trauma, *p. 258*

scene size-up, *p. 245*

SCENE SIZE-UP

Scene size-up is the first part of the patient assessment process. It begins as you approach the scene, surveying it to determine if there are any threats to your own safety or to the safety of your patients or bystanders, to determine the nature of the call, and to decide if you will need additional help. (See *Visual Guide: Scene Size-Up.*)

However, scene size-up is not confined to the first part of the assessment process. These considerations should continue throughout the call since emergencies are dynamic, always-changing events. You may find, for example, that patients, family members, or bystanders who were not a problem initially become increasingly hostile later in the call or that vehicles or structures that seemed stable suddenly shift and pose a danger.

After your initial scene size-up, you will become more directly involved in patient assessment and care. However, it is a good idea to remember the key size-up elements throughout the call to prevent dangerous surprises later.

You can obtain important information from just a brief survey of the scene. For example, you might see a downed electrical wire at the scene of a vehicle collision, a potentially deadly situation for you as the EMT, your patient, and bystanders. Further observations of the scene are likely to reveal more important information about the mechanism of injury. For example, damage to the steering wheel or windshield would be a strong indicator of potential chest, head, or neck injury caused by driver impact with those surfaces. A deployed air bag would cause you to assess for injuries air bags might cause, especially to an infant or child front-seat passenger (Figure 10-1).

Just as important as your observations will be the actions you take to obtain needed assistance and prevent further injury. For example, if there were two patients at a collision, you would request that a second ambulance be dispatched to the scene—more if you discovered that there were additional passengers. If there was also a downed wire at that scene, which poses a danger of fire, you would notify the fire department as well as the power company and the police department. In addition, you would take steps to keep bystanders clear of traffic, the collision, and the patients.

Scene Safety

The only predictable thing about emergencies is that they are often unpredictable and can pose many dangers if you are not careful.

>>>>>>

CORE CONCEPT ●
Identifying hazards at a scene

scene size-up
steps taken when approaching the scene of an emergency call: checking scene safety, taking Standard Precautions, noting the mechanism of injury or nature of the patient's illness, determining the number of patients, and deciding what, if any, additional resources to call for.

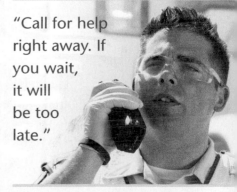

"Call for help right away. If you wait, it will be too late."

CHAPTER 10
Scene Size-Up

■ EXAMINE THE SCENE, MINIMIZE DANGERS, PLAN AHEAD

Identify hazards

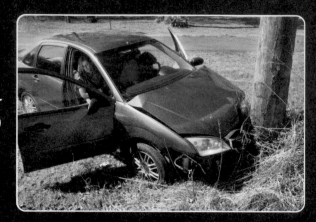

Examine for mechanism of injury or Nature of Illness (medical patient)

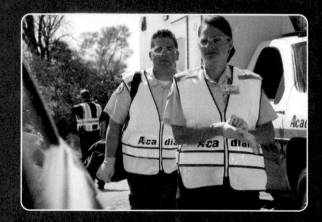

Take appropriate Standard Precautions

Determine number of patients

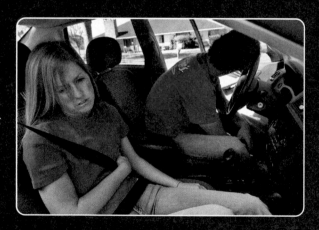

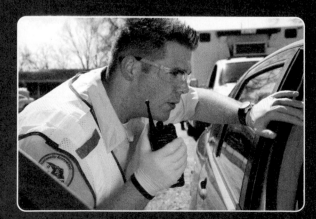

Radio for additional resources early

FIGURE 10-1 Clues such as (A) exterior damage, (B) a deployed air bag, or (C) a damaged windshield may lead you to suspect certain types of injuries. *(Photos A and B: © Daniel Limmer)*

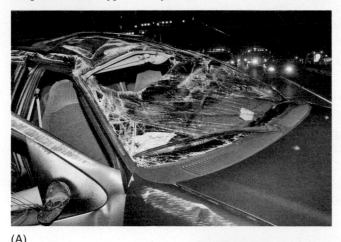

(A)

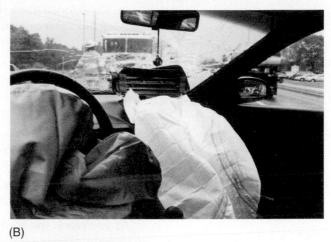

(B)

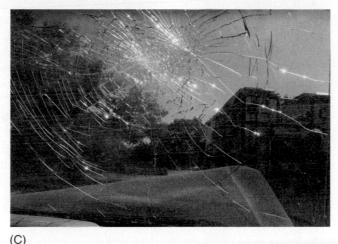

(C)

Before you arrive on-scene, the dispatcher may relay important information to you. A well-trained Emergency Medical Dispatcher (EMD) uses a set of questions to determine information that may affect you directly. For example, if the caller tells the EMD of particular hazards, you could immediately call for additional specialized assistance. You will learn more about the questions an EMD asks in Chapter 38, "EMS Operations."

Often you will arrive at a scene where there are police, fire, and even other ambulances already present. In a situation like this, do not assume that the scene is safe or that others have taken care of any hazards. Always perform your own size-up, no matter who arrives first. Scan for scene hazards, infection-control concerns, mechanisms of injury, and number of patients. The scene size-up begins even before the ambulance comes to a stop. Observe the scene while you approach and again before you exit the vehicle.

The following are scene size-up considerations you should keep in mind when you approach a crash or hazardous material emergency:

As you near the collision scene:

- Look and listen for other emergency service units approaching from side streets.
- Look for signs of a collision-related power outage, such as darkened areas which suggest that wires are down at the collision scene.
- Observe traffic flow. If there is no opposing traffic, suspect a blockade at the collision scene.
- Look for smoke in the direction of the collision scene—a sign that fire has resulted from the collision.

When you are within sight of the scene:

- Look for clues indicating escaped hazardous materials, such as placards, a damaged truck, escaping liquids, fumes, or vapor clouds. If you see anything suspicious, stop the ambulance

CORE CONCEPT

Determining if a scene is safe to enter

immediately and consult your hazardous-materials reference book or hazardous-materials team, if one is available. (See more information under "Establishing the Danger Zone.")

- Look for collision victims on or near the road. A person may have been thrown from a vehicle as it careened out of control, or an injured person may have walked away from the wreckage and collapsed on or near the roadway.

- Look for smoke not seen at a distance.

- Look for broken utility poles and downed wires. At night, direct the beam of a spotlight or handlight on poles and wire spans as you approach the scene. Keep in mind that wires may be down several hundred feet from the crash vehicles.

- Be alert for persons walking along the side of the road toward the collision scene. Curious onlookers (excited children in particular) are often oblivious to vehicles approaching from behind.

- Watch for the signals of police officers and other emergency service personnel. They may have information about hazards or the location of injured persons.

As you reach the scene:

- If personnel are at the scene and using the incident command/management system, follow the instructions of the person in charge. This may involve the positioning of the ambulance, wearing protective equipment and apparel, determining where to find the patients, or being aware of specific hazards. The Incident Commander may be able to provide you with lifesaving information regarding unstable conditions such as the stability of a building and the possibility of structural collapse.

  Don appropriate protective apparel, including head protection, a bunker coat (or similar clothing that will protect you from sharp edges), and a reflective vest that goes over your coat and meets the requirements of OSHA. You should have extrication gloves easily available in a pocket. When temperature and weather are significant factors, be sure to protect yourself with clothing that will keep you dry and at the appropriate temperature.

  Sniff for odors such as gasoline or diesel fuel or any unusual odor that may signal a hazardous material release.

Establishing the Danger Zone

danger zone
the area around the wreckage of a vehicle collision or other incident within which special safety precautions should be taken.

A **danger zone** exists around the wreckage of every vehicle collision, within which special safety precautions must be taken. The size of the zone depends on the nature and severity of collision-produced hazards (Scan 10-1). An ambulance should never be parked within the danger zone. Follow these guidelines in establishing the danger zone:

- **When there are no apparent hazards.** In this case, consider the danger zone to extend at least 50 feet in all directions from the wreckage. The ambulance will be away from broken glass and other debris, and it will not impede emergency service personnel who must work in or around the wreckage. When using highway flares to protect the scene, make sure that the person igniting them has been trained in the proper technique.

- **When fuel has been spilled.** In this case, consider the danger zone to extend a minimum of 100 feet in all directions from the wreckage and fuel. In addition to parking outside the danger zone, park upwind, if possible. (Note the direction of the wind by observing flags, smoke, and so on.) Thus, the ambulance will be out of the path of dense smoke if the fuel ignites. If fuel is flowing away from the wreckage, park uphill as well as upwind. If parking uphill is not possible, position the ambulance as far from the flowing fuel as possible. Avoid gutters, ditches, and gullies that can carry fuel to the ambulance. Do not use flares in areas where fuel has been spilled. Use orange traffic cones during daylight and reflective triangles at night.

- **When a vehicle is on fire.** In this case, consider the danger zone to extend at least 100 feet in all directions even if the fire appears small and limited to the engine compartment. If fire reaches the vehicle's fuel tank, an explosion could easily damage an ambulance parked closer than 100 feet.

- **When wires are down.** In this case, consider the danger zone as the area in which people or vehicles might be in contact with energized wires if the wires pivot around their points of attachment. Even though you may have to carry equipment and stretchers for

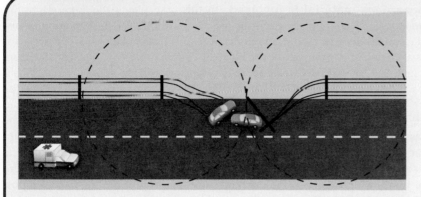

Downed Lines

In incidents involving downed electrical wires and damaged utility poles, the danger zone should extend beyond each intact pole for a full span and to the sides for the distance that the severed wires can reach. Stay out of the danger zone until the utility company has deactivated the wires, or until trained rescuers have moved and anchored them.

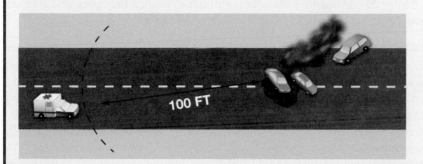

Vehicle on Fire

If no other hazards are involved, such as dangerous chemicals or explosives, the ambulance should park no closer than 100 feet (about 30 meters) from a burning vehicle. Park upwind.

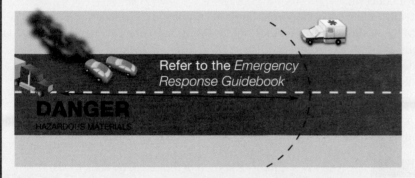

Hazardous Material Threatened by Fire

When hazardous materials are either involved in or threatened by fire, the size of the danger zone is dictated by the nature of the material. Use binoculars to read teh placard on the truck and refer to the *Emergency Response Guidebook* for a safe distance to establish your command post. Park upwind.

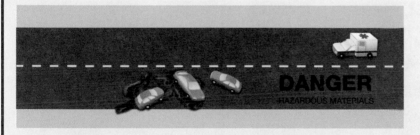

Spilled Fuel

The ambulance should be parked upwind from flowing fuel. If this is not possible, the vehicle should be parked as far from the fuel flow as possible, avoiding gutters, ditches, and gullies that may carry the spill to the parking site. Remember, your ambulance's catalytic converter is an ignition source over 1000 degrees Fahrenheit.

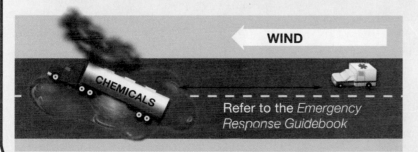

Hazardous Materials

Leaking containers of dangerous chemicals may produce a health as well as a fire hazard. When chemicals have been spilled, whether fumes are evident or not, the ambulance should be parked upwind. if the hazardous material is known, seek advice from experts such as CHEMTREC through the Incident Commander.

a considerable distance, the ambulance should be parked at least one full span of wires away from the poles to which broken wires are attached.

- **When a hazardous material is involved.** In this case, check the *Emergency Response Guidebook (ERG)*—published by the U.S. Department of Transportation, Transport Canada, and the Secretariat of Communications and Transportation of Mexico—for suggestions as to where to park, or ask the Incident Commander to request advice from an agency such as CHEMTREC (Chemical Transportation Emergency Center, Washington, DC, 24-hour hotline 800-424-9300 or 703-527-3887). In some cases you may be able to park 50 feet from the wreckage, as when no hazardous material has been spilled or released. In other cases, you may be warned to park 2,000 feet or more from the wreckage, as when there is the possibility that certain high explosives may detonate. In all cases, park upwind from the wreckage when you discover that a hazardous material is present at a collision site. Park uphill if a liquid is flowing, but on the same level if there are gases or fumes which may rise. Park behind some artificial or natural barrier if possible. (In Chapter 38, "EMS Operations," you will learn more about parking the ambulance. In Chapter 39, "Hazardous Materials, Multiple-Casualty Incidents, and Incident Management," you will learn more about hazardous materials.)

Crime Scenes and Acts of Violence

Another significant danger faced by the EMT is violence. Crime risks vary, but it is certain that EMTs working in the field are exposed to more dangerous situations than they were even a few years ago. Shootings at elementary and secondary schools, colleges, and shopping malls, as well as terrorist incidents, are now on the minds of EMS providers.

Although a majority of calls go by uneventfully, the EMT must be conscious of dangers from many sources, including other human beings (Figure 10-2). EMTs often envision violence as occurring at bar fights or on the street, but domestic violence (violence in the home) is also a cause for concern.

Protection from violence is as important as protection from the dangers at a vehicle collision. As an EMT, you should never enter a violent situation to provide care. Safety at a violent scene requires a careful size-up as you approach. Just as a downed wire signals danger at a collision site, there are many signals of danger from violence that you may observe as you approach the scene, such as:

- **Fighting or loud voices.** If you approach a scene and see or hear fighting, threatening words or actions, or the potential for fighting, there is a good chance that the scene will be a danger to you.

FIGURE 10-2 Crowds are a potential source of violence. *(© Mark C. Ide)*

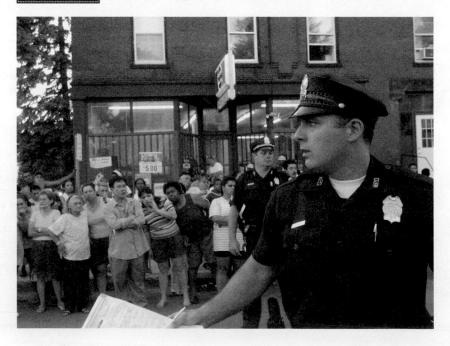

- **Weapons visible or in use.** Any time you observe a weapon, you must use an extreme amount of caution. The weapon may actually be in the hands of an attacker (a grave danger), or simply in sight. Weapons include knives, guns, and martial arts weapons as well as any other items that may be used as weapons.

- **Signs of alcohol or other drug use.** When alcohol or other drugs are in use, a certain unpredictability exists at any scene. It will not take long for you to observe unusual behavior from a person under the influence of one of these substances. This behavior may result in violence toward emergency personnel at the scene. Additionally, there are hazards associated with the drug culture, such as street violence and the presence of contaminated needles.

- **Unusual silence.** Emergencies are usually active events. A call that is "too quiet" should raise your suspicions. Although there may be a good reason for the silence, extra care should be taken.

- **Knowledge of prior violence.** If you or a member of your crew has been to a particular location for calls involving violence in the past, extra caution must be used on subsequent calls to the same location. Neighbors may sometimes volunteer information about previous incidents.

Whether the call is residential or in the street, observe the scene for the signs of danger listed previously and any others you may find (Figure 10-3). This brief danger assessment may be all that is required to prevent harm to you or your crew during the call.

FIGURE 10-3 Whether the call is to a residence or to the street, a variety of hazards may be present.

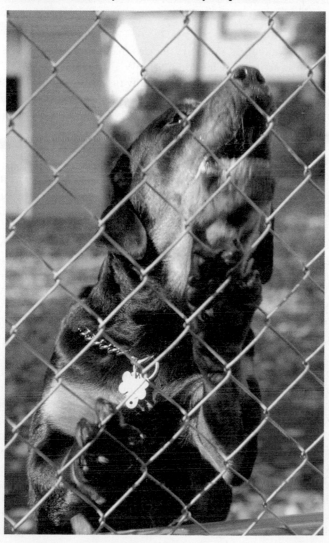

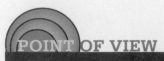

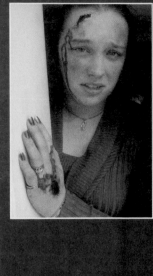

"I am still a relatively new EMT. Everyone always said you never know what you will find when you respond to a call. Well, I found out about this pretty early in my EMS career.

"My crew and I were sent to a 'fall' at a residence in a decent part of town. We pulled up to the house. Everything looked calm—but sometimes you just can't tell from the outside. We went to the door. We stood to the sides of the door like we were trained. We knocked. The woman came to the door and she looked like she had been through a war. I started to move like I was going into the house but she pushed the door closed a bit more and kind of peeked out. My first thought was to say, 'Come on. Let us in. We need to take care of you.' She put her weight behind the door and wouldn't let us in. Then it hit me. She didn't fall. Whatever had happened, she was trying to protect us.

"I asked her to step outside so we could talk but she refused. I motioned for my other crew members to get back to the rig and mouthed, 'Call for help.'

"I felt so helpless. I didn't want her to go back inside, but I was already on borrowed time and should be retreating. 'Come out here. Please!' I urged in a forced whisper. She looked behind her and then shut the door in my face.

"I moved rapidly to the rig, watching my back. We drove out of sight. Two police cruisers came by pretty quickly. I filled them in on what I saw. They went to the scene. About 5 minutes later the dispatcher radioed us to go back in. They had a man in handcuffs. The woman was crying. I'm still not sure whether she was crying because she was hurt or because he was arrested. The look in her eyes was so vacant.

"Always, always, always size-up the scene. I always wonder what would've happened if I wasn't cautious going to that call."

If you observe signs of danger, there are actions that you must take to protect yourself. You learned about these actions in Chapter 2, "The Well-Being of the EMT." To summarize: The specific actions you should take depend on many factors including your local protocols, the type of danger, and the help available to you. In general, you should retreat to a position of safety, call for help, and return only after the scene has been secured by police. Be sure to document the danger and your actions.

Standard Precautions

As you perform your initial size-up of the scene, there are many important points to consider. One very important aspect of personal protection—and one that you will need long after you have addressed any physical dangers—is Standard Precautions, also called body substance isolation (BSI).

You learned about Standard Precautions and personal protective equipment (PPE) in Chapter 2, "The Well-Being of the EMT." To summarize: Body substances include blood, saliva, and any other body fluids or contents. All body substances can carry viruses and bacteria. Your patient's body substances can enter your body through cuts or other openings in your skin. They can also easily enter your body through your eyes, nose, and mouth. You are especially at risk of being infected by a patient's body substances when the patient is bleeding, coughing, or sneezing, or whenever you make direct contact with the patient, as in mouth-to-mouth ventilation. Infection is a two-way street, of course. You can also infect the patient.

For example, at a vehicle collision that is likely to have caused severe injuries with bleeding, all personnel should wear protective gloves and eyewear. Since this potential hazard can be spotted before there is any contact with the patient, everyone should be wearing gloves before beginning patient care. If a patient requires suctioning or spits up blood, this would be another indication for protective eyewear and a mask. Whenever a patient is suspected of having tuberculosis or another disease spread through the air, wear an N-95 or high efficiency particulate air (HEPA) respirator to filter out airborne particles the patient exhales or expels.

A key element of Standard Precautions is always to have personal protective equipment readily available, either on your person or as the first items you encounter when opening a response kit. Remember that taking proper Standard Precautions early in the call and evaluating the need for such precautions throughout the call will prevent needless exposure later on.

Nature of the Call

After you have ensured scene safety and taken the appropriate Standard Precautions, it is important to determine the nature of the call by identifying the mechanism of injury or the nature of the patient's illness.

Mechanism of Injury

The **mechanism of injury** is what causes an injury (e.g., a rapid deceleration causes the knees to strike the dash of a car; a fall on ice causes a twisting force to the ankle) (Scan 10-2).

Certain injuries are considered "common" to particular situations. Injuries to bones and joints are usually associated with falls and vehicle collisions; burns are common to fires and explosions; penetrating soft-tissue injuries can be associated with gunshot wounds, and so on.

Even if you cannot determine the exact injury the patient has sustained, knowing the mechanism of injury may allow you to predict various injury patterns. For example, in many situations you will immobilize the patient's spine because the mechanism of injury, such as a forceful blow, is frequently associated with spinal injury. You do not need to know that the

CORE CONCEPT

Mechanisms of injury and how they relate to patient condition

mechanism of injury

a force or forces that may have caused injury.

SCAN 10-2 Mechanism of Injury and Affected Areas of the Body

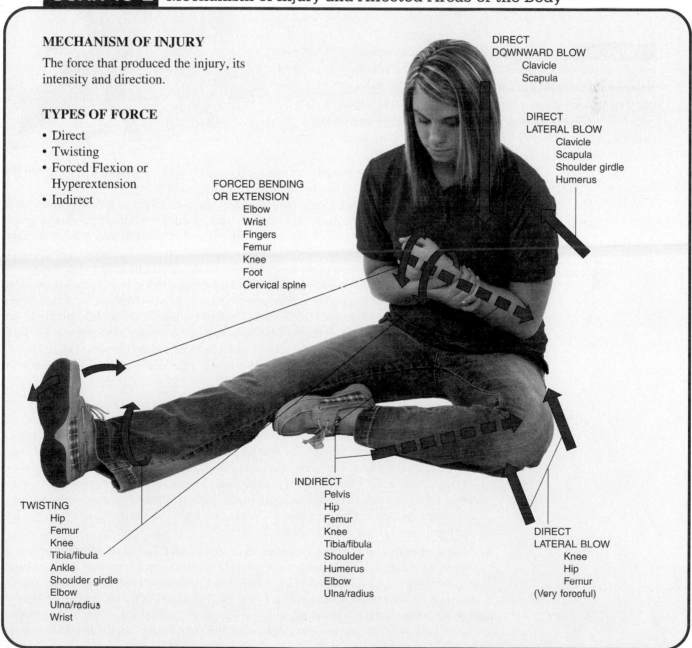

MECHANISM OF INJURY

The force that produced the injury, its intensity and direction.

TYPES OF FORCE

- Direct
- Twisting
- Forced Flexion or Hyperextension
- Indirect

FORCED BENDING OR EXTENSION
Elbow
Wrist
Fingers
Femur
Knee
Foot
Cervical spine

DIRECT DOWNWARD BLOW
Clavicle
Scapula

DIRECT LATERAL BLOW
Clavicle
Scapula
Shoulder girdle
Humerus

TWISTING
Hip
Femur
Knee
Tibia/fibula
Ankle
Shoulder girdle
Elbow
Ulna/radius
Wrist

INDIRECT
Pelvis
Hip
Femur
Knee
Tibia/fibula
Shoulder
Humerus
Elbow
Ulna/radius

DIRECT LATERAL BLOW
Knee
Hip
Femur
(Very forceful)

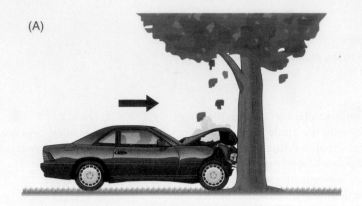

(A)

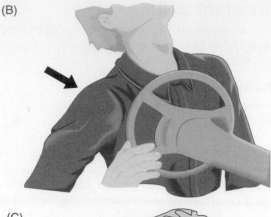

(B)

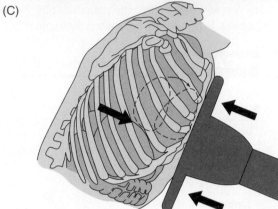

(C)

FIGURE 10-4 There are three collisions in a motor-vehicle crash: (A) a vehicle collision, when the vehicle strikes an object; (B) a body collision, when the person's body strikes the interior of the vehicle; and (C) an organ collision, when the person's organs strike interior surfaces of the body.

patient's spine is actually injured; you assume it is and treat accordingly. Knowing that the patient has fallen should tell you to check for an injured arm or leg.

Motor-Vehicle Collisions   Identifying the mechanism of injury is very important when dealing with motor-vehicle collisions. For example, a collapsed or bent steering column suggests that the driver has suffered a chest-wall injury with possible rib or even lung or heart damage. A shattered, blood-spattered windshield points to the likelihood of a forehead or scalp laceration and possibly a severe blow to the head that may have caused a head or spinal injury.

The law of inertia—that a body in motion will remain in motion unless acted upon by an outside force (e.g., being stopped by striking something)—explains why there are actually three collisions involved in each motor-vehicle crash. The first collision is the vehicle striking an object. The second collision is when the patient's body strikes the interior of the vehicle. The third collision occurs when the organs of the patient strike surfaces within the body (Figure 10-4).

Identifying the type of motor-vehicle collision also provides important information on potential injury patterns:

- **Head-on collisions.** These have a great potential for injury to all parts of the body. Two types of injury patterns are likely: the up-and-over pattern and the down-and-under pattern. In the first pattern, the patient follows a pathway up and over the steering wheel, commonly striking the head on the windshield (especially when he was not wearing a seat belt), causing head and neck injuries. Additionally, the patient may strike the chest and abdomen on the steering wheel, causing chest injuries or breathing problems and internal organ injuries. In the second pattern, the patient's body follows a pathway down and under the steering wheel, typically striking his knees on the dash, causing knee, leg, and hip injuries (Figures 10-5 and 10-6).

- **Rear-end collisions.** These are common causes of neck and head injuries. The law of inertia states not only that a body in motion will remain in motion unless acted on by an outside force (as discussed earlier), but also that a body at rest will remain at rest unless acted on by an outside force (such as being pushed or jerked). This explains why neck injuries are common in a rear-end collision—the head remains still as the body is pushed violently forward by the seat back, extending the neck backward, if a headrest was not properly placed behind the head (Figures 10-7 and 10-8).

FIGURE 10-5 A head-on impact.

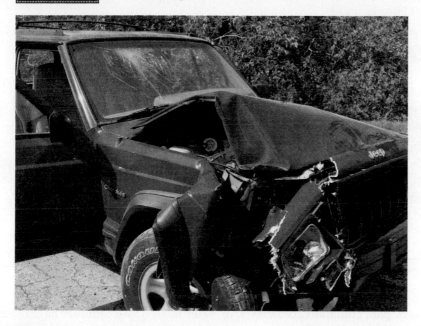

FIGURE 10-6 In a head-on collision, an unrestrained person is likely to travel in (A) an up-and-over pathway causing head, neck, chest, and abdominal injuries or in (B) a down-and-under pathway causing hip, knee, and leg injuries. (C) A deploying airbag can also cause injuries.

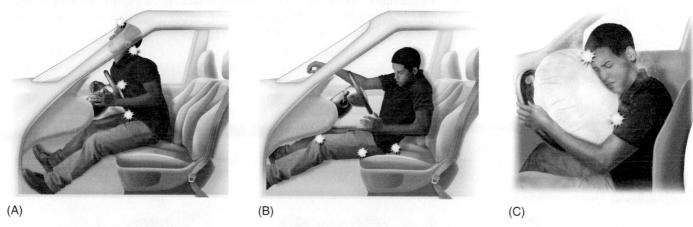

(A)   (B)   (C)

FIGURE 10-7 Rear impact. (© Edward T. Dickinson, MD)

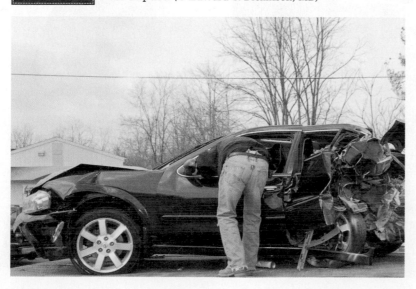

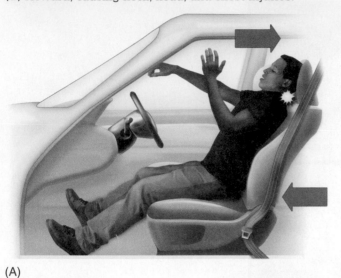

(A)

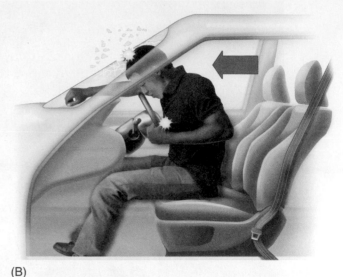

(B)

- **Side-impact collisions** *(broadside, or "T-Bone")*. These collisions have other injury patterns. The head tends to remain still as the body is pushed laterally, causing injuries to the neck. The head, chest, abdomen, pelvis, and thighs may be struck directly, causing skeletal and internal injuries (Figures 10-9 and 10-10).

- **Rollover collisions.** These are potentially the most serious because of the potential for multiple impacts. Rollover collisions frequently cause ejection of anyone who is not wearing a seat belt. Expect any type of serious injury pattern (Figures 10-11 and 10-12).

- **Rotational impact collisions.** These involve cars that are struck, then spin. The initial impact often causes subsequent impacts (the spinning vehicle strikes another vehicle or a tree). As in a rollover collision, this can cause multiple injury patterns.

FIGURE 10-10 A side-impact collision may cause head and neck injuries as well as injuries to the chest, abdomen, pelvis, and thighs.

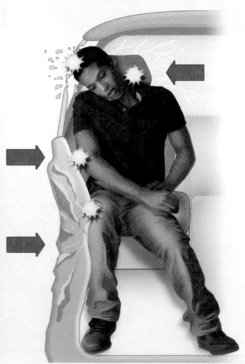

FIGURE 10-9 Side impact. *(© Edward T. Dickinson, MD)*

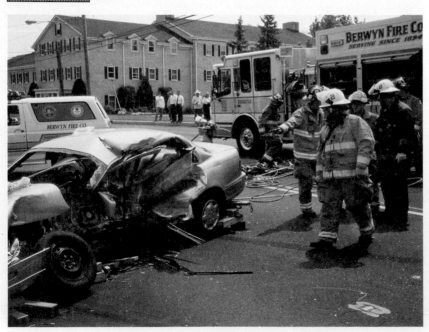

FIGURE 10-11 Rollover collision. *(© Daniel Limmer)*

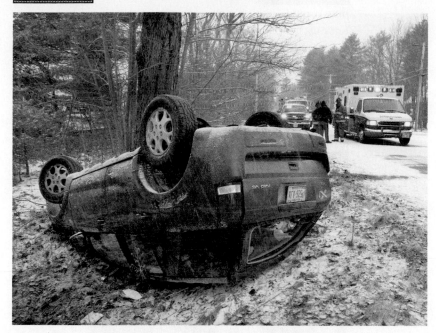

An important aspect of mechanism of injury determination is to find out where the patient was sitting in the vehicle and if he was wearing lap and shoulder belts. Note any deformities in the steering wheel, dash, pedals, or other structures within the vehicle.

You will often be able to observe important clues regarding mechanism of injury before you even exit the ambulance. At a head-on collision, for instance, you can anticipate up-and-over or down-and-under injury patterns for a driver who remains in his car and multiple injury patterns for a driver who is thrown from his car. For both patients, anticipate external injuries (from the collision of the body with auto interiors and pavement) and internal injuries (from collision of organs with the interior of the body as well as from external blunt-force or penetrating trauma). When a patient appears to have been the driver of a vehicle, look for damage to the windshield, steering wheel, dash, and pedals when you are able to do a close-up inspection. You should also observe for damage to other interior surfaces, which might indicate there were additional passengers/patients.

Injuries involving motorcycles and all-terrain vehicles also have the potential to be serious. These vehicles offer the operator and passengers little protection in the event of a

FIGURE 10-12 In a rollover collision, the unrestrained person will suffer multiple impacts and possible multiple injuries.

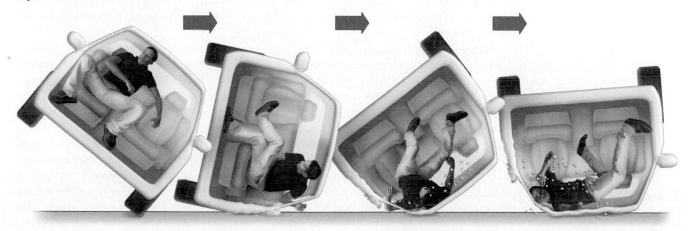

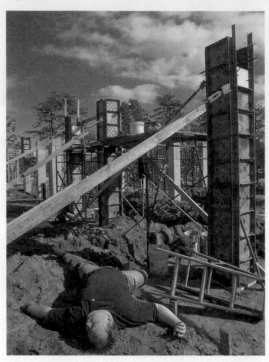

collision. Determine whether the patient was wearing a helmet that offered some protection from head injury. Also attempt to determine whether the patient was ejected. In some cases, the operator will be thrown from the bike and strike and severely injure his hips, thighs, or legs.

Falls   Falls are another cause of injury where the extent and pattern of damage may be determined by the characteristics of the fall (Figure 10-13). Important factors to consider are the height from which the patient fell, the surface the patient fell onto, the part of the patient that hit the surface, and anything that interrupts the fall.

In falls, injury to the part of the body that comes in contact with the ground or another hard surface is only the beginning of the trauma experienced by the patient. The force is also transmitted to adjoining parts of the body. For example, think of a person who dives head first into a shallow body of water and strikes his head. Although the head will be injured, the force travels on to the cervical and thoracic spine, very possibly resulting in severe spinal cord injury and paralysis. Similarly, when a patient jumps from a height and lands squarely on his feet, there is trauma to the feet but also to the ankles, legs, and even the pelvis. Always assess along the path of the energy. It is likely that you will find additional injuries.

The general guideline from the U.S. Department of Health and Human Services and the Centers for Disease Control and Prevention is that a fall of greater than 20 feet for an adult or greater than 10 feet for a child under age 15, or more than two to three times the child's height, is considered to be a severe fall for which transport to a trauma center is recommended. This is a reasonable guideline, but it doesn't guarantee a resulting injury (or rule out injury if the fall is less than this distance). It is important to look at all factors at the scene in combination with the patient's complaint, vital signs, and your physical examination findings. When in doubt, assign the patient a high priority for rapid packaging and prompt transport.

Penetrating Trauma   *Penetrating trauma*, or injury caused by an object that passes through the skin or other body tissue, also has characteristics that may help in determining the extent of injury. These wounds are classified by the velocity, or speed, of the item that caused the injury. Low-velocity items are those that are propelled by hand, such as knives.

penetrating trauma
injury caused by an object that passes through the skin or other body tissues.

FIGURE 10-14 Bullets cause damage in two ways: from the bullet itself (A and C) and from cavitation, which is the temporary cavity caused by the pressure wave (B).

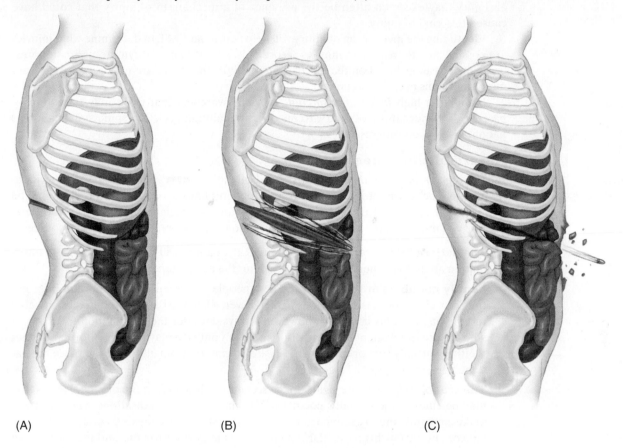

(A)   (B)   (C)

Low-velocity injuries are usually limited to the area that was penetrated. Remember that there can be multiple wounds, or the blade may have been moved inside the patient, so there can be damage to multiple vital organs.

Medium-velocity wounds are usually caused by handguns and shotguns. Some forcefully propelled items such as an arrow launched from a compound bow or a ballistic knife will also cause greater velocities than the same items propelled by hand.

Bullets propelled by a high-powered or assault rifle travel at a high velocity. Medium- and high-velocity injuries can cause damage almost anywhere in the body. Bullets cause damage in two ways (Figure 10-14):

- **Damage directly from the projectile.** The bullet itself will damage anything in its path. The damage depends on the size of the bullet, its path, or whether it fragments (breaks up into smaller projectiles), with the fragments taking different paths. The path of the bullet once it is inside the body is unpredictable since it may be deflected by bone or other tissue onto a totally different course. There is often damage to organs and tissues that are not in a straight line between the entrance and exit wounds.

- **Pressure-related damage, or cavitation.** This means that the energy of the bullet as it enters the body creates a pressure wave that causes a cavity considerably greater than the size of the bullet. This cavity is temporary, but it may damage items in its path.

Blunt-Force Trauma *Blunt-force trauma* is injury caused by a blow that strikes the body but does not penetrate the skin or other body tissues (e.g., when one is struck by a baseball bat or thrown against a steering wheel). The energy from a blunt-force blow will travel through the body, often causing serious injury to, and even rupture of, internal organs and vessels. The resulting compromise of body functions, hemorrhage, or spillage of organ contents into the body cavity may have more severe consequences for the patient than a penetrating injury. Yet signs of blunt-force trauma are often subtle and easy to overlook. The skin

blunt-force trauma
injury caused by a blow that does not penetrate the skin or other body tissues.

may appear reddened at the site of the blow, but in the prehospital setting the bluish coloration characteristic of a bruise may not have had time to appear. Your main clue that such an injury may exist will often be the presence of a mechanism of injury that could have caused this kind of injury.

Identifying the mechanism of injury will help you, as an EMT, to determine what injuries are possible and to treat these injuries accordingly, even if signs and symptoms are not present. Never assume, based on the mechanism of injury, that there are no injuries. Even very minor collisions may cause injuries.

Maintain a high *index of suspicion*—a keen awareness that there may be injuries—based on the mechanism of injury. Remember to maintain neck and spine stabilization as patient assessment progresses.

Nature of the Illness

Identifying the *nature of the illness* for a medical patient serves the same purpose as identifying the mechanism of injury for a trauma patient: finding out what is or what may be wrong with the patient. To begin identifying the nature of a patient's illness during the scene size-up, you must scan the entire scene. Information may be obtained from many sources:

- **The patient.** When conscious and oriented, the patient will be a prime source of information about his or her condition throughout the assessment process.
- **Family members or bystanders.** These people can also provide important information, especially for the unconscious patient. Even when the patient is conscious and able to tell you about his condition, however, always consider the information from others who are present. Patients who are disoriented or confused may provide information that is either partially true or even untrue. Use information from all sources to piece the patient assessment "puzzle" together.
- **The scene.** While you are sizing up the scene for safety, make note of other factors that may be clues to the patient's condition. You may observe medications, which you will make a mental note to examine later. You may be struck by dangerous or unsanitary living conditions for this particular patient. This is important to note and mention to the emergency department personnel later.

Number of Patients and Adequacy of Resources

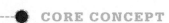

The final part of the scene size-up is determining if you have sufficient resources to handle the call. If, for example, you noted at a two-car collision that there were at least two patients—one driver still in his car and the other thrown to the pavement—you would immediately request an additional ambulance. As you approach the scene, you should actively look for clues that there may be additional patients—other passengers or pedestrians involved in the collision (Figure 10-15)—and if so, you should immediately call for additional ambulances.

Sometimes you may discover a need for additional resources even in a situation that, at first, would not seem to require them. For example, you may not feel that a single-patient medical call could tax your resources, but consider the following scenarios where you may find yourself needing extra help:

- Your ambulance is called to respond to an elderly woman with chest pain. You are greeted at the door by her husband, who does not look well. He denies any complaints but is sweaty and holding his chest. Your first patient tells you that her husband has a heart condition.
- A single patient experiences back pain. This is usually not a reason for additional assistance, but this patient is immobilized on a backboard in a third-floor apartment (no elevator) and weighs 425 pounds.
- Your ambulance is called for a patient with "general weakness." Upon the arrival of you and your partner, two more persons in the same family develop the same flu-like symptoms. You appropriately suspect carbon monoxide poisoning, since they admit that they have been having furnace problems.

In each of these situations, what appeared to be a routine one-patient call actually turned out to be more. An important part of scene size-up is to recognize these situations and call for help immediately. As the call progresses and you get more involved in patient care, it is

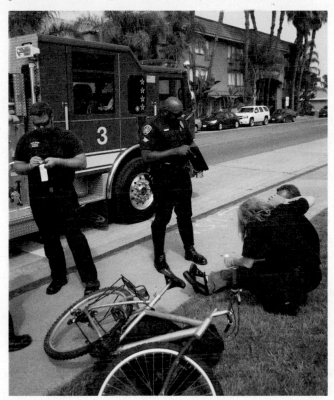

FIGURE 10-15 Actively look for any additional patients, such as pedestrians or cyclists. *(©Kevin Link)*

less likely that you will remember to call for the additional help. It may also be too late when the help arrives if you do not call immediately.

Your response can range from simply calling for another ambulance to care for the ill husband in the first situation, or extra personnel to help move the 425-pound man in the second, to activating a multiple-casualty incident for the family with carbon monoxide poisoning. (You will learn about multiple-casualty incidents in Chapter 39, "Hazardous Materials, Multiple-Casualty Incidents, and Incident Management.") Try to anticipate the maximum numbers of patients and radio for help accordingly. Follow local protocols.

CRITICAL DECISION MAKING

Determining Areas of Concern at the Scene

The scene size-up is a vital part of any call. For each of the following scenes, determine a few areas of concern you would want to check before proceeding to the patient. Remember each of the components of the scene size-up. You shouldn't try to think of every possibility, only the most likely ones. Practice the critical thinking process of evaluating a scene—something you will do on every call.

1. An 18-wheeler with an enclosed trailer slid off the road into a ditch in an ice storm. The vehicle is in the ditch, leaning to the right.

2. A van and a passenger car collided on an interstate highway.

3. You arrive at an office building and see people running out the front and side doors in a panic. One person appears bloody and is running toward your ambulance.

4. You respond to a residence with the fire department and arrive on-scene first. A resident meets you at the end of the driveway and tells you there is a strong smell of natural gas in his house.

5. You respond to a construction site for a fall.

CHAPTER REVIEW

Key Facts and Concepts

- Scene size-up is the first part of the patient assessment process.
- It is important during scene size-up to determine what, if any, threats there may be to your own safety and to the safety of others at the scene, and then to take appropriate Standard Precautions.
- Next, it is important to determine the nature of the call by identifying the mechanism of injury or the nature of the patient's illness.
- Finally, you must take into account the number of patients and other factors at the scene to determine if you will need additional help.

Key Decisions

- Is it safe to approach the scene?
- What precautions should my crew and I take to protect ourselves at the scene?
- What personal protective equipment should I put on and what should I have available?
- What does the scene suggest about the mechanism of injury?
- What is the nature of illness?
- How many patients are present and what additional assistance should I call?

Chapter Glossary

blunt-force trauma injury caused by a blow that does not penetrate the skin or other body tissues.

danger zone the area around the wreckage of a vehicle collision or other incident within which special safety precautions should be taken.

index of suspicion awareness that there may be injuries.

mechanism of injury a force or forces that may have caused injury.

nature of the illness what is medically wrong with a patient.

penetrating trauma injury caused by an object that passes through the skin or other body tissues.

scene size-up steps taken when approaching the scene of an emergency call: checking scene safety, taking Standard Precautions, noting the mechanism of injury or nature of the patient's illness, determining the number of patients, and deciding what, if any, additional resources to call for.

Preparation for Your Examination and Practice

Short Answer

1. For each of the following dangers, describe actions that must be taken to remain safe at a collision scene.
   - Leaking gasoline
   - Toxic or hazardous material spill
   - Vehicle on fire
   - Downed power lines

2. List several indicators of violence or potential violence at an emergency scene.

3. Describe several situations where it is appropriate to wear disposable gloves. Describe situations where you would additionally wear protective eyewear and mask. Describe situations where you would wear an N-95 or HEPA respirator.

4. Describe common mechanism-of-injury patterns.

5. List sources of information about the nature of a patient's illness.

6. List several medical and trauma situations where you may require additional assistance.

Thinking and Linking

Use the information you learned in earlier chapters to answer the following questions:

1. You respond to a head-on collision of two automobiles late at night. There are no apparent fluids leaking, no smoke involved, no wires down, and no abnormal smells. What PPE should you put on as you exit the ambulance? What PPE should you have available close by in case it is needed?

2. A patient has stab wounds to the lower anterior ribs and lower posterior ribs. What organs are most at risk of injury from the different wounds?

3. As you are assessing an alert passenger in a car that was hit from behind, you suddenly smell smoke. What technique should you use to remove the patient from the vehicle?

4. You responded to a call with possible domestic violence. Because the scene did not appear to be safe, you did not go into the house, but retreated and called for police assistance. Another EMT says that you committed abandonment when you did that. What is your response?

Critical Thinking Exercises

You can and should start planning your scene size-up en route, on the basis of dispatch information. The purpose of this exercise will be to apply this skill in the following situation.

1. You are called to the scene of a shooting at a fast food restaurant. En route, you plan your scene size-up strategy. What actions do you anticipate taking on arrival?

Pathophysiology to Practice

The following questions are designed to assist you in gathering relevant clinical information and making accurate decisions in the field.

1. A patient has stab wounds to the anterior lower ribs and the lower posterior ribs. What organs are most at risk of injury from the wounds located:
   - In the lower left lateral ribs?
   - In the lower right lateral ribs?
   - In the lower posterior ribs on either side?

2. Would any of your answers change if you discovered that the patient was in the fetal position, trying to defend himself, when he was stabbed?

Street Scenes

It is the middle of the night, and you are hoping to get a few hours of sleep. You are just getting relaxed when the monitor activates. "Ambulances Bravo 5 and Delta 2 with heavy rescue to the Avenue A off-ramp for Interstate 55 to the report of a two-vehicle crash."

You are the first EMS responder to arrive, and as you approach the scene, you see both vehicles: one a passenger vehicle, the other a truck with a placard. As you do a scene size-up, you try to get the "big picture." You are concerned about where to stage your ambulance because of traffic, safety of crews, possible gasoline leaking, and not knowing what the placard on the truck identifies. You notify the dispatcher that you are on the scene and request that the Highway Patrol be notified for traffic-control assistance. You find a location upwind about 100 yards from the scene. You place warning markers to alert traffic and to mark the staging area for other responding units. You are putting on your turnout gear with helmet, goggles, and gloves, including a reflective vest, when heavy rescue arrives. You talk with the captain, and he tells you that his crew will stabilize the vehicles and handle the battery disconnects and gasoline leaks. You point out the placard that needs to be checked out.

Street Scene Questions

1. What other scene size-up issues are left to consider?
2. Is this scene now safe or do other precautions need to be taken?
3. What Standard Precautions should be considered?

The crew from heavy rescue approaches the scene, stabilizes the vehicles, and then motions you forward. The Highway Patrol has closed off traffic and the captain from heavy rescue tells you that there is no hazardous material concern. On-scene, you determine that the drivers were the only occupants of the vehicles. You check one patient and, at the same time, your partner checks the other. Your patient has significant facial cuts and bruises and complains of leg pain. You realize that the extrication gloves you are wearing will not provide the proper Standard Precautions, so you put proper disposable gloves on immediately. After you try unsuccessfully to open the driver's side door next to your patient, you realize that he will require heavy rescue. The captain has already alerted his crew, and they are almost ready to use pry tools. You learn that your partner's patient is conscious and alert with no specific complaints.

Street Scene Questions

4. When the second ambulance arrives, where should it be located in relation to the collision scene?
5. What precautions should you take to protect the patients from any further harm while they are being extricated from the vehicle?
6. How should you plan to make sure that you can safely get the patient from the scene to the ambulance?

As heavy rescue finishes getting their tools ready, you set a protective cloth over your patient. You explain what is being done and stay next to him for reassurance. While this is going on, the second ambulance arrives, parks close to the second collision vehicle, and the crew takes over patient care. Your ambulance is relatively far away, so you ask your partner to bring it closer to prevent having to carry your patient a long distance. This makes packaging the patient for transport safer and easier. The remainder of the call is uneventful, with both patients transported safely to the hospital emergency department.

11 The Primary Assessment

STANDARD
Assessment (Primary Assessment)

COMPETENCY
Applies scene information and patient assessment findings (scene size-up, primary and secondary assessment, patient history, and reassessment) to guide emergency management.

CORE CONCEPTS
— Deciding on the approach to the primary assessment

— Manual stabilization of the head and neck

— The general impression

— Assessment of mental status using the AVPU scale

— The ABCs as part of the assessment process

— How to make a priority decision

EXPLORE Resource Central

OBJECTIVES

After reading this chapter you should be able to:

11.1 Define key terms introduced in this chapter.

11.2 Explain the purpose of the primary assessment. (p. 265)

11.3 Discuss the difference in first steps to assessment if the patient is apparently lifeless (C-A-B approach) or if the patient has signs of life, including a pulse (A-B-C approach). (pp. 265–267, 268–269, 273–278, 280–281)

11.4 Given several scenarios, do the following:
a. Form a general impression (pp. 267, 270–272)
b. Determine the chief complaint (pp. 271–272)
c. Determine the patient's mental status (pp. 272–273)
d. Assess the airway (p. 273)
e. Assess breathing (pp. 273–274, 278)
f. Assess circulation (p. 278)
g. Determine the patient's priority for transport (pp. 278–279)

(continued)

KEY TERMS

Usually, you will take the time to do a thorough assessment (patient evaluation), transporting your patient to the hospital only after the complete assessment is finished. But if the patient has an immediately life-threatening problem—such as a blocked airway, a stoppage of breathing or heartbeat, or severe bleeding—you must provide emergency care immediately. This is the major principle guiding the primary assessment. During the primary assessment, you will also be gaining critical information about the seriousness of your patient's condition, which will be the foundation for important decisions as you continue the care of your patient.

THE PRIMARY ASSESSMENT

The *primary assessment* is the portion of the patient assessment during which you will focus exclusively on life threats—specifically those that interfere with airway, breathing, and circulation. This chapter deals with this very vital part of the assessment process. You may also hear the primary assessment referred to as the *primary survey* or *initial assessment*. It is always the first element in the total assessment of the patient.

Approach to the Primary Assessment

As an EMT, you will see many different patients with varied medical and traumatic conditions. The primary assessment can—and should—vary depending on several factors that include the patient's condition, how many EMTs are on the scene, and other priorities you determine as you assess your patient.

Although it may seem easiest to assume that you will assess each patient in A-B-C order (airway, breathing, circulation), this is not necessarily the case in all patients. If you took a CPR course recently, you were likely taught a C-A-B (circulation (compressions), airway, breathing) approach to the first steps in your assessment of a patient who appears lifeless and has no pulse. In short, you will perform your primary assessment in the way your patient needs it most: A-B-C if the patient has signs of life; C-A-B if the patient appears lifeless and has no pulse (Figure 11-1).

Consider the following patient conditions and situations:

- You are called to a responsive patient who dropped a concrete block on his foot and is in considerable pain.

- You are eating in a restaurant and observe a man with what appears to be a complete airway obstruction.

primary assessment
the first element in a patient assessment; steps taken for the purpose of discovering and dealing with any life-threatening problems. The six parts of primary assessment are: forming a general impression, assessing mental status, assessing airway, assessing breathing, assessing circulation, and determining the priority of the patient for treatment and transport to the hospital.

CORE CONCEPT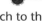

Deciding on the approach to the primary assessment

FIGURE 11-1 The approach to the patient: determining if the patient appears lifeless or if the patient has signs of life.

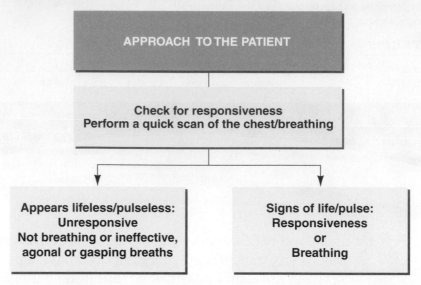

- You arrive at the side of a patient who had "passed out" and is now moaning. She has vomited.
- You are called for a "man down" and see a person on the ground who does not appear to be moving or breathing.
- You are called for an industrial accident and find a man who looks pale, sweaty, and about to pass out. He has blood spurting from his thigh.

In the responsive patient who dropped a block on his foot, you will perform a primary assessment, but little action will be required. The other patients will require you to perform many vital actions. The man who is choking needs to have his airway cleared as a first priority. The woman who passed out is in immediate need of suction. The "man down" will likely need CPR. For this patient, compressions and defibrillation are your first priorities. The man with spurting blood is essentially bleeding to death. In this case you must immediately take action to stop the bleeding.

Remember that you will not be alone on an ambulance. Professional rescuers (EMTs are included in this category) will often work in a team environment in which multiple tasks may be accomplished immediately and simultaneously. In this case there is no need to wonder whether you should open the airway first or stop the bleeding first, because both may be done at the same time. It is also possible that a friend, family member, or even the patient himself may be able to help control bleeding while you do other important tasks.

Decision Making in the Primary Assessment

The mnemonic A-B-C can help you remember the things you have to do in the primary assessment—but not the exact order in which you must perform them. To determine exactly what you will do and in what sequence during the primary assessment, there are certain general considerations you will take into account.

- Any vomit in the airway that enters the lungs is very serious—and often fatal. The stomach contents contain solids that may obstruct the airway as well as strong acids that can cause irritation within the airway. Some patients are saved by defibrillation but later die because of aspiration pneumonia or pneumonitis. *It is a vital component of the primary assessment to suction the airway as soon as needed and before ventilating.*
- Exsanguinating (very severe, life-threatening) bleeding must be stopped immediately. Damage to major vessels, especially arteries, can cause death extremely rapidly from bleeding. *Life-threatening bleeding must be controlled immediately.*
- Breathing and circulation are obviously vital for life. You must make sure your patient is breathing and breathing adequately to support life. *In cases where there appears to be*

no breathing or only very occasional, ineffective breaths (agonal breathing), you should check for a pulse and begin CPR if necessary.

- If immediate interventions such as bleeding control or CPR are not required, you will shift into an important but less urgent mode in which you will administer oxygen appropriate for the patient's condition and evaluate for shock.

Again, the order in which these interventions are performed depends on the patient's specific condition and the number and priority of the urgent conditions just listed that you are presented with. Remember: Multiple EMTs can accomplish multiple priorities simultaneously.

Performing the Primary Assessment

Keep in mind that the initial steps of the primary assessment will depend on your initial impression of the patient. As already noted, if the patient shows signs of life you will begin to work through the ABCs in an order dictated by your patient's priorities. If the patient appears lifeless—that is, not moving and apparently not breathing—you will take a different course of action and shift toward resuscitation beginning with chest compressions and preparation of the defibrillator if the patient is pulseless. (Review Figure 11-1.)

The primary assessment is actually considered to have six parts (See *Visual Guide to Primary Assessment*):

- Forming a general impression
- Assessing the patient's mental status (and manually stabilizing the patient's head and neck, when appropriate—Scan 11-1)
- Assessing the patient's airway
- Assessing the patient's breathing
- Assessing the patient's circulation
- Determining the patient's priority

> **NOTE:** *If during the primary assessment you discover any life-threatening condition, you must immediately perform the appropriate **interventions** (actions to correct those problems).*

Form a General Impression

Forming a ***general impression*** helps you to determine how serious the patient's condition is and to set priorities for care and transport. It is based on your immediate assessment of the environment and the patient's chief complaint and appearance (Figure 11-2).

The environment can provide a great deal of information about the patient. It frequently gives clues—to the EMT who looks for them—about the patient's condition and history. One of the most important things it can sometimes tell you is what happened. Is there an overturned ladder, indicating that the patient may have fallen? Has the patient been exposed to a cold outdoor environment for a long time? Or is there no apparent mechanism of injury, leading you to presume that the patient has a medical problem rather

CORE CONCEPT
Manual stabilization of the head and neck

interventions
actions taken to correct or manage a patient's problems.

CORE CONCEPT
The general impression

general impression
impression of the patient's condition that is formed on first approaching the patient, based on the patient's environment, chief complaint, and appearance.

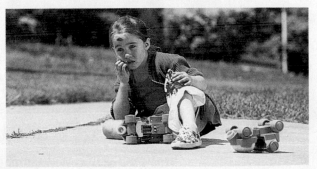

FIGURE 11-2 Forming a general impression includes your immediate assessment of the environment and the patient's chief complaint and appearance.

CHAPTER 11
Primary Assessment
Identify and Treat Life Threats

■ **GENERAL IMPRESSION:** Chief Complaint and *AVPU*

Key Decision

How does the patient look?

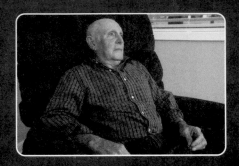
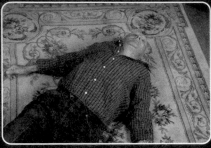

If the patient is apparently lifeless (no breathing or agonal breathing), go directly to a pulse check and the C-A-B approach.

You may perform **airway, breathing** and **circulation** in any order.

This is dependent on the patient's presentation and emergent needs. Multiple parts of the primary assessment can be performed simultaneously when more than one EMT is present.

■ **AIRWAY**

Key Decision

Open the Airway　　　　　*Suction If Necessary*　　　　　*Place an Oral or Nasal Airway If Indicated*

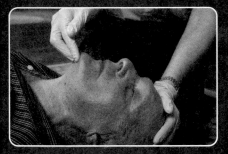
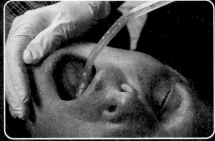
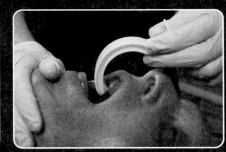

■ **BREATHING**

Key Decision

Is the patient breathing?　　　*Is the patient breathing adequately?*　　　*Is the patient hypoxic?*

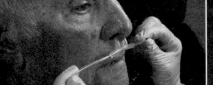
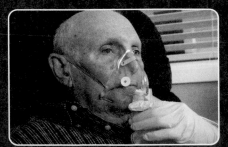
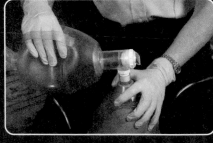

Mild distress　　　　　　Significant distress or hypoxia　　　　　Absent or inadequate breathing

■ CIRCULATION

Does the patient have a pulse?
Does the patient have signs of shock?
Does the patient have life-threatening bleeding?

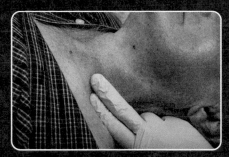

Unresponsive

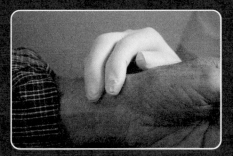

Responsive

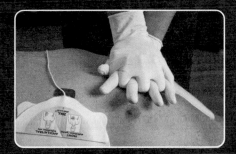

If pulseless, perform CPR and
apply defibrillator

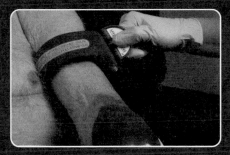

Control life-threatening bleeding
Treat for shock

■ PRIORITY DETERMINATION

How do I handle this patient from this point on?

Stable: slower place, more detailed secondary examination
Potentially unstable: expedite transport, fewer assessments and interventions on scene
Unstable: rapid transport, only life-saving assessment and interventions on scene

You should apply manual stabilization of the head and neck on first contact with any patient you suspect may have an injury to the spine based on mechanism of injury, or history, or signs and symptoms—that is, to virtually any trauma patient.

When you apply manual stabilization, your object is to hold the patient's head still in a neutral, in-line position. That is, the head should be facing forward and not turned to either side nor tilted forward or backward. You must be careful not to pull or twist the patient's head but rather to

hold it perfectly still and to remind the patient not to try to move it.

If your patient is in another position (for example, crumpled on his side) or is being moved by other EMS personnel, adapt the technique to the best of your ability to hold the head in a steady position in line with the spine. Some EMS systems have specific guidelines for when to use and when not to use spine immobilization. If this is the case in the system where you work, you should familiarize yourself with the local protocols and follow them.

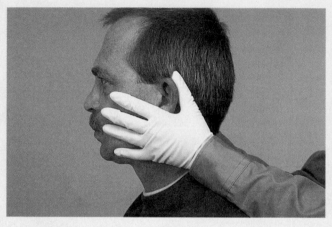

1 When your patient is sitting up, position yourself just behind the patient and hold the patient's head by spreading your fingers over the sides of the head and placing your thumbs behind the ears.

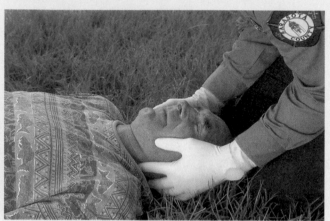

2 When your patient is supine, kneel behind the patient and spread your fingers and thumbs around the sides of the patient's head to hold it steady.

than trauma (an injury)? Although the EMT cannot rely completely on the patient's environment to rule out trauma, when combined with the chief complaint (e.g., the patient complaining of symptoms that sound more like a medical problem than an injury), environmental clues become extremely useful.

The "Look Test"

At this point, experienced providers often get a "feeling" about the patient's condition. This feeling comes from environmental observations as well as from the brief but valuable information obtained by that first look at the patient as the EMT approaches. Some call this the "look test." You will gain more of this instinctual approach to assessment as you gain experience.

Chapter 6, "Principles of Pathophysiology," explained many of the things listed next as clinical topics. This chapter will discuss how and why they play a part in your assessment. For now, we will tell you some of the things experienced EMTs use to identify patients who may be critical, such as:

- **Patients who appear lifeless.** Patients who appear to be lifeless—who have no movement or apparent evidence of breathing or have only gasping breathing—will be resuscitated by beginning CPR compressions and preparing your defibrillator as soon as possible if they are found to be pulseless.

- **Patients who have an obvious altered mental status.** An altered mental status can indicate many underlying conditions, from hypoxia to shock to diabetes to overdose to seizure. During the primary assessment, your concern is not the cause of the altered mental status; it is the impact it will have on your patient and your assessment and care decisions. In this case:

- Your primary assessment will be more aggressive because of a higher potential for life-threatening problems, including vomitus or secretions in the airway and the need for ventilation.
- Your subsequent assessments will likely be done more quickly to expedite transport.

- **Patients who appear unusually anxious and those who appear pale and sweaty.** These signs are indicators of possible shock. Recognizing these signs at the earliest possible moment will help you to identify this potentially serious condition early. In this case:
  - Recognizing anxiety, pallor, and sweatiness early will prompt you to look for other signs of shock as you complete your primary assessment, including observation of rapid pulse and respiratory rates.
  - Identification of shock will help you make the decision to classify the patient as unstable or potentially unstable and expedite your assessment and care.
  - Recognizing potential shock early in the call will help you perform appropriate assessments later. In cases of suspected trauma, you will match this information with the mechanism of injury, the patient's complaint, and assessment findings. In the medical patient, identifying shock may help you identify a body system to examine later (e.g., the gastrointestinal tract for indications of GI bleeding, or the cardiac system for signs and symptoms of a heart attack).

- **Obvious trauma to the head, chest, abdomen, or pelvis.** Experienced EMTs identify serious trauma to these areas as injuries that can cause airway problems, profound shock, or death.
  - Head injuries are serious because the brain is housed within the skull. Also, because the head bleeds a lot when injured, the airway may require significant attention and care.
  - The integrity of the chest is vital for breathing. When the chest is injured, normal adequate breathing may be disrupted by rib injury, collapsed lungs, and bleeding from the major blood vessels within the mediastinum.
  - The abdomen not only contains a rich blood supply, but it also contains many organs that may be injured during trauma.
  - Injury to the pelvis can cause severe—and even fatal—bleeding.

- **Specific positions indicate distress.** The tripod position (Figure 11-3) indicates significant difficulty breathing, whereas Levine's sign (Figure 11-4) indicates significant chest pain or discomfort.
  - Seeing either of these signs tells two things. The level of chest discomfort or respiratory distress is severe, and the patient's complaints (cardiac and respiratory) are among the most serious medical complaints, indicating a high priority.

The clinical clues just listed are not all-inclusive. There are many indications—some very subtle—that something is wrong with a patient. Something as seemingly simple as a statement that the patient "isn't himself" may indicate a serious problem. You should also remember that these signs are only part of the information you will gather. You will find unstable patients who present with none of these signs and patients with very minor complaints who look serious.

Most important, remember that the presence of any of these signs usually indicates a serious patient, but absence of these signs does not guarantee that the patient is stable.

The Chief Complaint

The *chief complaint* is the reason EMS was called, usually in the patient's own words. It may be as specific as abdominal pain or as vague as "not feeling good." In any case, it is the patient's description of why you were called.

chief complaint
in emergency medicine, the reason EMS was called, usually in the patient's own words.

You form a general impression by looking, listening, and smelling. You look for the patient's age and sex—which are easy to determine once the patient is in sight. You look at the patient's position to see if it indicates an injury, pain, or difficulty in breathing. You listen for sounds like moaning, snoring, or gurgling respirations. You sniff the air to detect any smells like hazardous fumes, urine, feces, vomitus, or decay.

Something that is more difficult to describe than your direct observations but just as important is the feeling or sense you get when you arrive at the scene or encounter the patient.

FIGURE 11-3 In cases of severe difficulty breathing, patients may assume the tripod position—sitting upright, leaning forward, and supporting themselves with arms locked in front of them.

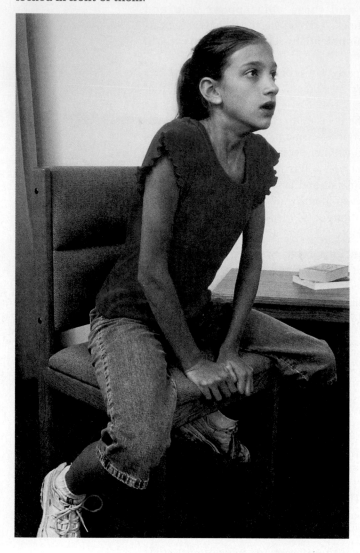

FIGURE 11-4 The classic sign of chest pain is Levine's sign, a fist clenched over the chest.

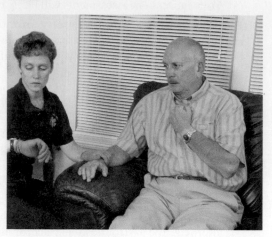

You may become anxious when you see a patient who exhibits no outward signs of illness or injury, yet "just doesn't look right" to you. Or you may feel reassured when you are dispatched to a "sick baby," but see that the infant is alert and smiling. After you gain some practice assessing and managing patients, you may develop a "sixth sense" that clues you in to the severity of a patient's condition. This is part of what is called *clinical judgment*, or judgment based on experience in observing and treating patients. Some people find it easier than others to cultivate this ability, but even those who have excellent clinical judgment do not depend on it alone. A systematic approach to finding threats to life is the best way to make sure they are not missed.

Assess Mental Status

Determining the patient's *mental status*, or level of responsiveness, will usually be easy, since most patients are alert and responsive; that is, they are awake and will talk and answer questions sensibly. Some, even if not awake, will still respond to verbal stimuli, such as talking or shouting. At a lower level of responsiveness, the patient will respond only to painful stimuli, such as pinching a toe or ear or squeezing the trapezius muscle between the neck and the shoulder. The lowest and most serious status is unresponsiveness, when the patient will not respond even to a painful stimulus. An easy way to keep these levels of responsiveness in mind is by remembering the letters *AVPU*, for *alert*, *verbal response*, *painful response*, and *unresponsive*.

● **CORE CONCEPT**
Assessment of mental status using the AVPU scale

mental status
level of responsiveness.

AVPU
a memory aid for classifying a patient's level of responsiveness or mental status. The letters stand for alert, verbal response, painful response, unresponsive.

A patient may be awake but confused. An awake patient's mental status can be described by specifying what he is "oriented to." Most EMS systems document orientation to person, place, and time. A patient who can speak clearly can almost always tell you his name (orientation to person). A few patients are oriented to person, but cannot tell you where they are (orientation to place). Some patients are oriented to person and place but cannot tell you the time, day, or date (orientation to time). A few EMS systems include additional questions to determine orientation.

A depressed mental status may indicate a life-threatening problem such as insufficient oxygen reaching the brain or shock. If the level of responsiveness is lower than alert, provide high-concentration oxygen by nonrebreather mask and consider the patient a high transport priority.

POINT OF VIEW

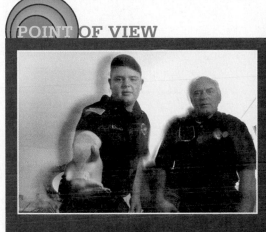

"I thought I'd just lay down for a nap. I wasn't feeling that well. Most everything from then on is really a blur. I remember my wife trying to wake me up. I can't even tell you how much time had passed.

"The next thing I knew here were these two big guys standing over me in dark clothes. I had a hard time focusing on them . . . or even hearing them. I know this sounds silly, but it was like everyone on Earth was walking through air and I was walking through Jell-O. It took me extra time to do everything—extra time to hear or think or do something simple like move my arms. They'd ask me a question, and I couldn't even think about the right answer, and they moved on to the next question. It felt like all I was doing was mumbling.

"All I can say is that it was one of the scariest things I have ever experienced. Turns out my blood sugar was off. I'm glad EMS was there to help, that's for sure, although my recollection of it is still fuzzy."

Assess the ABCs

You will always check the *ABCs*—airway, breathing, and circulation—as you look for life-threatening problems. Later in this chapter you will be introduced to four patients with various kinds of medical and traumatic complaints. You will see how the primary assessment differs for each of these patient types. Remember as you perform the primary assessment that there are two purposes: to identify and correct life threats with airway, breathing, and circulation and to gather information (e.g., indications of severity/priority; signs of illness or injury) that will help you later in your assessment.

You were introduced to the initial decision-making scheme earlier in the chapter. Figure 11-5 shows an expanded view of the primary assessment. Remember that you will use the primary assessment components listed in Figure 11-5 in the order that is most appropriate for your patient's condition (Scan 11-2 and Scan 11-3).

CORE CONCEPT

The ABCs as part of the assessment process

ABCs
airway, breathing, and circulation.

Airway

If the patient is alert and talking clearly or crying loudly, you know that the airway is open. If the airway is not open or is endangered (the patient is not alert, is supine, or is breathing noisily), take measures to open the airway, such as the jaw-thrust or head-tilt, chin-lift maneuver; suctioning; or insertion of an oropharyngeal or nasopharyngeal airway. If the airway is blocked, perform clearance procedures.

Breathing

Once an open airway is ensured, assess the patient's breathing. There are four general situations that call for assistance with breathing, listed here from more to less severe:

- **If the patient is in respiratory arrest,** perform rescue breathing.
- **If the patient is not alert and his breathing is inadequate (with an insufficient minute volume because of decreased rate or depth or both),** provide positive pressure ventilations with 100 percent oxygen.

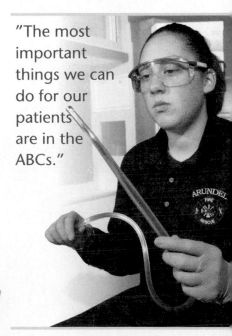

"The most important things we can do for our patients are in the ABCs."

FIGURE 11-5 The approach to the patient: two pathways.

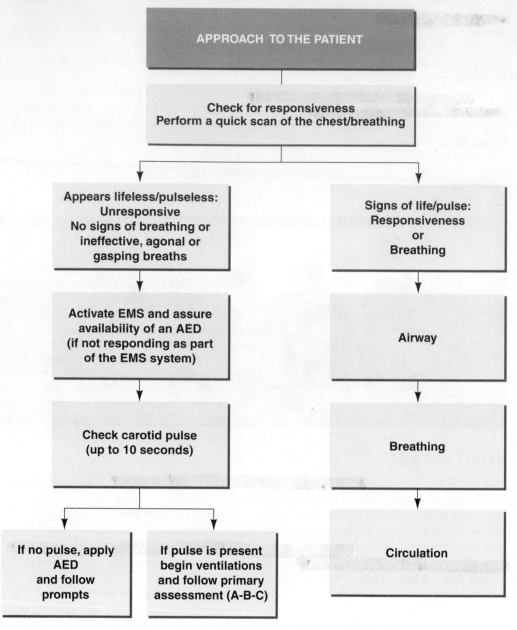

APPROACH TO THE PATIENT

Check for responsiveness
Perform a quick scan of the chest/breathing

Appears lifeless/pulseless:
Unresponsive
No signs of breathing or
ineffective, agonal or
gasping breaths

Signs of life/pulse:
Responsiveness
or
Breathing

Activate EMS and assure
availability of an AED
(if not responding as part
of the EMS system)

Airway

Check carotid pulse
(up to 10 seconds)

Breathing

If no pulse, apply
AED
and follow
prompts

If pulse is present
begin ventilations
and follow primary
assessment (A-B-C)

Circulation

NOTE:
The type of emergency or patient
(e.g., pediatric, drowning, trauma, severe bleeding)
may alter the procedures, priorities, or order of
assessment or interventions

Multiple rescuers will be able to handle
multiple initial priorities at the same time

- **If the patient has some level of alertness and his breathing is inadequate,** assist his ventilations with 100 percent oxygen. Synchronize your ventilations with the patient's own respirations so that they are working together, not against each other.
- **If the patient's breathing is adequate but there are signs or symptoms suggesting respiratory distress or hypoxia,** provide oxygen based on the patient's need as determined by your examination, the patient's complaint, and the pulse oximetry readings.

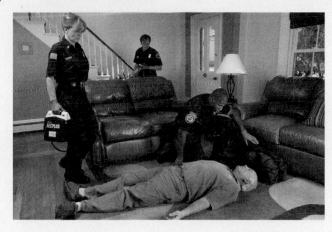

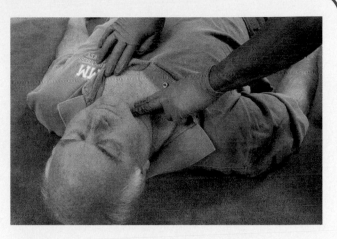

1 Look for signs of life including movement. Scan the chest for signs of breathing. If no signs of life such as breathing (or only gasping breathing) are found, check the pulse.

2 Check the pulse for no longer than 10 seconds.

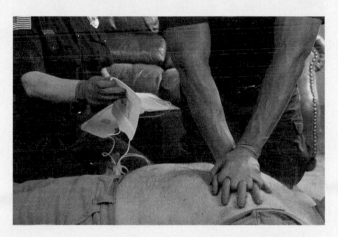

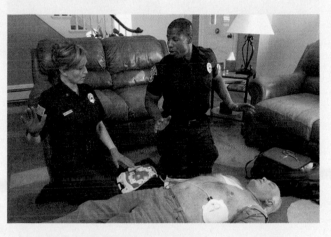

3 If no pulse, begin CPR compressions while the defibrillator is being readied.

4 Clear the patient. Apply the defibrillator and follow the voice prompts. (Use of the defibrillator will be discussed in depth in Chapter 20, "Cardiac Emergencies.")

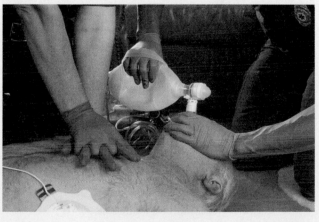

5 Continue resuscitation. Multiple rescuers can handle multiple assessment tasks simultaneously.

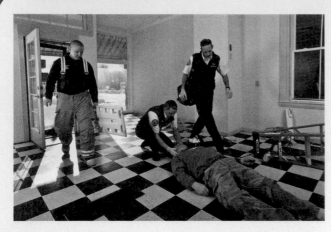

1 Develop a general impression and obtain a chief complaint. Take spinal precautions if trauma is suspected.

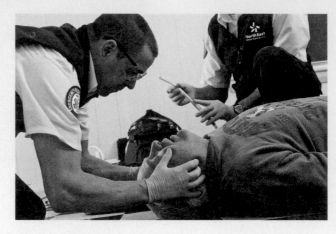

2 Open the airway.

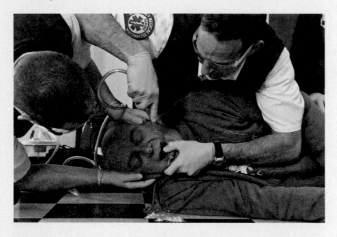

3 Suction if necessary.

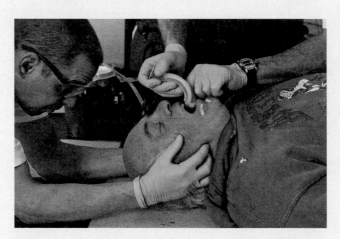

4 Insert an oral or nasal airway if required to maintain a patent airway.

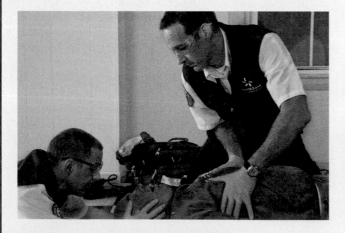

5 Evaluate breathing for rate and depth.

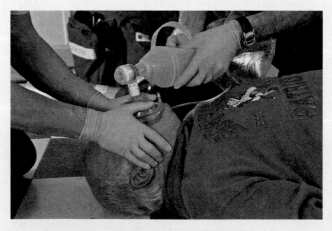

6 Apply positive pressure ventilation to patients who are not breathing or breathing inadequately.

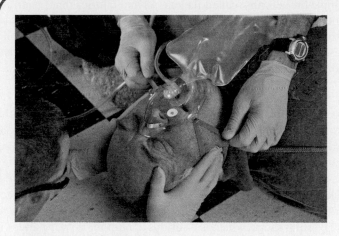

7 Provide oxygen based on patient complaint, condition, and pulse oximetry reading.

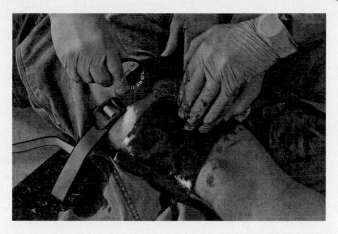

8 Identify and control life-threatening bleeding.

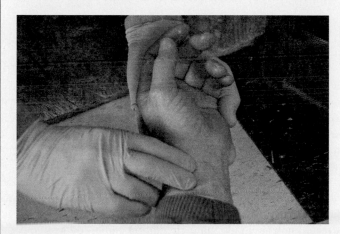

9 Evaluate circulation. Check the pulse.

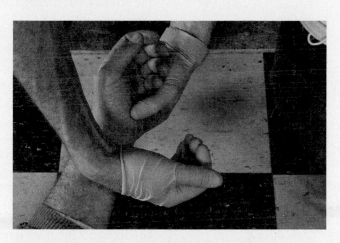

10 Evaluate circulation. Check skin color, temperature, and conditions.

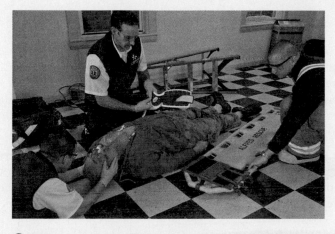

11 Make a status/transport priority decision.

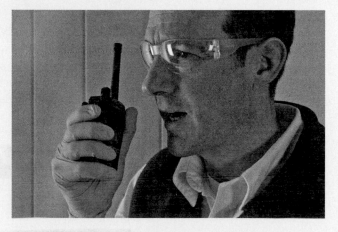

12 Request ALS or other assistance as necessary.

Part of the primary assessment includes correcting certain conditions you may find. Injuries to the chest can reduce the rate and depth of breathing and significantly impact the functioning of the lungs. Multiple broken ribs (called flail chest) and injuries that penetrate the chest, leaving an open wound, are examples of severe conditions you will look for. They are relatively easy to identify by observing and palpating the chest cavity. Although you won't be taught how to care for these chest injuries until later in the book, for now remember that it will be important to look for these life-threatening conditions in the primary assessment.

Circulation

Once any breathing problems are corrected, assess the patient's circulation. Begin by taking the patient's pulse. If the patient was lifeless on your initial approach you will have begun CPR at that point. Keep in mind, however, that cardiac arrest is not the only possible life-threatening circulation problem. Inadequate circulation and severe blood loss are also life threatening.

To evaluate circulation, assess pulse, skin, and bleeding. If the patient is light-skinned, you can check the pulse and skin at the same time. As you take the radial pulse, note whether the skin at the wrist is warm, pink, and dry—indicating good circulation—or pale and clammy (cool and moist)—suggesting shock, which is a serious condition. If your patient is dark-skinned, you can check the color of the lips or nail beds, which should be pink.

You don't have to take the pulse for a full 30 seconds and obtain an exact rate. During the primary assessment, there are only three possible results of the pulse check that you will be looking for:

- Within normal limits
- Unusually slow
- Unusually fast

Anything other than normal is concerning and may indicate a serious condition. You will get used to different pulse rates as you practice. This will allow you to identify these three types of pulse rates easily—especially in combination with other things (e.g., a very rapid pulse in the presence of trauma or a very slow pulse in a patient who has chest pain, both indicating an unstable, high-priority patient).

Also check for and control severe bleeding. If even one large vessel or several smaller ones are bleeding, a patient can lose enough blood in just a minute or two to die. Quick control of severe external bleeding can be lifesaving. Transport decisions should take into account the potential for shock resulting from inadequate circulation and blood loss.

Keep in mind that to perform a primary assessment, you must touch your patient. Even when you encounter an alert patient, you should still feel for a pulse, as well as for skin temperature and condition. These may help you identify shock early—a potentially lifesaving decision.

Determine Priority

CORE CONCEPT

How to make a priority decision

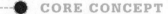

priority
the decision regarding the need for immediate transport of the patient versus further assessment and care at the scene.

Any life-threatening airway, breathing, or circulation problem must be treated as soon as it is discovered. Once life threats are under control, you will decide on the patient's *priority* for immediate transport versus further on-scene assessment and care.

A useful approach to decision making is to classify a patient as stable, potentially unstable, or unstable. Although there are few hard and fast rules for how to determine stability, several principles will help you.

- **To be stable, a patient needs to have vital signs that are in the normal range or just slightly abnormal.** If they are abnormal, they must be small deviations from normal or easily explained by factors other than injury and illness (e.g., sweating on a hot day). Stable vital signs are not the only requirement for a stable classification, but they are necessary.

- **A threat to the airway, breathing, or circulation, either actual or imminent, rules out stable.** This puts a patient in either the unstable or potentially unstable category, depending on the severity of the patient's condition.

- **There are many times when it is not crystal clear what a patient's problem is, so there will be many possible diagnoses, some more serious than others.** When a patient does not have any immediate threats to life, but you believe he may deteriorate because of the nature of the problem, you should consider the potentially unstable category for the patient. This means you will not delay transport, but it does not necessarily mean you will use lights and siren to transport the patient to the hospital.

- **A patient's priority can change.** For example, an unconscious diabetic patient with a low blood sugar would initially be unstable because of the threat to the airway. If the patient became awake enough to swallow oral glucose and then became alert and oriented, it would be appropriate to change this patient's priority to stable.

Although most patients do not need immediate transport, a few do. Therefore, you must be able to determine which patients fall into which category. *If any life-threatening problem cannot be controlled or threatens to recur, or if the patient has a depressed level of responsiveness, he has an immediate priority for transport to the hospital, with assessment and care continuing en route.*

A number of findings indicate a high priority for transport (Table 11-1) (i.e., the patient is categorized as unstable or potentially unstable). These are conditions for which, usually, there is little or no treatment that can be given in the field that will make a difference in how well the patient does. You will learn more about these conditions in later chapters.

Primary assessment steps and interventions are summarized in Table 11-2.

Table 11-1   High-Priority Conditions
• Poor general impression
• Unresponsive
• Responsive, but not following commands
• Difficulty breathing
• Shock
• Complicated childbirth
• Chest pain consistent with cardiac problems
• Uncontrolled bleeding
• Severe pain anywhere

CRITICAL DECISION MAKING

Determining Priority

At the end of the primary assessment you will make a priority determination. This determination is a key decision that will affect the rest of your assessment and care. Patients deemed a high priority will receive a streamlined assessment process leading to prompt transport. Patients who are not a high priority will receive their assessment and care at a slower (although not slow) pace. Determine whether each patient described here should be classified as a high or low priority at the end of the primary assessment.

1. A responsive patient who is sitting up and having difficulty breathing ~ High
2. A man who "passed out" at a wedding and is still unresponsive High
3. A responsive child who got his foot caught in bike spokes and may have broken the foot Not
4. A responsive patient who describes severe pain in his abdomen High
5. A patient who only moans (doesn't respond with words or actions) and appears to have ingested alcohol

Table 11-2 Primary Assessment Steps and Interventions

MEDICAL PATIENT		TRAUMA PATIENT	
RESPONSIVE	**UNRESPONSIVE**	**RESPONSIVE**	**UNRESPONSIVE**
1. *General impression:* Form general impression of patient's condition.	1. *General impression:* Form general impression of patient's condition.	1. *General impression:* Form general impression of patient's condition. Evaluate mechanism of injury. **Intervention:** Manual stabilization of head and neck.	1. *General impression:* Form general impression of patient's condition. Evaluate mechanism of injury. **Intervention:** Manual stabilization of head and neck.
2. *Mental status:* AVPU (alert)	2. *Mental status:* AVPU (responsive only to verbal or painful stimulus or not responsive) **Intervention:** High-concentration oxygen as soon as airway is open.	2. *Mental status:* AVPU (alert)	2. *Mental status:* AVPU (responsive only to verbal or painful stimulus or not responsive) **Intervention:** High-concentration oxygen as soon as airway is open.
3. *Airway* is open.	3. *Airway* is compromised. **Interventions:** Open airway with head-tilt, chin-lift maneuver; consider oro- or nasopharyngeal airway; suction as needed. For foreign body obstruction, use abdominal thrusts or other blockage-clearing technique.	3. *Airway* is open.	3. *Airway* is compromised. **Interventions:** Open airway with jaw-thrust maneuver; consider oro- or nasopharyngeal airway; suction as needed. For foreign body obstruction, use abdominal thrusts or other blockage-clearing technique.
4. *Breathing:* Look for rise and fall of chest, listen and feel for rate and depth of breathing. Look for work of breathing (use of accessory muscles, retractions). **Interventions:** If there is hypoxia, respiratory distress, or threat to the airway, ventilation, oxygenation, or circulation, administer high-concentration oxygen by nonrebreather mask. If breathing becomes inadequate, provide positive pressure ventilations and high-concentration oxygen.	4. *Breathing:* Look for rise and fall of chest, listen and feel for rate and depth of breathing. Look for work of breathing (use of accessory muscles, retractions). **Interventions:** If there is hypoxia, respiratory distress, or threat to the airway, ventilation, oxygenation, or circulation, administer high-concentration oxygen by nonrebreather mask. Position patient on side. If breathing is inadequate, provide positive pressure ventilations and high-concentration oxygen. If respiratory arrest develops, perform rescue breathing.	4. *Breathing:* Look for rise and fall of chest, listen and feel for rate and depth of breathing. Look for work of breathing (use of accessory muscles, retractions). **Interventions:** If there is hypoxia, respiratory distress, or threat to the airway, ventilation, oxygenation, or circulation, administer high-concentration oxygen by nonrebreather mask. If breathing becomes inadequate, provide positive pressure ventilations and high-concentration oxygen.	4. *Breathing:* Look for rise and fall of chest, listen and feel for rate and depth of breathing. Look for work of breathing (use of accessory muscles, retractions). Expose and palpate the chest for signs of trauma that will affect breathing. **Interventions:** If there is hypoxia, respiratory distress, or threat to the airway, ventilation, oxygenation, or circulation, administer high-concentration oxygen by nonrebreather mask. Position patient on side once spinal stability is assured. If breathing is inadequate, provide positive pressure ventilations and high-concentration oxygen. If respiratory arrest develops, perform rescue breathing.

Table 11-2 Primary Assessment Steps and Interventions (continued)

MEDICAL PATIENT		TRAUMA PATIENT	
RESPONSIVE	**UNRESPONSIVE**	**RESPONSIVE**	**UNRESPONSIVE**
5. *Circulation:* Pulse; bleeding; skin color, temperature, condition (capillary refill in infants and children under 6). **Interventions:** Control bleeding. Treat for shock. If cardiac arrest occurs, perform CPR.	5. *Circulation:* Pulse; bleeding; skin color, temperature, condition (capillary refill in infants and children under 6). **Interventions:** Control bleeding. Treat for shock. If cardiac arrest occurs, perform CPR.	5. *Circulation:* Pulse; bleeding; skin color, temperature, condition (capillary refill in infants and children under 6). **Interventions:** Control bleeding. Treat for shock. If cardiac arrest occurs, perform CPR.	5. *Circulation:* Pulse; bleeding; skin color, temperature, condition (capillary refill in infants and children under 6). **Interventions:** Control bleeding. Treat for shock. If cardiac arrest occurs, perform CPR.
6. *Priority:* A responsive patient's priority depends on chief complaint, status of ABCs, and other factors.	6. *Priority:* An unresponsive patient is automatically a high priority for immediate transport.	6. *Priority:* A responsive patient's priority depends on chief complaint, status of ABCs, and other factors.	6. *Priority:* An unresponsive patient is automatically a high priority for immediate transport.

Patient assessment takes different forms, depending on the following patient characteristics:

- Whether the patient has a medical problem or trauma (injury)
- Whether the patient does or does not have an altered mental status
- Whether the patient is an adult, a child, or an infant

How can the steps of primary assessment be applied to such varied types of patients? The following scenarios—plus some final paragraphs—will help to show you.

Patient Characteristics and Primary Assessment

■ Mr. Schmidt—*A Responsive Adult Medical Patient*

One afternoon, you are dispatched to "an elderly man whose stomach hurts." Mrs. Schmidt greets you at the door and leads you to her husband.

General Impression

As you approach the sofa where Mr. Schmidt is sitting, you see that he is an older male who appears ill and in pain. You see nothing around him to suggest that he has been injured. All of this suggests a medical problem rather than an injury.

Mental Status, Airway, and Breathing

You introduce yourself by saying, "Hello, Mr. Schmidt. I'm Gerry Jones (your name). I'm an emergency medical technician from the Fairfield Ambulance Service. How can I help you?" "My stomach hurts," he replies. As you ask questions, you note that Mr. Schmidt is alert and answering clearly. The fact that he is speaking in a normal way indicates that his airway is open. You can hear that his breathing is not labored. You look at his chest and note that his breathing is normal in rate and depth.

Circulation

"I'm going to check your pulse," you explain as you reach for his wrist. You quickly assess Mr. Schmidt's circulation by palpating his radial pulse, observing his skin, and looking for bleeding. Although you do not stop to count exactly how fast his pulse is, you can tell that it is normal in rate and strength and regular in rhythm. The skin at his wrist is pink, warm, and dry. No blood is evident anywhere around him.

Priority

With the information you have gathered in just a few seconds, you conclude that Mr. Schmidt has no problems that are likely to kill him in the next few minutes. There-fore, you decide he is probably stable. No immediate lifesaving measures are required, and neither is immediate transport to the hospital. You are able, instead, to move ahead with the next steps of your assessment as Mr. Schmidt continues to rest on the sofa. Note that categorizing a patient as stable does not mean you can sit back and have a leisurely conversation with the patient on the way to the hospital. There are many causes of abdominal pain, most of them not life threatening, but there is the possibility the patient will deteriorate. You will need to keep a close eye on him. You will learn more about this in Chapter 15, "Reassessment."

■ Mrs. Malone—*An Unresponsive Adult Medical Patient*

Your dispatcher sends you to an "unconscious" woman. Her daughter says she cannot wake her mother, Mrs. Malone, and leads you to the bedroom.

General Impression

An older woman in nightclothes is lying on her back in bed. Her eyes are closed and she is not moving.

Mental Status

You say loudly, "Mrs. Malone, can you hear me?" In response to your question, she moans a little, so you know she responds to a verbal stimulus. In your report, you will describe both the stimulus (verbal) and the response (moaning). If Mrs. Malone had not responded to verbal stimulus, you would have scanned her chest for indications of breathing. If she didn't appear to be breathing, you would check the pulse and begin compressions if necessary. If the patient is breathing, you should continue the primary assessment by inflicting a painful stimulus to try to get a response from her.

Airway and Breathing

Because she is lying on her back, Mrs. Malone's airway is threatened by her tongue. Since patients with depressed responsiveness are always at risk for airway problems, you know that you need to be aggressive about opening and maintaining her airway. Even though you haven't heard any sounds indicating partial airway obstruction (like snoring or gurgling), your partner (having ruled out trauma) removes the pillow, tilts her head back, and lifts her chin.

Next, you evaluate her breathing by bringing your ear next to her mouth and looking for movement of her chest and abdomen as you listen and feel for the movement of air with your ear. You determine the depth of Mrs. Malone's respirations and if her breathing rate is slow or fast. If you found that her breathing was inadequate, you would ventilate Mrs. Malone with 100 percent oxygen.

Her respirations are in the normal range, but you give Mrs. Malone high-concentration oxygen by nonrebreather mask anyway because her level of responsiveness is depressed. You put in a nasopharyngeal airway and move Mrs. Malone onto her side in order to help protect her airway.

Circulation

Mrs. Malone's pulse is strong, regular, and in the normal range for rate. You look for blood, but find none. The skin at her wrist is cool and dry. Because Mrs. Malone is dark-skinned, you assess for skin color at her lips and nail beds, which are pale. Although the pulse and bleeding check are normal, the pallor and coolness of her skin are slightly abnormal.

Priority

The priority of this patient is high because her mental status is depressed, her airway is at risk, and her skin indicates a circulation problem. You arrange immediate transport to the hospital for this unstable patient, and plan to continue assessment and care en route.

■ Clara Diller—*A Responsive Child Trauma Patient*

You respond to the scene where, the dispatcher says, a child has fallen.

General Impression

As you get out of the ambulance, you see a girl who is about 5 years old sitting on the sidewalk. She is crying and holding a bloody cloth on her knee. The mechanism of injury is apparent: a pair of skates indicates that she has probably taken a tumble while skating.

Mental Status, Airway, and Breathing

When you reach the patient, you kneel next to her and introduce yourself. You ask what happened. She confirms your suspicion that she fell down while trying out her new skates. When you ask her, she tells you her name is Clara Diller and that her head and knee hurt. Since she is crying and answers your question easily, you determine that her mental status is alert and her airway is clear.

Because there is a mechanism of injury indicating possible trauma, you explain to her that she should not move her head and that your partner is going to hold her head to help her keep it still. Her breathing is not labored and her respiratory rate and depth are in the normal range.

Circulation

You feel Clara's radial pulse. It is slightly rapid but strong and regular. You look around her and see no blood except on the cloth and on her knee. Since it is hard to tell how much bleeding may be under the cloth, you tell Clara you want to look at her knee. You see a 2-inch laceration which is oozing some blood, so you put the cloth back on and ask the neighbor who takes care of Clara to apply a little pressure to it. When you felt Clara's radial pulse, you noted that her skin is warm, pink, and dry. You also assess her capillary refill by pressing on the end of her fingernail. The color in the nail bed returns to pink in less than 2 seconds, so all indications are that Clara's circulation is good.

Priority

Based on the information you have gathered, you determine that Clara's priority for immediate transport is low. She has no significant mechanism of injury and no immediately life-threatening problems. There is no evidence that she was struck by a car or hit any object other than the sidewalk. However, since the sidewalk is a hard surface and she may have been moving fast, you maintain a high index of suspicion for possible cervical-spine injury. As soon as it is practical, you will apply a cervical collar and immobilize Clara on a backboard. You categorize her as stable.

PEDIATRIC NOTE

Because Clara is a child, several other factors were different in her case than they were for your adult patients, Mr. Schmidt and Mrs. Malone.

Since children are often shy or distrustful of strangers or adults, you made a special effort to gain Clara's trust by kneeling to her level as you talked with her. Responsive children need to have some trust in the EMT. This may take a minute or two, but the general impression will guide you in determining how long to spend developing a rapport with the child.

Infants and children breathe faster than adults and their hearts beat faster, which you kept in mind when you evaluated Clara's breathing and circulation.

A special part of checking circulation in infants and children is capillary refill. Nail beds are typically pink in healthy, normal people. When the end of the fingernail is gently pressed, it turns white. When the pressure is released, the nail bed turns pink again very quickly, usually in less than 2 seconds. In children, this may help you to evaluate the circulation of blood. In an infant or small child with small nail beds, press the back of the hand or top of the foot instead. Count, "one-one thousand, two-one thousand" or say "capillary refill." If the nail or skin regains its pink color in the time it takes to say one of these, it is probably normal. Abnormal responses include prolonged and absent capillary refill (taking too long to turn pink again, or not turning pink again at all). These usually indicate problems with circulation.

Capillary refill is not a reliable sign for adults, so it is used only in infants and young children. In some adults, especially in the elderly, it is normal for capillary refill to take longer than 2 seconds. Even in infants and young children, capillary refill can be affected by factors such as the weather. Cold temperatures will prolong capillary refill. In other words, it should be used as one factor to consider in determining the priority of the young patient, but not the only one.

Like adult trauma patients, child and infant trauma patients need to have their heads immobilized in order to prevent injury to the spinal cord.

An infant has an airway that is different from an adult's, so opening an infant's or child's airway means moving the head to a neutral position, not tilting it back the way an adult's airway is opened. The mental status of unresponsive infants is typically checked by talking to the infant and flicking the feet.

You will learn about other considerations in approaching and assessing pediatric patients in Chapter 35, "Pediatric Emergencies."

■ Brian Sawyer—*An Unresponsive Adult Trauma Patient*

At the scene of a motor-vehicle collision, you go to the aid of a young man who has been thrown from his car.

General Impression

The young man appears to be approximately 25 years old. His eyes are closed and he is not moving. As you approach, you can hear snoring respirations. The mechanism of injury, the collision, and the fact that he is quite a distance from his vehicle are obvious. A police officer who has retrieved the patient's wallet tells you that his name is Brian Sawyer.

Mental Status and Airway

Your partner moves to stabilize Brian's head and the two of you position him on his back. Your partner attends to Brian's airway as you begin to check his mental status. He doesn't respond to your calling his name, and he is unresponsive to a brisk rub of your knuckles on his sternum.

Your partner has started to treat the airway problem you both heard, snoring respirations that mean partial obstruction of the airway. Your partner manually stabilizes Brian's head at the same time that he does a jaw thrust, which relieves the snoring sound. You listen closely and hear no other noises from his airway. If you heard gurgling or saw fluid in Brian's airway, you would suction him.

Breathing and Circulation

To evaluate breathing, you look, listen, and feel. Brian has respirations that appear normal in rate and depth. Because he is unresponsive but has adequate respirations, you decide to give Brian high-concentration oxygen by nonrebreather mask as soon as you finish checking his circulation. You select an oropharyngeal airway and insert it, then apply a non-rebreather mask with 15 liters per minute of high-concentration oxygen.

You start to assess circulation by feeling the radial pulse. It is rapid and weak. There is no blood on or near the patient that you can see. His skin is pale, cool, and sweaty.

Priority

The priority you assign Brian is high. He is unresponsive to pain and his rapid, weak pulse and pale, clammy skin are signs of diminished circulation. You will spend as little time on the scene as possible with this unstable patient. You plan to monitor his airway, place a cervical collar on him, immobilize him on a backboard, and get him to an appropriate facility quickly. Since you and your partner will both be needed to care for this patient en route to the hospital, you radio for additional personnel to drive the ambulance.

COMPARING THE PRIMARY ASSESSMENTS

The four patients—Mr. Schmidt, Mrs. Malone, Clara Diller, and Brian Sawyer—were very different in their characteristics. Notably:

- Mr. Schmidt and Mrs. Malone were medical patients, whereas Clara Diller and Brian Sawyer had suffered trauma.
- Both Mr. Schmidt and Clara Diller were responsive and neither was a priority for immediate transport. However, both Mrs. Malone and Brian Sawyer had an altered mental status and airway and circulation problems that made them a high priority for immediate transport to the hospital.
- Clara Diller was a child, whereas the other three patients were adults.

There were a few obvious differences in the primary assessments of these patients. For example, both Clara Diller and Brian Sawyer, as trauma patients, required stabilization and immobilization of the head and spine. In contrast, Mr. Schmidt and Mrs. Malone, as medical patients with no evidence of any mechanism of injury, did not. For all four patients, the purpose of the primary assessment was to discover and correct any life-threatening problems. Mrs. Malone and Brian Sawyer had more problems to correct (mainly airway problems), so there were more actions to take. Therefore, the primary assessment of these two patients took a little longer than the primary assessment of Mr. Schmidt and Clara Diller.

In spite of these differences, the main thing to note is that the primary assessment steps were the same for all of them: forming a general impression; assessing mental status; checking airway, breathing, and circulation (and correcting any immediately life-threatening problems as soon as they were found); and making a priority decision regarding immediate transport vs. continued on-scene assessment and care.

These steps of the primary assessment must be followed systematically for every patient, no matter if that patient has a medical condition or trauma; is responsive or unresponsive; is an infant, child, or adult—and no matter how mild or serious that patient's condition may seem to be. If these steps are not followed consistently and systematically, it is very possible to overlook and neglect to manage a life-threatening problem.

To consider how the steps of the primary assessment are applied to responsive and unresponsive medical and trauma patients, review Table 11-2. For a summary of how the steps of the primary assessment are applied to adults, children, and infants, see Table 11-3.

Table 11-3	Primary Assessment of Adults, Children, and Infants		
	ADULTS	**CHILDREN 1–5 YEARS**	**INFANTS TO 1 YEAR**
Mental Status	AVPU: Is patient alert? Responsive to verbal stimulus? Responsive to painful stimulus? Unresponsive? If alert, is patient oriented to person, place, and time?	As for adults.	If not alert, shout as a verbal stimulus, flick feet as a painful stimulus. (Crying would be infant's expected response.)
Airway	Trauma: jaw-thrust maneuver. Medical: head-tilt, chin-lift maneuver. Both: Consider oro- or nasopharyngeal airway, suctioning.	As for adults, but see Chapter 8 and BCLS Review for special child airway techniques. If performing head-tilt, chin-lift maneuver, do so without hyperextending (stretching) the neck.	As for children, but see Chapter 8 and BCLS Review for special infant airway techniques.
Breathing	If respiratory arrest, perform rescue breathing. If depressed mental status and inadequate breathing (slower than 8 per minute), give positive pressure ventilations with 100 percent oxygen. If alert and respirations are more than 24 per minute, give 100 percent oxygen by nonrebreather mask.	As for adults, but normal rates for children are faster than for adults. (See Chapter 12 for normal child respiration rates.) Parent may have to hold oxygen mask to reduce child's fear of mask.	As for children, but normal rates for infants are faster than for children and adults. (See Chapter 12 for normal infant respiration rates.)
Circulation	Assess skin, radial pulse, and bleeding. If patient is in cardiac arrest, perform CPR. See Chapter 27 on how to treat for bleeding and shock.	Assess skin, radial pulse, bleeding, and capillary refill. See Chapter 12 for normal child pulse rates (faster than for adults). If patient is in cardiac arrest, perform CPR. See BCLS Review for child techniques. See Chapter 27 on how to treat for bleeding and shock.	Assess skin, brachial pulse, bleeding, and capillary refill. See Chapter 12 for normal child pulse rates (faster than for children and adults). If patient is in cardiac arrest, perform CPR. See BCLS Review for special infant techniques. See Chapter 27 on how to treat for bleeding and shock.

Key Facts and Concepts

- The primary assessment is a systematic approach to quickly finding and treating immediate threats to life.

- The general impression, although somewhat subjective, can provide extremely useful information regarding the urgency of a patient's condition.

- The determination of mental status follows the AVPU approach.

- Evaluating airway, breathing, and circulation quickly but thoroughly will reveal immediate threats to life that must be treated before the EMT proceeds further with assessment.

- Your approach to a patient will vary depending on how he presents. The American Heart Association recommends a C-A-B approach for patients who appear lifeless and appar-

ently are not breathing or have only agonal respirations. This begins with a pulse check and chest compressions if there is no pulse.

- If your patient shows signs of life (e.g., moving, moaning, talking) and is breathing, you will take a traditional A-B-C approach.

- Remember that the mnemonic A-B-C is a guide to interventions that may be taken. You will choose your interventions based on the patient's immediate needs.

- The patient's priority describes how urgent the patient's need to be transported is and how to conduct the rest of your assessment.

Key Decisions

- Is this patient medical or trauma; responsive or unresponsive; adult, child, or infant?

- Does this patient have any signs of life?

- Does my patient require a C-A-B approach (likely in cardiac arrest)? Does he therefore require chest compressions and defibrillation as my first priority?

- Do I need to stop and suction the airway, insert an artificial airway, administer oxygen, or ventilate the patient?

- Is the patient's condition stable enough to allow further assessment and treatment at the scene?

Chapter Glossary

ABCs airway, breathing, and circulation.

AVPU a memory aid for classifying a patient's level of responsiveness or mental status. The letters stand for alert, verbal response, painful response, unresponsive.

chief complaint in emergency medicine, the reason EMS was called, usually in the patient's own words.

general impression impression of the patient's condition that is formed on first approaching the patient, based on the patient's environment, chief complaint, and appearance.

interventions actions taken to correct or manage a patient's problems.

mental status level of responsiveness.

primary assessment the first element in a patient's assessment; steps taken for the purpose of discovering and dealing with any life-threatening problems. The six parts of primary assessment are: forming a general impression, assessing mental status, assessing airway, assessing breathing, assessing circulation, and determining the priority of the patient for treatment and transport to the hospital.

priority the decision regarding the need for immediate transport of the patient versus further assessment and care at the scene.

Preparation for Your Examination and Practice

Short Answer

1. List factors you will take into account in forming a general impression of a patient.

2. Explain how to assess a patient's mental status with regard to the AVPU levels of responsiveness.

3. Explain how to assess airway, breathing, and circulation during the primary assessment. Explain the interventions you will take for possible problems with airway, breathing, and circulation.

4. Explain the C-A-B approach to the primary assessment and explain the circumstances in which the C-A-B approach would be appropriate.

5. Explain the A-B-C approach to the primary assessment and explain the circumstances in which the A-B-C approach would be appropriate.

6. Explain what is meant by this statement in the chapter: "The order in which these interventions [Airway, Breathing, Circulation] are performed depends on the patient's specific condition and the number and priority of urgent conditions that you are presented with."

7. Explain what is meant by this statement in the chapter: "Multiple EMTs can accomplish multiple priorities simultaneously."

8. Explain what is meant by the term *priority decision*.

9. Explain what special interventions are required in the following situations.
   - If a patient has suffered trauma
   - If a patient is unresponsive

Thinking and Linking

Think back to Chapter 9, "Respiration and Artificial Ventilation," and link information from that chapter (regarding oxygen administration and artificial ventilation) with information from this chapter as you consider the following situation:

- Your patient, injured in a car crash, is breathing at 6 breaths/minute. Would you administer oxygen by nonrebreather mask or provide artificial ventilations? Describe the technique you would use.

Critical Thinking Exercises

Determining a patient's priority status is a critical skill within the primary assessment. For each of the following patients, state whether the patient's priority is stable, potentially unstable, or unstable—and explain your reasoning:

1. A 26-year-old male found unresponsive on the ground outside a bar who is now waking up after you attempted to insert a nasopharyngeal airway

2. A 60-year-old female complaining only of weakness who appears pale and sweaty, is alert, has no problem with the ABCs, but just "looks" to you as though she is very sick

3. A 6-month-old infant who vomited but appears happy and is reacting appropriately to the people and things around her now

4. For each of the following patients, determine which portion of the primary assessment would be performed first (C-A-B approach or A-B-C approach) and explain your reasoning.
   - A patient who is unresponsive with arterial bleeding coming from his neck
   - A patient with a broken ankle and no other apparent injury
   - A patient who is not moving and does not appear to be breathing
   - A patient who tells you that she has severe difficulty breathing
   - A patient who has ingested too much alcohol and is vomiting
   - A patient who is doubled over, screaming because of abdominal pain

Pathophysiology to Practice

The following questions are designed to assist you in gathering relevant clinical information and making accurate decisions in the field.

1. Describe how administration of oxygen to an unresponsive patient might lead you to change a patient's priority.

2. An elderly patient with Alzheimer's disease is acting abnormally, according to his family. He is alert and oriented to name, but not place or time. His family says this is his normal mental status. What priority should you assign him and why?

3. A middle-aged male is lying on the street after he was hit by a car. He appears unresponsive as you approach. You notice that he is bleeding from a laceration on his forearm and making gurgling sounds from his airway. If you are alone, what factors do you consider in deciding what to do first? Why?

Street Scenes

Your patient is a 78-year-old unconscious male, who was shaving with his electric razor when he fell to the floor. You hear snoring respirations as you manually stabilize his head and neck and determine that the patient responds to painful stimuli. You then perform a jaw-thrust maneuver, continue to assess the airway and breathing, and confirm that the patient has snoring respirations. With the help of your partner, you insert an oropharyngeal airway, reassess breathing, and observe labored respirations and cyanosis around the lips. After you give the patient high-concentration oxygen by nonrebreather mask, you assess his circulation. In a minute or so, the patient regains consciousness and his skin color improves. He tells you his name is Danya and explains that he had suddenly felt lightheaded, sat down, and must have passed out. Later, during transport, you keep the patient on oxygen, take another set of vital signs, and gather a patient history.

Street Scene Questions

1. What should be done immediately upon contact with an unconscious patient who has fallen? *Stabilize neck*

2. What are some considerations when opening the airway of an unconscious patient? *Jaw thrust*

3. Using the AVPU scale, what is the level of responsiveness of a patient who responds to you calling out his name?

When you return to quarters, you hope to get a short break, but it's just minutes before you receive a call for a 7-year-old patient reported to be unresponsive at the Mount Hope Elementary School. Upon arrival, you are directed to the athletic field where the coach and school nurse tell you that Joey Sullivan had a seizure for the second time this month. His eyes are closed, he is not moving, and his skin color appears normal. Your partner gets down next to the patient to assess his mental status. "Hey, Joey!" she calls out. He does not respond. She rubs his sternum briskly with her knuckles. There is still no response. "Unresponsive to pain," she says to you. When she tilts Joey's head back, there is a good deal of saliva visible in his mouth. Suctioning removes it without difficulty, and you administer oxygen to the patient by nonrebreather mask. You turn Joey onto his side and get a complete set of vital signs as your partner gets the stretcher. By the time you place Joey on the stretcher, he is becoming more responsive. Because of his improving mental status, you downgrade his priority and transport him along with the school nurse.

Street Scene Questions

4. Would knowing the cause of Joey's seizures change how you perform his primary assessment?

5. For Joey, what is the best position to prevent airway problems from occurring?

6. How did Joey's priority change during this call?

Vital Signs and Monitoring Devices

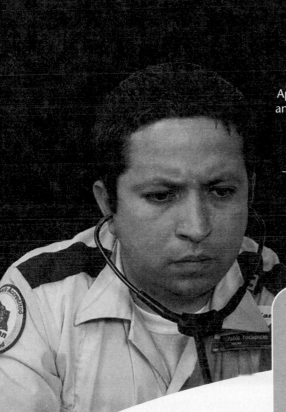

STANDARD
Assessment (Monitoring Devices)

COMPETENCY
Applies scene information and patient assessment findings (scene size-up, primary and secondary assessment, patient history, and reassessment) to guide emergency management.

CORE CONCEPTS
— How to obtain vital signs, including pulse, respirations, blood pressure, skin, temperature, and pupils

— How to document vital signs on a prehospital care report

— How to use various monitoring devices

EXPLORE Resource Central

To access Resource Central, follow directions on the Student Access Card provided with this text. If there is no card, go to **www.bradybooks.com** and follow the Resource Central link to Buy Access from there. Under Media Resources, you will find:

▶ **Official Trauma System Agenda for the Future**
Learn about the purpose of a trauma system, what the fundamental components are of trauma care, and what role EMS has in responding to trauma.

▶ **Trauma**
Watch a video on trauma and learn why traumatic injuries can become a distraction for the EMT and what your role is in assessing and managing a trauma patient.

▶ **Trauma Scenarios**
Learn why it is important for you to perform an assessment on every trauma patient and what information you should give to a trauma team to help continue the patient's care.

OBJECTIVES

After reading this chapter you should be able to:

12.1 Define key terms introduced in this chapter.

12.2 Identify the vital signs used in prehospital patient assessment. (pp. 291, 292)

12.3 Explain the use of vital signs in patient care decision making. (p. 291)

12.4 Integrate assessment of vital signs into the patient assessment process, according to the patient's condition and the situation. (pp. 290–291)

12.5 Discuss the importance of documenting vital signs and the times they were obtained in the patient care record. (p. 291)

(continued)

12.6 Demonstrate assessment of:
  a. Pulse (pp. 291, 293–294)
  b. Respirations (pp. 295–296)
  c. Skin (pp. 297–298)
  d. Pupils (pp. 298–299, 300)
  e. Blood pressure (pp. 299–305)
  f. Oxygen saturation (pp. 307–309)
  g. Blood glucose (pp. 309–312)

12.7 Integrate assessment of mental status and ongoing attention to the primary assessment while obtaining vital signs. (p. 291)

12.8 Differentiate between vital signs that are within expected ranges for a given patient, and those that are not. (pp. 293, 296, 297, 300, 301)

12.9 Compare and contrast the techniques of assessment and expected vital sign values for pediatric and adult patients. (pp. 293, 296, 298, 301, 305, 312)

KEY TERMS

auscultation, *p. 302*
blood pressure, *p. 299*
blood pressure monitor, *p. 302*
brachial artery, *p. 302*
brachial pulse, *p. 294*
bradycardia, *p. 293*
carotid pulse, *p. 294*

constrict, *p. 298*
diastolic blood pressure, *p. 299*
dilate, *p. 298*
oxygen saturation (SpO$_2$), *p. 307*
palpation, *p. 302*
pulse, *p. 291*

pulse oximeter, *p. 307*
pulse quality, *p. 294*
pulse rate, *p. 293*
pupil, *p. 298*
radial pulse, *p. 294*
reactivity, *p. 298*
respiration, *p. 295*
respiratory quality, *p. 295*

respiratory rate, *p. 295*
respiratory rhythm, *p. 296*
sphygmomanometer, *p. 301*
systolic blood pressure, *p. 299*
tachycardia, *p. 293*
vital signs, *p. 291*

Following the primary assessment and control of any immediate life threats, you will begin a more thorough assessment of your patient. An essential element of this assessment will be measuring vital signs. Vital signs are measurable things like pulse, blood pressure, and respirations. Because they reflect the patient's condition—and changes in the patient's condition—you will take them early and repeat them often.

GATHERING THE VITAL SIGNS

When you begin to assess a patient, some things are obvious or easy to discover. For example, the most important part of patient assessment is the chief complaint, the reason the patient called for EMS. Usually, the patient will tell you his complaint. Other parts of assessment that are usually apparent as soon as you see and talk to the patient are age, sex, and general alertness. However, not all parts of your assessment are so obvious or so easy to find out. The vital signs, for example, are major components of assessment that will take a few minutes to complete.

Vital signs are gathered on virtually every EMS patient. Occasionally, a patient will be so seriously injured or ill that you are not able to get this information because you are too busy treating immediate threats to life. This is the exception, however. The vast majority of patients you will encounter as an EMT should have an assessment that includes vital sign measurement. If you do not get this information, you may remain unaware of important conditions or trends in patient conditions that require you to provide particular treatments in the field or prompt transport to a hospital.

Where do vital signs fit into the sequence of patient assessment? After the primary assessment to find and treat immediate life threats (which was the subject of Chapter 11, "The Primary Assessment") you will conduct a more thorough assessment that includes a secondary assessment (which will be the subject of Chapter 13, "Assessment of the Trauma

Patient," and Chapter 14, "Assessment of the Medical Patient"). Vital signs will be obtained during this part of the assessment process.

VITAL SIGNS

Vital signs are outward signs of what is going on inside the body. They include pulse; respiration; skin color, temperature, and condition (plus capillary refill in infants and children); pupils; and blood pressure. Although it is not considered to be a vital sign, many EMS providers include oxygen saturation with their consideration of the vital signs. (See Visual Guide: Vital Signs Evaluation.)

Evaluation of these indicators can provide you, as an EMT, with valuable information. The first measurements you obtain are called the baseline vital signs. You can gain even more valuable information when you repeat the vital signs and compare them to the baseline measurements. This allows you and other members of the patient's health care team to see trends in the patient's condition and to respond appropriately.

Another sign that gives important information about a patient's condition is mental status. Although it is not considered one of the vital signs, you should assess the patient's mental status whenever you take the vital signs. Chapter 11, "The Primary Assessment," described how to evaluate mental status.

NOTE: *It is essential that you record all vital signs as you obtain them, along with the time at which you took them.*

Pulse

The pumping action of the heart is normally rhythmic, causing blood to move through the arteries in waves, not smoothly and continuously at the same pressure like water flowing through a pipe. A fingertip held over an artery where it lies close to the body's surface and crosses over a bone can easily feel the characteristic "beats" as the surging blood causes the artery to expand. What you feel is called the *pulse*. When taking a patient's pulse, you are concerned with two factors: rate and quality (Figure 12-1).

CORE CONCEPT

How to obtain vital signs, including pulse, respirations, blood pressure, skin, temperature, and pupils

vital signs
outward signs of what is going on inside the body, including respiration; pulse; skin color, temperature, and condition (plus capillary refill in infants and children); pupils; and blood pressure.

pulse
the rhythmic beats felt as the heart pumps blood through the arteries.

FIGURE 12-1 Assess pulse rate and quality. Count for 30 seconds and multiply by 2.

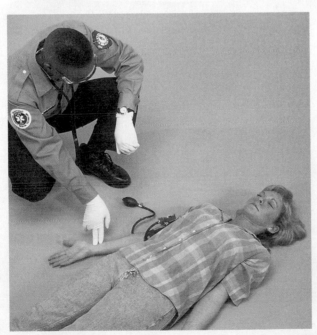

CHAPTER 12

Obtaining Vital Signs

■ THE SIX VITAL SIGNS

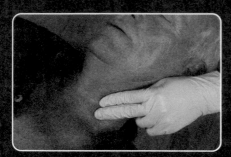

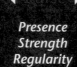

◄ Pulse ►

Presence
Strength
Regularity

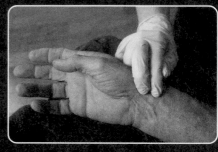

Unresponsive

Responsive Patient

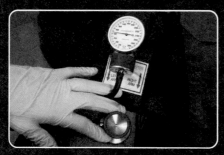

◄ Blood Pressure ►

Systolic
―――
Diastolic

Palpation – systolic only

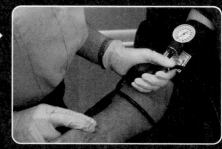

Auscultation

Palpation

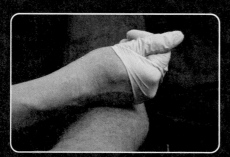

◄ Respiratory

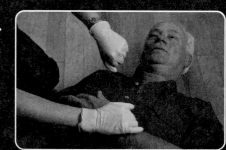

Skin ◄

Color, temperature
and condition

Rate and depth

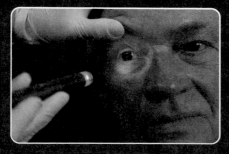

Pulse ►
Oximetry

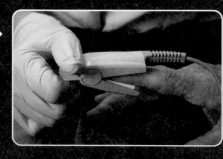

Pupils ◄

Size and reactivity

CRITICAL DECISION MAKING

Solving Assessment Problems

An accurate set of vital signs is an important foundation for critical decision making. For each of the common EMS situations that follow, describe how you would solve the problem you are faced with. In some cases, you may think of more than one potential solution.

1. You are trying to count the respiratory rate of a very talkative middle-aged male. Every time you think you're beginning to get an accurate count, he starts talking again.

2. You are about to put a blood pressure cuff on a 40-year-old male when he says that you can't put the cuff on that arm. He is a kidney dialysis patient and says he has a "shunt" in that arm. Because of the small room he is in, you can't get over to his other side.

3. The patient is an unconscious 32-year-old female who was thrown from a car when it flipped over. When you attempt to check the pulse at the patient's wrist, you search and search but can't find it.

Pulse Rate

The *pulse rate* is the number of beats per minute. The number you get will allow you to decide if the patient's pulse rate is normal, rapid, or slow (Table 12-1).

Pulse rates vary among individuals. Factors such as age, physical condition, degree of exercise just completed, medications or other substances being taken, blood loss, stress, and body temperature all have an influence on the rate. The normal rate for an adult at rest is between 60 and 100 beats per minute. Any pulse rate above 100 beats per minute is rapid, whereas a rate below 60 beats per minute is slow. A rapid pulse is called *tachycardia*. In contrast, a slow pulse is called *bradycardia*. An athlete may have a normal at-rest pulse rate

pulse rate
the number of pulse beats per minute.

tachycardia (TAK-uh-KAR-de-uh)
a rapid pulse; any pulse rate above 100 beats per minute.

bradycardia (BRAY-duh-KAR-de-uh)
a slow pulse; any pulse rate below 60 beats per minute.

Table 12-1 Pulse

NORMAL PULSE RATES (BEATS PER MINUTE, AT REST)	
Adult	60 to 100
Infants and children	
Adolescent 11 to 14 years	60 to 105
School age 6 to 10 years	70 to 110
Preschooler 3 to 5 years	80 to 120
Toddler 1 to 3 years	80 to 130
Infant 6 to 12 months	80 to 140
Infant 0 to 5 months	90 to 140
Newborn	120 to 160
PULSE QUALITY	**SIGNIFICANCE/POSSIBLE CAUSES**
Rapid, regular, and full	Exertion, fright, fever, high blood pressure, first stage of blood loss
Rapid, regular, and thready	Shock, later stages of blood loss
Slow	Head injury, drugs, some poisons, some heart problems, lack of oxygen in children
No pulse	Cardiac arrest (clinical death)
Infants and Children: A high pulse in an infant or child is not as great a concern as a low pulse. A low pulse may indicate imminent cardiac arrest.	

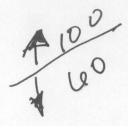

between 40 and 50 beats per minute. This is a slow pulse rate, but it is certainly not an indication of poor health. However, the same pulse rate in a non-athletic or elderly person may indicate a serious condition. You should be concerned about the typical adult whose pulse rate stays above 100 or below 60 beats per minute.

In an emergency, it is not unusual for this rate to temporarily be between 100 and 140 beats per minute. If the pulse rate is higher than 150, or if you take a patient's pulse several times during care on-scene and find him maintaining a pulse rate above 120 beats or below 50 beats per minute, consider this a sign that something may be seriously wrong with the patient and transport as soon as possible.

Pulse Quality

pulse quality
the rhythm (regular or irregular) and force (strong or weak) of the pulse.

Two factors determine **pulse quality**: rhythm and force. *Pulse rhythm* reflects regularity. A pulse is said to be regular when intervals between beats are constant. When the intervals are not constant, the pulse is irregular. You should report and document irregular pulse rhythms.

Pulse force refers to the pressure of the pulse wave as it expands the artery. Normally, the pulse should feel as if a strong wave has passed under your fingertips. This is a strong or full pulse. When the pulse feels weak and thin, the patient has a thready pulse. Many disorders can be related to variations in pulse rate, rhythm, and force (Table 12-1).

radial (RAY-de-ul) **pulse**
the pulse felt at the wrist.

Pulse rate and quality can be determined at a number of points throughout the body. During the determination of vital signs, you should initially find a **radial pulse** in patients 1 year of age and older. This is the wrist pulse, named for the radial artery found on the lateral (thumb) side of the forearm. In an infant who is 1 year old or less, you should find the **brachial pulse** in the upper arm (Figure 12-2) rather than the radial pulse. If you cannot measure the pulse on one arm, try the pulse of the other arm. When you cannot measure the radial or brachial pulse, use the **carotid pulse**, felt along the large carotid artery on either side of the neck. Be careful when palpating a carotid pulse in a patient. Excessive pressure on the carotid artery can result in slowing of the heart, especially in older patients. If you have difficulty finding the carotid pulse on one side, try the other side, but *do not assess the carotid pulses on both sides at the same time.*

brachial (BRAY-key-al) **pulse**
the pulse felt in the upper arm.

carotid (kah-ROT-id) **pulse**
the pulse felt along the large carotid artery on either side of the neck.

In order to measure a radial pulse, find the pulse site by placing your first three fingers on the thumb side of the patient's wrist just above the crease (toward the shoulder). Do not use your thumb. It has its own pulse that may cause you to measure your own pulse rate. Slide your fingertips toward the thumb side of the patient's wrist, keeping one finger over the crease. Apply moderate pressure to feel the pulse beats. If the patient has a weak pulse, you may need to apply greater pressure. But take care—if you press too hard you may press the artery shut. Remember: If you experience difficulty, try the patient's other arm.

Count the pulsations for 30 seconds and multiply by 2 to determine the beats per minute. While you are counting, judge the rhythm and force. Record the information: for example, "Pulse 72, regular and full," and the time of determination.

• **CORE CONCEPT**
How to document vital signs on a prehospital care report

If the pulse rate, rhythm, or force is not normal, continue with your count and observations for a full 60 seconds.

FIGURE 12-2 Palpating a brachial pulse in an infant.

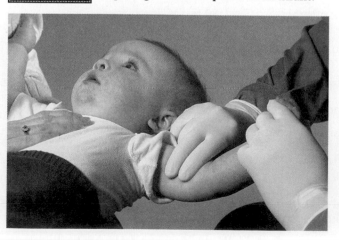

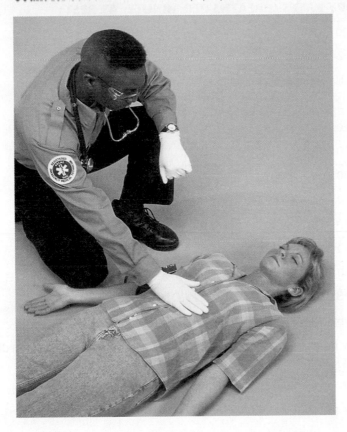

Respiration

The act of breathing is called **respiration**. A single breath is considered to be the complete process of breathing in (called *inhalation* or *inspiration*) followed by breathing out (called *exhalation* or *expiration*). For the determination of vital signs, you are concerned with two factors: rate and quality (Figure 12-3).

Respiratory Rate

The **respiratory rate** is the number of breaths a patient takes in 1 minute (Table 12-2). The rate of respiration is classified as *normal*, *rapid*, or *slow*. The normal respiration rate for an adult at rest is between 12 and 20 breaths per minute. Keep in mind that age, sex, size, physical conditioning, and emotional state can all influence breathing rates. For example, fear and other emotions experienced during an emergency can cause an increase in respiratory rate. However, if you have an adult patient maintaining a rate above 24 (rapid) or below 8 breaths per minute (slow), you must administer high-concentration oxygen and be prepared to assist ventilations.

Respiratory Quality

Respiratory quality, the quality of a patient's breathing, may fall into any of four categories: *normal*, *shallow*, *labored*, or *noisy*. Normal breathing means that the chest or abdomen moves an average depth with each breath and the patient is not using his accessory muscles (look for pronounced movement of the shoulder, neck, or abdominal muscles) to breathe. How can you tell if breathing is normal? Normal depth of respiration is something you can learn to judge by watching healthy people breathe when at rest.

Shallow breathing occurs when there is only slight movement of the chest or abdomen. This is especially serious in the unconscious patient. It is important to look not only at the chest but also at the abdomen when assessing respiration. Many resting people breathe more with their diaphragm (the muscle between the chest and the abdomen) than with their chest muscles.

respiration (res-puh-RAY-shun)
the act of breathing in and breathing out.

respiratory rate
the number of breaths taken in 1 minute.

respiratory (RES-puh-ruh-tor-e)
quality
the normal or abnormal (shallow, labored, or noisy) character of breathing.

Table 12-2 Respirations

NORMAL RESPIRATORY RATES (BREATHS PER MINUTE, AT REST)	
Adult	12 to 20
	Above 24: Serious
	Below 10: Serious
Infants and Children	
Adolescent 11 to 14 years	12 to 20
School age 6 to 10 years	15 to 30
Preschooler 3 to 5 years	20 to 30
Toddler 1 to 3 years	20 to 30
Infant 6 to 12 months	20 to 30
Infant 0 to 5 months	25 to 40
Newborn	30 to 50
RESPIRATORY SOUNDS	**POSSIBLE CAUSES/INTERVENTIONS**
Snoring	Airway blocked/open patient's airway; prompt transport
Wheezing	Medical problem such as asthma/assist patient in taking prescribed medications; prompt transport
Gurgling	Fluids in airway/suction airway; prompt transport
Crowing (harsh sound when inhaling)	Medical problem that cannot be treated on the scene/prompt transport

Labored breathing can be recognized by signs such as an increase in the work of breathing (the patient has to work hard to move air in and out), the use of accessory muscles, nasal flaring (widening of the nostrils on inhalation), and retractions (pulling in) above the collarbones or between the ribs, especially in infants and children. You may also hear stridor (a harsh, high-pitched sound heard on inspiration), grunting on expiration (especially in infants), or gasping.

Noisy breathing is obstructed breathing (when something is blocking the flow of air). Sounds to be concerned about (Table 12-2) include snoring, wheezing, gurgling, and crowing. A patient with snoring respirations needs to have his airway opened. Wheezing may respond to prescribed medication the patient has and that you may be able to assist the patient in taking. Gurgling sounds usually mean that you need to suction the patient's airway. Crowing (a noisy, harsh sound when breathing in) may not respond to any treatment you give. The patient who is crowing needs prompt transport—as do all patients with difficulty breathing.

Respiratory Rhythm

respiratory rhythm
the regular or irregular spacing of breaths.

Respiratory rhythm is not important in most of the conscious patients you will see. This is because the regularity of an awake patient's breathing is affected by his speech, mood, and activity, among other things. If you observe irregular respirations in an unconscious patient, however, you should report and document it.

Start counting respirations as soon as you have determined the pulse rate. Many individuals change their breathing rate if they know someone is watching them breathe. For this reason, do not move your hand from the patient's wrist or tell the patient you are counting the respiratory rate. After you have counted pulse beats, immediately begin to watch the patient's chest and abdomen for breathing movements. Count the number of breaths taken by the patient during 30 seconds and multiply by 2 to obtain the breaths per minute. While counting, note the rate, quality, and rhythm of respiration. Record your results; for example, "Respirations are 16, normal, and regular." Then record the time of your assessment.

Table 12-3 Skin Color

SKIN COLOR	SIGNIFICANCE/POSSIBLE CAUSES
Pink	Normal in light-skinned patients; normal at inner eyelids, lips, and nail beds of dark-skinned patients
Pale	Constricted blood vessels possibly resulting from blood loss, shock, hypotension, emotional distress
Cyanotic (blue-gray)	Lack of oxygen in blood cells and tissues resulting from inadequate breathing or heart function
Flushed (red)	Exposure to heat, emotional excitement
Jaundiced (yellow)	Abnormalities of the liver
Mottled (blotchy)	Occasionally in patients with shock

Skin

The color, temperature, and condition of the skin can provide valuable information about your patient's circulation. There are many blood vessels in the skin. Since the skin is not as important to survival as some of the other organs (like the heart and brain), the blood vessels of the skin will receive less blood when a patient has lost a significant amount of blood or the ability to adequately circulate blood. Constriction (growing smaller) of the blood vessels causes the skin to become pale. For this reason, the skin can provide clues to blood loss as well as a variety of other conditions.

The best places to assess skin color in adults are the nail beds, the inside of the cheek, and the inside of the lower eyelids. Tiny blood vessels called capillaries are very close to the surface of the skin in all of these places, so changes in the blood are quickly reflected at these sites. They are also more accurate indicators than other sites in adults with dark complexions. In infants and children, the best places to look are the palms of the hands and the soles of the feet. In patients with dark skin, you can check the lips and nail beds.

Ordinarily, the color you see (Table 12-3) in any of these places is pink. Abnormal colors include pale, cyanotic (blue-gray), flushed (red), and jaundiced (yellow). Pale skin frequently indicates poor circulation of blood. A common cause of this in the field is loss of blood. Cyanotic skin is usually a result of not enough oxygen getting to the red blood cells. Flushed skin may be caused by exposure to heat. Jaundice is a yellowish tint to the skin from liver abnormalities. An uncommon skin coloration is mottling, a blotchy appearance that sometimes occurs in patients, especially children and the elderly, who are in shock.

To determine skin temperature (Table 12-4), feel the patient's skin with the back of your hand. A good place to do this is the patient's forehead (Figure 12-4). Note if the skin feels normal (warm), hot, cool, or cold. If the patient's skin seems cold, then further assess by placing the back of your hand on the abdomen beneath the clothing. At the same time, notice the patient's condition—is the skin dry (normal), moist, or clammy (both cool and moist)? Look for "goose pimples," which are often associated with chills. Many patient problems are exhibited

Table 12-4 Skin Temperature and Condition

SKIN TEMPERATURE/CONDITION	SIGNIFICANCE/POSSIBLE CAUSES
Cool, clammy	Sign of shock, anxiety
Cold, moist	Body is losing heat
Cold, dry	Exposure to cold
Hot, dry	High fever, heat exposure
Hot, moist	High fever, heat exposure
"Goose pimples" accompanied by shivering, chattering teeth, blue lips, and pale skin	Chills, communicable disease, exposure to cold, pain, or fear

FIGURE 12-4 Determining skin temperature.

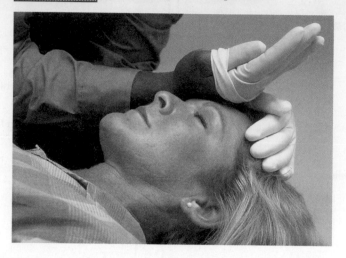

by changes in skin temperature and condition. Continue to be alert for major temperature differences on various parts of the body. For example, you may note that the patient's trunk is warm but his left arm feels cold. Such a finding can reveal a problem with circulation.

PEDIATRIC NOTE

In infants and children under 6 years of age, you should also evaluate capillary refill. Press on the nail bed—or the top of the hand or foot—and watch how long it takes for the normal pink color to return after you release it. Normally, this takes no more than 2 seconds. If it takes longer, the patient's blood is probably not circulating well. Abnormal responses include prolonged and absent capillary refill. This sign is not reliable in infants and children who have been exposed to cold temperatures.

pupil
the black center of the eye.

dilate (DI-late)
get larger.

constrict (kon-STRIKT)
get smaller.

reactivity (re-ak-TIV-uh-te)
in the pupils of the eyes, reacting to light by changing size.

Pupils

The **pupil** is the black center of the eye. One of the things that cause it to change size is the amount of light entering the eye. When the environment is dim, the pupil will **dilate** (get larger) to allow more light into the eye. When there is a lot of light, it will **constrict** (get smaller). Therefore, you will check a patient's pupils by shining a light into them (Figures 12-5 and 12-6). When you check pupils, you should look for three things: size, equality, and **reactivity** (reacting to light by changing size). Under ordinary conditions, pupils are neither large nor small, but midpoint. Dilated pupils are extremely large. In fact, it is usually difficult to tell what color eyes the

FIGURE 12-5 Examining the pupils.

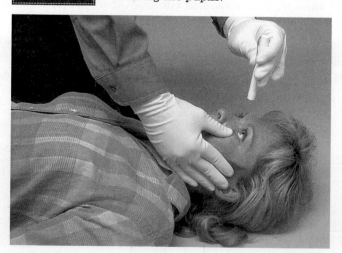

FIGURE 12-6 (A) Constricted, (B) dilated, and (C) unequal pupils.

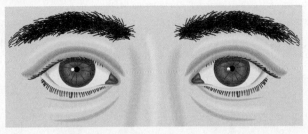

(A)   Constricted pupils

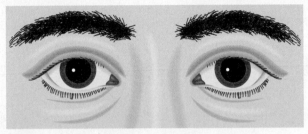

(B)   Dilated pupils

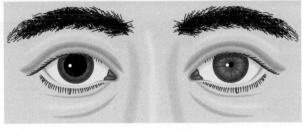

(C)   Unequal pupils

patient has if his pupils are dilated. Both pupils are normally the same size, and when a light shines into them, they react by constricting. The rate at which they constrict should be equal. Nonreactive (fixed) pupils do not constrict in response to a bright light.

To check the patient's pupils, first note their size before you shine any light into them. Next, cover one eye as you shine a penlight into the other eye. The pupil should constrict when the light is shining into it and enlarge when you remove the light. Repeat this process with the other eye. When performing this test, you should cover the eye you are not examining because light entering one eye usually affects the size of the pupils in both eyes. When you are examining a patient in direct sunlight or very bright conditions, initially cover both eyes. After a few seconds, uncover one eye and evaluate it. Cover it again and repeat with the other eye.

Pupils that are dilated, constricted to pinpoint size, unequal in size or reactivity (Figure 12-7), or nonreactive may indicate a variety of conditions (Table 12-5) including drug influence, head injury, or eye injury. Any deviations from normal should be reported and documented.

Blood Pressure

Each time the ventricle (lower chamber) of the left side of the heart contracts, it forces blood out into the circulation. The force of blood against the walls of the blood vessels is called *blood pressure*. The pressure created when the heart contracts and forces blood into the arteries is called the *systolic blood pressure*. When the left ventricle relaxes and refills, the pressure remaining in the arteries is called the *diastolic blood pressure*. These two pressures indicate the amount of pressure against the walls of the arteries and together are known as the blood pressure. When you take a patient's blood pressure, you report the systolic pressure first, the diastolic second; for example, as "120 over 80," or "120/80."

blood pressure
the force of blood against the walls of the blood vessels.

systolic (sis-TOL-ik) *blood pressure*
the pressure created when the heart contracts and forces blood out into the arteries.

diastolic (di-as-TOL-ik) *blood pressure*
the pressure remaining in the arteries when the left ventricle of the heart is relaxed and refilling.

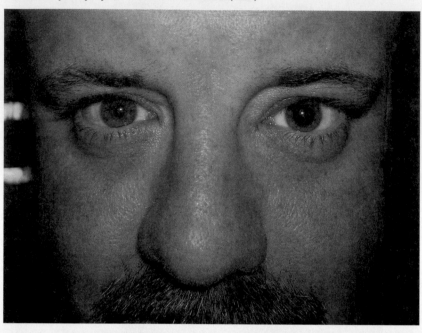

FIGURE 12-7 Unequal pupils can be a sign of the influence of a topical drug (one placed directly on the eye, such as an eye drop) or of head or eye injury. (© Edward T. Dickinson, MD)

Table 12-5 Pupils

PUPIL APPEARANCE	SIGNIFICANCE/POSSIBLE CAUSES
Dilated (larger than normal)	Fright, blood loss, drugs, prescription eye drops
Constricted (smaller than normal)	Drugs (narcotics), prescription eye drops
Unequal	Stroke, head injury, eye injury, artificial eye, prescription eye drops
Lack of reactivity	Drugs, lack of oxygen to brain

One blood pressure reading in isolation may not be very meaningful. You will need to take several readings over a period of time while care is provided at the scene and during transport. Changes in blood pressure can be very significant. The patient's blood pressure may be normal in the early stages of some very serious problems, only to change rapidly in a matter of minutes.

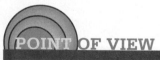

POINT OF VIEW

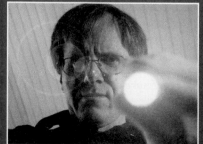

"I have to tell you, people are glad when the ambulance shows up, but it is intimidating as hell. Pardon my language and everything, but I remember when I hit my head and passed out. It was like the cavalry came into my kitchen.

"My sister-in-law is an EMT. She talks about medical things like other people talk about going shopping. Really easy, like something you do every day. But when the EMTs came to my house I was a little intimidated. They started doing this and checking that. It was hard enough to focus after just getting my bell rung. I couldn't even start to answer their questions, and to make things worse they kept shining a flashlight in my eyes.

"On the way to the hospital it got better. Actually, I think my head got clearer and it turns out they were worried about me. Something about 'altered mental status.' Maybe that means I was kind of nuts. We had a nice talk and they told me it was good news that my pupils looked OK (Aha! That's why they were shining that light in my eyes . . .) and also good news that I was talking with them now.

"I just finally felt like I had some control over what was going on."

Table 12-6 Blood Pressure

BLOOD PRESSURE NORMAL RANGES	SYSTOLIC	DIASTOLIC
Adults	Less than or equal to 120	Less than or equal to 80
Infants and children	Approx. 80 + 2 × age (yrs)	Approx. 2/3 systolic
Adolescent 11 to 14 years	Average 114 (88 to 120)	Average 76
School age 6 to 10 years	Average 105 (80 to 115)	Average 69
Preschooler 3 to 5 years	Average 99 (78 to 104)	Average 65
BLOOD PRESSURE	**SIGNIFICANCE/POSSIBLE CAUSES**	
High blood pressure	Medical condition, exertion, fright, emotional distress, or excitement	
Low blood pressure	Athlete or other person with normally low blood pressure; blood loss; late sign of shock	

Infants and Children: Blood pressure is usually not taken on a child under 3 years, although this may vary from system to system. In cases of blood loss or shock, a child's blood pressure will remain within normal limits until near the end, then fall swiftly.

Pulse and respiratory rates vary among individuals, but blood pressure is a little different (Table 12-6). A normal blood pressure is a systolic pressure of no greater than 120 millimeters of mercury (mmHg) and a diastolic pressure of no greater than 80 mmHg. *Millimeters of mercury* refers to the units on the blood pressure gauge. If an adult has a systolic pressure of 140 mmHg or greater or a diastolic pressure of 90 mmHg or greater, the person has hypertension (high blood pressure). Readings between these limits (121 to 139 mmHg systolic and 81 to 89 mmHg diastolic) indicate a condition sometimes called prehypertension. This means the patient is at risk of developing some of the complications of hypertension like heart disease, stroke, or kidney disease.

Serious low blood pressure is generally considered to exist when the systolic pressure falls below 90 mmHg. Many individuals under stress (like that caused by having the ambulance come to their home) will exhibit a temporary rise in blood pressure. More than one reading will be necessary to decide if a high or low reading is only temporary. If the blood pressure drops, your patient may be developing shock (however, other signs are usually more important early indicators of shock). Report any major changes in blood pressure to emergency department personnel without delay.

To measure blood pressure with a ***sphygmomanometer*** (the cuff and gauge), first place the stethoscope around your neck. Position yourself at the patient's side and place the blood pressure cuff on his arm (Figure 12-8). The cuff should cover two-thirds of the upper arm,

sphygmomanometer

(SFIG-mo-mah-NOM-uh-ter)
the cuff and gauge used to measure blood pressure.

FIGURE 12-8 Positioning blood pressure cuff.

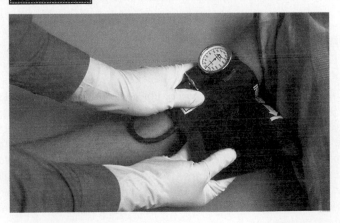

FIGURE 12-9 Measuring blood pressure by auscultation.

FIGURE 12-10 Measuring blood pressure by palpation.

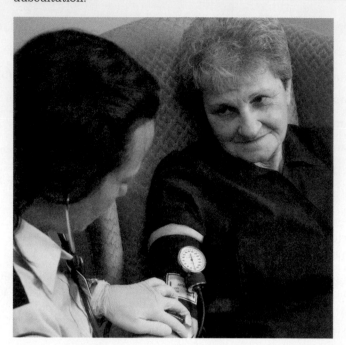

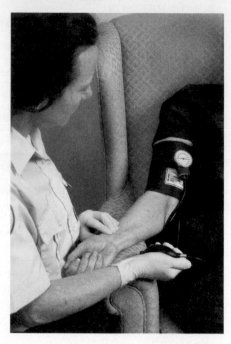

brachial artery
the major artery of the arm.

auscultation (os-kul-TAY-shun)
listening. A stethoscope is used to
auscultate for characteristic sounds.

palpation
touching or feeling. A pulse or blood
pressure may be palpated with the
fingertips.

blood pressure monitor
machine that automatically inflates a
blood pressure cuff and measures
blood pressure.

elbow to shoulder. Be certain that there are no suspected or obvious injuries to this arm. There should be no clothing under the cuff. If you can expose the arm sufficiently by rolling the sleeve up, do so, but make sure that this roll of clothing does not become a constricting band.

Wrap the cuff around the patient's upper arm so that the lower edge of the cuff is about 1 inch above the crease of the elbow. The center of the bladder must be placed over the **brachial artery**, the major artery of the arm. The marker on the cuff (if provided) should indicate where you place the cuff in relation to the artery. However, many cuffs do not have markers in the correct location. Tubes entering the bladder are not always in the right location, either. According to the American Heart Association, the only accurate method is to find the bladder center. Apply the cuff so it is secure but not overly tight. You are now ready to begin your determination of the patient's blood pressure.

Three common techniques are used to measure blood pressure with a sphygmomanometer: (1) **auscultation**, when a stethoscope is used to listen for characteristic sounds (Figure 12-9); (2) **palpation**, when the radial pulse or brachial pulse is palpated (felt) with the fingertips (Figure 12-10); and (3) **blood pressure monitor**, when a machine controls inflation of the cuff and detects changes in blood flow in the artery (Figures 12-11 and 12-12). Palpation is not as accurate as auscultation, since only an approximate systolic pressure can be determined. Palpation is used when there is too much noise around a patient to allow the use of the stethoscope. Blood pressure monitors are improving in quality and many emergency departments and EMS agencies use them.

Determining Blood Pressure by Auscultation

1. **Prepare.** The patient should be seated or lying down. If the patient has not been injured, support his arm at the level of his heart.

2. **Position the cuff and the stethoscope.** Place the cuff snugly around the upper arm so that the bottom of the cuff is just above the elbow. With your fingertips, palpate the brachial artery at the crease of the elbow (Figure 12-13). Place the ear pieces of the stethoscope in your ears (the ear pieces should be pointing forward in the direction of your ear canals). Position the diaphragm of the stethoscope directly over the brachial pulse or over the medial anterior elbow (front of the elbow) if no brachial pulse can be found. Do not place the head of the stethoscope underneath the cuff, since this will give you false readings.

FIGURE 12-11 An automatic blood pressure monitor.

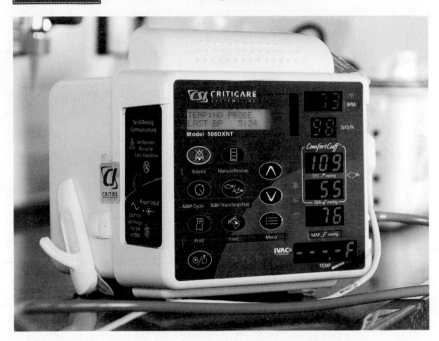

FIGURE 12-12 (A and B) Automated blood pressure cuff as part of an ECG monitor. (C and D) Stand-alone automated blood pressure cuff.

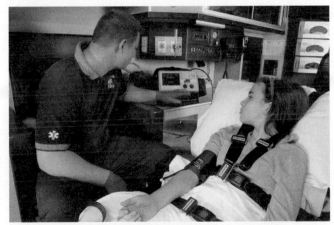

(A)

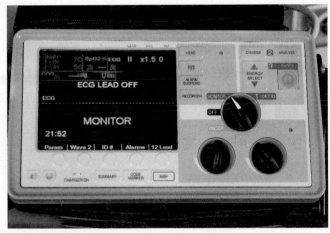

(B)

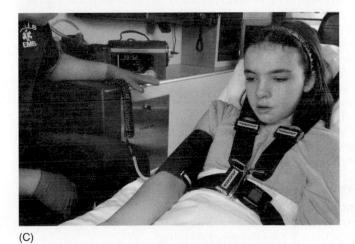

(C)

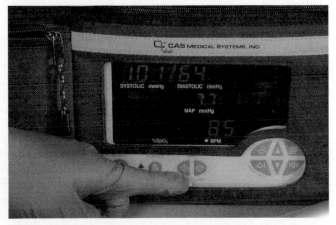

(D)

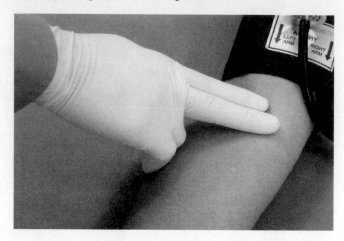

FIGURE 12-13 When measuring blood pressure by auscultation, locate the brachial artery by palpation before placing the stethoscope.

3. **Inflate the cuff.** With the bulb valve (thumb valve) closed, inflate the cuff. As you do so, you soon will be able to hear pulse sounds. Inflate the cuff, watching the gauge. At a certain point, you will no longer hear the brachial pulse. Continue to inflate the cuff until the gauge reads 30 mm higher than the point where the pulse sound disappeared.

4. **Obtain the systolic pressure.** Slowly release air from the cuff by opening the bulb valve, allowing the pressure to fall smoothly at the rate of approximately 5 to 10 mm per second. Listen for the start of clicking or tapping sounds. When you hear the first of these sounds, note the reading on the gauge. This is the systolic pressure.

5. **Obtain the diastolic pressure.** Continue to deflate the cuff, listening for the point at which these distinctive sounds fade. When the sounds turn to dull, muffled thuds, the reading on the gauge is the diastolic pressure. Sometimes you will not be able to hear a change in these sounds. When this happens, the point at which the sounds disappear is the diastolic pressure.

6. **Record measurements.** After obtaining the diastolic pressure, let the cuff deflate rapidly. Record the measurements and the time. For example, "Blood pressure is 140/90 at 1:10 p.m." Blood pressure is reported in even numbers. If a reading falls between two lines on the gauge, use the higher number.

If you are not certain of a reading, repeat the procedure. You should use the other arm or wait 1 minute before re-inflating the cuff. Otherwise, you will tend to obtain an erroneously high reading. If you are still not sure of the reading, try again or get some help. Never make up vital signs!

> **NOTE:** *Some patients who have high systolic blood pressures will have the pulse sounds disappear as you deflate the cuff, but reappear as you continue with deflation. When this happens, false readings may be obtained. If you determine a high diastolic reading, wait 1 to 2 minutes and take another reading. As you inflate the cuff, feel for the disappearance of the radial pulse to ensure that you are not measuring a false diastolic pressure. Listen as you deflate the cuff down into the normal range. The diastolic pressure is the reading at which the last clear sound takes place.*
>
> *When the heartbeat is irregular, the interval between heartbeats can vary a great deal. You may obtain an artificially low blood pressure reading if you pass the systolic or diastolic pressure between two widely separated beats, especially if you deflate the cuff quickly. If the patient's heartbeat is irregular, you should deflate the cuff a little more slowly and listen even more carefully to obtain an accurate reading.*

Determining Blood Pressure by Palpation

1. **Position the cuff and find the radial pulse.** Apply the cuff as described for auscultation. Then find the radial pulse on the arm to which the cuff has been applied. If a radial pulse cannot be palpated, find the brachial pulse.

2. **Inflate the cuff.** Make certain that the adjustable valve is closed on the bulb and inflate the cuff to a point where you can no longer feel the radial pulse. Note this point on the gauge and continue to inflate the cuff 30 mmHg beyond this point.

3. **Obtain and record the systolic pressure.** Slowly deflate the cuff, noting the reading at which the radial pulse returns. This reading is the patient's systolic pressure. Record your findings as, for example, "blood pressure 140 by palpation" or "140/P" and the time of the determination. (You cannot determine a diastolic reading by palpation.)

Determining Blood Pressure by Blood Pressure Monitor

1. **Position the cuff.** Apply the cuff as described for auscultation.

2. **Inflate the cuff.** Press the button that tells the monitor to begin inflating the cuff.

3. **Obtain and record the blood pressure.** After the monitor has finished deflating the cuff, it will indicate the patient's blood pressure on a screen. If it cannot get a blood pressure, it will tell you. Some monitors will give not only the systolic and diastolic pressures but also the mean arterial pressure (MAP). As this is not typically used in prehospital care, do not let it distract you from the numbers you are seeking.

CORE CONCEPT ●----------

How to use various monitoring devices

PEDIATRIC NOTE

Obtain a blood pressure on every patient who is more than 3 years old. Blood pressures are difficult to obtain with any accuracy on infants and children younger than 3 and have little bearing on the patient's field management. You can get more useful information about the condition of an infant or very young child by observing for conditions such as a sick appearance, respiratory distress, or unconsciousness. Follow your local protocols.

Unless medical direction advises otherwise, the first blood pressure you get should be with the auscultation method. Although the quality of blood pressure monitors has been improving, these machines still make errors and occasionally fail. This may be more likely to happen in the prehospital environment. The blood pressure obtained by auscultation is the standard that other blood pressures will be compared against. If a reading from the blood pressure monitor is very different from the auscultated blood pressure, check the blood pressure yourself by auscultation or palpation.

Many blood pressure monitors have timers you can set to take the blood pressure every 5 minutes, every 15 minutes, or at some other interval determined by the operator. This can provide a useful reminder to the EMT when it is time to check the rest of the vital signs again.

It is important that the EMT follow the manufacturer's directions and local medical direction in using an automated blood pressure monitor or any other device used in patient assessment.

Vital signs are usually taken more than once. How frequently they should be repeated depends on the patient's condition and your interventions. Stable patients need repeat vital signs at least every 15 minutes. Unstable patients need repeat vital signs at least every 5 minutes. Also repeat vital signs after every medical intervention. Record every reading of the vital signs (Figure 12-14), because if you don't write them down, you probably won't remember them.

Temperature

The human body continuously generates and loses heat but manages to maintain a temperature within a narrow range that allows chemical reactions and other activities to take place inside the body. For most patients an EMT encounters, the temperature will not be important, although for some it may be. This includes cases where the patient may be hypothermic or hyperthermic (with a below normal or above normal temperature, often from a change in the environment), febrile (feverish), or suffering from a generalized infection (septic).

One very important use for temperature is in screening for influenza. Since many EMS systems now record patient data electronically, this has allowed health departments to evaluate EMS data during flu season to see if there has been an outbreak of the disease in a particular area. By looking for patients with signs and symptoms consistent with influenza, including fever, public health specialists may be able to detect outbreaks earlier than ever before.

FIGURE 12-14 The prehospital care report (run sheet) provides spaces for recording vital signs.

Time	Pulse	Respirations	Blood Pressure
1410	88 str, reg	28	132/84

Pupils	Skin Color	Skin Temperature	Skin Condition
Equal ☑ Unequal ☐	Normal ☐	Cold ☐	Moist ☑
Reactive (L) (R)	Pale ☑	Cool ☑	Dry ☐
Nonreactive L R	Cyanotic ☐	Warm ☐	
Dilated ☐	Flushed ☐	Hot ☐	
Normal Size ☑	Jaundiced ☐		
Constricted ☐			

You learned earlier in this chapter about skin color, temperature, and condition. In this section, we are dealing not with the surface temperature of the skin, but with the body's core temperature, or the closest we can get to measuring it. The core temperature reflects the level of heat inside the trunk, where the heart, lungs, and digestive organs function. Since it is usually not practical to place a thermometer inside someone's heart or stomach, we measure the closest substitute available. Traditionally, this is either an oral or rectal temperature, but it is also possible to get an axillary temperature in the armpit (axilla).

Although glass thermometers are usually accurate, the conditions EMTs encounter in the field make them undesirable. Putting a piece of glass into the patient's mouth and then traveling over bumpy roads in the back of a moving ambulance risks injuring the patient from broken glass. A quicker way to get an oral temperature is to use an electronic thermometer (Figure 12-15), which usually provides a reading in just a few seconds. This is also

FIGURE 12-15 An electronic thermometer is safer, more hygienic, and quicker to produce a reading than a glass thermometer. (© Welch Allyn)

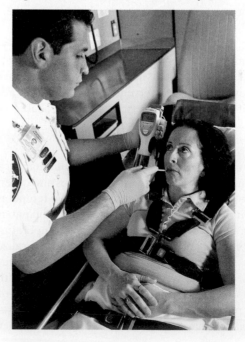

safer and more hygienic, since these machines usually employ metal probes with disposable plastic covers. To get a temperature with an electronic thermometer, put a new plastic cover over the probe, insert it under the patient's tongue, and follow the manufacturer's instructions. When an oral temperature is not practical, you can sometimes get an axillary temperature. Rectal temperatures are not usually practical or necessary in the field.

Tympanic thermometers that measure the temperature in the ear are commercially available and frequently used but are not accurate enough for EMS use. Numerous evaluations of these devices have consistently found that the margin of error is quite wide. Many patients are misclassified as having abnormally high or low temperatures by tympanic devices. Forehead thermometers, strips placed on the forehead, are also not accurate enough for EMTs to use.

A normal temperature is not necessarily 98.6°F (37°C). A person's normal temperature depends on the time of day, activity level, age, where the temperature is measured, and simple genetics—some people just have a higher or lower normal temperature than other people. Temperature rises and falls at different times of the day and night and usually rises with increased physical activity. Older people tend to have lower temperatures than younger people. A rectal temperature is often about one degree higher than an oral temperature, and an axillary temperature is frequently about a degree lower. Most people have a typical temperature somewhere near 98.6°F or 37°C, but many healthy people walk around with temperatures that are not "normal" by these traditional measures. In general, a healthy, normal person will have a temperature greater than 96°F and less than 100°F.

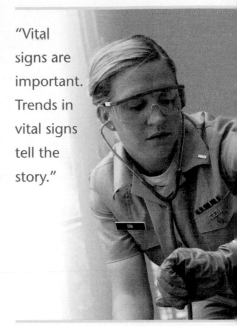

"Vital signs are important. Trends in vital signs tell the story."

Oxygen Saturation

EMTs and other health care providers commonly measure the level of oxygen circulating through a patient's blood vessels. A measurement of oxygen saturation is not a vital sign, but many EMS providers incorporate it into their gathering of vital signs. Your EMS system may have specific guidance on when to perform this measurement.

The device that measures oxygen saturation of the blood, called a ***pulse oximeter*** (Figure 12-16), sends different colors of light into the tissue at the end of a finger or on an earlobe and measures the amount of light that returns. The machine then determines the proportion of oxygen in the blood and displays the ***oxygen saturation*** percentage, also called the **SpO₂**.

A different kind of oximeter uses different wavelengths of light that allow it to measure carbon monoxide (CO) as well as oxygen. For this reason, it is sometimes called a

pulse oximeter
an electronic device for determining the amount of oxygen carried in the blood, known as the oxygen saturation or SpO_2.

oxygen saturation (SpO₂)
the ratio of the amount of oxygen present in the blood to the amount that could be carried, expressed as a percentage.

FIGURE 12-16 A pulse oximeter with sensor applied to the patient's finger.

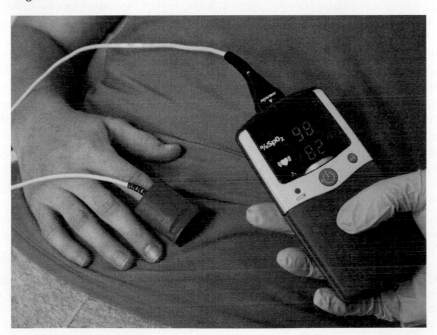

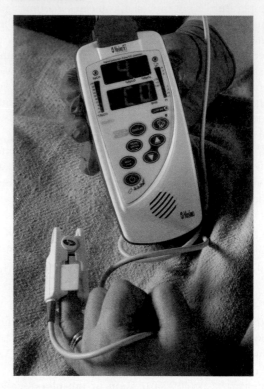

CO-oximeter (Figure 12-17). Future versions of this device will very likely be more accurate, less expensive, and easier to use than early models. Interpreting CO-oximeter readings in a particular clinical situation can be challenging, so if you use a CO-oximeter, be sure to follow your local protocols regarding its application and interpretation.

When to Use a Pulse Oximeter

If your service has a pulse oximeter, you should have a protocol describing when to use it. Generally, this will include all patients complaining of respiratory problems. When used properly, the device can help you to assess the effectiveness of artificial respirations, oxygen therapy, and bronchodilator (inhaler) therapy. Some services recommend its use in other patients as well. Follow your local protocols.

Interpreting Pulse Oximeter Readings

The oxygen saturation, or SpO_2, is typically 96 to 100 percent in a normal healthy person. A value less than 96 percent may sound good, but that is not really the case. A reading of 91 to 95 percent indicates mild hypoxia, 86 to 90 percent indicates significant or moderate hypoxia, and 85 percent or less indicates severe hypoxia. The lower the oxygen saturation reading you get, the more aggressive your management should be. Any indication of hypoxia is reason to administer high-concentration oxygen by nonrebreather mask. For very low readings, you will need to look at the patient's clinical condition and decide whether to ventilate the patient with high-concentration oxygen. You should try to get the SpO_2 up to at least 96 percent.

The reverse situation is not true; that is, a reading above 96 percent does NOT mean you should withhold oxygen from a patient with signs and symptoms that indicate the need for oxygen.

NOTE: *Never deprive a patient in respiratory distress of supplemental oxygen while attempting to obtain an accurate pulse oximetry reading. For these patients, providing supplemental oxygen, or even assisting ventilations, is a far more important intervention than documenting their "room air" saturation of oxygen.*

Cautions The following cautions apply to interpreting pulse oximetry readings.

- The oximeter is inaccurate with patients in shock and hypothermic patients (those whose body temperatures have been lowered by exposure to cold) because not enough blood is flowing through the capillaries for the device to get an accurate reading.

- The oximeter will produce falsely high readings in patients with carbon monoxide and certain other uncommon types of poisoning. This is because carbon monoxide binds with hemoglobin in the blood, producing the red color read by the device. Cigarettes produce carbon monoxide, so chronic smokers may have 10 to 15 percent of their hemoglobin bound to carbon monoxide. This means their oxygen saturation readings will be higher than the actual oxygen saturation.

- Excessive movement of the patient can cause inaccurate readings; so can nail polish, if the device is attached to a finger. Carry acetone wipes to quickly remove the nail polish from a patient's fingernail before attaching the oximeter. Anemia, hypovolemia, and certain kinds of poisoning are other potential causes of falsely high oxygen saturation readings.

- The accuracy of the pulse oximeter should be checked regularly, following the manufacturer's recommendations. The batteries used to power the device must be in good condition and the probe needs to be kept clean to get accurate readings.

- Pulse oximetry is most useful in two situations: evaluating the effect of an intervention you have instituted (when you hope the SpO_2 goes up or remains high) and alerting you to a deterioration in the patient's oxygen saturation (when the SpO_2 starts going down). Like any other device, the pulse oximeter can distract you from the patient. Keep pulse oximetry in its proper place in the assessment. Remember, the oximeter is just another tool. Do not rely on it solely for indications of the patient's condition. Treat the patient, not the device.

Determining Oxygen Saturation

1. Connect the sensor lead to the monitor and clip it onto a fingertip (toe or distal foot in an infant).

2. Turn the device on. After a few seconds the device should display the SpO_2 and heart rate. Make sure the heart rate displayed on the monitor screen is the same as the patient's pulse rate (which you palpated already). If the heart rate shown on the pulse oximeter does not match the pulse rate that you have determined, it is likely that the oxygen saturation will not be an accurate reading either.

3. If you get a poor signal or "trouble" indicator, try repositioning the sensor on the finger or moving it to a different finger.

4. Once you get an accurate reading, check the oximeter reading every 5 minutes. A convenient time to do this is when you check the patient's vital signs.

Blood Glucose Meters

One of the many advances in managing diabetes in the last few years has been the development of portable, reliable blood glucose meters. The portability, low cost, and accuracy of blood glucose meters has made it practical to carry them on the ambulance. They are easy to use, and since they are routinely used by patients (Figure 12-18), many EMS systems allow EMTs to use blood glucose meters that are carried on the ambulance. Your protocols will tell you whether you are allowed to carry and use a glucose meter.

People with diabetes now routinely test the level of glucose in their blood at least once a day, and sometimes as often as five or six times a day. By determining the amount of glucose in their blood, they can determine very precisely how much insulin they should take and how much and how often they should eat. Keeping blood glucose levels as close to normal as possible leads to significantly fewer diabetes-related complications (heart disease, blindness, and kidney failure, to name a few), so a person with diabetes has a strong motivation to keep his blood glucose level within the normal range.

A blood glucose meter is used by placing a drop of the patient's blood on a test strip. The blood is traditionally obtained from pricking a finger, although some glucose meters allow patients to obtain the blood from other areas, like the forearm. The glucose meter evaluates the change in chemical composition of the material on the strip and displays a number that

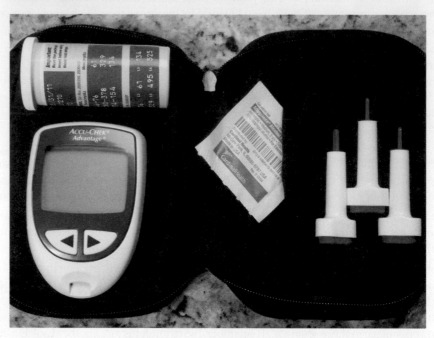

correlates to the glucose concentration in the person's blood. In the United States, this number usually shows the amount of glucose in milligrams per deciliter (100 mL) of blood (expressed as mg/dL), also called milligrams percent. Outside of the United States, the meter may use a different system of measuring glucose to report results.

Using a Blood Glucose Meter

NOTE: *EMTs must have permission from medical direction or by local protocol to perform blood glucose monitoring using a blood glucose meter.*

If the patient has a glucose meter, the patient or a family member can use it to determine the patient's blood glucose level. Generally, EMTs should not use a patient's glucose meter. There are many different types of these devices on the market, each with its own instructions for use, which may be very different from device to device. Additionally, there is no way for the EMT to know whether the test strips have been stored properly or when the device was last calibrated. These facts are very important if the reading is to be accurate.

If you have blood glucose monitors on the ambulance, they must be calibrated and stored according to the manufacturer's recommendations. Take Standard Precautions. When using the glucose meter (Scan 12-1), you will follow these steps:

1. Prepare the device including a test strip and lancet.

2. Use an alcohol prep to cleanse the patient's finger.

3. After allowing the alcohol to dry, use the lancet to perform a finger stick on the patient. Wipe away the first drop of blood that appears. Squeeze the patient's finger if necessary to get a second drop of blood. Holding the patient's hand lower than the heart and warming the hand may increase blood flow.

4. Apply the blood to the test strip. This is often done by holding the strip up to the finger and then drawing the blood into the strip.

5. The blood glucose meter analyzes the sample and provides a reading—usually in less than a minute.

A normal blood glucose level is usually at least 60 to 80 mg/dL (milligrams per deciliter) and no more than 120 or 140 (depending on the manufacturer's instructions and local protocols). You will learn in Chapter 21, "Diabetic Emergencies and Altered Mental Status," how to interpret this information and apply it to the patient's care.

NOTE: *EMTs must have permission from medical direction or by local protocol to perform blood glucose monitoring using a blood glucose meter.*

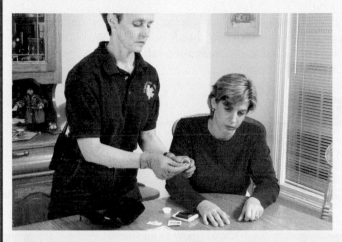

1 Prepare the blood glucose meter, including a test strip and a lancet.

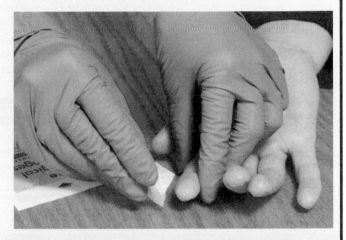

2 Cleanse the skin with an alcohol preparation. Allow the alcohol to dry before performing the finger stick.

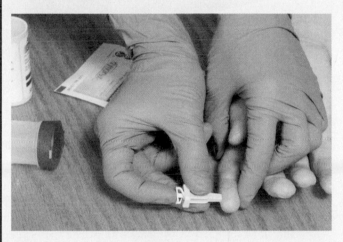

3 Use the lancet to perform a finger stick. Wipe away the first drop of blood that appears. Squeeze the finger if necessary to get a second drop of blood.

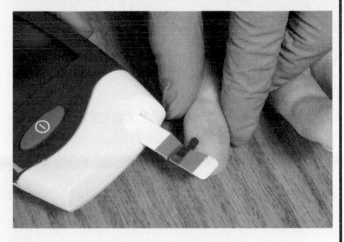

4 Apply the blood to the test strip. This may be done by holding the strip to the finger to draw the blood into the strip.

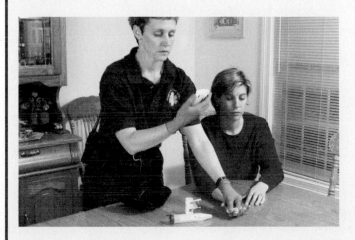

5 Read the blood glucose level displayed on the glucose meter. (It may take 15 to 60 seconds for the device to provide a reading.) Assess the puncture site and apply direct pressure or a bandage to the site if bleeding continues.

Although many people use blood glucose meters appropriately and accurately, it is quite common to get an inaccurate reading, especially when the device is not used properly. It is critical for any health care provider who is using a blood glucose meter to test a patient's blood to have the proper training in use of the device and be thoroughly familiar with its care and maintenance. Calibration and testing on a regularly scheduled basis are essential if the device is to give accurate results.

Remember that the blood glucose monitor is just one tool in your patient assessment. Blood glucose monitoring, or any other examinations, should never be done before performing a thorough primary assessment. Some areas recommend that the blood glucose measurements be done while en route to the hospital.

PEDIATRIC NOTE

One of the most important factors that determines the normal range of vital signs is age. Infants and children have faster pulse and respiratory rates and lower blood pressures than adults. Compare the ranges for infants and children with those for adults as displayed in the tables in this chapter.

CHAPTER REVIEW

Key Facts and Concepts

- You can gain a great deal of information about a patient's condition by taking a complete set of baseline vital signs, including pulse, respirations, skin, pupils, and blood pressure.

- The EMT must become familiar with the normal ranges for pulse, respirations, and blood pressure in adults and children.

- Trends in the patient's condition will become apparent only when vital signs are repeated, an important step in continuing assessment.

- How often you repeat the vital signs will depend on the patient's condition: at least every 15 minutes for stable patients and at least every 5 minutes for unstable patients.

Key Decisions

- Do I have time to obtain vital signs, or is the patient so unstable I should get them en route to the hospital?

- When should I apply a pulse oximeter to a patient with difficulty breathing? Without difficulty breathing?

- Are abnormal vital signs a result of an illness or injury or are they the result of some other factor?

- Under what circumstances might it be appropriate to check vital signs on a stable patient every 5 minutes?

Chapter Glossary

auscultation (os-kul-TAY-shun) listening. A stethoscope is used to auscultate for characteristic sounds.

blood pressure the force of blood against the walls of the blood vessels.

blood pressure monitor machine that automatically inflates a blood pressure cuff and measures blood pressure.

brachial (BRAY-key-al) *artery* the major artery of the arm.

brachial pulse the pulse felt in the upper arm.

bradycardia (BRAY-duh-KAR-de-uh) a slow pulse; any pulse rate below 60 beats per minute.

carotid (kah-ROT-id) *pulse* the pulse felt along the large carotid artery on either side of the neck.

constrict (kon-STRIKT) get smaller.

diastolic (di-as-TOL-ik) *blood pressure* the pressure remaining in the arteries when the left ventricle of the heart is relaxed and refilling.

dilate (DI-late) get larger.

oxygen saturation (SpO₂) the ratio of the amount of oxygen present in the blood to the amount that could be carried, expressed as a percentage.

palpation touching or feeling. A pulse or blood pressure may be palpated with the fingertips.

pulse the rhythmic beats felt as the heart pumps blood through the arteries.

pulse oximeter an electronic device for determining the amount of oxygen carried in the blood, known as the oxygen saturation or SpO₂.

pulse quality the rhythm (regular or irregular) and force (strong or weak) of the pulse.

pulse rate the number of pulse beats per minute.

pupil the black center of the eye.

radial (RAY-de-ul) *pulse* the pulse felt at the wrist.

reactivity (re-ak-TIV-uh-te) in the pupils of the eyes, reacting to light by changing size.

respiration (res-puh-RAY-shun) the act of breathing in and breathing out.

respiratory (RES-puh-ruh-tor-e) *quality* the normal or abnormal (shallow, labored, or noisy) character of breathing.

respiratory rate the number of breaths taken in 1 minute.

respiratory rhythm the regular or irregular spacing of breaths.

sphygmomanometer (SFIG-mo-mah-NOM-uh-ter) the cuff and gauge used to measure blood pressure.

systolic (sis-TOL-ik) *blood pressure* the pressure created when the heart contracts and forces blood out into the arteries.

tachycardia (TAK-uh-KAR-de-uh) a rapid pulse; any pulse rate above 100 beats per minute.

vital signs outward signs of what is going on inside the body, including respiration; pulse; skin color, temperature, and condition (plus capillary refill in infants and children); pupils; and blood pressure.

Preparation for Your Examination and Practice

Short Answer

1. Name the vital signs.
2. Explain why vital signs should be taken more than once.

Thinking and Linking

Think back to Chapter 9, "Respiration and Artificial Ventilation," and link information from that chapter (regarding oxygen administration and artificial ventilation) with information from this chapter (regarding oxygen saturation) as you consider the following situations:

1. You are assessing a patient who complains of "feeling dizzy." On primary assessment, her breathing appears to be adequate, but when you apply the pulse oximeter during vital signs measurement, you note that her blood oxygen saturation reading is 93 percent. You know that a normal reading would be at least 96 percent. What intervention should you take to improve this patient's oxygen saturation? What technique and equipment would you use?

2. At the scene of a motor-vehicle collision, you are caring for a patient with multiple injuries. Because his breathing was obviously inadequate (shallow and rapid), you initiated artificial ventilation with a bag-valve-mask unit. However, a subsequent reading on this pulse oximeter shows his blood oxygen saturation level—even with assisted ventilations—is only 90 percent. What can you do to attempt to improve his oxygen saturation level?

Critical Thinking Exercises

Vital signs assessments are a critical part of patient assessment. The purpose of this exercise will be to consider how you might deal with the following challenges to obtaining accurate vital signs.

1. How much time should the EMT spend looking for a pulse when the radial pulse is absent or extremely weak?

2. How should you react when the blood pressure monitor gives a reading that is extremely different from previous readings you got?

3. How can you get an accurate pulse oximeter reading on a patient with thick artificial nails?

Pathophysiology to Practice

The following questions are designed to assist you in gathering relevant clinical information and making accurate decisions in the field.

- Sometimes a patient's heart will have an electrical problem and beat more than 200 times a minute. Why is the pulse so weak in such a patient?

- When someone has lost a significant amount of blood, the adrenal glands secrete epinephrine (adrenaline), which causes pale, sweaty skin. What effect does epinephrine have on blood vessels, leading to this condition?

- Why is chronically high diastolic pressure strongly associated with heart disease?

You are just sitting down to relax when the dispatcher calls to notify you of a 73-year-old female patient with abdominal pain at 19 Oakwood Lane. Before getting to the scene, you and your partner agree that you will do the patient interview and he will assess vital signs. When you arrive, you find the patient sitting at her kitchen table. She tells you her name is Ms. Socorro Alvarez. She says she has stomach pain, "But I don't need to go to the hospital."

As you look at this patient, you find that you aren't confident that this is a good decision. You start to think ABCs and realize that her airway is obviously open and clear, but her breathing seems a little rapid.

Street Scene Questions

1. What is your primary concern for this patient?
2. What vital signs should be taken even if a no transport decision is being considered?
3. Ideally, what should the patient history include?

You mention to Ms. Alvarez that since she called EMS, she must be concerned. Then you ask her permission to assess her vital signs and ask her a few questions. She consents. "Tell me about the abdominal pain you had today," you begin. She explains that the pain was pretty bad and worse than the pain she had yesterday. "It is a sharp pain," she says. "It got much worse when I had a bowel movement." She tells you that her stools are black and tarry, she hasn't eaten today, and she was cleaning the kitchen when this last "attack" came on.

After your partner takes the patient's vital signs, he tells you that her pulse is 110 and thready, respirations are 28, and blood pressure is 100/70. You ask the patient if she knows her usual blood pressure, and she tells you 150/90.

Street Scene Questions

4. What other patient history information should be obtained?
5. Should you take another set of vital signs?
6. How might you get the patient to rethink her decision not to be transported?

You ask the patient if she is taking any medication. When she hands you two bottles from the kitchen table, you notice that her skin is pale and clammy. You write down the names of the medications and ask if she has any allergies. She tells you she is allergic to penicillin. You tell the patient that you think she really needs to go to the hospital and be seen by a doctor. You explain that her pulse is high and some of the other information she has provided needs to be evaluated. Your partner takes another set of vital signs and reports that the pulse is now 120 and thready. The other vital signs have not changed. Finally, after a bit more talk, the patient gives consent for transport.

You load the patient onto a stretcher and provide oxygen. The transport to the hospital is less than 10 minutes and uneventful. En route, your partner gives the radio report and you obtain another set of vital signs. After you transfer patient care to the emergency department personnel and are doing your paperwork, you notice a great deal of activity around her. After a while, a woman approaches and tells you that she is Mrs. Alvarez's daughter. "The doctor told me that mama is bleeding internally," she says, "and that she needed immediate medical attention. Thank you."

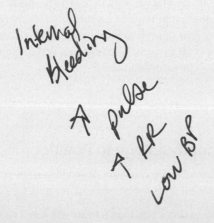

Assessment of the Trauma Patient

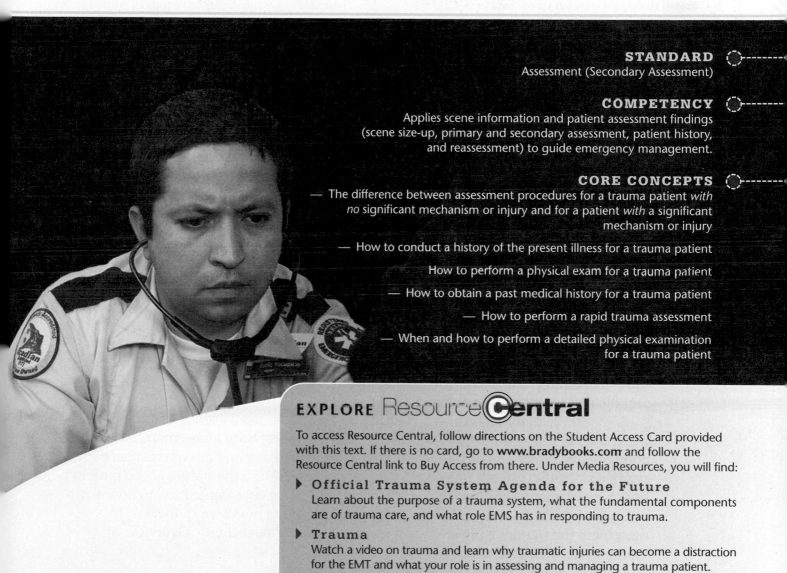

STANDARD ○------
Assessment (Secondary Assessment)

COMPETENCY ○------
Applies scene information and patient assessment findings (scene size-up, primary and secondary assessment, patient history, and reassessment) to guide emergency management.

CORE CONCEPTS ○------
— The difference between assessment procedures for a trauma patient *with no* significant mechanism or injury and for a patient *with* a significant mechanism or injury

— How to conduct a history of the present illness for a trauma patient

How to perform a physical exam for a trauma patient

— How to obtain a past medical history for a trauma patient

— How to perform a rapid trauma assessment

— When and how to perform a detailed physical examination for a trauma patient

EXPLORE Resource**C**entral

To access Resource Central, follow directions on the Student Access Card provided with this text. If there is no card, go to **www.bradybooks.com** and follow the Resource Central link to Buy Access from there. Under Media Resources, you will find:

▶ **Official Trauma System Agenda for the Future**
Learn about the purpose of a trauma system, what the fundamental components are of trauma care, and what role EMS has in responding to trauma.

▶ **Trauma**
Watch a video on trauma and learn why traumatic injuries can become a distraction for the EMT and what your role is in assessing and managing a trauma patient.

▶ **Trauma Scenarios**
Learn why it is important for you to perform an assessment on every trauma patient and what information you should give to a trauma team to help continue the patient's care.

OBJECTIVES

After reading this chapter you should be able to:

13.1 Define key terms introduced in this chapter.

13.2 Differentiate between trauma patients with a significant mechanism or injury and those without a significant mechanism or injury. (pp. 316–317, 320)

13.3 Conduct a systematic secondary assessment of the trauma patient with no significant mechanism or injury. (pp. 317–322)

13.4 Select the appropriate physical examination for a patient with no significant mechanism or injury. (pp. 320–321)

(continued)

13.5 Recognize patients for whom manual stabilization of the cervical spine and application of a cervical collar are indicated. (pp. 332–336)

13.6 Conduct a systematic secondary assessment of an unstable or potentially unstable trauma patient, or patient with a significant mechanism or injury. (pp. 336–340)

13.7 Explain the purpose of the rapid trauma assessment. (p. 332)

13.8 Recognize significant findings in the rapid trauma assessment. (pp. 332–340)

13.9 Recognize situations in which you should consider requesting advanced life support personnel to assist with the management of a trauma patient. (pp. 317, 326, 331–332)

13.10 Incorporate a detailed physical examination of the unstable or potentially unstable trauma patient at the appropriate time for a given scenario. (pp. 342–343)

KEY TERMS

crepitation, *p. 332*
detailed physical exam, *p. 342*
distention, *p. 336*
history of the present illness (HPI), *p. 317*

jugular vein distention (JVD), *p. 334*
paradoxical motion, *p. 335*
past medical history (PMH), *p. 321*

priapism, *p. 337*
rapid trauma assessment, *p. 332*
SAMPLE, *p. 321*

stoma, *p. 335*
tracheostomy, *p. 335*
trauma patient, *p. 316*

For the trauma patient—especially one whose injuries are serious—time must not be wasted at the scene. This patient needs to get to a hospital as quickly as possible. However, you must spend enough time at the scene to adequately assess the patient and give proper emergency care. How can you strike the right balance between care and speed? The key is focus. Instead of performing a time-consuming, comprehensive assessment on every patient, the EMT focuses in on what is important for a particular patient.

Since the primary assessment is what you do first, it makes sense that the next major step is called the secondary assessment. The secondary assessment has several components: history gathering to determine the symptoms and circumstances of the patient's current concern (history of the present illness) and the nature of the patient's health problems in the past (past medical history), physical examination to find signs of injury and illness, and vital signs, including the use of monitoring devices, to determine the patient's physiological condition. (See Visual Guide: Overview of Trauma Assessment.)

>>>>>>

SECONDARY ASSESSMENT OF THE TRAUMA PATIENT

Immediately following the primary assessment for immediate life threats (which was discussed in Chapter 11, "The Primary Assessment"), you will conduct a *secondary assessment*, sometimes called a *secondary survey*. This assessment takes somewhat different paths for trauma and medical patients. In this chapter we will discuss the secondary assessment of the **trauma patient**.

trauma patient
a patient suffering from one or more physical injuries.

Remember that *trauma* means "injury." Injuries can range from slight to severe, from a cut finger to a massive wound. Often you will not be able to see the injury or how serious it

Table 13-1   Secondary Assessment—Trauma Patient

NO SIGNIFICANT MECHANISM OF INJURY	SIGNIFICANT MECHANISM OF INJURY
AFTER SCENE SIZE-UP AND PRIMARY ASSESSMENT:	*AFTER SCENE SIZE-UP AND PRIMARY ASSESSMENT:*
1. Determine the chief complaint and elicit information about how the patient was injured (history of the present illness).	1. Determine the chief complaint and rapidly elicit information about how the patient was injured (history of the present illness).
2. Perform secondary assessment based on the chief complaint and mechanism of injury.	2. Continue manual stabilization of the head and neck.
3. Assess baseline vital signs.	3. Consider requesting advanced life support personnel.
4. Obtain a past medical history.	4. Perform rapid trauma assessment.
	5. Assess baseline vital signs.
	6. Obtain a past medical history.

is, especially if it is internal. Usually, however, you will be able to identify the mechanism of injury (MOI). If the MOI is significant, you will do the secondary assessment differently than if the mechanism of injury is not significant. If you can see that there is an obvious major injury or signs of major injury (or injuries), you will use the same expedited approach. Examples of a major injury include serious bleeding or penetrating injury to the neck, chest, or abdomen. Signs of a major injury include altered mental status or lack of a patent airway. Although it is important to consider mechanism *OF* injury, a better and more accurate way to look at this is to consider mechanism *OR* injury. This is because not just the mechanism of injury must be assessed, but also actual injuries to the patient must be assessed in forming a complete evaluation of the severity or potential severity of the patient's condition.

Since you learned about vital signs in Chapter 12, "Vital Signs and Monitoring Devices," this chapter will focus on how to conduct a secondary assessment for a trauma patient. The procedures for a trauma patient who does not have a significant mechanism or injury are discussed in the following section. The procedures for a patient who does have a significant mechanism or injury will be discussed later in the chapter. Table 13-1 lists and contrasts the procedures for these two categories of trauma patient.

CORE CONCEPT

The difference between assessment procedures for a trauma patient *with no* significant mechanism or injury and for a patient *with* a significant mechanism or injury

Trauma Patient with No Significant Mechanism or Injury

When the patient has no significant mechanism or injury, the steps of the secondary assessment are appropriately simplified. Instead of examining the patient from head to toe, you focus your assessment on just the areas that are clearly injuried or that the patient tells you are painful or that you suspect may be injured because of the mechanism of injury. The assessment will include a history of the present illness, physical exam, a set of baseline vital signs, and a past medical history.

Determine the Chief Complaint

The chief complaint is what the patient tells you is the matter. For example, one patient may tell you he has cut his finger. Another may complain of pain after twisting his ankle.

Conduct a History of the Present Illness

Although the phrase *history of the present illness (HPI)* suggests only problems related to sickness, it is used frequently in health care with the word *illness* meaning both nontrauma medical problems and injuries from trauma. When getting the HPI for a trauma patient, gather information on how the injury occurred in addition to relevant details. For example, if the patient was in a motor-vehicle collision, find out where the patient was in the vehicle, whether the patient was wearing lap and shoulder belts, and the speeds of the vehicles involved. If the patient was on a bicycle or motorcycle, ask whether the patient was wearing a helmet when the incident occurred. If the patient was stabbed or shot, find out the size and type of knife or type of gun and ammunition (only if it is possible to do so safely). A much

CORE CONCEPT

How to conduct a history of the present illness for a trauma patient

history of the present illness (HPI)
information gathered regarding the symptoms and nature of the patient's current concern.

CHAPTER 13
Trauma Assessment
Rapidly Identify and Correct Life Threats

Identify critical patients promptly and provide rapid transport to a trauma center

■ SIZE UP THE SCENE

Provide c-spine stabilization based on mechanism of injury and/or complaint of pain

■ PRIMARY ASSESSMENT

Airway

Breathing

Circulation

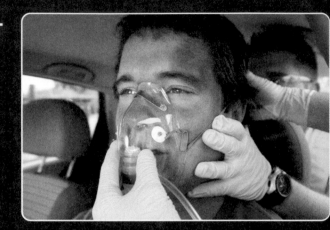

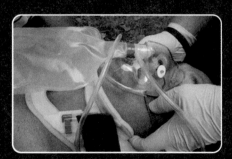

Maintain the airway

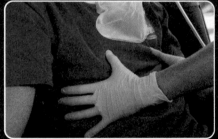

Assess for injuries that could affect breathing. Apply Oxygen or ventilate as needed.

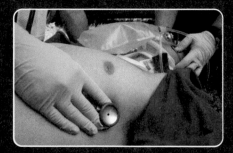

Listen for and compare lung sounds bilaterally

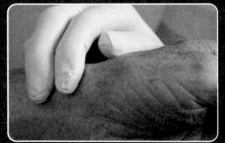

Check for signs of shock

■ PRIORITY DETERMINATION

Does my patient have serious injury requiring prompt transport from the scene

OR

Does the patient have minor and/or isolated non-life-threatening injury

ON SCENE EXAMINATION

Serious or multiple injuries

Rapid head-to-toe exam
Head, neck, chest, abdomen, pelvis, extremities, posterior

Minor or isolated injury

Slower, focused exam

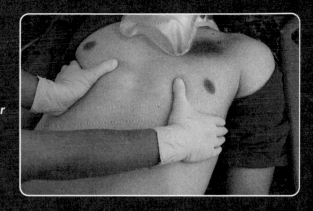

TRANSPORT

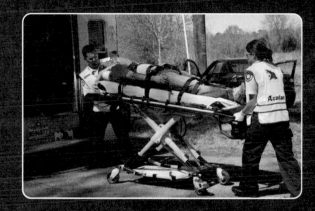

PERFORM DETAILED ASSESSMENT AND REASSESSMENTS ENROUTE

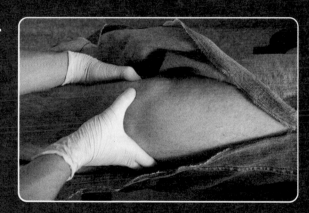

NOTIFY RECEIVING HOSPITAL

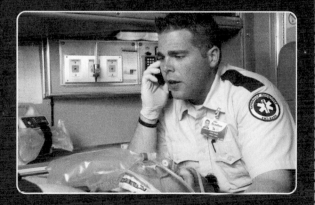

VISUAL GUIDE

more important question in shootings is, "How many shots did you hear?" (This is more important than ammunition and such details, because it tells you whether you need to worry about one hole or lots of potential holes.)

In general, what you should try to find out in the history of the present illness for a trauma patient is:

- The nature of the force involved (blunt, like hitting the steering wheel; penetrating, such as from a knife or a saw; crushing, such as something heavy falling on the patient)
- The direction and strength of the force
- Equipment used to protect the patient
- Actions taken to prevent or minimize injury
- Areas of pain and injuries resulting from the incident

If the patient is unable to provide this information because of an altered mental status, use the procedures described later in this chapter on how to assess a patient with a significant mechanism or injury.

The HPI for a medical patient looks quite different from the HPI for a trauma patient. You will learn more about this in Chapter 14, "Assessment of the Medical Patient."

Perform a Physical Exam

● CORE CONCEPT
How to perform a physical exam
for a trauma patient

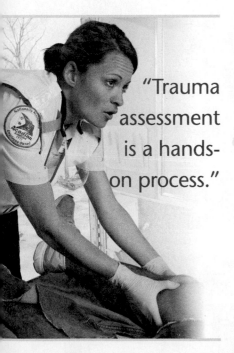

"Trauma assessment is a hands-on process."

Your decision on which areas of a patient's body to assess will depend partly on what you can see (e.g., the cut on the patient's finger) and what the patient tells you (the chief complaint, perhaps "My ankle hurts"). But you will not rely just on these obvious signs and symptoms. You will also pay attention to potential injuries the mechanism of injury causes you to suspect. For example, if the patient with the painful ankle suffered his injury by falling down a flight of steps, you should suspect that he may have more than just an ankle injury—including a potential spine injury that would require stabilization and, later, immobilization of the patient's head and spine.

There are three techniques of physical examination that an EMT must master: inspection, palpation, and auscultation. When you *inspect*, you look for abnormalities in symmetry (e.g., differing chest expansion on one side as compared to the other), color (e.g., pale, flushed, black-and-blue, blisters.), shape (e.g., swelling, deformity, lacerations, punctures, penetrations), and movement (e.g., strength and equality of hand grip strength, ability to raise an arm). When you *palpate*, you press on possibly injured or affected areas to determine abnormalities in shape, temperature (e.g., hot, cool), texture (e.g., smooth, wet, abraded), and sensation (e.g., tenderness, ability to detect touch). Although *auscultation* means listening, in the context of emergency care, it usually refers to listening with a stethoscope. You will listen to a patient's chest for abnormalities such as decreased or absent breath sounds, typically comparing one side of the chest to the other.

There are many signs of trauma an EMT may detect on physical exam. Which irregularities you search for will depend on the circumstances of the patient and the situation. This chapter will introduce you to the basics of inspection, palpation, and auscultation in the physical exam. In later chapters on specific injuries and illnesses, you will learn more about how to evaluate specific areas and what to search for.

One aid some EMTs use when performing a physical exam is the acronym DCAP-BTLS, which stands for deformities, contusions, abrasions, punctures and penetrations, burns, tenderness, lacerations, and swelling. Although this memory aid may be helpful, it does not include all of the abnormalities an EMT may encounter and so must be used with caution, if at all.

Deformities are just what they sound like, parts of the body that no longer have the normal shape. Common examples are broken or fractured bones that push up the skin over the bone ends. *Contusions* is the medical term for bruises. *Abrasions*, or scrapes, are some of the most common injuries you will see. *Punctures and penetrations* are holes in the body, frequently the result of gunshot wounds and stab wounds. When they are small, they are easy to overlook. *Burns* may be reddened, blistered, or charred-looking areas. *Tenderness* means that an area hurts when pressure is applied to it, as when it is palpated. Pain (which is present even without any pressure) and tenderness frequently, but not always, go together. *Lacerations* are cuts, open wounds that sometimes cause significant blood loss. *Swelling* is a very common result of injured capillaries bleeding under the skin.

Wounds, tenderness, and deformities is a classification that is simpler to remember than DCAP-BTLS but that covers a similar range of signs and symptoms you should watch for in the patient with trauma or suspected trauma. Wounds, tenderness, and deformities are the categories that will be summarized later in Table 13-4 and that will referred to throughout the physical examination portions of this chapter.

In order to find these signs and symptoms, you will need to expose the patient. This means removing or cutting away clothing so you can see and palpate the area or areas of the body you are assessing. Compare normal to injured areas to determine if an abnormality exists. Be sure to tell the patient what you are doing and offer reassurance as necessary. Protect the patient's privacy, and take steps to prevent unnecessarily long exposure to cold.

Obtain Baseline Vital Signs and a Past Medical History

For a trauma patient, first conduct a history of the present illness and a physical exam to assess his injuries. Next, assess his baseline vital signs and take a past medical history.

An EMT can gain two kinds of information about the patient's problem: signs and symptoms. A sign is objective—something you see, hear, feel, and smell when examining the patient. The vital signs are, of course, signs, as are sweaty skin, staggering, and vomiting, for example. A symptom is subjective—an indication you cannot observe but that the patient feels and tells you about. Such things as chest pain, dizziness, and nausea are considered symptoms.

An important part of the information you should gain on all of your patients is information about the ***past medical history (PMH)*** (Figure 13-1). The past medical history is often referred to in EMS as the ***SAMPLE*** history because the letters in SAMPLE stand for elements of the history: signs and symptoms, allergies, medications, pertinent past history, last

past medical history (PMH)
information gathered regarding the patient's health problems in the past.

SAMPLE
a memory aid in which the letters stand for elements of the past medical history: signs and symptoms, allergies, medications, pertinent past history, last oral intake, and events leading to the injury or illness.

FIGURE 13-1 Taking the past medical history.
(© Mark C. Ide)

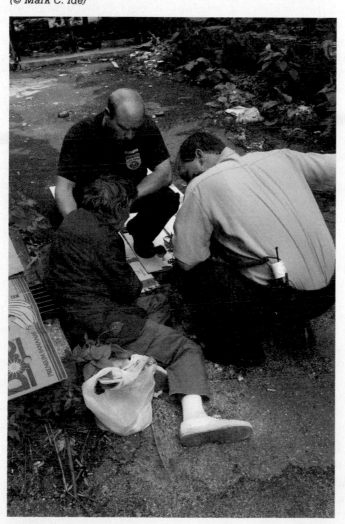

oral intake, and events leading to the injury or illness. To obtain the past medical history, ask your patient (or, if the patient is unconscious, ask the family and bystanders) these questions:

- **Signs and symptoms.** What's wrong? This is a reminder to get the history of the present illness.

- **Allergies.** Are you allergic to medications, foods, or do you have environmental allergies? Is there a medical identification tag describing your allergies?

- **Medications.** What medications are you currently taking or are you supposed to be taking (prescription, over-the-counter, or recreational)? Are you on birth control pills? Is there a medical identification tag with the names of medications on it? Do you take any herbal supplements or medications?

- **Pertinent past history.** Have you been having any medical problems? Have you been feeling ill? Have you recently had any surgery or injuries? Have you been seeing a doctor? What is your doctor's name?

- **Last oral intake.** When did you last eat or drink? What did you eat or drink? (Food or liquids can cause symptoms or aggravate a medical condition. Also, if a patient will need to go to surgery, the hospital staff must know when he last had anything to eat or drink, since stomach contents can be vomited while a patient is under anesthesia, which is a very dangerous occurrence.)

- **Events leading to the injury or illness.** What sequence of events led up to today's problem (e.g., the patient passed out, then got into a car crash versus got into a car crash and then passed out)?

Applying a Cervical Collar

Apply a cervical collar to any patient who may have an injury to the spine based on mechanism of injury, history, or signs and symptoms. (Remember that signs are what you observe; symptoms are what the patient tells you he feels.)

When is it appropriate to apply a cervical collar? There is a simple principle you can follow: If the mechanism of injury exerts significant force on the upper body or if there is any soft-tissue damage to the head, face, or neck from trauma (such as a cut or bruise from being thrown against a dashboard), you may then assume that there is a possible cervical-spine injury. Any blow above the clavicles (collarbones) may damage the cervical spine, as may a fall from a height, even if the patient landed on his feet. Some patients cannot communicate because of a depressed level of responsiveness, intoxication with alcohol or other drugs, or an inability to speak your language. Similarly, a painful injury in an area other than the neck may limit the patient's ability to sense neck pain and communicate that to you. In cases like these, if injury cannot be ruled out—even if the mechanism of injury is not known—suspect cervical-spine injury. When any of these conditions exists, apply a cervical collar. It should also be noted that patients with penetrating trauma such as gunshot wounds do not require placement of a cervical collar unless there are signs or symptoms of neurological injury or if the patient is unconscious and cannot be fully assessed for these findings.

Several types of cervical-spine immobilization devices are on the market. It is important that you select one that is rigid (stiff, not easily movable) and that is the right size. The traditional soft collar that you occasionally see someone wearing on the street has no role in immobilizing a prehospital patient's cervical spine.

The wrong size immobilization device may actually harm the patient by making breathing more difficult or obstructing the airway. Whatever device is used must not obstruct the airway. If the proper size collar is not available, it is better to place a rolled towel around the neck (to remind the patient not to move his head) and tape the patient's head to the backboard.

The techniques for selecting the right size cervical collar and for applying a cervical collar are presented in Scan 13-1. As you study the scan and practice applying a cervical collar, consider the following:

- Make certain that you have completed the primary assessment and that you have cared for all life-threatening problems before you apply the collar.

- Use the mechanism of injury, level of responsiveness, and location of injuries to determine the need for cervical immobilization. Apply a rigid cervical collar whenever any of these factors leads you to believe that spine injury is a possibility.

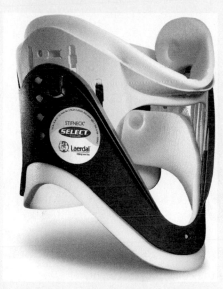

STIFNECK®SELECT™ *(© Laerdal Medical Corporation)*

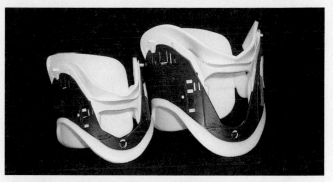

Philadelphia Cervical Collar™ Patriot Adult and Pediatric. *(© Philadelphia Collar Corporation)*

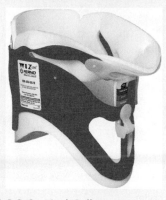

WIZLOC Cervical Collar. *(© Ferno Corporation)*

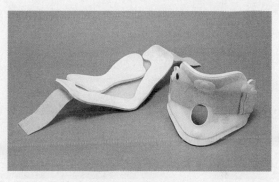

NEC-LOC™ rigid extrication collar, opened. Rigid cervical collars are applied to protect the cervical spine. DO NOT apply a soft collar.

SIZING A CERVICAL COLLAR

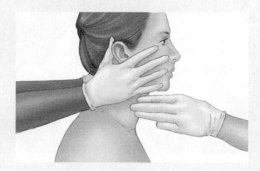

❶ Measure the patient's neck.

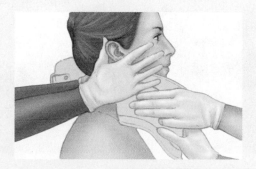

❷ Measure the collar. The chin piece should not lift the patient's chin and hyperextend the neck. Make sure the collar is not too small or tight, which would make the collar act as a constricting band.

(continued)

APPLYING AN ADJUSTABLE COLLAR TO A SEATED PATIENT

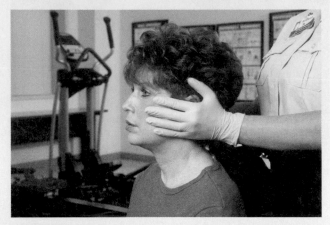

1 Stabilize the head and neck from the rear.

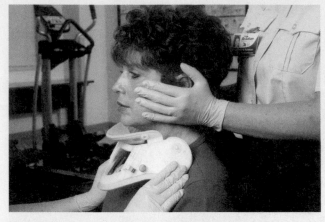

2 Properly angle the collar for placement.

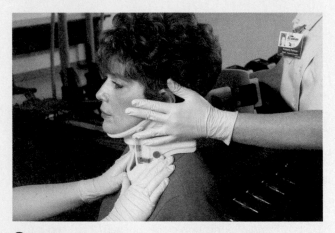

3 Position the collar.

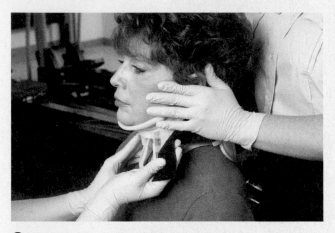

4 Begin to secure the collar.

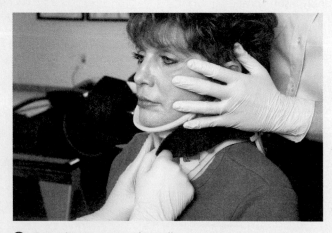

5 Complete securing the collar.

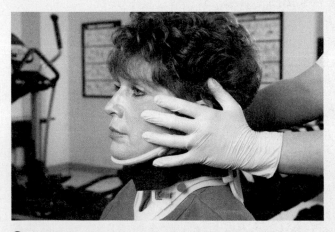

6 Maintain manual stabilization of the head and neck.

APPLYING AN ADJUSTABLE COLLAR TO A SUPINE PATIENT

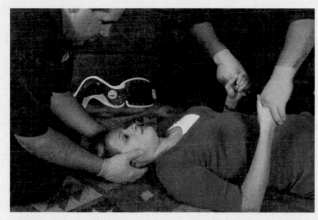

1 Kneel at the patient's head and stabilize the head and neck.

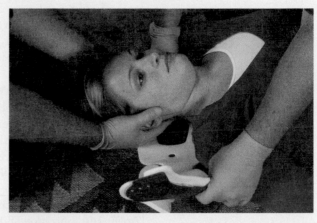

2 Set the collar in place.

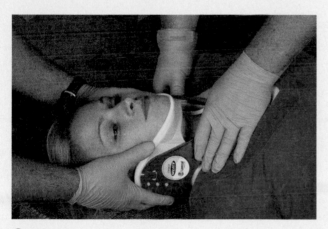

3 Secure the collar.

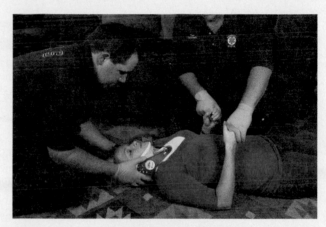

4 Continue to manually stabilize the head and neck.

- Assess the patient's neck prior to placing the collar. Once the collar is in place, you will not be able to inspect or palpate the back of the neck.

- Reassure the patient. Having a cervical collar applied around your neck can be a constricting and frightening experience. Explain the procedure to the patient.

- Make sure the collar is the right size for the patient. The proper size rigid collar depends more on the length of the patient's neck than on the width. A large patient may not be able to wear a large collar. A small patient with a long neck may need your largest collar. The front height of the collar should fit between the point of the chin and the chest at the suprasternal (jugular) notch—the U-shaped dip where the clavicle and sternum meet. Once in place, the collar should rest on the clavicles and support the lower jaw. It should not stretch the neck (too high), it should not support the chin (too short), and it should not constrict the neck (too tight).

- Remove the patient's necklaces and large earrings before applying the collar.

- Keep the patient's hair out of the way

- Keep the patient's head in the in-line anatomical position (a neutral position with head facing front, not tilted forward or back or turned to either side) when applying manual stabilization and the collar.

Cervical collars alone do not provide adequate in-line immobilization. In fact, applying the collar is not the first step. Whenever there is the possibility of a spine injury, you must manually stabilize the patient's head and neck immediately upon first patient contact, before applying the collar (as you learned in Chapter 11, "The Primary Assessment"). Continue to manually stabilize the head and neck, both before and after applying the cervical collar, until the patient is completely immobilized and secured to a backboard. (You learned about immobilization on a backboard in Chapter 3, "Lifting and Moving Patients," and will learn more in Chapter 31, "Trauma to the Head, Neck, and Spine," and in Chapter 40, "Highway Safety and Vehicle Extrication.")

Trauma Patient with a Significant Mechanism or Injury

When you have a patient you have determined is unstable or potentially unstable because of problems found in the primary assessment or because of a significant mechanism or injury, you will do all of the following: continue manual stabilization of the head and neck, consider requesting advanced life support (ALS) personnel, and perform a rapid trauma assessment. (Review Table 13-1 and see Scan 13-2.)

Note that there are several additional steps for the patient with a significant mechanism or injury compared to the steps for the patient with no significant mechanism or injury (manual stabilization and ALS request consideration). Also note that instead of a physical exam focused just on the area of injury, the patient with a significant mechanism or injury receives a complete, head-to-toe rapid trauma assessment.

PEDIATRIC NOTE

Infants and children are more fragile than adults. This means that a child may sustain the same injury as an adult, but from less force. For this reason, there are additional mechanisms of injury that the EMT needs to consider significant when children and infants are concerned. (Review Table 13-2.)

Some patients who undergo experiences like those listed in Table 13-2 will escape without serious injury, but many more will not be so lucky. For this reason, you should provide rapid assessment and treatment to any patient with a mechanism of injury listed in Table 13-2.

Although the mechanism of injury can provide a lot of information about the kinds of injuries a patient may have, there is still the possibility that patients will have "hidden injuries." These injuries are considered to be hidden because patients may have no signs or symptoms initially but nevertheless have serious conditions that may become apparent only later.

Table 13-2   Field Triage: Significant Mechanisms of Injury

GUIDELINES FOR FIELD TRIAGE OF INJURED PATIENTS
Transport to a trauma center if any of the following are identified:

- Falls
  - Adults: fall >20 feet (one story = 10 feet)
  - Children aged <15 years: fall >10 feet or two to three times child's height
- High-risk auto crash
  - Intrusion: >12 inches to the occupant site or >18 inches to any site
  - Ejection (partial or complete) from automobile
  - Death in same passenger compartment
  - Vehicle telemetry data consistent with high risk of injury
- Auto versus pedestrian/bicyclist thrown, run over, or with significant (>20 mph) impact;

or

- Motorcycle crash >20 mph.

Source: Centers for Disease Control and Prevention, Guidelines for Field Triage of Injured Patients, Recommendations of the National Expert Panel on Field Triage, Morbidity and Mortality Weekly Report (MMWR), January 23, 2009, Vol. 58, No. RR-1.

Reassess the mechanism of injury and actual injury. If the mechanism or injury is not significant (e.g., patient has a cut finger), focus the physical exam only on the injured part. If the mechanism or injury is significant:

- Continue manual stabilization of the head and neck.
- Consider requesting ALS personnel.
- Reconsider transport decision.

- Reassess mental status.
- Perform a rapid trauma assessment.

HISTORY OF THE PRESENT ILLNESS
Rapidly determine what happened to the patient to cause injury.

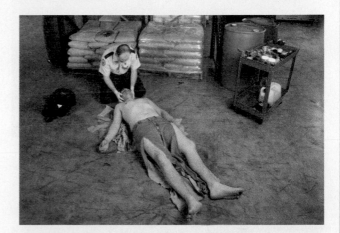

RAPID TRAUMA ASSESSMENT
Rapidly assess each part of the body.

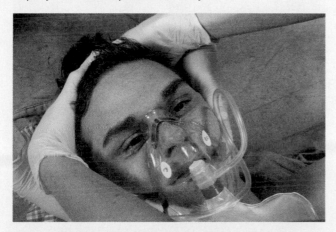

HEAD: Check for WOUNDS, TENDERNESS, AND DEFORMITIES plus crepitation.

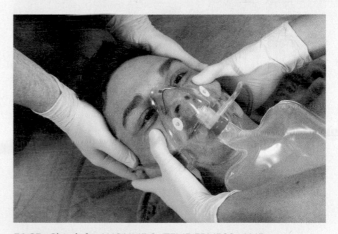

FACE: Check for WOUNDS, TENDERNESS, AND DEFORMITIES.

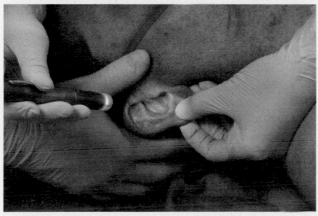

EARS: Check for WOUNDS, TENDERNESS, AND DEFORMITIES plus drainage of blood or clear fluid.

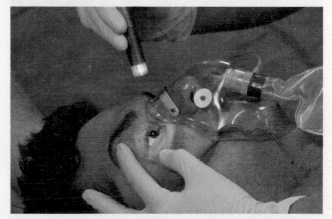

EYES: Check for WOUNDS, TENDERNESS, AND DEFORMITIES plus discoloration, unequal pupils, foreign bodies, and blood in the anterior chamber.

(continued)

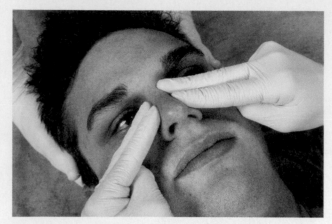

NOSE: Check for WOUNDS, TENDERNESS, AND DEFORMITIES plus drainage of blood or clear fluid.

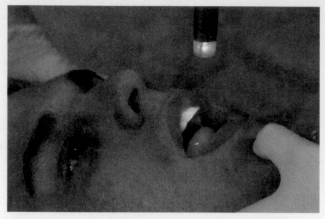

MOUTH: Check for WOUNDS, TENDERNESS, AND DEFORMITIES plus loose or broken teeth, objects that could cause obstruction, swelling or laceration of the tongue, unusual breath odor, or discoloration.

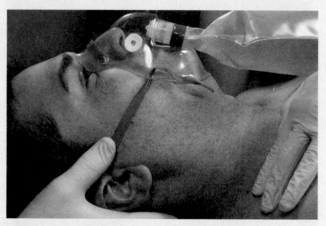

NECK: Check for WOUNDS, TENDERNESS, AND DEFORMITIES plus jugular vein distention and crepitation.

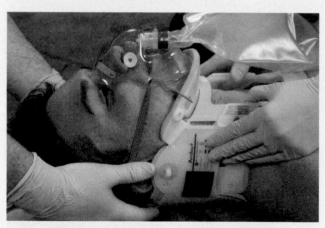

APPLICATION OF COLLAR: Once the neck has been examined, apply the cervical collar.

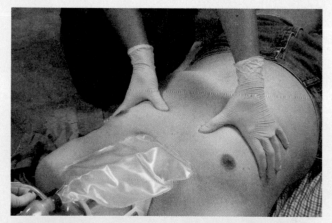

CHEST: Inspect and palpate for WOUNDS, TENDERNESS, AND DEFORMITIES plus crepitation and paradoxical motion.

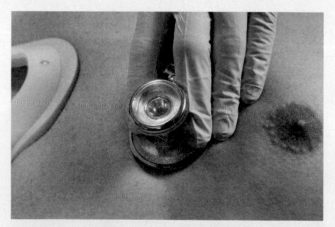

CHEST: Auscultate for BREATH SOUNDS (presence, absence, and equality).

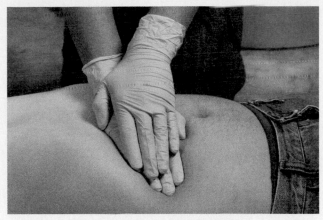

ABDOMEN: Check for WOUNDS, TENDERNESS, AND DEFORMITIES plus firm, soft, and distended areas.

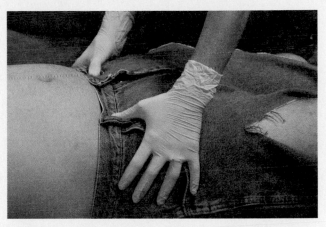

PELVIS: Check for WOUNDS, TENDERNESS, AND DEFORMITIES using gentle compression for tenderness or motion.

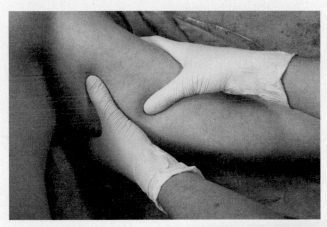

UPPER EXTREMITIES: Check for WOUNDS, TENDERNESS, AND DEFORMITIES.

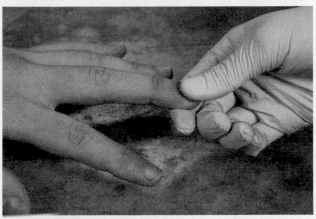

UPPER EXTREMITIES: Check for CIRCULATION, SENSATION, AND MOTOR FUNCTION.

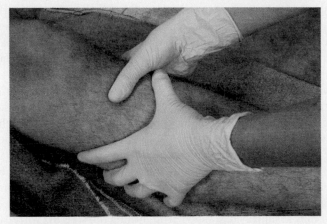

LOWER EXTREMITIES: Check for WOUNDS, TENDERNESS, AND DEFORMITIES.

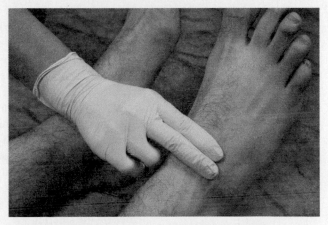

LOWER EXTREMITIES: Check for CIRCULATION, SENSATION, AND MOTOR FUNCTION.

(continued)

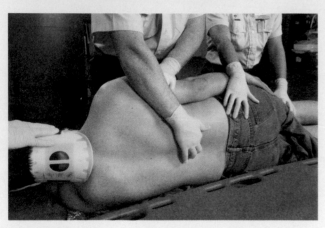

POSTERIOR: Check for WOUNDS, TENDERNESS, AND DEFORMITIES. (To examine posterior, roll patient using spinal precautions.)

VITAL SIGNS

Assess the patient's baseline vital signs:

- Respiration
- Pulse
- Skin color, temperature, condition (capillary refill in infants and children)
- Pupils
- Blood pressure
- Oxygen saturation (if directed by local protocol)

PAST MEDICAL HISTORY

Interview patient or (if patient is unresponsive) family and bystanders to get as much information as possible about the patient's problem. Ask about:

Signs and symptoms
Allergies
Medications
Pertinent past history
Last oral intake
Events leading to problem

INTERVENTIONS AND TRANSPORT

Contact on-line medical direction and perform interventions as needed.
Package and transport the patient.

Seat belt injuries are a good example. There is no doubt that, when properly used, seat belts save lives by preventing drivers and passengers from hitting hard objects inside a vehicle and by preventing them from being ejected. But seat belts can also cause injuries. When patients are in high-velocity collisions, the force of being thrown forward against buckled seat belts will occasionally cause injury to the bowel and other abdominal organs. Similarly, patients with seat belt marks on the upper chest and side of the neck may sustain trauma to the major arteries in the neck that supply the brain. These injuries may not become apparent for several hours or even days. It is important to realize that even people who were wearing seat belts may have sustained serious injuries.

Air bags may also save lives; however, they do not provide total protection from injury (Figure 13-2). Air bags prevent occupants from going through the windshield and hitting hard objects inside the vehicle. However, they only protect occupants once, even if the vehicle sustains collisions with several other vehicles or objects. They are most effective when used in combination with seat belts. In a few instances, especially with a small driver or passenger (particularly a child), or when the front seat is pulled far forward, or when a seat belt is not in place to keep the person from being thrown forward, the expanding air bag may cause injury. Also, the driver may sustain an arm injury because of improper positioning of hands on the steering wheel or may sustain a chest injury from hitting the steering wheel after the bag deflates. When inspecting a vehicle in which an air bag has deployed, you should look at the steering wheel. Whenever you see a bent or broken steering wheel, you should treat the patient like every other patient who has a significant mechanism of injury. A good way to find this kind of damage is to remember to "lift and look" under the air bag after the patient has been removed from the vehicle.

Using mechanism of injury as a tool for determining your assessment has significant limitations. Study in this area is still needed to indicate more clearly which patients will benefit from expedited assessment, treatment, and transport. Determining whether a patient has a

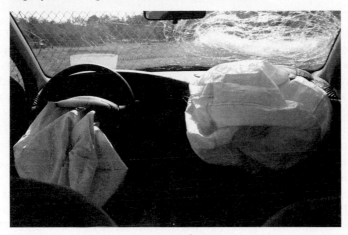

FIGURE 13-2 An air bag can prevent injuries. However, once deployed, it can also conceal important information about the patient's mechanism of injury. When you see a deployed air bag, remember to "lift and look."

significant MOI when he has an obviously critical injury will not make a difference in your decision making. Although you will note the MOI for potential use by hospital staff, you will do a rapid trauma assessment for the patient with a significant injury whether or not he has a significant MOI. Table 13-3 lists some examples of significant injuries and signs of significant injuries.

Continue Spinal Stabilization

During the primary assessment, make sure that someone is manually stabilizing the patient's head to prevent any cervical-spine injury from becoming a paralyzing spinal-cord injury. Manual stabilization must continue throughout the assessment until the patient is fully immobilized on a backboard.

Consider a Request for Advanced Life Support Personnel

Some areas of the country, particularly urban and suburban areas, have advanced life support (ALS) personnel—paramedics who respond with EMTs when they are transporting patients who might benefit from the additional interventions paramedics can provide. If this is the case where you practice as an EMT, you should familiarize yourself with your local protocols. Rural EMTs do not always have this option, but they may have other means by which to improve the patient's care before arrival at a hospital.

In some areas that are very distant from hospitals, local clinics arrange to provide advanced care to certain kinds of patients. For example, if an ambulance is an hour away from the closest hospital, but a local clinic is only 10 minutes away, the ambulance may be able to stop there with a patient in cardiac arrest. There are limits, though, on what can be done at health care centers like these. Many of them would not be able to provide additional care that is worth a delay in transport for awake trauma patients.

Table 13-3   Significant Injuries and Signs of Significant Injuries
Unresponsive or altered mental status
Penetrating wound of the head, neck, chest, or abdomen (e.g., stab and gunshot wounds)
Airway that is not patent
Respiratory compromise
Pallor, tachycardia, and other signs of shock

If arrangements like these exist where you work as an EMT, you must be familiar with the types of patients your clinic can help. The arrangements should be in writing in order to reduce confusion and prevent loss of precious time with critical patients. In any case, the patient with serious trauma must ultimately, if at all possible, be transported to a trauma center.

Perform a Rapid Trauma Assessment

● **CORE CONCEPT**

How to perform a rapid trauma assessment

rapid trauma assessment
a rapid assessment of the head, neck, chest, abdomen, pelvis, extremities, and posterior of the body to detect signs and symptoms of injury.

A patient with a significant mechanism or injury needs a quickly performed physical exam, known as the ***rapid trauma assessment***. This requires only a few moments and should be performed at the scene, before loading the patient into the ambulance, even if the patient is a high priority for transport. The care that you provide en route will be based on the results of this rapid assessment, and you will obtain valuable information to relay to the hospital staff so that they can be prepared for your patient.

During the rapid trauma assessment, you will be able to detect injuries that may later threaten life or limb. You may also find life-threatening injuries that you did not find during the primary assessment. When dealing with a responsive patient, you should ask the patient before and during the trauma assessment about any symptoms.

To perform the rapid trauma assessment, you will use your sense of sight to inspect and your sense of touch to palpate different areas of the body. You may also use your sense of hearing to detect abnormal sounds, not just from the airway but also from other areas, such as the sound of broken bones rubbing against each other. You may use your sense of smell, as well, to detect odors like gasoline, urine, feces, or vomitus. You will evaluate the patient from head to toe, in the sequence described next.

The signs and symptoms you will assess each area for are summarized in Table 13-4. Remember, however, that this is a quick evaluation, so you will not spend a lot of time on any one area.

crepitation (krep-uh-TAY-shun)
the grating sound or feeling of broken bones rubbing together.

Rapid Assessment of the Head   Gently palpate the cranium for wounds, tenderness, and deformities, as well as the sound or feel of broken bones rubbing against each other, known as ***crepitation***. Run your gloved fingers through the patient's hair and palpate gently. A good way to check the back of the head in a supine patient is to start with your fingers at the top of the neck and carefully slide them upward toward the top of the patient's head. If there is blood on your gloves, there is an open wound. However, if you do not see any blood on the floor or ground, then you do not need to apply a dressing to the wound right away.

Inspect and palpate the face for wounds, tenderness, and deformities by looking and then gently palpating the cheekbones, forehead, and lower jaw. The bones in the face are fragile and may break when subjected to significant forces.

Inspect and palpate the ears, searching for wounds, tenderness, and deformities, as well as drainage of blood or other fluid. If these are found, they are important pieces of information to pass on to the emergency department staff because they may be indications of injury to the skull (Figure 13-3). Also gently bend each ear forward to look for any bruising. A bruise behind the patient's ear is called Battle's sign and is another important sign of skull injury to tell hospital staff about.

Table 13-4   Physical Exam/Trauma Assessment

BODY PART	WOUNDS, TENDERNESS, AND DEFORMITIES	PLUS
Head	Wounds, tenderness, and deformities	Crepitation
Neck	Wounds, tenderness, and deformities	Jugular vein distention, crepitation
Chest	Wounds, tenderness, and deformities	Paradoxical motion, crepitation, breath sounds (present, absent, equal)
Abdomen	Wounds, tenderness, and deformities	Firmness, softness, distention
Pelvis	Wounds, tenderness, and deformities	Pain, tenderness, motion
Extremities	Wounds, tenderness, and deformities	Distal circulation, sensation, motor function
Posterior	Wounds, tenderness, and deformities	

FIGURE 13-3 Cerebrospinal fluid draining from the ear of a trauma patient. *(© Edward T. Dickinson, MD)*

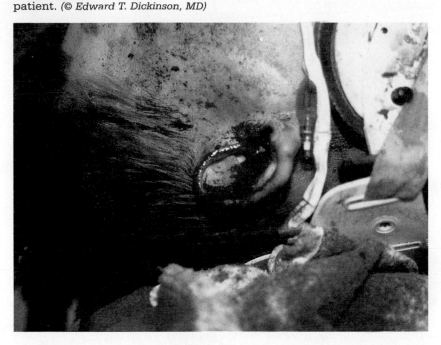

Next assess the eyes, inspecting for the usual wounds, tenderness, and deformities, as well as discoloration, unequal pupils, foreign bodies, and blood in the anterior chamber (front) of the eye. Blood in the anterior chamber is not common; however, when present, it is a sign that the eye sustained significant force and is bleeding inside (Figure 13-4).

Inspect and palpate the nose for injuries or signs of injury. Look not only for wounds, tenderness, and deformities but also for drainage and bleeding.

When assessing the ears and nose, you may find blood or clear fluid draining from them. Blood may be from a laceration of that area or it may be coming from inside the skull. Clear fluid may be just from a runny nose or it may be cerebrospinal fluid (CSF). You should prevent an ear or nose that is draining blood or clear fluid from getting any dirtier than it is at that point. CSF surrounds the brain and spinal cord, and if it is leaking out then bacteria can get into the brain. Similarly, a wound from inside the skull that is leaking blood can also provide a route for bacteria to get in. Figure 13-5A summarizes signs of brain injury. Figure 13-5B is a photo of a patient with Battle's sign and Figure 13-5C is a CT scan of that same Battle's sign patient.

FIGURE 13-4 Blood in the anterior chamber of the eye is a sign that the eye has sustained considerable force. *(Photo: © Edward T. Dickinson, MD)*

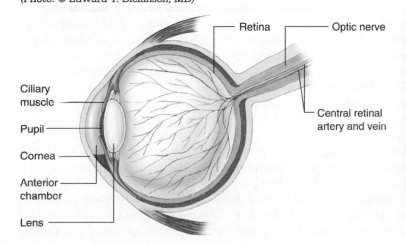

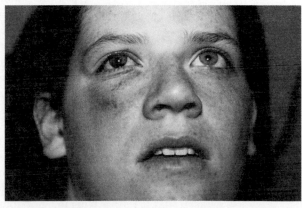

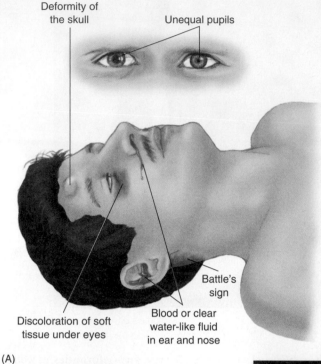

Deformity of the skull

Unequal pupils

Battle's sign

Blood or clear water-like fluid in ear and nose

Discoloration of soft tissue under eyes

(A)

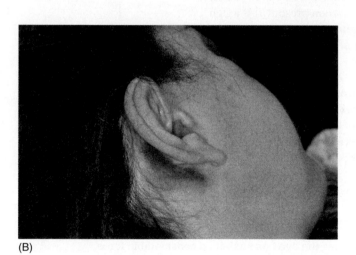

(B)

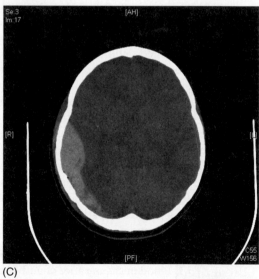

(C)

Open the patient's mouth and look for wounds, tenderness, and deformities; loose or broken teeth; other objects that could cause obstruction; swelling or laceration of the tongue; unusual breath odor; and discoloration. A foreign body like a broken tooth is a potential source of airway obstruction and must be removed as soon as possible from the patient's mouth. The most common unusual breath odor is from alcoholic beverages. Other conditions besides alcohol, though, can cause similar odors.

Rapid Assessment of the Neck   Assess the neck for wounds, tenderness, deformities, and *jugular vein distention (JVD)* (Figure 13-6). Jugular vein distention is present when you can see the patient's neck veins bulging. The neck veins are usually not visible when the patient is sitting up. If they are bulging when the patient is upright, it means that blood is backing up in the veins because the heart is not pumping effectively. This could be the result of a tension pneumothorax (air trapped in the chest) or cardiac tamponade (blood filling the sac around the heart). However, it is normal to see bulging of the neck veins when the patient is lying in a horizontal position or with his head down. Flat neck veins in a patient who is lying down may be a sign of blood loss, showing that there is not enough blood to fill them.

jugular (JUG-yuh-ler) *vein distention (JVD)*
bulging of the neck veins.

FIGURE 13-6 Jugular vein distention. *(© Edward T. Dickinson, MD)*

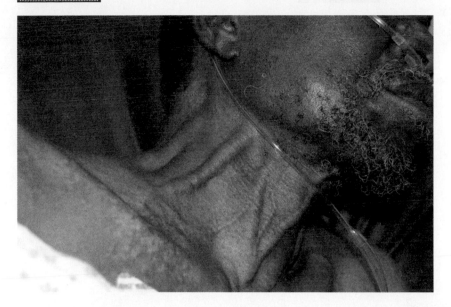

When you see *flat* neck veins in a *flat* patient, think "blood loss." To summarize, *either* neck veins that are bulging when the patient is sitting up *or* neck veins that are flat when the patient is flat are abnormal and should be noted during the exam.

Another thing you might find when assessing the patient's anterior neck is a surgical opening. A *stoma* is a permanent surgical opening in the neck through which the patient breathes. A *tracheostomy* is a surgical incision held open by a metal or plastic tube. If the patient requires artificial ventilation, you may need to provide it through the stoma, as described in Chapter 9, "Respiration and Artificial Ventilation."

You may also find a medical identification medallion on a necklace when assessing the neck. Note the information on the necklace if you find one.

Application of a Cervical Collar After you assess the patient's head and neck, size and apply a rigid cervical spine immobilization collar. Use the principles and methods that were described earlier in this chapter and in Scan 13-1.

Rapid Assessment of the Chest Next, assess the chest for wounds, tenderness, deformities, crepitation, breath sounds, and paradoxical motion. ***Paradoxical motion***, or movement of part of the chest in the opposite direction from the rest of the chest, is a sign of a serious injury. It usually occurs when several ribs have broken at two ends and are "floating" free of the rest of the rib cage. (This condition is sometimes known as "flail chest.") The opposite motion of the broken section is obvious during respiration, moving inward when the lungs expand with air and outward when the lungs empty (Figure 13-7). Paradoxical motion also indicates that a great deal of force was applied to the patient's chest; in other words, there was a significant mechanism of injury.

You can check for crepitation and paradoxical motion of the chest at the same time. Start by palpating the patient's clavicles (collarbones). Next, gently feel the sternum (breastbone). Position your hands on the sides of the chest and feel for equal expansion of both sides of the chest. During this process you may feel broken bones or floating paradoxical segments.

Palpate the entire rib cage for deformities. Use your hands to apply gentle pressure to the sides of the rib cage. If there is an injured rib and the patient is able to respond, he will tell you that it hurts. Occasionally, you may detect a crackling or crunching sensation under the skin from air that has escaped from its normal passageways. This is called subcutaneous emphysema.

Listen for breath sounds (Scan 13-3) just under the clavicles in the mid-clavicular line and at the bases of the lungs in the mid-axillary line. Notice whether the breath sounds are present and equal. A patient who has breath sounds that are absent or very hard to hear on one side may have a collapsed lung or other serious respiratory injury. There are many other characteristics of breath sounds, but in the trauma patient, presence and equality are the two things to look for at this time.

stoma (STO-ma)
a permanent surgical opening in the neck through which the patient breathes.

tracheostomy (TRAY-ke-OS-to-me)
a surgical incision held open by a metal or plastic tube.

paradoxical (pair-uh-DOCK-si-kal) ***motion***
movement of a part of the chest in the opposite direction to the rest of the chest during respiration.

FIGURE 13-7 Paradoxical motion.

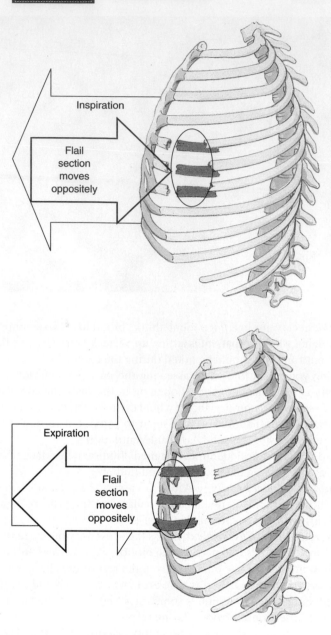

Inspiration

Flail
section
moves
oppositely

Expiration

Flail
section
moves
oppositely

It is important to remember that when you reach the point of examining the patient's chest in the rapid trauma assessment, you need to expose the chest if you have not already done so. However, keep the weather and the patient's privacy in mind when doing this.

Rapid Assessment of the Abdomen When you assess the abdomen for wounds, tenderness, and deformities, also check for firmness, softness, and distention. The term ***distention*** is another way of saying the abdomen appears larger than normal. One of its causes can be internal bleeding. Whether the abdomen is abnormally distended or not may be a very difficult judgment to make, so do not spend a lot of time on it. You may also see a colostomy or ileostomy when you inspect the abdomen. This is a surgical opening in the abdominal wall with a bag in place to collect excretions from the digestive system. If you see such a bag, leave it in place and be careful not to cut it if you cut clothing away.

Palpate the abdomen by gently pressing down once on each abdominal quadrant. (Picture the abdomen divided into four segments—upper left, upper right, lower left, lower right—and press on each quadrant in turn.) If the patient tells you he has pain in a specific area of the abdomen, palpate that site last. When practical, make sure your hands are warm. Press in on the abdomen with the palm side of your fingers, depressing the surface about

distention (dis-TEN-shun)
a condition of being stretched, inflated, or larger than normal.

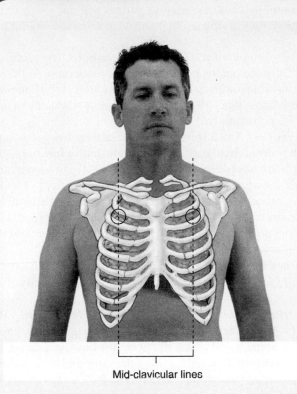

Mid-clavicular lines

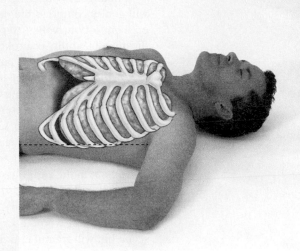

Mid-axillary line

Listen at the mid-clavicular line.

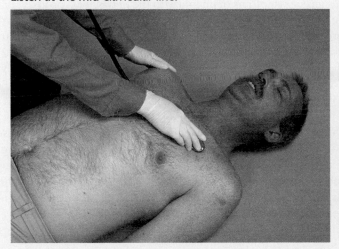

Listen at the mid-axillary line.

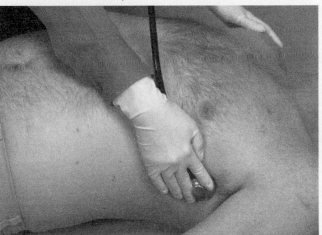

Listen at the mid-clavicular and the mid-axillary lines on both sides of the chest. Is air entry present? Absent? Equal on both sides?

1 inch. Many EMTs prefer to use two hands, one on top of the other at the fingertips. Normally the abdomen is soft. Firmness of the abdomen can be a sign of injury to the organs in the abdomen and internal bleeding.

Another finding you may occasionally come across when palpating a patient's abdomen is a pulsating mass. This may be an enlarged aorta. If you do feel such pulsations, do not press any farther into the abdomen. Doing so could cause further injury to a weakened blood vessel.

Rapid Assessment of the Pelvis Next, assess the pelvis for wounds, tenderness, and deformities. You may observe bleeding or ***priapism***, a persistent erection of the penis that can result from spinal cord injury or certain medical problems. If the patient is awake, palpate

priapism (PRY-ah-pizm) persistent erection of the penis that may result from spinal injury and some medical problems.

the pelvis gently, stopping as soon as the patient identifies pain in the pelvis. Consider the complaint of pain as reason enough to treat the patient for an injury to the pelvis. Continuing to palpate or compress the painful pelvis of a conscious patient will not give you any more useful information, but it can produce excruciating pain and, if done too strenuously, may injure the patient.

An unconscious patient, however, cannot tell you if his pelvic area hurts. Therefore, you will gently compress the pelvis of the unconscious patient to detect tenderness (if there is enough responsiveness to pain to cause him to flinch or groan) and motion of the bones (indicating instability or broken bones). These signs will help you determine whether you need to treat the unconscious patient for a pelvic injury.

Rapid Assessment of the Extremities Quickly assess all four extremities for wounds, tenderness, and deformities, as well as distal circulation, sensation, and motor function—that is, whether a pulse is present, the patient has feeling in his hands and feet, and he can move his hands and feet (Scan 13-4). In a conscious patient, you will touch the patient's hand or foot and ask whether he can feel your touch. If you are not sure whether the patient is telling you the truth, you can ask where on the hand or foot you are touching him. You can also test movement in the extremities of a conscious patient by asking him to squeeze your fingers in his hands and to move his feet against your hands.

If you find a deformity, diminished function, or other indication of injury to an extremity in a patient who is a high priority for transport, you will not splint the extremity at the scene but will treat it en route.

Rapid Assessment of the Posterior Body and Immobilization on a Backboard Roll the patient onto his side as a unit (you will learn how to do a log-roll maneuver in Chapter 31, "Trauma to the Head, Neck, and Spine") and assess the posterior body, inspecting and palpating for wounds, tenderness, and deformities in the area of the spine and to the sides of the spine, the buttocks, and the posterior extremities. Meanwhile, have someone slide a backboard next to the patient so that, when you roll the patient back into a supine position, he is on the backboard.

If the patient has shown signs or symptoms of an injury to the pelvis, local protocol may direct you to place a pneumatic anti-shock garment (PASG) on the board before you roll the patient onto it. Local protocol may direct you to place the anti-shock garment on the backboard for other kinds of trauma, too. (You will learn about the PASG in Chapter 27, "Bleeding and Shock.") A newer method of stabilizing an injured pelvis is forming a pelvic wrap from a folded sheet. (You will learn about how to apply a pelvic wrap in Chapter 30, "Musculoskeletal Trauma.") Become familiar with how local medical direction wishes you to manage these patients.

Obtain Baseline Vital Signs and Past Medical History Quickly obtain a set of baseline vital signs, as discussed in Chapter 12, "Vital Signs and Monitoring Devices." If using a pulse oximeter is part of your assessment, apply it now (or earlier, if your local protocol suggests doing so). If the patient is unresponsive, you will not be able to get a past medical history from him. If there is a friend or family member nearby, that person may be able to give you information about the patient's medical history.

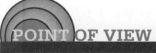

POINT OF VIEW

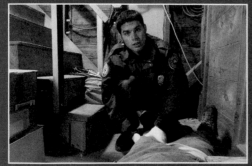

"I was putting some boxes up in the loft in our barn. I must've missed a step. I fell down the first few stairs and felt a 'crack' in my leg. I heard it, but man, I really felt it snap. If that wasn't proof enough, it hurt more than anything I ever felt before. It was broken!

"The EMTs came. They were great, but I gotta tell you, even when they said they'd be careful, they made horrible pain even worse. When the one EMT examined my leg, I thought I was going to jump out of my skin. Any little movement was just so painful.

"They put a splint on and took me to the hospital. I won't even tell you how much the bumps hurt on the ride to the hospital. I don't want to be a complainer, but, well, it hurts to break your leg. Let me tell you."

Assess all four extremities for distal circulation, sensation, and motor function. Diminished function may be a sign of injury that has compromised circulation, motor function, or nerve function. Distal function should be checked both before and after any interventions such as splinting, bandaging, and immobilization, and at intervals during transport, to be sure such interventions are not interfering with distal function. If distal function has become compromised, adjust your interventions as necessary.

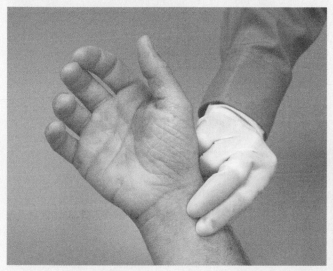

1 Assess distal circulation in the upper extremities by feeling for radial pulses.

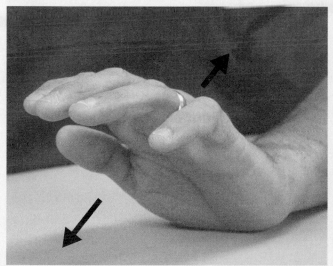

2 Assess distal motor function by checking the patient's ability to move both hands.

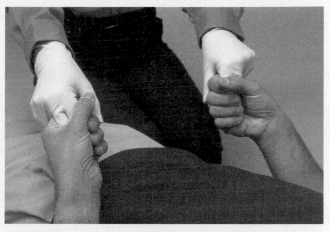

3 Assess strength in the hands by asking the patient to squeeze your fingers.

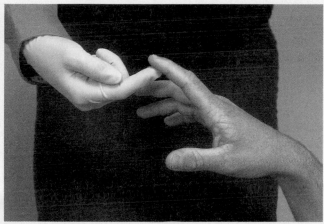

4 Assess distal sensation to the upper extremities by asking the patient, "Which finger am I touching?" (Be sure the patient cannot see which finger.)

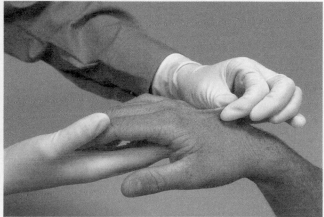

If the patient is unresponsive, check distal sensation in the upper extremities by pinching the back of the hand. Watch and listen for a response.

(continued)

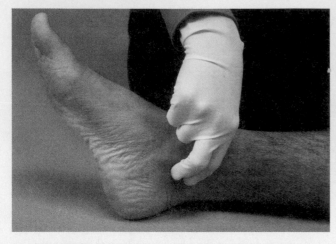

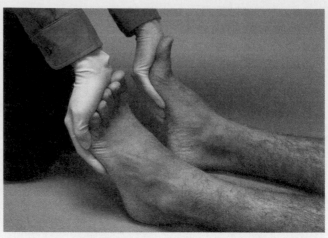

5 Check distal circulation in the lower extremities by feeling the posterior tibial pulse just behind the medial malleolus of the ankle, or . . .

7 Assess strength in the feet and legs by asking the patient to push against your hands.

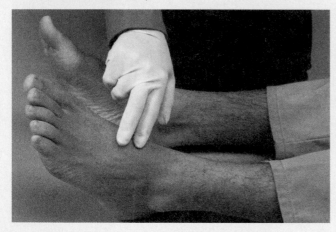

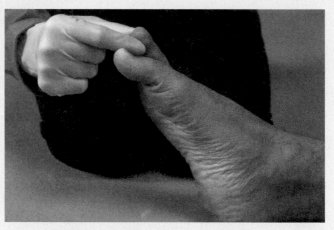

. . . feel the dorsalis pedis pulse at the top of the foot.

8 Assess distal sensation in the lower extremities by asking the patient, "Which toe am I touching?" (Be sure the patient cannot see which toe.)

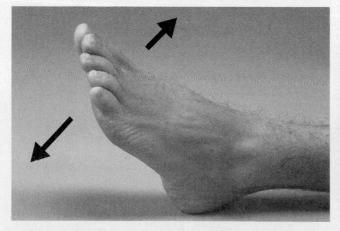

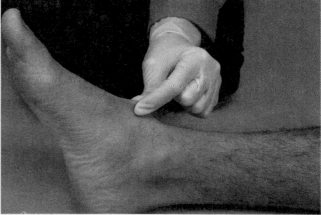

6 Assess distal motor function by checking the patient's ability to move his feet.

If the patient is unresponsive, check distal sensation in the lower extremities by pinching the top of the foot. Watch and listen for a response.

Rapid Trauma or Focused Exam?

For each of the following patients, determine if you should perform a head-to-toe rapid trauma assessment or, instead, a physical exam focused on a specific area or injury.

1. Your patient was found ejected from a vehicle in a rollover collision.

2. Your patient tripped and believes he broke his wrist. He complains of no other injuries.

3. Your patient only complains of minor neck pain after a frontal impact accident in which there was considerable damage and airbag deployment.

4. Your patient fell about 6 feet from a tree and believes he broke his ankle. Bystanders tell you he briefly lost consciousness.

Some General Principles

Several important principles to remember when examining a patient, which are mentioned throughout the chapter, are summarized in the following list:

- **Tell the patient what you are going to do.** In particular, let the patient know when there may be pain or discomfort. Stress the importance of the examination and work to build the patient's confidence. Ask the patient if he understands what you are doing, and explain your actions again if needed.

- **Expose any injured area before examining it.** By exposing areas, you can see such things as bruises and puncture wounds. Let the patient know when you must lift, rearrange, or remove any article of clothing. Do all you can to ensure the patient's privacy.

- **Try to maintain eye contact.** Do not turn away while you are talking or while the patient is answering your questions.

- **Assume spinal injury.** Unless you are sure that you are dealing with a patient who does not have a spine injury (e.g., a medical patient with no mechanism or injury or reason to suspect trauma), assume the patient has such injuries. Always assume that the unconscious trauma patient has a spine injury. Manually stabilize the head and neck on first contact with the patient, fit the patient with a properly sized cervical collar as soon as you have examined the head and neck, and fully immobilize the patient to a spine board before transport to the hospital.

- **During the physical exam, you may stop or alter the assessment process to provide care that is necessary and appropriate for the priority of the patient.** For a patient who is not a priority for rapid transport, you may pause to bandage a bleeding wound, even if the bleeding is not life threatening, or to splint an injured extremity.

- **During the rapid trauma assessment, apply a cervical collar if spine injury is suspected.** For a patient who is a priority for rapid transport, treatments such as controlling non-life-threatening bleeding or splinting an injured extremity may take place en route to the hospital if time and the patient's condition permit.

PEDIATRIC NOTE

The secondary assessment of the pediatric (infant or child) trauma patient is very similar to the secondary assessment of the adult patient. One important difference is that you may need to spend more time reassuring children and explaining procedures to them. You will want to kneel or find another way to get on the same level with the child as you speak with him. Young children may be less frightened if you begin your assessment at the toes and work toward the head instead of proceeding in the usual head-to-toe direction. (Assessment of infants and children will be discussed in greater detail in Chapter 35, "Pediatric Emergencies.")

A child's airway is narrower than an adult's and more susceptible to being closed. A cervical collar that is too tight can easily constrict a child's airway, and a collar that is too high can close the airway by stretching the neck. Therefore, it is especially important to choose the correct size cervical collar for a child.

DETAILED PHYSICAL EXAM

CORE CONCEPT

When and how to perform a detailed physical examination for a trauma patient

detailed physical exam
an assessment of the head, neck, chest, abdomen, pelvis, extremities, and posterior of the body to detect signs and symptoms of injury. It differs from the rapid trauma assessment only in that it also includes examination of the face, ears, eyes, nose, and mouth during the examination of the head. It may be done less rapidly, and it may be done en route to the hospital after earlier on-scene assessments and interventions are completed.

The primary assessment and the rapid trauma assessment are done quickly because of the necessity of getting the seriously injured or ill patient into the ambulance and to the hospital without delay. En route to the hospital, you may have time to do a more complete patient assessment known as the ***detailed physical exam***. If you are not on a transporting unit and the ambulance has not arrived, you may do the detailed physical exam at the scene.

The purpose of the detailed physical exam is to gather additional information about the patient's injuries and conditions. Some of this information may help you to determine the proper treatment for the patient, and some of the information you gather in the detailed physical exam will assist the emergency department staff.

The detailed physical exam is performed most often on the trauma patient with a significant injury or mechanism of injury, less often on a trauma patient with no significant injury or mechanism of injury, and seldom on a medical patient.

Trauma Patient with a Significant Injury or Mechanism of Injury

For a trauma patient who is not responsive or has a significant injury or an unknown mechanism of injury, you will have assessed almost the entire body during the rapid trauma assessment—but very quickly. For this patient, a detailed physical exam may reveal signs or symptoms of injury that you missed or that have changed since the rapid trauma assessment.

Before Beginning the Detailed Physical Exam

It is important to remember that you should perform the detailed physical exam only after you have performed all critical interventions. The best way to ensure this is to repeat your primary assessment before you begin the detailed physical exam. To do this, reassess your general impression of the patient, focusing on his mental status, plus airway, breathing, and circulation.

If you are treating a severely injured patient, you may be too busy to begin or complete the detailed physical exam at all. This is not a failure on your part. Your responsibility is to give the patient the best care possible under the difficult conditions found in the field. If you do not do a complete assessment, but you keep a critical patient's airway, breathing, and circulation intact, you have helped the patient far more than if you had done the complete assessment. *Performing a detailed physical exam is always a lower priority than addressing life-threatening problems.* Table 13-5 shows the place of the detailed physical exam among the priorities and sequence of assessment.

Performing the Detailed Physical Exam

If you have not already exposed the patient, you need to do so now. Since you are now in the enclosed ambulance, it is much easier to protect the patient's privacy and protect him from exposure to the environment.

The detailed physical exam will look a lot like the rapid trauma assessment that you did during the secondary assessment. You will look for the familiar signs of wounds, tenderness, and deformity.

Table 13-5 Detailed Physical Exam in the Sequence of Assessment Priorities
1. Scene size-up.
2. Primary assessment and critical interventions for immediately life-threatening problems.
3. History of the present illness, rapid physical exam, vital signs, plus interventions as needed.
4. Repeat primary assessment for immediately life-threatening problems. Provide critical interventions as needed.
5. Detailed physical exam (time and critical-care needs permitting).
6. Reassessment for life-threatening problems, plus reassessment of vital signs. Provide critical interventions as needed.

The detailed physical exam is similar to the rapid trauma assessment—with some important differences:

- The exam usually takes place in the ambulance, en route. Noise and motion may interfere with some procedures.

- Since immobilization devices have been applied, you must work around them; for example, examining the ears through holes in the head immobilizer or below head tape, examining the neck through openings in the rigid collar, and examining only as much of the posterior as you can reach.

There are only a few differences in the rest of the exam compared to what you did in the rapid trauma assessment. These differences result from either the different environment (the back of the ambulance) or from the treatment you have already given to the patient (e.g., cervical collar and immobilization on a backboard).

When you assess the neck you will be limited by the cervical collar that you placed on the patient during the secondary assessment (rapid trauma assessment). You will not be able to inspect or palpate the back of the neck, but you will be able to assess for wounds, tenderness, deformities, jugular vein distention (JVD), and crepitation through the openings in the collar. You should make sure the collars you use have these openings. Remember that some degree of JVD may be a normal finding in a supine patient but is always an abnormal finding in a seated patient.

Reassessing the chest can be a challenge in a moving ambulance. You can reassess for anything you can palpate, such as crepitation or flail chest. However, because of road noise, breath sounds may be difficult to hear. Just keep in mind that you are auscultating for the presence and equality of breath sounds in your trauma patient, not the different kinds of abnormal sounds that are more common in medical patients. If you are unable to hear breath sounds because of road noise, it is generally better to continue transporting the patient to the hospital. It makes little sense to stop the ambulance and delay transport unless you can do something to treat an abnormality you find. Reassess the abdomen and pelvis as in the rapid assessment.

Any deformities or other indications of a musculoskeletal injury to an extremity found during the rapid trauma assessment will most likely have been temporarily immobilized by securing the patient to the spine board. It is unlikely that taking time to splint such injuries would have been appropriate at the scene when rapid transport was a priority. En route to the hospital, if the patient's other injuries are not keeping you too busy, it may be a good time to apply a splint to an injured extremity after you perform the detailed physical exam. You will learn splinting techniques in Chapter 30, "Musculoskeletal Trauma."

When it comes to reassessing the posterior body it would, of course, be inappropriate to roll the patient up off the backboard. By having the patient immobilized on a backboard, you are already treating for possible spine injury, so your primary concern at this point is to evaluate as much of the posterior body as you can reach for other injuries that may have been missed earlier. Simply reassess the flanks (sides) and as much of the spinal area as you can touch without moving the patient.

Although the rest of the detailed physical exam is essentially the same as the rapid trauma assessment, you have more time, so you can be more thorough. This is especially true with long transports in rural or wilderness areas.

Your next priority is to make sure that the emergency department is ready for your patient by using the ambulance radio or cellular phone to notify the emergency department of the patient's condition. Depending on how far you are from the hospital and what your local protocols say, you may do this step before the detailed physical exam. If you have not yet notified the hospital, you should do it now. You will learn more about what to say to hospital personnel and how to say it in Chapter 17, "Communication and Documentation."

Trauma Patient with No Significant Injury or Mechanism of Injury

When caring for a trauma patient who is responsive and has no significant injury or mechanism of injury, you will have focused your assessment on just the areas the patient tells you hurt plus those areas that you suspect may be injured based on the mechanism of injury.

This kind of patient received all the assessment he needed while still at the scene. He does not generally need a detailed physical exam. It is important to keep a high index of suspicion, though. When in doubt, do a detailed physical exam. Be aware of the responsive trauma patient's fear and need for emotional support.

You should perform a detailed physical exam on a trauma patient who has a significant injury (or mechanism of injury) and on any patient who has an unclear or unknown mechanism of injury. However, the detailed physical exam typically takes a different form in medical patients. This is because there are usually few signs an EMT can find in the physical exam of a medical patient that are significant or about which you can or should do anything. Most of the assessment information on medical patients comes from the history and vital signs.

Occasionally, you may come across a patient who could be either medical or trauma, or both. For example, imagine you have responded to an elderly man who is found alone and unconscious, slumped over the steering wheel of his car. The car is off the road and there is no damage to it. Did the patient lose consciousness first and then drive his car off the road, or did he drive off the road and then get knocked out from a blow to the head? The safest and best thing to do for a patient like this is generally to treat him as a trauma patient who gets a rapid trauma assessment and, if there is time, a detailed physical exam—but whenever possible, also get a history from any witnesses you can find.

COMPARING ASSESSMENTS

Following are two scenarios that may help you see the difference between assessment of a trauma patient with a significant mechanism or injury and assessment of a trauma patient with no significant mechanism or injury:

■ **Clara Diller**—*Responsive Child with No Significant Mechanism or Injury*

You have been dispatched to a 5-year-old girl, Clara, who has fallen while skating. She is crying and holding a bloody cloth to her knee. After completing the scene size-up and primary assessment, and deciding that she is stable and not a priority for immediate transport, you begin the secondary assessment for a trauma patient.

Chief Complaint

"Where do you hurt, Clara?" you ask her. You are not surprised when she says, "My knee hurts," because you can see that her knee is bleeding. Then she adds, "My head hurts, too." So you know that she may have struck her head. Based on the mechanism of injury—a fall to a hard surface—you suspect that she may have injured her spine as well. Therefore, you now focus your assessment according to the chief complaint and mechanism of injury. You focus not on Clara's whole body, but on her head, neck, spine, and knee.

Physical Exam

You look at Clara's head and the back of her neck, searching for injuries such as contusions, abrasions, punctures or penetrations, and lacerations. You find only some swelling on her forehead. Next, you gently press on her head and cervical spine, starting at the top, then moving to the back of her head and going down her neck to the large bump that indicates the lower end of the neck. You find no deformities, tenderness, or swelling. You now determine the proper cervical collar for a child Clara's size. You put it around her neck without moving her head or neck while your partner continues to hold her head.

During the primary assessment, you controlled the bleeding from Clara's knee. Now you tell her, "Clara, I need to lift up that cloth and look underneath. I'm going to feel around your knee, too. If it hurts, you can tell me. Okay?" Clara agrees, and you look at her knee for wounds, tenderness, and deformities. There is only the laceration you found earlier. It is bleeding very slowly and does not appear to be deep. You palpate the area around the knee. You find no deformities or swelling, but the lateral side of the knee is tender. You place a sterile dressing over the wound in place of the cloth Clara was holding.

Baseline Vital Signs

Next, you assess Clara's vital signs. Her pulse is 104 per minute, strong and regular. She has respirations of 24 per minute. They are normal in depth. You check her skin by looking at the palm of her hand and see that it is pink. You feel it and determine that it is warm and dry. You squeeze the end of her fingernail and find that her capillary refill is normal. After telling Clara what you are going to do, you shine a light into her eyes and find that her pupils are equal and reactive. Again, you tell Clara what to expect before you inflate a pediatric cuff on her arm and find her blood pressure is 90/60.

History

While you are doing the physical exam, you ask Clara for more information in order to get the history of the present illness. She is 5 years old, she tells you, and very scared because "my mommy told me not to try my new skates till later." The neighbor who takes care of Clara says, "I called Clara's mother at work when I saw her fall." You ask, "Did you see if Clara got knocked out? Even for a moment?" The neighbor tells you Clara did not lose consciousness.

Just now, Clara's mother arrives on-scene. You reassure her that Clara seems to have just an injury to her knee and a slight bump on her head. You also explain that you have put a special collar on her just in case she injured her neck and that she will be placed on a spine board for the ride to the hospital.

Clara's mother is a better source of medical information than a 5-year-old, so you interview her for the past medical history. You have already asked Clara what symptoms she has, so you ask her mother if Clara has any allergies or takes any medicines. You also ask about pertinent past history. She tells you that Clara has no allergies, takes no medicines, and is healthy. The neighbor tells you Clara's last food or drink was lunch a couple of hours ago. When you ask her about events leading to the injury, she tells you Clara has been feeling fine and acting normal today.

Detailed Physical Exam and Further Care

You immobilize Clara on a backboard and transport her to the emergency department. Although she has no significant mechanism or injury, there is time on the way to the hospital to do a detailed physical exam. You take special care in examining her head, since she had a bump on her forehead. You discover no new significant findings.

Clara's visit to the hospital is brief. The hospital staff rules out any serious head or spine injury. She gets some ointment and a cartoon bandage for her knee, and then talks excitedly about her ambulance ride all the way home.

■ Brian Sawyer—*Unresponsive Adult with Significant Mechanism of Injury*

You are caring for a young man who has been thrown to the pavement during a vehicle collision. After completing the scene size-up, you conducted a primary assessment during which you checked Brian's mental status, took steps to correct an airway problem, checked breathing and circulation, and applied high-concentration oxygen. Because your primary assessment revealed that he was unresponsive to pain and showed signs of diminished circulation (rapid, weak pulse and pale, clammy skin), you determined he was unstable and so assigned Brian a high priority for rapid transport. You now take just a few moments to conduct a rapid version of the secondary assessment for a trauma patient.

History of the Present Illness

You have no opportunity to take a closer look at the car Brian was in because it is 20 feet away. Instead, you ask a police officer to inspect the car for any deformities that would indicate where Brian might have struck interior surfaces. The officer reports that there are no deformities in the interior of the car. However, the fact that Brian appears to have been thrown from the car is a significant mechanism of injury.

Manual Stabilization of the Head and Neck

Your partner started manual stabilization during the primary assessment. He continues to hold the patient's head and neck in a neutral in-line position and keep the airway open.

Advanced Life Support Request

If you are in an area where paramedics are available to respond, this would be a good time to call them. However, in your area, you do not have this option, so you continue your secondary assessment.

Rapid Trauma Assessment

The physical exam you perform on Brian is different from the one you did on Clara. Clara did not have a significant mechanism or injury. She was able to tell you where she hurt, and you were able to focus your exam on just the parts identified by her complaint and mechanism of injury. You examined only her head, neck, and knee. Then you put on a cervical collar and dressed and bandaged her knee.

Brian, however, is unresponsive to pain and cannot tell you what hurts. Even if he could, you would want to give him a more thorough exam because he had a significant mechanism of injury. Being thrown from a car during a collision is likely to produce more than just a localized cut or scrape. Yet, your examination of Brian must be speedy. You must do a more comprehensive exam than you did for Clara, but you must do it rapidly so that you can get Brian into the ambulance and en route to the hospital without delay.

Therefore, you now perform a rapid trauma assessment. As you inspect and palpate each part of his body, you look and feel for wounds, tenderness, and deformities. In addition, with particular areas of Brian's body, you also look for certain signs. You expose each part of the body as necessary. Your rapid trauma assessment of Brian goes as follows:

- **Head.** You assess Brian's head for wounds, tenderness, deformities, and crepitation (the sound or feel of broken bones rubbing against each other). You find a laceration on the back of his head that is not bleeding.
- **Neck.** You assess the neck for wounds, tenderness, deformities, crepitation, and bulging or flat neck veins. There is no response from Brian when you palpate along his cervical spine. Brian's neck veins are flat, indicating possible blood loss, but no other abnormalities.
- **Stabilization.** You now size and apply a cervical collar. Your partner continues to hold manual stabilization as well.
- **Chest.** Next, you open Brian's shirt and assess his chest for wounds, tenderness, deformities, crepitation, breath sounds, and paradoxical motion (movements of part of the chest in a direction that is different from the rest of the chest). You find no abnormalities.
- **Abdomen.** When you cut open Brian's trousers and assess his abdomen for tenderness and deformities, you also check for firmness, softness, and distention. Brian's abdomen is very firm but does not look distended.
- **Pelvis.** Next, you assess Brian's pelvis for wounds, tenderness, and deformities. You find no abnormalities. Since he is not able to complain of any pain in the pelvis, you compress it gently to determine tenderness or motion. You find nothing unusual, except for confirming that his mental status is still such that he does not respond to any pain from compression.
- **Extremities.** Now you quickly assess all four extremities for wounds, tenderness, and deformities, plus distal circulation, sensation, and motor function. You find a deformity in Brian's right lower leg. You do not pause to splint the leg now but will tend to it en route to the hospital. He has weak pulses in all extremities and does not respond to a pinch there. Since he is not responsive, you cannot determine whether he has sensation or motor function.
- **Posterior and immobilization.** A firefighter has gotten a backboard from your ambulance and places it next to Brian. You and your partner roll Brian onto his side as a unit and cut away his clothing to assess his posterior body, inspecting and palpating for wounds, tenderness, and deformities. You find nothing abnormal. The firefighter places the board next to Brian and you roll him onto the board.

You have been able to conduct the entire assessment in just a few moments. If any life-threatening problem had been discovered before or during the rapid trauma assessment, you would have altered the procedure as needed to allow for treatment of the problem.

Baseline Vital Signs

You quickly assess Brian's baseline vital signs. He has a pulse of 120, regular and weak. His respirations are 20 per minute. His skin is pale, cool, and sweaty. His left pupil is dilated and slow to react (the right pupil reacts normally to light). He has a blood pressure of 130/80. His oxygen saturation is 96 percent.

Past Medical History

No one is available to give you a past medical history. You did not come across any medical identification bracelet or necklace when you assessed Brian's extremities and neck.

Detailed Physical Exam

Inside the ambulance, before conducting a detailed physical exam on Brian, you first ensure that any critical interventions are performed. You accomplish this by repeating your primary assessment. Your general impression is that he appears to have serious injuries. His mental status is still unresponsive to pain. You are now managing his airway with an oropharyngeal airway and suction. You are giving him high-concentration oxygen, but he is breathing adequately and you do not need to ventilate him. A check of his circulation shows that his radial pulse is still rapid and weak, there is no external bleeding, and his skin is pale, cool, and sweaty.

After you feel certain that Brian's ABCs are under control, you have time to undertake the detailed physical exam. You reassess his head. You find no wounds, tenderness, or deformities. You go on to reassess Brian's neck, chest, abdomen, pelvis, extremities, and posterior body as you did during the rapid trauma assessment. You find no changes.

The last step in the detailed physical exam is to repeat Brian's vital signs. You obtain a pulse of 136, regular and weak; respirations of 14 per minute; skin that is still cool, pale, and sweaty; a left pupil that is still dilated and slow to react; and a blood pressure of 100/70—indicating a more rapid pulse, slower respirations, and a lower blood pressure than during the rapid trauma assessment at the scene. Your EMS agency uses an automatic blood pressure machine and has guidelines on how and when to use it, so you applied it to Brian and it saved you a little bit of time. You also applied the pulse oximeter and obtained a reading of 99 percent.

You continue to care for Brian as the ambulance proceeds toward the hospital.

CHAPTER REVIEW

Key Facts and Concepts

- The patient without a significant mechanism or injury receives a history of the present illness and physical exam focused on areas that the patient complains about and areas that you think may be injured based on the mechanism of injury.

- Next, gather a set of baseline vital signs and a past medical history.

- For the patient with a significant injury or MOI, ensure continued manual stabilization of the head and neck, consider whether to call advanced life support personnel (if available), get a brief history of the present illness, and then perform a rapid trauma assessment.

- In the rapid trauma assessment, look for wounds, tenderness, and deformities, plus certain additional signs appropriate to the part being assessed (as summarized in Table 13-4). Systematically examine the head, neck, chest, abdomen, pelvis, extremities, and posterior body.

- After assessing the neck, apply a cervical collar. After completing the physical assessment, immobilize the patient to a spine board and get a baseline set of vital signs and a past medical history.

- After you have performed the appropriate critical interventions and begun transport, the patient may receive a detailed physical exam en route to the hospital.

- The detailed physical exam is very similar to the rapid trauma assessment, but there is time to be more thorough in the assessment. The detailed physical exam does not take place before transport unless transport is delayed.

- The detailed physical exam is most appropriate for the trauma patient who is unresponsive or has a significant injury or unknown MOI.

- A responsive trauma patient with no significant injury or MOI will seldom require a detailed physical exam.

Key Decisions

- Does this patient have an injury or mechanism of injury severe enough to suggest a rapid trauma assessment is appropriate?

- Should we apply a cervical collar to this patient?

- How should the task of assessment be divided when there are two EMTs at the scene?

Chapter Glossary

crepitation (krep-uh-TAY-shun) the grating sound or feeling of broken bones rubbing together.

detailed physical exam an assessment of the head, neck, chest, abdomen, pelvis, extremities, and posterior of the body to detect signs and symptoms of injury. It differs from the rapid trauma assessment only in that it also includes examination of the face, ears, eyes, nose, and mouth during the examination of the head. It may be done less rapidly, and it may be done en route to the hospital after earlier on-scene assessments and interventions are completed.

distention (dis-TEN-shun) a condition of being stretched, inflated, or larger than normal.

history of the present illness (HPI) information gathered regarding the symptoms and nature of the patient's current concern.

jugular (JUG-yuh-ler) **vein distention (JVD)** bulging of the neck veins.

paradoxical (pair-uh-DOCK-si-kal) **motion** movement of a part of the chest in the opposite direction to the rest of the chest during respiration.

past medical history (PMH) information gathered regarding the patient's health problems in the past.

priapism (PRY-ah-pizm) persistent erection of the penis that may result from spinal injury and some medical problems.

rapid trauma assessment a rapid assessment of the head, neck, chest, abdomen, pelvis, extremities, and posterior of the body to detect signs and symptoms of injury.

SAMPLE a memory aid in which the letters stand for elements of the past medical history: signs and symptoms, allergies, medications, pertinent past history, last oral intake, and events leading to the injury or illness.

stoma (STO-ma) a permanent surgical opening in the neck through which the patient breathes.

tracheostomy (tray-ke-OS-to-me) a surgical incision held open by a metal or plastic tube.

trauma patient a patient suffering from one or more physical injuries.

Preparation for Your Examination and Practice

Short Answer

1. Explain how the secondary assessment of a trauma patient with a significant mechanism or injury differs from that of a trauma patient with no significant mechanism or injury.

2. List the steps of the rapid trauma assessment and describe the kind of patient for whom the rapid trauma assessment is appropriate.

3. List the areas covered in the detailed physical exam. What do you look and feel for as you assess each of these areas?

Thinking and Linking

Think back to Chapter 10, "Scene Size-Up," and link information from that chapter with information from this chapter as you consider the following situation:

1. You have been dispatched to the scene of a car that struck a light pole. You have gained access to the front seat and are beginning your assessment of an adolescent female who appears to be seriously injured. From the corner of your eye, you suddenly notice that the transformer is starting to spark. What should you do?

Critical Thinking Exercises

Trauma can take many forms and vary from minor to critical. The purpose of this exercise will be to consider how you might deal with the following situations.

1. You are assessing a patient who fell three stories. He is unresponsive and bleeding into his airway. The driver of the ambulance is positioning the vehicle and bringing equipment to you. How do you balance the patient's need for airway control (hc requires frequent suctioning) with your need to assess his injuries?

2. As an EMT, how would you balance the need for appropriate on-scene assessment and treatment with the need for speed in getting the patient to the hospital in each of the following situations?
   - You arrive at the residence to find a patient who explains that he has accidentally cut his finger with a kitchen knife. The cut is bleeding profusely.

- You arrive at a schoolyard to find a girl who bystanders say was shot by a rival gang member. She is lying in a pool of blood but is able to speak to you.
- You are called to respond to a man who has been found unconscious on a sidewalk next to an apartment building in the middle of the night. There were no witnesses to explain what may have happened to him.

Pathophysiology to Practice

The following question is designed to assist you in gathering relevant clinical information and making accurate decisions in the field.

- A patient with a chest injury may have a lung collapse. Why are the breath sounds on the injured side typically decreased or absent when the chest cavity is filled with air, which usually transmits sounds very well?

It's Saturday night, and you've been assigned to one of the ambulances that covers downtown, where there is usually some kind of excitement going on. As you sit in quarters, you're listening to the scanner. The police seem to be busy with a variety of calls—disturbances, domestics, and larcenies, to name a few. Then you hear on the police frequency: "Dispatch, we need an ambulance ASAP. We have a stabbing here." You don't wait for your pager to activate before you're in the ambulance bay with your partner. The pager follows shortly: "Delta 55, respond to 1512 Broadway, outside, for a stabbing. Police on the scene, and scene is secure."

Your response takes only a few minutes. When you arrive, you see a male in his twenties lying on the sidewalk. "What happened?" you ask him.

"Some punks punched me in the face and threw me into the street when they stole my wallet."

At this point, you tell the patient not to move his head and that you will help by manually stabilizing it. The patient continues: "When I tried to fight them off, they stabbed me in the chest."

The patient's airway is open, but he is out of breath and his breathing is rapid and shallow. You check the chest and see the entrance wound. You listen for breath sounds. There is silence on the side of the wound. You put on an occlusive dressing and administer oxygen by nonrebreather mask. You then rapidly check for external bleeding.

Street Scene Questions

1. What is the priority of this patient?
2. What should be done next?
3. When should vital signs be taken?

You and your partner agree that this patient needs to be rapidly transported to the trauma center. You are still maintaining manual stabilization of the patient's head and neck, so your partner gets a backboard and cervical collar. You perform a rapid physical exam from head to toe. The patient has abrasions on the left cheek, the left wrist is swollen with pain on movement, and there is tenderness in both lower abdominal quadrants. Your partner takes a set of vital signs. You decide to do the past medical history in the ambulance. You immobilize the patient to the backboard with the head immobilizer in place. During this transfer, you check the patient's back for any wound, bleeding, or tenderness.

Once the patient is loaded in the ambulance, your partner starts toward the hospital with red lights and siren. The patient is still conscious, but he is having trouble talking in complete sentences. He reports a lot of discomfort. You think there may be pressure building up in his chest because of an injury to the lung.

Street Scene Questions

4. What should you do next?
5. What should be done for the detailed physical exam, if there is time before reaching the trauma center?

You are confident that you need to treat the patient's worsening difficulty breathing. You lift the corner of the occlusive dressing and hear some air escape. The patient starts to breathe easier almost immediately. You take another set of vital signs. Then you secure the bandage over the chest wound again, but only on three sides. You turn your attention to the detailed exam, starting at the head, then moving to the chest and abdomen, and finally ending with all four extremities and as much of the back as you can reach. With each location, you check for wounds, tenderness, and deformities.

The remainder of the transport is uneventful. You transfer the patient to the hospital with an updated prehospital care report that includes the latest set of vital signs.

14

Assessment of the Medical Patient

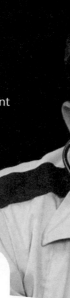

- - - - - - ◯ **STANDARD**
Assessment (Secondary Assessment)

- - - - - - ◯ **COMPETENCY**
Applies scene information and patient assessment findings (scene size-up, primary and secondary assessment, patient history, and reassessment) to guide emergency management.

- - - - - - ◯ **CORE CONCEPTS**
— The difference between assessment procedures for a responsive medical patient and for an unresponsive medical patient

— How to perform a secondary assessment for a responsive medical patient

— How to tailor the physical exam for a responsive medical patient using a body systems approach

— How to perform a secondary assessment for an unresponsive medical patient

EXPLORE Resource**Central**

To access Resource Central, follow directions on the Student Access Card provided with this text. If there is no card, go to **www.bradybooks.com** and follow the Resource Central link to Buy Access from there. Under Media Resources, you will find:

▶ **Medical Emergencies**
Watch this video to find out what systems may be involved with a medical emergency and why it is important to link a patient's symptoms back to the body system involved.

▶ **Techniques Used during a Physical Assessment**
Observe techniques used during a physical assessment. Why should an area be inspected before it is palpated? What areas of the body should be auscultated? Find out in this video!

▶ **Patient Interviews**
Communication is key in patient care. Learn why you should use open-ended questions and how past injuries and illnesses may relate to the current emergency call.

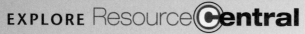

OBJECTIVES

After reading this chapter you should be able to:

14.1 Define key terms introduced in this chapter.

14.2 Adapt the secondary assessment process to both responsive and unresponsive medical patients. (pp. 351–365)

14.3 Collect a systematic history of the present illness. (pp. 354, 356–357, 364–365)

14.4 Collect a relevant past medical history. (pp. 356–357)

14.5 Adapt the secondary assessment process to specific patient complaints. (pp. 357, 360)

(continued)

14.6 Adapt your approach to secondary assessment of the medical patient to overcome challenges, according to the circumstances. (pp. 357, 360)

14.7 Conduct a rapid physical examination for the unresponsive medical patient. (pp. 362–364)

14.8 Explain the importance of checking baseline vital signs in the unresponsive medical patient. (p. 364)

14.9 Recognize situations in which you should consider requesting the assistance of advance life support personnel for a medical patient. (p. 364)

14.10 Identify other sources of patient information for the unresponsive or uncooperative medical patient. (pp. 364–365)

KEY TERMS

medical patient, *p. 351*   *OPQRST, p. 356*

T he key to moving from the primary assessment into the secondary assessment is reconsideration of the mechanism of injury as well as of the patient's complaint. If there is a mechanism of injury or actual injury, you will perform the secondary assessment for the trauma patient, which was described in Chapter 13, "Assessment of the Trauma Patient." When the patient has a complaint that is medical in nature, and you have confirmed that there is no significant mechanism of injury or actual injury, you will perform the secondary assessment for the medical patient—the subject of this chapter. (See Visual Guide: Overview of Medical Assessment.)

SECONDARY ASSESSMENT OF THE MEDICAL PATIENT

$<<<<<<$

Assessment procedures for a responsive *medical patient* are discussed in the following section. The procedures for an unresponsive medical patient will be discussed later in the chapter.

Table 14-1 lists and contrasts the procedures for these two categories of medical patient.

medical patient
a patient suffering from one or more medical diseases or conditions.

Responsive Medical Patient

As you learned in Chapter 11, "The Primary Assessment," it makes a great deal of difference in the assessment process whether the patient is responsive or unresponsive. This is especially true of the medical patient. In trauma patients, there are often many external signs of trauma, or injury, but this is not true of a patient with a medical condition. The most important source of information about a medical patient's condition is what the patient can tell you. This is why, when the patient is awake and responsive, obtaining the patient's history comes first.

A good example of the kind of patient you will see often is one who is awake and has a medical problem with no immediately life-threatening problems. After you finish the primary assessment for this patient, perform a secondary assessment. This will tell you what you need to know in order to administer the proper treatment.

The secondary assessment for a medical patient has four parts: history of the present illness, past medical history, physical exam, and baseline vital signs (Scan 14-1 and Table 14-1).

CORE CONCEPT
The difference between assessment procedures for a responsive medical patient and for an unresponsive medical patient

CORE CONCEPT
How to perform a secondary assessment for a responsive medical patient

Medical Patient Assessment

VISUAL GUIDE

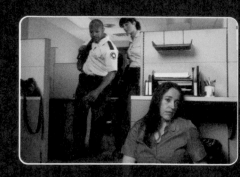

■ DEVELOP A GENERAL IMPRESSION

PRIMARY ASSESSMENT

Responsive

Unresponsive

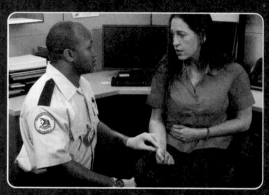

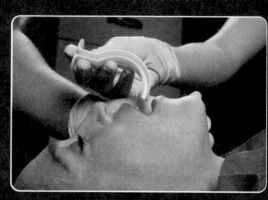

Assure adequate breathing
Check pulse and skin for signs
of shock

Aggresive ABCs
Suction
Airway adjuncts
Ventilate if necessary
Circulation

■ OXYGEN

NOTE: *Upon approach if patient appears lifeless and without breathing,*
begin with circulation and a pulse check as part of C-A-B

Determine Priority

SECONDARY ASSESSMENT

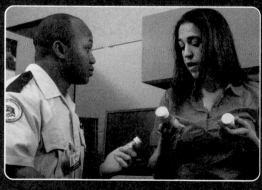

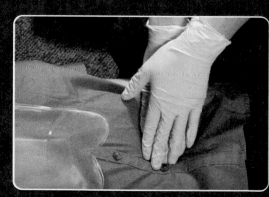

History first
Body systems exams as appropriate

Body systems exams first
History
Expedited pace

■ VITAL SIGNS

Interventions (done enroute for serious or unstable patients)

Timing, priority, and destination based on patient's condition

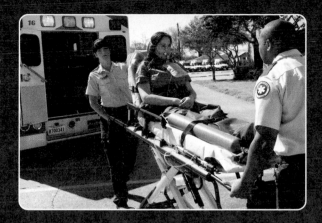

About every 5 minutes for unstable patients
About every 15 minutes for stable patients
Repeat primary assessment
Reassess chief complaint
Check interventions
Repeat vital signs

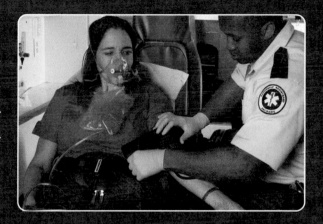

Provide a concise report

Notify any specialized teams:
Cardiac (syspected myocardial infarction/chest pain) Stroke

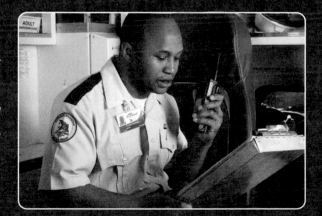

■ THROUGHOUT THE CALL

Provide comfort and reassurance
Be alert for changes in the patient's condition

VISUAL GUIDE

RESPONSIVE MEDICAL PATIENT	UNRESPONSIVE MEDICAL PATIENT
1. Gather the history of the present illness (OPQRST) from the patient: Onset Provokes Quality Radiation Severity Time	1. Conduct a rapid physical exam: Head Neck Chest Abdomen Pelvis Extremities Posterior
2. Gather a past medical history from the patient: Allergies Medications Pertinent past history Last oral intake Events leading to the illness	2. Obtain baseline vital signs: Respirations Pulse Skin Pupils Blood pressure Oxygen saturation*
3. Conduct a physical exam (focusing on the area the patient complains about).	3. Gather the history of the present illness (OPQRST) from family or bystanders: Onset Provokes Quality Radiation Severity Time
4. Obtain baseline vital signs: Respirations Pulse Skin Pupils Blood pressure Oxygen saturation*	4. Gather a past medical history from bystanders or family: Allergies Medications Pertinent past history Last oral intake Events leading to the illness

*As directed by local protocol

Note: This table shows the general order of steps. You may alter this order in accordance with the situation and the number of EMTs available and when the patient's condition warrants immediate action due to immediate life threats.

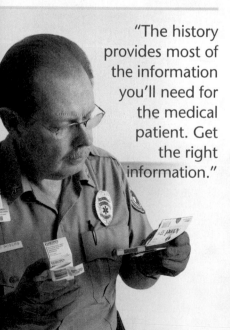

"The history provides most of the information you'll need for the medical patient. Get the right information."

Take a History of the Present Illness

The interview you do with a patient is similar to the interview a physician conducts before a physical examination. It is a conversational information-gathering effort. Not only will you gain needed information from the interview, but you will also reduce the patient's fear and promote cooperation.

Although relatives and bystanders may serve as sources of information, the most important source is the patient. Do not interview relatives and bystanders before you interview the patient unless the patient is unconscious or unable to communicate. You may gain information from bystanders and medical identification devices later, while you are conducting the physical examination.

One purpose of talking to the patient is to find out his chief complaint, the one thing that seems most seriously wrong to him. When you ask the patient what is wrong, he may tell you that several things are bothering him. If this happens, ask what is bothering him most. Find out if the patient is in pain and where he hurts. Unless the pain of one injury or medical problem masks that of another, most people will be able to tell you of painful areas.

Try to ask open-ended questions, or questions that the patient answers with responses other than "Yes" or "No." For example, do not ask, "Is your chest pain dull and crushing?" Ask instead, "How would you describe your pain?" In this way, you will avoid giving the patient the impression that you want a particular answer. If the patient says that he cannot describe his pain, you can try giving him several choices: "Is your pain dull, or sharp, or burning?"

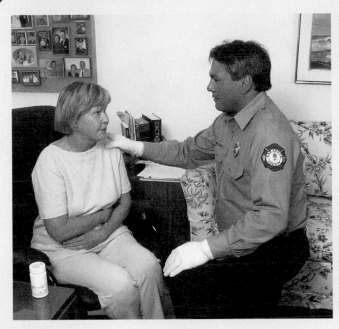

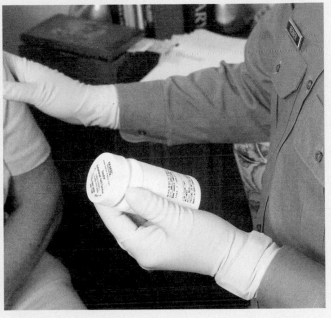

1 **HISTORY OF PRESENT ILLNESS.** Ask the OPQRST questions:
Onset
Provokes
Quality
Radiation
Severity
Time

2 **PAST MEDICAL HISTORY.** Ask the SAMPLE questions:
Signs and symptoms
Allergies
Medications
Pertinent past history
Last oral intake
Events leading to the illness

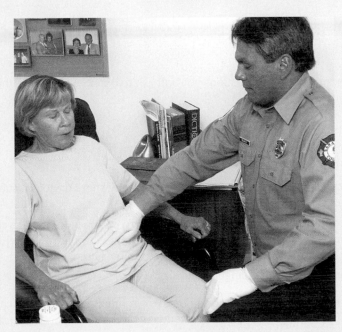

3 **PHYSICAL EXAM.** Perform a quick assessment of the affected body part or system:
Head
Neck
Chest
Abdomen
Pelvis
Extremities
Posterior

(continued)

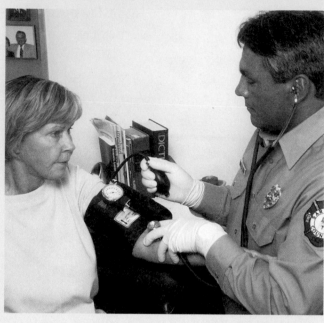

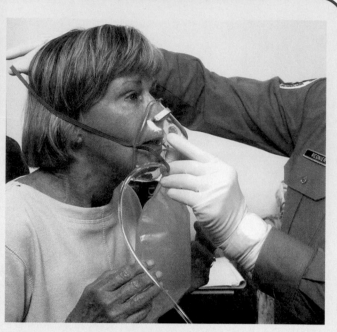

4 **VITAL SIGNS.** Assess the patient's baseline vital signs:
Respiration
Pulse
Skin color, temperature, condition (and capillary refill in infants and children)
Pupils
Blood pressure
Oxygen saturation (if appropriate for the patient's chief complaint)

5 **INTERVENTIONS AND TRANSPORT.** Perform interventions as needed and transport the patient. Contact on-line medical direction as needed.

OPQRST
a memory aid in which the letters stand for questions asked to get a description of the present illness: onset, provokes, quality, radiation, severity, time.

An easy way to remember most of the questions you will ask to obtain a history of the present illness is to use the letters **OPQRST**:

- **Onset.** What were you doing when it started?
- **Provokes.** Can you think of anything that might have triggered this pain?
- **Quality.** Can you describe it for me?
- **Radiation.** Where exactly is the pain? Does it seem to spread anywhere or does it stay right there?
- **Severity.** You look uncomfortable. How bad is the pain? If zero was no pain and 10 was the worst pain you can imagine, what number would you assign to your pain? (Use the system of determining pain severity recommended by local protocols.)
- **Time.** When did the pain start? Has it changed at all since it started?

You should also inquire about accompanying conditions. For example, a patient with severe chest pain may be so apprehensive that he doesn't tell you about his moderate shortness of breath until you ask him about it specifically. There are certain chief complaints that by their nature suggest the possibility of other symptoms. This chapter will describe some of the more common ones.

Take a Past Medical History

After finding out the patient's age, you should then get the rest of the past medical history and the name of his personal physician. Using the SAMPLE letters, as defined in Chapter 13,

"Assessment of the Trauma Patient," the "S" (symptoms) were explored during the history of the present illness, as just described. (Signs will be discovered during the physical exam and vital signs measurements.) For the past medical history, continue with the rest of the SAMPLE questions, as follows:

- **Allergies.** Are you allergic to anything?

- **Medications.** What medicines do you take? What do you take those for? Are there any other medicines you are supposed to take, but don't?

- **Pertinent past history.** Do you have any other medical problems? Have you ever had this kind of problem before? Who is your doctor?

- **Last oral intake.** When was the last time you ate or drank anything? What did you eat or drink?

- **Events leading to the illness.** How have you felt today? Have you experienced anything out of the ordinary?

Tailoring the Physical Exam for Specific Chief Complaints

If you obtain the history of the present illness and the past medical history as they have been described up until now, you will obtain a great deal of information. Many times, however, you can gain additional important information by tailoring the history to the patient's chief complaint. This means asking questions pertinent to that complaint.

Body Systems Approach You learned in earlier chapters that discussed anatomy, physiology, and pathophysiology (Chapter 5, "Medical Terminology and Anatomy and Physiology," and Chapter 6, "Principles of Pathophysiology") about the different systems of the body and how they work. Part of the reason for studying anatomy, physiology, and pathophysiology is to be able to use this knowledge to guide your assessment. When an illness or other nontraumatic condition occurs, it frequently affects not just one particular organ or part of the body but a system of the body. For example, when you get an upper respiratory infection, you may have signs and symptoms related to the nose, throat, and chest. These are all part of the respiratory system. Sometimes more than one body system may be affected, as when problems with the respiratory system affect the cardiovascular system or vice versa.

To get the most information about the medical patient's problem, you should focus your questioning and physical examination of the medical patient on the particular body system or systems most likely to be involved.

For example, if a patient is having difficulty breathing, you should inquire about whether the patient has had a fever or chills (which can be associated with pneumonia) or a cough (which can be associated with not just pneumonia, but also upper respiratory infections, asthma, cystic fibrosis, and many other conditions). You should also ask whether the patient's physician has prescribed an inhaler for the patient. This may significantly affect the treatment you administer.

However, with the patient who complains of difficulty breathing you should also consider the cardiovascular system. You will learn that difficulty breathing is often a sign of heart attack. When assessing a patient with difficult breathing you should also assess for signs of fluid build-up (this may be seen in the ankles—or in the lower back of a bedridden patient). You should ask about chest pain or discomfort as well as other signs that the heart could be involved in the breathing difficulty.

Altered mental status is a complaint that could be associated with many body systems. If the patient has an altered mental status, you may assess the endocrine system for blood sugar problems, the neurological system for signs of a stroke, and possibly other systems, depending on the patient's presentation.

Table 14-2 lists some of the questions and physical examination steps for some of the most common chief complaints you will encounter as an EMT. Also see Visual Guide: A Body Systems Approach.

There are many other questions you can and should ask when gathering a history for certain conditions. You will find more questions to ask about specific complaints in the chapters on various medical conditions in the "Medical Emergencies" section.

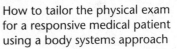

CORE CONCEPT

How to tailor the physical exam for a responsive medical patient using a body systems approach

CHAPTER 14
Medical Body System Exams

■ **WHERE YOU PERFORM THE EXAM DEPENDS ON PATIENT PRIORITY AND STATUS**
UNSTABLE PATIENT—IN THE AMBULANCE; STABLE PATIENT—ON SCENE

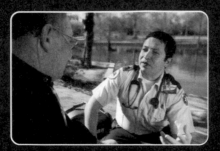

First, perform a history

The body system exam(s) you choose are based on the information you obtain in the history

Body Systems Exam: Respiratory

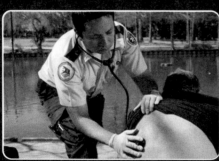

Work of breathing and position
Pedal and sacral edema
Lung sounds
Pulse oximetry

Respiratory Specific History
Dyspnea on exertion
Orthopnea
Weight gain

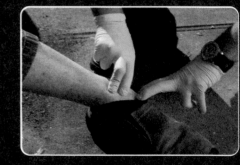

Body Systems Exam: Cardiovascular

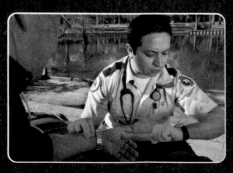

Check pulse
(presence/rate/regularity)

Skin color/temperature/condition

Blood pressure

Orthostatic blood pressure changes

JVD

Many components of the respiratory exam also apply to the cardiovascular system

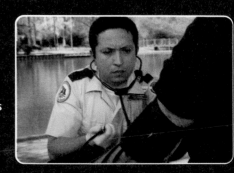

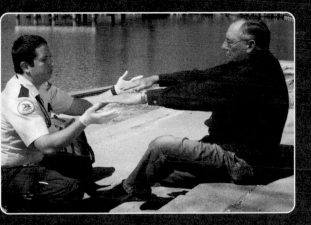

Body Systems Exam: ## Neurological

Cincinatti Prehospital Stroke Scale (or other approved scale)
Pupils
Monitoring mental status changes over time

Endocrine
Body Systems Exam:

Blood glucose monitoring
Skin color/temperature/condition
Breath odors
Excessive hunger, thirst or urination

Diabetic specific history
Oral intake
Medication history/use
Recent illness

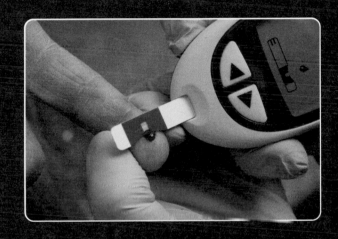

Body Systems Exam: ## GI/GU

Palpation of abdominal quadrants

GI/GU specific history
Input/output amount and frequency
Question or observe for bright red or digested blood in vomit, stool, or urine
Menstrual history and pregnancy where appropriate

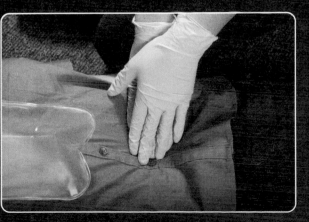

VISUAL GUIDE

Table 14-2 Secondary Assessment: Specific Medical Complaints

TYPE OF COMPLAINT	ADDITIONAL HISTORY	PHYSICAL EXAM
Respiratory	Cough Fever or chills Dyspnea on exertion Weight gain (indicates fluid) Have a prescribed bronchodilator?	Lung sounds (presence and equality) Wheezing Work of breathing and position Pulse oximetry (oxygen saturation)
Cardiovascular (cardiac and respiratory systems closely related)	Have prescribed nitroglycerin? Taking aspirin?	Skin color, temperature, and condition Blood pressure Pulse (including strength and regularity) Lung sounds (presence and equality) Jugular vein distention Ankle edema Oxygen saturation
Neurological	Headache Seizure	**FAST** (Face-Arm-Speech-Test—Includes components of the Cincinnati Prehospital Stroke Scale) **Face**–does one side of the patient's face droop (ask the patient to smile)? **Arms**—can the patient hold both arms in front of him? **Speech**—is the patient's speech clear and understandable? **Test**—oxygen saturation
Allergic (involves components of the cardiovascular and respiratory systems)	Time of exposure Time of symptom onset	Stinger Hives (urticaria) Lung sounds (presence and equality) Face and neck edema Oxygen saturation
Abdominal/gastrointestinal	Fever Nausea and vomiting Diarrhea or constipation Blood in vomit or bowel movements; may be bright red (fresh) or dark (digested) Menstrual history	Inspect and palpate all four quadrants of the abdomen
Endocrine	Oral intake Medication history History of recent illness Excessive hunger, thirst, urination	Blood glucose monitoring Skin color, temperature, and condition Mental status Unusual breath odors

Perform a Physical Exam

With responsive medical patients, the EMT's physical exam is usually brief. You will gather most of the important assessment information in this type of patient from the history and vital signs. Table 14-2 lists some of the physical exam steps you should take when evaluating patients with certain chief complaints. For example, if your patient has difficulty breathing, you should listen to the patient's chest with a stethoscope for the presence and equality of breath sounds. If you have received additional education on recognizing specific types of breath sounds, you should attempt to do so. For a patient who is at risk for hypoxia, like this one, you should also check oxygen saturation. If your patient has a complaint that does not fit into any of the categories you learned in your EMT course, you should focus the exam on the body part that the patient has a complaint about. For example, if the patient complains of thigh pain, you will inspect and palpate his thigh.

Although there are a few other steps you can take in the physical exam, most of the useful information in medical patients comes from the history.

CRITICAL DECISION MAKING

Challenges in History Gathering

Obtaining a history is a key part of the assessment of the medical patient. However, some patients are easier to get a history from than others. Consider what you might say and do to improve your history gathering in the following circumstances:

1. A 79-year-old female keeps talking, saying a lot about things that have nothing to do with the problem you are there for.

2. A 16-year-old female is surrounded by her family. She has abdominal pain that you suspect may be from a pregnancy, but you have not yet asked her if she might be pregnant.

3. A 32-year-old male with diabetes has not eaten lately, according to his family. He is sometimes combative, sometimes quiet. When you ask him questions, he gives you a vacant stare and says nothing.

4. A 22-year-old male college student, his roommate tells you, has been acting strangely the last few weeks. The patient is now sitting on his bed with his knees drawn up against his chest, rocking back and forth, saying things that don't make sense to you.

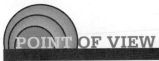

PEDIATRIC NOTE

When gathering a history from a child, be sure to kneel or find another way to get on the same level with the child. Put questions in simple language the child can understand. Note that much of the history for a child and all of the information for an infant will need to be gathered from the parents, guardian, or other adult caretaker.

Obtain Baseline Vital Signs

A complete set of baseline vital signs taken during the secondary assessment is essential to the assessment of a medical patient. Later assessments of the vital signs will be compared against this baseline set of vital signs to determine trends in the patient's condition. If you have an automated blood pressure monitoring device, use it in accordance with local protocol. Typically, this means getting a manual blood pressure first, then using the machine to obtain repeat vital signs.

POINT OF VIEW

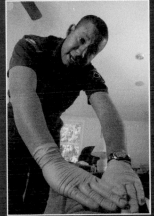

"At first I thought it might be a stomach bug. You know how your belly gets kind of achy? But then it got worse. The pain was strong. And came in waves. I curled up in a ball and asked my husband to call the ambulance. I knew something was really wrong.

"By the time the ambulance got to the house I had vomited. But it still was painful. And it still wasn't the flu. I could tell.

"The EMT was very nice. He asked where it hurt and then pushed on my belly. He was pretty gentle but it hurt anyhow. He also asked me questions. Everything from if I thought I had a fever to if I was pregnant to when I ate last . . . even when I pooped last. He sure was thorough.

"Well, I can look back at it now and laugh . . . now that they took out my appendix and I'm walking around again. But it sure wasn't funny then."

Administer Interventions and Transport the Patient

In later chapters, you will learn when to provide treatment for specific medical conditions. The only treatment you have learned about so far that might be appropriate for a responsive patient is oxygen.

Unresponsive Medical Patient

CORE CONCEPT

How to perform a secondary assessment for an unresponsive medical patient

The sequence of assessment for an unresponsive medical patient differs from the sequence of assessment for a responsive medical patient. If the patient were responsive, the first step of your secondary assessment would be talking with the patient to obtain the history of his present illness and the past medical history, followed by the physical exam and baseline vital signs. For an unresponsive patient, the process is reversed (Table 14-1 and Scan 14-2). Since you cannot obtain a history from the patient, you will begin with the physical exam and baseline vital signs. After these procedures, you will gather as much of the patient's history as you can from any bystanders or family members who may be present.

Another difference between the secondary assessment for the responsive and for the unresponsive patient is the nature of the physical exam. For a responsive patient, you will be able to focus your exam on just the part of the body the patient mentions in his complaint. Since an unresponsive patient cannot tell you where the problem is, you will need to do a rapid assessment of the entire body.

Perform a Rapid Physical Exam

The physical exam of an unresponsive medical patient will be almost the same as the head-to-toe physical exam for a trauma patient. You will rapidly assess the patient's head, neck, chest, abdomen, pelvis, extremities, and posterior. As you assess each area, you will look for signs of injury. Other things to look for in the medical patient include:

- **Neck.** Jugular vein distention, medical identification devices
- **Chest.** Presence and equality of breath sounds
- **Abdomen.** Distention, firmness, or rigidity
- **Pelvis.** Incontinence of urine or feces
- **Extremities.** Pulse, motor function, sensation, oxygen saturation, medical identification devices

Medical ID Devices Medical identification devices can provide important information. One of the most commonly used medical identification devices is the Medic Alert emblem shown in Figure 14-1. Over 1 million people wear a medical identification device in the

FIGURE 14-1 A medical identification device.

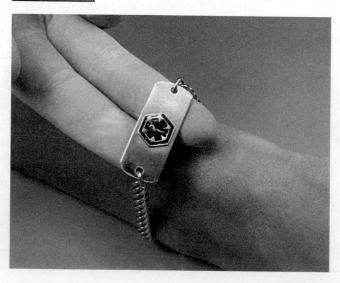

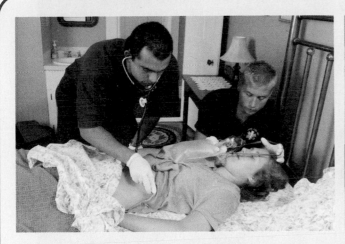

1 RAPID PHYSICAL EXAM. Perform a rapid assessment of the entire body:

Head	Pelvis
Neck	Extremities
Chest	Posterior
Abdomen	

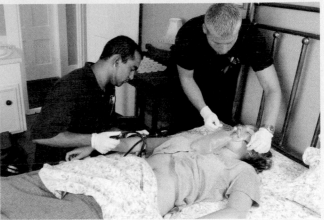

2 VITAL SIGNS. Assess the patient's baseline vital signs:
Respiration
Pulse
Skin color, temperature, condition (and capillary refill in infants and children)
Pupils
Blood pressure
Oxygen saturation (if directed by local protocol)

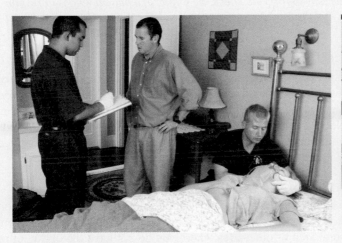

3 PAST MEDICAL HISTORY. Interview family and bystanders for information about the present illness (OPQRST) and also the SAMPLE history:

Signs and symptoms	Last oral intake
Allergies	Events leading to the
Medications	illness
Pertinent past history	

4 INTERVENTIONS AND TRANSPORT. Contact on-line medical direction as needed. Perform interventions as needed and transport the patient.

form of a necklace or a wrist or ankle bracelet. One side of the device has a Star of Life emblem. The patient's medical problem is engraved on the reverse side, along with a telephone number to call for additional information.

When doing the physical exam, look for necklaces and bracelets or wallet cards. Never assume you know the form of every medical identification device. Check any necklace or bracelet carefully, taking care when moving the patient or any of his extremities. You should alert the emergency department staff when you arrive that the patient is wearing

FIGURE 14-2 A pulse oximeter.

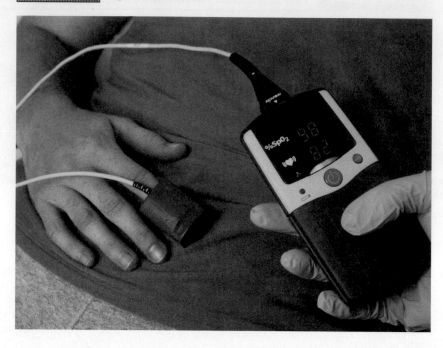

or carrying medical identification and tell them what is on it (diabetes or heart condition, for example). **NOTE:** *It is easy to forget to check the pupils of a patient who is unresponsive. Try to keep in mind that the most important time to check the pupils is when the patient's eyes are closed!*

Obtain Baseline Vital Signs

Assess the patient's pulse, respirations, skin, pupils, and blood pressure and note any abnormalities. Determine the patient's oxygen saturation if you can (Figure 14-2). Be sure to record your observations so later vital sign assessments can be compared with these baseline observations. If you have an automated blood pressure monitoring device, use it after you have obtained a manual blood pressure or in accordance with local protocol. This will allow you to be confident that the machine reading is correct.

Consider a Request for ALS Personnel

In accordance with local protocols, and if advanced life support personnel are available, consider at this time if the additional services paramedics can provide would benefit your patient.

If you are serving in a rural area or other area where you do not have the option of requesting advanced life support, and if you are very distant from a hospital, there may be a closer local clinic or other health facility that has an arrangement to provide advanced care. Consider if it is worth a delay to stop at such a facility for the special care that may help stabilize your patient before you continue transporting the patient to the hospital.

If arrangements like these exist where you work as an EMT, you must be familiar with the types of patients this facility can help. The arrangements should be in writing in order to reduce confusion and prevent loss of precious time with critical patients.

Take a History of the Present Illness and a Past Medical History

Since an unresponsive patient cannot talk, you will have to interview bystanders to get as much information as possible. When interviewing bystanders, determine if any are relatives or friends of the patient. They usually have more information to provide about past problems than other bystanders would have. See which of the bystanders saw what happened. When questioning bystanders, you should ask:

- **What is the patient's name?** If the patient is obviously a minor, ask if the parent or guardian is present or if he or she has been contacted.

- **What happened?** You may be told that the patient fell off a ladder, appeared to faint, fell to the ground and began seizing, was hit on the head by a falling object, or other possible clues.

- **Did you see anything else?** For example, was the patient clutching his chest or head before he fell?

- **Did the patient complain of anything before this happened?** You may learn of chest pain, nausea, concern about odors where he was working, or other clues to the problem.

- **Does the patient have any known illnesses or problems?** This may provide you with information about heart problems, alcohol abuse, allergies, or other problems that could cause a change in the patient's condition.

- **Is the patient taking any medications?** Be sure to use the word *medications* or *medicines*. If you say "drugs" or some other term, bystanders may not answer you, thinking that you are asking questions as part of a criminal investigation. In rare cases, you may feel that the bystanders are holding back information because the patient was abusing drugs. Remind them that you are an EMT and you need all the information they can give you so proper care can begin.

While gathering the patient's history, you should also see if there is a "Vial of Life" or similar type of sticker on the main outside door, closest window to the main door, or the refrigerator door. If so, patient information and medications can usually be found in the refrigerator. (The Vial of Life is not used in some regions.)

Administer Interventions and Transport the Patient

There is not usually much information gained from the secondary assessment of an unresponsive medical patient that will change treatment in the field. The most important thing to look for is a mechanism of injury or signs that would make you suspect a spine injury. Either of these would mean that you need to immobilize the patient's spine. Most of the time, the information you gather in your assessment of unresponsive medical patients will be particularly helpful to the staff in the emergency department. Emergency physicians and nurses depend on EMTs to evaluate the scene carefully and to gather as much useful information as possible that they cannot get in the hospital.

COMPARING ASSESSMENTS

The following text contains two scenarios that may help you see the difference between assessment of a responsive medical patient and assessment of an unresponsive medical patient.

■ Mr. Schmidt—*Responsive Adult Medical Patient*

You have been dispatched to an older man who is complaining of stomach pain. After completing the scene size-up, you conduct the primary assessment. You determine that Mr. Schmidt is alert and that his airway, breathing, and circulation are not compromised. You decide that he is a medical patient with no immediately life-threatening problems and you proceed to the secondary assessment for a medical patient.

History

You tell Mr. Schmidt that you need to get some information about his condition. You start by asking him questions that will give you the history of the present illness:

You: *When did the pain start, Mr. Schmidt?*
Mr. Schmidt: *About 2 hours ago.*
You: *Can you describe it for me?*
Mr. Schmidt: *It's kind of a burning pain.*
You: *Has it changed at all since it started?*
Mr. Schmidt: *It's gotten worse, especially in the last hour.*
You: *Where exactly is the pain?*
Mr. Schmidt: *(points to his upper abdomen) Right here.*

You: *Does it seem to spread anywhere or does it stay right there?*
Mr. Schmidt: *It just stays right here.*
You: *What were you doing when it started?*
Mr. Schmidt: *I was talking with my wife.*
You: *Can you think of anything that might have triggered this pain?*
Mr. Schmidt: *No, not really.*
You: *You look uncomfortable. How bad is the pain?*
Mr. Schmidt: *Pretty bad. I've never had a pain this bad.*
You: *If zero was no pain and 10 was the worst pain you can imagine, what number would you assign to your pain?*
Mr. Schmidt: *Probably a 6.*

Now that you have the history of the present illness, you can find out the patient's age and proceed with the rest of the past medical history:

You: *How old are you, Mr. Schmidt?*
Mr. Schmidt: *I'm 68.*
You: *Have you had any other symptoms?*
Mr. Schmidt: *Well, I've been sick to my stomach.*
You: *Do you have any pain in your chest, arms, neck, or shoulders?*
Mr. Schmidt: *No.*
You: *Have you vomited?*
Mr. Schmidt: *No.*
You: *Have you had any diarrhea?*
Mr. Schmidt: *No.*
You: *Are you allergic to anything?*
Mr. Schmidt: *Just cats.*
You: *What medicines do you take?*
Mr. Schmidt: *Ibuprofen and Minipress.*
You: *What do you take those for?*
Mr. Schmidt: *I have arthritis and high blood pressure.*
You: *Do you have any other medical problems?*
Mr. Schmidt: *No.*
You: *Have you ever had this kind of problem before?*
Mr. Schmidt: *No.*
You: *Who is your doctor?*
Mr. Schmidt: *Dr. Anderson.*
You: *When was the last time you ate or drank anything?*
Mr. Schmidt: *I had dinner about 3 hours ago.*
You: *How have you felt today? Anything out of the ordinary?*
Mr. Schmidt: *No, it was a pretty normal day.*

Physical Exam

The next step in assessment is a physical exam. Since Mr. Schmidt is complaining of abdominal pain, you unbutton his shirt to expose his abdomen so you can inspect and palpate it. His abdomen does not appear distended, but there is some tenderness in both upper quadrants.

Vital Signs

Next, you assess Mr. Schmidt's baseline vital signs. His pulse is 92, regular and full. Respirations are 20 and unlabored. Skin is normal (warm, pink, and dry). Blood pressure is 140/86. Because his complaint is of abdominal pain, which has no direct relationship to the brain, you do not check his pupils.

Together, the primary assessment, history, physical exam, and vital signs did not give you any reason to believe that Mr. Schmidt needed oxygen. (If your protocols had told you to, however, or if you wished, you could have given Mr. Schmidt oxygen. It would not harm him.) Throughout the exam you reassured Mr. Schmidt and tried to calm his fears. Now you move Mr. Schmidt to your stretcher and put him in the position in which he is most comfortable: sitting. You and your partner move him to the ambulance and begin the trip to the hospital.

■ Mrs. Malone—*Unresponsive Adult Medical Patient*

You arrive at the home of an older woman whose daughter has reported that she cannot waken her mother. After completing the scene size-up, you conduct the primary assessment. You find that Mrs. Malone only responds to verbal stimulus by moaning. Her airway is endangered because of her depressed level of responsiveness and the fact that she is supine. Your partner performs a head-tilt, chin-lift maneuver to open and protect the airway and you provide high-concentration oxygen by nonrebreather mask. Her circulation is normal. Because of her depressed level of responsiveness and threatened airway, you determine that Mrs. Malone is unstable and a high priority for transport to the hospital. However, before loading her into the ambulance, you will quickly conduct the secondary assessment for a medical patient.

Rapid Physical Exam

Because Mrs. Malone is unresponsive, you have no way of knowing what part of her body to focus on. Therefore, you do a rapid assessment of her head, neck, chest, abdomen, pelvis, extremities, and posterior in just the same way as you would for an unresponsive trauma patient. As you assess each area of her body, you remove enough clothing to be able to inspect and palpate it, then quickly replace the clothing. You find no abnormalities.

Vital Signs

Your partner finds that Mrs. Malone has a pulse of 92, strong and regular. Her respirations are 20, full and unlabored. Skin is cool and dry. Pupils are equal and reactive. Blood pressure is 160/90. Her oxygen saturation is 98 percent when she is on 15 liters per minute of oxygen by nonrebreather mask. Everything is in the normal range except for her high blood pressure. You note this, but it does not require any action on your part.

You have placed Mrs. Malone in the recovery position, and you now check her airway again. Since you turned her on her side, you have not heard any abnormal sounds from her airway like snoring or gurgling. This, and the fact that she is breathing adequately, means that her airway is open. You check the oxygen and confirm that you are administering oxygen at 15 liters per minute by nonrebreather mask.

History

Because Mrs. Malone has a decreased level of responsiveness and you could not get a history by interviewing her, you need to depend on others to provide as much of this information as possible. The family member who met you at the door is Mrs. Malone's daughter, Florence. You question her to find out what happened and what medical history her mother has.

You: *What happened?*
Florence: *I think she had a convulsion.*
You: *What happened to make you say that?*
Florence: *Well, I heard some choking sounds from the room next door, and when I came in her arms and legs were moving around.*
You: *Was it both arms and both legs?*
Florence: *Yes, I think so.*
You: *Was anyone with her when this started?*
Florence: *No, no one else was home.*
You: *When did this happen?*
Florence: *About 10 minutes ago, just before I called 911.*
You: *How long did you see her arms and legs moving?*
Florence: *I think it was only about a minute, but it felt like a lot longer when it was happening.*
You: *Has she ever had anything like this happen before?*
Florence: *I don't think so, but my mother lives alone, so I'm not sure.*
You: *How old is your mother?*
Florence: *She's 60.*
You: *Is she allergic to anything?*
Florence: *Not that I know of.*
You: *Does she take any medicines?*
Florence: *No, I don't think so.*

You: *Is she generally healthy?*

Florence: *Yes, although sometimes she gets migraines.*

You: *Does she take any medicine for her migraines?*

Florence: *No, she used to, but she had to stop taking it because it made her feel so tired.*

You: *When did she stop taking the medicine?*

Florence: *Oh, that was months ago.*

You: *Do you know when she last ate?*

Florence: *We had lunch about 4 hours ago—just a cheese sandwich and some tomato soup. I was starting to make dinner when this happened.*

You: *Can you think of anything unusual that happened today that might explain what happened to your mother?*

Florence: *No, it seemed like a normal day until just a little while ago.*

You: *I think you were right when you said she had a convulsion, or seizure. What you described sounds a lot like a seizure. We're going to take her to the hospital to be checked by a doctor in the emergency department.*

Florence: *Thank you. Should I come with you or drive to the hospital myself?*

You: *You're welcome to come with us, but it might be easier for you to get home if you drive.*

Florence: *OK. I'll meet you there.*

You: *Don't follow the ambulance too closely. Take your time and be careful.*

Having completed the secondary assessment, you move Mrs. Malone to your stretcher and take her to the ambulance for transport to the hospital. You will not do a detailed physical exam en route because there is no reason to suspect injuries of the kind that a detailed physical exam would assess. Since Mrs. Malone is unresponsive, however, you maintain a high index of suspicion and remain ready to do a more detailed exam en route if anything about her condition should change so as to cause you to suspect that she may have been injured.

Mrs. Malone's condition is potentially very serious. At the hospital, she will be scheduled for a series of tests and referred to a specialist.

CHAPTER REVIEW

Key Facts and Concepts

- The secondary assessment of the medical patient takes two forms, depending on whether the patient is or is not responsive.

- You assess the responsive patient by getting a history of the present illness and a past medical history, then performing a physical exam of affected parts of the body before getting baseline vital signs.

- Since unresponsive medical patients cannot communicate, it is appropriate to start the assessment with a rapid physical exam. Baseline vital signs come next, and then you interview bystanders, family, and friends to get any history that can be obtained.

- You may not change any field treatment as a result of the information gathered here, but the results of the assessment may be very important to the emergency department staff.

Key Decisions

- Is the patient responsive enough to provide a history?

- If a patient cannot provide a history, can someone present at the scene do so?

- What kind of secondary assessment does the patient's chief complaint suggest?

Chapter Glossary

medical patient a patient with one or more medical diseases or conditions.

OPQRST a memory aid in which the letters stand for questions asked to get a description of the present illness: onset, provokes, quality, radiation, severity, time.

Preparation for Your Examination and Practice

Short Answer

1. Explain how and why the secondary assessment for a medical patient differs from the secondary assessment for a trauma patient.

2. Explain how and why the secondary assessment for a responsive medical patient differs from the secondary assessment for an unresponsive medical patient.

Thinking and Linking

Think back to Chapter 10, "Scene Size-Up," and link information from that chapter with information from this chapter as you consider the following situation.

1. You are at the home of an elderly man whose wife called 911 because her husband was complaining of chest pain. While assessing your patient, the wife begins to complain of shortness of breath. Now you have two patients. What should you do?

Critical Thinking Exercises

Getting a history from a medical patient can require a good deal of skill. The purpose of this exercise will be to consider how you might obtain a history in the following situations.

1. What questions would you ask to get a history of the present illness from a patient with a chief complaint of chest pain?

2. You are trying to get information from the very upset son of an unresponsive man. He is the only available family member. He is so upset that he is having difficulty talking to you. How can you quickly get him to calm down and give you his father's medical history?

3. You are interviewing a very pleasant older man. Unfortunately, your assessment is taking a long time because he does not answer your questions and instead starts talking about other things. He lives alone and appears to be lonely. How should you handle this?

Pathophysiology to Practice

The following question is designed to assist you in gathering relevant clinical information and making accurate decisions in the field.

- A patient has a history as a three-pack-a-day smoker. How is this likely to affect the patient's blood pressure? Why?

Street Scenes ------------------------------

Just as you are about to sit down to eat lunch, your ambulance is dispatched to a local health club for a 50-year-old female having an asthma attack. Upon arrival, you find the scene to be safe. Taking Standard Precautions, you are directed to the women's locker room where you find your patient sitting on a workout bench.

"Hello. How can we help you today?" you ask. Your general impression is of an alert middle-aged woman in moderate respiratory distress.

"Oh, I'm having an asthma attack," she says. You can see her airway is open, but her breathing is rapid and moderately labored. You observe no bleeding, find her skin to be normal, and determine her radial pulse to be slightly rapid but strong and regular.

Street Scene Questions

1. What priority is this patient?

2. What are the next steps in the management of this patient?

Satisfied there are no life threats for which you have to provide immediate intervention, you determine this patient's priority to be medium in severity with the potential to get worse.

"What's your name?" you ask. She replies that her name is Andrea.

"What were you doing when the difficulty breathing started?" you ask. It turns out she had been exercising on the treadmill. You note that she is speaking in complete sentences and does not have to stop every few words to catch her breath. You ask Juan, your partner, to begin administering oxygen by way of a nonrebreather mask. While Juan is doing that, you continue your examination.

Street Scene Questions

3. What part of the secondary assessment should follow next?

4. What signs or symptoms would you look for to determine if the patient was getting better or worse?

"What do you think caused your shortness of breath?" you ask. She replies that she's had a mild case of asthma for about 10 years and that it is exercise induced. You ask how long she has been having trouble breathing with this episode. "About 10 minutes," she replies.

You know that many asthmatics carry their own medication for asthma, so you ask what medications she is taking. "I have an inhaler, but I left it at home. I think it's called Al Butterball or something like that." You suggest the name "albuterol" and she nods her head.

Meanwhile, Juan places the oxygen mask on Andrea's face. You ask if she is allergic to anything and she shakes her head no. While you listen to lung sounds, Juan obtains baseline vitals. You note that the lung sounds are equal but noisy, like a whistling sound. Juan informs you that her pulse is 120 and regular; skin is warm and dry; respirations are 24 and slightly labored; and her blood pressure is 130/70. Her oxygen saturation is 96 percent.

Andrea accepts your offer to transport her to the emergency department, so you put her on the stretcher in her position of comfort, sitting up. During the short trip to the hospital, you use the radio to inform the emergency department of your patient's condition and treatment, take another set of vital signs, and reassess the patient. She appears to be a little better, but her breathing is still slightly labored and a little noisy. She does not have any signs suggesting that she is getting worse, things like retractions above the clavicles and between the ribs, the ability to speak only a few words at a time, and cyanosis, particularly of the lips and nail beds. After you transfer Andrea to the care of the emergency department staff, you return to service.

Reassessment

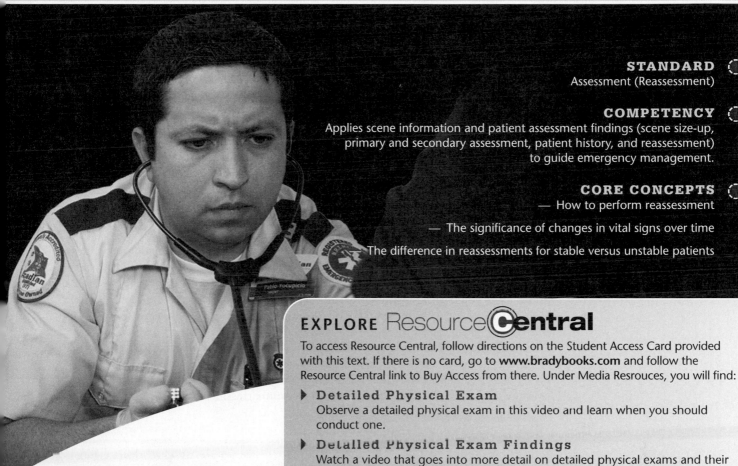

Assessment (Reassessment)

COMPETENCY ○------
Applies scene information and patient assessment findings (scene size-up, primary and secondary assessment, patient history, and reassessment) to guide emergency management.

CORE CONCEPTS ○------
— How to perform reassessment

— The significance of changes in vital signs over time

— The difference in reassessments for stable versus unstable patients

EXPLORE Resource Central

To access Resource Central, follow directions on the Student Access Card provided with this text. If there is no card, go to **www.bradybooks.com** and follow the Resource Central link to Buy Access from there. Under Media Resrouces, you will find:

▶ **Detailed Physical Exam**
Observe a detailed physical exam in this video and learn when you should conduct one.

▶ **Detailed Physical Exam Findings**
Watch a video that goes into more detail on detailed physical exams and their findings.

▶ **Ongoing Assessment**
View a video of an ongoing assessment and learn its purpose, steps you should perform, and what equipment you need.

OBJECTIVES

After reading this chapter you should be able to:

15.1 Define key terms introduced in this chapter.

15.2 Explain the importance of reassessment. (p. 372)

15.3 Identify the proper points in the patient care process at which reassessment should be performed. (p. 372)

15.4 Discuss the purpose of each of the components of reassessment. (pp. 372–375)

15.5 Adapt the reassessment process and frequency of reassessment based on patients' conditions. (pp. 375–376)

15.6 Recognize both obvious and subtle changes in the patient's condition. (pp. 372–376)

15.7 Assign meaning to trends in the patient's condition over time. (pp. 375–376)

KEY TERMS

reassessment, *p. 372*   trending, *p. 375*

An appropriate assessment at the scene and en route to the hospital allows you to detect and treat injuries and illnesses. Your job does not stop there, though. The patient's condition can change, either gradually or suddenly. You will be able to detect these changes by performing a series of steps called **reassessment**.

REASSESSMENT

It is important to observe and re-observe your patient, not only to determine his condition when you first see him, but also to detect any changes. The patient may exhibit an obvious change, like loss of consciousness, or more subtle differences, such as restlessness, anxiety, or sweating. These may indicate a change in circulation. Some patients may take a turn for the worse before they reach the hospital, although this is uncommon. In some cases, you may see patient improvement, possibly in response to interventions you perform.

You will perform reassessment on every patient after you have finished performing lifesaving interventions and, often, after you have done the detailed physical exam. Sometimes you may skip doing a detailed physical exam because you are too busy taking care of life-threatening problems, or you have a medical or noncritical trauma patient for whom the detailed physical exam would not yield useful information. *Reassessment, however, must never be skipped except when lifesaving interventions prevent you from doing it.* Even in the latter situation, one partner can often perform the reassessment while the other continues lifesaving care.

Throughout the assessment procedures that take place on the way to the hospital, remember to explain to a conscious patient what you are doing, talk in a reassuring tone, and consider the patient's feelings, such as anxiety or embarrassment.

PEDIATRIC NOTE

Remember to maintain eye contact with a conscious child, stay on the child's level as much as possible, and explain what you are doing in a quiet and reassuring voice.

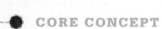

CORE CONCEPT

How to perform reassessment

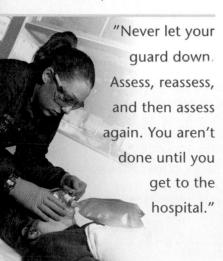

"Never let your guard down. Assess, reassess, and then assess again. You aren't done until you get to the hospital."

Components of Reassessment

During the reassessment, you will repeat key elements of assessment procedures you have already performed. For example, you will repeat the primary assessment (to check for life-threatening problems), reassess vital signs, repeat the physical exam related to the patient's specific complaint or injuries, and check any interventions you have performed (see Scan 15-1).

Repeat the Primary Assessment

Begin reassessment by repeating the primary assessment to recheck for life-threatening problems:

- Reassess mental status.
- Maintain an open airway.
- Monitor breathing for rate and quality.
- Reassess the pulse for rate and quality.
- Monitor skin color and temperature.
- Reestablish patient priorities.

Remember, life-threatening problems that were not present or were brought under control during the primary assessment may develop or redevelop before the patient reaches the hospital. For example, the mental status of the patient who was responsive and alert may begin to deteriorate, which is a significant trend and worrisome sign. The airway that was open may become

SCAN 15-1 Reassessment

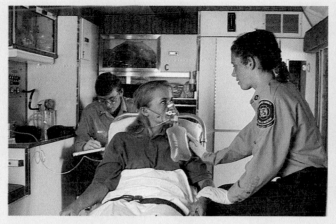

1 Repeat the primary assessment.

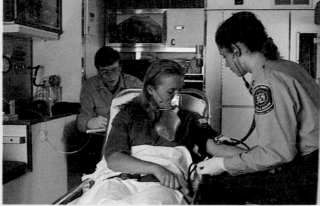

2 Reassess and record vital signs.

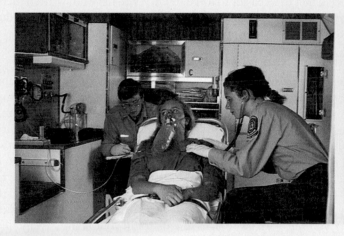

3 Repeat pertinent parts of the secondary assessment.

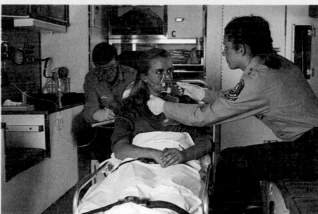

4 Check interventions.

occluded, the patient who was breathing adequately on his own may now require respiratory support, and other signs—such as a rapid pulse, cool skin, and pallor—may indicate the onset of shock. Life threats must be continually watched and managed immediately when discovered.

PEDIATRIC NOTE

The mental status of an unresponsive child or infant can be checked by shouting (verbal stimulus) or flicking the feet (painful stimulus). Crying would be an expected response from a child with an adequate mental status.

Reassess and Record Vital Signs

During the secondary assessment, you took and recorded a set of baseline vital signs: pulse, respiration, skin, pupils, and blood pressure. During reassessment, you will reassess and record the vital signs, comparing the results with the earlier baseline measurements and any other vital sign measurements you may have taken (for example, during the detailed physical exam, if you conducted one). Reevaluate oxygen saturation if you previously assessed it.

It is especially important to record each vital sign measurement as soon as you obtain it. In this way, you will not need to worry about remembering the different numbers you get for pulse rate, blood pressure, respiratory rate, and oxygen saturation. When you have more

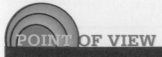
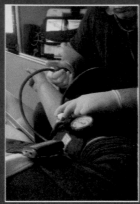

than one set of vital signs, it becomes even easier to forget them if you have not written them down. Another reason to document your reassessment is so that you can see trends in the patient's condition, which we will discuss later in this chapter.

Repeat Pertinent Parts of the History and Physical Exam

A patient's chief complaint may change over time, especially with regard to its severity. Ask the patient about changes in symptoms, especially ones that you anticipate because of treatments you have administered. At the same time, be careful not to suggest particular answers to the patient.

You may also find changes as you repeat the physical exam. For example, a chest injury may become apparent as muscles get tired and you see paradoxical motion that was not present or noticeable when you first assessed the patient (paradoxical motion is present when a part of the chest goes in as the patient inhales and goes out as the patient exhales, opposite to the motion of the rest of the chest). The abdomen may become distended, a sign that you are especially likely to see if you have a long transport. As you learn more about specific injuries and illnesses in later chapters, you will learn more signs to look for in your reassessment.

Check Interventions

Whenever you check the interventions that you have performed for a patient, try to take a fresh look at the patient. Attempt to see the patient as though you had never seen him before. This may help you to evaluate the adequacy of your interventions more objectively and to adjust them as necessary. Always do the following:

- Ensure adequacy of oxygen delivery and artificial ventilation.
- Ensure management of bleeding.
- Ensure adequacy of other interventions.

Situations change. The fact that you put the patient on oxygen initially does not prevent the tank from running out later, or the tubing from becoming kinked or disconnected. A good habit to develop is to check the entire path of the oxygen from the tank to the patient. This means looking at the regulator on the tank and confirming that it has sufficient oxygen and that the flowmeter is set to the proper flow. Make sure that the tube is firmly connected to the regulator. Follow the tubing and make sure there are no kinks that would prevent the flow of oxygen. Look at the mask. Make sure the tubing is connected to it, and that it is the proper mask. Confirm that it is snug on the patient's face and, if it is a nonrebreather mask, that the nonrebreather bag does not completely deflate when the patient inhales. Increase the flow rate if it does. With practice, this sequence of steps will take just a few seconds.

Wounds that stopped bleeding can start bleeding again, so it is important to check them as part of reassessment. Check any bandage you have applied and make sure it is dry with no blood seeping through. When an unbandaged wound is in a location where you cannot see it, gently palpate it with gloved hands and check your gloves for blood.

Also be sure to check other interventions, such as cervical collars, backboard straps, and splints. Any of these can slip and need adjustment.

Observing Trends

Because reassessment is a means of determining trending (changes over time) in the patient's condition, you will need to repeat the reassessment steps frequently. Be sure to record your findings and compare them to earlier findings. It is important to notice and document any changes or trends. In later chapters, you will learn about specific trends to look for in patients' vital signs. For example, when you reach Chapter 27, "Bleeding and Shock," you will learn about trends in the pulse rate and blood pressure as signs of shock.

CRITICAL DECISION MAKING

Trending Vital Signs

Observing a trend in vital signs—*trending*—is more valuable than getting an individual set of vital signs. Observing trends is essential for making accurate decisions regarding transport destination and whether ALS may be necessary. Look at the following sets of vital signs for three patients and determine the trend for each patient.

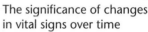

CORE CONCEPT

The significance of changes in vital signs over time

trending
changes in a patient's condition over time, such as slowing respirations or rising pulse rate, that may show improvement or deterioration, and that can be shown by documenting repeated assessments.

1. A 32-year-old male fell about 15 feet from a roof and has multiple injuries. His vital signs have been:

TIME	PULSE	BLOOD PRESSURE	RESPIRATORY RATE	SKIN
2140	88	120/90	20, shallow	Pale but dry
2155	84	100/80	18, shallow	Pale but dry
2200	80	90/60	16, full	Pale but dry

How would you describe the trend of his vital signs: deteriorating, essentially unchanged, returning to normal, or not possible to determine?

2. A 64-year-old female fell to the floor and is complaining of hip pain. Her vital signs have been:

TIME	PULSE	BLOOD PRESSURE	RESPIRATORY RATE	SKIN
1330	108	160/90	24, shallow	Pale but dry
1345	112	150/90	20, shallow	Pale but dry
1350	96	140/80	20, full	Pale but dry

How would you describe the trend of her vital signs: deteriorating, essentially unchanged, returning to normal, or not possible to determine?

3. A 19-year-old female injured her left ankle and lower leg in a soccer game. Her vital signs have been:

TIME	PULSE	BLOOD PRESSURE	RESPIRATORY RATE	SKIN
1922	108	126/96	20, shallow	Pale and sweaty
1930	116	110/80	22, shallow	Pale and sweaty
1935	124	90/70	22, full	Pale and sweaty

How would you describe the trend of her vital signs: deteriorating, essentially unchanged, returning to normal, or not possible to determine?

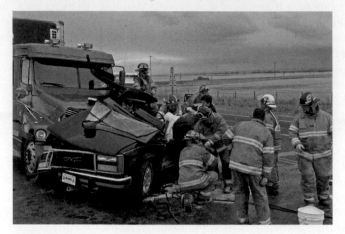

FIGURE 15-1 In rural EMS, long transport distances and times may dictate many reassessments—at least every 15 minutes for a stable patient, at least every 5 minutes for an unstable patient. (© *Kevin Link*)

Based on your findings, you may need to institute new treatments or adjust treatments you have already started. Your findings, in particular any trends you have noted, will also be important information for the hospital staff and will let them know if the patient's condition is improving or deteriorating.

Reassessment for Stable and Unstable Patients

-----------● CORE CONCEPT

The difference in reassessments
for stable versus unstable
patients

The patient's condition, as well as the length of time you spend with the patient, will determine just how often you will conduct the reassessment. The more serious the patient's condition, the more often you will do it. Unless your protocols direct you to do otherwise, reassess your patient at these intervals:

- Every 15 minutes for a stable patient, such as a patient who is alert, has vital signs in the normal range, and has no serious injury.

- Every 5 minutes for an unstable or potentially unstable patient, such as a patient who has an altered mental status; difficulty with airway, breathing, or circulation, including severe blood loss; or a significant mechanism of injury.

Whenever you believe there may have been a change in the patient's condition, repeat at least the primary assessment. In this way, you will detect signs of life-threatening conditions as soon as possible. When in doubt, repeat reassessment every 5 minutes or as frequently as possible (Figure 15-1).

COMPARING ASSESSMENTS

The following text contains two scenarios that may help you see the difference between a reassessment of a responsive medical patient and reassessment of an unresponsive trauma patient.

■ Mr. Schmidt—*Responsive Adult Medical Patient*

You have been dispatched to an older man who is complaining of stomach pain. You complete the scene size-up and primary assessment. You determine that there is no mechanism of injury; that Mr. Schmidt is alert; and that his airway, breathing, and circulation are not compromised. Since he is alert and has no immediate life threats, he is stable and not a priority for immediate transport. You conduct the secondary assessment, discovering that Mr. Schmidt is suffering a burning pain localized to his upper abdomen that started about

2 hours ago and is getting worse. He reports no history of any similar disorder. The physical exam reveals some tenderness in the upper quadrants but no distention. His vital signs are normal. You load him into the ambulance for transport to the hospital, placing him in a position he finds comfortable, sitting up. Deciding that a detailed physical exam will not be useful, you proceed with reassessment en route.

Reassessment—Stable Medical Patient

To begin reassessment, you repeat the primary assessment to check for any immediately life-threatening problems. You get a general impression of an older man who is in discomfort. By talking to him, you confirm that his mental status is alert and his airway and breathing are adequate. You check circulation by feeling his radial pulse and looking for external bleeding. His radial pulse is normal in rate and strength and regular in rhythm. The skin at his wrist is warm, pink, and dry. You do not see any blood around him. You conclude that Mr. Schmidt's condition has not changed and he is still stable.

Next, you repeat and record the vital signs. Mr. Schmidt has a pulse of 88, regular and full, respirations 20 and unlabored, skin normal (warm, pink, and dry), and blood pressure 134/88. His pulse and blood pressure are somewhat lower than when you assessed them during the secondary assessment, but well within normal ranges, probably indicating that he is somewhat calmer than before. You record your new findings.

Now you repeat the pertinent parts of the history and physical exam. When you ask Mr. Schmidt about his abdominal pain, he tells you there has been no change. He is still a little nauseated, but does not feel as though he will vomit. Nevertheless, you anticipate that he may vomit, so you keep a basin nearby. You very gently palpate his abdomen again. He reports no change in the amount of tenderness present, and you find no firmness or distention.

Next, you check the interventions you have performed. In Mr. Schmidt's case, the only intervention that was appropriate was positioning. You ask Mr. Schmidt whether you can make him more comfortable, but he says he is fine sitting up.

The trip to the hospital takes about 20 minutes, so 15 minutes after you leave the scene, you repeat the reassessment and find no changes in Mr. Schmidt's condition.

At the hospital, after you drop off another patient, you see Mr. Schmidt as he is leaving the emergency department. He tells you the doctor diagnosed a probable ulcer, gave him a prescription for medication, and advised him to follow-up for further tests with Dr. Anderson, his regular physician.

■ Brian Sawyer—Unresponsive Adult Trauma Patient

You have responded to a collision in which Brian, the driver, was thrown from his car. You complete the scene size-up and primary assessment, determining that there is a significant mechanism of injury and that Brian is unresponsive with a compromised airway. Your partner stabilizes Brian's spine and performs a jaw-thrust maneuver. You insert an oral airway and administer high-concentration oxygen. You decide that Brian is critical and therefore a high priority for transport. You quickly complete a rapid trauma assessment, finding a head laceration, flat neck veins, and a deformity to his right leg. You apply a cervical collar during the rapid trauma assessment. As soon as the assessment is finished, you immobilize Brian to a backboard, load him into the ambulance, and conduct a detailed physical exam en route, during which you make no further significant findings. You then proceed immediately to reassessment.

Reassessment—Unstable Trauma Patient

You and your partner both need to be with this critically injured patient on the way to the hospital. Fortunately during your primary assessment, when you realized how seriously injured Brian might be, you asked dispatch to send another qualified driver so the two of you could continue to work on Brian en route to the hospital. In accordance with your local protocol, you told the driver to drive to the closest hospital able to provide quality trauma care.

You start reassessment by repeating the primary assessment to check for life-threatening problems. First, you reassess Brian's mental status. When he does not respond to your shouting his name, you pinch his shoulder. There is no response. You reevaluate his airway by putting your ear next to his mouth and listening for abnormal sounds like snoring, gurgling, or stridor. There is a little bit of gurgling, so you suction his mouth. When you listen again, you hear no more abnormal sounds. You also look in Brian's mouth. You see nothing that could cause his airway to become obstructed. Next, you look at Brian's breathing. It is now slow (approximately 8 breaths per minute) and shallow, so you get the flow-restricted, oxygen-powered ventilation device for your partner, who starts to ventilate Brian at a rate of 12 breaths per minute. Brian's pulse is rapid and weak. His skin is still pale, cool, and sweaty. You reconfirm that Brian is a high-priority patient. In fact, his condition is even more serious than before, because you now need to assist his ventilations.

The next step in reassessment is to repeat and record his vital signs. Brian has a pulse of 132, regular and weak; respirations of 8 and shallow; a blood pressure of 100 by palpation; and an oxygen saturation of 96 percent. As you record these findings, you note that his pulse and blood pressure have not changed from your earlier readings, but—as you noted when repeating the primary assessment of respiration—his breathing has now slowed to a dangerous level that requires assisted ventilations.

Next, you repeat the trauma assessment. You palpate the laceration on the back of Brian's head and check your gloves but find no fresh blood. The deformity to his right leg is temporarily stabilized by his immobilization on the backboard. You find no additional injuries.

Finally, you check the interventions you performed for Brian. You confirm that oxygen is running into the flow-restricted, oxygen-powered ventilation device and that Brian's chest is rising with each ventilation. There is no bleeding to control. Now you check the other interventions: the cervical collar, straps, and long backboard. The collar is the right size and is in the right place (sometimes cervical collars can slip). The straps are snug, and Brian has not moved on the board. You find time now to splint his injured leg.

During the ride to the hospital, you repeat your reassessment every 5 minutes (performing any needed interventions), recording your findings and noting any trends in his condition.

The importance of reassessment became clear in Brian's case. Unlike Mr. Schmidt, the medical patient whose condition improved somewhat during the trip to the hospital, Brian took a turn for the worse. Because you closely reevaluated his airway, you discovered that he had some fluid in his pharynx (which caused the gurgling sound), and so you suctioned him. His respiratory rate had decreased to the point where his breathing was inadequate, and so your partner began to assist his ventilations with a flow-restricted, oxygen-powered ventilation device.

The value of looking at trends also became apparent. If you look at Brian's vital signs (Table 15-1), you can see that his respiratory rate was decreasing, which is a bad sign in an unresponsive patient. During the course of Brian's recovery, your Quality Improvement officer checks with hospital personnel from time to time to see how he's doing. You are told that the quick work you and your partner did in opening Brian's airway and assisting his ventilations have prevented any brain damage that might have occurred. Brian is transferred to the rehabilitation institute and, after several months, returns to work.

Table 15-1 Vital Sign Trends for Brian Sawyer				
ASSESSMENT STEP	PULSE	RESPIRATIONS	BLOOD PRESSURE	OXYGEN SATURATION
Secondary assessment	120, regular and weak	14 and normal	110/80	96 percent
Reassessment	132, regular and weak	8 and shallow	100/P (by palpation)	95 percent

CHAPTER REVIEW

Key Facts and Concepts

- Reassessment is the last step in your patient assessment.
- You should reassess a stable patient at least every 15 minutes and an unstable patient at least every 5 minutes.
- Elements of reassessment include repeating the primary assessment, repeating and recording vital signs, repeating pertinent parts of the history and physical exam, and checking the interventions you performed for the patient.
- Interventions you need to check include oxygen, bleeding, spine immobilization, and splints.

Key Decisions

- Has the patient's condition changed in any way that indicates the need for new interventions? Is the airway clear? Is breathing adequate? Is circulation intact?
- Are the interventions I performed functioning as they should?
- Do I need to adjust any of the interventions I initially applied?

Chapter Glossary

reassessment a procedure for detecting changes in a patient's condition. It involves four steps: repeating the primary assessment, repeating and recording vital signs, repeating the physical exam, and checking interventions.

trending changes in a patient's condition over time, such as slowing respirations or rising pulse rate, that may show improvement or deterioration, and that can be shown by documenting repeated assessments.

Preparation for Your Examination and Practice

Short Answer

1. Name the four steps of reassessment and list what assessments you will make during each step.
2. Explain the value of recording, or documenting, your assessment findings, and explain the meaning of the term *trending*.

Thinking and Linking

Think back to Chapter 6, "Principles of Pathophysiology," and link information from that chapter with information from this chapter as you consider the following situation.

- You are transporting an 80-year-old man with general weakness that, according to his description, has been coming and going all morning. His initial vital signs were pulse 84, blood pressure 130/80, respirations 18 and full, SpO_2 98 percent. En route, he tells you that he's having one of his "weak spells" and that he's also dizzy. You check his vital signs again and find the following: pulse 180, blood pressure 90/70, respirations 22 and full, SpO_2 95 percent. How would an extremely rapid pulse cause such a change in vital signs and his chief complaint?

Critical Thinking Exercises

The reassessment must be conducted with the same care and attention to needed interventions as in the primary and secondary assessments. The purpose of this exercise will be to consider how you might manage certain situations you might discover during reassessment.

- What do you need to do if your reassessment turns up one of these findings?
  1. Gurgling respirations
  2. Bag on nonrebreather mask collapses completely when the patient inhales
  3. Snoring respirations

Pathophysiology to Practice

The following question is designed to assist you in gathering relevant clinical information and making accurate decisions in the field.

- Your patient is having an asthma attack. Her breathing rate is normal at 12 breaths per minute, but her blood oxygen level (SpO_2) is too low. Why?

You receive a call for an elderly woman with a possible stroke. After taking the appropriate Standard Precautions, you ensure scene safety and enter the house. An older man, identifying himself as the patient's husband, meets you at the door. As he leads you to the kitchen, he explains that he came home after being out for a while and found his wife unable to stand up. When you reach the kitchen, you find Althea Stokes sitting in a chair.

Your general impression is of an elderly woman who appears awake but is slumped onto her left side. As you introduce yourself, you notice the patient's eyes are open and she appears awake, but her speech is slow and slurred. She does not appear to be in pain. A small amount of saliva is drooling onto her blouse. Her airway is open (at least for the moment); breathing appears normal and unlabored; there is no sign of bleeding; and her radial pulse is strong, slightly rapid, and very irregular. You assign Mrs. Stokes a medium priority as a medical patient. In your BLS system, calling for advanced life support is not an option.

Street Scene Questions

1. How does the patient's mental status affect the way you maintain the patient's airway?
2. What questions should you ask the patient and her husband?

You wipe the saliva away from the patient's mouth and consider how to maintain her airway. If she loses consciousness, you should be prepared to suction. In the meantime, you make a mental note to keep an eye on further potential threats to her airway.

Since the patient is having difficulty speaking, you get most of the history from Mr. Stokes. His 82-year-old wife is usually alert and very active, he informs you. She was fine when he left about 4 hours ago, but when he came home, she was slumped over in the chair and couldn't seem to move her left arm and leg. When you ask Mrs. Stokes if she is having any pain or difficulty breathing, she slowly responds with slurred speech, "No, I'm not." As your partner gathers vital signs, you look at the patient more carefully. The right side of her face seems to be drooping, especially her cheek and upper eyelid. When you ask her to hold her arms out in front of her, she picks up her right arm, but can barely move her left one. When you ask her to smile, only the left side of her face moves. Her pupils are equal and reactive to light. Her vital signs are pulse 92 and irregular, blood pressure 180/96, respirations 20 and unlabored.

According to Mr. Stokes, the only medical problem his wife has is high blood pressure, for which she takes just one medication, Vasotec. She has no allergies to medications. She is a patient of Dr. Newman and has not been hospitalized recently.

Because her brain might not be getting enough oxygen, you give her 12 liters per minute by nonrebreather mask even though

she has an oxygen saturation of 98 percent. You take special care to put Mrs. Stokes on her left side on the stretcher so she is able to still move her right arm and saliva will not obstruct her airway.

Street Scene Question

3. How should you perform a reassessment on this patient?

En route, you contact the receiving hospital and report on the patient's condition and treatment. You repeat her vital signs and this time get a pulse of 88 and irregular, blood pressure of 170 by palpation, and respirations of 22 and unlabored. When you ask the patient how she feels now, she replies in a clear voice, "Why, much better, young man." Surprised at this sudden improvement, you proceed to assess her again. She can now hold both arms up in front of her with her eyes closed. When she smiles, there is no longer any sign of a deficit. Cheered up by this turn of events, you confirm that her husband's version of events is accurate. You also learn that Mrs. Stokes has led an interesting life, having been a history teacher for 40 years.

About 5 minutes after this improvement, you notice that the patient seems to be having trouble speaking again. When you ask her to hold her arms out in front of her, she is able to pick both of them up, but her left arm drifts off and falls down. Her smile barely shows her teeth. When you ask her to repeat the phrase, "The sky is blue in Cincinnati," she can get only the first few words out and only with great difficulty. Concerned about these changes in the patient's condition, you call the hospital again and advise them of the developments.

When you arrive at the emergency department a few minutes later, Mrs. Stokes' condition has not changed again. The nurse undresses her and the emergency physician assesses her as you prepare the ambulance for the next call and complete your patient care report. Just as you are finishing the report, the doctor comes out of the patient's room. "Well, I'm glad you brought this patient here," he says. "She's not a candidate for clot-busting drugs, but since this is a teaching hospital, we can offer Mrs. Stokes the opportunity to participate in a research project evaluating a new experimental treatment for stroke."

"Do you think she's really having a stroke?" you ask. "Her condition kept changing, getting better and then getting worse again."

Knowing that understanding the manifestations of a disease in a patient is an important part of Quality Improvement, the doctor tells you, "We often see changes in the condition of stroke patients in the first few hours of the episode. It can make assessment a real challenge. I'm glad you were able to detect the changes and let us know about them."

With a new appreciation for the value of a reassessment, you return to your service area, ready for another call.

Critical Thinking and Decision Making

16

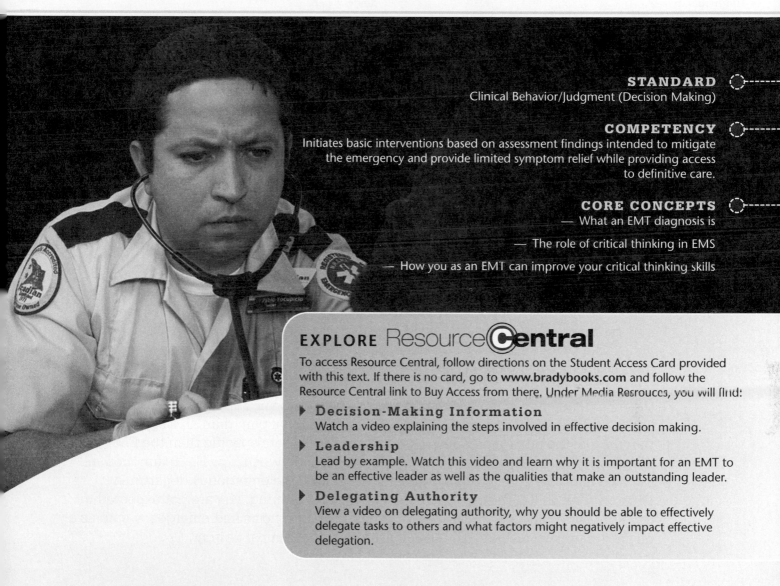

STANDARD ⊙------
Clinical Behavior/Judgment (Decision Making)

COMPETENCY ⊙------
Initiates basic interventions based on assessment findings intended to mitigate the emergency and provide limited symptom relief while providing access to definitive care.

CORE CONCEPTS ⊙------
— What an EMT diagnosis is
— The role of critical thinking in EMS
— How you as an EMT can improve your critical thinking skills

EXPLORE Resource**Central**

To access Resource Central, follow directions on the Student Access Card provided with this text. If there is no card, go to **www.bradybooks.com** and follow the Resource Central link to Buy Access from there. Under Media Resrouces, you will find:

▶ **Decision-Making Information**
Watch a video explaining the steps involved in effective decision making.

▶ **Leadership**
Lead by example. Watch this video and learn why it is important for an EMT to be an effective leader as well as the qualities that make an outstanding leader.

▶ **Delegating Authority**
View a video on delegating authority, why you should be able to effectively delegate tasks to others and what factors might negatively impact effective delegation.

OBJECTIVES

After reading this chapter you should be able to:

16.1 Define key terms introduced in this chapter.

16.2 Compare and contrast EMTs' and physicians' diagnoses. (p. 382)

16.3 Explain the relationship between critical thinking and diagnosis. (pp. 382–383)

16.4 Explain typical steps used in the basic approach to reaching diagnoses. (pp. 383–384)

16.5 Explain how diagnosis in emergency situations may differ from traditional approaches to diagnosis. (pp. 384–385)

16.6 Identify some of the special challenges to EMS providers in the diagnostic process. (pp. 385–386)

16.7 Discuss the relationship between diagnosis and treatment in emergency situations. (pp. 385–386)

(continued)

16.8 Discuss the benefits and pitfalls of diagnostic shortcuts (heuristics). (pp. 386–389)

16.9 Identify heuristics commonly used by highly experienced physicians. (pp. 386–389)

16.10 Describe ways in which EMTs can improve their critical thinking processes. (pp. 389–390)

KEY TERMS

critical thinking, *p. 383*
diagnosis, *p. 382*

differential diagnosis, *p. 383*

EMS diagnosis/EMT diagnosis, *p. 383*

red flag, *p. 384*

For years, EMTs have heard, "EMTs don't diagnose." In reality, there are conditions that EMTs have to diagnose, like cardiac arrest. There are also conditions that EMTs don't diagnose, like tetanus. However, paramedics and emergency physicians don't typically make the diagnosis of tetanus, either. What's the difference between the **diagnosis** an EMT makes and the diagnosis other health care providers make?

Cardiac arrest is at one end of a spectrum of diagnoses that stretches all the way from minor conditions like a cut finger to liver lacerations and lung cancer and beyond. EMTs learn enough to diagnose a few things, although the EMT's conclusion may be a very generalized diagnosis. For example, an EMT may say that a patient has abdominal pain of unknown cause. Although this sounds vague, it is the same diagnosis emergency physicians may use when, after both laboratory and radiologic testing, the cause of a patient's abdominal pain still cannot be determined. Of course, the emergency physician has the training, experience, and resources to rule out (exclude) and diagnose many more causes of abdominal pain than an EMT does. For that reason, the emergency physician's diagnosis is more specific than the EMT's diagnosis. Nonetheless, there are some similarities between how EMTs function in the field and how emergency physicians function in the emergency department. Obviously, as an EMT with only about 150 hours of training, you are not expected to have the same depth of knowledge or expertise in diagnosis and emergency care as a physician with thousands of hours of classroom and clinical training.

>>>>>> EMT DIAGNOSIS AND CRITICAL THINKING

diagnosis
a description or label for a patient's condition that assists a clinician in further evaluation and treatment.

An EMT's diagnosis is a description or label for a patient's condition, based on the patient's history, physical exam, and vital signs, that assists the EMT in further evaluation and treatment. It may be referred to by other names: *EMS diagnosis, EMT diagnosis*, field diagnosis, presumptive diagnosis, or working diagnosis. Regardless of the name, they all refer to how EMTs come to a conclusion, after assessing a patient, about the nature of the patient's condition (or sometimes what it is not). The process of reaching a diagnosis involves a great deal of simultaneous activity, both physical and intellectual. It is sometimes difficult to determine in the field how much information to get and when to get it. The process that assists the EMT in doing this is called *critical thinking*.

● **CORE CONCEPT**
What an EMT diagnosis is

 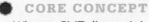

There are many descriptions of critical thinking. It is an analytical process that can help someone think through a problem in an organized and efficient manner. It is also thinking that is reflective, reasonable, and focused on deciding what to do in a particular situation. Some people describe it as an attitude of inquiry that involves the use of facts, principles, theories, and other pieces of information. All of these descriptions contain some truth. However, this chapter is going to focus primarily on critical thinking as an analytical process that can help someone think through a problem in an organized and efficient manner.

For example, suppose an EMT is assessing a patient with abdominal pain. He does a primary assessment, gathers the history of the present illness and past medical history, performs a pertinent physical exam, and institutes treatment and transport. After completing all of these steps, the EMT still is unsure of what is causing the patient's condition. The patient might have an abdominal aortic aneurysm, pancreatitis, gallstones, a duodenal ulcer, or any of a variety of other conditions. Although a physician may be able to diagnose many of these specific conditions, that ability usually requires a significant amount of training, experience, clinical skill, laboratory tests, imaging, and perhaps even consultation with a specialist. How would a clinician determine what is wrong with this patient?

HOW A CLINICIAN REACHES A DIAGNOSIS

Different clinicians have different levels of training and experience, time, technology, and other resources. Despite all of these differences, they all have to reach some kind of conclusion about what is wrong with the patient and what kind of treatment to administer. All clinicians begin with the same basic approach: gather information, consider possibilities, and reach a conclusion. The way they implement these steps, however, varies significantly.

The Traditional Approach to Diagnosis in Medicine

The first step in the traditional approach to diagnosis is assessing the patient (Figure 16-1). Next, the clinician draws up a list of conditions or diagnoses that could be causing the patient's condition. This list is called a *differential diagnosis* or just "the differential." To determine which of the potential diagnoses is correct, the patient receives further evaluation and perhaps some tests to rule in or rule out the diagnoses on the list. Once the results of the assessment and tests are known, the clinician considers those results and excludes conditions that are unlikely to be correct. In the end, this results in a diagnosis (or, in some cases, a few

EMS diagnosis/EMT diagnosis
a description or label for a patient's condition, based on the patient's history, physical exam, and vital signs, that assists the EMT in further evaluation and treatment. An EMS diagnosis is often less specific than a traditional medical diagnosis.

critical thinking
an analytical process that can help someone think through a problem in an organized and efficient manner.

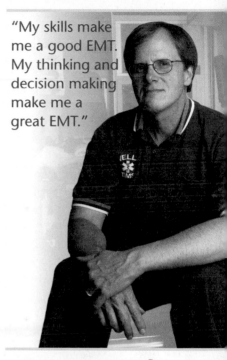

"My skills make me a good EMT. My thinking and decision making make me a great EMT."

CORE CONCEPT

The role of critical thinking in EMS

differential diagnosis
a list of potential diagnoses compiled early in the assessment of the patient.

FIGURE 16-1 The traditional approach to reaching a diagnosis includes interviewing the patient in the controlled environment of a clinic or office.

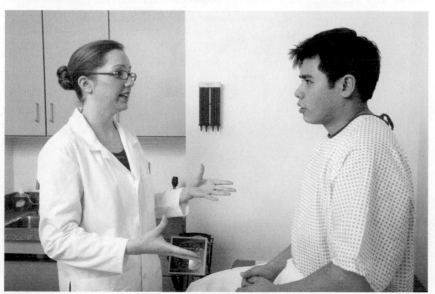

FIGURE 16-2 The traditional approach to diagnosis in medicine.

TRADITIONAL APPROACH TO DIAGNOSIS IN MEDICINE

Patient assessment (history, physical exam, vital signs, tests)

List of possible causes/diagnoses (differential diagnosis)

↓

Further evaluation

↓

Consider results of evaluation

↓

Narrow the list (may have to consider additional possibilites before reaching a diagnosis)

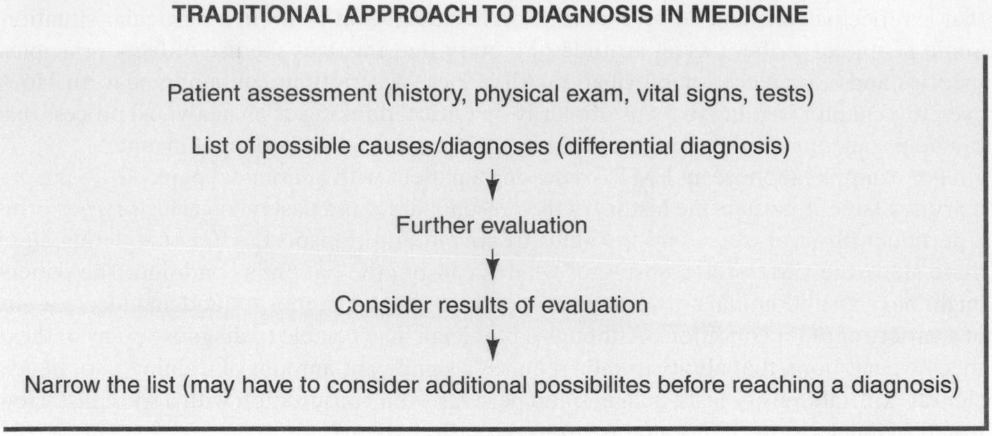

possible diagnoses). Sometimes, as a result of the additional assessment, the list becomes longer before it can be narrowed down (Figure 16-2).

The Emergency Medicine Approach to Diagnosis

The emergency physician often does not have the time or the resources to use the traditional approach to reach a diagnosis. Instead, because of the unique circumstances and environment of the emergency department, his goals are ruling out life-threatening conditions, narrowing the range of possible diagnoses, and instituting urgent treatment. Part of the treatment may often be referral to the patient's own physician or a specialist to conduct further evaluation once the emergency physician determines that the patient's condition does not require admission to the hospital.

The first step in the emergency department, therefore, is to quickly rule out or identify and treat immediate life threats. Once that is done, the physician gathers information from the patient, family, and friends and performs a physical exam (Figure 16-3). The focus of much of the questioning and assessment is to rule out the worst-case scenarios (i.e., the conditions that may threaten the patient's life or quality of life later on). The emergency physician looks for *red flags*, which are signs or symptoms that suggest the possibility of a particular problem that is very serious. For example, sudden onset of tearing pain in the abdomen that radiates to the back is a red flag that suggests an abdominal aortic aneurysm.

red flag
a sign or symptom that suggests the possibility of a particular problem that is very serious.

FIGURE 16-3 The emergency physician assesses patients in the busy, hectic atmosphere of an emergency department. *(©Edward T. Dickinson)*

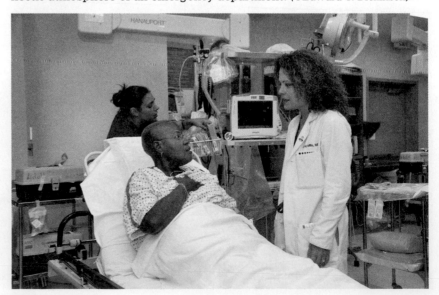

FIGURE 16-4 The emergency medicine approach to reaching a diagnosis.

EMERGENCY MEDICINE APPROACH TO DIAGNOSIS

Primary assessment to find and treat immediate threats to life

Patient assessment (history, physical exam, vital signs, tests) with special attention to looking for red flags

Consider the most serious conditions associated with the patient's presentation and rule them in or out (rule out the worst case scenario)

List of possible causes/diagnoses (differential diagnosis)

↓

Further evaluation in light of time and resources available in the ED

↓

Consider results of evaluation

↓

Narrow the list (may have to re-state the chief complaint as the diagnosis)

The information obtained from the secondary assessment guides the clinician in formulating a differential diagnosis, leading him to ask further questions and order particular tests. However, not every test is available to the physician in the ED. A patient with a 4-week-old knee injury will probably have to wait to get an MRI (magnetic resonance imaging) to see what is going on inside the joint. The emergency physician is therefore working with less information than the physician in an office environment. Once additional information is available from the laboratory and other tests, the physician considers it and comes to a diagnosis and disposition. The diagnosis may be very specific, like appendicitis, or it may be as general as abdominal pain of unknown cause (Figure 16-4).

All of this occurs in the busy, hectic environment of the emergency department, where the physician may be caring for four or five (or more) patients simultaneously and is frequently being interrupted with additional information or questions.

The EMS Approach to Diagnosis

The EMT has a lot in common with the emergency physician. He has limited resources available, has few treatment options (although those he does have are very important), and knows time is of the essence. Unlike the emergency physician, however, the EMT cannot usually care for four or five patients simultaneously. Since the EMT has to go to the patient, the EMT is unavailable for other patients until that first patient has been delivered to another clinician. This puts pressure on the EMT to be very efficient; the sooner he completes his duties with one patient, the sooner he can get to the next. The EMT also works in an uncontrolled environment (Figure 16-5). For example, the emergency physician does not usually have to worry about being bitten by a patient's dog. However, emergency physicians do occasionally encounter violent patients in the ED, just as the EMT does in the field.

The tools the EMT has available in the field differ, too. Although the amount of technology used in the field has increased tremendously over the last 10 to 20 years, EMTs have nowhere near the resources available in an ED. An EMT can merely evaluate a patient's vital signs and oxygen level of the blood, whereas the emergency physician can order multiple blood tests and imaging studies like X-rays, ultrasound, and CT (computed tomography) scans. The EMT's education focuses narrowly on certain conditions that have high statistical morbidity (illness) or mortality (death), whereas the emergency physician completes at least 3 years of postgraduate training after 4 years of medical school. Most important, much of that education is spent seeing thousands of patients and learning assessment and management skills under supervision.

All of this means that although the EMT will follow many of the same steps the emergency physician does in reaching a diagnosis, most of the EMT's diagnostic steps will be abbreviated or limited. The EMT's primary assessment finds and treats the patient's immediate life threats.

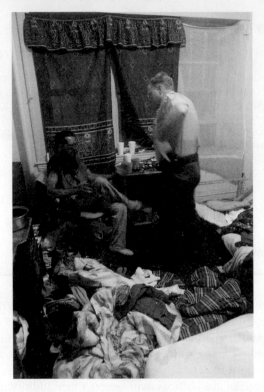

FIGURE 16-5 The EMT assesses a patient in the uncontrolled environment of the field. (© *Mark C. Ide*)

Secondary assessment—consisting of the patient's history, physical exam, vital signs and a few tests—comes next, with special attention devoted to looking for red flags. Simultaneously, the EMT begins treatment that may be beneficial and is not harmful. The most common example of this is administering oxygen.

The EMT then considers the most serious conditions associated with the patient's presentation that can be treated in the field and quickly rules them in or out, so that important treatment can be administered as quickly as possible. If the patient has no life-threatening conditions and no red flags, the EMT creates a mental list of possible causes or diagnoses (a differential diagnosis). This list will often be short (e.g., in a patient with abdominal pain, the differential may be abdominal aortic aneurysm, gastrointestinal bleeding, dehydration, and all other causes of abdominal pain).

Next, depending on the situation, there may be further evaluation limited by the time and resources available in the field. This further evaluation may take place while en route to the hospital. After considering the results of any additional evaluation, the EMT may be able to narrow the list of possible diagnoses. In many cases, this may simply be a restatement of the chief complaint (e.g., abdominal pain) as the diagnosis (Figure 16-6).

Although all three of these approaches to diagnosis—traditional, emergency medicine, and EMS—have a lot in common, some differences clearly exist (Table 16-1).

The Highly Experienced Physicians' Approach to Diagnosis

Very experienced physicians do not always use the traditional approach of drawing up an extensive list and narrowing it down. Instead, they have learned "shortcuts" (also called heuristics) that speed up the process of reaching a diagnosis. These shortcuts, based on pattern recognition, help make physicians better, more efficient clinicians. The expert clinician can quickly recognize certain features of a patient's presentation that significantly narrow the diagnostic possibilities. The experienced physician can also quickly determine what further evaluation is necessary to rule in or rule out certain possibilities. As a result, highly experienced physicians can reach difficult diagnoses or conclusions more quickly than newer physicians who need more time to consider the possibilities.

FIGURE 16-6 The EMS approach to reaching a diagnosis.

EMS APPROACH TO DIAGNOSIS

Primary assessment to find and treat immediate threats to life

Patient assessment (history, physical exam, vital signs, tests) with
special attention to looking for red flags
Simultaneously, the EMT begins treatment that may be beneficial
and is not harmful, e.g., oxygen

Consider the most serious conditions associated with the patient's
presentation that can be treated in the field and rule them in or out

List of possible causes/diagnoses (differential diagnosis) if time
allows
↓
Further evaluation in light of limited time available and restricted
resources present in the field
↓
Consider results of evaluation
↓
Narrow the list (may have to re-state the chief complaint as the
diagnosis)

Shortcuts to diagnosis have limitations, of course. Experienced clinicians understand this and keep in mind avoidable traps so that their conclusions are as accurate as possible.

As you gain experience in the medical field, you can start to develop shortcuts like experienced physicians do. In doing so, however, you will need to understand the advantages and shortcomings of shortcuts, or heuristics. Here are some of the more common heuristics and their biases.

 Representativeness. Representativeness means that when you encounter a patient with a certain group of signs and symptoms that resemble a particular condition, you assume the patient has that condition. Representativeness is at the heart of pattern recognition and is

Table 16-1	Approaches to Reaching a Diagnosis		
	TRADITIONAL APPROACH	**EMERGENCY MEDICINE APPROACH**	**EMS APPROACH**
Goal	Reach definitive diagnosis and institute treatment	Rule out life-threatening conditions, narrow range of possible diagnoses, and institute urgent treatment	Rule out life-threatening conditions, narrow range of possible diagnoses, institute treatment important to patient survival and comfort, and transport for more extensive assessment and treatment
Pace	Leisurely	Efficient	Urgent
Thoroughness	Very thorough	Focused	Limited
Assessment Tools and Tests	Wide range of tests patient can be sent for	Limited to pertinent tests that are available at the time of the patient's presentation	A few tools pertinent to finding serious conditions quickly, like BP cuff and pulse oximeter
Extent of Patient Rapport	Significant	Limited	Limited with short transport times, greater with long transport times
Range of Possible Diagnoses	Extensive	Moderate	Limited

an important heuristic. What is its disadvantage? Patients don't always present with the typical signs and symptoms of a condition. As a result, when a patient doesn't fit the classic pattern, it's easy for the health care provider to mistakenly conclude the patient doesn't have that condition. For example, older patients with myocardial infarctions sometimes deny chest pain and complain instead of shortness of breath or weakness as their chief complaint.

To avoid this trap, remain aware of its possibility. Remind yourself that patients don't read the textbooks and can present with uncommon or atypical signs or symptoms.

A way to summarize representativeness is to think of the saying, "If it looks like a duck and quacks like a duck, it must be a duck—except when it isn't."

- **Availability.** Availability is the urge to think of things because they are more easily recalled, often because of a recent exposure. For example, if an EMT has a patient with chest pain who is diagnosed with a dissecting thoracic aneurysm, the next time he sees a patient with chest pain, he is more likely to think of dissecting thoracic aneurysm as a possibility, even though the condition is much less common than angina and myocardial infarctions. Because of his recent exposure to this condition, he may overestimate its frequency.

  You can reduce your chances of falling into this trap by asking yourself just how common the particular condition is that you're considering and whether you're considering it mainly because it matches information that is easily available. One way to think of the problem of availability is the EMT's tendency to say, "You have the same thing my last patient had!"

- **Overconfidence.** Being an EMT requires a significant degree of confidence. Without it, the EMT is unable to function in a chaotic environment. Overconfidence, however, can work against the EMT. Thinking you know more than you really do can lead to many problems. A good way to avoid this tendency is to be aware of the limits of your knowledge and ability. Be careful in your assessment, however. Surveys consistently show that people think they know more than they actually do.

  When faced with a clinical situation, try to be as objective as possible when evaluating how much evidence has been gathered and whether it has been gathered in a logical and thorough fashion. Try to keep your ego out of this self-evaluation as much as possible. You can summarize the problem of overconfidence as, "Of course I know what to do. I'm an EMT!"

- **Confirmation bias.** A clinician commits confirmation bias when he primarily looks for evidence that supports the diagnosis he already has in mind. By doing so, he may very well overlook evidence that refutes or reduces the probability of that diagnosis. This commonly occurs when the patient's presentation includes a lot of information and the clinician feels it's easier to go with one diagnosis rather than look for others.

  To avoid this pitfall, look for data that refutes the diagnosis you have in mind or reduces the likelihood of it. In other words, look for contrary data and consider competing hypotheses. The tendency to look only for information that supports what you already think is reflected in the saying, "It must be right—I thought of it!"

- **Illusory correlation.** Human beings are able to draw conclusions about how the world works because they are able to see how one thing causes another. However, this human tendency can be misleading sometimes. Very often, one event may appear to cause another when, in fact, the two events are either coincidental or both caused by the same thing, leading to illusory correlation. For example, some believe that fluoridated water causes cancer. It is true that communities that have fluoridated their water have a higher rate of cancer than rural areas. Therefore, it would be very easy to conclude that one caused the other. However, when you look more closely at the data, you discover that cities are more likely than rural areas to fluoridate their water. Cities have higher rates of cancer than rural areas in general. Furthermore, cities that fluoridate have the same incidence of cancer as cities that do not fluoridate. Therefore, the appearance of cause and effect in this case is an illusion.

  To avoid this illusion, be skeptical about instances where one thing appears to cause another. Consider how the appearance of two things together may be just coincidence or, alternatively, consider that they may both have the same cause. An easy way to remember illusory correlation is to think of this: "Most ice cream is eaten during the summer. Most drownings occur in the summer. Therefore, ice cream causes drowning."

- **Anchoring and adjustment.** In this situation, an EMT considers a particular condition to be likely, and his later thinking is anchored to that hypothesis. He may adjust it in time, but sometimes not as much as he should because of his starting point. For example, an EMT may initially think that an unconscious intoxicated person is unconscious because "he's just drunk." When information appears that the patient may have sustained head trauma, the EMT may cling to the hypothesis that the patient's real problem is just intoxication.

  To avoid this, be careful not to jump to conclusions and determine a diagnosis on the basis of just a few signs or symptoms. Do a thorough assessment. The tendency to cling to your first conclusion is exemplified in the saying, "You only get one chance to make a first impression."

- **Search satisfying.** It can be very satisfying to finally determine what is causing a patient's problem. However, once that happens, it becomes very easy to stop looking for other causes of potential problems. This is called "search satisfying." The problem with search satisfying is that you can miss a secondary diagnosis (many EMS patients have more than one problem) or just be mistaken in the primary diagnosis. If you don't look for other problems, you will probably not detect them.

  A good way to prevent this problem is to keep an open mind about other possibilities and to evaluate each diagnosis before accepting it. This principle is well stated in the saying, "Don't count your chickens before they hatch."

HOW AN EMT CAN LEARN TO THINK LIKE AN EXPERIENCED PHYSICIAN

The following list features attitudes and understandings you can develop to help you think like an expert.

CORE CONCEPT
How you as an EMT can improve your critical thinking skills

- **Learn to love ambiguity.** This is at the core of EMS. Working in EMS means you are going out into unknown situations armed with limited education and experience (compared to physicians and many other clinicians) and equipped with limited tools and treatments. You are expected to make decisions, including some life-or-death decisions, in a very short period of time before you transport the patient to definitive care. You will not be able to gather the same amount of information that staff does in a hospital and you have a limited range of treatments to provide your patients. No matter how conscientious and knowledgeable you are, you will run into situations where you just can't find a definitive answer to the question of why a patient is sick. That is the nature of EMS. By accepting that uncertainty is a natural part of what you do, you will actually become a better provider, able to understand the limitations of your knowledge and how this affects your patient care.

- **Understand the limitations of technology and people.** No one is perfect. Every human being makes errors. Some people go about procedures in ways you would never think of doing. Once you accept this, you will find it easier to work in the everyday world where things don't always go as you planned. When you get information from someone else, whether a crew member, patient, or bystander, consider the source. How accurate and reliable do you judge the source to be? Is there a potential source of bias that might affect the way that person reports information? Is there a limited skill level or lack of familiarity with EMS that should make you consider how to process information from someone else?

  Similarly, no piece of equipment is perfect. Every mechanical or electronic device is subject to failure, whether from low batteries, inappropriate use, or excessive wear. When you get a reading from a device that doesn't make sense for the clinical picture in front of you, don't accept it as necessarily correct. If possible, have the device repeat the reading. Consider how the unexpected result could affect your management of the patient. In the end, you may need to make a decision regarding whether to accept an anomalous reading or go with your clinical judgment. Whether you made the correct decision is often not clear until later.

- **Realize that no one strategy works for everything.** No matter how experienced and skilled you become, you will encounter situations that don't work well for your particular approach to EMS calls. In cases like this, it is important to be flexible and able to use more than just a single tactic. Times like this are when experts think like new clinicians. They have to formulate a longer list than usual of differential diagnoses and rule them in or out.

- **Form a strong foundation of knowledge.** Expert clinicians may use different approaches to thinking through problems, but one thing they all have in common is a strong foundation of knowledge. They are extremely familiar with the signs and symptoms of conditions they are expected to be familiar with. They are also very aware of conditions that can mimic those diseases. They keep up-to-date with new information on associated conditions that sometimes accompany those diseases. They have both the tools (the thinking processes) and the supplies (the knowledge to apply those tools to).

- **Organize the data in your head.** Create what experts call elaborated knowledge. Once you can list the signs and symptoms of a disease, work in the other direction. Take signs and symptoms and consider what other diseases they may be associated with. This actually creates new connections in your brain and provides practice for what you actually will do in the field. Reflect on how the presence or severity of a particular sign or symptom changes the probability of a particular disease or condition. At first, concentrate on a few diseases that have similar chief complaints. Study them until you know the signs and symptoms of each and then work from the signs and symptoms back to the problem.

- **Change the way you think.** Once you have mastered the presentations of several conditions, compare and contrast them. Determine what features the conditions have in common and what features set them apart from each other. Rephrase the symptoms a patient provides so that they match more closely the way a disease is described. For instance, if a patient complains of 9/10 pain in the middle of his stomach that hit him like a thunderbolt, characterize this as the sudden onset of severe pain in the center of the abdomen.

- **Learn from others.** Your EMT class is only part of your education. Take advantage of the exposure you get to expert clinicians and ask them to think out loud when they are solving problems. This will familiarize you with the ways an expert looks for information, processes it, and uses it to reach a diagnosis.

- **Reflect on what you have learned.** An essential part of being an expert clinician is learning from your experiences. Contrary to popular belief, people don't learn only from their mistakes. People learn even more from their successes. When someone succeeds in a venture, this reinforces the behavior that led to the success and leads to good habits. After a patient contact, especially a challenging one, evaluate your behavior. What did you do well? What can you do better? What did you learn that you didn't know before? What knowledge do you need to be more accurate and efficient in the future?

Keep in mind that once you have reached a possible diagnosis, your work is not necessarily over. You should continue looking for data that will help to rule in or rule out the conditions you are considering. A patient may have more than one thing wrong with him, so don't stop looking for causes too early. Your conclusion may also be wrong, so it is good to continue thinking about what may be wrong with the patient.

These steps can be used not only with reaching an EMT diagnosis, but also with many other problems. Being aware of how you think gives you a powerful tool for improving your information gathering and thought processes. Keep in mind that when you are faced with an unfamiliar situation you should go back to the basics. Do your assessment and follow the general principles outlined in your EMT course.

Reaching an EMT diagnosis is a process that you can learn. However, be careful not to expect too much of yourself at the beginning—the process of thinking critically is developed through study, practice, and reflection. It will take time to develop this skill. In the meantime, don't let anyone force you to go further than your level of competence. Know the boundaries of your knowledge, skill, and judgment. Overconfidence can be dangerous. Strive to learn more by study and observation of more experienced providers. Most important, don't let attempts to reach a diagnosis delay patient care that is safe and appropriate.

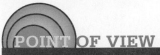
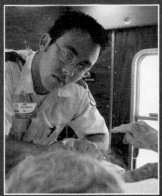

"Probably the best lesson I learned about critical thinking was to listen. You can't figure out what is going on without the facts. Sometimes it's the little pieces of information you could easily overlook. Other times it is the thought between the words that doesn't come out but you know it is there. Sure, you'll assess and take vitals. But trust me. You'll never find what you need to know unless you listen."

CHAPTER REVIEW

Key Facts and Concepts

- EMTs make some diagnoses in the field, although they are not as extensive or detailed as physicians' diagnoses.

- The traditional approach to reaching a diagnosis is to assess the patient, draw up a list of differential diagnoses, assess further to rule in or rule out different conditions, and narrow the list until you reach a conclusion.

- Highly experienced physicians don't always use the traditional approach. They use heuristics (shortcuts), in combination with their experience and training, which speed up the process of reaching a diagnosis.

- Shortcomings of heuristics include representativeness, anchoring and adjustment, overconfidence, confirmation bias, illusory correlation, and search satisfying.

- Learn to think more critically by accepting the ambiguity of EMS working conditions, understanding limitations of people and technology, forming a strong foundation of knowledge, and organizing the data in your mind.

- When considering the cause of a patient's condition, don't let your search for a cause delay your treatment of the patient.

Key Decisions

- Have I addressed life threats before beginning the assessment and diagnostic process?

- Does this patient have an obvious problem or do I need to think more critically?

- Are there other causes besides the obvious one for this patient's condition?

- Have I considered other reasonable possibilities?

- What other information should I get to confirm or refute the working diagnosis?

- How specific does my field diagnosis have to be to determine the right treatment?

- What is best for the patient?

Chapter Glossary

critical thinking an analytical process that can help someone think through a problem in an organized and efficient manner.

diagnosis a description or label for a patient's condition that assists a clinician in further evaluation and treatment.

differential diagnosis a list of potential diagnoses compiled early in the assessment of the patient.

EMS diagnosis/EMT diagnosis a description or label for a patient's condition, based on the patient's history, physical exam, and vital signs, that assists the EMT in further evaluation and treatment. An EMS diagnosis is often less specific than a traditional medical diagnosis.

red flag a sign or symptom that suggests the possibility of a particular problem that is very serious.

Preparation for Your Examination and Practice

Short Answer

1. How would you describe critical thinking?

2. What are the differences in the way an emergency physician reaches a diagnosis compared to the way an EMT reaches a diagnosis?

3. What are "search satisfying" and "confirmation bias"?

4. How can "overthinking" (considering too many possibilities) make it more difficult for an EMT to determine what to do for a patient?

Thinking and Linking

Think back to the chapters on pathophysiology and patient assessment, and link information from those chapters with the information in this chapter as you answer the following questions.

1. Why are patients who are *pale and sweaty* considered more serious than patients who aren't? How will seeing pale and sweaty patients affect your critical thinking and decision making?

2. Why are patients who are *anxious and restless* considered more serious than patients who aren't? How will seeing anxious and restless patients affect your critical thinking and decision making?

3. Why are patients with an *altered mental status* considered more serious than patients who aren't? How will seeing an altered mental status affect your critical thinking and decision making?

Critical Thinking Exercises

For the following patients, determine how the critical thinking process will interact with the patient assessment process you learned in the previous chapters. First, determine your priorities. Then, describe what information you may want to obtain for EMT diagnosis where appropriate.

1. A 52-year-old man complains of chest pain while sitting at his desk at work. He appears alert and oriented. He tells you he thinks it may "just be stress."

2. You are called to a 67-year-old man who was reportedly "acting unusually" when he became unresponsive. His wife said he complained of an odd feeling in his arm and his speech was slurred before he became unresponsive.

3. An 18-year-old snowboarder took a fall and thinks he may have broken his ankle.

4. A 41-year-old woman has difficulty breathing and a little pain when she breathes in deeply. She is alert but a little anxious.

Street Scenes

You are called to a patient with an altered mental status at an assisted living facility. The staff tells you that Mr. Ronson is normally very active and vibrant, "like the mayor of this place." But today he just isn't himself. He just sits in the chair and doesn't talk. "It is so unlike him," they say.

You arrive at the patient's side and introduce yourself. The patient turns his head toward you and acknowledges you with a grunting noise. His color appears OK. He is breathing deeply and regularly. His radial pulse is strong at about 60/minute and regular. You quickly check his pulse oximetry reading and it is 96 percent. You place him on 2 liters of oxygen via nasal cannula.

The attendant gives you a list of medications taken by the patient. They tell you he is diabetic and has had two heart attacks and one stroke. He also has high blood pressure and high cholesterol.

Street Scene Questions

1. Assuming that your primary assessment is completed, what would be your next assessment steps?
2. What body systems may be involved in causing this altered mental status?
3. How do the medications impact your history taking and decision making?

You further find that Mr. Ronson lives alone. He was fine when he went to bed last night, and was laughing and joking with the staff. His vital signs are pulse 58, strong and regular; respirations 22 and adequate; blood pressure 164/92; pupils equal and reactive; skin warm and slightly moist.

His medications all seem to match the conditions the staff reported. He has taken the meds with assistance from the staff. He has no known allergies and last ate yesterday afternoon. No one saw Mr. Ronson after he went to bed last night, so the events leading up to the current incident are unclear. He does appear to be able to follow your directions but not able to answer questions.

Street Scene Questions

4. What assessments would you perform on this patient and why?
5. What is your transport priority for the patient?
6. At what point would you call for an ALS intercept?

Mr. Ronson is able to perform a Cincinnati Prehospital Stroke Scale and does not show signs of stroke. Checking his blood glucose levels, you find a level of 32 mg/dL, which is significantly below normal. Because of his mental status you are concerned about his ability to swallow, so you notify ALS and request an intercept. Fortunately, they are close and respond before you leave the scene. They begin an IV and administer 50 percent dextrose. Mr. Ronson was joking again before he reached the hospital.

The medics commend you for figuring out what was wrong and for the initial report when they got to the scene.

Communication and Documentation

17

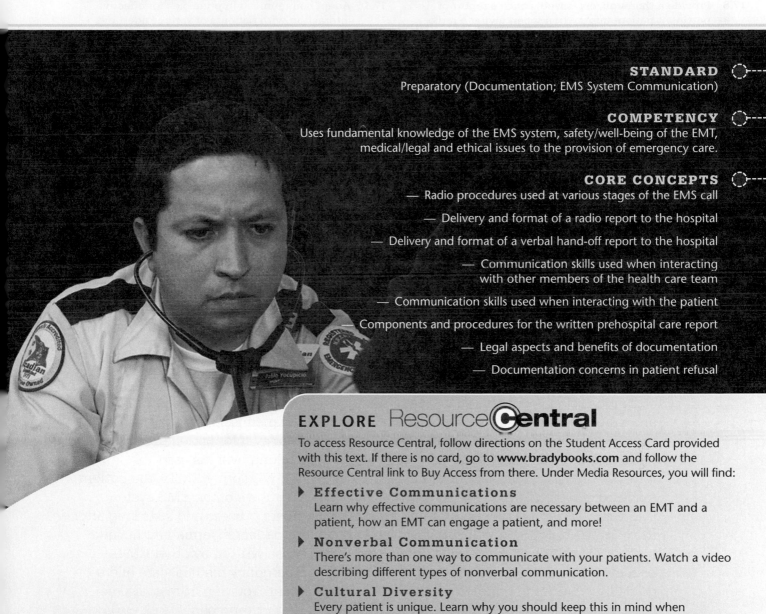

STANDARD ⊙-----
Preparatory (Documentation; EMS System Communication)

COMPETENCY ⊙-----
Uses fundamental knowledge of the EMS system, safety/well-being of the EMT, medical/legal and ethical issues to the provision of emergency care.

CORE CONCEPTS ⊙-----
— Radio procedures used at various stages of the EMS call

— Delivery and format of a radio report to the hospital

— Delivery and format of a verbal hand-off report to the hospital

— Communication skills used when interacting with other members of the health care team

— Communication skills used when interacting with the patient

— Components and procedures for the written prehospital care report

— Legal aspects and benefits of documentation

— Documentation concerns in patient refusal

EXPLORE Resource**Central**

To access Resource Central, follow directions on the Student Access Card provided with this text. If there is no card, go to **www.bradybooks.com** and follow the Resource Central link to Buy Access from there. Under Media Resources, you will find:

▶ **Effective Communications**
Learn why effective communications are necessary between an EMT and a patient, how an EMT can engage a patient, and more!

▶ **Nonverbal Communication**
There's more than one way to communicate with your patients. Watch a video describing different types of nonverbal communication.

▶ **Cultural Diversity**
Every patient is unique. Learn why you should keep this in mind when approaching your patient and why you should be sensitive to your patients' different cultural beliefs and values.

OBJECTIVES

After reading this chapter you should be able to:

17.1 Define key terms introduced in this chapter.

17.2 Describe the role of communication technology in EMS systems. (p. 394)

17.3 Describe various types of communication devices and equipment used in EMS system communication. (pp. 394–396)

(continued)

KEY TERMS

You will learn about several types of communication in this chapter: radio communication, the verbal report at the hospital, interpersonal communication, and documentation. As the name implies, radio communication is conducted by radio. Technology has allowed the use of cell phones and other equipment to be used in areas where radio transmissions were previously the only choice. The verbal report is your chance to convey information about your patient directly to the hospital personnel who will be taking over his care. Interpersonal communications are important in dealing with other EMTs, the patient, family and bystanders, medical direction, and other members of the EMS system.

Documentation is an important part of the patient care process and lasts long after the call. The report you write will become a part of the patient's permanent hospital record. As records of your agency, your reports and those written by other EMTs become a valuable source for research on trends in emergency medical care and a guide for continuing education and quality improvement. Your report may also be used as evidence in a legal case. Documentation has short-term benefits as well. Noting vital signs and a patient's history will help you remember important facts about the patient during the course of the call.

>>>>>>

COMMUNICATIONS SYSTEMS AND RADIO COMMUNICATION

Radio equipment is often taken for granted since it is now so common (Figure 17-1). However, the development of radio links between dispatchers, mobile units, and hospitals has been one of the key contributors to improvement in EMS over the years. Imagine if you had to call the dispatcher by phone every few minutes to see if there is a call! Without radio transmissions from ambulances, hospitals would be unable to prepare for the arrival of patients, as they do now.

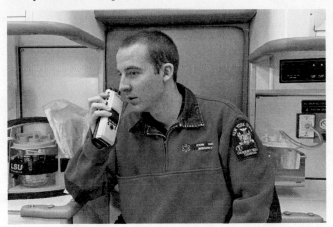

FIGURE 17-1 Communication from the ambulance can be by radio or cell phone.

Communications Systems

There are a number of components to any radio or communications system: base stations, mobile radios, portable radios, repeaters, cell phones, and other devices.

- **Base stations** are two-way radios that are at a fixed site such as a hospital or dispatch center.
- **Mobile radios** are two-way radios that are used or affixed in a vehicle. Most are actually mounted inside the vehicle. These devices have lower transmitting power than base stations. The unit used to measure output power of radios is the *watt*. The output of a mobile radio is generally 20–50 watts with a range of 10–15 miles.
- **Portable radios** are handheld two-way radios with an output of 1–5 watts. This type of radio is important because it will allow you to be in touch with the dispatcher, medical direction, and other members of the EMS system while you are away from the ambulance.
- **Repeaters** are devices that are used when transmissions must be carried over a long distance. Repeaters may be in ambulances or placed in various areas around an EMS system. The repeater picks up signals from lower-power units, such as mobile and portable radios, and retransmits them at a higher power. The retransmission is done on another frequency (Figure 17-2).
- **Cell phones** are phones that transmit through the air to a cell tower. In many areas where the distances or expense is too great to set up a conventional EMS radio system, cell phones allow EMS communications through an already established commercial system. Cell phones are not always a solution to the problem of radio communication, however, because a cell phone needs to be able to reach a cell tower or site. As the number of cell towers increases, the ability to use these devices should improve.

New technology is developing almost constantly. For example, microwave radio transmissions are used in some areas. In others, radio communications are carried via phone lines for part of the signal's journey from one point to another. Digital radio equipment permits transmission of some standard messages, such as ambulance identification or arrival at the scene, by punching a key. The messages are transmitted in a condensed form that helps keep busy frequencies less crowded.

Since radios are so important to EMS today, many systems have backup radios. This means that in the event of power failure or malfunction, another option is available. For example, if the base station fails, there may be a backup radio or alternative power supply available. If the mobile radio in your ambulance malfunctions, portable radios or phones may be used in its place.

Note that radio systems require preventive maintenance and repair, just like the ambulance and your EMS equipment. Radio equipment must be treated with care on a daily basis and not mishandled.

base station
a two-way radio at a fixed site such as a hospital or dispatch center.

mobile radio
a two-way radio that is used or affixed in a vehicle.

watt
the unit of measurement of the output power of a radio.

portable radio
a handheld two-way radio.

repeater
a device that picks up signals from lower-power radio units, such as mobile and portable radios, and retransmits them at a higher power. It allows low-power radio signals to be transmitted over longer distances.

cell phone
a phone that transmits through the air instead of over wires so that the phone can be transported and used over a wide area.

FIGURE 17-2 Example of an EMS communication system using repeaters.

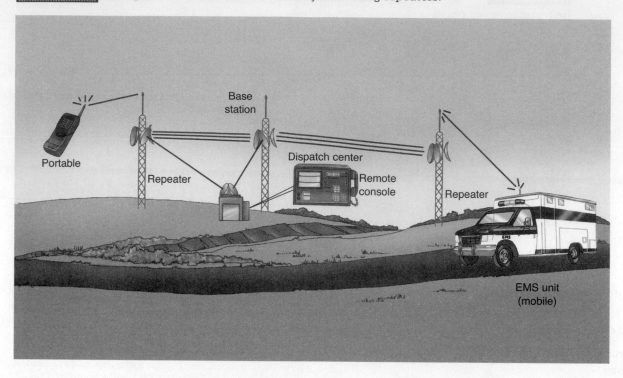

Radio Communication

EMS is just one of many public services that use radio communication. To maintain order on the airwaves, the Federal Communications Commission (FCC) assigns and licenses radio frequencies. This prevents two or more agencies from trying to use the same frequency and interfering with each other's communications. There are also strict rules about interfering with emergency radio traffic and prohibiting profanities or offensive language.

Some general rules for radio transmissions should always be followed. These rules prevent delays and allow all persons to use the frequencies. Although there may be some minor variations within your EMS system, always keep in mind the principles shown in Table 17-1.

Radio Transmissions throughout the Call

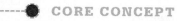

CORE CONCEPT

Radio procedures used at various stages of the EMS call

The initial call for help received by the Emergency Medical Dispatcher (EMD) most often comes via telephone but may also be radioed from another agency, such as the police. After proper information is obtained, the EMD dispatches the units. The following is a sample flow of information between the dispatcher and units in the field. You are the EMT on ambulance number 6:

Dispatcher: Ambulance 6. . . .

You: Ambulance 6. Go ahead.

Dispatcher: Ambulance 6, respond to 1243 Magnolia Boulevard—that's one-two-four-three Magnolia Boulevard—for an assault. The police are en route. Stand by at the corner of Magnolia and Third until the police report the scene secure.

You: Ambulance 6 received that. Will stand by at Magnolia and Third.

Without a prompt and efficient receipt and dispatch of information, the ambulance could easily be sent to the wrong location. In this situation, the dispatcher also relayed important safety information. Since the call was for an assault, the dispatcher "staged" the ambulance, or ordered it to stand by, until the scene was safe.

You respond to the assigned location, reporting your arrival to the dispatcher:

You: Dispatcher, Ambulance 6 is arriving at the staging area.

Dispatcher: Message received, Ambulance 6. I will advise you when the scene is secure.

Most scenes are safe. However, in this case the dispatcher has decided, from the nature of the call and other information he was able to obtain, that it is not. Police arrive at the scene

Table 17-1   Principles of Radio Communication

FOLLOW THESE PRINCIPLES WHEN USING THE EMS RADIO SYSTEM:

- Make sure that your radio is on and the volume is adjusted properly.
- Reduce background noise by closing the vehicle window when possible.
- Listen to the frequency and ensure that it is clear before beginning a transmission.
- Press the "press to talk" (PTT) button on the radio, then wait 1 second before speaking. This prevents cutting off the first few words of your transmission.
- Speak with your lips about 2 to 3 inches from the microphone.
- When calling another unit or base station, use their unit number or name, followed by yours. "Dispatcher, this is Ambulance 2."
- The unit being called will signal that the transmission should start by saying, "Go ahead" ("Ambulance 2, this is the dispatcher. Go ahead") or another regionally accepted term. If the unit you are calling tells you to "Stand by," wait until they tell you they are ready to take your transmission.
- Speak slowly and clearly.
- Keep the transmissions brief. If it takes longer than 30 seconds, stop at that point and pause for a few seconds so that emergency traffic can use the frequency if necessary.
- Use plain English. Avoid codes.
- Do not use phrases like "be advised." These are implied and serve no purpose.
- Courtesy is assumed, so there is no need to say "Please," "Thank you," and "You're welcome."
- When transmitting a number that might be unclear (15 may sound like 16 or 50), give the number, then repeat the individual digits. Say "15, one-five."
- Anything said over the radio can be heard by the public on a scanner. Do not use the patient's name over the radio. For the same reason, do not use profanities or statements that tend to slander any person. Use objective, impartial statements.
- Use "we" instead of "I." As an EMT, you will rarely be acting alone.
- "Affirmative" and "Negative" are preferred over "Yes" and "No" because the latter are difficult to hear.
- Give assessment information about your patient, but avoid offering a field diagnosis of the patient's problem. For example, say "Patient complains of chest pain" rather than "Patient is probably having a heart attack."
- After transmitting, say "Over." Wait for acknowledgment that the person to whom you were speaking heard your message.
- Avoid slang or abbreviations that are not authorized.
- Use EMS frequencies only for authorized EMS communication.

and separate the parties involved in the assault. The police radio the dispatcher and advise that the scene is secure. The next transmission is to your ambulance:

Dispatcher: Ambulance 6, the police report that the scene is secure. Respond in.

You: Message received by Ambulance 6. (You drive two blocks to the scene and report to the dispatcher.) Dispatcher, Ambulance 6 is at the scene.

Dispatcher: Ambulance 6 at the scene (gives the time on the 24-hour clock) at 1310 hours.

The dispatcher records all the times: the time of the original call, the time the ambulance was dispatched, the time when the ambulance reached the staging area, and finally the time when the ambulance arrived at the scene. Should this case go to court, the records of the dispatch center, your care report, and the dispatch audio tape of the call may be subpoenaed. Unless there is a need for medical direction or assistance from the scene, the next call will be when you are en route to the hospital:

You: Dispatcher, Ambulance 6 is en route to Mercy Hospital with one patient.

Dispatcher: Ambulance 6 en route to Mercy Hospital at 1323 hours.

You will call the hospital via radio or phone to advise them of the status of your patient and the estimated time of arrival (ETA). When arriving at the hospital, you again advise the dispatcher:

You: Ambulance 6 is arriving at Mercy Hospital.

Dispatcher: Ambulance 6 at Mercy at 1334 hours.

You will note that the dispatcher gives the time after most transmissions. This will allow you to record times if they are required on your patient care record. The dispatcher also usually acknowledges by briefly repeating the message to ensure that he has acknowledged the right unit. If two units happened to transmit at exactly the same time and the dispatcher simply acknowledged a transmission, both units would think that the dispatcher heard them when, actually, only one unit was able to get through.

After turning the patient over to the hospital staff and preparing the ambulance for the next run, you will advise the dispatcher that you are leaving the hospital. You may also find it part of your local procedure to advise the dispatcher when you are back in your district or area and when you are back in quarters (the station or ambulance garage).

A majority of these transmissions were made between the mobile radio within the ambulance and the dispatcher at a base station. Remember, when you have one available, bring your portable radio with you whenever you leave the ambulance. You may need to call for assistance during scene size-up if hazards or multiple patients are found, and the portable radio allows you to do that without running back to the ambulance to make the call on the fixed unit.

Radio Medical Reports

 CORE CONCEPT

Delivery and format of a radio report to the hospital

Reports must be made to medical personnel as part of almost every call. These reports may be by radio, verbally (in person), in writing, or in all three ways. The radio report is specifically structured to present pertinent facts about the patient without telling more detail than necessary. Too much detail ties up the radio frequency and takes up the time of hospital personnel.

In an effort to protect patient privacy, some hospitals encourage EMTs to use the telephone at the patient's house or a cell phone en route to the emergency department rather than the radio. Follow your local protocols.

Experienced EMTs try to "paint a picture" of the patient in words. This requires knowledge of radio procedure and practice. If you have a critical patient, your radio report should make that clear. This can be done by describing the chief complaint, injuries, vital signs, treatments, and mechanism of injury. Even with critical patients you must keep a clear, steady tone to your voice. Resist the urge to talk fast or appear excited as it will prevent effective communication.

A medical radio report has 12 parts (Table 17-2). The following example, broken into its individual parts, shows a report you might make to the hospital:

1. **Unit identification and level of provider**
   Memorial Hospital, this is Community BLS Ambulance 6 en route to your location . . .

2. **Estimated time of arrival**
   . . . with a 15-minute ETA.

3. **Patient's age and sex**
   We are transporting a 68-year-old male patient . . .

4. **Chief complaint**
   . . . who complains of pain in his abdomen.

Table 17-2   Radio Medical Report
TWELVE PARTS OF A RADIO MEDICAL REPORT
1. Unit identification and level of provider
2. Estimated time of arrival
3. Patient's age and sex
4. Chief complaint
5. Brief, pertinent history of the present illness
6. Major past illnesses
7. Mental status
8. Baseline vital signs
9. Pertinent findings of the physical exam
10. Emergency medical care given
11. Response to emergency medical care
12. Contact made with medical direction if required or if you have questions

5. Brief, pertinent history of the present illness

Onset of pain was 2 hours ago and is accompanied by slight nausea.

6. Major past illnesses

The patient has a history of high blood pressure and arthritis.

7. Mental status

He is alert and oriented, never lost consciousness.

8. Baseline vital signs

His vital signs are pulse 88 regular and full, respirations 20 and unlabored, skin normal, and blood pressure 134 over 88; SpO$_2$ is 98 percent.

9. Pertinent findings of the physical exam

Our exam revealed tenderness in both upper abdominal quadrants. They did not appear rigid.

10. Emergency medical care given

For care, we have placed him in a position of comfort.

11. Response to emergency medical care

The level of pain has not changed during our care. Mental status has remained unchanged. Vital signs are basically unchanged.

12. Contact medical direction if required or if you have questions

Does medical direction have any orders?

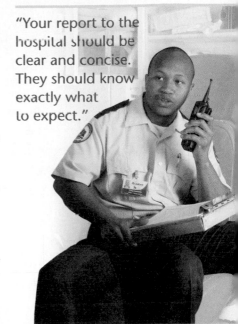

"Your report to the hospital should be clear and concise. They should know exactly what to expect."

After giving this information, you will continue with reassessment of the patient en route to the hospital. During that time, additional vital signs will be taken, there may be changes in the patient's condition, or you may discover new information about the patient, particularly on long transports. In some systems, you should radio this additional information to the hospital in a follow-up radio call while en route (follow local protocols).

When you contact medical direction, you may be given orders. The on-line physician may order you to assist in administering the patient's own medication, or order the administration of a medication you carry on the ambulance, or give other orders. In any case, the communication between you and medical direction must be clear and concise to avoid misinterpretations that can inadvertently harm the patient. For example, a patient may have a medication for chest pain called nitroglycerin. This medication, as you will learn in Chapter 18, "General Pharmacology," is one that you may assist the patient in taking (according to local protocols). The medication should be given only if the patient's blood pressure is above a certain level. If there is a misunderstanding between you and the physician and this medication is ordered improperly, harm may come to the patient.

To avoid misunderstanding and miscommunication, use the following guidelines when communicating with medical direction:

- Give the information to medical direction clearly and accurately. Speak slowly and clearly. The physician's orders will be based on what you report.

- After receiving an order for a medication or procedure, repeat the order word for word. You may also ask to do a procedure or give a medication and be denied by medical direction. Repeat this also.

- If an order is unclear, ask the physician to repeat it. After you have a clear understanding of the order, repeat it back to the physician.

- If an order appears to be inappropriate, question the physician. There may have been a misunderstanding, and your questioning may prevent the inappropriate administration of a medication. If the physician verifies the order, he may explain to you why he has given you that particular order.

THE VERBAL REPORT

At the hospital, you will give a written report on your patient to hospital personnel, as explained later in the chapter. However, since it will take some time to complete your written report, the first information you give to hospital personnel will be your verbal report.

As you transfer your patient to the care of the hospital staff, introduce the patient by name. Then summarize the same kind of information you gave over the radio, pointing out

CORE CONCEPT ●
Delivery and format of a verbal hand-off report to the hospital

Communication Challenges

Communication may take various forms in EMS: for example, written, face-to-face verbal, or by radio. Make your decisions based on the following scenarios.

1. You are en route to a call of unknown nature for an elderly patient. Emergency Medical Responders arrived at the scene about 5 minutes ago and you are still 10 minutes from the scene. Dispatch has not called you on the radio with an update on the patient's condition. What are some of the reasons why this might be the case? How should you proceed?

2. A 17-year-old male drank a large amount of alcohol and then "passed out," according to his friends, who called 911. When you arrive, you find the patient initially unresponsive to painful stimuli, then a few minutes later able to slur some words when you ask him questions. A few minutes after that, he withdraws when you apply a painful stimulus. How should you describe his mental status to the hospital while you are en route?

3. You are at the scene of a two-car motor-vehicle collision and would like to give the local hospital some warning that you will be transporting a severely injured patient in a few minutes. Unfortunately, when you try to call the hospital on the radio, they are unable to understand what you are saying. How should you proceed?

4. You have just arrived at the scene of a 34-year-old diabetic male who is "out of it," according to what the caller told dispatch. One of his friends, trying to be helpful, tells you that he thinks the patient is "conscious but unresponsive." Confused as to what this might mean, you proceed to the patient and find him sitting in a chair, staring straight ahead, not saying anything. When you ask him a question, he doesn't answer and doesn't even look at you. When you pinch his arm, he looks down at his arm but doesn't respond in any other way. How can you describe this patient's mental status in a way that will give the hospital an accurate impression of what is going on? *Hint*: Describe what you observe instead of trying to attach labels to this patient.

any information that is updated or different from your last radio report. Include the following in your verbal report:

- Chief complaint
- History that was not given previously
- Additional treatment given en route
- Additional vital signs taken en route

INTERPERSONAL COMMUNICATION

Team Communication

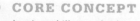

CORE CONCEPT

Communication skills used when interacting with other members of the health care team

As an EMT, you are part of a team of health care professionals. For example, at the scene, you may need to communicate with first responders (trained Emergency Medical Responders or others who have reached the scene and provided care before your arrival) or with advanced providers (Advanced EMTs or Paramedics) (Figure 17-3). On many medical calls, a home health care aid or family member may be at the scene who can provide you with valuable information about the patient and the present emergency (Figure 17-4). You will need to speak candidly and respectfully with these members of the health care team in order to gather important information about the patient and in order to complete any necessary and appropriate transfer of care.

Therapeutic Communication

CORE CONCEPT

Communication skills used when interacting with the patient

Although communication between two or more human beings is a skill that you have learned over the years, many people still do not communicate as well as they could. Communicating with patients and others who are in crisis is even more difficult (Figure 17-5). Al-

FIGURE 17-3 You may need to communicate with Emergency Medical Responders or advanced EMS personnel at the scene.

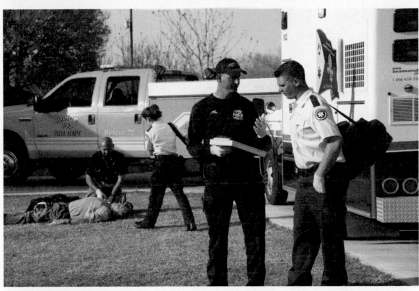

FIGURE 17-4 You may need to communicate with a home health aide or family member about the patient's condition and present emergency.

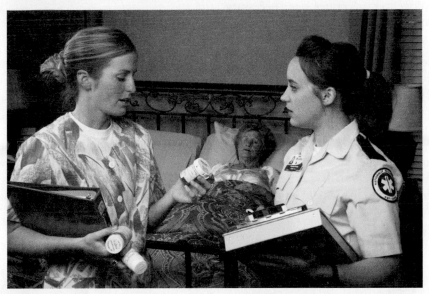

though interpersonal communication could be presented as a course in itself, the following guidelines will help when dealing with patients, families, friends, and bystanders:

- **Use eye contact.** Make frequent eye contact with your patient. It shows that you are interested in your patient and that you are attentive. Failure to make eye contact signals that you feel uneasy around the patient. (If your patient is avoiding eye contact, consider that in some cultures eye contact is considered rude. You may want to match your behavior to the patient's in this situation.)

- **Be aware of your position and body language.** Your positioning in respect to the patient is important. If you are higher than the patient, you may appear intimidating. If possible, position yourself at or below the patient's eye level (Figure 17-6). This will be less threatening to the patient. Body language is also important. Standing with your arms crossed or not directly facing the patient (a closed stance) sends a signal to the patient that you are not interested. Use a more open stance (arms down, facing the patient), when it can be done safely, to communicate a warmer attitude.

FIGURE 17-5 Communicating with patients and others who are in crisis requires skill and tact.

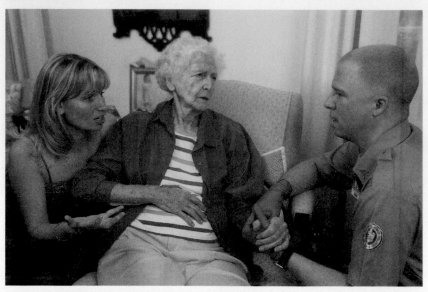

A closed or more serious stance may sometimes be beneficial, however, when you need to calm or direct bystanders at the scene. Standing above a patient may convey authority and can be done to gain control when necessary.

Watch the patient's body language to see how your communication with him is going. If the patient uses a closed stance, your communication efforts may not be working.

- **Use language the patient can understand.** Speak slowly and clearly. Do not use medical or other terms that the patient will not understand. Explain procedures before they are performed, to prevent anxiety.

- **Be honest.** Honesty is important. You will frequently be asked questions that you will not have the answer to: "Is my leg broken?" "Am I having a heart attack?" At other times you will know the answer to the question, but it is not pleasant: "Will it hurt when you put that splint on?" If the answer is "Yes," tell the truth. Explain that you will do it as gently as possible to reduce pain, but some pain may be experienced. It is much worse to lie to the patient and have him find out that you were not being truthful. This

FIGURE 17-6 Position yourself at or below the patient's eye level to be less intimidating and to aid communication.

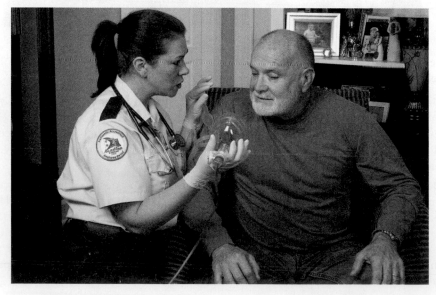

will erode the patient's confidence in you as well as in other EMTs and medical personnel the patient may meet later on.

- **Use the patient's proper name.** Especially with senior citizens and other adults, do not assume familiarity. As a general rule, call patients as they introduce themselves to you. If a person many years older than you introduces himself as William Harris, it might be best to call him Mr. Harris as a sign of respect. Immediately calling him "Bill" when he clearly stated his name was "William" would be disrespectful. If, after you call him "Mr. Harris," he says "Please call me Bill," you have shown respect and can then use the less formal name. If in doubt, ask the patient what he would like to be called.

- **Listen.** If you ask the patient a question, get an answer, then have to ask again, it will show the patient that you were not listening. If you are not listening, the patient will feel that you are not interested in what he has to say, or that you just don't care. If you ask a question, wait for the answer. Then write it down so you will not forget.

If a person has a mental disability or is hard of hearing, speak slowly and clearly. Do not talk down to the patient. If the patient has a hearing disability, he may read lips. In any case, seeing your lips may help him understand what you are saying. Therefore, be sure that a deaf or hearing-impaired person can see your mouth when you talk.

Remember that a person who is blind or has a visual deficit can usually hear, so do not give in to the temptation to speak to him loudly or unnaturally. For the visually impaired person, you will want to take extra effort to explain anything that is happening that he cannot see.

You may also find people who do not speak the same language as you. In this case, use an interpreter (for example, a family member or friend who speaks both languages) or a manual that provides translations. Family members are not always familiar with medical terminology, so you should be cautious using them. It is usually possible to get a professional translator through the phone company. You may also find that your communications center or medical direction has someone available who speaks the patient's language.

The elderly are a rapidly growing segment of the population who often need EMS care. These older patients may have medical problems simply because of their age. They may also be more prone to falls and serious injury from trauma due to the condition of their bones and body systems.

Many elderly patients are well oriented and physically able. Others, however, may have problems with hearing, sight, or orientation that have come on with age. These patients may seem confused or may simply find it difficult to communicate. In spite of their sensory limitations, of course, these patients still have needs and feelings. They deserve patience, kindness, and understanding—along with proper emergency care (Figure 17-7).

FIGURE 17-7 Be considerate of the elderly patient.

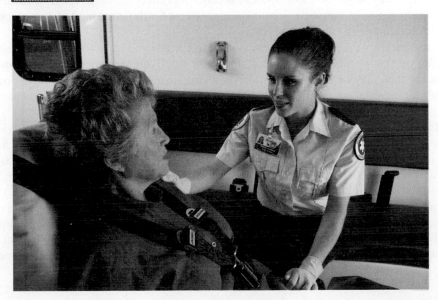

Since children sometimes can be difficult to assess and communicate with, it is often best to involve the parents of the child when communicating. Two rules of communication are critically important to children:

- Always come down to the child's level (Figure 17-8). Never stand above a child, as you will literally tower over the child and appear very intimidating. Crouching down reduces the size difference and greatly improves communication. If the child is not critically ill, you might even take the time to sit on the floor and get slightly below the child in the beginning.

- Children often sense lies even faster than adults. It is important to tell the truth to children. Remember, you may be the first contact from the EMS system that the child has ever had. Work to make it positive.

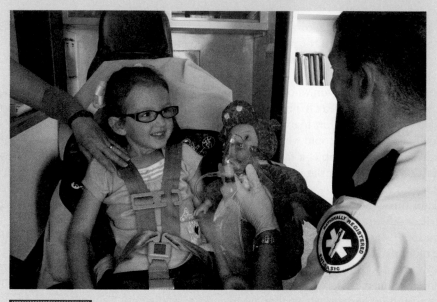

FIGURE 17-8 Stay at a child's eye level or lower.

PREHOSPITAL CARE REPORT

The record that you produce during a call is called a prehospital care report or, informally, a PCR. Your region or service may use a different name for the same kind of document, such as trip sheet, run report, or another name.

Prehospital care reports vary from system to system and state to state. Although the information that is required to complete each is relatively similar, the method used to record the data may be somewhat different. Written reports are those that have portions with narrative areas, areas to record vital signs in written number form, and check boxes (Figure 17-9).

Many, perhaps most, prehospital care reports are now done by direct data entry (Figure 17-10A and Figure 17-10B). This can take several forms. An electronic clipboard is a computer in a clipboard format. The computer is able to recognize handwriting and convert it to computer text. The data are stored and eventually downloaded to a larger computer. More commonly used tools are laptop or pen-based computers in the ambulance (Figure 17-11). They allow the EMT to enter information about a call directly into a database. One of the most popular methods is the web-based approach. With this increasingly popular method, the EMT signs on to a secure web site and enters the data through a keyboard. With all of these methods, the EMS uses a printer at a receiving hospital to print out a hard copy of the report for the emergency department staff.

MAINE ★EMS   **PRESS DOWN, YOU ARE MAKING THREE COPIES.**

RUN REPORT # **746118**	Mo.	Day	Year	M T W Th	F S Sun	SERVICE NAME		SERVICE NO.	VEHICLE NO.	ALS ☐ Performed ☐ Back-up called	SERVICE RUN NO.

NAME _____ BILLING INFORMATION

STREET OR R.F.D. _____

CITY/TOWN _____ STATE _____ ZIP _____

AGE/DATE OF BIRTH _____ ☐ Male ☐ Female   PHONE _____

INCIDENT LOCATION: _____ ADDRESS _____ CITY/TOWN _____

TRANSPORTED TO: _____ TREATING/FAMILY PHYSICIAN _____ CREW LICENSE NUMBERS _____

TRANSPORTATION/COMMUNICATIONS PROBLEMS _____

☐ Medical
  ☐ Cardiac
  ☐ Poisoning/OD
    ☐ Respiratory
  ☐ Behavioral
    ☐ Diabetic
  ☐ Seizure
    ☐ CVA
  ☐ OB/Gyn
    ☐ Other _____

☐ Trauma
  ☐ Multi-Systems Trauma
  ☐ Head
  ☐ Spinal
  ☐ Burn
  ☐ Soft Tissue Injury
  ☐ Fractures
  ☐ Other _____

☐ Code 99

☐ MEDICATIONS   ☐ ALLERGIES

CHIEF COMPLAINT:

R	L	LUNG SOUNDS
☐	☐	CLEAR
☐	☐	ABSENT
☐	☐	DECREASED
☐	☐	RALES
☐	☐	WHEEZE
☐	☐	STRIDOR

TYPE OF RUN
☐ Emergency Transport
☐ Routine Transfer
☐ Emergency Transfer
☐ No Transport
☐ Refused Transport

TIME	CODE		ODOMETER
		Call Received	
		Enroute	
		At Scene	
		From Scene	
		At Destination	
		In Service	

TIME	PULSE	RESP	BP	PUPILLARY RESPONSE	SKIN	VERBAL RESPONSE	MOTOR RESPONSE	EYE-OPENING RESPONSE	CAPILLARY REFILL
						5 4 3 2 1	6 5 4 3 2 1	4 3 2 1	☐ Normal ☐ None ☐ Delayed
						5 4 3 2 1	6 5 4 3 2 1	4 3 2 1	☐ Normal ☐ None ☐ Delayed
						5 4 3 2 1	6 5 4 3 2 1	4 3 2 1	☐ Normal ☐ None ☐ Delayed

☐ MVA   ☐ Concern AOB/ETOH   SEAT BELTS: ☐ Used ☐ Not Used ☐ N/A ☐ Helmet Used

MUTUAL AID: Assisted/Assisted by Service # _____   Time Called: _____

(narrative lines)

PATIENT'S SUSPECTED PROBLEM: **746118**		☐ Medication Administered	☐ Defib Lic.# _____	MEDICAL CONTROL	☐ Written Order/Protocol ☐ Verbal Order/Protocol

		☐ Monitor	☐ Chest Decomp	IV ☐ SUC LIC.# _____ ☐ UNSUC LIC.# _____	Total Attempts
		☐ Pacing	☐ Caricothyrotomy		

Cleared Airway	Extrication	EOA ☐ SUC LIC.# _____ ☐ UNSUC LIC.# _____	Total Attempts	ET ☐ SUC LIC.# _____ ☐ UNSUC LIC.# _____	Total Attempts
Artificial Respiration/BVM	Cervical Immobilization				
Oropharyngeal Airway	KED/Short Board				
Nasopharyngeal Airway	Long Board				

CPR–Time:	Restraints	LIC #	EKG RHYTHM	TIME	MEDS/DEFIB/C-VERT	DOSE W/S	ROUTE
Bystander CPR	Traction Splinting						
AED	General Splinting						
Suction	Cold Application						
Oxygen–LPMin ___ ☐ Nasal ☐ Mask	MAST Inflated						
Pulse Oximetry							
Autovent							

NAME OF E.D. TREATING PHYSICIAN _____   SIGNATURE OF CREW MEMBER IN CHARGE _____   COPY 1 HOSPITAL

FIGURE 17-10 (A) Printout of an electronic prehospital care report. (B) As an electronic report appears on the computer screen. (© Courtesy of ImageTrend, Inc.)

Patient Name: Miller, George

Prehospital Care Report

XYZ
XYZ
Burlington, VT 05401

Incident Date: 06/07/2010 | Call #: SB-10612 | Patient Care #: 1
Medical Record #: -25

Patient Information

Name: Miller, George	Age: 57 Years	D.O.B: 06/15/1952 (mm/dd/yyyy)
	Gender: Male	SSN:
Address: 124 Cyprus St	Weight: KG / LB	Race: White
Arlington, Tarrant, TX 76001	Phone:	Ethnicity: Not Hispanic or Latino

Closest Relative/Guardian

Name: ,	Relationship: Not Applicable
Address: Not Applicable, Not Applicable	Phone #:

Provider Impression

Primary Impression	Secondary Impression
Chest Pain/Discomfort	Not Applicable

Narrative

Summary of Events

Chief complaint: "My chest hurts."

HPI: 57 year old male developed sudden onset of crushing substernal pain radiating to the left shoulder and arm while watching TV. The pt. states this pain is "exactly the same as when I had a heart attack 2 years ago." He denies loss of consciousness or difficulty breathing. Pain has not changed since it started.

PMH: History of heart attack 2 years ago. Meds Cardizem. Allergic to aspirin.

Physical exam: Alert 57 year old male found sitting on couch. No jugular vein distention. Skin pale and sweaty. Lung sounds clear and equal. No pedal edema.

Treatment: Oxygen by nonrebreather mask at 15 lpm. Transported sitting. No change in condition en route.

Prior Aid

Prior Aid	Performed By	Outcome
	N/A,	N/A

Past Medical History

MEDICATION ALLERGIES	Generic Name	Description
	Aspirin	

Patient Medications	Generic Name	Dosage
Cardizem		Not Applicable

Medical Surgery History
Not Known

History Primarily Obtained From	Pregnancy	Advanced Directives	Practitioner Name
	N/A		,

Assessment Exam

Patient Condition

Chief Complaint: Chest pain X 2 Hours
Secondary Complaint: Difficulty breathing X 2 Hours
Alcohol/Drug Use: No Apparent Alcohol/Drug Use

Injury Onset	Injury Cause	Injury Mechanism	Injury Intent	Ht. of Fall
05:00 06/07/2010	Not Applicable	Not Applicable	Not Applicable	

Primary Symptom	Other Associated Symptoms
Chest Pain	Not Applicable

Patient Vitals

Time	B/P	Pulse	Rhythm	Resp.	Effort	SpO2	SpO2 Qual.	EtCO2	GCS	Pain	Stroke Scl	PTA	B.G.	RTS	Limb	Patient Position
07:30	144/86	84	RR	18	Normal		High O2		15					12	Left Arm	Sitting
07:45	144/86	88	RR	20	Normal		High O2		15					12	Left Arm	Sitting
07:24	148/88	88	RR	18	Normal		Rm. Air		15					12	Left Arm	Sitting

Patient Name: Miller, George

ECG Monitor

Time	ECG Type	ECG Lead	ECG Interpretation		ECG Ectopy	Cause For Change

Procedures and Treatments

Time	Crew	Name	Location	Size of Equipment	Attempts	Response	Success	Comments

Intubation Confirmation - Initial/Final

Time	Size	Depth	Lung Sounds	Chest Rise	EDD	Abdomen Assessment	Tube Misting	Recheck	ETCO2 Color	Secured By

Medication Administered

Time	Crew	Medication	Route	Dosage	Response	PTA	Comments
07:19		Oxygen (non-rebreather mask)	NRB/PRB	15 LPM	Unchanged	N/A	

Injury Details

Patient Safety Equipment Used

Not Applicable

Patient Transport/Positioning

Patient Moved To Ambulance	Patient's Position In Transport	Patient Moved From Ambulance
Stretcher	Sitting	Stretcher

Call Type and Location / Call Disposition / Response Times and Mileage

Call Type: Chest Pain
Resp. Mode: Lights and Sirens
Urgency: Immediate
Response: 911 Response
Location: Home/Residence
Address: 124 Cyprus St
Arlington, Tarrant,
TX 76001

Disposition: Treated, Transported by EMS (BLS)
Resp. Mode: No Lights or Sirens
Destination: COLUMBIA HOSPITAL AT, MEDICAL CITY DALLA S , 7777 FOREST LN , DALLAS , TX 75230
Dest. Determ.: Closest Facility
Diverted From: Not Applicable
Response Delay: None
Scene Delay: None
Transport Delay: None

1st Resp. Arr.:
PSAP:
Disp. Notified: 07:05
Unit Disp.: 07:05
Enroute: 07:07
At Scene: 07:19
At Patient: 07:19
Depart: 07:38
Arrive Dest: 07:54
In Service: 08:10
Cancelled:
In Quarters: 08:32

Incident #: SB-10612
Call Sign: Not Applicable
Veh. #: Ambulance 12
Start Miles:
Scene Miles: To Scene:
Dest. Miles: To Dest:
End Miles: To End:

Unit Personnel

Crew Member	Level of Certification	Role
Not Applicable ()	Not Applicable	Not Available
Not Applicable ()	Not Applicable	Not Available

Billing Information

Payment Method:	Work Related?

Patient Occupation Information

Occupation	Industry
Not Known	Not Known

Service-Defined Questions

Did you leave Equip at the Hosp
Did you attempt to use a King airway?
Were you successful with the King airway?

Valuables

Valuables: Not Applicable

Inc. Date: 06/07/2010 | Patient Name: Miller, George | XYZ | Page: 1
Incident #: SB-10612 | Call #: SB-10612 | | Date Printed: 06/07/2010 23:49

Inc. Date: 06/07/2010 | Patient Name: Miller, George | XYZ | Page: 2
Incident #: SB-10612 | Call #: SB-10612 | | Date Printed: 06/07/2010 23:49

(A)

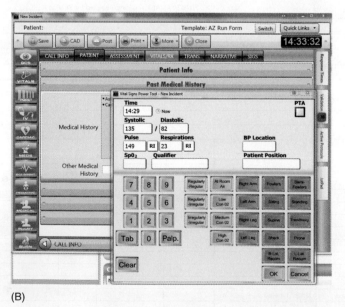

(B)

FIGURE 17-11 Direct data devices as documentation tools: (A) a laptop pen-based computer, and (B) a pen-based computer with PCR form on the screen.

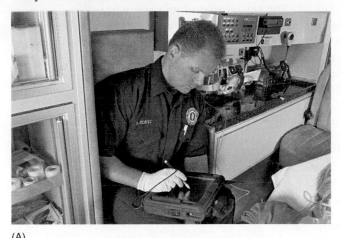

(A)

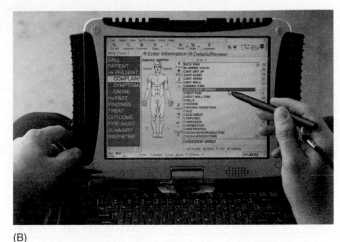

(B)

Whenever possible, you should complete the PCR while you are still at the receiving facility with fresh memory of the call (Figure 17-12). Since it is not always possible to complete the PCR before a crew has to leave, many EMS agencies using electronic data collection employ a ***drop report or transfer report***. This is an abbreviated report containing the minimum data set, described later.

drop report (or transfer report) an abbreviated form of the PCR that an EMS crew can leave at the hospital when there is not enough time to complete the PCR before leaving.

Functions of the Prehospital Care Report

The prehospital care report has many functions. It is the record of patient care, serves as a legal document, provides information for administrative functions, aids education and research, and contributes to quality improvement. These functions are discussed in the following paragraphs.

Patient Care Record

The prehospital care report conveys important information about the patient to members of the EMS system and beyond. Although you provide a verbal report to the hospital staff before you leave the patient, your written record allows emergency department personnel to see the status of the patient when you arrived on-scene, the care you gave, and how the patient's status may have changed during your care. An example of this would be the emergency department staff looking back at your original set of vital signs to compare the patient's current condition with the patient's condition when he was first found at the scene.

A copy of the prehospital care report becomes part of the patient's permanent hospital record.

FIGURE 17-12 An EMT completes her prehospital care report, using a computer in the receiving hospital ED.

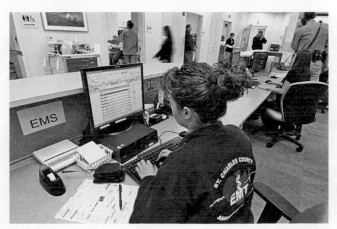

Legal Document

The prehospital care report also serves as a legal document, which may be called for at any legal proceeding resulting from the call. The person who wrote the report will ordinarily go to court with the form. If the patient was the victim or perpetrator of a crime, the report and the writer may be called into court to testify about the call during criminal proceedings. Civil law proceedings for negligence in injuries (e.g., if a patient falls in a shopping mall and sues) are another reason that your report may be examined.

Unfortunately, there may be a time when the report is being examined because you are the subject of a lawsuit. Fortunately, this is rare and usually preventable. In a case like this, the report in which you documented the circumstances and the care you gave will be very important.

Administrative Purposes

Depending on the service you belong to, you may have to obtain insurance and billing information from the patient or patient's family. This may be recorded on your prehospital care report, on a separate form, or on both.

Education and Research

Your report may be examined later as part of a research project. Analysis of statistics compiled from prehospital care reports can reveal patterns and trends in EMS management and care. For example, analysts may see instances in which response time could be improved or different ways of scheduling and deploying units to prepare for busy areas and times. Statistics also may justify a request for additional resources.

Prehospital care reports can help management keep track of each EMT's experience and skills. Extra practice may be scheduled during continuing education sessions for skills that the reports reveal are underutilized, for instance. When an unusual or uncommon type of call takes place, the prehospital care report may be used as a demonstration of how to document such a case after it is stripped of data that might identify the patient.

Quality Improvement

Most organizations have a Quality Improvement (QI)—also known as a Quality Assurance (QA) or Continuous Quality Improvement (CQI)—system in place by which calls are routinely reviewed for conformity to current medical and organizational standards. Examination of prehospital care reports is one major way of conducting this review. At times, QI evaluations reveal excellent care by an EMT team that deserves special recognition and a "pat on the back."

Elements of the Prehospital Care Report

Data Elements

Each individual box in the prehospital care report is called a data element. Although some elements may seem insignificant, each is actually an important part of the report and the description of the patient and response. These elements are necessary for research as well as for documenting the call.

POINT OF VIEW

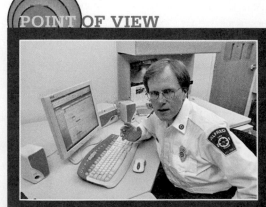

"I remember the day I found out the right way to do documentation.

"I turned in a run report one evening. When I came in to work the next day the chief called me in. He wasn't happy. And, looking back, he had reason not to be. It wasn't my best work. I had listened to my partner. He has been around for 25 years. He told me to just put down a couple of sentences and the vitals. Said it was a 'no brainer.'

"Now I know that if I got sued it would've looked bad. But the thing that really got me is when the chief told me it looked like I was doing a poor job. I know I took good care of that patient. And I even helped contact her family on the cell phone so someone would be at the hospital for her.

"I don't want a bad report to go to the QI committee—or to court—but most important I am proud of what I do. The chief made me realize my reports should reflect that pride. And believe me, now they do."

Table 17-3 NHTSA Minimum Data Set

PATIENT INFORMATION

This information is gathered at the time of the EMT's initial contact with a patient upon arrival at the scene, following all interventions, and upon arrival at the medical facility:

- Chief complaint
- Level of responsiveness (AVPU)—mental status
- Systolic blood pressure for patients greater than 3 years old
- Skin perfusion (capillary refill) for patients less than 6 years old
- Skin color and temperature
- Pulse rate
- Respiratory rate and effort

ADMINISTRATIVE INFORMATION

- Time of incident report
- Time unit notified
- Time of arrival of patient
- Time unit left scene
- Time of arrival at destination
- Time of transfer of care

To aid in evaluation and research across states and regions, the National Highway Traffic Safety Administration (NHTSA) has developed a data set of over 400 elements. There is a standardized definition of what each element means so that regions and states can consolidate and compare their data. There is also a minimum data set containing a much smaller number of elements that all prehospital care reports should have nationwide. The NHTSA data set has been widely adopted by states, which are in the process of implementing it. The minimum data set is briefly summarized in Table 17-3.

The prehospital care report can be broken down into two sections: run data and patient information. The format for data varies, depending on whether it is a paper report or an electronic report as well as the specific information required by your service. Formats you may encounter may include check boxes, short answers, and narrative sections for longer answers. Review Figure 17-9 (a paper report) and Figure 17-10 (an electronic report) as you read about the following report elements.

Run Data

Spaces for run data, which may be provided at the beginning or end of the report form, include the agency name, date, times, call number, unit personnel and levels of certification, and other basic information as mandated by your service. Times recorded must be accurate and synchronous (by clocks or watches that show the same time). Be sure to use the time as given by the dispatcher when noting times on your report. Unless your watch or the ambulance clock displays exactly the same time as the dispatch center, the times on your report will not match. There may be a difference of several minutes between the time displayed on your watch and the dispatch center's official time.

This time difference may seem insignificant but is actually very important in such areas as determining how long a patient has been in cardiac arrest, trends in patient condition, or measurement of system efficiency in response times.

Patient Information

This section contains information about the patient. Specifically, it typically includes:

- Patient's name, address, and phone number
- Patient's gender, age, and date of birth
- Patient's weight

- Patient's race and/or ethnicity
- Billing and insurance information (in many jurisdictions)

Information Gathered during the Call

Following the run data and basic patient information, prehospital care reports provide areas for information about the entire call. This information may include:

- Your general impression of the patient
- A narrative summary of events throughout the call, including the chief complaint, history of the present illness, past medical history, physical exam, and care
- Specific sections to detail prior aid, past medical history, physical exam results, vital signs, ECG results, procedures and treatments, medications administered, and other information about the call as required by your service
- Transport information

Narrative Sections

The narrative section or sections of a prehospital care report are less structured than the fill-in or check-box sections. It provides space to write information about the patient that cannot fit into fill-in blanks or check-off boxes. In a paper report, the space provided for narratives is still somewhat limited. In an electronic report, however, the space for the narrative will typically expand as needed. Even though the electronic space is expandable, and you want to include all important information, you should still strive to write clearly and concisely as a courtesy to those who will need to read your report.

Experienced EMTs consider a good prehospital care report as one that "paints a picture" of their patient. The report, as mentioned previously, is read by many people and is a vital part of the patient's record. When hospital personnel or your Quality Improvement team reads your report, it should tell the patient's story fully and appropriately.

Remember, you were involved throughout the call and are familiar with the patient, his chief complaint, and the care you gave. The people who read your report will have no prior knowledge of the call or the patient. It is imperative that you provide complete, accurate, and pertinent information about your patient and present the information in a logical order.

> **NOTE:** *The simple fact that there is no pain or complaint of difficulty does not mean that the patient should not be treated. If the patient's medical condition or mechanism of injury so indicates, treat the patient despite his absence of pain or other symptoms.*

The following guidelines will help you prepare narrative portions of your prehospital care reports.

- **Include both objective and pertinent subjective information.** Objective statements are those that are observable, measurable, or verifiable, such as, "The patient has a swollen, deformed extremity." This is backed up by your visual observation. An objective statement might also be, "The patient's blood pressure was 110/80," based on a measurement you took. Or it might be "Patient uses a prescribed inhaler," a verifiable fact provided by the patient.

    Subjective information is information from an individual point of view. It may be provided by the patient as a symptom ("I feel dizzy"). It also may be provided by the EMT, such as your general impression of the patient ("Patient appears to have difficulty breathing"). Avoid subjective statements that are merely opinions, are beyond your level of training or scope of practice ("I do not believe that the leg is broken" or "Patient is probably having a heart attack"), or are irrelevant ("Patient's daughter was rude").

    Prehospital care reports are designed to be factual documents. Use objective statements whenever possible and only pertinent subjective statements. If you record something you did not observe yourself, put it in quotation marks (e.g., a bystander stated that, "The patient passed out at the wheel before crashing"). Placing a statement in quotation marks and identifying the source lets readers of the report know where the information came from.

    The chief complaint is another piece of information that is usually given in quotes. If a patient is conscious and oriented, he will usually tell you why he or someone else called you

("My chest hurts"). If the patient is not conscious or oriented, the person who called EMS may provide the chief complaint (She said he "felt faint and then passed out"). Since the chief complaint is in someone else's words, it should be placed in quotes.

In documenting your assessment procedures, remember to document important observations about the scene, such as suicide notes, weapons, and any other facts that would be important for patient care but not available to the emergency department personnel.

- **Include pertinent negatives.** These are examination findings that are negative (things that are not true), but are important to note. For example, if a patient has chest pain, you will ask that patient if he has difficulty breathing. If the patient says he does not have difficulty in breathing, that statement is an important piece of negative information. On your prehospital care report, you would note, "The patient denies difficulty breathing." Negative information often applies to trauma patients. For example, if the mechanism of injury indicates that there may be an injury to the arm but the patient says he feels no pain, you would note, "The patient denies pain in right arm." Documenting pertinent negatives lets other medical professionals know that you thought to examine these areas and that the findings were negative. Not documenting them might leave the reader wondering if this area was explored at all.

- **Avoid radio codes and nonstandard abbreviations.** Codes you may use on the radio may not be familiar to hospital personnel, so do not use them in written documentation. Abbreviations, when used properly, make writing efficient and accurate. However, using nonstandard abbreviations will cause confusion and possibly lead to errors in patient care.

- **Write legibly and use correct spelling.** A prehospital care report will have absolutely no value if it cannot be read, so take the time to make your handwriting readable. Unclear writing, misread by others, may cause errors that could harm the patient. Additionally, your QI team will be unable to read the report for review, and it will have no value for research or training. Spelling is also important. If you cannot properly spell a word, look it up (many ambulances and emergency departments have medical dictionaries) or use another word.

- **Use medical terminology correctly.** Be sure that any medical terms you use are used correctly. If you are not sure of the meaning of a term, look it up in a medical dictionary or use everyday language to describe the condition instead. Careless use of medical terms could make your report unclear or cause a misunderstanding that might result in harm to the patient.

- **If it's not written down, you didn't do it.** This is a statement that you will most likely hear from your instructor and experienced EMTs in the field. It explains an important concept of EMS documentation. Make sure that you document all your interventions thoroughly. If you did not document them, it will appear as if they were never performed when the call is later reviewed.

The prehospital care report's most important function is to present an accurate representation of the patient's condition throughout the call, the patient's history and vital signs, treatments performed, and changes or lack of changes in the patient's condition following treatments.

SPECIAL DOCUMENTATION ISSUES

Legal Issues

There are several legal issues pertaining to prehospital care reports and other documents you may be asked to complete. These include issues of confidentiality, patient refusals, falsification, and error correction.

CORE CONCEPT
Legal aspects and benefits of documentation

Confidentiality

The prehospital care report itself and the information it contains are strictly confidential. The information must not be discussed with or distributed to unauthorized persons. The Health Insurance Portability and Accountability Act (HIPAA) requires ambulance services that are covered by the law to take certain steps to safeguard patient confidentiality (Figure 17-13). This

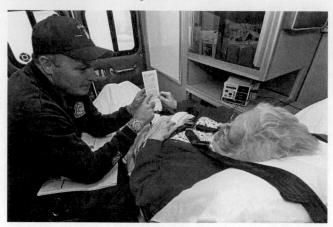

FIGURE 17-13 An EMT explains a HIPAA privacy information leaflet to a patient.

CRITICAL DECISION MAKING

Choosing How and What to Document

Documentation is an important and challenging duty of the EMT. The documentation you produce may be looked at years later in criminal and civil cases—as well as being reviewed by your QI committee. You will need to make decisions about how and what you document . . . as you will see in the following scenarios.

1. After the police secure the scene, you treat a man and woman who apparently had a dispute. Neither sustained any life-threatening injuries, so you have time to gather more information at the scene. Even though you and your partner evaluate them in different rooms, they are still angry and trading insults. The boyfriend claims she is a two-timing slut who has syphilis and chlamydia. The girlfriend claims he is an alcoholic and a drug addict. How much of this should you document on the PCR? How should you phrase any information you obtained in this way?

2. Three years from now, you receive a notice to appear for a deposition regarding a call you had a long time ago. So much time has passed that you don't remember the call. Are you allowed to look at the PCR before you go? Why or why not?

3. When you treat a 3-year-old girl for an arm injury, you suspect she has been abused. How do the privacy rules of HIPAA affect what you may and should do with regard to reporting this situation to the authorities?

typically includes placing completed PCRs into a locked box. HIPAA, state, and local regulations will indicate to whom the information may be distributed. Obviously, the receiving hospital must receive patient care information so they can treat the patient properly. Most reports have a copy that will be left at the hospital. Confidentiality issues were discussed in Chapter 4, "Medical, Legal, and Ethical Issues."

Patient Refusals

CORE CONCEPT

Documentation concerns in patient refusal

Chapter 4, "Medical, Legal, and Ethical Issues," discussed the issue of liability when patients refuse treatment. It is one of the foremost causes of liability for EMTs and their EMS systems. Chapter 4 presented several suggestions on what to do when a patient refuses care or transportation.

Document all actions you take to persuade the patient to go to the hospital. Additionally, you will have to make notes on the patient's competency, or his ability to make an informed, rational decision on his medical needs. If the patient is not capable of making this determination for any reason—including age, intoxication (alcohol and/or other drugs), mental competency, or as a result of the patient's medical condition—you must document any actions you take to protect the patient. The patient must be informed of the potential results of not going to the hospital or of refusing your care.

The fact that a patient refuses transport to a hospital does not mean that you should not perform an assessment. If the patient greets you with a statement such as, "I don't know why my daughter called, because I'm not going anywhere," you may still be able to persuade the patient to get "checked out." Perform as much of a secondary assessment as possible, including vital signs. Document all of your findings and emergency care given on the prehospital care report. This information will be important to give to medical direction when you talk to them. Be sure to consult medical direction, according to your local protocols, whenever there is a patient refusal.

Most EMS agencies have a refusal-of-care form to use in the event that you have done your best to persuade the patient to accept care or transport and the patient still refuses. This form may be part of either the prehospital care report or a separate document. You should make sure the patient reads and signs this form (Figure 17-14). It is rare that a patient will refuse to sign the form. If he does, be sure to document this, as well, and note the names of witnesses to the refusal. If possible, when a patient refuses to sign a refusal form, get the witnesses to sign a statement confirming that the patient has refused care or transport.

You should also include information about the patient refusal in the narrative section of the prehospital care report. Figure 17-15 shows a handwritten sample documentation of a patient refusal that might go into the narrative portion of the prehospital care report.

You will note that the narrative shown in Figure 17-15 contains many points of information, including pertinent negatives. The report states that the patient "denies" chest pain or difficulty in breathing. Statements from the patient's daughter are noted as to the source: "according to her daughter . . ." and "The daughter denies seeing any seizure activity."

Before you leave the patient who has refused care or transport, be sure to make alternative care suggestions, such as encouraging him to seek care from a doctor, and document them. Try to be sure that a responsible family member or friend remains with the patient. Make sure that person also understands that the patient should seek care. Never convey the impression that you are annoyed about being called to the scene "for nothing." Make certain the patient understands that if his condition worsens or if he changes his mind, he can call EMS and you or another EMT team will gladly come back.

Falsification

Prehospital care reports document the information obtained and the care rendered during the call. False entries or misrepresentations on a report are usually intended to cover up serious flaws in assessment or in care. However, falsification may actually make the problem look worse when it is uncovered.

Two types of errors may be committed during a call: omission and commission. Errors of omission are those in which an important part of the assessment or care was left out. An example is oxygen. If a patient is experiencing chest pain, oxygen is an appropriate treatment. If it is overlooked for any reason, never write that oxygen was administered when it was not.

Occasionally, because of events during transport to a hospital, an EMT may only be able to get one set of vital signs. Never be tempted to write down an extra set of vital signs when none were taken. Just don't do it! Document only the vital signs that were taken. If there is a reason why you have only taken one set, document the reason (e.g., "The patient became combative and disoriented en route, preventing a second set of vital signs").

Errors of commission are actions performed on the patient that are wrong or improper. An example of this is incorrect administration of medication. There are certain medications that you will be able to administer or assist the patient in administering to himself. This is a great responsibility. If a medication was administered when it was not indicated, it is important to tell medical direction and document the incident on the prehospital care report. Failure to document exactly what happened may have a negative effect on the patient's care. The hospital may think that the patient's condition is due to some other cause. In other situations, the hospital may readminister the medication, not realizing that it had already been given.

Document the situation surrounding any error of omission or commission and explain exactly what happened. Document what was done to correct the situation, including advising medical direction and verbally notifying hospital personnel.

FIGURE 17-14 Example of a refusal information sheet.

GUIDELINES

REFUSAL INFORMATION SHEET

PLEASE READ AND KEEP THIS FORM!

This form has been given to you because you have refused treatment and/or transport by Emergency Medical Services (EMS). Your health and safety are our primary concern, so even though you have decided not to accept our advice, please remember the following:

1) The evaluation and/or treatment provided to you by the EMS providers is not a substitute for medical evaluation and treatment by a doctor. We advise you to get medical evaluation and treatment.

2) Your condition may not seem as bad to you as it actually is. Without treatment, your condition or problem could become worse. If you are planning to get medical treatment, a decision to refuse treatment or transport by EMS may result in a delay which could make your condition or problem worse.

3) Medical evaluation and/or treatment may be obtained by calling your doctor, if you have one, or by going to any hospital Emergency Department in this area, all of which are staffed 24 hours a day by Emergency Physicians. You may be seen at these Emergency Departments without an appointment.

4) If you change your mind or your condition becomes worse and you decide to accept treatment and transport by Emergency Medical Services, please do not hesitate to call us back. We will do our best to help you.

5) DON'T WAIT! When medical treatment is needed, it is usually better to get it right away.

I have received a copy of this information sheet.

PATIENT SIGNATURE: _____ DATE: _____

WITNESS SIGNATURE: _____ DATE: _____

AGENCY INCIDENT #: _____ AGENCY CODE: _____

NAME OF PERSON FILLING OUT FORM: _____

G 11A

> The 49 year old female patient, according to her daughter, "passed out" suddenly. She was in that condition for about 3-5 minutes. The daughter stated that the patient "came to" gradually. Upon our arrival she was fully conscious and oriented. The daughter denies observing any seizure activity. She states that the patient passed out in a chair and did not fall or injure herself as a result of the incident. The patient denies any problems such as chest pain or difficulty breathing. She denies allergies. Her last oral intake was about 2 hours ago (sandwich and coffee). The patient denies any past medical history or current medications.
>
> Vital signs noted above show no abnormalities between two sets taken at a 15 minute interval. The patient refuses transportation to the hospital and has signed the refusal form attached to this report. Her daughter is present with her at her residence and witnessed the refusal. The patient appears competent and oriented. She was advised to call back at any time should she need our assistance or transportation to the hospital of her choice. She was also advised that her failure to go to the hospital may result in a return or worsening of the previous symptoms which, depending on the underlying cause, could result in a serious medical problem or even death.
>
> The patient's daughter will stay with her for several hours and then provide follow-up calls throughout the evening to make sure the patient is all right. The patient was encouraged to contact her family physician for follow-up care as soon as possible. Since the patient did not have one, a sticker listing our phone number was placed on her phone. We contacted medical direction about the situation and spoke to Dr. Baker at Mercy Hospital. She had no further suggestions.

Falsification or misrepresentation on a prehospital care report leads to poor patient care because the facts were not documented, and hospital personnel may be misled about the patient's condition and the care he received. Falsification or misrepresentation may also lead to the suspension or revocation of your certification or license as an EMT.

You will avoid falsifications if you follow this rule: Write everything important that did happen and nothing that didn't.

Correction of Errors

Prehospital care reports are not always written in ideal circumstances. You may even find yourself being dispatched to another call before you finish writing up your last one. In situations such as this, you may inadvertently write incorrect information on the report.

COMMENTS PATIENT COMPLAINS OF PAIN IN HIS ~~RIGHT~~ ^DL^ LEFT SHOULDER THAT RADIATES TO THE LEFT ARM.

Any time there is incorrect information on the report, it must be corrected. If the report is still intact (all copies attached and not yet distributed), draw a single horizontal line through the error, initial it, then write the correct information beside it (Figure 17-16). Do not completely cross out the error or obliterate it. This may appear to be an attempt to cover up a mistake in patient care.

If the error is discovered at a later date, after the report has been submitted, draw a single line through the error, mark the area with your initials and the date, and add the correct information to the end of the report or on a separate note. This should be done in a different color ink when possible so the change will be obvious. Copies of the report may have already been distributed to other agencies, your Quality Improvement committee, insurance companies, or attorneys, and a corrected copy may need to be sent. Make sure that you place the date on the changes so the most recent copy is identifiable. If information has been omitted and you wish to add it, be sure also to date this information and place your initials by the added information.

If you have a direct data entry system instead of paper forms, you will simply log in to the system and make the correction. Electronic data systems log every change made to a report, including the identity of the person making the change, so the process is relatively simple.

Whether you need to submit a copy of the revised form to the receiving hospital will probably depend on the seriousness of your change. Follow your agency's procedures for correction of errors.

Special Situations

Multiple-Casualty Incidents

An incident in which there are many patients or injuries—such as a multiple-vehicle collision, a major fire, or a plane crash—causes many logistical problems for an EMS system. Documentation of information for each individual patient may be difficult. A patient in a multiple-casualty incident (MCI) will probably be moved from one treatment area to another at the scene and then receive transport to a hospital. Patients may be transported to several different hospitals. It is very important to keep the information with the patient as he moves through the system. This is often done through the use of a triage tag (Figure 17-17). This tag is affixed to the patient and used to record the patient's chief complaint and injuries, vital signs, and treatments given. At a point later in the emergency, the tag will be used to complete a traditional prehospital care report.

When completing a prehospital care report for a patient involved in a multiple-casualty incident, it will not be possible to provide the detail that you would normally provide for a

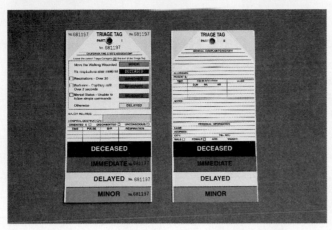

FIGURE 17-17 During a multiple-casualty incident, triage tags are used to document information for each patient.

single-patient call. This is an understandable consequence of the MCI. Your region or agency may have requirements for what information must be completed on the report during an MCI.

Special Situation Reports

Many states use a supplemental form for advanced life support (ALS) calls or additional documentation for calls that were complex or involved (Figure 17-18).

Your activities as an EMT may also take you to some unusual situations that will require documentation on a form other than a prehospital care report. Such forms are usually specific to a local agency rather than mandated statewide (Figure 17-19). Some examples of situations that might require this kind of special report include:

- Exposure to infectious disease
- Injury to yourself or another EMT
- Hazardous or unsafe scenes to which other crews should be alerted
- Referrals to social service agencies for elderly or other patients in need of home care
- Mandatory reports for child or elderly abuse

This list is not all-inclusive. If there is any situation that requires extra documentation, the special report form may be the place to note it. It is important to remain accurate and objective when filling out this type of report, especially in an unusual or emotional situation. Follow local guidelines for the documentation of confidential information in these reports and for distribution of copies to appropriate agencies or persons.

FIGURE 17-18 Example of a supplemental form.

FIGURE 17-19 Example of a special situation report.

Special Incident Report

Town of Colonie
Department of Emergency Medical Services ————————

EMERGENCY MEDICAL SERVICES
TOWN OF COLONIE

Date of Incident: _____ Time: _____ REMO #: _____

Town Run #: _____ Reported by: _____ Zone: _____

Type of Incident: ☐ MCI ☐ Rescue ☐ Personnel Matter ☐ Injury ☐ Accident with an EMS vehicle
☐ Infectious Disease Exposure ☐ Scene Conflict ☐ Other _____

Total # of Patients: ☐ #P-1: _____ ☐ #P-2: _____ ☐ #P-3: _____ ☐ #P-0: _____
Elapsed Scene Time: *(First unit arrival to last unit to hospital)* _____
Total Time of Incident: _____

Describe the Incident Below:
Attach any additional documentation such as news clipppings and the pre-hospital care report.
Attach additional sheets if necessary.

_____
_____
_____
_____
_____
_____
_____
_____
_____
_____
_____
_____
_____
_____
_____
_____
_____
_____
_____

Signature: _____ Date: _____

- -

Office Use Only
This incident relates to: ☐ Day Operation: TOT ☐ Night Operations: TOT: ☐ Administration: TOT:
_____ _____ _____

Disposition: _____
_____
Date:

Notifications/Copies: ☐ Director ☐ Deputy Director ☐ Supervisors
☐ Deputy Supervisors ☐ Senior Medics ☐ Zone Coordinator(s)
☐ Other _____ Zone: ☐ 2 ☐ 3 ☐ 4

Key Facts and Concepts

- When calling in patient information, include these elements:
  - Unit identification and level of provider
  - Estimated time of arrival
  - Patient's age and sex
  - Chief complaint
  - Brief, pertinent history of the present illness
  - Major past illnesses
  - Mental status
  - Baseline vital signs
  - Pertinent findings of the physical exam
  - Emergency medical care given
  - Response to emergency medical care
  - Contact made with medical direction if required or if you have questions
- When completing the prehospital care report, or PCR, include the following:
  - Patient's name, address, date of birth, age, sex
  - Billing and insurance information (in many jurisdictions)

- Nature of the call
- Mechanism of injury
- Location where the patient was found
- Treatment administered before arrival of the EMT (by bystanders, Emergency Medical Responders, or others)
- Signs and symptoms, baseline and subsequent vital signs
- Secondary assessment
- Care administered and the effect that the care had on the patient (e.g., improved, no change)
- Changes in condition throughout the call

- A PCR may be a legal document in a court proceeding.
- Data from PCRs may help determine future treatments, trends, research, and quality improvement.
- Your report should "paint a picture" of your patient and his condition, accurately describing your contact with the patient throughout the call.

Key Decisions

- What radio procedure should I follow at this (or any) stage of the call?
- What elements should I include in the medical radio report?
- What information about this patient must I include in the care report?
- What steps must I take to avoid legal issues during communication and documentation for this call?

Chapter Glossary

base station a two-way radio at a fixed site such as a hospital or dispatch center.

cell phone a phone that transmits through the air instead of over wires so that the phone can be transported and used over a wide area.

drop report/transfer report an abbreviated form of the PCR that an EMS crew can leave at the hospital when there is not enough time to complete the PCR before leaving.

mobile radio a two-way radio that is used or affixed in a vehicle.

portable radio a handheld two-way radio.

repeater a device that picks up signals from lower-power radio units, such as mobile and portable radios, and retransmits them at a higher power. It allows low-power radio signals to be transmitted over longer distances.

watt the unit of measurement of the output power of a radio.

Preparation for Your Examination and Practice

Short Answer

1. List the steps of a medical radio report and describe the communication that may be necessary during each part.

2. List several guidelines for effective interpersonal communication with patients.

3. Explain what is meant by "objective" and "subjective" information in the narrative portion of the prehospital care report. Explain what is meant by "a pertinent negative."

4. Explain how spelling and the use of codes, abbreviations, and medical terms relate to writing a clear and accurate narrative report.

5. List some important steps to take and information to include when documenting a patient refusal.

Thinking and Linking

Think back to Chapter 12, "Vital Signs and Monitoring Devices," and link information from that chapter with information from this chapter as you consider the following situation:

- Five minutes before arrival at the hospital, you obtain a pulse of 108 on your critically injured patient. As you are writing up your prehospital care report, your partner tells you that just as you arrived, he was taking the patient's pulse and got a rate of 59. You are slightly stunned. How could the patient's pulse have dropped from 108 to 59? Then common sense kicks in. "You forgot to multiply by 2," you tell him. "The pulse must have been 118." How did you figure out that the rate of 59 had not been multiplied by 2? What is the reason for multiplying by 2?

Critical Thinking Exercises

It is important to be able to organize your radio and written reports correctly. The purpose of this exercise will be to consider how you might organize the information provided.

1. The following information, describing a patient, is in random order. Organize the information and present a medical radio report as if you were radioing the hospital.
   - Chest pain radiating to the shoulder
   - 56 years old
   - Oxygen applied at 15 liters per minute via nonrebreather
   - Alert and oriented
   - Female
   - Came on 20 minutes ago while mowing the lawn
   - History of high blood pressure and diabetes
   - ETA 20 minutes
   - Pulse 86, respirations 22, skin cool and moist, blood pressure 110/66, SpO_2 96 percent
   - Oxygen relieved the pain slightly
   - Denies difficulty breathing
   - You are requesting orders from medical direction
   - You are on Community BLS Ambulance 4
   - Lung sounds equal on both sides
   - Placed in a position of comfort

2. Write a narrative report for the same call. What did you include in the narrative that you did not include in the radio report? Why?

Street Scenes

You and your partner have just finished a call involving a motor-vehicle crash with two vehicles. It was the first call of the day, just after you had checked out the ambulance but before you had time for breakfast. It is now 9:30 a.m. and you are sitting at a desk in the emergency department doing the prehospital care report. Although the patient didn't seem to be hurt badly, he had been complaining of lower back pain. Based on the patient complaint and the patient assessment, you decided to do a full immobilization.

Street Scene Question

1. What information is important to include in the prehospital care report?

Although your partner is hurrying you, you write a very complete and thorough prehospital care report. You detail the patient's pulses, motor function, and sensation in all extremities before and after immobilization, including the fact that you observed the patient had difficulty moving his left foot and that it felt numb. The patient also told you that he was wearing only a lap-style seat belt at the time of the crash, and that he had a considerable amount of pain. He had not moved from the vehicle prior to the arrival of EMS.

Street Scene Questions

2. What is the importance of doing an accurate and thorough prehospital care report?

3. Should you have your partner read and comment on the prehospital care report before considering it complete?

4. What are the ramifications of having a prehospital care report in the hospital record that is different from the original copy on file with your EMS agency?

After writing your prehospital care report, your partner reviews it and you leave a copy at the hospital for inclusion with the hospital chart. You manage to make it to breakfast, and you put this call behind you.

A few months later the director of your ambulance service stops you and asks if you remember this call. You think for a moment but only have a vague recollection. He informs you that the patient has started a lawsuit and claims that he sustained damage as the result of prehospital care. The prehospital care report has been reviewed by the ambulance service's lawyer, who believes that it will be a very good defense and the case will probably be dismissed. The director lets you read a copy of the prehospital care report. As you read it, you start to remember the call. You had forgotten about the patient's complaint of pain and other symptoms.

As he walks away, the director tells you that good documentation will make all the difference in how this case gets decided. This is very different from a case he had a few years ago when an EMT changed the service's copy of the PCR after he left a copy at the hospital. The lawyer for the plaintiff noticed the discrepancies and made things very difficult for the service.

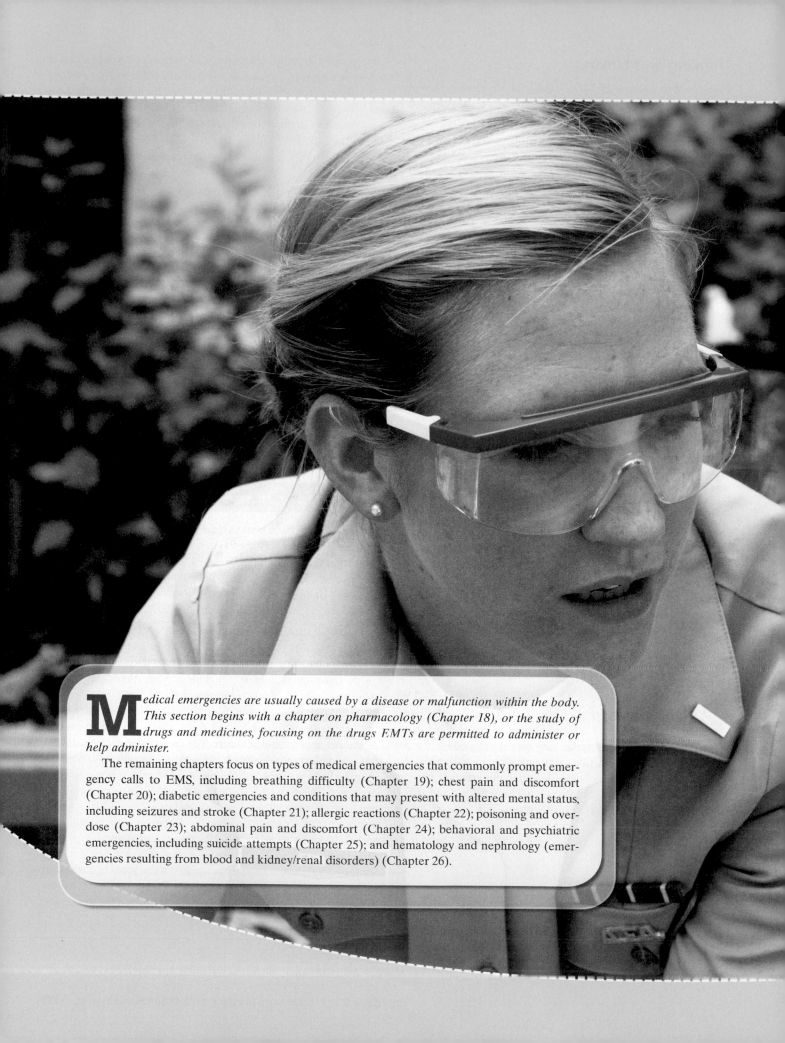

Medical emergencies are usually caused by a disease or malfunction within the body. This section begins with a chapter on pharmacology (Chapter 18), or the study of drugs and medicines, focusing on the drugs EMTs are permitted to administer or help administer.

The remaining chapters focus on types of medical emergencies that commonly prompt emergency calls to EMS, including breathing difficulty (Chapter 19); chest pain and discomfort (Chapter 20); diabetic emergencies and conditions that may present with altered mental status, including seizures and stroke (Chapter 21); allergic reactions (Chapter 22); poisoning and overdose (Chapter 23); abdominal pain and discomfort (Chapter 24); behavioral and psychiatric emergencies, including suicide attempts (Chapter 25); and hematology and nephrology (emergencies resulting from blood and kidney/renal disorders) (Chapter 26).

Medical Emergencies

General Pharmacology

STANDARDS
Pharmacology (Principles of Pharmacology; Medication Administration; Emergency Medications)

COMPETENCY
Applies fundamental knowledge of the medications that the EMT may assist with/administer to a patient during an emergency.

CORE CONCEPTS
— Which medications may be carried by the EMT

— Which medications the EMT may help administer to patients

— What to consider when administering any medication

— The role of medical direction in medication administration

— How the EMT may assist in IV therapy

EXPLORE ResourceCentral

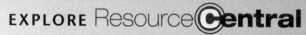

To access Resource Central, follow directions on the Student Access Card provided with this text. If there is no card, go to **www.bradybooks.com** and follow the Resource Central link to Buy Access from there. Under Media Resources, you will find:

▶ **Information on Prescribed Drugs**
Learn why you should obtain a list of medications from every patient and why an EMT should have a basic understanding of how different types of prescribed medications work.

▶ **Oral Medication**
Learn how to administer medication to a child, what the difference is between oral and buccal administration, and why you must assess the patient after administering a medication. All this and more in this video!

▶ **Epinephrine Auto-Injector Actions and Use**
Here's an animation detailing how to use an epinephrine auto-injector and see what changes the medication causes in the body.

OBJECTIVES

After reading this chapter you should be able to:

18.1 Define key terms introduced in this chapter.

18.2 List the drugs in your scope of practice. (pp. 425–430)

18.3 For each medication you may administer or assist a patient in self-administering, describe the following:
  a. Generic and common trade names (p. 431)
  b. Indication(s) (p. 432)
  c. Contraindications (p. 432)

  d. Side effects and untoward effects (p. 432)
  e. Form(s) (p. 432)
  f. Route(s) of administration (pp. 433–434)

18.4 Follow principles of medication administration safety, including the five rights of medication administration. (pp. 432–433)

18.5 Discuss the importance of looking up medications and requesting information from medical direction when needed. (p. 432)

(continued)

18.6 Identify the type of medical direction (on-line or off-line) required to administer each medication in the scope of practice. (p. 433)

18.7 Describe the characteristics of the oral, sublingual, inhaled, intravenous, intramuscular, subcutaneous, and endotracheal routes of administration. (pp. 433–434)

18.8 Identify special considerations in medication administration related to patients' ages and weights. (p. 434)

18.9 Explain the importance of accurate documentation of drug administration and patient reassessment following drug administration. (p. 434)

18.10 Discuss the importance of having readily available references to identify drugs commonly taken by patients. (pp. 434–437)

18.11 Discuss the steps an EMT may take in assisting with IV therapy. (pp. 437–440)

KEY TERMS

As an EMT, you will be trusted with the task of administering medications in emergency situations. This important responsibility requires you to use critical decision-making skills and pay attention to detail. Although in many cases these medications may be lifesaving, there is the potential to do significant harm to the patient when they are administered incorrectly.

The study of drugs—their sources, characteristics, and effects—is called ***pharmacology***. This chapter introduces the terminology, basic principles, and rules regarding pharmacology. We will discuss medications EMTs carry on the ambulance and review prescribed medications you may assist the patient in taking with approval from medical direction. You will learn the forms of medications your patients may be taking as well as the names for common types of medications and why they are used.

Although you will learn many facts and terms regarding medications, remember that nothing replaces good judgment and proper decision making. As always, the most important tool you carry is your brain.

NOTE: *Although EMS personnel use the terms medications and drugs interchangeably, the public often associates the word drugs with illegal or abused substances. When dealing with the public, therefore, use the terms medicines or medications.*

MEDICATIONS EMTS CAN ADMINISTER

>>>>>>

You will be able to administer or assist with six medications in the field: aspirin, oral glucose, oxygen, prescribed bronchodilator inhalers, nitroglycerin, and epinephrine auto-injectors. The information that follows is a brief introduction to each of these drugs.

Your local system may allow additions to this medication list. It is beyond the scope of this chapter, however, to include all the potential possibilities. However, if your system uses medications that are not covered here, be sure to obtain the appropriate information and education for those medications before administering them to a patient.

pharmacology

(FARM-uh-KOL-uh-je)
the study of drugs, their sources, their characteristics, and their effects.

FIGURE 18-1 Aspirin is administered to patients with chest pain of a suspected cardiac origin.

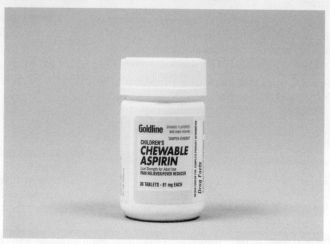

Medications on the Ambulance

As an EMT, you will carry aspirin, oral glucose, and oxygen on the ambulance. Under specific circumstances that will be described later, you will be able to administer these medications to patients.

Aspirin

aspirin
a medication used to reduce the clotting ability of blood to prevent and treat clots associated with myocardial infarction.

Many of you have taken a simple *aspirin* to relieve a headache or treat a fever. In the world of EMS, however, aspirin has a much more important role. As an EMT, you will administer aspirin to patients with chest pain of a suspected cardiac origin (Figure 18-1). In the event a heart attack is occurring, aspirin reduces the blood's ability to clot and works to prevent the clot formation that causes damage to the heart. It is an exceptionally important medication under these circumstances. Fortunately, it is also very simple to administer. As ambulances typically do not carry drinking water, most services will carry chewable children's aspirin and the patient will simply be asked to chew and swallow the appropriate dose. There are very few reasons not to administer aspirin to a patient having chest pain of a suspected cardiac origin. However, some patients do have allergies and others have gastrointestinal bleeding that can be made worse by the administration of aspirin. Always follow your local protocols for administration guidelines.

Oral Glucose

oral glucose (GLU-kos)
a form of glucose (a kind of sugar) given by mouth to treat an awake patient (who is able to swallow) with an altered mental status and a history of diabetes.

Glucose is a kind of sugar. *Oral glucose* is a form of glucose that can be taken by mouth as a treatment for a conscious patient (who is able to swallow) with an altered mental status and a history of diabetes. Poorly managed diabetes often leads to low blood sugar. The brain is very sensitive to low levels of sugar, and this is commonly a cause of altered mental status. Oral glucose usually comes as a tube of gel (Figure 18-2) that you can apply to a tongue depressor and place between the patient's cheek and gum or under the tongue. This allows the patient to swallow the glucose so it can be easily absorbed into the digestive tract and bloodstream, which carries it to the brain. This action may begin to reverse the patient's potentially life-threatening condition. The procedure for administering oral glucose will be found in Chapter 21, "Diabetic Emergencies and Altered Mental Status."

Oxygen

oxygen
a gas commonly found in the atmosphere. Pure oxygen is used as a drug to treat any patient whose medical or traumatic condition may cause him to be hypoxic, or low in oxygen.

Oxygen is a gas commonly found in the atmosphere. Pure oxygen is used as a drug to treat any patient whose medical or traumatic condition causes him to be hypoxic (low in oxygen) or in danger of becoming hypoxic (Figure 18-3). Throughout this text, you have learned—and will continue to learn—many situations in which a patient should be given oxygen. Spe-

FIGURE 18-2 Oral glucose may help a patient with diabetes.

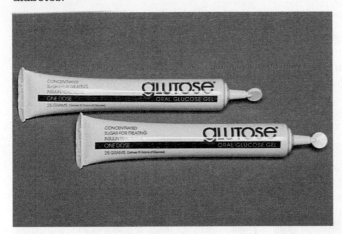

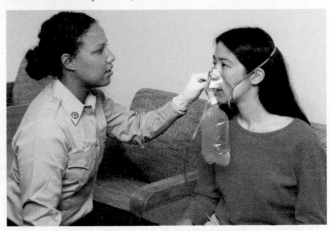

cific methods of administering oxygen were explained in Chapter 9, "Respiration and Artificial Ventilation."

NOTE: *Many systems allow the administration of activated charcoal. Therefore, although it is technically not one of our six commonly carried medications, we will discuss it here. Always consult local protocol to confirm which medications you are allowed to carry and administer.*

Activated charcoal is a powder prepared from charred wood, usually premixed with water to form a slurry for use in the field (Figure 18-4). It is used to treat a poisoning or overdose when a substance is swallowed and is in the patient's digestive tract. Activated charcoal will absorb some poisons (bind them to the surfaces of the charcoal) and help prevent them from being absorbed by the body. The procedure for administering activated charcoal will be found in Chapter 23, "Poisoning and Overdose Emergencies."

FIGURE 18-4 Activated charcoal is sometimes used in poisoning cases.

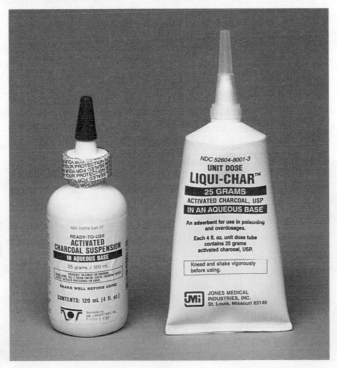

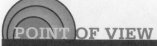
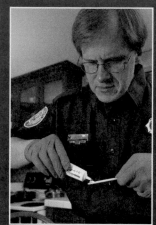
Prescribed Medications

● **CORE CONCEPT**
Which medications the EMT may help administer to patients

The three medications described next—prescribed inhaler, nitroglycerin, and epinephrine auto-injector—are drugs that you, as an EMT, may assist the patient in taking if they have been prescribed for the patient by a physician.

Bronchodilator Inhalers

inhaler
a spray device with a mouthpiece that contains an aerosol form of a medication that a patient can spray into his airway.

Patients can carry various medications to help them through a period of difficulty breathing. Most often patients with diseases like asthma, emphysema, or chronic bronchitis carry a "bronchodilator," a medication designed to enlarge constricted bronchial tubes, making breathing easier. Many of these medications can be carried in an *inhaler*, which contains an aerosol form of a medication the patient can spray directly into his airway (Figure 18-5). Examples of these medications include albuterol (Ventolin, Proventil, Volmax) and levalbuterol (Xopenex).

FIGURE 18-5 (A) A prescribed inhaler may help a patient who has respiratory problems. (B) A spacer attached to the inhaler helps the patient by allowing the medication to be released into the spacer where it remains airborne for a time so the patient can inhale it without feeling rushed—as he would be if inhaling it directly, without the spacer.

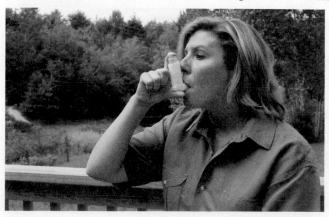

(A)

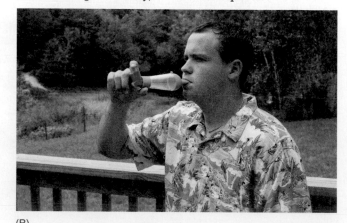

(B)

Since many bronchodilators also have an effect on the heart, an increased heart rate and patient jitteriness are common side effects of treatment.

Be sure to determine that the inhaler is actually the patient's and not that of a family member or bystander. You may need to have permission from medical direction to help a patient self-administer a prescribed inhaler. This permission from medical direction may come by phone or radio, or there may be a standing medical order that permits you to assist a patient with this kind of medication. *Always comply with the protocols of your EMS system.* More details on the use of a prescribed inhaler will be found in Chapter 19, "Respiratory Emergencies."

Nitroglycerin

Many patients with problems such as recurrent chest pain or a history of heart attack carry *nitroglycerin* pills or spray. Nitroglycerin (Figure 18-6) is a drug that helps to dilate the coronary vessels, which supply the heart muscle with blood. It is often called just "nitro." A common trade name is Nitrostat.

nitroglycerin (NYE-tro-GLIS-uh-rin) a drug that helps to dilate the coronary vessels that supply the heart muscle with blood.

This drug is taken by the patient when he begins to have chest pain he believes to be cardiac in origin. It is not uncommon for EMTs to treat patients who have already taken a nitroglycerin pill or who are carrying a bottle of nitroglycerin tablets and have not thought to try one. (Many patients are instructed by their physician to take up to three nitroglycerin pills for their chest pain and, if the chest pain persists, to call EMS.)

Be sure to determine that the nitroglycerin is actually the patient's and not that of a family member or bystander. Also determine whether the patient has recently taken anything to treat erectile dysfunction, such as sildenafil (Viagra), vardenafil (Levitra), tadalafil (Cialis), or similar medication. If so, he should not take nitroglycerin because of the possibility of a serious negative interaction with these drugs.

Since nitroglycerin causes a dilation of blood vessels, a drop in the patient's blood pressure is always a potential side effect of administration. If this should occur, you may also need to lay the patient flat as you contact medical direction again for advice.

You may need to seek permission from medical direction by phone or radio, or there may be a standing medical order that permits you to assist a patient with nitroglycerin administration. *Always comply with the protocols of your EMS system.* More information on assisting a patient in taking nitroglycerin will be found in Chapter 20, "Cardiac Emergencies."

Epinephrine Auto-Injectors

When a patient is highly allergic to something like shellfish, penicillin, or a bee sting, he may have a very severe reaction that may cause life-threatening changes in the airway and circulation. The reaction can be reversed by using *epinephrine*, a medication that will help to constrict the blood vessels and relax airway passages.

epinephrine (ep-uh-NEF-rin) a drug that helps to constrict the blood vessels and relax passages of the airway. It may be used to counter a severe allergic reaction.

Because severe allergic reactions may reach a life-threatening stage in a very short time, epinephrine must be administered quickly. Many patients who are prone to severe allergic reactions carry an epinephrine auto-injector (Figure 18-7). This is a syringe with a spring-loaded needle that will release and inject epinephrine into the muscle when the auto-injector is pushed

FIGURE 18-6 Nitroglycerin is often prescribed for chest pain. Forms of nitroglycerin include (A) tablets or (B) a spray.

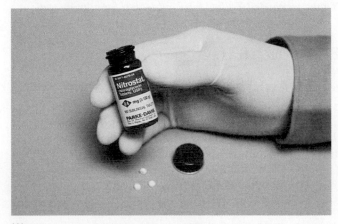

(A)

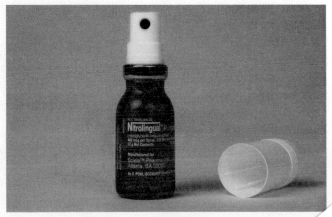

(B)

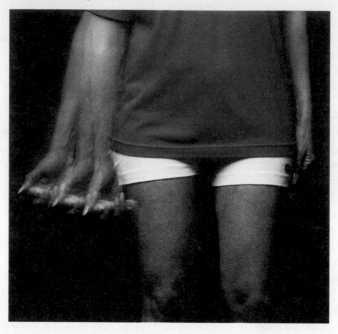

FIGURE 18-7 An epinephrine auto-injector can reverse a severe allergic reaction.

against the thigh. Epi-Pen® is the trade name of a commonly carried epinephrine auto-injector. Twinject® is the trade name of an auto-injector that contains two doses of epinephrine. If you need to assist a patient with the use of an epinephrine auto-injector, be sure to determine that the auto-injector is actually the patient's and not that of someone else.

Since epinephrine has a potent effect on the heart and vascular system, increased heart rate and blood pressure commonly occur after its administration to the patient.

You may need to seek permission from medical direction by phone or radio, or there may be a standing medical order that permits you to assist a patient with an epinephrine auto-injector. *Always comply with the protocols of your EMS system*. More information on assisting a patient in using an epinephrine auto-injector will be found in Chapter 22, "Allergic Reaction."

NOTE: *An increasing number of states are expanding the scope of practice to allow the basic-level EMT to carry and use an epinephrine auto-injector to treat life-threatening allergic reactions. The authority to administer epinephrine to the patient, rather than to assist a patient in the use of his own auto-injector, is normally granted by the Medical Director only after the EMT has received additional education and testing.*

Many systems also carry "force protection medications" such as atropine in auto-injector form to treat responders in the event of a chemical weapons attack. Typically, you would administer these medications to yourself and your partner if you found yourself exposed to certain weapons of mass destruction like nerve gas. Local protocols will determine which of these medications (if any) are carried. Follow local guidelines for administration.

CRITICAL DECISION MAKING

ALS Is on the Way. Should I Assist the Patient with Her Inhaler?

You are treating a 21-year-old asthma patient. She has been having an "asthma attack" for about 20 minutes. The patient complains of severe shortness of breath and your assessment confirms her difficulties. You have completed a thorough patient assessment, administered high-concentration oxygen, and called for ALS. The patient has a prescribed albuterol inhaler that you are allowed to assist her with based on your protocols. However, you note that ALS is only 5–8 minutes away. Should you assist with the medication or simply wait for the paramedics to arrive?

Inside/Outside

Medications are valuable tools to help patients in the most serious of medical emergencies. Some medications are carried by EMTs whereas others belong to the patients. You may be allowed to assist patients with taking their medications.

This section discusses the pathophysiology of two common emergency presentations, asthma and anaphylaxis, and explains how medications available to the EMT work.

CONDITION	PATHOPHYSIOLOGY	ACTION OF MEDICATIONS
Asthma	Small airways become reactive and constrict. Air does not move in and out easily although exhaling is more difficult. This results in air trapping. Upon auscultation of a full respiratory cycle, you will notice that the expiratory phase is prolonged. "Triggers" such as exercise, allergens, respiratory viruses, and even aspirin and non-steroidal anti-inflammatory drugs (NSAIDs) cause this reaction.	Albuterol is a medication very commonly used during asthma attacks. It is available in an inhaler and in a small volume nebulizer (SVN). Albuterol must actually enter the smaller airways—it acts upon contact. Albuterol acts on the (beta$_2$) receptors of the sympathetic nervous system, which results in dilation of the airways. The fact that albuterol acts primarily on the specific receptors means there will be limited cardiac side effects (such as rapid heart rate).
Anaphylaxis	Anaphylaxis is a life-threatening response of the immune system. Anaphylaxis affects major systems such as the circulatory and respiratory systems and, if untreated, can cause death. Anaphylaxis begins when the body overreacts to an antigen. Common causes of anaphylaxis are bee stings, peanut butter, and medication allergies. The allergic reaction (begun when an antigen meets antibodies within the body) causes the body to release a variety of substances, including histamine, which cause vasodilatation and shock as well as bronchoconstriction. These substances also alter vascular permeability, allowing fluid to enter and swell the airways, lips, tongue, and throat.	The epinephrine auto-injector carried by patients and on many ambulances provides immediate and significant benefit to those suffering from anaphylaxis. Epinephrine causes vasoconstriction (which reverses shock) by acting on the alpha receptors of the sympathetic nervous system. It reduces vascular permeability and the edema found in the face and airways. Epinephrine also causes bronchodilation to open constricted bronchioles through the beta receptors in the sympathetic nervous system.

GENERAL INFORMATION ABOUT MEDICATIONS

Drug Names

Every drug or medication is listed in a comprehensive government publication called the *U.S. Pharmacopoeia* (USP). Each drug is listed by its generic name (a general name that is not the brand name of any manufacturer). However, each drug actually has at least three names: the chemical name, the generic name, and one or more trade (brand) names given the drug by various manufacturers. For example, *epinephrine* is a generic drug name. Its chemical name is B-(3, 4 dihydroxyphenyl)-a-methylaminoethanol. (Chemical names are technical formulas used only by scientists or manufacturers.) As mentioned earlier, Epi-Pen® is the trade name of an epinephrine auto-injector.

What You Need to Know When Giving a Medication

Every drug has an indication or *indications*, that is, specific signs, symptoms, or circumstances under which it is appropriate to administer the drug to a patient. For example, nitroglycerin is indicated when a patient has chest pain or squeezing, dull pressure. Each drug also has *contraindications*, or specific signs, symptoms, or circumstances under which it is not appropriate, and may be harmful, to administer the drug to the patient. For example, nitroglycerin is contraindicated (should not be given) if the patient has low blood pressure, because nitroglycerin, in dilating the arteries, causes a slight drop in the systolic blood pressure. As noted earlier, nitroglycerin is also contraindicated if the patient has recently taken Viagra or a similar medication because of possible serious negative interactions.

A *side effect* is any action of a drug other than the desired action. Some side effects are predictable, like the drop in blood pressure from nitroglycerin. If you were not aware of the side effect of a drop in blood pressure and gave the drug to a patient who started out with low blood pressure, the results could be devastating. The patient's blood pressure might "bottom out"—which is definitely not a desirable effect for a cardiac patient. Often medications have unintended effects; that is, effects that occur in addition to the specific reason the drug was administered. Occasionally, such an effect can be classified as an *untoward effect*, or an effect that is not only unexpected, but also potentially harmful to the patient.

Medications come in many different forms. A few examples are:

- Compressed powders or tablets, such as nitroglycerin pills.
- Liquids for use outside the digestive tract, such as in an injection. This route is called the *parenteral* route and refers to bypassing the GI tract. An example of this type of medication would be epinephrine from an auto-injector.
- Liquids to be taken orally (like a cough syrup). This route utilizes the digestive tract to reach the bloodstream and is known as an *enteral* route.
- Liquid that is vaporized, such as a fixed-dose nebulizer.
- Gels, such as the paste in a tube of oral glucose.
- Suspensions, such as the thick slurry of activated charcoal in water.
- Fine powder for inhalation, such as that in a prescribed inhaler.
- Gases for inhalation, such as oxygen.
- Sublingual (under-the-tongue) sprays such as a nitroglycerin spray.

Medication Safety and Clinical Judgment

Administering or assisting with medications is a serious responsibility, since if medications are given incorrectly they can cause serious harm to the patient. As an EMT, you need to use good judgment and carefully consider any medication you administer.

The back of an ambulance is a dynamic place. There are many distractions and many decisions you will have to make. However, when it comes time to make decisions about medications, you need to focus. Medication administration should only be undertaken after a thorough patient assessment. You must see all the factors that go in to safe medication administration. You must understand not only how this medication will impact the patient in general, but also how it will impact your current patient under the current, specific circumstances.

Know the medication. If you are unsure about it, look it up. Never guess. Medical direction may be required for permission, but it may also be contacted for assistance. Ask questions. An EMT must multitask routinely, but when it comes to medication administration you need to be singular of focus. This is the time to think only about the task at hand.

Once the medication is administered you cannot take it back. Focus, clear thinking, and good judgment—all will help assure a proper and safe treatment.

Medication Authorization

As an EMT, you are authorized to administer medications by your Medical Director. This Medical Director may be service level, regional level, or even state level. The authorization to administer medications can come in two different manners:

CORE CONCEPT

What to consider when administering any medication

indications
specific signs or circumstances under which it is appropriate to administer a drug to a patient.

contraindications (KON-truh-in-duh-KAY-shunz)
specific signs or circumstances under which it is not appropriate, and may be harmful, to administer a drug to a patient.

side effect
any action of a drug other than the desired action.

untoward (un-TORD) *effect*
an effect of a medication in addition to its desired effect that may be potentially harmful to the patient.

parenteral (pair-EN-tur-al)
referring to a route of medication administration that does not use the gastrointestinal tract, such as an intravenous medication.

enteral (EN-tur-al)
referring to a route of medication administration that uses the gastrointestinal tract, such as swallowing a pill.

CORE CONCEPT

The role of medical direction in medication administration

 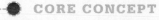

- **Off-line medical direction.** In this case, you will not actually speak to a physician to ask permission. Off-line medical direction uses "standing orders"; that is, orders written down in the form of protocols. Providers learn these protocols and administer medications guided by the specific circumstances and conditions previously outlined in their rules and regulations.

- **On-line medical direction.** In this case, you will need to speak directly to a physician (or his designee) to obtain verbal permission to administer a medication. Verbal confirmation is required. As an EMT, you should always be diligent to ensure you have heard and correctly understand the instructions. A useful technique to employ is the "echo technique." In this technique, you will listen to the order and then repeat the order back. The physician then should give you a verbal confirmation that what you have heard is correct. Use of this process significantly reduces medication errors. If at any time you are confused or have a question, speak up. Asking for clarification while on-line always is appropriate.

The Five Rights

Before administering a drug to any patient, confirm the order and write it down. Then check the "five rights" by asking yourself the following questions as you select the medication and confirm that it is not expired:

- **Do I have the right patient?** Does this medication belong to the patient? Is this the same patient medical direction approved a medication order for?

- **Is it the right time to administer this medication?** Have I made the right decision to administer the medication based on what I am seeing? Is it appropriate under these circumstances to give this particular medication?

- **Is this the right medication?** Did I pick up the right bottle? Am I sure this is the correct medication?

- **Is this the right dose?** Have I double checked? Am I sure I am giving the correct amount?

- **Am I giving this medication by the right route of administration?**

Routes of Administration

The route by which the drug is administered affects the rate that the medication enters the bloodstream and arrives at its target organ to achieve its desired effect. EMTs use the following routes of administration:

- **Oral, or swallowed.** This route is very safe and has few complications associated with administration. However, since the medication must be digested to take effect, it also takes longer for the medication to become effective. Oral medications are typically given in pill or capsule form; however, liquids are also a possible option. Patients simply swallow the medication. In EMS, most oral medications are given in chewable pill form (such as aspirin), since water for swallowing pills is often not available.

- **Sublingual, or dissolved under the tongue.** This route also accesses the body through the mouth; however, in this case the medication is typically placed under the tongue and allowed to dissolve. As it dissolves, the medication is absorbed by the vascular soft tissue of the mouth. This route is faster than swallowing pills, but absorption sometimes is difficult if circulation is poor (as in shock). (More information on assisting a patient with sublingual nitroglycerin can be found in Chapter 20, "Cardiac Emergencies").

- **Inhaled, or breathed into the lungs, usually as tiny aerosol particles (such as from an inhaler) or as a gas (such as oxygen).** Inhaled medications are breathed in through the respiratory system, and the medication is absorbed into the bloodstream through the alveoli. This is typically a simple process of putting a mask on your patient (as with oxygen). However, inhaled medications can be delivered via inhalers or nebulizers as well. (More details on the use of a prescribed inhaler will be found in Chapter 19, "Respiratory Emergencies.")

- **Intravenous, or injected into a vein.** The intravenous route is beyond the scope of the EMT level. However, you should know that this is a fast and precise way to administer medications into the body by directly accessing the bloodstream through a vein.

- **Intramuscular, or injected into a muscle.** The intramuscular route injects medication directly into the muscle. There, blood vessels can rapidly absorb the medication and transfer it to other parts of the body. This method of administration is very fast and allows for the effects of medication to rapidly occur. It can, however, be affected by poor circulation (as in shock) and also has a much higher complication rate than the oral or sublingual routes. This route typically uses a needle, as in an auto-injector, to deliver the medication. When you break the integrity of the skin's defenses with the needle, infections are somewhat common. More information on assisting a patient in using an auto-injector can be found in Chapter 22, "Allergic Reaction."

- **Subcutaneous, or injected under the skin.** Subcutaneous injections are very similar to intramuscular injections except that they deliver medications into the layers of the skin rather than into the muscle. This results in a slightly slower absorption than with intramuscular injections.

- **Intraosseous, or injected into the bone marrow cavity.** New technology (the "IO gun" or "IO drill") allows rapid placement of a rigid needle into the bone marrow cavities of long bones such as the tibia. This technology, with compelling research that shows medications and fluids injected into the marrow reach the central circulation as fast as those given IV, has made the IO route popular among ALS providers and emergency physicians in emergency situations such as cardiac arrests.

- **Endotracheal, or sprayed directly into a tube inserted into the trachea.** This route is used in some ALS systems. Endotracheal medications are administered through a tube inserted into the trachea to be absorbed by the tissue of the lungs. Recent evidence has questioned the effectiveness of this route, however, because lung tissue has very unpredictable absorption rates. Yet you may find this route still used as a last resort.

Age- and Weight-Related Considerations

pharmacodynamics
(FARM-uh-KO-die-nam-ICS)
the study of the effects of medications on the body.

Pharmacodynamics is the study of the effects of medications on the body. It is important to consider pharmacodynamics anytime you administer a medication. You should ask questions like: What effect will this medication have? How will it affect my patient? Remember that patient-specific factors can change how a medication will work. For example, a smaller, lighter patient, like a pediatric patient, will require less medication to achieve the desired effect. Often, geriatric patients will have difficulty eliminating medications and therefore feel the effects of medications longer. Consider age- and weight-related dose changes, and always understand how the medication will affect your specific patient before administering it.

Reassessment and Documentation

After administering any medication you must reassess your patient. Essentially, you should begin your patient assessment again and look for any changes—improvements, deteriorations, or unintended effect—that the medication might have caused. Reassessment should occur immediately and be frequently repeated, especially with medications that take time to be effective.

It is also important to clearly document the medications you have administered. Good documentation must include the name of the medication (spelling counts), the dose of the medication, the route by which you administered it (be specific, as in "injected into the right upper thigh"), the time of administration, and any effects you noted. Remember that the hospital will continue to give the patient medications and must know what has already been administered in order to carry out a safe treatment plan.

MEDICATIONS PATIENTS OFTEN TAKE

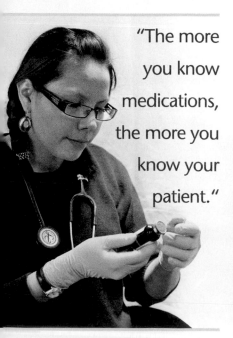

"The more you know medications, the more you know your patient."

It would be impossible to learn and carry around in your head all the types of medications you might discover your patients are taking. However, the medications a patient is taking may be a clue to a preexisting medical condition or, if improperly used, a cause of the patient's current problem. For example, a patient who is taking antihypertensives and antidiabetics might also be taking or misusing other medications that can contribute to an altered mental status—perhaps Dilantin to control seizures, codeine for pain, or Inderal for a heart rhythm disorder.

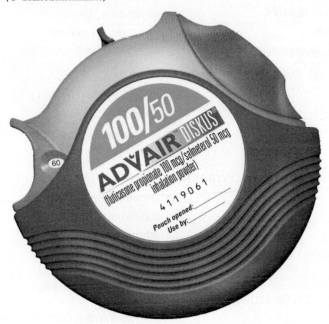

FIGURE 18-8 Advair™ is a medication that may be prescribed to a patient for daily management of a respiratory disease. It should not be used for emergency treatment of an acute attack or breathing difficulty.
(© GlaxoSmithKline)

Some medications that may be prescribed to a patient for daily use in managing a respiratory condition (one example would be beclomethasone, another would be Advair, Figure 18-8) should not be used to reverse an acute attack or to alleviate breathing difficulty.

It is a good idea to have a resource from which you can find out additional information about a patient's medications en route to the hospital. Many ambulances carry a *Physician's Desk Reference*, or *PDR*, for this purpose. Most EMTs carry with them, or have easily available access to, a pocket guide that contains useful information such as commonly used drug abbreviations. These pocket guides usually list the most commonly prescribed medications along with the general category of that medication to help you understand what the medication may be used for. A high-tech version of this guide is available that can be carried on an Internet-capable phone or even a personal digital assistant (PDA). This high-tech version is often more comprehensive than the paper version and more easily updated over the Internet. Several Internet-based or PDA-compatible programs are available, some of them at very little or no cost. However, remember that your main purpose in finding out what medications the patient is taking is not to make a field diagnosis but to report this information to medical direction and hospital personnel.

Table 18-1 lists the seven most common categories of medications you will find in the field that are relevant to patient care, with a few examples of medications in each category. Table 18-2 lists some common herbal agents patients sometimes take. A sizable number of people use these preparations, but they do not always think of them as medications that they should tell you about when you ask them what medications they take. Some of these agents have powerful effects, both intended and unintended, and should be recorded on the prehospital care report. Many also have interactions with prescription or over-the-counter medications. There are many other drugs and drug categories in addition to those listed in the table.

After any medication is given to a patient, it is important that you reassess the patient to see how the drug has affected him. Obtain another set of vital signs and compare them to the vital signs that you took before administering the medication. Ongoing patient assessment should include an evaluation of the changes in the patient's condition and vital signs after administration of medication. Be sure to document the patient's response to each drug intervention; for example, "The patient's respiratory distress decreased after 5 minutes of high-concentration oxygen by nonrebreather mask."

Table 18-1 Medications Patients Often Take

ANALGESICS: DRUGS PRESCRIBED FOR PAIN RELIEF

- propoxyphene
- nalbuphine (Nubain)
- morphine (Astramorph PF, Duramorph, MS Contin, Roxanol)
- acetaminophen (Anacin-3, Panadol, Tempra, Tylenol)
- Ibuprofen (Actiprofen, Advil, Excedrin IS, Motrin, Novoprofen, Nuprin)
- aspirin (Ecotrin, Emprin)
- codeine
- oxycodone (OxyContin)
- naproxen (Naprosyn)
- indomethacin (Indocin)

ANTIDYSRHYTHMICS: DRUGS PRESCRIBED FOR HEART RHYTHM DISORDERS

- digoxin (Lanoxin)
- propranolol (Inderal)
- Verapamil (Calan, Calan SR, Isoptin, Isoptin SR, Verelan)
- procainamide (Procan SR, Promine, Pronestyl)
- disopyramide (Norpace)
- carvedilol (Coreg)
- metoprolol (Lopressor, Toprol XL)

ANTICONVULSANTS: DRUGS PRESCRIBED FOR PREVENTION AND CONTROL OF SEIZURES

- carbamazepine (Epitol, Tegretol)
- phenytoin (Dilantin)
- primidone (Mysoline)
- phenobarbital (Phenobarbital, Phenobarbital Sodium, Solfoton)
- valproic acid (Depakene)
- lamotrigine (Lamictal)
- topiramate (Topamax)
- ethosuximide (Zarontin)
- gabapentin (Neurontin)
- levetiracetam (Keppra)

ANTIHYPERTENSIVES: DRUGS PRESCRIBED TO REDUCE HIGH BLOOD PRESSURE

- captopril (Capoten)
- clonidine (Catapres)
- guanabenz (Wytensin)
- Hydralazine (Apresoline, Hydralazine HCL)
- hydrochlorothiazide (Esidrix, HydroDiuril, Oretic)
- methyldopa (Aldomet)
- nifedipine (Adalat, Adalat CC, Procardia)
- prazosin (Minipress)

BRONCHODILATORS: DRUGS THAT RELAX THE SMOOTH MUSCLES OF THE BRONCHIAL TUBES. THESE MEDICATIONS PROVIDE RELIEF OF BRONCHIAL ASTHMA AND ALLERGIES AFFECTING THE RESPIRATORY SYSTEM

- albuterol (Proventil, Ventolin, Volmax)
- isoetharine (Bronkometer, Bronkosol)
- metaproterenol (Alupent, Metaproterenol sulfate, Metaprel)
- Terbutaline (Brethaire, Brethine, Bricanyl)
- ipratropium (Atrovent)
- salmeterol (Serevent)
- albuterol/ipratropium (Combivent, DuoNeb)
- montelukast (Singulair)
- zafirlukast (Accolate)
- levalbuterol (Xopenex)

ANTIDIABETIC AGENTS: DRUGS PRESCRIBED TO DIABETIC PATIENTS TO CONTROL HYPERGLYCEMIA (HIGH BLOOD SUGAR)

- glipizide (Glucotrol)
- Glyburide (DiaBeta, Glynase PresTab, Micronase)
- insulin (Humulin, Novolin, NPH, Humalog)
- metformin (Glucophage)
- glimepiride (Amaryl)
- rosiglitazone maleate (Avandia)

ANTIDEPRESSANT AGENTS: DRUGS PRESCRIBED TO HELP REGULATE THE EMOTIONAL ACTIVITY OF THE PATIENT TO MINIMIZE THE PEAKS AND VALLEYS IN THEIR PSYCHOLOGICAL AND EMOTIONAL STATE

- amitriptyline (Elavil)
- amoxapine
- bupropion (Wellbutrin)
- clomipramine (Anafranil)
- venlafaxine (Effexor)
- escitalopram (Lexapro)
- fluoxetine (Prozac)
- imipramine (Tofranil, Tripamine)
- nefazodone (Serzone)
- nortriptyline (Aventyl, Pamelor)
- paroxetine (Paxil)
- protriptyline (Vivactil)
- sertraline (Zoloft)
- trimipramine (Surmontil)
- citalopram (Celexa)

Note: Generic names are lowercase. Trade names are capitalized.

Table 18-2   Herbal Agents and What They Are Sometimes Used For

HERBAL AGENT	SOMETIMES USED FOR
Gingko or gingko biloba	Dementia, poor circulation to the legs, ringing in the ears
St. John's wort	Depression
Echinacea	Prevention and treatment of the common cold
Garlic	High cholesterol
Ginger root	Nausea and vomiting
Saw palmetto	Swollen prostate
Hawthorn leaf or flower	Heart failure
Evening primrose oil	Premenstrual syndrome
Feverfew leaf	Migraine prevention
Kava kava	Anxiety
Valerian root	Insomnia

ASSISTING IN IV THERAPY

Setting Up an IV Fluid Administration Set

IV therapy is an advanced life support procedure. In this procedure, an intravenous (IV) catheter is inserted into a vein so that blood, fluids, or medications can be administered directly into the patient's circulation. A blood transfusion is almost always given at the hospital, whereas an infusion of other fluids and many medications can be done in the field.

There are two ways fluids and medications may be administered into the vein. One of these is through a heparin or saline lock (Figure 18-9). In this case, a catheter is placed into the vein. A small cap or lock is placed over the end of the catheter that protrudes from the skin. This

CORE CONCEPT

How the EMT may assist in IV therapy

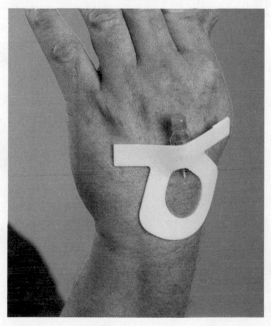

FIGURE 18-9 A saline or heparin lock can be used when fluid is not likely to be administered but medication administration or IV access may be needed later on.

lock contains a port through which you can administer medication. There is no IV bag attached to a saline lock. It is used in cases where fluid isn't likely to be administered but the administration of medications and/or the need for IV access later on is likely.

The second way fluids can be administered is through the traditional IV bag, which hangs above the patient and constantly flows fluids and medications into the patient.

The bag of fluid that feeds the IV is usually a clear plastic bag that collapses as it empties. The administration set is the clear plastic tubing that connects the fluid bag to the needle, or catheter. There are three important parts to this tubing:

- The *drip chamber* is near the fluid bag. There are two basic types: the micro drip (also sometimes called mini drip) and the macro drip. The micro drip is used when minimal flow of fluid is needed (with children, for example). For example, 60 small drops from the tiny metal barrel in the drip chamber equal 1 cubic centimeter (cc) or 1 milliliter (mL). The macro drip is used when a higher flow of fluid is needed (for a multitrauma patient in shock, for example). There is no little barrel in the drip chamber of the macro drip, and just 10 to 15 large drops equal 1 cc or 1 mL.

- The *flow regulator* is located below the drip chamber. It is a device that can be pushed up or down to start, stop, or control the rate of flow.

- The *drug or needle port* is below the flow regulator. The paramedic can inject medication into this opening.

An extension set includes an extra length of tubing, which can make it easier to carry or disrobe the patient without accidentally pulling out the IV. Extension sets are sometimes not used with the macro drip set because lengthening tubing reduces the flow rate.

In most cases, a paramedic will insert the IV into the patient's vein. However, you may be enlisted to help set up the IV administration set. If so, you will need to do the following steps.

1. Take out and inspect the fluid bag (Figure 18-10). The bags come in a protective wrapping to keep them clean. If you are setting up the IV, you must remove the wrapper, then inspect the bag to be sure it contains the fluid that has been ordered. Check the expiration date to make sure the fluid is usable, and look to see that the fluid is clear and free of particles. Squeeze the bag to check for leaks. Occasionally, the fluid comes in a bottle. If so, be sure it is free of cracks. If anything is wrong, report the problem and inspect another bag or bottle.

2. Select the proper administration set. Uncoil the tubing, and do not let the ends touch the ground (Figure 18-11).

3. Connect the extension set to the administration set, if an extension set is to be used.

4. Make sure the flow regulator is closed. To do this, roll the stopcock away from the fluid bag.

FIGURE 18-10 Inspect the IV bag to be sure it contains the solution that was ordered, it is clear, it does not leak, and it has not expired.

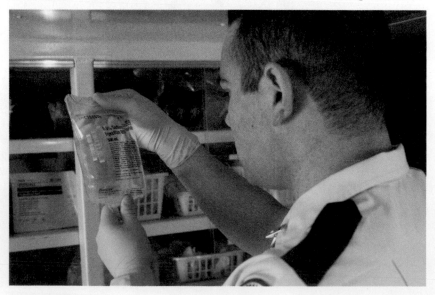

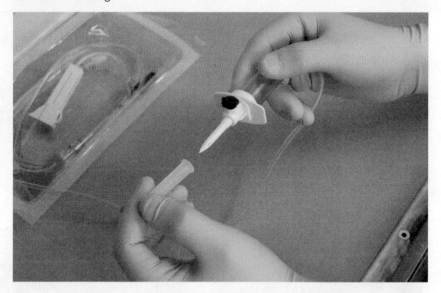

5. Remove the protective covering from the port of the fluid bag and the protective covering from the spiked end of the tubing. Insert the spiked end of the tubing into the fluid bag with a quick twist (Figure 18-12). Do this carefully. Maintain sterility. If these parts touch the ground, they must not be used. Introducing germs or dirt directly into a patient's bloodstream can be extremely serious, if not fatal.

6. Hold the fluid bag higher than the drip chamber. Squeeze the drip chamber a time or two to start the flow. Fill the chamber to the marker line (approximately one-third full).

7. Open the flow regulator and allow the fluid to flush all the air from the tubing (Figure 18-13). You may need to loosen the cap at the lower end to get the fluid to flow. Maintain the sterility of the tubing end and replace the cap when you are finished. Most sets can be flushed without removing the cap. Be sure that all air bubbles have been flushed from the tubing to avoid introducing a dangerous air embolism into the patient's vein.

8. Turn off the flow (Figure 18-14).

Make certain that the setup stays clean until the paramedic removes the needle and connects the IV tubing to the catheter inside the patient's vein. Occasionally, the paramedic will draw blood from the vein to obtain samples before inserting the IV. You may be asked to assist by placing the blood in sample tubes and labeling the tubes with the patient's name and any other information that your hospital requires. Remember that these tubes are potential carriers of pathogens. Be sure to take Standard Precautions. Carry the blood tubes to a safe place where they will not be in danger of breaking.

Do not be surprised if you are asked to hold up the patient's arm for a few minutes during a cardiac arrest. During cardiac arrest, medications can be more effective if the arm is temporarily raised after a drug is injected into the IV.

Maintaining an IV

An IV must continue to flow at the proper rate once it has been inserted into the patient's vein. However, a number of things may interrupt the flow. If you are charged with maintaining an IV, be sure to check for and correct the following problems:

- The constricting band used to raise the vein for insertion of the needle may have been mistakenly left on the patient's arm, perhaps covered by a sleeve.
- The flow regulator may be closed.
- The clamp may be closed on the tubing.
- The tubing may kink.
- The tubing may get caught under the patient or the backboard.

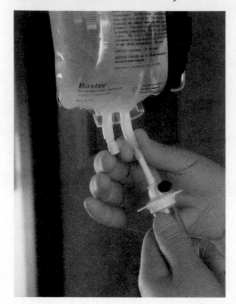

FIGURE 18-12 Insert spiked end of tubing into fluid bag. Squeeze drip chamber to fill about halfway.

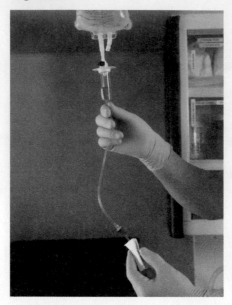

FIGURE 18-13 Open the flow regulator.

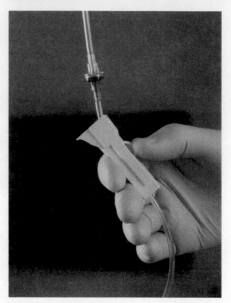

FIGURE 18-14 Once the fluid reaches the end of the tubing, turn off the flow.

The position of the IV or of the patient's arm also may need to be adjusted. Some IVs only flow when the patient's arm or IV site is in a certain position. Adjusting, or even splinting, the arm may be helpful as long as the splint is not too tight. Since the IV flow usually depends on gravity, be sure that the bag is held well above the IV site and the patient's heart.

Insufficient flow can cause blood to clot in the catheter. This can be prevented by adjusting the flow to an adequate "keep the vein open" or KVO rate. Although the KVO rate varies, it is usually about 30 drops per minute for a micro drip and 10 drops per minute for a macro drip set. If the drip chamber is overfilled, clamp the tubing, invert the drip chamber, and pump some fluid back into the bag.

An IV with a flow rate that is too fast is called a "runaway IV." It can rapidly overload the patient with fluid and cause serious problems, especially in an infant or child.

An infiltrated IV is one where the needle has either punctured the vein and exited the other side or has pulled out of the vein. In either case, the fluid is flowing into the surrounding tissues instead of into the vein. An unnoticed infiltrated IV can be very dangerous. Certain high-concentration medications (such as 50 percent dextrose) can cause the death of the surrounding tissue. In addition to complaining of pain, the patient will show swelling at the site (noticeable in all but some obese patients). The person in charge of maintaining the IV

CRITICAL DECISION MAKING

How or Whether to Assist with Medications

Your decisions on how to assist patients with their medications—or whether to assist them at all—are a critical part of your practice as an EMT. The following questions will test your knowledge and decision making in this vital area.

1. You are treating a patient who has chest pain. He tells you his wife has nitroglycerin. He asks if he should take her pills. What should you tell him?

2. You are treating a patient who is diabetic. She appears very sleepy and only responds to loud verbal stimulus by briefly opening her eyes. The patient's sister says, "Give her some sugar!" Should you? Why or why not?

3. Your COPD patient is breathing 48 times per minute shallowly. His wife believes his "lung problems" have been acting up. Would the patient's inhaler help him?

must stop the flow and discontinue the IV according to local protocol. If you are not authorized to do this, report the problem immediately to the paramedic or medical direction.

If you learn how to help advanced life support personnel start an IV, set up an administration set, label blood tubes, and maintain an IV, valuable time can be saved at the scene and during transport.

CHAPTER REVIEW

Key Facts and Concepts

- Aspirin, oral glucose, and oxygen are medications carried on the ambulance that the EMT may administer to a patient under specific conditions.

- Prescribed inhalers, nitroglycerin, and epinephrine in auto-injectors are medications that, if prescribed for the patient, the EMT may assist the patient in taking.

- You may need to have permission from medical direction to administer or assist the patient with a medication. Follow local protocols.

- There is a wide variety of medications that a patient may be taking. You will try to find out what medications a patient is taking when you take the SAMPLE history. These drugs may be identified by a variety of generic and trade names. Your main purpose in finding out what medications the patient is taking is to report this information to your Medical Director or hospital personnel.

Key Decisions

- Should I administer aspirin?
- Should I assist the patient with his prescribed medication?
- What medications is my patient taking and what information about his current condition can I obtain based on those medications?

- How do the patient's medications potentially affect his current condition?

Chapter Glossary

aspirin a medication used to reduce the clotting ability of blood to prevent and treat clots associated with myocardial infarction.

contraindications (KON-truh-in-duh-KAY-shunz) specific signs or circumstances under which it is not appropriate, and may be harmful, to administer a drug to a patient.

enteral (EN-tur-al) referring to a route of medication administration that uses the gastrointestinal tract, such as swallowing a pill.

epinephrine (ep-uh-NEF-rin) a drug that helps to constrict the blood vessels and relax passages of the airway. It may be used to counter a severe allergic reaction.

indications specific signs or circumstances under which it is appropriate to administer a drug to a patient.

inhaler a spray device with a mouthpiece that contains an aerosol form of a medication that a patient can spray into his airway.

nitroglycerin (NYE-tro-GLIS-uh-rin) a drug that helps to dilate the coronary vessels that supply the heart muscle with blood.

oral glucose (GLU-kos) a form of glucose (a kind of sugar) given by mouth to treat an awake patient (who is able to swallow) with an altered mental status and a history of diabetes.

oxygen a gas commonly found in the atmosphere. Pure oxygen is used as a drug to treat any patient whose medical or traumatic condition may cause him to be hypoxic, or low in oxygen.

parenteral (pair-EN-tur-al) referring to a route of medication administration that does not use the gastrointestinal tract, such as an intravenous medication.

pharmacodynamics (FARM-uh-KO-die-nam-ICS) the study of the effects of medications on the body.

pharmacology (FARM-uh-KOL-uh-je) the study of drugs, their sources, their characteristics, and their effects.

side effect any action of a drug other than the desired action.

untoward (un-TORD) *effect* an effect of a medication in addition to its desired effect that may be potentially harmful to the patient.

Preparation for Your Examination and Practice

Short Answer

1. Name the drugs that are commonly carried on the ambulance and may be administered by the EMT under certain circumstances.

2. Name the drugs that the EMT may assist the patient in taking if they have been prescribed for him and with approval by medical direction.

3. Medications may take the form of tablets. Name several other forms in which medications may appear.

4. Describe the difference between on-line medical direction and off-line medical direction. Provide examples of each.

5. Name several routes by which medications may be administered.

Thinking and Linking

Medication administration is a key intervention the EMT may perform during patient assessment and transpsort. Think back to Chapters 13 through 15 on Assessment of the Trauma Patient and Medical Patient and Reassessment as you answer the following question.

- List the "five rights" of medication administration and discuss why each is important. What would the potential risk to the patient be if each were not checked prior to administration?

Critical Thinking Exercises

Administering medications to the patient is a serious responsibility. How would you act in the following situation?

- A patient is complaining of chest pain. "Here's some nitroglycerin," says a family member. "Give him that." What do you do?

Pathophysiology to Practice

The following question is designed to assist you in gathering relevant clinical information and making accurate decisions in the field.

- In this chapter, we have discussed the need to reassess the patient after the administration of any medication. What elements would you reassess? What findings might be significant?

Street Scenes

It is winter and cold, so you are not too surprised when the dispatcher tells you to respond to the mall for a 62-year-old male patient with chest pain. During winter, many cardiac patients walk for exercise in the mall, and this is not the first cardiac call you have had there. When you arrive, you find the patient sitting in a chair. You introduce yourself and your partner, ask the patient his name, and then say, "Well, Mr. Edwards, why was EMS called?"

"I was doing my usual morning walk," he explains, "when I started to get chest pain. I thought it might go away but it didn't. I got concerned and asked the security guard to call 911."

As your partner administers oxygen by nonrebreather mask and takes a set of vital signs, you ask the patient: "On a scale of 1 to 10, with 10 being the worst pain you've ever had, how would you rate the chest pain you're having now?" He tells you that it is a 7. You ask him to describe the pain and to point to where it is located. He says that it feels like a dull pain and points to the center of his chest. He also says the pain does not radiate. The patient seems pale, and his skin is dry. After a bit more questioning, he tells you the last time this happened he took nitro for relief.

Street Scene Questions

1. What additional patient history should you obtain?
2. Should you let the patient take nitroglycerin? Why, or why not?
3. Are vital signs important if nitroglycerin is going to be taken by the patient?

You ask Mr. Edwards if he has nitroglycerin with him now. He says his wife has it, but she went to a store in another part of the mall and should be back shortly. You then ask about other medications, and the patient tells you he is on propranolol and a diuretic. Next, you ask if he has ever had a heart attack. The patient tells you that he had one about a year and a half ago that was treated with an angioplasty. Vital signs are: pulse 90, blood pressure 120/90, and respirations of 24 and labored. When his wife shows up, she attempts to administer a pill, but you ask her to wait.

Street Scene Questions

4. What information do you want to know about the nitroglycerin?
5. How should the nitroglycerin be administered?
6. When should vital signs be taken again?

At your request, the patient's wife gives you the nitroglycerin bottle so you can check the expiration date. At the same time, you check to make sure that it is the patient's specific prescription. It all checks. According to standing orders in your system, if a patient has these signs and symptoms, including a systolic blood pressure over 100, you may give a nitro without having radio contact with medical direction. You tell the patient that you are going to put the pill under his tongue and he should let it dissolve. You specifically tell Mr. Edwards not to swallow.

About a minute after you give Mr. Edwards the pill, he complains of a slight headache. You tell him this is a possible side effect of taking nitro and not to be concerned. After another minute goes by, you ask the patient to rate the chest pain on a scale of 1 to 10 again. "About a 2," he replies. "In fact, the pain is almost gone," he tells you. Your partner takes another set of vital signs, since a patient's blood pressure can drop when taking nitro, but there is no change. You package the patient for transport and move to the ambulance, making sure you keep the AED close by. You give Mrs. Edwards a short update and explain to her that you will take the nitroglycerin bottle with the patient. The transport to the hospital is uneventful, and you take another set of vital signs en route.

Respiratory Emergencies

19

STANDARD ○-------
Medicine (Respiratory)

COMPETENCY ○-------
Applies fundamental knowledge to provide basic emergency care
and transportation based on assessment findings for an acutely ill patient.

CORE CONCEPTS ○-------
— How to identify adequate breathing

— How to identify inadequate breathing

— How to identify and treat a patient with breathing difficulty

— Use of continuous positive airway pressure (CPAP) to relieve
difficulty breathing

— Use of a prescribed inhaler and how to assist a patient with one

— Use of a prescribed small-volume nebulizer and how to assist
a patient with one

EXPLORE Resource Central

To access Resource Central, follow directions on the Student Access Card provided
with this text. If there is no card, go to **www.bradybooks.com** and follow the
Resource Central link to Buy Access from there. Under Media Resources, you will find:

▶ **Breath Sounds and Assessment Tips**
Listen to breath sounds and learn how to differentiate among them and find out
what assessment findings may be present in patients complaining of respiratory
distress.

▶ **Chronic Obstructive Pulmonary Diseases**
View an animation on COPD and learn some of the causes associated with this
disease.

▶ **Information on Pulmonary Edema**
Learn what causes pulmonary edema, some signs and symptoms, and why a
patient with pulmonary edema should receive oxygen therapy.

OBJECTIVES

After reading this chapter you should be able to:

19.1 Define key terms introduced in this chapter.

19.2 Describe the anatomy and physiology of
respiration. (pp. 444–445)

19.3 Differentiate between adequate and inadequate
breathing based on the rate, rhythm, and quality of
breathing. (pp. 445–448)

19.4 Discuss differences between the adult and pediatric
airways and respiratory systems. (p. 447)

19.5 Recognize signs of inadequate breathing in
pediatric patients. (p. 447)

19.6 Provide supplemental oxygen and assisted
ventilation as needed for patients with inadequate
breathing. (p. 448)

(continued)

KEY TERMS

A s an EMT, you will encounter some patients who are having breathing difficulty but who nevertheless are breathing adequately. You will provide oxygen by nonrebreather mask to these patients and complete an on-scene assessment before transporting them to the hospital. At other times, you will encounter patients whose respiratory problems are more severe. They may be having such extreme difficulty moving air in and out of their lungs that their breathing is no longer adequate to support life. These patients will require much more rapid care, which will probably include assisted ventilations.

The difference between adequate and inadequate breathing is one of the most important concepts covered in this chapter.

>>>>>> RESPIRATION

Respiratory Anatomy and Physiology

You learned about the respiratory system in Chapter 5, "Medical Terminology and Anatomy and Physiology"; Chapter 6, "Principles of Pathophysiology"; Chapter 8, "Airway Management"; and Chapter 9, "Respiration and Artificial Ventilation." In preparation for this chapter, you should review those chapters and make sure you are familiar with the following structures of the respiratory system: nose, mouth, oropharynx, nasopharynx, epiglottis, trachea, cricoid cartilage, larynx, bronchi, lungs, alveoli, and diaphragm.

The diaphragm is a muscular structure that separates the chest cavity from the abdominal cavity. During a normal respiratory cycle, the diaphragm and other parts of the body work together to allow the body to inhale (breathe in) and exhale (breathe out) air. The respiratory cycle progresses as follows (Figure 19-1):

inspiration (IN-spuh-RAY-shun) an active process in which the intercostal (rib) muscles and the diaphragm contract, expanding the size of the chest cavity and causing air to flow into the lungs.

- **Inspiration.** The active process that uses the contraction of several muscles to increase the size of the chest cavity is called *inspiration*. In this process, the intercostal (rib) muscles and the diaphragm contract. The diaphragm lowers and the ribs move upward and outward. The expanding size of the chest cavity then causes air to flow into the lungs. Another term for inspiration is *inhalation*.

- **Expiration.** A passive process, *expiration* involves the relaxation of the rib muscles and diaphragm. The ribs move downward and inward, while the diaphragm rises. This movement causes the chest cavity to decrease in size and causes air to flow out of the lungs. Another term for expiration is *exhalation*.

Review in Chapter 5, "Medical Terminology and Anatomy and Physiology," how oxygen and carbon dioxide are exchanged through the alveoli and capillaries of the lungs, and through the capillaries and cells throughout the body. The exchange of oxygen and carbon dioxide, both in the lungs and in the body's cells, is critical to support life. There are many things that can go wrong within the body that will alter this vital exchange. Primarily, these are problems with the respiratory system or the circulatory system, as were described in Chapter 6, "Principles of Pathophysiology." This chapter will further discuss the respiratory system as well as problems with breathing and their effects on the body. Problems with the circulatory system will be discussed in greater detail in Chapter 20, "Cardiac Emergencies."

Adequate Breathing

It is easy to take breathing for granted. Fortunately, we do not consciously have to tell ourselves to inhale and exhale. The brain does that automatically.

As you learned in Chapter 9, "Respiration and Artificial Ventilation," breathing may be classified as adequate or inadequate. Simply stated, adequate breathing is breathing that is sufficient to support life. Inadequate breathing is not. Your assessment of the adequacy of a patient's breathing may be vital to his survival.

Adequate breathing falls within certain ranges that are considered "normal." The patient will not appear to be in distress. He will be able to speak full sentences without having to catch his breath. His color, mental status, and orientation will be normal. Normal breathing may be determined by observing for rate, rhythm, and quality:

- **Rate.** Rates of breathing that are considered normal vary by age. For an adult, a normal rate is 12–20 breaths per minute. For a child, it is 15–30 breaths per minute. For an infant, it is 25–50 breaths per minute.

- **Rhythm.** Normal breathing rhythm will usually be regular. Breaths will be taken at regular intervals and will last for about the same length of time. Remember that talking and other factors can make normal breathing slightly irregular.

- **Quality.** Breath sounds, when auscultated with a stethoscope, will normally be present and equal when the lungs are compared to each other. When observing the chest cavity, both sides should move equally and adequately to indicate a proper air exchange. The depth of the respirations must be adequate.

inhalation (IN-huh-LAY-shun) another term for inspiration.

expiration (EK-spuh-RAY-shun) a passive process in which the intercostal (rib) muscles and the diaphragm relax, causing the chest cavity to decrease in size and forcing air from the lungs.

exhalation (EX-huh-LAY-shun) another term for expiration.

CORE CONCEPT
How to identify adequate breathing

FIGURE 19-1 The process of respiration.

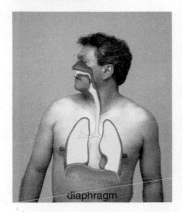 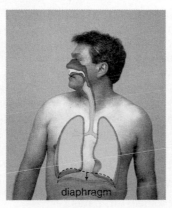 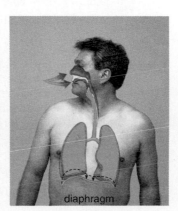 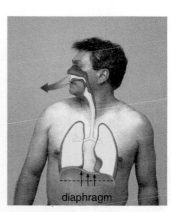

RELAXED

CONTRACTION
Inspiration begins

INSPIRATION

RELAXED
Passive expiration begins

Table 19-1 Adequate and Inadequate Breathing

	ADEQUATE BREATHING	INADEQUATE BREATHING
Rate	Adult: 12–20/Minute; Child: 15–30/Minute; Infant: 25–50/minute	Above or below normal rates for the patient's age group
Rhythm	Regular	May be irregular
Quality Breath Sounds Chest Expansion Effort of Breathing	Present and equal Adequate and equal Unlabored, normal respiratory effort	Diminished, unequal, or absent Inadequate or unequal Labored: increased respiratory effort; use of accessory muscles (may be pronounced in infants and children and involve nasal flaring, seesaw breathing, grunting, and retractions between the ribs and above the clavicles and sternum)
Depth	Adequate	Too shallow

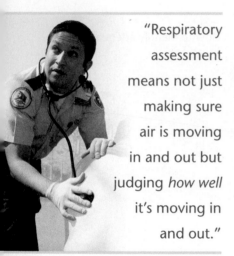

"Respiratory assessment means not just making sure air is moving in and out but judging *how well* it's moving in and out."

● CORE CONCEPT

How to identify inadequate breathing

Inadequate Breathing

Inadequate breathing is breathing that is not sufficient to support life. If left untreated, this condition will surely lead to death. One of your most important tasks as an EMT is to identify and treat patients with inadequate breathing. Begin assessment and treatment early in the call and continue them throughout your time with the patient. Patients who are breathing adequately at first may deteriorate into inadequate breathing later on (Table 19-1).

PATIENT ASSESSMENT

Inadequate Breathing

If the patient is not breathing adequately to support life, you may see any of the following conditions:

- **Rate.** The patient with inadequate breathing will have a breathing rate that is out of the normal ranges. Very slow breaths and very rapid breaths may not allow enough air to enter the lungs, resulting in not enough oxygen being distributed throughout the body.

    Agonal respirations (also called dying respirations) are sporadic, irregular breaths that are usually seen just before respiratory arrest. They are shallow and gasping with only a few breaths per minute. This breathing pattern is clearly a sign of inadequate breathing.

- **Rhythm.** The rhythm of inadequate breathing may be irregular. However, rhythm is not an absolute indicator of adequate or inadequate breathing. Remember that someone who is talking or is aware that you are observing his respirations may have slight irregularities, even though his breathing is adequate. However, a patient may have a regular rate, even when his breathing is inadequate.

- **Quality.** When breathing is inadequate, breath sounds may be diminished or absent. The depth of respirations (tidal volume) will be inadequate or shallow. Chest expansion may be inadequate or unequal and respiratory effort increased. You may note the use of accessory muscles (e.g., muscles of the neck and abdomen) in breathing. Since oxygenation of the body's tissues is reduced, the skin may be pale or cyanotic (blue) and feel cool and clammy to the touch.

    In patients with diminished responsiveness, sounds such as snoring and gurgling also indicate a serious airway problem that requires immediate intervention.

Decision Points

- Is the patient breathing?
- Is the patient breathing adequately?
- Do I have an intervention to help this patient?
- Will this patient benefit from ALS?

Respiratory problems can be very serious in infants and children. Although children rarely have heart attacks or other problems of adulthood, respiratory conditions are a leading killer of infants and children. With this in mind, you must begin respiratory treatment of infants and children with a thorough and accurate assessment and prompt, proper care.

The structure of infants' and children's airways differs somewhat from that of adults:

- **Airway.** All airway structures are smaller in an infant or child than in an adult and therefore are more easily obstructed.
- **Tongue.** Infants' and children's tongues are proportionately larger and therefore take up more space in the mouth than an adult's tongue.
- **Trachea.** The trachea is smaller, softer, and more flexible in infants and children, which may lead to obstruction from swelling or trauma more easily than in adults. The cricoid cartilage is less developed and less rigid.
- **Diaphragm.** Infants and children depend more heavily on the diaphragm for respiration since the chest wall is softer. This is why infants and small children in respiratory distress exhibit "seesaw breathing" in which the movement of the diaphragm causes the chest and abdomen to move in opposite directions.

Be aware that some signs of inadequate breathing are unique to, or more prominent in, infants and children. Therefore, be on the lookout for these signs:

- Nasal flaring (widening of the nostrils)
- Grunting
- Seesaw breathing
- Retractions (pulling in of the muscles) between the ribs (intercostal), above the clavicles (supraclavicular), and above the sternum (suprasternal)

PATIENT CARE

Inadequate Breathing

There is a wide range of function between adequate respirations and complete stoppage of breathing (respiratory arrest). You must pay careful attention to the patient's breathing throughout the call. It is not enough to simply make sure he is breathing. The patient must be breathing adequately! If at any time you find that he is not breathing adequately, the treatment of this condition is your first patient-care priority (Table 19-2).

When you determine, by the signs that were discussed under the previous Patient Assessment feature, that a patient's breathing is inadequate, you will provide assisted ventilation with supplemental oxygen. In order of preference, the means of providing assisted ventilation are:

1. Pocket face mask with supplemental oxygen
2. Two-rescuer bag-valve mask with supplemental oxygen
3. Flow-restricted, oxygen-powered ventilation device
4. One-rescuer bag-valve mask with supplemental oxygen

The means of providing artificial ventilation were discussed in Chapter 9, "Respiration and Artificial Ventilation." Make sure that you are properly trained with the device that you are using for ventilation. If supplemental oxygen is not immediately available, begin artificial ventilation without supplemental oxygen and attach the oxygen supply to the mask as soon as it is available.

If you are uncertain about whether a patient's breathing is inadequate and requires artificial ventilation, provide artificial ventilation. In the rare circumstance when a patient with inadequate breathing is conscious enough to fight artificial ventilation, transport immediately and consult medical direction.

Table 19-2 Respiratory Conditions with Appropriate Interventions

CONDITION	SIGNS	EMT INTERVENTION	
ADEQUATE BREATHING Patient breathing adequately but needs supplemental oxygen due to a medical or traumatic condition.	• Rate and depth of breathing are adequate. • No abnormal breath sounds. • Air moves freely in and out of the chest. • Skin color normal.	Oxygen by nonrebreather mask or nasal cannula.	
INADEQUATE BREATHING Patient is moving some air in and out but it is slow or shallow and not enough to live.	• Patient has some breathing but not enough to live. • Rate and/or depth outside of normal limits. • Shallow ventilations. • Diminished or absent breath sounds. • Noises (crowing, stridor, snoring, gurgling, or gasping). • Blue (cyanosis) or gray skin color. • Decreased minute volume.	Assisted ventilations (air put into the lungs under pressure) with a pocket face mask, bag-valve mask, or FROPVD. See chapter text about adjusting rates for rapid or slow breathing. *Note: A nonrebreather mask requires adequate breathing to pull oxygen into the lungs. It DOES NOT provide ventilation if patient is not breathing or is breathing inadequately.*	
PATIENT IS NOT BREATHING AT ALL	• No chest rise. • No evidence of air being moved from the mouth or nose. • No breath sounds.	Immediately verify a pulse. If pulse present, provide ventilations with a pocket face mask, bag-valve mask, or FROPVD at 12/minute for an adult and 20/minute for an infant or child. If pulse absent, immediately begin chest compressions followed by ventilations and apply an AED. *Note: DO NOT use oxygen-powered ventilation devices on infants or children.*	

Adequate and Inadequate Artificial Ventilation

Like breathing, artificial ventilation can be adequate or inadequate. When adequate, the chest will rise and fall with each artificial ventilation. The adequate rate for artificial ventilation is 12 breaths per minute for adults and 20 per minute for infants and children.

When you provide artificial ventilation without chest compressions (patient has a pulse), monitor the pulse carefully. With adequate artificial ventilation, the rate should return to normal or near normal. Since the pulse in adults will usually increase when there is a lack of

Pediatric patients differ from adults in many ways. There are few differences that are more important in emergency care than those within the respiratory system. When adult patients experience a decrease in oxygen in the bloodstream (hypoxia), their pulse increases.

In infants and children with respiratory difficulties, you may observe a slight increase in pulse early, but soon the pulse will drop significantly. A low (or bradycardic) pulse in infants and small children in the setting of a respiratory emergency usually means trouble! This is a sharp contrast from adults where it is a good sign when their pulse lowers to a more normal level.

If you observe a pulse below the expected rates for infants and children, evaluate your ventilations or oxygen therapy thoroughly. In ventilations, make sure that you have an open airway and that the chest rises with each breath. Nothing is more important for infants and children than adequate airway care! In any situation, make sure that the oxygen tank has not run out and that the tubing has not kinked or slipped off the delivery device or oxygen cylinder.

For any patient—adult, child, or infant—if the chest does not rise and fall with each artificial ventilation, or the pulse does not return to normal, increase the force of ventilations. If the chest still does not rise, check that you are maintaining an open airway by the head-tilt, chin-lift maneuver (if there is no suspected spine injury) or by the jaw-thrust maneuver (if spine injury is possible). Insert an oropharyngeal or nasopharyngeal airway as needed to prevent the tongue from blocking the airway. Suction fluids and foreign matter from the airway as necessary, or perform abdominal thrusts and finger sweeps as needed to clear large airway obstructions. (Deliver alternating series of back blows and chest thrusts to clear airway obstructions in infants. Do not perform blind finger sweeps—remove only visible objects—in infants and children.) If you are using supplemental oxygen, check that all connections are secure and that the tubing has not kinked.

In infants and children, it is especially important to distinguish between an upper airway obstruction and a lower airway disease if there appears to be a blockage of the airway. If the airway is blocked by the tongue, blood, secretions, or debris, consider suctioning, performing finger sweeps, or inserting an oropharyngeal or nasopharyngeal adjunct to help maintain an open airway.

Infants and children are also subject to respiratory infections (e.g., croup) that may result in swelling of the airway passages. In such cases, probing or placing anything in the patient's mouth or pharynx may set off spasms along the airway.

Refrain from placing anything in the patient's mouth, administer oxygen, and transport as quickly as possible if you see any signs of a serious respiratory problem such as:

- Wheezing, stridor, or grunting
- Increased breathing effort
- Flared nostrils or retracted muscles of breathing
- Rapid breathing
- Pale or cyanotic lips or mouth

For more information about assessing and treating respiratory conditions in infants and children, see Chapter 35, "Pediatric Emergencies."

oxygen, a pulse that remains the same or increases may indicate inadequate artificial ventilation. Naturally, if the pulse disappears this indicates that the patient is in cardiac arrest and needs chest compressions (CPR).

BREATHING DIFFICULTY

Breathing difficulty is a frequent chief complaint, representing a patient's feeling of labored, or difficult, breathing. Although there are objective signs associated with breathing difficulty (as the following text will show), the "difficulty" the patient reports to you is a subjective perception of the patient. The amount of distress the patient feels may or may not reflect the actual severity of his condition. His breathing may be more adequate or less adequate than he feels it is. Therefore, you should not rely entirely on the patient's report to decide the seriousness of the condition. Perform an assessment to help you make that determination.

It is important to remember that a patient with breathing difficulty may have either adequate or inadequate breathing. You may encounter two patients, at different times, who tell you that they are having difficulty breathing ("I can't catch my breath" or a similar complaint). One patient may be having minor difficulty due to a preexisting respiratory condition

CORE CONCEPT ●
How to identify and treat a
patient with breathing difficulty

but still have adequate breathing. His condition is not life threatening. The other patient, who has offered exactly the same complaint, may be having a problem such as an allergic reaction and severe difficulty breathing. Your examination of this patient may reveal inadequate breathing that requires immediate artificial ventilation.

Difficulty in breathing may have many causes ranging from ongoing medical conditions to illnesses such as pneumonia and other infections, to cardiac problems that cause disturbances in the respiratory system.

PATIENT ASSESSMENT

Breathing Difficulty

The secondary assessment for patients with respiratory emergencies involves an appropriate interview and an examination of the chest and respiratory structures. The OPQRST memory aid is very useful for gathering a history when the chief complaint is pain, but needs to be adapted when the chief complaint is difficulty breathing:

O—**Onset.** When did it begin?

P—**Provocation.** What were you doing when this came on? Have you been short of breath when exerting yourself?

Q—**Quality.** Do you have a cough and are you bringing anything up with it?

R—**Radiation.** Do you have pain or discomfort anywhere else in your body? Does it seem to spread to any other part of your body?

S—**Severity.** On a scale of 1 to 10, how bad is your breathing trouble? (10 is worst, 1 best)

T—**Time.** How long have you had this feeling?

Associated symptoms. Have you noticed any weight gain in the last few days?

Ask if the patient has taken any prescribed medications or done anything else to help relieve his condition. This may affect the treatment provided by you and the treatment provided later at the hospital.

After assessing the adequacy of respirations, you should gather vital signs and perform a physical exam focused on the respiratory system. This includes (see also Figure 19-2) the following:

Observing

- Altered mental status, including restlessness, anxiety, or depressed level of consciousness
- Unusual anatomy (barrel chest)
- The patient's position:
  - Tripod position (patient leaning forward with hands on knees or another surface)
  - Sitting with feet dangling, leaning forward
- Work of breathing, including
  - Retractions
  - Use of accessory muscles to breathe
  - Flared nostrils
  - Pursed lips
  - The number of words the patient can say without stopping, described as one-word dyspnea, two-word dyspnea, for example
- Pale, cyanotic, or flushed skin
- Pedal edema, swelling around the calves, ankles, and feet
- Sacral edema, swelling around the low back in bedridden patients
- Noisy breathing, which may be described as:
  - Audible wheezing (heard without stethoscope)
  - Gurgling
  - Snoring
  - Crowing
  - Stridor (harsh, high-pitched sound during breathing, usually due to upper airway obstruction)
  - Coughing

Auscultating

- Lung sounds on both sides during inspiration and expiration

FIGURE 19-2 Signs and symptoms of breathing difficulty.
(© *Ray Kemp/911 Imaging*)

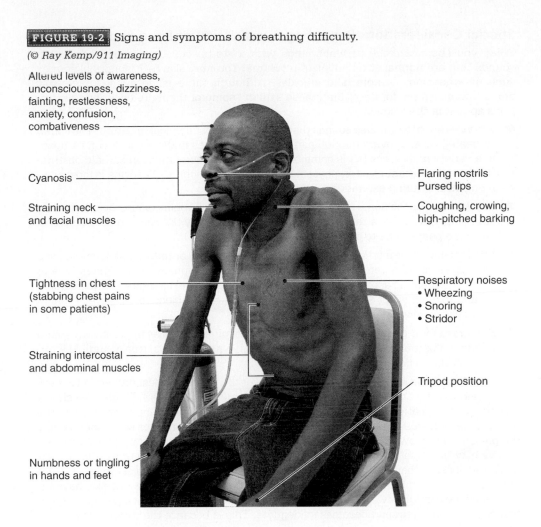

Altered levels of awareness, unconsciousness, dizziness, fainting, restlessness, anxiety, confusion, combativeness

Cyanosis

Straining neck and facial muscles

Tightness in chest (stabbing chest pains in some patients)

Straining intercostal and abdominal muscles

Numbness or tingling in hands and feet

Flaring nostrils
Pursed lips

Coughing, crowing, high-pitched barking

Respiratory noises
• Wheezing
• Snoring
• Stridor

Tripod position

Evaluating Vital Sign Changes, Which May Include:

■ Increased pulse rate

■ Decreased pulse rate (especially in infants and children)

■ Changes in the breathing rate (above or below normal levels)

■ Changes in breathing rhythm

■ Hypertension or hypotension

■ Oxygen saturation, or SpO$_2$, reading of less than 95 percent on the pulse oximeter

Special Considerations Regarding Pulse Oximeter Readings

Chapter 12, "Vital Signs and Monitoring Devices," discussed use of the pulse oximeter to determine the oxygen saturation of the patient's blood and identify hypoxic patients (patients with less than adequate oxygenation). Although the other signs and symptoms listed previously are certainly enough to identify hypoxia, the pulse oximeter will allow you to obtain a precise numerical reading.

If you have a pulse oximeter immediately available, place the sensor on the patient's finger before applying oxygen. This will give you a "room air" reading and give you the patient's saturation before you apply oxygen. When you apply oxygen to the patient, the reading should improve. Document both readings on the report. *Never delay administration of oxygen to obtain a reading. If the pulse oximeter is not immediately available, apply oxygen immediately and apply the pulse oximeter when it becomes available.*

Although an oximeter reading between 96 and 100 percent is normal, *oxygen should be administered to all patients with respiratory distress regardless of their oxygen saturation readings. Even a patient with a saturation reading of 100 percent should receive oxygen if he has any signs of respiratory distress.*

Special Considerations Regarding Auscultation of Lung Sounds

When you auscultate the patient's lungs with a stethoscope, you may hear breath sounds that are normal or diminished in volume. You may also hear abnormal sounds such as wheezing, rhonchi, and crackles. Although there is no single universally agreed-upon system for describing these sounds, some of the more common descriptions appear in the following list.

- *Wheezes* are high-pitched sounds that will seem almost musical in nature. The sound is created by air moving through narrowed air passages in the lungs. It can be heard in a variety of diseases but is common in asthma and sometimes in chronic obstructive lung diseases such as emphysema and chronic bronchitis. Wheezing is most commonly heard during expiration.

- *Crackles* are (as the name indicates) a fine crackling or bubbling sound heard upon inspiration. The sound is caused by fluid in the alveoli or by the opening of closed alveoli. Some people refer to crackles as rales.

- *Rhonchi* are lower-pitched sounds that resemble snoring or rattling. They are caused by secretions in larger airways as might be seen with pneumonia or bronchitis or when materials are aspirated (breathed) into the lungs. The difference between crackles and rhonchi is not always obvious and is somewhat subjective. However, rhonchi generally are louder than crackles.

- *Stridor* is a high-pitched sound that is heard on inspiration. It is an upper-airway sound indicating partial obstruction of the trachea or larynx. Stridor is usually audible without a stethoscope.

Listen for these lung sounds on both sides over the patient's chest (upper and lower), at the mid-axillary line, and over the patient's back (upper and lower). Figure 19-3 shows locations on the patient's body where you should listen for lung sounds. Listening to the lungs in several areas may help to localize the patient's problem, since some sounds may be present in the lower lobes (e.g., crackles from early congestive heart failure) whereas others may be present throughout the lungs (e.g., wheezes from an asthma attack). You may also observe changes over time when listening to lung sounds. An asthmatic patient who has used his inhaler may feel that he is breathing easier and the wheezes have diminished. Be careful, however. Sometimes the wheezes will also disappear when a patient worsens and his breathing becomes inadequate. This is because the patient is not moving enough air in and out of the lungs any more to create the wheezing.

Although lung sounds can be useful, they are only a rough indicator of what is going on inside the patient's chest. Only movement or vibrations that are strong enough to be transmitted through the tissue of the chest are audible with your stethoscope. Remember that your patient's overall status is more important than his lung sounds.

FIGURE 19-3 Auscultate for breath sounds on the upper and lower chest, the upper and lower back, and at the mid-axillary line.

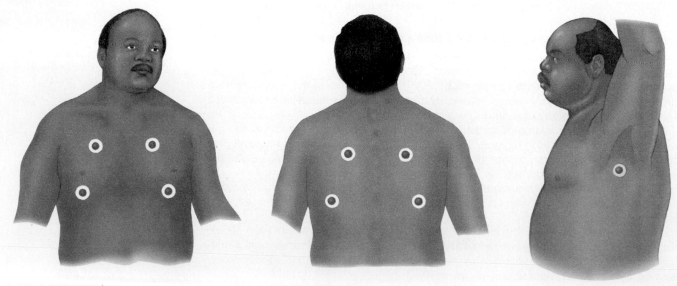

Breathing Difficulty

When a patient is suffering from breathing difficulty, provide the following care:

- **Assessment.** Assess the airway during the primary assessment and then frequently throughout the call. Assist respiration with artificial ventilations and supplemental oxygen whenever the patient has or develops inadequate breathing.

- **Oxygen.** Oxygen is the main treatment for any patient in respiratory difficulty. If the patient is breathing adequately, use a nonrebreather mask at 15 liters per minute to provide oxygen. Use a nasal cannula only in cases where the patient will not tolerate a mask. If the patient has inadequate breathing, provide supplemental oxygen while performing artificial ventilation.

- **Positioning.** If the patient is experiencing breathing difficulty but is breathing adequately, place him in a position of comfort. Most patients with breathing difficulty feel they can breathe better sitting up. However, this is not possible if the patient has inadequate breathing, since the patient would need to be supine to receive assisted ventilations.

- **Prescribed inhaler.** If the patient has a prescribed inhaler, you may be able to assist the patient in taking this medication. This would be done after consultation with medical direction, often during transportation to the hospital. (More information will be provided on prescribed inhalers later in this chapter.)

- **Continuous positive airway pressure (CPAP).** See the discussion of CPAP that follows.

Continuous Positive Airway Pressure (CPAP)

The use of noninvasive positive pressure ventilation (NPPV) was discussed in Chapter 9, "Respiration and Artificial Ventilation." The most common NPPV, available in some EMS systems for use in relieving difficulty breathing, is **continuous positive airway pressure (CPAP)**. It consists of a mask and a means of blowing oxygen or air into the mask at relatively low pressures. Patients with obstructive sleep apnea sometimes have these devices at home and use them at night to prevent the airway from collapsing during sleep. They are also used in health care settings in some patients with respiratory failure.

A CPAP device works through some simple principles: Blowing oxygen or air continuously at a low pressure into the airway prevents the alveoli from collapsing at the end of exhalation, and it can also push fluid out of the alveoli back into the capillaries that surround them.

Portable CPAP is relatively new, so the indications for its use are evolving. Common uses include pulmonary edema and drowning, in which there is fluid in the alveoli that can be pushed out of the alveoli and back into the capillaries; asthma and COPD, in which the alveoli are at risk of closing at the end of exhalation; and in some EMS systems, respiratory failure in general.

Contraindications generally fall into two classes: anatomic-physiologic and pathologic. Anatomic-physiologic contraindications include mental status so depressed that the patient cannot protect his airway or follow instructions; lack of a normal, spontaneous respiratory rate (CPAP increases the volume of air the patient breathes, but does not increase the patient's respiratory rate); inability to sit up; hypotension, generally considered to be less than 90 mmHg; and inability to get and maintain a good mask seal.

Pathologic contraindications include nausea and vomiting; penetrating chest trauma, particularly when a pneumothorax is possible; shock; upper gastrointestinal bleeding or recent gastric surgery; and any condition that would prevent a good mask seal, such as congenital facial malformations, trauma, or burns.

There are other conditions in which, even though CPAP may not be contraindicated, the EMT nevertheless needs to exercise caution: claustrophobia or inability to tolerate the mask and seal; history of inability to use CPAP; secretions so copious that they need to be suctioned; and a history of pulmonary fibrosis.

> **CORE CONCEPT**
> Use of continuous positive airway pressure (CPAP) to relieve difficulty breathing
>
> **continuous positive airway pressure (CPAP)**
> a form of noninvasive positive pressure ventilation (NPPV) consisting of a mask and a means of blowing oxygen or air into the mask to prevent airway collapse or to help alleviate difficulty breathing.

Although CPAP is frequently effective in relieving patients' difficulty breathing, it has some side effects the EMT needs to be aware of. Since CPAP works by maintaining a positive pressure throughout the respiratory cycle, less blood is able to return to the heart through the veins. Ordinarily, when inspiration occurs, the pressure in the thoracic cavity decreases enough that it promotes the return of blood to the heart. When CPAP is being used, the pressure in the lungs causes less blood to return to the heart, so the cardiac output decreases, frequently resulting in a drop in blood pressure. In some patients, the drop may be enough to make the patient hypotensive. For this reason, the patient needs to have a systolic blood pressure of at least 90 mmHg.

When the lungs are subject to continuous positive pressure, there is a risk that the pressure may cause a weak area to rupture, leading to lung collapse (pneumothorax). This risk is increased in patients with chronic respiratory conditions such as COPD and asthma. However, COPD patients with difficulty breathing are commonly treated with BiPAP in the emergency department.

Patients who are vomiting (or nauseated, putting them at risk of vomiting) have an increased risk of aspiration because positive pressure can push air into the stomach, resulting in gastric distention. This can lead to vomiting and blowing of the vomitus into the airway and lungs.

A less dangerous side effect, though very uncomfortable for the patient, is drying of the corneas of the eyes. Even a small leak at the top of the mask can lead to a high volume of air blowing directly into the eyes, especially if transport time is long.

Different models of CPAP devices are available. One uses a battery-powered machine to blow oxygen and air at an adjustable pressure. This has the advantage of using only as much oxygen as the patient needs; however, its disadvantage is that it needs a charged battery in order to operate. Another model has no machine, but instead uses the Venturi principle. As oxygen goes through specially shaped channels in the plastic mask, a certain flow rate creates a particular pressure. Higher flow rates produce higher pressures. This has the advantages of lighter weight and no need for a battery; however, its disadvantage is that it uses oxygen quickly.

To apply CPAP (Scan 19-1), explain to the patient that you are applying a mask that is going to push air into his lungs. It may feel strange but, within a couple of minutes, he should feel better. If the patient has never had CPAP before, it may help to allow him to hold the mask initially. Once he gets used to it and starts to feel some improvement, you can attach the straps that will hold the mask in place. Start with a low level of CPAP. Many systems start between 2 and 5 centimeters of water (cm H_2O). Reassess the patient's mental status, vital signs, and level of dyspnea frequently. Raise the level of CPAP if there is no relief within a few minutes. If the patient's mental status or respiratory condition deteriorates, remove the CPAP and begin ventilating the patient with a bag mask.

Follow your local protocols as to when to apply CPAP, how much to start with, how frequently to increase it, and how high to go.

RESPIRATORY CONDITIONS

Although treatment in the field is very similar for different respiratory diseases, the EMT may find it useful to understand some of the more common causes of this complaint, along with the signs and symptoms associated with them.

Chronic Obstructive Pulmonary Disease (COPD)

Emphysema—as well as chronic bronchitis, black lung, and many undetermined respiratory illnesses that cause the patient problems like those seen in emphysema—are all classified as chronic obstructive pulmonary disease (COPD).

COPD is mainly a problem of middle-aged or older patients (Figure 19-4). This is because these disorders take time to develop as tissues in the respiratory tract react to irritants. Cigarette smoking causes the overwhelming majority of cases of COPD. Occasionally other irritants such as chemicals, air pollutants, or repeated infections cause this condition.

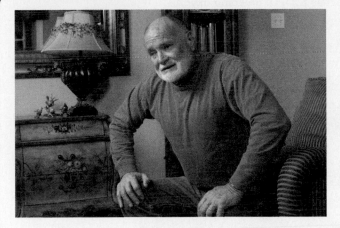

1 Assess the patient and ensure that he meets the criteria for CPAP.

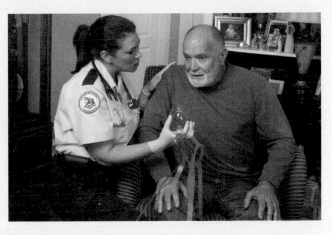

2 Explain the device to the patient. The mask and snug seal may initially cause the patient to feel smothered and anxious.

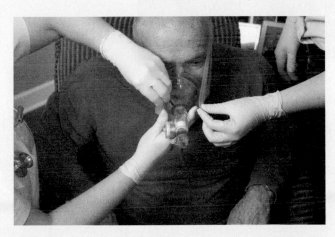

3 Apply the mask to the patient's face. Continue to calm and reassure the patient.

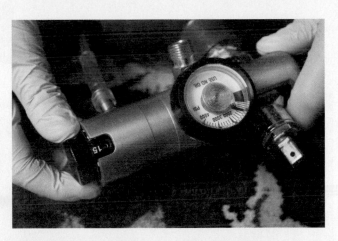

4 Use settings as defined in your protocols.

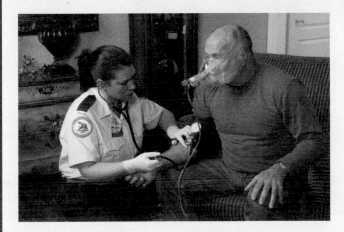

5 Reassess and monitor the patient.

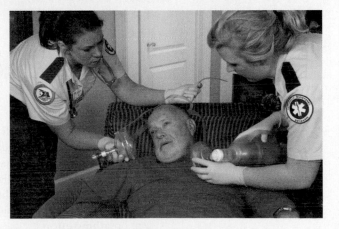

6 Discontinue CPAP and ventilate the patient if breathing becomes inadequate.

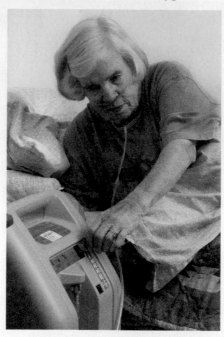

FIGURE 19-4 A patient with chronic obstructive pulmonary disease (COPD) on home oxygen.

FIGURE 19-5 Chronic bronchitis and emphysema are chronic obstructive pulmonary diseases.

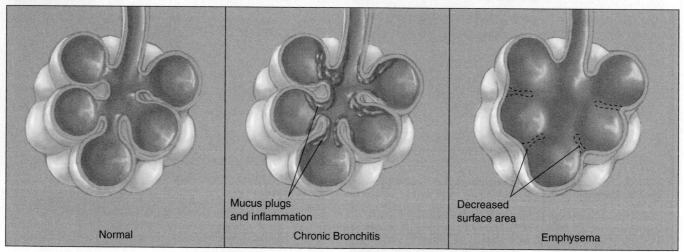

Mucus plugs and inflammation

Decreased surface area

Normal   Chronic Bronchitis   Emphysema

Chronic bronchitis and emphysema are compared in Figure 19-5. In chronic bronchitis, the bronchiole lining is inflamed and excess mucus is formed. The cells in the bronchioles that normally clear away accumulations of mucus are not able to do so. The sweeping apparatus on these cells, the cilia, have been damaged or destroyed.

In emphysema, the walls of the alveoli break down, greatly reducing the surface area for respiratory exchange. The lungs begin to lose elasticity. These factors combine to allow stale air laden with carbon dioxide to be trapped in the lungs, reducing the effectiveness of normal breathing efforts.

Many COPD patients will exhibit characteristics of both emphysema and chronic bronchitis. Usually the reason a COPD patient calls the ambulance is that a recent upper respiratory infection has caused an acute worsening of his chronic disease. This may cause the patient to experience a fever and cough up green or dark sputum.

A very few COPD patients develop a hypoxic drive to trigger respirations. In patients without COPD, the brain determines when to breathe based on increased levels of carbon dioxide in the blood. Since COPD patients develop a tolerance to their body's high levels of carbon dioxide, the brain learns to rely, instead, on low oxygen levels as the trigger to breathe. The higher oxygen levels that result from oxygen administration may, in rare cases, signal the COPD patient to reduce breathing or even to stop breathing (develop respiratory arrest).

In most cases, however, the hypoxic drive will not be a problem in the prehospital setting. (Indeed, many patients with COPD are on continuous home oxygen by nasal cannula because of chronic hypoxia.) The patient's need for oxygen will outweigh any risk involved with administration. If the patient has a possible heart attack or stroke, is developing shock, or has respiratory distress, a higher concentration of oxygen will be required in spite of the potential problems. If oxygen is required by the COPD patient, do not withhold it.

Constantly monitor the patient. If the patient's breathing becomes inadequate or stops, be prepared to assist respirations through artificial ventilation, and then contact medical direction.

Asthma

Seen in young and old patients alike, asthma is a chronic disease that has episodic exacerbations or flares (a disease that only seems to affect the patient at irregular intervals). This is far different from chronic bronchitis and emphysema, both of which continually afflict the patient. Asthma also differs from chronic bronchitis and emphysema in that it does not produce a hypoxic drive. An asthma attack or flare can be life threatening. Between episodes, the asthmatic patient can lead a normal life. Many use steroid inhalers for their chronic condition with albuterol administered only for a "rescue" during a flare.

Attacks can be precipitated by insect stings, air pollutants, infection, strenuous exercise, or emotional stress. When an asthma attack occurs, the small bronchioles that lead to the air sacs of the lungs become narrowed because of contractions of the muscles that make up the airway. To complicate matters, there is an overproduction of thick mucus. The combined effects of the contractions and the mucus cause the small passages to practically close down, severely restricting air flow.

The air flow is mainly restricted in one direction. When the patient inhales, the expanding lungs exert an outward pull, increasing the diameter of the airway and allowing air to flow into the lungs. During exhalation, however, the opposite occurs and the stale air becomes trapped in the lungs. This requires the patient to exhale the air forcefully, producing the characteristic wheezing sounds associated with asthma.

There is no known way to prevent asthma, but episodes of distress can often be prevented by use of appropriate medications and careful attention to avoiding items that trigger attacks.

Pulmonary Edema

Patients with congestive heart failure (CHF) may experience difficulty breathing because of fluid that accumulates in the lungs, preventing them from breathing adequately. The abnormal accumulation of fluid in the alveoli of the lungs is known as pulmonary edema. It typically occurs because the left side of the heart has been damaged, often by a myocardial infarction (heart attack) or chronic hypertension. Since the left side of the heart receives blood from the lungs, the inability to pump blood out results in pressure building up and going back to the lungs. Since there is only one layer of cells lining the alveolus and one layer of cells covering the adjoining capillaries, when pressure builds up, it is relatively easy for fluid to cross this thin barrier and accumulate in the alveoli. If fluid occupies the lower airways, it is difficult for oxygen to reach the blood and the patient experiences dyspnea.

Patients with CHF often have both left-sided heart failure and right-sided heart failure. Since the right side of the heart receives its blood from the systemic circulation (everything besides the lungs), pressure backs up into the systemic circulation. This becomes visible as edema in the lower parts of the body, typically the lower legs. In bedridden patients, the legs are not the lowest part of the body. Instead, fluid accumulates in the sacral area of the lower back. Sometimes, the CHF patient will also have jugular vein distention (JVD), bulging of the neck veins, and accumulation of fluid in the abdominal cavity.

When the patient lies down at night to sleep, the fluid in the body moves back into the circulation. This means it can easily overload the system and leak into the lungs, leading at first to mild dyspnea that can be relieved by sleeping propped up on one pillow, then two pillows or even three pillows. At some point, the amount of fluid becomes too much and the patient awakens acutely short of breath, with the feeling that he is drowning.

If the patient can speak, he may be able to tell you that he has been feeling a little worse each night for the last several days. He may also have noticed a weight gain of several pounds in just a few days, perhaps accompanied by the need for a larger belt. Other signs and symptoms include anxiety, pale and sweaty skin, tachycardia, hypertension, respirations that are rapid and labored, and a low oxygen saturation. In severe cases, you may hear a gurgling sound from the lungs, even without a stethoscope, each time the patient breathes. When you auscultate the lungs, you will usually hear crackles or sometimes wheezes. In severe cases, the patient may cough up frothy sputum, which is usually white but sometimes pink-tinged.

Treatment includes high-concentration oxygen by mask unless the patient's breathing is inadequate and you need to ventilate the patient. If at all possible, keep the patient's legs in a dependent position (hanging down). Bringing the legs up may push more fluid into the already overloaded circulatory system and make matters worse. As noted earlier, CPAP may be very useful in these patients since it can physically push the fluid back out of the lungs and into the capillaries where it belongs.

Although most cases of pulmonary edema you see will be the result of heart failure or MI, there are some noncardiac causes. Some people, for example, when exposed to the low atmospheric pressure of high altitudes, may develop pulmonary edema. In this case, the heart is fine. The most important treatment for these patients is to bring them back to normal altitude and atmospheric pressure. You should administer high-concentration oxygen until this can be accomplished.

Although traditionally called congestive heart failure, this condition is now called simply heart failure to reflect the reality that many patients don't develop the congestion (with blood) of the body's organs. This condition, whatever it is called, is quite common and is fortunately much more treatable than it used to be. Many patients who wouldn't have survived more than a year or two just a decade ago are now living active lives, thanks to strict diet modification (low sodium), modern pharmacology, and, in some cases, the use of advanced electronic pacemakers that make the heart beat more efficiently.

Pneumonia

Pneumonia is an infection of one or both lungs caused by bacteria, viruses, or fungi. It results from the inhalation of certain microbes that grow in the lungs and cause inflammation. People with COPD or other respiratory diseases are more likely to get pneumonia. People with chronic health problems are also at higher risk.

Some of the most common signs and symptoms of pneumonia include coughing (mucus can be greenish, yellow, or occasionally bloody), fever, chest pain, and severe chills. Most, but not all, patients complain of shortness of breath, either with or without exertion; chest pain that is sharp and pleuritic (worsens on inhalation); headache; pale, sweaty skin; fatigue; and confusion, especially in the elderly. Sometimes an older person will have only a few other signs or symptoms besides confusion. When you auscultate the chest, you may hear crackles on one side in just one region.

Prehospital care consists of supportive treatment that you would administer to any patient with difficulty breathing. If the pneumonia is thought to be bacterial, the patient will receive antibiotics at the emergency department. The cause of the pneumonia, severity of the patient's condition, and the patient's state of general health will determine whether the patient needs to be admitted to the hospital.

Immunization with a vaccine that prevents the most common types of bacterial pneumonia is an important and effective part of prevention for the elderly and those with chronic health conditions.

Spontaneous Pneumothorax

When a lung collapses without injury or any other obvious cause, it is called a spontaneous pneumothorax. This is usually the result of rupture of a bleb, a small section of the lung that is weak. Once the bleb ruptures, the lung collapses and air leaks into the thorax. Certain conditions and activities place patients at higher risk of a spontaneous pneumothorax. Tall, thin people, for example, are more likely to have a weak spot that can rupture with just a cough. Smoking destroys lung tissue, so smokers are also at higher risk of this condition.

The patient with a collapsed lung typically has sharp, pleuritic chest pain and shortness of breath, although these may be mild when the pneumothorax is small. When the area involved is larger, the patient will often tire easily, be tachycardic, breathe fast, have a low oxygen saturation, and exhibit cyanosis.

In the patient with a classic spontaneous pneumothorax, auscultation will reveal breath sounds that are decreased or absent on the side with the injured lung. This test is not reliable, however, as some patients with a pneumothorax may have perfectly normal breath sounds.

Administer oxygen and treat the patient like anyone else who is short of breath. As mentioned earlier, CPAP is contraindicated in patients with a suspected pneumothorax. Most patients with a pneumothorax will need to have a small catheter or a larger plastic chest tube inserted between the ribs, then into the pleural space around the collapsed lung. The catheter will help remove the air, allowing the lung to re-expand.

Pulmonary Embolism

Blood usually travels through the vessels in the lung, eventually getting to the capillaries, where oxygen and carbon dioxide are exchanged. When something that is not blood—like a blood clot, air, or fat—tries to go through these blood vessels, it gets stuck and blocks an artery in the lungs. This is a dangerous condition known as a pulmonary embolism.

The most common example of a pulmonary embolism is a blood clot that starts in a vein, often a vein in the leg or in the pelvis. This dangerous type of clot is called a deep vein thrombosis (DVT). DVT can occur in a variety of situations. The three factors that increase the risk of DVT are limb immobility, local trauma to an extremity, and/or abnormally fast blood clotting. Patients at increased risk for developing a DVT include women on birth control pills, patients with cancer, patients with lower extremity injuries (such as casted fractures), and anyone who is in the same position for a long period of time (such as transcontinental air travelers).

Other things can block the pulmonary arteries, though not as often as a blood clot. A significant amount of air introduced into a vein can cause great harm and even death. If fat gets into the circulation—for example, from the marrow of a fractured bone—the same results can occur.

The signs and symptoms of a pulmonary embolus are extremely variable, making this one of the most difficult conditions to detect. The typical patient has sudden onset of sharp, pleuritic chest pain; shortness of breath; anxiety; a cough (sometimes with bloody sputum); sweaty skin that is either pale or cyanotic; tachycardia; and tachypnea. Unfortunately, few patients with a pulmonary embolism present in this way. The patient may also complain of feeling lightheaded or dizzy, with pain and swelling in one or both legs. Wheezing is sometimes heard on auscultation of the chest. If the clot is large, the patient may be hypotensive or go into cardiac arrest.

Administer oxygen and treat the patient like anyone else who is short of breath. Keep a high index of suspicion for pulmonary embolism in patients with recent immobilizations or those with a previous history of DVT. Pulmonary embolus can sometimes be prevented by avoiding long periods of inactivity, refraining from smoking, taking appropriate medication when there is a high risk of forming clots, and getting early care for DVT.

Epiglottitis

When an infection inflames the area around and above the epiglottis, the tissue swells. If it swells enough, it can actually occlude, or close off, the airway. Epiglottitis used to be a disease of children, but it is now much less common in children than in adults in the United States. This is primarily the result of childhood vaccination against *Haemophilus influenzae* type B, the bacterium that used to cause most cases of epiglottitis in children.

The typical adult with epiglottitis is a male in his forties who may have had a recent cold. Symptoms include sore throat and painful or difficult swallowing. The patient is typically in the tripod position to increase the glottic opening. Other signs may include a sick appearance, muffled voice, fever, and drooling because of the pain and difficulty in swallowing. An alarming sign is stridor. This indicates the airway already has a significant degree of obstruction.

In contrast to the slower onset of symptoms in adults, children who have this disease often experience a sudden onset. Although children between 2 and 7 years of age used to be the most likely to experience epiglottitis, it can now appear in a child of any age. The presentation of a still child leaning forward in the tripod position, drooling, and appearing to be in distress should alert the EMT to the possibility of this disease.

Treatment for epiglottitis includes doing as much as possible to make the patient calm and comfortable. This means you should NOT inspect the throat. Administer high-concentration oxygen if you can do it without alarming the patient. Transport as soon as possible to an emergency department capable of dealing with this type of patient. Be sure to advise the staff when you expect to arrive so that the proper personnel can be there. Because of the possibility of sudden closure of the airway, use of light and siren is justified for a patient like this unless you are very close to the hospital. If untreated, up to 10 percent of children with this disease may die. Adults can tolerate the swelling better but still bear the risk of losing the airway.

Childhood epiglottitis can be prevented by administration of the *Haemophilus influenzae* type B vaccine. Adult epiglottitis can result from infection by many different microbes, so there is no known way to prevent it in adults.

Cystic Fibrosis

A genetic disease that typically appears in childhood, cystic fibrosis (CF) causes thick, sticky mucus that accumulates in the lungs and digestive system. The mucus can cause life-threatening lung infections and serious problems with digestion. Signs and symptoms may include:

- Coughing with large amounts of mucus from the lungs
- Fatigue
- Frequent occurrences of pneumonia, characterized by fever, more coughing than usual, worse shortness of breath than usual, more sputum than usual, and loss of appetite
- Abdominal pain and distention
- Coughing up blood
- Nausea
- Weight loss

If you encounter a patient with CF, the patient or parent will be able to tell you about how the disease affects the child. Although most patients with this disease are children, many of these patients are now surviving to adulthood, something that was almost unheard of a generation ago. The patient or parent will be very familiar with the disease and what usually works for the patient. Use their knowledge to your advantage.

There is no known way to prevent cystic fibrosis, although a great deal of research is going on in this area.

Viral Respiratory Infections

One of the most common afflictions a person may get is a viral respiratory infection. There are many presentations, but it often starts with a sore or scratchy throat with sneezing, a runny nose, and a feeling of fatigue. There may be a fever and chills. The infection can spread into the lungs, causing shortness of breath, especially in those who have chronic health conditions. The cough can be persistent and may produce sputum that is yellow or greenish. Symptoms usually persist for 1 to 2 weeks.

Because the signs and symptoms of a respiratory infection resemble those of so many other diseases, the EMT should administer oxygen and care for the patient like any other patient with respiratory distress.

Because the infection is viral, antibiotics do not help and may worsen things by promoting antibiotic resistance. This happens when a patient receives an unnecessary antibiotic, resulting in killing off bacteria except for the ones that are resistant to that antibiotic.

Good hygiene can help prevent viral respiratory infections. Before touching your hand to your nose or eyes, be sure it is clean. If you have shaken hands with someone who is carrying the virus, it can be transmitted to you and then introduced into your system through the mucous membranes of the nose and eyes. Alcohol-based hand sanitizer can be very helpful. Avoiding the spray of a sick person who is sneezing or coughing will also reduce your risk of contracting a viral respiratory infection.

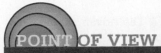
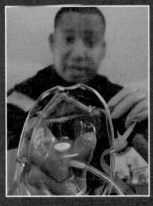

"I couldn't breathe. I mean I really couldn't breathe. I felt like I couldn't get air in and out and I was pretty sure I was going to die.

"I tell you this because I feel bad about how I yelled at the EMT. I can't remember everything, but I seem to remember being downright nasty. You see, I have asthma but have never had an attack like that before.

"My husband called the EMTs and they came to the house pretty quickly. But my breathing was getting worse and worse and, well, like I said, I wasn't sure I'd live through this one. It makes you crazy.

"When the EMT tried to put that mask on my face, I felt like I was being smothered. Even though I know it's supposed to help, I couldn't stop myself from lashing out at the EMT. I pushed his hand away and yelled. I can't imagine what it must've looked like . . . or what was going through his mind while I was yelling at him.

"He finally got me to put the mask on. He was very patient and calm. The oxygen did help me, but it wasn't easy. By the time we got to the hospital I felt a little better. And I apologized to him. He told me not to worry about it. But I do.

"I really hope this never happens again."

THE PRESCRIBED INHALER

A patient with asthma, COPD, or similar chronic illness may have an inhaler prescribed by a physician. You will need to get permission from medical direction to help the patient use the inhaler. This may be accomplished by phone/radio or by standing order, depending on your local protocols. Keep in mind that a patient may overuse the inhaler prior to your arrival, so it is important to determine exactly when and how many times the inhaler has been used. Be sure to give this information to medical direction.

The metered-dose inhaler gets its name from the fact that each activation of the inhaler provides a metered, or exactly measured, dose of medication. Most patients simply refer to the device as their "inhaler" or "puffer." The inhaler is prescribed for patients with respiratory problems that cause **bronchoconstriction** (constriction, or blockage, of the bronchi that lead from the trachea to the lungs) or other types of lung obstructions. The inhalers contain a drug that dilates, or enlarges, the air passages, making breathing easier. These drugs are in the form of a fine powder. The timing of the activation of the inhaler in relation to a deep breath is very important to prevent the fine powder from coming to rest on the moist inner surface of the mouth. The medication will work only if it comes in contact with lung tissue directly. Studies have shown that inhalers can be very beneficial—but only when used properly.

Spacer devices (Figure 19-6) make the exact timing necessary to use an inhaler less critical. The inhaler is activated into the spacer device (sometimes called an Aerochamber™). The medication stays airborne inside the chamber and can then be inhaled directly into the lungs.

When patients use an inhaler, they often are excited or nervous because they are short of breath. Many do not use their inhaler properly. Some people have never had proper instruction in use of their inhaler. Make sure to calm the patient the best you can and coach him to use the inhaler properly, as follows:

1. As with any medication, ensure that you have the right patient, the right time, the right medication, the right dose, and the right route. Check the expiration date. Make sure the inhaler is at room temperature or warmer. Shake the inhaler vigorously several times.

2. Make sure that the patient is alert enough to use the inhaler properly. Use a spacer device if the patient has one available.

3. Make sure the patient first exhales deeply.

4. Have the patient put his lips around the opening and press the inhaler to activate the spray as he inhales deeply.

5. After the patient inhales, make sure he holds his breath as long as possible so the medication can be absorbed. This may be difficult with a patient who is anxious, but unless the medication is held in the lungs, it will have minimal or no value.

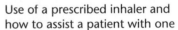

CORE CONCEPT
Use of a prescribed inhaler and how to assist a patient with one

bronchoconstriction
constriction, or blockage, of the bronchi that lead from the trachea to the lungs.

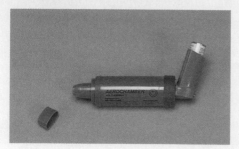

FIGURE 19-6 A spacer between the inhaler and patient makes the timing during inhaler use less critical.

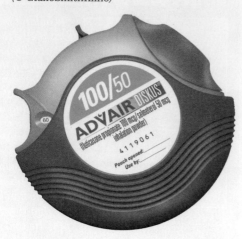

FIGURE 19-7 The Advair inhaler.
(© GlaxoSmithKline)

Your role will involve more coaching than actually administering the medication. The proper sequence for administration of a prescribed inhaler is shown in Scan 19-2. Inhalers are described in detail in Scan 19-3. Follow local protocols and consult medical direction, if required, before assisting a patient with an inhaler.

> **NOTE:** *There are many types of drugs used in prescribed inhalers. The so-called "rescue inhalers" act immediately in an emergency to reverse airway constriction. Fast-acting emergency inhalers include inhalers that contain albuterol (Ventolin, Proventil, Volmax), levalbuterol (Xopenex), and combination inhalers containing albuterol and ipratropium (Combivent and DuoNeb). Other inhalers are not for use in emergencies; rather, they are used daily to help reduce inflammation and prevent attacks. These medications (e.g., beclomethasone, Flovent, Advair—Figure 19-7) should not be used to reverse an acute attack, nor should they be used in the event of breathing difficulty or airway constriction. Fast-acting emergency inhalers include albuterol inhalers (Ventolin, Proventil) and combination inhalers (Combivent).*

CRITICAL DECISION MAKING

Assisting with a Prescribed Inhaler

As an EMT, you may be allowed to assist a patient in using his prescribed inhaler. Certain inhalers deliver a medication that relaxes narrowed airways and provides tremendous benefit to the patient when they are used properly.

For each of the following situations, decide whether you should or should not assist the patient with the inhaler.

1. You are called to a 14-year-old patient who complains of difficulty breathing. He tells you he has a history of asthma. The patient's pulse is 104, strong and regular; respirations 28 with audible wheezes; blood pressure 130/84; skin warm and dry. The patient's parents are present. The inhaler is prescribed to the patient.

2. You are called to a 67-year-old patient who complains of difficulty breathing. The patient tells you she has a history of breathing problems but doesn't know specifically which ones. Her vital signs are pulse 122, strong and regular; respirations 28 with audible wheezes; blood pressure 104/64; skin cool and dry. The patient's daughter presents an inhaler, saying, "This is mine, but it's what I use when I'm wheezing."

3. You are called to a 24-year-old female who was exercising when she developed difficulty breathing. She has a history of asthma. You find her looking tired and weak. Her vital signs are pulse 142, respirations 42 and shallow, blood pressure 96/56, skin cool and moist. You do not hear any wheezes. A friend ran and got the patient's inhaler from her car.

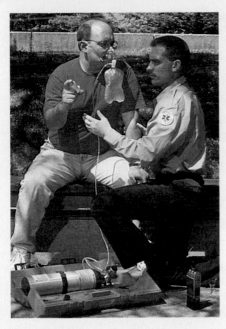

❶ The patient has the indications for use of an inhaler: signs and symptoms of breathing difficulty and an inhaler prescribed by a physician.

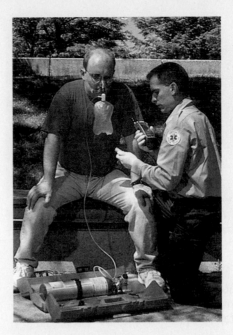

❷ Contact medical direction and obtain an order to assist the patient with the prescribed inhaler.

❸ Ensure the five "rights":
- Right patient
- Right time
- Right medication
- Right dose
- Right route

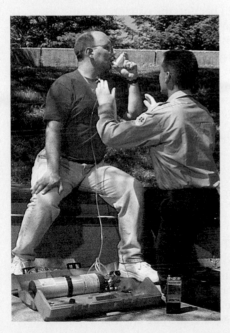

❹ Coach the patient in the use of an inhaler. Tell him he should exhale deeply, press the inhaler to activate the spray, inhale, and hold his breath in so medication can be absorbed.

    Check the expiration date, shake the inhaler, make sure the inhaler is room temperature or warmer, and make sure the patient is alert.

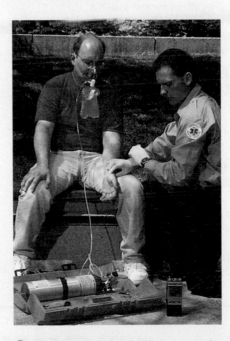

❺ After use of the inhaler, reassess the patient: take vital signs, perform a focused exam, and determine if breathing is adequate.

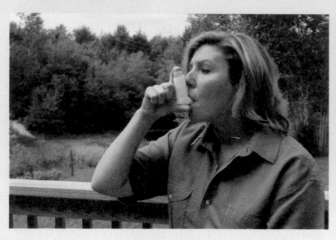
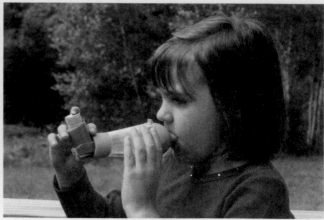

MEDICATION NAME

1. Generic: albuterol, isoetharine, metaproterenol
2. Trade: Proventil, Ventolin, Bronkosol, Bronkometer, Alupent, Metaprel

INDICATIONS

Meets all the following criteria:

1. Patient exhibits signs and symptoms of respiratory emergency.
2. Patient has physician-prescribed handheld inhaler.
3. Medical direction gives specific authorization to use.

CONTRAINDICATIONS

1. Patient is unable to use the device (e.g., not alert).
2. Inhaler is not prescribed for the patient.
3. No permission has been given by medical direction.
4. The patient has already taken the maximum prescribed dose prior to the EMT's arrival.

MEDICATION FORM

Handheld metered-dose inhaler.

DOSAGE

Number of inhalations based on medical direction's order or physician's order.

ADMINISTRATION

1. Obtain an order from medical direction, either on-line or off-line.
2. Ensure the right patient, right time, right medication, right dose, right route, and patient is alert enough to use the inhaler.
3. Check the expiration date of the inhaler.
4. Check if the patient has already taken any doses.

5. Ensure the inhaler is at room temperature or warmer.
6. Shake the inhaler vigorously several times.
7. Have the patient exhale deeply.
8. Have the patient put her lips around the opening of the inhaler.
9. Have the patient depress the handheld inhaler as she begins to inhale deeply.
10. Instruct the patient to hold her breath for as long as she comfortably can so the medication can be absorbed.
11. Put the oxygen back on the patient.
12. Allow the patient to breathe a few times and repeat the second dose if so ordered by medical direction.
13. If the patient has a spacer device for use with her inhaler (device for attachment between inhaler and patient to allow for more effective use of medication), it should be used.

ACTIONS

Beta-agonist bronchodilator dilates bronchioles, reducing airway resistance.

SIDE EFFECTS

1. Increased pulse rate
2. Tremors
3. Nervousness

REASSESSMENT STRATEGIES

1. Gather vital signs.
2. Perform a focused reassessment of the chest and respiratory function.
3. Observe for deterioration of the patient; if breathing becomes inadequate, provide artificial respirations.

THE SMALL-VOLUME NEBULIZER

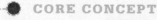

CORE CONCEPT

Use of a prescribed small-volume nebulizer and how to assist a patient with one

The medications used in metered-dose inhalers can also be administered by a small-volume nebulizer (SVN). Nebulizing a medication involves running oxygen or air through a liquid medication. The patient breathes the vapors created. Small-volume nebulizers are used in hospitals and ambulances; they are also prescribed to patients. Patients with chronic respiratory conditions such as asthma, emphysema, or chronic bronchitis may have these devices in their homes.

Unlike the inhaler, which is used in only one breath, a nebulizer produces a continuous flow of aerosolized medication that can be taken in during multiple breaths over several minutes, giving the patient a greater exposure to the medication.

Some states have begun to allow EMTs to carry and administer nebulized medications such as albuterol, whereas other states may allow EMTs to assist with a home nebulizer when allowed by medical direction. Scan 19-4 demonstrates the use of an oxygen-powered nebulizer similar to ones carried on ambulances. Follow your local protocols regarding the use of nebulized medications.

The side effects and precautions with nebulized medications are the same as noted in Scan 19-3 for prescribed inhalers. Patients may experience an increased pulse rate, tremors, nervousness, or a "jittery" feeling. Patients who are not breathing adequately will not benefit from a nebulizer, since they are not breathing deeply enough to get the medication into their lungs.

SCAN 19-4 Small-Volume Nebulizer (SVN)—Patient Assessment and Management

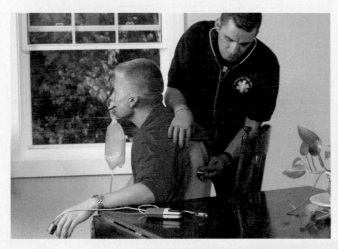

1 Identify the patient as a candidate for nebulized medication per protocol (e.g., history of asthma with respiratory distress). Administer oxygen and assess vital signs. Be sure the patient is not allergic to the medication.

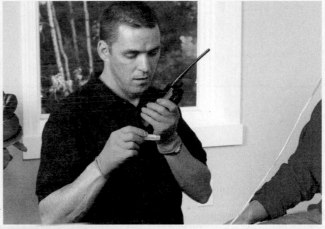

2 Obtain permission from medical direction to administer or assist with the medication.

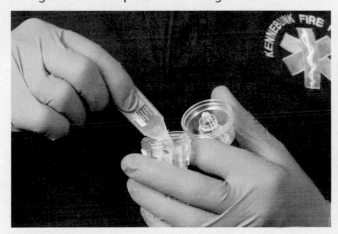

3 Ensure the five rights (right patient, right time, right medication, right dose, right route). Prepare the nebulizer. Put the liquid medication in the chamber. Attach the oxygen tubing and set the oxygen flow for 6 to 8 liters per minute (or according to manufacturer's recommendations).

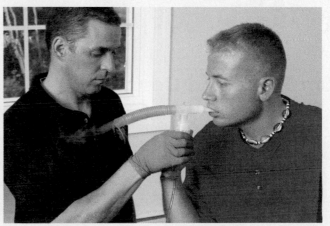

4 Have the patient seal his lips around the mouthpiece and breathe deeply. Instruct the patient to hold his breath for 2 to 3 seconds if possible. Continue until the medication is gone from the chamber.

(continued)

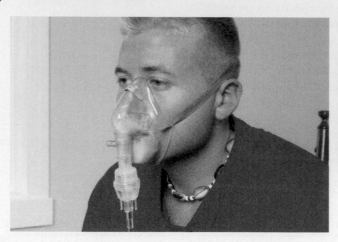

5 Use an alternative device—a mask delivers the medication.

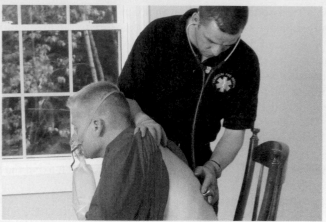

6 Reassess the patient's level of distress and vital signs. Additional doses may be authorized by medical direction if the patient continues to be in distress and the patient is not having adverse effects from the medication.

CHAPTER REVIEW

Key Facts and Concepts

- Respiratory emergencies are common complaints for EMTs. It is important to understand the anatomy, physiology, pathophysiology, assessment, and care for patients experiencing these emergencies.

- Patients with respiratory complaints (which are closely related to cardiac complaints) may exhibit inadequate breathing. Rapid respirations indicate serious conditions including hypoxia, cardiac and respiratory problems, and shock.

- Very slow and shallow respirations are often the endpoint of a serious condition and are a precursor to death.

- The history usually provides significant information about the patient's condition. In addition to determining a perti-nent past history and medications, determine the patient's signs and symptoms with a detailed description including OPQRST and events leading up to the episode.

- Important physical examination points include checking the patient's work of breathing, inspecting accessory muscle use, gathering pulse oximetry readings, assuring adequate and equal lung sounds bilaterally, examining for excess fluid (lungs, ankles, and abdomen), and gathering vital signs.

- Several medications are available that may help correct a patient's difficulty in breathing.

Key Decisions

- Is the patient's breathing adequate, inadequate, or absent?
- What are the appropriate oxygenation or ventilation therapies?
- Should I assist a patient with, or administer, any medications?
  - Do I have protocols and medications that may help this patient?
- Does the patient have a presentation and condition that may fit these protocols?
- Are there any contraindications or risks to using medications in my protocols?

Chapter Glossary

bronchoconstriction constriction, or blockage, of the bronchi that lead from the trachea to the lungs.

continuous positive airway pressure (CPAP) a form of non-invasive positive pressure ventilation (NPPV) consisting of a mask and a means of blowing oxygen or air into the mask to prevent airway collapse or to help alleviate difficulty breathing.

exhalation (EX-huh-LAY-shun) another term for expiration.

expiration (EK-spuh-RAY-shun) a passive process in which the intercostal (rib) muscles and the diaphragm relax, causing the chest cavity to decrease in size and force air from the lungs.

inhalation (IN-huh-LAY-shun) another term for inspiration.

inspiration (IN-spuh-RAY-shun) an active process in which the intercostal (rib) muscles and the diaphragm contract, expanding the size of the chest cavity and causing air to flow into the lungs.

Preparation for Your Examination and Practice

Short Answer

1. What would you expect a patient's respiratory rate to do when the patient gets hypoxic? Why?
2. What would you expect a patient's pulse rate to do when the patient gets hypoxic? Why?
3. List the signs of inadequate breathing.
4. Would you expect to assist a patient with his prescribed inhaler when he is experiencing congestive heart failure? Why or why not?
5. List some differences between adult and infant/child respiratory systems.
6. List the signs and symptoms of breathing difficulty.

Thinking and Linking

Think back to Chapter 3, "Lifting and Moving Patients," Chapter 8, Airway Management," and Chapter 9, "Respiration and Artificial Ventilation," and link information from those chapters with information from this chapter as you consider the patients listed.

Assume that each patient is on the second floor of the house and that your wheeled stretcher will not go beyond the front door. For each, decide in which position and via which device you would transport the patient down a flight of stairs. You will consider both the patient's comfort and clinical needs in the decision.

Once you choose the transportation device, explain how you will also safely transport a "D" cylinder of oxygen down the stairs with the patient.

1. A 15-year-old patient having an asthma attack
2. A 77-year-old man in minor distress who reports he has a slight fever and believes his phlegm has changed color
3. A 44-year-old woman who overdosed on sleeping pills and is not breathing
4. An 82-year-old woman who is barely responsive, appears sleepy, and has slow, shallow breaths
5. A 69-year-old man with difficulty breathing and severely swollen ankles who has to sleep propped up by two pillows whose wife states has been diagnosed with congestive heart failure.

Critical Thinking Exercises

Being able to determine if breathing is or is not adequate is a critical skill. For each of the following patients, state whether the patient's breathing seems adequate or inadequate—and explain your reasoning.

1. A 45-year-old male patient experiences severe difficulty in breathing. His respirations are 36/minute and very shallow. He has minimal chest expansion and can barely speak.
2. A 65-year-old female tells you that she has trouble breathing. Her respirations are 20/minute and slightly labored. Her respirations are regular and there appears to be good chest expansion.
3. A 3-year-old patient recently had a respiratory infection. Her parents called because she is having difficulty breathing. You observe retractions of the muscles between the ribs and above the collarbones as well as nasal flaring. The child seems drowsy. Respirations are 40/minute.

Pathophysiology to Practice

The following questions are designed to assist you in gathering relevant clinical information and making accurate decisions in the field.

1. Is it possible to have fluid in a patient's lungs without having swollen ankles? Why or why not?

2. Would you expect a longer inspiratory cycle or expiratory cycle in an asthma patient? Explain your answer.

3. Can a patient experience respiratory distress when his pulse oximetry reading is 98 percent? Why or why not?

For each of the following patients, decide which condition is most likely. Although minimal information is presented for each patient, your knowledge of the conditions will guide you to the correct choice and help hone your decision making and intuition in the field.

A. COPD
B. Congestive heart failure
C. Asthma

4. 10-year-old patient

5. 82-year-old patient who recently finds she can't sleep lying down

6. 76-year-old patient who reports difficulty breathing with fever and increased mucus production

7. A patient who has had a prior heart attack with difficulty breathing who reports gaining 5 pounds in the past 2 to 3 days

8. A very skinny elderly man who is constantly on a nasal cannula at 2 liters per minute at home

9. A 35-year-old man who has difficulty breathing while playing racquetball

Street Scenes

Your pager is activated, and the only information the dispatcher provides is: "A female patient with difficulty breathing." The dispatcher also advises you that the ALS response unit is unavailable. Upon arrival, you find Mrs. Carmela Bartolone in a lawn chair with her husband and neighbor standing next to her, trying to get her to slow her breathing. You ask some quick medical questions and realize that the neighbor saw what happened, the husband has the medical history, and the patient can't talk in full sentences because of severe dyspnea.

Street Scene Questions

1. What is the first thing you should do for this patient?
2. What questions should you ask the husband? The neighbor?

After you perform a primary assessment, you decide to get patient information from the husband. He states that Mrs. Bartolone has emphysema from many years of smoking two packs of cigarettes a day. He says this same type of attack happened once before about 6 months ago. At that time, she was taken to the hospital and needed to be intubated and placed on a ventilator. She is on a number of medications, which he needs to get from inside the house. He reports no known allergies or other medical history.

From what you can gather, Carmela Bartolone spends many days housebound on a home oxygen unit. On this particular spring day, she felt that she should work in her flower garden. As she started to pull weeds, she failed to realize how much her rate of breathing was picking up. She soon found herself unable to catch her breath and was unable to get back to the house. The neighbor who saw Carmela's breathing problem asked if she needed anything. Carmela's response was, "Get help!"

Street Scene Questions

3. What is the significance of the medical history provided by the husband?
4. How much oxygen should the patient receive?

The fact that Mrs. Bartolone had to be put on a ventilator makes you realize that this patient is at risk of deteriorating very

quickly. As you evaluate her breathing again, you note her respiration rate is still rapid. Your partner counts it at 36. You notice the patient's lips are bluish, her nostrils are flaring, and she is pushing herself up in the chair to make it easier to breathe. Your partner informs you that the patient is using the muscles of the chest and stomach to help her breathe. Mrs. Bartolone is becoming less restless because she is getting drowsy, a sign that action is needed. Your partner recommends that you assist ventilations with a bag-valve mask and you concur. As you start to hook up the oxygen reservoir, the husband returns with Carmela's inhalers and tells you she only gets 2 liters per minute on her home unit. He also tells you that the doctor stressed she should not get more than that.

Street Scene Questions

5. Is the patient a good candidate for use of an inhaler?
6. Should this patient be considered a high priority with lights and siren for transport to the hospital?

You and your partner agree that this patient needs ventilations assisted with high-concentration oxygen and transport without delay. Her normal 2 liters per minute of oxygen are not enough to oxygenate her in this condition. You transport the patient while assisting ventilations. You would like to help her use her inhaler but your protocol requires the patient to be alert (she is drowsy). In addition, you know you are doing the patient a lot of good by ventilating her with high-concentration oxygen.

While en route, your partner notifies the hospital by radio of the patient's condition, treatment being provided, and an ETA of 10 minutes. You are able to ventilate the patient well by yourself, but that also means you are unable to get repeat vital signs. Keeping your priorities in mind, you continue ventilating Carmela and estimate her pulse rate by checking it quickly and frequently between ventilations. The patient seems more alert as you arrive at the emergency department. There you provide a prehospital care report to the waiting physician, which includes the patient history you obtained from the husband. As you start to leave the patient area, the doctor thanks you for being aggressive in assisting ventilations.

Cardiac Emergencies

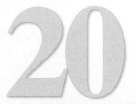

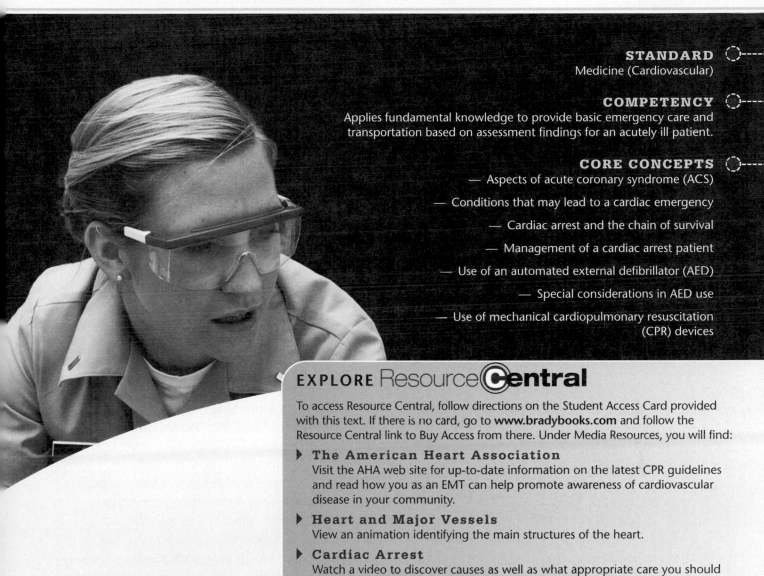

STANDARD
Medicine (Cardiovascular)

COMPETENCY
Applies fundamental knowledge to provide basic emergency care and transportation based on assessment findings for an acutely ill patient.

CORE CONCEPTS
— Aspects of acute coronary syndrome (ACS)
— Conditions that may lead to a cardiac emergency
— Cardiac arrest and the chain of survival
— Management of a cardiac arrest patient
— Use of an automated external defibrillator (AED)
— Special considerations in AED use
— Use of mechanical cardiopulmonary resuscitation (CPR) devices

EXPLORE ResourceCentral

To access Resource Central, follow directions on the Student Access Card provided with this text. If there is no card, go to **www.bradybooks.com** and follow the Resource Central link to Buy Access from there. Under Media Resources, you will find:

▶ **The American Heart Association**
Visit the AHA web site for up-to-date information on the latest CPR guidelines and read how you as an EMT can help promote awareness of cardiovascular disease in your community.

▶ **Heart and Major Vessels**
View an animation identifying the main structures of the heart.

▶ **Cardiac Arrest**
Watch a video to discover causes as well as what appropriate care you should provide if you witness a patient in cardiac arrest.

OBJECTIVES

After reading this chapter you should be able to:

20.1 Define key terms introduced in this chapter.

20.2 Describe the anatomy and physiology of the cardiovascular system. (pp. 470–471)

20.3 Define acute coronary syndrome and discuss its most common signs and symptoms. (pp. 471–472)

20.4 Discuss the management of a patient with acute coronary syndrome. (pp. 472–475)

20.5 Discuss the indications, contraindications, dosage, and administration of nitroglycerin to a patient with chest pain. (p. 476)

20.6 Discuss the indications (including conditions that must be met), contraindications, and administration of aspirin to a patient with chest pain. (p. 477)

20.7 Discuss the following conditions and how each may lead to a cardiac emergency:
  a. Coronary artery disease (CAD) (p. 478)
  b. Aneurysm (pp. 478–479)
  c. Electrical malfunctions of the heart (p. 479)
  d. Mechanical malfunctions of the heart (p. 479)
  e. Angina pectoris (pp. 479–480)
  f. Acute myocardial infarction (AMI) (pp. 480–481)
  g. Congestive heart failure (CHF) (p. 481)

469

20.8 Discuss the following factors in the chain of survival and how each may contribute to patient survival of cardiac arrest:
  a. Immediate recognition and activation (p. 483)
  b. Early cardiopulmonary resuscitation (CPR) (pp. 483–484)
  c. Rapid defibrillation (p. 484)
  d. Effective advanced life support (pp. 484–485)
  e. Integrated post-cardiac arrest care (p. 485)

20.9 List the skills necessary for the EMT to manage a patient in cardiac arrest. (pp. 485–486)

20.10 Discuss types of automated external defibrillators (AEDs) and how AEDs work. (pp. 486–488)

20.11 Discuss the effective coordination of CPR and AED for a patient in cardiac arrest. (pp. 489–495)

20.12 Discuss special considerations for AED use, including general principles, coordination with others, and post-resuscitation care. (pp. 495–500)

20.13 Discuss the purpose and use of mechanical CPR devices. (pp. 500–501)

KEY TERMS

acute coronary syndrome (ACS), *p. 471*
acute myocardial infarction (AMI), *p. 480*
agonal breathing, *p. 493*
aneurysm, *p. 478*
angina pectoris, *p. 479*

apnea, *p. 493*
cardiopulmonary resuscitation (CPR), *p. 470*
cardiovascular system, *p. 470*
congestive heart failure (CHF), *p. 481*

coronary artery disease (CAD), *p. 478*
defibrillation, *p. 470*
dyspnea, *p. 471*
dysrhythmia, *p. 479*
edema, *p. 481*
embolism, *p. 478*

occlusion, *p. 478*
pedal edema, *p. 481*
pulmonary edema, *p. 481*
sudden death, *p. 480*
thrombus, *p. 478*

EMTs may often encounter patients who complain of chest discomfort. Sometimes this discomfort will be the result of a cardiac (heart) problem—possibly a heart attack, possibly some other cardiac disorder. As an EMT, you will be able to provide these patients with oxygen, which is the most important drug in the treatment of heart problems. You may also be able to assist patients with taking nitroglycerin and aspirin. Most patients with chest pain will not be having heart attacks. In fact, they may not have a heart problem at all. Nonetheless, oxygen will not harm patients who are not having heart problems and may be of benefit to those who are.

Occasionally, you will encounter a patient who is in cardiac arrest—whose normal heartbeat and circulation of blood have completely stopped. *Cardiopulmonary resuscitation (CPR)* can help postpone death for a short time, but defibrillation must be performed as quickly as possible. *Defibrillation*, which will be covered in the second part of this chapter, is the application of an electrical shock to the chest in order to restart the heart's normal action. Cardiac arrest is a situation in which you may actually be able to save someone's life by acting quickly and efficiently.

>>>>>>

CARDIAC ANATOMY AND PHYSIOLOGY

cardiopulmonary resuscitation (CPR)
actions taken to revive a person by keeping the person's heart and lungs working.

defibrillation
delivery of an electrical shock to stop the fibrillation of heart muscles and restore a normal heart rhythm.

You learned about the *cardiovascular system* (made up of the heart and the blood vessels) and circulation of the blood in Chapter 5, "Medical Terminology and Anatomy and Physiology." Before continuing through this chapter on cardiac emergencies, you should review that material. In particular, you should review:

- Flow of blood through the chambers of the heart (the atria and ventricles), and the cardiac conductive system (the electrical impulses and specialized muscles that cause the heart to contract)

- Composition of the blood (red and white blood cells, platelets, and plasma)
- Flow of blood through the arteries, veins, arterioles, venules, and capillaries, and the names and positions of major blood vessels
- Circulation of blood between the heart and the lungs and between the heart and the rest of the body
- How heart function and the circulation of blood relate to pulse (review the peripheral and central pulses) and blood pressure (review systolic and diastolic pressure; also review Chapter 12, "Vital Signs and Monitoring Devices")
- Shock (hypoperfusion)

You may also wish to review the diagrams of the heart, the cardiovascular system, the cardiac conductive system, and the circulatory system in Chapter 5, "Medical Terminology and Anatomy and Physiology."

cardiovascular system
the heart and the blood vessels.

ACUTE CORONARY SYNDROME

Acute coronary syndrome (ACS), sometimes called *cardiac compromise*, is a blanket term that refers to any time the heart may not be getting enough oxygen. There are many different ways in which patients' hearts show that they are in trouble. One reason for this is that there are many different kinds of problems the heart can experience. A coronary artery may become narrowed or blocked, a one-way valve may stop working properly, or the specialized tissue that carries electrical impulses may function abnormally.

Just as there are many different problems the heart can experience, there is a very wide variety of signs and symptoms associated with these problems. Most of these signs and symptoms can also result from problems that have nothing to do with the heart. Many patients with heart trouble will complain of pain in the center of the chest. Others may have only mild chest discomfort or no pain at all. Some may experience difficulty breathing, while still others have only the sudden onset of sweating, nausea, and vomiting.

Since the signs and symptoms of a heart problem can vary so greatly, it is much safer for the EMT to treat all patients with certain signs and symptoms as though they are having a heart problem—ACS—instead of trying to decide whether or not the patient has a particular type of heart problem. Some common cardiovascular disorders will be discussed later in this chapter to assist you in recognizing and treating the symptoms associated with such disorders. Definitive diagnosis and care will be provided at the hospital.

The best known symptom of a heart problem is chest pain. Typically, a patient describes this pain as crushing, dull, heavy, or squeezing. Sometimes the patient will vehemently deny having pain but may admit to some pressure. Some patients will describe this sensation as just a discomfort. This is a good example of why you should have a patient describe in his own words how he is feeling. If you ask some of these patients whether they are having chest pain, they will tell you they are not, because to them it is not pain. When a patient is having difficulty describing the sensation, try suggesting several choices, as you learned in Chapter 14, "Assessment of the Medical Patient."

The pain, pressure, or discomfort associated with cardiac compromise commonly radiates along the arms, down to the upper abdomen, or up to the jaw. Patients complain of radiation to the left arm more than the right, but either (or both) is possible.

Another frequent complaint (and sometimes the only complaint in a patient with cardiac compromise) is difficulty breathing, called *dyspnea*. If the patient does not complain of difficulty breathing, specifically ask him about it. Sometimes the pain is so intense that patients focus their attention on that and do not mention other important symptoms.

A patient with ACS is often anxious. In some patients, this takes the form of a feeling of impending doom, which the patient may express to you or others. Occasionally, you will see a patient whose anxiety displays itself through irritability and a short temper.

Other common symptoms in patients with cardiac compromise are nausea and pain or discomfort in the upper abdomen (epigastric pain). Some of these patients also vomit. A less common finding is loss of consciousness. This may result from the heart beating too fast or too slow to adequately supply the brain with oxygenated blood. Usually, the patient regains consciousness quickly.

CORE CONCEPT
Aspects of acute coronary syndrome (ACS)

acute coronary syndrome (ACS)
a blanket term used to represent any symptoms related to lack of oxygen (ischemia) in the heart muscle. Also called *cardiac compromise*.

dyspnea (DISP-ne-ah)
shortness of breath; labored or difficult breathing.

There are also several signs you will see in some of these patients, including the sudden onset of sweating and an abnormal pulse or blood pressure. Many patients who have sudden onset of sweating think they are coming down with the flu, but this may result from the denial that is common in these patients. They refuse to acknowledge, at least consciously, that they may be having heart problems. The pulse may be abnormally slow (slower than 60 beats per minute, called **bradycardia**) or abnormally fast (faster than 100 beats per minute, called **tachycardia**) and will frequently be irregular. Some patients complain of palpitations, which are irregular or rapid heartbeats they feel as a fluttering sensation in the chest. A few patients are hypotensive (systolic blood pressure less than 90), whereas others are hypertensive (systolic greater than 150 or diastolic greater than 90).

Patients with cardiac compromise have many different presentations. Most commonly, the patient complains of pressure or pain in the chest with difficulty breathing and a history of heart problems. Others may have just mild discomfort that they ignore for several hours or that goes away and returns. Between one-quarter and one-third do *not* have the typical presentation of chest discomfort. This is especially true in older patients and women—women primarily because they are older when they have cardiac problems. In this case, you may see a patient who complains of difficulty breathing, sudden onset of sweating, or a sudden, unusual feeling of fatigue without chest discomfort. Because of these many possibilities and because of the potentially severe complications of heart problems, it is important to have a high index of suspicion and treat patients with any of these signs and symptoms for cardiac compromise. The treatment will not hurt them and may help them.

Management of Acute Coronary Syndrome

The management of a patient with ACS is detailed in the following text and in Scan 20-1.

PATIENT ASSESSMENT

Acute Coronary Syndrome

After performing your primary assessment, perform a history and physical exam. Get a history of the present illness by asking the OPQRST questions (inquire about onset, provocation, quality, radiation, severity, and time). Also get a past medical history (allergies, medications the patient may be taking, pertinent past history, last oral intake, events leading to the present emergency). Then take baseline vital signs.

The following signs and symptoms are often associated with ACS:

- Pain, pressure, or discomfort in the chest or upper abdomen (epigastrium)
- Difficulty breathing
- Palpitations
- Sudden onset of sweating and nausea or vomiting
- Anxiety (feeling of impending doom, irritability)
- Unusual generalized weakness
- Abnormal pulse (rapid, slow, or irregular)
- Abnormal blood pressure

PATIENT CARE

Acute Coronary Syndrome

Follow these steps for the emergency care of a patient with suspected ACS:

1. Place the patient in a position of comfort, typically sitting up. This is especially true of patients with difficulty breathing. Patients who are hypotensive (systolic blood pressure less than 90) will usually feel better lying down. This position allows more blood to flow to the brain. Occasionally, you will see a patient who has both difficulty breathing and hypotension. It may be very difficult to find a good position in this case. The best way to determine the proper position is to ask the patient what position will relieve his breathing difficulty without making him weak or lightheaded.

2. Apply high-concentration oxygen through a nonrebreather mask if not already done. This is especially important if the patient is hypoxic, as reflected in his signs and

bradycardia (bray-di-KAR-de-ah) when the heart rate is slow, usually below 60 beats per minute.

tachycardia (tak-e-KAR-de-ah) when the heart rate is fast, above 100 beats per minute.

FIRST TAKE STANDARD PRECAUTIONS.

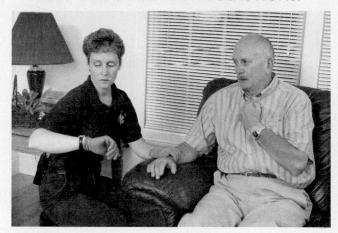

1 Perform the primary assessment.

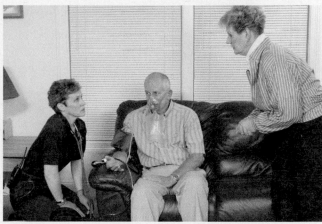

2 Provide high-concentration oxygen by nonrebreather mask. Perform the history and physical exam for a medical patient. Document the findings.

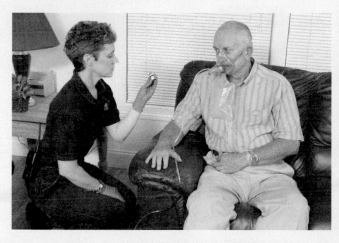

3 If the patient meets nitroglycerin criteria and has prescribed nitroglycerin, ask him about the last dose taken.

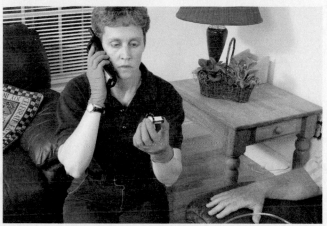

4 Check the five rights: right patient, right time, right drug, right dose, and right route. Check the expiration date. Follow local protocols and consult medical direction before assisting the patient with taking medication.

(continued)

symptoms, including the oxygen saturation level. Keep the patient's oxygen saturation at a level of at least 94 percent.

Although oxygen has never been proven to benefit "stable" patients with cardiac compromise, this does not mean oxygen is useless. There are many interventions that have never been proven to help patients, but are felt by authorities and the health care community to have little risk and potentially significant benefits. For example, no one has proven that direct pressure is a safe and effective means of controlling bleeding. The consensus is that, nonetheless, direct pressure is the first and most important step in controlling hemorrhage. Similarly, the traditional teaching has been to administer oxygen to any patient, even a stable one, with potential cardiac compromise.

Another reason to administer oxygen to these patients is the difficulty of determining who is "stable." It is often easy to tell that some patients are unstable, like the elderly man clutching his chest who has cyanosis around his lips and in his nail beds. It is much more difficult, and sometimes impossible, to determine definitively that a patient is stable, so the best thing to do is generally to administer oxygen to the patient with potential cardiac compromise.

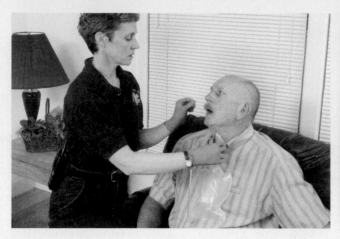

5 Remove the oxygen mask. Ask the patient to open his mouth and lift his tongue.

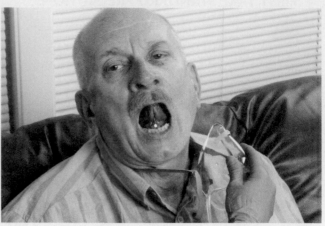

6 A. Place the nitroglycerin tablet under the tongue, or . . .

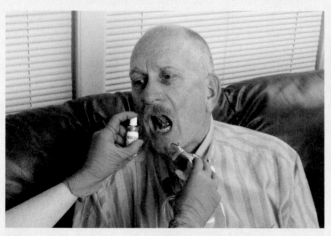

6 B. If the nitroglycerin is in spray form, spray the medication under the tongue according to label directions.

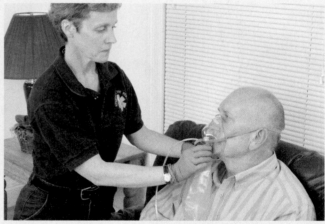

7 Have the patient close his mouth and hold the nitroglycerin under his tongue, where the medication will be quickly absorbed. Replace the oxygen mask.

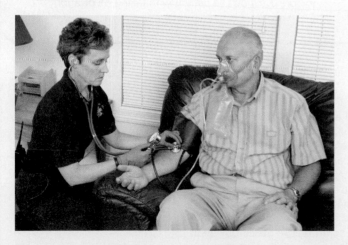

8 Reassess the patient, and document the findings.

If the patient already has a normal reading on the pulse oximeter while breathing room air, has stable vital signs, and has vague or unclear symptoms that might or might not be associated with cardiac compromise, many EMS systems recommend providing high-concentration oxygen by nonrebreather mask, although some may allow EMTs to give low-concentration oxygen by means of a nasal cannula. This is an area that needs further study, so follow your local protocols.

If the patient has or develops an altered mental status, you will need to open and maintain the patient's airway. If the patient is not breathing adequately, you will also need to ventilate him. Always be prepared for the patient to go into cardiac arrest. (Procedures for cardiac arrest will be discussed later in this chapter.)

3. Transport immediately if the patient has any one of the following:
   - No history of cardiac problems
   - History of cardiac problems, but does not have nitroglycerin
   - Systolic blood pressure below 90 to 100

4. If you are trained, equipped, and authorized to do so, obtain a 12-lead electrocardiogram (ECG). Follow local protocol with regard to whether you should transmit it to a hospital or physician for interpretation. Determining whether the patient has an ST-elevation myocardial infarction (STEMI) may be extremely important in determining the kind of treatment the patient may benefit from and where you will transport the patient.

   In areas with more than one hospital, there may be one or two facilities with special treatment available for cardiac patients. Almost all hospitals can administer an intravenous drug to dissolve the clot that is causing insufficient oxygenation of the heart. A more effective way to unclog the coronary artery is to insert a catheter with a balloon at the tip into the arterial system and thread it into the coronary arteries. When the balloon reaches the narrow section of the artery, it is inflated, compressing the obstructive material against the side of the blood vessel and opening up circulation to the heart muscle again. This is called percutaneous coronary intervention (PCI) and is often better than the "clotbuster drug" approach when it is done early (within a few hours of onset of symptoms). Only hospitals with special facilities and available staff can do this, however. If your EMS system has the ability to transport patients to a hospital with this capability, there will be a local protocol that you should follow describing when, where, and how you should transport patients with certain signs and symptoms.

5. Give the patient (or help the patient take) nitroglycerin (Scan 20-2) if all of the following conditions are met:
   - Patient complains of chest pain
   - Patient has a history of cardiac problems
   - Patient's physician has prescribed nitroglycerin (NTG)
   - Patient has the nitroglycerin with him
   - Systolic blood pressure meets your protocol criteria (usually greater than 90 to 100 systolic)
   - Patient has not taken Viagra or a similar drug for erectile dysfunction within 48 to 72 hours
   - Medical direction authorizes administration of the medication

6. After giving one dose of the nitroglycerin, give a repeat dose in 5 minutes if all of the following conditions are met:
   - Patient experiences no relief or only partial relief
   - Systolic blood pressure remains greater than 90 to 100 systolic
   - Medical direction authorizes another dose of the medication

   Administer a maximum of three doses of nitroglycerin, reassessing vital signs and chest pain after each dose. If the blood pressure falls below 90 to 100 systolic, treat the patient for shock (hypoperfusion). Transport promptly.

7. Give the patient (or help the patient take) aspirin if *all* of the following conditions are met:
   - Patient complains of chest pain.
   - Patient is not allergic to aspirin.
   - Patient has no history of asthma.
   - Patient is not already taking any medications to prevent clotting. (Since some of these patients may still benefit from aspirin, consult your local protocol or medical direction in this case.)
   - Patient has no other contraindications to aspirin (Scan 20-3).
   - Patient is able to swallow without endangering the airway.
   - Medical direction authorizes administration of the medication.

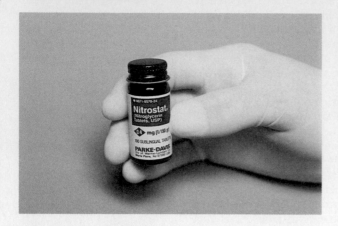

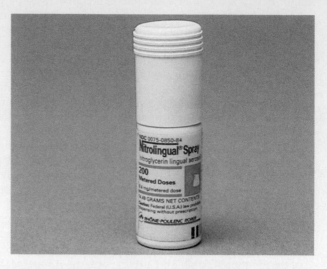

MEDICATION NAME
1. Generic: nitroglycerin
2. Trade: Nitrostat™, Nitrolingual®

INDICATIONS
All the following conditions must be met:
1. Patient complains of chest pain.
2. Patient has a history of cardiac problems.
3. Patient's physician has prescribed nitroglycerin (NTG).
4. Systolic blood pressure is greater than 90 to 100 systolic.
5. Medical direction authorizes administration of the medication.

CONTRAINDICATIONS
1. Patient has hypotension, or a systolic blood pressure below 90 to 100.
2. Patient has a head injury.
3. Patient is an infant or child.
4. Patient has already taken the maximum prescribed dose.
5. Patient has recently taken Viagra, Cialis, Levitra, or another drug for erectile dysfunction.

MEDICATION FORM
Tablet, sublingual (under-the-tongue) spray

DOSAGE
One dose. Repeat in 5 minutes, if less than complete relief, if systolic blood pressure remains above 90 to 100, and if authorized by medical direction, up to a maximum of three doses.

ADMINISTRATION
1. Perform a focused assessment for the cardiac patient.
2. Take the patient's blood pressure. (Systolic pressure must be above 90 to 100.)
3. Contact medical direction, if no standing orders.
4. Ensure the right patient, right time, right medication, right dose, and right route. Check the expiration date.
5. Ensure the patient is alert.
6. Question the patient on the last dose taken and effects. Ensure understanding of the route of administration.
7. Ask the patient to lift his tongue, and place the tablet or spray dose under the tongue (while wearing gloves) or have the patient place the tablet or spray under the tongue.
8. Have the patient keep his mouth closed with the tablet under the tongue (without swallowing) until dissolved and absorbed.
9. Recheck the patient's blood pressure within 2 minutes.
10. Record the administration, route, and time.
11. Reassess the patient.

ACTIONS
1. Relaxes blood vessels
2. Decreases workload of heart

SIDE EFFECTS
1. Hypotension (lowers blood pressure)
2. Headache
3. Pulse rate changes

REASSESSMENT STRATEGIES
1. Monitor blood pressure.
2. Ask patient about effect on pain relief.
3. Seek medical direction before readministering.
4. Record assessments.

PEDIATRIC NOTE

Children usually have very healthy hearts, so it is rare for an EMT to see a pediatric patient with a cardiac problem. Most such problems are congenital; that is, the child is born with them, so they are discovered before the newborn leaves the nursery. You may see a child who has had cardiac surgery or has learned to live with his problem through changes in lifestyle or medication. In cases like these, parents are frequently very well informed and can be of great assistance.

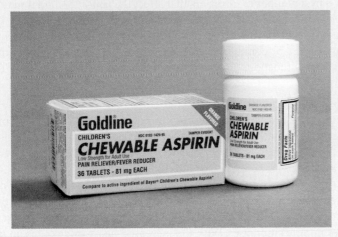

MEDICATION NAME
1. Generic: aspirin
2. Trade: many available

INDICATIONS
All of the following conditions must be met:
1. Patient complains of chest pain.
2. Patient is not allergic to aspirin.
3. Patient has no history of asthma.
4. Patient is not already taking any medications to prevent clotting.
5. Patient has no other contraindications to aspirin.
6. Patient is able to swallow without endangering the airway.
7. Medical direction authorizes administration of the medication.

CONTRAINDICATIONS
1. Patient is unable to swallow without endangering the airway.
2. Patient is allergic or sensitive to aspirin.
3. Patient has a history of asthma (many people with asthma are allergic to aspirin).
4. Patient has gastrointestinal ulcer or recent bleeding.
5. Patient has a known bleeding disorder.
6. Medical direction may decide if the benefit of giving aspirin to a patient who has one of the following conditions outweighs the risk:
   a. Is already taking medication to prevent clotting (including aspirin)
   b. Pregnancy
   c. Recent surgery

MEDICATION FORM
Tablet; many EMS systems use baby aspirin, usually supplied as 81 mg chewable tablets.

DOSAGE
162 to 324 mg (two to four 81 mg tablets of chewable baby aspirin). Aspirin does not usually need to be administered more than once in the early treatment of cardiac problems.

ADMINISTRATION
1. Gather a history and perform a physical exam appropriate for a cardiac patient.
2. Contact medical direction, if no standing orders.
3. Ensure the right medication, right patient, right time, right dose, and right route. Check the expiration date.
4. Ensure the patient is alert.
5. Ask the patient to chew (if directed by protocol) and swallow tablets.
6. Record the administration, route, and time.
7. Perform reassessment.

ACTIONS
1. Prevents blood from clotting as quickly, leading to increased survival after myocardial infarction.
2. When administered to cardiac patients, aspirin is not being used to relieve pain.

SIDE EFFECTS
1. Nausea
2. Vomiting
3. Heartburn
4. If patient is allergic, bronchospasm and wheezing
5. Bleeding

REASSESSMENT STRATEGIES
1. Perform reassessment.
2. Evaluate the patient for new onset of difficulty breathing from bronchospasm.
3. Any bleeding resulting from the aspirin is very unlikely to occur before the patient arrives at a hospital.
4. Record the assessments.

NOTE: *Transportation of a patient with a heart condition must be carried out in a thoughtful, calm, and careful fashion. A rough ride with sudden starts, stops, and turns and siren wailing is likely to increase the patient's fear and apprehension, placing additional stress on the heart. Speed is important, as the patient must reach the hospital quickly. However, the judicious use of siren or horn must be balanced against the possibility of worsening the patient's condition.*

CAUSES OF CARDIAC CONDITIONS

CORE CONCEPT

Conditions that may lead to a cardiac emergency

Heart problems can be caused by a number of disorders that affect the condition and function of the blood vessels and the heart. The majority of cardiovascular emergencies are caused, directly or indirectly, by changes in the inner walls of arteries. These arteries can be part of the systemic (total body), pulmonary (lung), or coronary (heart) circulatory systems. Problems with the heart's electrical and mechanical functions also cause cardiovascular emergencies.

Coronary Artery Disease

The heart is a muscle—a very active muscle. Like all other muscles, it needs oxygen to contract. The blood that is pumped through the chambers of the heart does not provide oxygen to the heart itself. Instead, the heart muscle is supplied with oxygenated blood by special blood vessels: the coronary arteries.

When the coronary arteries are narrowed or blocked, blood flow is reduced, thereby reducing the amount of oxygen delivered to the heart. This might not be noticed when the body is at rest or at a low activity level. However, when the body is subject to stress or exertion, the heart rate (beats per minute) increases. With the increased heart rate comes an increased need for oxygen. Arteries that are narrowed or blocked cannot supply enough blood to meet the heart's demands.

coronary artery disease (CAD)
diseases that affect the arteries of the heart.

Conditions that narrow or block the arteries of the heart are commonly called **coronary artery disease (CAD)**. Coronary artery disease is a serious health problem that results in hundreds of thousands of deaths yearly in the United States.

CAD is often the result of the buildup of fatty deposits on the inner walls of arteries. This buildup causes a narrowing of the inner vessel diameter, restricting the flow of blood. Fats and other particles combine to form this deposit, known as plaque. As time passes, calcium can be deposited at the site of the plaque, causing the area to harden.

thrombus (THROM-bus)
a clot formed of blood and plaque attached to the inner wall of an artery or vein.

occlusion (uh-KLU-zhun)
blockage, as of an artery by fatty deposits.

embolism (EM-bo-lizm)
blockage of a vessel by a clot or foreign material brought to the site by the blood current.

This restricts the amount of blood passing through the artery. The rough surface formed inside the artery can facilitate formation of blood clots, which narrow the artery even more. The clot and debris from the plaque form a **thrombus**. A thrombus can reach a size where it causes an **occlusion** (cutting off) of blood flow, or it may break loose to become an **embolism** and move to occlude the flow of blood somewhere downstream in a smaller artery. In cases of partial or complete blockage, the tissues beyond the point of blockage will be starved of oxygen and may die. If this blockage involves a large area of the heart (as in a heart attack) or the brain (causing one kind of stroke), the results may be quickly fatal.

Some factors that put a person at risk of developing CAD, such as heredity (a close relative who has CAD) and age, cannot be changed. However, there are also many risk factors that can be modified to reduce the risk of coronary artery disease. These include hypertension (high blood pressure), obesity, lack of exercise, elevated blood levels of cholesterol and triglycerides, and cigarette smoking.

Many patients have more than one of these risk factors. Fortunately, the damage caused by the second group of risk factors may be reversed or slowed by changing behavior. Smokers can return to the risk level of a nonsmoker soon after quitting. Medication and weight loss can lower high blood pressure. Improved diet and exercise can help the other controllable factors.

In the majority of cardiac-related medical emergencies, the reduced blood supply to the myocardium (heart muscle) causes the emergency. The most common symptom of this reduced blood supply is chest pain. Patients may have symptoms that range anywhere from mild chest pain to cardiac arrest. Angina pectoris (chest pain), acute myocardial infarction (heart attack), and congestive heart failure—all conditions that can be related to CAD—are discussed later in this chapter.

Aneurysm

aneurysm (AN-u-rizm)
the dilation, or ballooning, of a weakened section of the wall of an artery.

Another cause of cardiovascular system disorder stems from weakened sections in the arterial walls. Each weak spot that begins to dilate (balloon) is known as an **aneurysm**. This weakening can be related to other arterial diseases, or it can exist independently. When a weakened section of an artery bursts, there can be rapid, life-threatening internal bleeding (Figure 20-1). Tissues beyond the rupture can be damaged because the oxygenated blood they need is escaping and not reaching them. If a major artery ruptures, death from shock

FIGURE 20-1 A weakened area in the wall of an artery will tend to balloon out, forming a sac-like aneurysm, which may eventually burst.

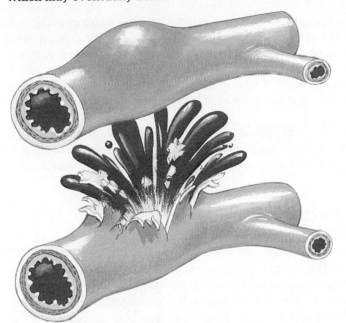

FIGURE 20-1 A weakened area in the wall of an artery will tend to balloon out, forming a sac-like aneurysm, which may eventually burst.

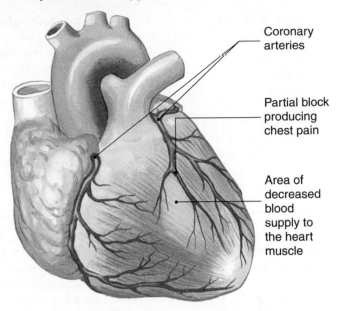

FIGURE 20-2 Angina pectoris, or chest pain, results when a coronary artery is blocked, depriving an area of the myocardium of oxygen.

Coronary arteries

Partial block producing chest pain

Area of decreased blood supply to the heart muscle

can occur very quickly. The two most common sites of aneurysms that you will encounter in emergency situations are the aorta (see Chapter 24, "Abdominal Emergencies") and the brain (see Chapter 21, "Diabetic Emergencies and Altered Mental Status"). When an artery in the brain ruptures, a severe form of stroke occurs. The severity is dependent on the site of the stroke and the amount of blood loss.

Electrical Malfunctions of the Heart

Electrical impulses generated within the heart are responsible for the heart's rhythmic beating that pumps blood throughout the body. A malfunction of the heart's electrical system will generally result in a *dysrhythmia*, an irregular, or absent, heart rhythm. Dysrhythmias include bradycardia (abnormally slow, less than 60 beats per minute), tachycardia (abnormally fast, greater than 100 beats per minute), and rhythms that may be present when there is no pulse (in cardiac arrest) including ventricular fibrillation, ventricular tachycardia, pulseless electrical activity, and asystole (described later in this chapter).

dysrhythmia (dis-RITH-me-ah) a disturbance in heart rate and rhythm.

Mechanical Malfunctions of the Heart

Another complication sometimes seen with a myocardial infarction, or heart attack, is mechanical pump failure. In this situation, a lack of oxygen causes the death of a portion of the myocardium. The dead area can no longer contract and pump. If a large enough area of the heart dies, the pumping action of the whole heart will be affected. This can lead to cardiac arrest, shock, pulmonary edema (fluids "backing up" in the lungs), or congestive heart failure (discussed later in this chapter). A few heart attack patients suffer cardiac rupture as the dead tissue area of the heart muscle bursts open. This occurs days after a heart attack.

Deterioration or malfunction of the heart valves is also a common component of cardiovascular disorders such as congestive heart failure.

Angina Pectoris

Angina pectoris means, literally, a pain in the chest. In this condition, coronary artery disease has narrowed the arteries that supply the heart. During times of exertion or stress, the heart works harder. The portion of the myocardium supplied by the narrowed artery becomes starved for oxygen. When the myocardium is deprived of oxygen, chest pain—angina pectoris—is the most frequent result (Figure 20-2). This pain is sometimes called an angina attack.

angina pectoris (AN-ji-nah [or an-JI-nah] PEK-to-ris) pain in the chest, occurring when blood supply to the heart is reduced and a portion of the heart muscle is not receiving enough oxygen.

Since the pain of angina pectoris comes on after stress or exertion, the pain will frequently diminish when the patient stops the exertion. As the oxygen demand of the heart returns to normal, the pain subsides. Seldom does this painful attack last longer than 3 to 5 minutes.

Possession of *nitroglycerin* is another indication that the patient has a history of this condition. Nitroglycerin is a medication that dilates the blood vessels. This results in more blood staying in the veins of the body, so there is less blood coming back to the heart. With less blood to pump out, the heart does not have to work as hard. Nitroglycerin is available in tablets that are placed under the patient's tongue to dissolve, as well as sprays and patches. The patches have adhesive that keeps them on the skin. They gradually release nitroglycerin throughout the day.

Most angina patients are advised by their doctors to take nitroglycerin for their chest pain. Patients are usually told to rest and are allowed to take three nitroglycerin doses over a 10-minute period. If there is no relief of symptoms after that time, they are instructed to call for help.

Acute Myocardial Infarction

The condition in which a portion of the myocardium (heart muscle) dies as a result of oxygen starvation is known as *acute myocardial infarction (AMI)* (Figure 20-3). Often called a heart attack by laypersons, AMI is brought on by the narrowing or occlusion of the coronary artery that supplies the region with blood. Rarely, the interruption of blood flow to the myocardium may be due to the rupturing of a coronary artery (aneurysm).

Over a million cases of AMI occur in the United States each year and cardiovascular disease causes hundreds of thousands of deaths annually. A major portion of these deaths are cases of *sudden death*, a cardiac arrest that occurs within 2 hours of the onset of symptoms. In most cases, sudden death occurs outside of hospitals. The patient may have no prior symptoms of coronary artery disease. Nearly 25 percent of these individuals have no previous history of cardiac problems.

A variety of factors can cause an AMI. Coronary artery disease is usually the underlying reason for the incident. However, for some patients, factors often regarded as harmless, such as chronic respiratory problems, unusual exertion, or severe emotional stress, may trigger an AMI.

The treatment of AMI has changed radically over recent years. Previously, patients were admitted to coronary care units where they were observed and, when emergencies occurred, treated with varying degrees of success. Now, some patients receive treatment with medications called *fibrinolytics* to dissolve the clot that is blocking the coronary artery. To be most effective, these medications must be administered early. With each hour

nitroglycerin (NTG)
a medication that dilates the blood vessels.

acute myocardial infarction (AMI) (ah-KUTE MY-o-KARD-e-ul in-FARK-shun)
the condition in which a portion of the myocardium dies as a result of oxygen starvation; often called a heart attack by laypersons.

sudden death
a cardiac arrest that occurs within 2 hours of the onset of symptoms. The patient may have no prior symptoms of coronary artery disease.

FIGURE 20-3 (A) Cross-section of a myocardial infarction and (B) a heart with normal and infarcted tissue.

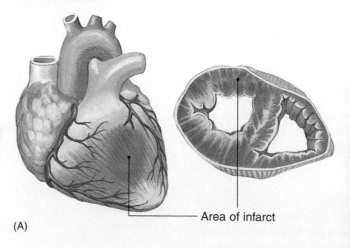

(A)

Area of infarct

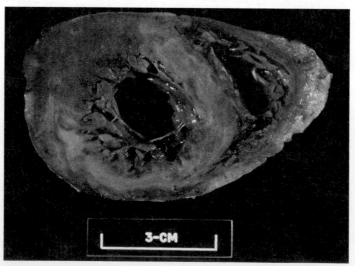

3-CM

(B)

that passes before they are administered, they become less and less likely to dissolve the clot. As noted earlier, an even more effective way to unclog the coronary artery is to insert a catheter with a balloon that can be inflated to reopen circulation to the heart, a procedure known as *balloon angioplasty* or *balloon catheterization*. Many patients with myocardial infarctions are not candidates for these treatments, but those who are must reach the hospital quickly.

A patient who leaves the hospital after an AMI will usually be told to take aspirin every day to prevent another episode. He will also probably be told to take a medication known as a *beta blocker*. This group of medications slows the heart and makes it beat less strongly. This would not usually be considered a good thing, but in these patients it results in a decrease in the work the heart has to do. This actually benefits the heart and leads to longer and better lives for these patients.

Congestive Heart Failure

Congestive heart failure (CHF) is a condition of excessive fluid buildup in the lungs and/or other organs and body parts because of the inadequate pumping of the heart. The fluid buildup causes *edema*, or swelling. The disorder is traditionally termed *congestive* because the fluids congest, or clog, the organs. It is termed *heart failure* because the congestion both results from and also aggravates failure of the heart to function properly. The congestion may also result from and aggravate failure of the lungs to function properly.

Congestive heart failure may be brought on by diseased heart valves, hypertension, or some form of obstructive pulmonary disease such as emphysema. CHF is often a complication of AMI. Congestive heart failure often progresses as follows:

1. A patient sustains an AMI. Myocardium in the area of the left ventricle dies. (Recall the function of the heart: The left is the side of the heart that receives oxygenated blood from the lungs and pulmonary circulation and pumps it to the rest of the body.)

2. Because of the damage to the left ventricle, blood backs up into the pulmonary circulation and then the lungs. Fluid accumulation in the lungs is called *pulmonary edema*. This edema causes a poor exchange of oxygen between the lungs and the bloodstream, and the patient experiences shortness of breath, or dyspnea. Listening to this patient's lungs with a stethoscope may reveal crackling or bubbly lung sounds called crackles (rales). Some patients cough up blood-tinged sputum from their lungs.

3. Left heart failure, if untreated, commonly causes right heart failure. The right side of the heart (which receives blood from the body and pumps it to the lungs) becomes congested because the clogged lungs cannot receive more blood. In turn, fluids may accumulate in the dependent (lower) extremities, the liver, and the abdomen. Accumulation of fluid in the feet or ankles is known as *pedal edema*. The abdomen may become noticeably distended. In a bedridden patient, fluid collects in the sacral area of the spine.

    The signs and symptoms of CHF may include:
- Tachycardia (rapid pulse, 100 beats per minute or more)
- Dyspnea (shortness of breath)
- Normal or elevated blood pressure
- Cyanosis
- Diaphoresis (profuse sweating), or cool and clammy skin
- Pulmonary edema, sometimes coughing up of frothy white or pink sputum
- Anxiety or confusion due to hypoxia (inadequate supply of oxygen to the brain and other tissues) caused by poor oxygen/carbon dioxide exchange
- Pedal edema
- Engorged, pulsating neck veins (late sign)
- Enlarged liver and spleen, with abdominal distention (late sign)

The CHF patient is probably on several medications for this condition. Often patients will tell you that they take a water pill for fluid buildup. This refers to a diuretic, a medication that helps remove fluid from the circulatory system. Other medications may decrease the heart's workload, leading to improvement in the patient's condition.

congestive heart failure (CHF) the failure of the heart to pump efficiently, leading to excessive blood or fluids in the lungs, the body, or both.

edema (eh-DEEM-uh) swelling resulting from a buildup of fluid in the tissues.

pulmonary edema accumulation of fluid in the lungs.

pedal edema accumulation of fluid in the feet or ankles.

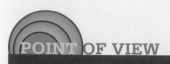
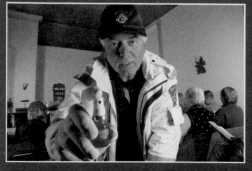

"I couldn't believe I was having chest pain. How cruel was it that I'd prayed I wouldn't have another heart attack—and where do I get chest pain again? Church. Not only did my chest hurt, but I was so embarrassed.

"I was so embarrassed and worried that I forgot I had the nitro spray with me. The EMTs came and checked me over and asked me if I'd ever had pain like this before. That was when I remembered. I never had to use it before. They put a spray under my tongue before they wheeled me out of church, because it was quite a ways to get down and to the ambulance. It actually helped.

"When we got to the ambulance I told them that my pain felt better. When they found out that I still had some pain they checked me again and then gave me another spray. I have to say I relaxed a bit when the pain went away.

"When you have chest pain, you think you are going to die. It is a great feeling suddenly realizing that the pain is gone. You really think you have a chance of living. Wow."

CRITICAL DECISION MAKING

Meeting Sublingual Nitroglycerin Criteria

You are treating a patient with chest pain. For each scenario provided, decide whether this patient meets the general criteria for sublingual nitroglycerin administration. Each of the patients has nitroglycerin prescribed by his cardiologist.

1. You are treating an 84-year-old patient with chest pain. His wife tells you that he began having a sensation in his chest he thought was indigestion about 2 hours ago. The patient is very pale and sweaty and appears sleepy. His pulse is 104 and slightly irregular, respirations 28 and adequate, and blood pressure 94/66.

2. You are treating a 68-year-old male patient who has a history of angina pectoris. He tells you that he began having chest discomfort just after eating dinner. The discomfort is in the center of his chest and is described as a heavy feeling. It feels like the last time he had a heart problem. His vital signs are pulse 92, strong and regular; respirations 20 and adequate; blood pressure 138/92; and skin warm and moist.

3. You are treating a 49-year-old male patient complaining of pain in his "stomach." He states the pain is below his diaphragm and radiates to the left side. He has taken one nitroglycerin spray without relief. The patient states this pain is not like his one heart attack. His vital signs are pulse 68, strong and regular; respirations 18 and adequate; blood pressure 112/68; and skin warm and dry.

CARDIAC ARREST

CORE CONCEPT

Cardiac arrest and the chain of survival

In a typical ambulance service, only 1 to 2 percent of emergency calls are cardiac arrests. Furthermore, most patients with heart problems do not go into cardiac arrest while they are under your care. Nonetheless, EMS systems exert a great deal of time and energy on attempts to resuscitate these patients. The odds of bringing a cardiac-arrest patient back to life have increased considerably over the last 15 or 20 years. As the problem of cardiac arrest has received more attention, EMS researchers, physicians, administrators, and providers have learned more about what is effective and what is not.

Chain of Survival

The American Heart Association has summarized the most important factors that affect survival of cardiac arrest patients in its chain of survival concept. The chain (Figure 20-4) has five

elements: (1) immediate recognition and activation, (2) early CPR, (3) rapid defibrillation, (4) effective advanced life support, and (5) integrated post-cardiac arrest care. An EMS system where each of these links is strong is much more likely to bring back a patient from cardiac arrest than a system with weaknesses anywhere along the chain. This has been shown in systems that tried to strengthen just one link (early defibrillation) without strengthening the other links.

An underlying theme of the chain of survival is teamwork. Although many of the actions you should take to resuscitate someone are described as though you are alone or working with very little help, you will usually have at least one other person, if not more, to work with you. It is essential that you and your teammates work together in a coordinated fashion to maximize the chance of your patient's survival. The need for teamwork also extends to others beyond the first ambulance crew at the scene, including ALS teams, Emergency Medical Responders, public safety officers, emergency department physicians and staff, cardiac catheterization lab staff, and others.

Because so many people are working to help the patient, it is not only possible, but desirable, for many things to happen simultaneously or nearly simultaneously. There must be coordination for these combined activities to work in the patient's favor. Having clear expectations that everyone is aware of goes a long way toward achieving that goal. This will allow simple things like primary assessment to be more efficient as one person checks the pulse and another gets equipment ready and positioned properly. It also allows complex activities such as getting the patient to the cardiac catheterization lab at the right time so that the appropriate people are present and prepared. This teamwork is essential to the success of a resuscitation effort and EMTs are a vital part of it.

Immediate Recognition and Activation

Immediate recognition and activation means that the person who sees someone collapse or finds someone unresponsive calls a dispatcher who quickly gets EMS responding to the emergency. Unfortunately, this is easier said than done. The lay public, unlike EMS providers, are not used to recognizing emergencies. It takes longer for them to realize that an emergency exists and that they should call for help right away. Even when a layperson does decide to make the call for help, there may still be obstacles.

Many areas still do not have 911 service. This means that emergency services have seven-digit telephone numbers that laypeople cannot be expected to remember. Even though many phone companies list emergency numbers on the inside cover of their directories, this adds an extra step to the process and delays even further the call for help. Many EMS agencies in this position have public information programs that include the distribution of telephone stickers with emergency numbers on them. Since Americans change residence frequently (and buy new telephones more often than that), emergency services must make these stickers available frequently and easily.

Early CPR

Early CPR can increase survival significantly. About the only time it does not help is when defibrillation reaches the patient within approximately 2 minutes or less. Since this rarely happens in real life, EMS agencies need to address this factor. There are at least three ways in which CPR can be delivered earlier: get CPR-trained professionals to the patient faster, train laypeople in CPR, and train dispatchers to instruct callers in how to perform CPR.

An efficient way to get CPR to patients faster in many areas is to send CPR-trained professionals to the scene. This may mean police, firefighters, security officers, or lifeguards. These professionals need to receive notification of the possible need for CPR as soon as possible. They also need to be in the right place so they can respond quickly to where they are needed.

Some EMS agencies have CPR courses for the lay public as part of their public information and education programs, but too many do not. It is especially important to train the right laypeople. Teaching CPR to elementary and high school students is good, especially in the long run, but these students are not usually present when someone goes into cardiac arrest. The typical cardiac arrest patient is a male in his 60s, so it is not surprising to learn that the typical witness of a cardiac arrest is a woman in her 60s. Middle-age and older people need CPR courses at least as much as children and adolescents.

A surprisingly effective way to get a layperson to perform CPR is for a dispatcher to instruct the caller over the phone. This has been done in a number of areas and has produced significant increases in the survival rate from cardiac arrest. The quality of CPR done by untrained laypeople instructed by dispatchers is comparable to CPR done by laypeople who were previously trained in CPR. This appears to be true even when laypeople perform chest compressions without ventilating the patient. Emergency Medical Dispatchers (EMDs) are trained to give such instructions. Prearrival dispatch instructions are available to guide other dispatchers in this step.

Rapid Defibrillation

Early defibrillation has received a great deal of attention because it is the single most important factor in determining survival from cardiac arrest.

Although a lot of emphasis has been put on defibrillation, there is often not enough attention paid to early defibrillation. With a few thousand dollars or less, an agency can purchase an automated defibrillator. The hard part is getting this equipment to the patient in cardiac arrest early enough to be effective. If the response time of the defibrillator (time from call received to arrival of the defibrillator) is longer than 8 minutes, virtually no patients survive cardiac arrest. This is often true even if early CPR is performed. Although 8 minutes is really the maximum response time for effective defibrillation, the sooner the defibrillator arrives, the more likely it is that a patient will survive cardiac arrest. In this case, it is literally true that every minute counts.

One way to get around long ambulance response times is to provide defibrillators to other emergency services providers. Some EMS systems have used innovative ways to make sure that a defibrillator arrives in time. In urban and suburban areas, for example, police officers and firefighters have sometimes been equipped with the machines since they may arrive on scene before the ambulance. In rural areas, some EMTs and Emergency Medical Responders carry defibrillators in their personal vehicles so that the patient who needs a defibrillator gets it in time.

Another way to get defibrillation to patients earlier is to have nontraditional responders use them. There are well-documented cases where nonemergency responders have resuscitated patients in cardiac arrest. These cases share certain characteristics: Patients or potential patients are under constant observation so that a witnessed arrest can be detected and reported immediately (e.g., in an airport terminal or a casino), the responders are employees who receive initial and refresher training in CPR and use of an AED (e.g., flight attendants or casino security officers), and the areas in which the employees and AEDs are deployed are high volume or high risk areas where cardiac arrests occur on a regular basis.

Training laypeople to use an AED and administer CPR has become very popular and may have the potential to improve survival from cardiac arrest.

Effective Advanced Life Support

Effective advanced life support is second only to defibrillation in the drama and excitement it stirs in laypeople. Putting a breathing tube into someone's throat (endotracheal intubation), putting a needle into someone's arm (starting an intravenous line), and administering medications into an IV line are all activities that laypeople may not understand, but they are actions that the public has come to expect. They may also lead to a higher survival rate.

The most common way for patients to get advanced cardiac life support (ACLS) is through EMT-Paramedics who either respond to the scene or rendezvous with a basic life support unit en route to the hospital. In some areas, there are EMTs who have more training than basic-level EMTs but less than paramedics. Their level of practice is frequently called EMT-Cardiac, EMT-Critical Care, EMT-Intermediate, or Advanced EMT. They may be able to perform interventions that can improve survival of these patients. Another method that is not quite as fast is for EMTs to transport patients not to a hospital, but to a clinic or other medical facility that is closer. Any such arrangements need to be made before they are actually needed and should be in writing in the form of protocols. These protocols should be approved by your Medical Director.

Integrated Post-Cardiac Arrest Care

Integrated post-cardiac arrest care means coordinating numerous different means of assessment and interventions that, together, maximize the patient's chance of neurologically intact survival. Elements of this approach include maintaining adequate oxygenation, avoiding hyperventilation, performing a 12-lead ECG, finding and managing treatable causes of the arrest, determining the appropriate destination for the patient, possibly inducing hypothermia, and several other advanced interventions.

As researchers continue to evaluate new interventions to improve cardiac resuscitation, they are also evaluating treatments to improve cerebral or brain resuscitation. Most patients who regain a spontaneous pulse after a short period of ventricular fibrillation wake up with little or no brain damage. Some patients, however, especially those who had prolonged down times, have significant brain damage that prevents them from returning to normal activities or even from regaining consciousness.

One intervention that appears to reduce brain damage in some resuscitated patients is controlled hypothermia. Cooling a patient's body to around 90°F to 93°F (32°C to 34°C) and maintaining that temperature for up to 24 hours has led to more survivors and less brain damage than in patients who did not receive the treatment.

Although therapeutic hypothermia has improved neurologically intact survival, inducing it can be challenging. Different EMS systems have different approaches to this treatment, most involving advanced life support providers. If some of your local hospitals employ this treatment and others don't, it may be appropriate to transport your post-cardiac arrest patient to a facility that can provide it. Follow your local protocols.

EMS systems that have immediate recognition and activation, early CPR, rapid defibrillation, effective advanced life support, and integrated post-cardiac arrest care have survival rates from cardiac arrest that are higher than systems with weaknesses in one or more of the links in the chain of survival.

CORE CONCEPT ●-----------
Management of a cardiac arrest patient

Management of Cardiac Arrest

As an EMT, you can provide two links in the chain of survival: early CPR and rapid defibrillation. You can review CPR in Appendix A, "Basic Cardiac Life Support Review," at the end of this book.

The rest of this chapter will emphasize the role of defibrillation in treating cardiac arrest patients. Managing a patient in cardiac arrest means you need to be able to:

- Perform one- and two-rescuer CPR (Ordinarily, you will do two-rescuer CPR when you are on duty, but you must be able to perform one-rescuer CPR while your partner is preparing equipment or while you are en route to a medical facility.)
- Use an automated external defibrillator
- Request advanced life support (when available) to continue the chain of survival
- Use a bag-valve-mask device with oxygen
- Use a flow-restricted, oxygen-powered ventilation device
- Lift and move patients
- Suction a patient's airway
- Use airway adjuncts (oropharyngeal and nasopharyngeal airways)
- Take Standard Precautions to protect yourself (and patients)
- Interview bystanders and family members to obtain facts related to the arrest

Although most of the patients you see with chest pain or difficulty breathing will remain alert and in good condition while you are assessing or treating them, a few will go into cardiac arrest before you arrive at the hospital. For this reason, you must be prepared for

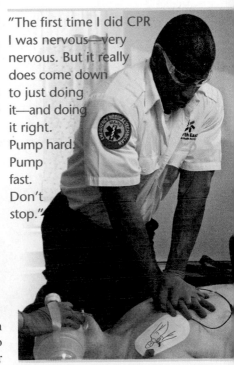

"The first time I did CPR I was nervous—very nervous. But it really does come down to just doing it—and doing it right. Pump hard. Pump fast. Don't stop."

cardiac arrest whenever you have a patient with chest discomfort or difficulty breathing. This means bringing the defibrillator to the scene when you are dispatched to one of these calls and having the defibrillator nearby while you are transporting.

Automated External Defibrillator (AED)

Types of AEDs

CORE CONCEPT

Use of an automated external defibrillator (AED)

There are two ways someone can defibrillate. The older method (manual defibrillation) is for the operator to look at the patient's heart rhythm on a screen, decide the rhythm is shockable, lubricate and charge two paddles, and deliver a shock to the patient's chest. An automated defibrillator, in contrast, contains a computer that analyzes the patient's heart rhythm after the operator applies two monitoring–defibrillation pads to the patient's chest (Figure 20-5).

There are two types of automated external defibrillators: semiautomatic and fully automatic. Semiautomatic defibrillators, the more common type, advise the EMT to press a button that will cause the machine to deliver a shock through the pads. Semiautomatic defibrillators are sometimes called "shock advisory defibrillators." Fully automated defibrillators do not advise the EMT to take any action. They deliver the shock automatically once enough energy has been accumulated. All the EMT has to do to use a fully automatic defibrillator is assess the patient, turn on the power, and put the pads on the patient's chest. The following information about how to operate an AED applies principally to a semiautomatic AED.

Another way in which AEDs can be classified is by the type of shock they deliver. The traditional monophasic defibrillator sends a single shock (this is what monophasic means) from the negative pad or paddle to the positive pad or paddle. A biphasic defibrillator sends the shock in one direction and then the other. This kind of machine also typically measures the impedance or resistance between the two pads and adjusts the energy accordingly, delivering more energy when the impedance is higher and less when it is lower. These features allow biphasic AEDs to use less energy and perhaps cause less damage to the heart. Use of biphasic AEDs does not result in higher survival rates, but they are at least as good as monophasic machines and have other advantages. Because the battery doesn't need to deliver as much energy, they are smaller and lighter than monophasic AEDs, a significant factor when an EMT has to carry several heavy pieces of equipment at once.

How AEDs Work

Like all muscles, the heart produces electrical impulses. By putting two monitoring electrodes on the patient's chest, it is possible to "see" the heart's electrical activity. An AED can analyze this cardiac rhythm and determine whether or not it is a rhythm for which a shock is indicated. The microprocessors and the computer programs used to do this have been tested extensively and have been very accurate, both in the laboratory and in the field. Today's AEDs are very reliable in distinguishing between rhythms that need shocks and rhythms that do not need shocks.

FIGURE 20-5 Automated external defibrillators (AEDs) are available from various manufacturers in a variety of models. (A) SMART Biphasic Automated External Defibrillator, Model FR2+. (B) Pediatric pads for the pediatric version of the Model FR2+. *(© Philips Medical Systems)*

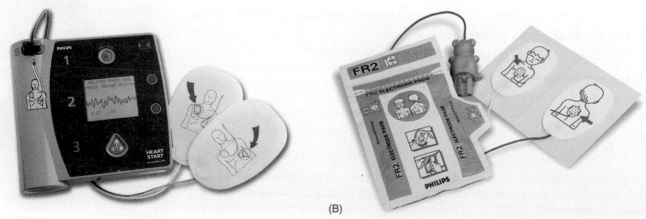

(A)   (B)

When AEDs deliver shocks inappropriately, it is almost always the result of human error. This occurs because the operator did not assess the patient properly (AEDs are designed only for use on patients in cardiac arrest), did not use the AED properly, or did not maintain the machine. The chance of mechanical error is always present, but it is small. Maintaining the AED in good operating order; attaching an AED only to unresponsive, pulseless, nonbreathing patients; practicing frequently; and following your local protocols are the best ways to avoid making an error that could affect a patient.

Often, a cardiac event such as a spasm or blockage of a coronary artery (myocardial infarction or heart attack) is associated with a disturbance of the heart's electrical, or conduction, system, which must function normally if the heart is to continue to beat with a regular rhythm. The most common conditions that result in cardiac arrest are shockable rhythms:

- Ventricular fibrillation
- Ventricular tachycardia

The primary electrical disturbance resulting in cardiac arrest is **ventricular fibrillation (VF)**. Up to 50 percent of all cardiac arrest victims will be in VF if EMS personnel arrive in the first 8 minutes or so. The heart in VF may have plenty of electrical energy, but it is totally disorganized. Chaotic electrical activity originating from many sites in the heart prevents the heart muscle from contracting normally and pumping blood. If you could see a heart in VF, it would appear to be quivering like a bag of worms. VF is considered a "shockable rhythm"; that is, VF is a rhythm for which defibrillation is effective.

Automated external defibrillators are also designed to shock a rhythm known as **ventricular tachycardia (V-tach)** if it is very fast. In ventricular tachycardia (an unusual cardiac arrest rhythm observed in less than 10 percent of all out-of-hospital cases), the heart rhythm is organized, but it is usually quite rapid. The faster the heart rate, the more likely it is that ventricular tachycardia will not allow the heart's chambers to fill with enough blood between beats to produce blood flow sufficient to meet the body's needs, especially that of the brain. Pulseless V-tach is considered a shockable rhythm.

Some patients with ventricular tachycardia are awake, even with very fast heart rates. If an AED is attached to one of these patients, it will charge up and advise a shock. Since the patient has a pulse and is awake, this action would be inappropriate. This is one of the reasons the AED should be attached only to patients in cardiac arrest.

Nonshockable rhythms include:

- Pulseless electrical activity (PEA)
- Asystole

In 15 to 20 percent of cardiac arrest victims, the rhythm is called **pulseless electrical activity (PEA)**; that is, the heart muscle itself fails even though the electrical rhythm remains relatively normal. This condition of relatively normal electrical activity but no pumping action means that the heart muscle is severely and almost always terminally sick. Or it may mean that the patient has lost too much blood. The heart could pump if it had something to pump, but there is no fluid in the system. Defibrillation cannot help these people because their heart's electrical rhythm is already organized and slow (unlike ventricular tachycardia, where the rhythm is organized but very fast). PEA is not considered a shockable rhythm.

In the remaining 20 to 50 percent of cardiac arrest victims, the heart has ceased generating electrical impulses altogether. This condition is called **asystole**. When this happens, there is no electrical stimulus to cause the heart muscle to contract, and so it does not. As a result, there is no blood flow, and the patient has no pulse or respirations and is unconscious. (This condition is commonly called *flatline*, because the wavy line displayed on an ECG when there is electrical activity goes flat with asystole.) This condition can be the result of untreated ventricular fibrillation, a sick heart, a terminal illness, or severe blood loss. Asystole is not considered a shockable rhythm.

By adding up the numbers, you can see that automated defibrillators will shock, at most, only about 6 or 7 of every 10 cardiac arrest patients to whom they are attached: those suffering from the disturbed rhythms of ventricular fibrillation and ventricular tachycardia. For patients suffering from pulseless electrical activity (heart muscle failure) or asystole (complete lack of electrical activity), defibrillation will not be effective.

ventricular fibrillation (VF)
(ven-TRIK-u-ler fib-ri-LAY-shun) a condition in which the heart's electrical impulses are disorganized, preventing the heart muscle from contracting normally.

ventricular tachycardia (V-tach) (ven-TRIK-u-ler tak-i-KAR-de-uh) a condition in which the heartbeat is quite rapid; if rapid enough, ventricular tachycardia will not allow the heart's chambers to fill with enough blood between beats to produce blood flow sufficient to meet the body's needs.

pulseless electrical activity (PEA)
a condition in which the heart's electrical rhythm remains relatively normal, yet the mechanical pumping activity fails to follow the electrical activity, causing cardiac arrest.

asystole (ay-SIS-to-le)
a condition in which the heart has ceased generating electrical impulses.

FIGURE 20-6 AED cardiac arrest treatment sequence.

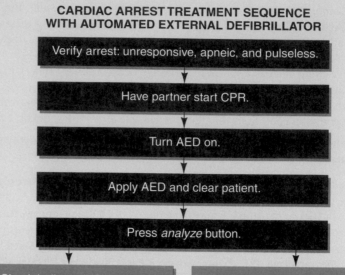

**CARDIAC ARREST TREATMENT SEQUENCE
WITH AUTOMATED EXTERNAL DEFIBRILLATOR**

Verify arrest: unresponsive, apneic, and pulseless.

↓

Have partner start CPR.

↓

Turn AED on.

↓

Apply AED and clear patient.

↓

Press *analyze* button.

Shock indicated (SI)	No shock indicated (NSI)
• Deliver 1 shock if AED gives *SI* message.	• Perform CPR for 2 minutes (5 cycles).
• If patient does not wake up, perform 2 minutes (5 cycles) of CPR.	• Press *analyze* button.
• Press *analyze* button.	• No shock indicated *(NSI)*.
• If *SI*, deliver 1 more shock if AED gives *SI* message.	• Perform 2 minutes (5 cycles) of CPR.
• After 3 shocks, prepare for transport. Follow local protocols for additional shocks.	

Check pulse. If none, do CPR and transport.

Notes:

Whenever a *no shock indicated (NSI)* message appears, begin 2 minutes (5 cycles) of CPR.

If the patient regains a pulse, check breathing. Ventilate with high-concentration oxygen, or give oxygen by nonrebreather mask as needed.

If you initially shock the patient and then receive an *NSI* message before giving six shocks, follow the steps in the above right-hand column.

If you initially receive an *NSI* message and then on a subsequent analysis receive a *shock indicated (SI)* message, follow the steps in the above left-hand column.

Occasionally you may need to shift back and forth between the two columns. If this happens, follow the steps until one of the indications for transport (described below) occurs.

Transport as soon as one of the following occurs:

• You have administered three shocks.

• You have received three consecutive *NSI* messages (separated by 2 minutes of CPR).

• The patient regains a pulse.

If you shock the patient out of cardiac arrest and he arrests again, start the sequence of shocks from the beginning.

You should do no more than three cycles of analyze, shock/no shock advised, and CPR before beginning transport. Your local protocols may recommend initiating transport earlier in the sequence.

Coordinating CPR and AED for a Patient in Cardiac Arrest

You should interrupt CPR only when absolutely necessary and for as short a period as possible. Since you will be using a defibrillator on patients in cardiac arrest, you need to understand some additional circumstances when you should interrupt CPR.

If you are touching the patient when the AED is analyzing the rhythm, there can be interference from the electrical impulses of your heart and from movement of the patient's muscles. This can fool the AED's computer into believing there is a shockable rhythm when there really isn't one or vice versa. It is also true that if a shock is delivered when you are touching the patient, the shock can be transmitted to you. Although this shock is not likely to cause you serious harm, you could be injured.

For these reasons, no one should ventilate, do chest compressions, or in any way touch the patient when the rhythm is being analyzed or a shock is being delivered.

Defibrillation is more effective than CPR in restoring a patient's pulse, so briefly stopping CPR to allow for rhythm analysis and defibrillation is actually better for the patient. Resume CPR immediately after delivering a shock (Figure 20-6 and Scan 20-4).

SCAN 20-4 Assessing and Managing a Cardiac Arrest Patient

NOTE: *At earliest opportunity, call for an ALS intercept.*

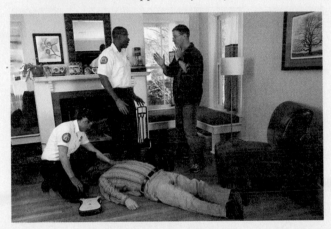

1 If the patient appears lifeless, do a quick scan for breathing. Obtain a quick history of events from family or bystanders.

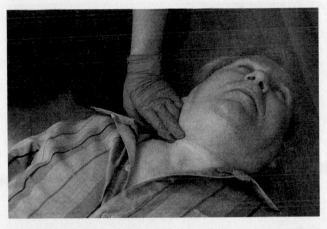

2 Verify the absence of a spontaneous pulse. Check for no longer than 10 seconds.

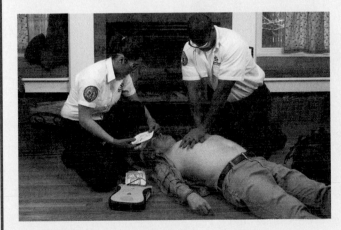

3 Provide CPR while another EMT sets up the AED.

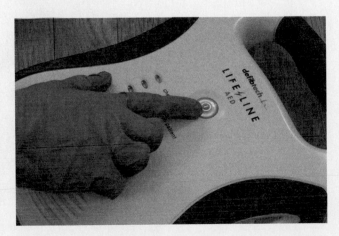

4 Turn on the AED power.

(continued)

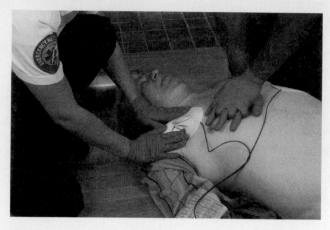

⑤ Apply pads to the patient's chest. Remove the backing. Place one pad on the upper right chest, one on the lower left ribs.

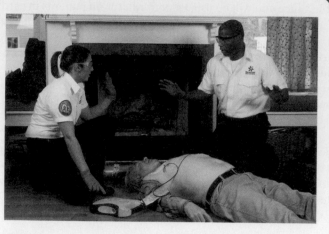

⑥ Say "Clear!" Ensure that all individuals are clear of the patient.

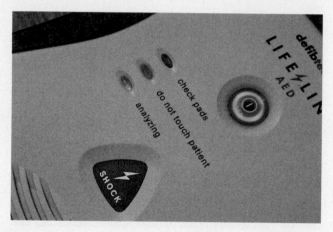

⑦ Press "analyze" if you AED has that button. Remain clear of the patient while the AED analyzes.

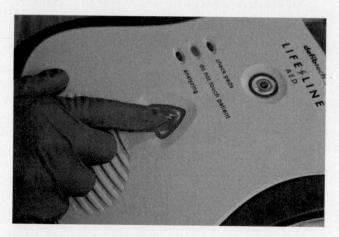

⑧ If advised by the AED, press the button to deliver a shock. Immediately perform compressions.

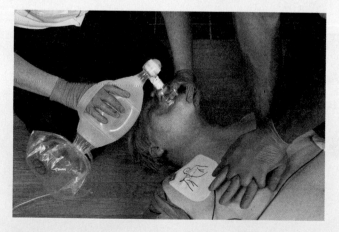

⑨ Perform CPR for 2 minutes (5 cycles), unless the patient wakes up, moves, or begins to breathe. Follow AED prompts.

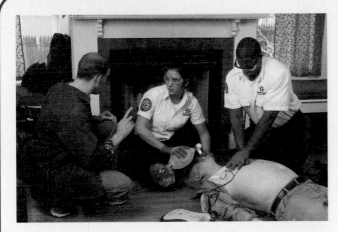

10 Gather additional information on the arrest events.

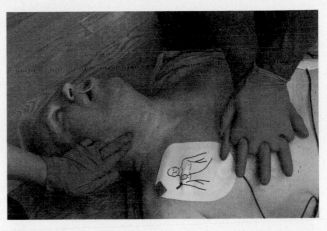

11 Check the patient's pulse during CPR to confirm the effectiveness of compressions.

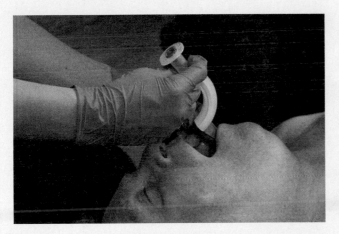

12 Direct insertion of the airway adjunct.

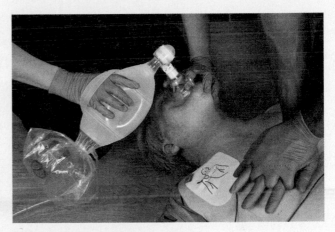

13 Direct ventilation of the patient with high-concentration oxygen.

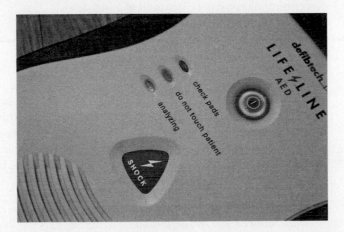

14 After 2 minutes of CPR, have all individuals stand clear and reanalyze with the AED.

(continued)

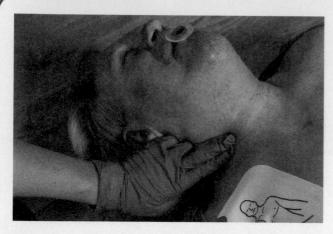

⑮ Check the patient's carotid pulse (maximum 10 seconds).

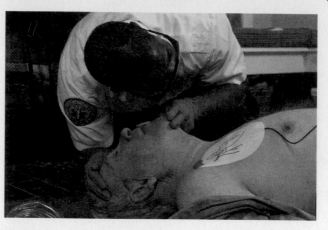

⑯ If there is a spontaneous pulse, check the patient's breathing. Note that in many cases, even when a pulse has returned, the patient will require ventilatory assistance.

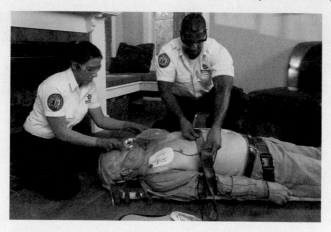

⑰ If breathing is adequate, provide high-concentration oxygen by nonrebreather mask. If breathing is inadequate, ventilate the patient with high-concentration oxygen. Transport without delay.

Researchers have evaluated whether it is better in the case of an unwitnessed arrest to start CPR first or to shock first. Although early studies suggested a brief period of CPR might increase survival, further evaluation has found that this provides little or no difference in outcomes. Some EMS systems stress CPR before defibrillation for unwitnessed arrests, whereas others have a second provider perform CPR only until an AED is available. For the sake of simplicity and ease of learning, this text follows the latter approach, though either is acceptable. Follow your local protocols.

NOTE: *As an EMT, you cannot diagnose heart ailments or causes of cardiac arrest. You must initiate CPR and defibrillation as rapidly as possible and, if defibrillation is not successful in restoring heart function, continue CPR to prevent biological death until the patient's care can be taken over at a medical facility or by those with advanced skills.*

NOTE: *The proper dose of electricity for the shock depends on the type of unit you are using. For monophasic units the dose should be 360 joules (J). The ideal dose using a biphasic defibrillator is the dose at which the device has been shown to be effective in terminating VF. Biphasic defibrillators use energy levels between 120 to 200 J, depending on the device.*

PATIENT ASSESSMENT

Cardiac Arrest

As with all calls, you should protect yourself from infectious diseases by using personal protective equipment and taking Standard Precautions. This is especially important in the case of a cardiac arrest where blood and other body fluids are commonly found. Patient assessment includes the following:

- Perform the primary assessment. If a bystander is doing CPR when you arrive, have the bystander stop. Spend no more than 10 seconds to verify pulselessness (no carotid pulse), *apnea* (no breathing) or *agonal breathing* (irregular, gasping breaths), and absence of other signs of life (e.g., movement). Look for external blood loss.

    NOTE: *In most patients you will encounter, the sequence of steps for patient assessment and treatment is A-B-C (airway, breathing, circulation). However, for patients in cardiac arrest, the sequence of treatment will actually be C-A-B (circulation/compression, airway, breathing.)*

    To determine whether a patient is a candidate for immediate CPR, you must rapidly evaluate the patient as you approach, looking for any signs of life: responsiveness or movement of the chest that might indicate the presence of breathing.

    If the patient has signs of life, you perform the head-tilt or jaw-thrust (airway) maneuver and check for respiration (breathing) and a pulse (circulation)—that is, A-B-C sequence. But if the patient appears to be lifeless (is unconscious, not moving, and not breathing, or has gasping breathing, and is pulseless), the first intervention you will perform is chest compressions followed by opening the airway and providing breathing—that is, C-A-B sequence.

    In short, you should do what is best for the patient—A-B-C or C-A-B—based on what you find in your assessment.

- Resume CPR immediately, gather a history, and perform a physical exam. Inquire about onset, trauma, and signs and symptoms that were present before the patient collapsed. Get a past medical history if you can. However, do not let history gathering interfere with or slow down defibrillation or chest compressions.

Decision Points

- Does my patient have signs of life? Should I go immediately to compressions or should I take the A-B-C approach?
- Do I have a defibrillator immediately available? How will I integrate defibrillation

apnea (AP-ne-ah)
no breathing.

agonal breathing
irregular, gasping breaths that precede apnea and death.

PATIENT CARE

Cardiac Arrest

Refer to Scan 20-4 as you read the following steps:

1. Begin or resume high-quality CPR.
2. Apply the AED in the following manner:
   - If the patient is an adult (defined by the American Heart Association as reaching puberty or older), analyze and defib if shock is indicated.
   - If the patient is a child or infant (defined as up to puberty), analyze and defib using an AED designed to provide shocks to children and infants. If such an AED is not available, apply an ordinary AED. In infants, you may need to apply one pad to the chest and the other to the back to prevent the pads from touching each other.

    NOTE: *If the patient already has an AED attached when you arrive, your actions will be slightly different. You will need to evaluate the performance of the person operating the machine. If the person is analyzing or shocking and is doing it properly, allow the person to continue until the next good time for a switch occurs, usually the next time it is appropriate to do CPR. Encourage the person as needed. If the operator is not performing adequately, however, you will need to intervene, either with corrections and encouragement if the problems are easily corrected or by taking over if the operator cannot, or does not wish to, perform the steps correctly. Patient care is your highest priority, keeping in mind that roughly interrupting a smoothly functioning operation does not benefit the patient or the layperson trying to assist.*

Inside/Outside

■ Inside

When the heart stops suddenly, oxygenated blood is present not only in the circulatory system but also in the brain and the muscles that control respiration—in particular, the intercostal muscles and the diaphragm. Since there is still some oxygen in the medulla, it is able to send occasional impulses through the nervous system to stimulate the respiratory muscles. As the patient inhales, the pressure in the thorax decreases. This encourages more blood to return to the heart. When the patient exhales, the pressure in the thorax increases. This promotes the movement of blood into the coronary arteries. Since the heart and arteries have one-way valves to push blood in one direction, it also increases blood flow to the aorta, carotid arteries, and the brain. This small amount of oxygen may actually allow the medulla to continue to send out some impulses to the respiratory muscles again, leading to a cycle in which the body attempts to resuscitate itself.

Unfortunately, this cannot go on forever. The amount of oxygen delivered to the medulla decreases with time, leading to a decrease in the number of breaths and then a downward spiral ending in death unless someone intervenes to improve perfusion (through CPR) and restart the heart's electrical rhythm (through defibrillation). The word *agonal* refers to something that occurs just before death, so these respirations are traditionally referred to as *agonal respirations*.

■ Outside

When someone suddenly goes into cardiac arrest and collapses in front of a witness, up to half the time the patient may exhibit irregular, gasping breaths (agonal respirations) that do not look normal, but can still be confusing. These are the body's attempts to prevent death, but they will last at most a few minutes, usually less. They are usually less frequent than normal respirations (even just a couple of times a minute in some cases) and more sudden and dramatic, not smooth and natural like normal breaths, although sometimes they are very brief and weak. Patients who exhibit agonal respirations have a high probability of survival when resuscitative measures (CPR, defibrillation) are provided, probably because agonal respirations are more often associated with shockable rhythms. In addition, they are an indication of the presence of oxygen in key areas like the heart and brain.

When you encounter a patient who exhibits agonal respirations, you should not let these respirations confuse you into thinking that the patient is breathing and therefore does not require CPR and defibrillation. If you don't feel a pulse (or you are not sure you feel a pulse), perform chest compressions. It is these patients, who have just gone into cardiac arrest, that have the greatest chance of survival with immediate high-quality chest compressions and rapid defibrillation.

An even more confusing situation may occur during your resuscitation efforts. You may be compressing the chest when the patient suddenly takes a spontaneous, gasping breath. If this happens, check the patient. Unless you are sure you feel a pulse, resume compressions. Take this as a good sign, however: You are providing enough oxygen to the brain, heart, and muscles for some impulses to get through to the respiratory muscles.

3. Bare the patient's chest and, if necessary, quickly shave the area where the pads will be placed if the patient has a lot of chest hair.
4. Turn on the AED.
5. Attach the monitoring/defibrillation electrode pads to the cables and then to the patient according to the instructions on the pads (upper right chest and lower left ribs). Many of these pads come already attached to the cables. It is helpful to remember "white to right and red to ribs."
6. Once the electrode pads are properly attached to the patient, advise all rescuers, "Stop CPR; we are analyzing."

   The AED will search for ventricular fibrillation and, if found, automatically charge the unit. Once fully charged, it will advise the EMT to clear the patient and deliver the shock to the patient.

   If the AED does not find a shockable ECG rhythm, it will advise the EMT that no shock is indicated and to resume CPR immediately.
7. If the AED advises to deliver a shock, the EMT should ensure no one is touching the patient and then deliver a single shock.

NOTE: *As stated earlier, about half of all patients in cardiac arrest have nonshockable heart rhythms. If this is the case, when you press the "analyze" button, the AED will give a "No shock" message. In other cases, the AED may provide a "Deliver shock" message and then, after one or more shocks are delivered, give a "No shock" message on a subsequent try. (When the AED gives a "No shock" message, it may be very bad news—the patient has a nonshockable heart rhythm and cannot be helped by the defibrillator. Or* *it may be very good news—the electrical rhythm of the patient's heart has responded successfully to earlier shocks. In the latter case, even though the heart's electrical activity has recovered, another stint of CPR may be required to get enough oxygen into the muscle cells of the heart to start it beating again.)*

8. Immediately begin CPR after delivering the shock. Sometimes a defibrillation will be immediately successful in generating the return of spontaneous circulation (ROSC), and the patient may wake right up. In most cases of a successful defibrillation, the patient may no longer be in VF but is still in cardiac arrest (most likely a period of non-perfusing rhythm) and needs CPR compressions to "keep the pump primed and circulation flowing."

9. Reassess the patient—after providing 2 minutes or 5 cycles of CPR, reassess the patient (if the patient is waking up, check the pulse; if not waking up, repeat steps 6 to 8).

If the patient wakes or begins to move, get a set of baseline vital signs, ensure high-concentration oxygen administration, and prepare to transport the patient to the most appropriate ED. If an ALS unit will be arriving shortly, consider waiting for them or otherwise try to arrange for an "intercept" somewhere between the scene and the ED. Research has shown that CPR performed while moving and/or transporting a patient is not of the best quality.

Whenever providing CPR, it is essential to remember: (1) compressions must not be interrupted for any longer than 10 seconds (e.g., reassessment, pulse checks, or placement of advanced airways), (2) compressions should be at least 2 inches deep for an adult and at least one-third the depth of the chest for infants and children (about 2 inches for children and 1/2 inch for infants) with full chest recoil, (3) the rate should be at least 100 per minute, and (4) personnel should rotate through the position of compressor to prevent rescuer fatigue.

If the patient does not have return of spontaneous circulation after three shocks or two consecutive analyses without a shock, prepare to transport the patient to the most appropriate ED.

NOTE: *If at any time you get a "No shock" message from the AED and determine that the patient has a pulse, check the patient's breathing. If breathing is adequate, provide high-concentration oxygen by nonrebreather mask and transport. If breathing is inadequate, provide artificial ventilations with high-concentration oxygen and transport.*

Special Considerations for AED Use

General Principles

The following are general principles that apply to the use of an AED:

CORE CONCEPT ●---------
Special considerations in AED use

- One EMT operates the defibrillator, while another does CPR. This prevents the EMT who is operating the defibrillator from being distracted.
- Remember that CPR must include high-quality compressions.
- Defibrillation comes first. Do not hook up oxygen or do anything that delays analysis of the rhythm or defibrillation.
- You must be familiar with the particular model of AED used in your area.
- All contact with the patient must be avoided during analysis of the rhythm.
- State "Clear!" and be sure everyone is clear of the patient before delivering every shock.
- No defibrillator is capable of working without properly functioning batteries. Check the batteries at the beginning of your shift and carry a spare.
- If you have delivered three shocks (a rare occurrence) and you have no ALS backup, prepare the patient for transport. You may deliver additional shocks at the scene or en route if local medical direction approves.
- An AED cannot analyze a rhythm accurately in a moving emergency vehicle. You must completely stop the vehicle in order to analyze the rhythm if more shocks are ordered.
- Pulse checks should not occur during rhythm analysis.

Coordination with ALS Personnel

You do not need to have an advanced life support (ALS) team at the scene in order to use an AED. However, the sooner the patient receives advanced cardiovascular life support (ACLS), the greater the patient's chance of survival. If you have an ALS team available, notify them of the arrest as soon as possible (preferably before you even arrive on scene). Your Medical Director-approved local protocols should state whether you postpone transport and wait for the ALS team at the scene or start transport and rendezvous with them. Your actions may depend on the location of the arrest and the estimated time of arrival of the ALS team.

If the ALS team arrives before you have finished the first shock, they should allow you to complete the shock. They should then institute the advanced care that they can give. The ALS team may allow you to defibrillate later, but that will be their decision. Since they are the most highly trained providers at the scene, the ALS team is responsible for the patient's overall care.

> **NOTE:** *The ALS personnel will initially focus on obtaining IV access to administer emergency medications and passing an advanced airway (e.g., ET tube, LMA, or Combitube®). Once an advanced airway has been inserted, you will be asked to switch the compressions and ventilations from cycles of 30:2 to an asynchronous procedure. When providing the compressions and ventilations in this manner, the compressor will push hard and fast with full chest recoil at a constant (i.e., with no interruptions) rate of at least 100 per minute while the ventilator provides a ventilation of 1-second duration to achieve visible chest rise at a rate of 8 to 10 per minute or every 8 seconds.*

Coordination with Others Who Defibrillate before You Arrive

Emergency Medical Responders, police officers, security officers, and others may defibrillate the patient before you arrive. If this happens, you should let the operator of the AED complete the shock before you take over care of the patient. After the shock is delivered, or a "No shock" message is received, work with the operator to bring about an orderly transfer of care.

In some areas, you may need to take the first AED to the hospital with the patient so that data can be retrieved from the machine. Your protocols should address this. They also should tell you whether or not to switch from the first AED to your own.

Post-Resuscitation Care

After you have run through the AED protocol, the patient will be in one of three conditions: (1) The patient has a pulse. In this case, you will need to keep a close eye on his airway and be aggressive in keeping it open. Keep the defibrillator on the patient during transportation in case the patient goes back into arrest. En route, assess the patient based on what he tells you is bothering him, and reassess frequently, approximately every 5 minutes. (2) If the patient has no pulse, the AED will have given you a "No shock indicated" message, or (3) the AED may be prompting you to analyze the rhythm because it "thinks" there is a shockable rhythm. In any case, you will need to resume CPR. (You will not perform further defibrillation once you have completed the initial shocks of the AED protocol unless the patient has recovered a pulse and then, later, goes back into cardiac arrest.)

Part of your post-cardiac arrest care is to ensure adequate ventilation and oxygenation, but do not hyperventilate the patient. Ventilating a patient too many times a minute has very bad effects and can significantly decrease the chance of neurologically intact survival. If your system provides therapeutic hypothermia after cardiac arrest, start the procedure or call for personnel who can.

For all of these patients, you will need to use the techniques of lifting and moving that you learned in Chapter 3, "Lifting and Moving Patients." You will also need to consider how and where to meet ALS personnel (if available).

Patients Who Go Back into Cardiac Arrest

A patient who has been resuscitated from cardiac arrest is at high risk of going back into arrest. This change may be difficult to detect since most patients who have just been resuscitated are unconscious and many of them will need assisted ventilation. Since you are breathing for the patient, you may not notice that he no longer has a pulse. This is why, on unconscious patients who have recovered a pulse, you should check the pulse frequently (approximately every 30 seconds). The AED may alert you that it "thinks" the patient has a shockable rhythm. If you get such a prompt from the defibrillator, check for a pulse immediately. If you find that there is no pulse, follow these steps:

1. If you are en route, stop the vehicle.
2. Have someone else start CPR, if the AED is not immediately ready.
3. Analyze the rhythm.
4. Deliver a shock if indicated.
5. Continue with two shocks separated by 2 minutes (5 cycles) of CPR or as your local protocol directs.

Witnessed Arrests in the Ambulance

Occasionally, you will be transporting a conscious patient with chest pain who becomes unconscious, pulseless, and apneic (not breathing). Although there are no guarantees, you have a very good chance of getting this patient back because you can defibrillate very shortly after the patient goes into a shockable rhythm. If this happens, stop the vehicle and treat him like any other patient in cardiac arrest.

Single Rescuer with an AED

Some EMTs will be alone or have no one else nearby who can do CPR when they reach the patient. If this happens, the sequence of steps to take changes slightly. If no one else is available to perform CPR, apply the AED and defibrillate immediately. Once you have delivered a shock or received a "No shock indicated" message from the device, begin chest compressions and then ventilations. After about 2 minutes of CPR, check the rhythm again and shock as needed. Resume CPR for another 2 minutes and check the rhythm one more time. If you are still alone, continue in this fashion as your protocol directs until advanced help or transport arrives.

Contraindications

The only contraindication to using a defibrillator is if the pads won't fit on the patient without touching each other. There are patients for whom defibrillation will not be the best or only remedy, however. An example is trauma. If a patient has a serious traumatic injury and is in cardiac arrest (unless the arrest preceded the trauma), this is most likely caused by severe blood loss or damage to one or more vital organs. Even if the patient were defibrillated, chances of success are unlikely. Also, you should spend as little time as possible at the scene of a serious traumatic injury because the patient requires immediate transport to a facility where surgery can be performed.

Another case where defibrillation may not always be effective is hypothermia (very low body temperature). Patients who are severely hypothermic are usually warmed in a controlled setting before defibrillation is performed. Some systems recommend shocks in the event of cardiac arrest. If this does not work, the patient should be transported immediately.

PEDIATRIC NOTE

Unlike adults, infants have healthy hearts and go into shockable rhythms less often. Cardiac arrest in infants is more often caused by respiratory problems like foreign body airway obstruction or drowning. For this reason, aggressive airway management and artificial ventilation with chest compressions are the best way to resuscitate these patients.

AEDs are now on the market that can be adapted to pediatric use in infants and children through reducing the energy delivered and attaching smaller pads designed for their chests (smaller pads and smaller shocks). If your service has such an AED, you should follow the protocol for its use.

If an adult-sized AED is the only one available and the pads fit on the patient's chest without touching each other, it is better to use the adult AED on the child or infant than to continue CPR without using it.

NOTE: *When you defibrillate a patient, you are delivering electrical current through the patient's chest. That current can be carried or conducted to you under certain conditions. Although it is unlikely to put you into cardiac arrest, this electricity can harm you. You*

FIGURE 20-7 Be alert to safety hazards when using an AED. Do not defibrillate a patient who is wet or in contact with metal. Before defibrillation, remove a nitroglycerin patch if it is on the patient's chest. Do not defibrillate until everyone is clear of the patient.

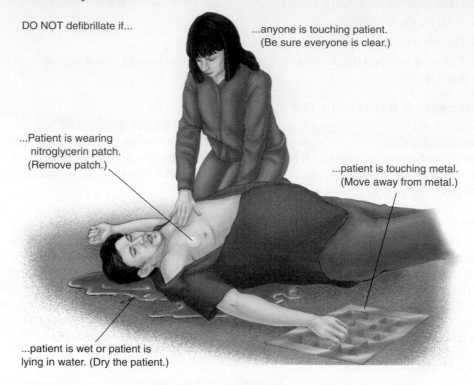

DO NOT defibrillate if...

...anyone is touching patient. (Be sure everyone is clear.)

...Patient is wearing nitroglycerin patch. (Remove patch.)

...patient is touching metal. (Move away from metal.)

...patient is wet or patient is lying in water. (Dry the patient.)

can prevent this and other potentially harmful effects from occurring by following a few basic principles (Figure 20-7).

Do not defibrillate a soaking-wet patient. Water is a very good conductor of electricity, so either dry the patient's chest or move him out of the wet environment (bring him inside, away from the rain, for example).

Do not defibrillate the patient if he is touching anything metallic that other people are touching. Metal is also a very good conductor of electricity. This means that you must be careful if the patient is on a metal floor or deck, and you must make sure no one is touching the stretcher when you deliver a shock. It is also a good idea to make sure no one is touching anything, including a bag-valve mask, that is in contact with the patient.

If you see a nitroglycerin patch on the patient's chest, remove it carefully before defibrillating. The plastic in the patch (not the nitroglycerin) may explode from the rapid melting that a defibrillatory shock can cause. This problem has been reported only when the patch is on the chest. Be sure to wear gloves when you remove the patch, as it is designed to release nitroglycerin through the skin, and it will not discriminate between the patient's skin and yours. One thing you don't need at a cardiac arrest is a headache from nitroglycerin.

Be absolutely sure that before every shock you say "Clear!" and look from the patient's head to his toes to ensure no one is touching the patient or any conductive material that the patient is touching.

Ask your instructor or refer to your local protocols for guidelines for defibrillating patients who have experienced trauma or are severely hypothermic. As new technology and information become available, your EMS system will keep you advised of these updates and may alter future protocols for AED use.

Advantages of Automated External Defibrillation

Until 30 years ago, it was unthinkable for EMTs to defibrillate patients in cardiac arrest. Now, EMTs are expected to be trained and equipped to perform this potentially lifesaving intervention. The biggest reason this situation has changed is the improvement in technology that allows defibrillators to quickly and accurately determine whether a patient's rhythm is shockable,

This means that initial training and continuing education are much easier and simpler than that required for manual defibrillation in which the operator has to be able to read and analyze the heart rhythms that the AED does automatically. This is especially true in areas where EMTs see few cardiac arrests, such as in rural areas. Automated defibrillation is actually easier to learn and remember than CPR. However, this does not mean that EMTs are "well programmed robots." You still must carefully perform a primary assessment to ensure that the patient is in cardiac arrest, you must memorize the treatment sequence, and you must always act with the safety of the patient and others in mind.

Automation also requires that the operator defibrillate through adhesive pads instead of paddles. This is safer and allows for more accurate and consistent electrode placement. Since the operator does not have to hold paddles on the patient's chest, there is almost no chance of "arcing," the passage of electrical current outside the chest from too little paddle pressure. Certainly, the EMT's level of anxiety is lower when he can push a button to deliver a shock instead of holding charged paddles on a patient's chest.

Some AEDs may allow for monitoring of the rhythm of patients who are not in cardiac arrest. This can be confusing for the EMT, since he is not trained in rhythm recognition and cannot treat nonshockable rhythms. A rhythm screen can be very distracting and take attention away from the patient. If you monitor patients with chest pain or difficulty breathing, make sure that this is allowed by your Medical Director.

Implants and Surgeries

With the rapidly expanding medical technology available, the EMT may be presented with patients who have undergone surgeries or had special electronic devices implanted in the body. The ABCs, including CPR and appropriate oxygen delivery, will not change because of prior surgery or conditions. Defibrillation can be performed on such a patient, although the positioning of defibrillation pads on the patient's chest may need to be adjusted to avoid contact with an implanted device.

Some of the devices and surgeries you may observe in the field include the following:

- **Cardiac pacemaker** (Figure 20-8). When the heart's natural pacemaker does not function properly, an artificial pacemaker can be surgically implanted to perform the same function. This pacemaker helps the heart beat in a normal, coordinated fashion. It is

FIGURE 20-8 (A) An implanted pacemaker is visible in this patient's left chest. (B) A combination implanted cardioverter defibrillator/pacemaker is noticeable in this patient's left chest. *(A)(© Dept. of Clinical Radiology, Salisbury District Hospital/Science Photo Library/Photo Researchers, Inc.) (B) (© Michael F. O'Keefe)*

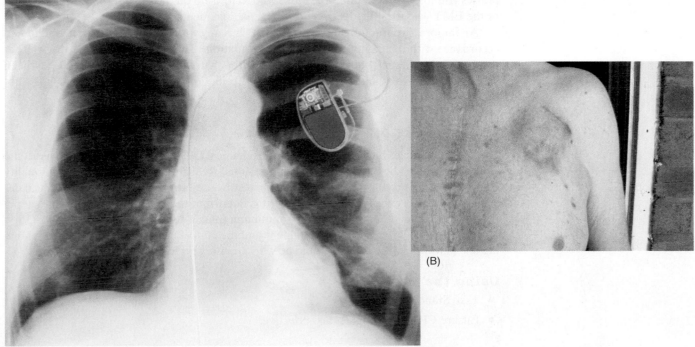

(A)

(B)

often placed below one of the clavicles, is visible as a small lump, and can be palpated. If you notice a lump under a clavicle, do not put a defibrillation pad over it. Try to put the pad at least several inches away while staying in the general area where you want the pad.

Occasionally pacemakers malfunction. Although this situation is rare, it is life threatening when it occurs. A malfunctioning pacemaker usually results in a slow or irregular pulse. The patient may have signs of shock due to the fact the heart is not beating properly. Remember that care for patients with implanted pacemakers and signs of a cardiac emergency are the same as for those without a pacemaker. You should arrange for an ALS intercept and transport the patient immediately.

- **Implanted defibrillator.** Cardiologists are sometimes able to identify patients who are at high risk of going into ventricular fibrillation. They sometimes receive a miniature defibrillator surgically implanted in the chest or abdomen. When the patient develops a lethal cardiac rhythm, the implanted defibrillator detects it and shocks the patient. Often an implanted defibrillator is actually a defibrillator and pacemaker. The number of patients receiving these devices will probably increase as it becomes easier to determine who is at risk of going into ventricular fibrillation. Since the implanted defibrillator is directly attached to the heart, low energy levels are needed for each shock. Many implanted defibrillators are also pacemaker functions. The presence of the implanted defibrillator should not pose a threat to the EMT. Emergency care, CPR, and defibrillation for this patient are the same as for other cardiac patients.

- **Cardiac bypass surgery.** The coronary artery bypass has become a relatively common procedure in cardiac surgery. A blood vessel from another part of the body is surgically implanted to bypass an occluded coronary artery. This helps restore blood flow to a section of the myocardium. Should a patient with a suspected myocardial infarction tell you that he has had bypass surgery, or if you observe a midline surgical scar on the chest of an unconscious patient, provide the same emergency care, including CPR and defibrillation, as for any other patient.

Quality Improvement

There are many ways you can evaluate and improve your ability to resuscitate patients in cardiac arrest. These methods should be part of your service's quality improvement (QI) program. The defibrillation part of your QI program involves a number of things, including medical direction, initial training, maintenance of skills, case review, trend analysis, and strengthening the links in the chain of survival. Every participant in the EMS system has a role to play in QI, whether it is the patient who comes back to thank you, the physician who praises you for a job well done, the nurse who follows up on the patient's in-hospital course, or the EMT who uses the defibrillator and then documents the call.

An important part of making sure an AED is ready when you need it is to maintain it in accordance with the manufacturer's recommendations. This includes checking the AED at the beginning of each shift. You should confirm that the battery in the AED has been charged if necessary and that monitoring–defibrillation pads are present that have not passed their expiration date.

Mechanical CPR Devices

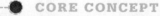
CORE CONCEPT
Use of mechanical cardiopulmonary resuscitation (CPR) devices

Some EMS agencies have chosen to utilize mechanical CPR compressor devices to assist the EMTs with providing high-quality compressions. Realizing how important high-quality compressions are to the success of cardiac arrest resuscitation and that the mechanical devices can provide excellent compressions, it is important that a system be in place to apply the device early in the arrest with only a minimum (maximum of 10 seconds) of interruption in the CPR. Two devices are the Thumper® and the Auto-Pulse™ (Figure 20-9). The following text shows how the devices would be worked into a typical cardiac arrest situation.

Using the Thumper®
- Take Standard Precautions.
- Ensure CPR is in progress and effective.

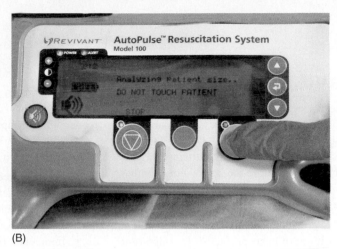

(B)

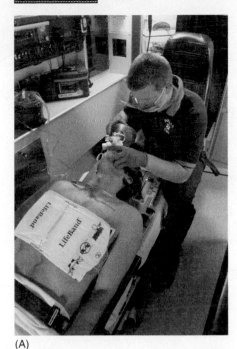

(A)

- Attach the Thumper® base plate to a long backboard.
- Stop CPR to slide the long backboard under the patient.*
- Restart CPR and attach shoulder straps to the patient.
- Slide the Thumper® piston plate into position on the base plate (away from the chest).
- Stop CPR and quickly pivot the piston arm into place, measuring anterior/posterior and middle sternum placement.*
- Slowly adjust the depth of compression to the appropriate diagram.
- Adjust ventilations.
- Turn off the compressions temporarily for pulse checks and defibrillation.*
- Upon termination of arrest or return of spontaneous circulation, power down the unit.**

NOTE: *Always limit interruptions in chest compressions to 10 seconds or less.*
    ***Always store with the compression depth turned down to the minimum setting.*

Using the Auto-Pulse™

- Take Standard Precautions.
- Ensure CPR is in progress and effective.
- Align the patient on the Auto-Pulse™ platform.*
- Close the Lifeband chest band over the patient's chest.
- Press start (Auto-Pulse™ is designed to do the compressions automatically).
- Provide bag-mask ventilation at a rate of two ventilations for every 30 compressions. Each ventilation should be given over 1 second to provide visible chest rise.
- If an advanced airway is in place (ETT, LMA, or Combitube®), there are no longer cycles of compressions to ventilations. The compression rate is a continuous 100/min., and the ventilation rate is 8 to 10/min.
- After 2 minutes of CPR, reassess for pulse and/or shockable rhythm.*

NOTE *Always limit interruptions in chest compressions to 10 seconds or less.*

Key Facts and Concepts

- Patients with acute coronary syndrome (ACS), or cardiac compromise, can have many different presentations. Some complain of pressure or pain in the chest with difficulty breathing and a history of heart problems. Others may have just mild discomfort that they ignore for several hours or that goes away and returns. Between 10 and 20 percent of patients having heart attacks have no chest discomfort at all.

- Because of the many possible presentations and the potentially severe complications of heart problems, it is important to have a high index of suspicion and treat patients with these symptoms for ACS. The treatment will not hurt them and may help them.

- Patients with suspected ACS need high-concentration oxygen and prompt, safe transportation to definitive care. You may be able to assist patients who have their own nitroglycerin in taking it, thereby relieving pain and anxiety.

- To provide excellent care and the maximum chance of survival for patients in cardiac arrest, EMS agencies must strengthen their performance of the five elements of the chain of survival:
  - Immediate recognition and activation
  - Early CPR
  - Rapid defibrillation
  - Effective advanced life support
  - Integrated post-cardiac arrest care.

Key Decisions

- Is this patient with possible acute coronary syndrome (ACS) a candidate for aspirin or nitroglycerin?
- What is the best hospital destination for this patient with possible ACS?

- What kind of cardiac arrest is this—respiratory (making airway and breathing top priorities) or cardiac (making circulation and compressions top priorities)?
- Are we providing effective CPR (i.e., compressing fast and hard, changing compressors frequently, avoiding hyperventilation, minimizing interruptions)?

Chapter Glossary

acute coronary syndrome (ACS) a blanket term used to represent any symptoms related to lack of oxygen (ischemia) in the heart muscle. Also called *cardiac compromise*.

acute myocardial infarction (AMI) (ah-KUTE MY-o-KARD-e-ul in-FARK-shun) the condition in which a portion of the myocardium dies as a result of oxygen starvation; often called a heart attack by laypersons.

agonal breathing irregular, gasping breaths that precede apnea and death.

aneurysm (AN-u-rizm) the dilation, or ballooning, of a weakened section of the wall of an artery.

angina pectoris (AN-ji-nah [or an-JI-nah] PEK-to-ris) pain in the chest, occurring when blood supply to the heart is reduced and a portion of the heart muscle is not receiving enough oxygen.

apnea (AP-ne-ah) no breathing.

asystole (ay-SIS-to-le) a condition in which the heart has ceased generating electrical impulses.

bradycardia (bray-di-KAR-de-ah) when the heart rate is slow, usually below 60 beats per minute.

cardiac compromise *see* acute coronary syndrome.

cardiopulmonary resuscitation (CPR) actions taken to revive a person by keeping the person's heart and lungs working.

cardiovascular system the heart and the blood vessels.

congestive heart failure (CHF) the failure of the heart to pump efficiently, leading to excessive blood or fluids in the lungs, the body, or both.

coronary artery disease (CAD) diseases that affect the arteries of the heart.

defibrillation delivery of an electrical shock to stop the fibrillation of heart muscles and restore a normal heart rhythm.

dyspnea (DISP-ne-ah) shortness of breath; labored or difficult breathing.

dysrhythmia (dis-RITH-me-ah) a disturbance in heart rate and rhythm.

edema (eh-DEEM-uh) swelling resulting from a buildup of fluid in the tissues.

embolism (EM-bo-lizm) blockage of a vessel by a clot or foreign material brought to the site by the blood current.

nitroglycerin (NTG) a medication that dilates the blood vessels.

occlusion (uh-KLU-zhun) blockage, as of an artery by fatty deposits.

pedal edema accumulation of fluid in the feet or ankles.

pulmonary edema accumulation of fluid in the lungs.

pulseless electrical activity (PEA) a condition in which the heart's electrical rhythm remains relatively normal, yet the mechanical pumping activity fails to follow the electrical activity, causing cardiac arrest.

sudden death a cardiac arrest that occurs within 2 hours of the onset of symptoms. The patient may have no prior symptoms of coronary artery disease.

tachycardia (tak-e-KAR-de-ah) when the heart rate is fast, above 100 beats per minute.

thrombus (THROM-bus) a clot formed of blood and plaque attached to the inner wall of an artery or vein.

ventricular fibrillation (VF) (ven-TRIK-u-ler fib-ri-LAY-shun) a condition in which the heart's electrical impulses are disorganized, preventing the heart muscle from contracting normally.

ventricular tachycardia (V-tach) (ven-TRIK-u-ler tak-i-KAR-de-uh) a condition in which the heartbeat is quite rapid; if rapid enough, ventricular tachycardia will not allow the heart's chambers to fill with enough blood between beats to produce blood flow sufficient to meet the body's needs.

Preparation for Your Examination and Practice

Short Answer

1. What position is best for a patient with:
   a. Difficulty breathing and a blood pressure of 100/70?
   b. Chest pain and a blood pressure of 180/90?

2. Describe how to "clear" a patient before administering a shock.

3. List three safety measures to keep in mind when using an AED.

4. List the steps in the application of an AED.

Thinking and Linking

Think back to Chapter 3, "Lifting and Moving Patients," and link information from that chapter with information from this chapter as you consider the following situation:

- Your patient is experiencing difficulty breathing, chest pressure, and a blood pressure of 160/100. What is the best way to transfer her down a flight of stairs?

Think back to Chapter 4, "Medical, Legal, and Ethical Issues," and link information from that chapter with information from this chapter as you consider the following situation:

- Your patient complains of crushing pain to the center of the chest, radiating to the left shoulder. His vital signs are within normal limits. He is alert. You tell him that he needs to go the hospital, but he says he doesn't want to go. You explain that he has signs and symptoms of a heart attack and that if he doesn't go to the hospital he could die. He says, "I understand that, but I'm not going to the hospital. Period." What should you do now?

Critical Thinking Exercises

The chain of survival as defined by the American Heart Association has five factors: immediate recognition and activation, early CPR, rapid defibrillation, effective advanced life support, and integrated post-cardiac arrest care. The purpose of this exercise is to apply these factors to the system where you work or live.

1. Evaluate the system you work or live in with respect to the chain of survival. Which links are strong and which need work?

2. How successful is your system in resuscitating patients from cardiac arrest?

Pathophysiology to Practice

The following questions are designed to assist you in gathering relevant clinical information and making accurate decisions in the field.

1. A 66-year-old male is complaining of excruciating central chest pain radiating to his back. His doctor said he has a "bubble" on a blood vessel in his chest. His pulse is 64 and regular, blood pressure 126/82, respirations 16 and unlabored. What medical condition is the patient most likely describing? What are the risks and benefits of administering aspirin and nitroglycerin in this situation?

2. You are treating an elderly male with congestive heart failure (CHF) who is complaining of severe difficulty breathing that has worsened over the last few nights. He takes numerous medications, but admits that he ran out of his "water pill" a few days ago. Since then, he has noticed that his weight has increased by several pounds and his belt has been getting tighter. He has also awakened short of breath and needs to sleep propped up on two pillows. How are these signs and symptoms related to the patient's CHF?

Mary Anderson is an active 70-year-old who lives by herself in an apartment. She just returned home from shopping and is sitting down eating lunch when she feels some chest discomfort that she believes is indigestion. She thinks it will go away, but it doesn't. She stops eating and goes into the living room to sit on the couch, which makes her feel out of breath. She thinks about calling her doctor but doesn't want to be a bother. Unfortunately, the discomfort is now turning into pain and she feels numbness in her left arm. So, she finally calls her doctor and asks what to do. After hearing the symptoms, her doctor calls 911 to have an ambulance take her to the hospital. Almost 2 hours have passed since Mary started having signs and symptoms.

You are having a late lunch, which you have only half finished, when a tone comes over your radio. "Ambulance 32, respond to a 70-year-old cardiac at the Maple Tree Apartments, #2-D, a third-party call from a physician's office."

When you arrive on scene, your partner says he knows a stair chair will be needed to get the patient from the second floor. He gets the stair chair, and you get the first-in bag.

Street Scene Question

1. What type of emergency equipment needs to be taken to the side of every potential cardiac patient?

You proceed to the patient's apartment. As you enter, you notice the patient sitting on the couch looking pale and anxious. You ask her why EMS was called. She responds by telling you about her discomfort and her trouble breathing. She also mentions that the pain has become worse. You ask the patient on a scale of 1 to 10 (with 10 being the worst pain she can imagine) what the pain was initially and what it is now. She answers, "3 in the beginning, but now it is 8." Your partner comes through the door with the AED and you give him a quick overview. You both agree that the

ALS unit needs to be requested. You radio the dispatcher, who gives you an ETA of 5 minutes.

Street Scene Questions

2. What are the treatment priorities for this patient?
3. What assessment information do you need to obtain next?

Your partner gets a set of vital signs, and you place the patient on a nonrebreather mask at 15 liters per minute. You get a history, with the most significant additional information being high blood pressure, for which she takes medication and has been compliant. Your partner has just finished taking vital signs when the patient gasps and appears to go unconscious.

Street Scene Question

4. What should you do next?

The patient is found to be unresponsive and without a pulse. As your partner applies the defib pads, you turn on the AED and hit the "analyze" button. The AED indicates the need to shock. You and your partner stand clear. The AED discharges. After 2 minutes of CPR, you check the pulse and find it to be slow. You check respirations and continue assisting ventilations. As you start to check the blood pressure, the EMT-Paramedic arrives.

The paramedic starts an intravenous line and administers medication. The patient starts to breathe on her own. You prepare for transport and 20 minutes later you arrive in the emergency department with a conscious patient. A few weeks later you learn from your agency's quality improvement coordinator that Mrs. Anderson has recovered fully and is expected to return to an active lifestyle.

Some of the material in this chapter on defibrillation and the AED has been adapted from material written by Kenneth R. Stults, M.S., former Director of the University of Iowa Hospitals and Clinics, Emergency Medical Services Learning Resources Center.

Diabetic Emergencies and Altered Mental Status

STANDARD
Medicine (Endocrine Disorders; Neurology)

COMPETENCY
Applies fundamental knowledge to provide basic emergency care and transportation based on assessment findings for an acutely ill patient.

CORE CONCEPTS
— General approaches to assessing the patient with an altered mental status

— Understanding the causes, assessment, and care of diabetes and various diabetic emergencies

— Understanding the causes, assessment, and care of seizure disorders

— Understanding the causes, assessment, and care of stroke

— Understanding the causes, assessment, and care of dizziness and syncope

EXPLORE Resource Central

To access Resource Central, follow directions on the Student Access Card provided with this text. If there is no card, go to **www.bradybooks.com** and follow the Resource Central link to Buy Access from there. Under Media Resources, you will find:

▶ **Capturing Manifest Destiny**
See 19th-century photographer Timothy O'Sullivan's iconic images of the American West.

▶ **Abraham Lincoln, True Crime Writer**
Read President Lincoln's strange-but-true tale of a presumed murder.

▶ **Engineers of the Forest**
Discover the workaholic beaver's essential role in shaping its environment.

OBJECTIVES

After reading this chapter you should be able to:

21.1 Define key terms introduced in this chapter.

21.2 Consider several possible causes of altered mental status when given scenarios involving patients with alterations in mental status. (p. 506)

21.3 Describe the basic physiological requirements for maintaining consciousness. (p. 506)

21.4 Perform primary and secondary assessments on patients with altered mental status. (p. 507)

21.5 Describe the pathophysiology of diabetes and diabetic emergencies. (pp. 507–511)

21.6 Determine a patient's blood glucose level using a blood glucose meter, as allowed by local protocol. (pp. 511–513)

21.7 Develop a plan to manage patients with diabetic emergencies involving hyperglycemia and hypoglycemia. (pp. 513–516)

21.8 Recognize the signs, symptoms, and history consistent with other causes of altered mental status, including seizures, stroke, dizziness, and syncope. (pp. 516–527)

(continued)

21.9 Given a variety of scenarios involving patients with seizures, search for potential underlying causes. (pp. 516–518)

21.10 Develop a plan to assess and manage patients who are having or who have just had a seizure. (pp. 518–520)

21.11 Explain the causes of strokes. (p. 520)

21.12 Develop a plan to assess and manage patients who are exhibiting signs and symptoms of a stroke. (pp. 521–524)

21.13 Given a scenario of a patient complaining of dizziness or syncope, search for potential underlying causes. (pp. 524–526)

21.14 Develop a plan to assess and manage patients with complaints of dizziness and syncope. (pp. 526–527)

KEY TERMS

aura, *p. 516*
diabetes mellitus, *p. 508*
diabetic ketoacidosis (DKA), *p. 509*
epilepsy, *p. 518*

generalized seizure, *p. 516*
glucose, *p. 507*
hyperglycemia, *p. 509*
hypoglycemia, *p. 508*
insulin, *p. 508*

partial seizure, *p. 516*
postictal phase, *p. 516*
reticular activating system (RAS), *p. 506*
seizure, *p. 516*

status epilepticus, *p. 519*
stroke, *p. 520*
syncope, *p. 524*
tonic-clonic seizure, *p. 516*

Altered mental status is a term used to describe a broad spectrum of abnormal behavior that ranges from unconsciousness to slight anxiety. These changes often result from a lack of oxygen; a brain-related problem, like a seizure; a stroke; or other serious medical issues such as a diabetic emergency. As an EMT, you should always consider altered mental status to be a serious finding and a potential concern. Although sometimes it may be a normal state for the patient, altered mental status can be the most important sign of a life-threatening condition. Use a thorough patient assessment to rapidly identify and treat life threats and use a good secondary assessment to help determine the cause of the unusual behavior. Remember, treating life threats is always more important than finding the overall cause of altered mental status.

>>>>>>

PATHOPHYSIOLOGY

reticular (ruh-TIK-yuh-ler)
activating system (RAS)
series of neurologic circuits in the brain that control the functions of staying awake, paying attention, and sleeping.

Normal consciousness is regulated by a series of neurologic circuits in the brain that comprise the *reticular activating system (RAS)*. The RAS is essentially responsible for the functions of staying awake, paying attention, and sleeping.

The brain tissue of the RAS has simple requirements to function properly and, thereby, keep a person alert and oriented. Oxygen is needed to perfuse brain tissue, glucose is needed to nourish brain tissue, and water is needed to keep brain tissue hydrated. A lack of any of these can lead to rapid and serious alterations of function and result in altered mental status. In addition to deficiencies in any of these basic needs, other causes such as trauma, infection, and chemical toxins (as in overdoses and substance abuse) can also harm brain tissue.

Altered mental status can result from a primary brain problem, like a stroke; but it may also be a symptom of a problem within another system, like hypoxia due to an asthma attack. Often, altered mental status is rapidly correctable by treating the underlying cause.

ASSESSING THE PATIENT WITH ALTERED MENTAL STATUS

Later in the chapter we will discuss the assessment of specific disorders that may lead to altered mental status. However, there are some general approaches to assessing the altered mental status patient that are important regardless of the cause.

CORE CONCEPT

General approaches to assessing the patient with an altered mental status

Safety

A patient with altered mental status often can be dangerous to responders. Always consider the safety of yourself and your team prior to approaching a patient who is not acting appropriately. Use law enforcement when necessary.

Primary Assessment

One of the most common causes of altered mental status is hypoxia. Even simple anxiety and combativeness may be the result of a failing respiratory system. Always consider the possibility of an airway and/or breathing problem in a patient with altered mental status. Although you should complete a thorough primary assessment on every patient, be especially attentive in the event of altered mental status.

Remember that the purpose of the primary assessment is to identify and treat life-threatening problems as found. You will begin oxygen to the patient with an altered mental status during the primary assessment (or ensure that another is doing so). Be alert to the need for positioning and suction if the patient requires it or if the patient's mental status worsens.

"Altered mental status cases are the detective cases of EMS."

Secondary Assessment

Often, altered mental status is a subtle sign. Although you may rule out immediate life threats, even a slightly altered mental status indicates serious underlying issues. Any patient exhibiting new, unusual behavior must be examined thoroughly. A body systems exam and complete history may reveal important information about the suspected cause of the altered mental status. Based on this exam you may find that field treatments are available, including administering glucose in the case of a hypoglycemia or prompt transport to an appropriate facility for stroke. Consider interviewing family members and bystanders who may be able to tell you if the patient's behavior and mental condition are or are not normal for him and provide information the patient may not be able to give you himself. Review the patient's medicines to point to relevant medical history, and look for clues such as medic alert bracelets and other health-related items at the scene.

PEDIATRIC NOTE

Young children may not be able to answer questions in the same manner as adults, and therefore their mental status is often difficult to establish. In these cases, use parents or caregivers to identify their baseline level of consciousness by asking, "Are they acting differently than normal?" Most often parents are the best judge of their child's current mental status.

DIABETES

Glucose and insulin are key elements in human physiology. The condition known as diabetes mellitus occurs as a result of an alteration in either of these substances or in the interaction between them.

CORE CONCEPT

Understanding the causes, assessment, and care of diabetes and various diabetic emergencies

Glucose and the Digestive System

Glucose, a form of sugar, is the body's basic source of energy. The cells of the body require glucose to remain alive and create energy. We take sugars into our body from the foods we eat, either sugar itself or other carbohydrates that the body's digestive system will convert to

glucose (GLU-kos)
a form of sugar, the body's basic source of energy.

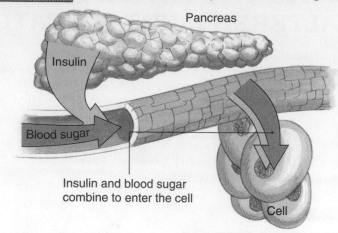

FIGURE 21-1 Insulin is needed to help the cells take in glucose.

Pancreas

Insulin

Blood sugar

Insulin and blood sugar
combine to enter the cell

Cell

glucose. After the digestive system converts sugar and other carbohydrates into glucose, the glucose is absorbed into the bloodstream. The glucose molecule is large and will not pass into the cell without the assistance of insulin (described next). The pancreas secretes insulin when the blood glucose rises above about 90 mg/dL. Insulin binds to receptor sites on cells—especially those in the liver and muscles—and allows the large glucose molecule to pass into the cells.

Patients who are diabetic (1) don't produce insulin, (2) don't produce enough insulin, or (3) have a body that has become resistant to the insulin that is produced. Medications taken by diabetics are designed to overcome these conditions.

Insulin and the Pancreas

The pancreas is an organ found along the midline of the upper abdomen. The pancreas has a variety of functions, but one of its most important roles is the production of the hormone *insulin*. Within the pancreas, specialized clusters of cells called the islets of Langerhans secrete insulin. Insulin secreted by the pancreas is then used by the body to help transfer glucose from the blood across cell membranes into the cells. The insulin-glucose relationship has been described as a "lock and key" mechanism. Consider insulin the key. Without the insulin "key," glucose cannot enter the locked cells (Figure 21-1). When sugar intake and insulin production are balanced, the body can effectively use sugar as an energy source.

Diabetes Mellitus

About 16 million Americans, or roughly 1 in 17 people, have a condition called *diabetes mellitus*. Generally speaking, this condition results either from an underproduction of insulin by the pancreas or from an inability of the body's cells to use insulin properly.

There are two types of diabetes, type 1 and type 2. *Type 1 diabetes* (formerly known as insulin-dependent diabetes) occurs when pancreatic cells fail to function properly and insulin is not secreted normally. A type 1 diabetic simply does not have enough insulin in his system to transfer circulating glucose into the cells. If left untreated, glucose levels will build up in the blood while the cells of the body starve for sugar—too much glucose in the blood, not enough in the cells. A type 1 diabetic typically would be prescribed synthetic insulin to supplement his inadequate naturally occurring insulin.

Type 2 diabetes (formerly known as non-insulin-dependent diabetes) occurs when the body's cells fail to utilize insulin properly. The pancreas may be secreting enough insulin, but the body is unable to use it to move glucose out of the blood and into the cells. Patients with type 2 diabetes can often control their condition with diet and/or oral antidiabetic medications.

Diabetic Emergencies

The most common medical emergency for the diabetic is *hypoglycemia*, or low blood sugar. (*Hypo* means "less than normal" or "deficient." *Glyc* means "sugar.") Hypoglycemia is caused when the diabetic does any one of the following:

insulin (IN-suh-lin)
a hormone produced by the pancreas or taken as a medication by many diabetics.

diabetes mellitus
(di-ah-BEE-tez MEL-i-tus)
also called "sugar diabetes" or just "diabetes," the condition brought about by decreased insulin production or the inability of the body cells to use insulin properly. The person with this condition is a diabetic.

hypoglycemia
(HI-po-gli-SEE-me-ah)
low blood sugar.

- Takes too much insulin (or, less commonly, takes too much of an oral medication used to treat diabetes), thereby transferring glucose into the cells too quickly and causing a rapid depletion of available sugar
- Reduces sugar intake by not eating
- Overexercises or overexerts himself, thus using sugars faster than normal
- Vomits a meal, emptying the stomach of sugar as well as other food

When blood sugar is thus reduced, brain cells, as well as other cells of the body, starve. Even when the cause is too much insulin, the rapid uptake of sugar into the cells soon depletes the available supply in the bloodstream. Altered mental status, possibly unconsciousness, and even permanent brain damage can occur quickly if the sugar is not replenished.

The brain and body do not tolerate low levels of sugar. Because of this fact, hypoglycemia typically has a very rapid onset. Abnormal behavior that often mimics a drunken stupor is very common. Other signs of hypoglycemia include pale, sweaty skin; tachycardia; and even seizures. Quick replenishment of blood sugar, often in the form of oral glucose, is critical to this patient's outcome. When it can be given without threatening the patient's airway, oral glucose should be administered promptly, before the patient becomes unconscious.

Hyperglycemia is high blood sugar. (*Hyper* means "more than normal" or "excessive." *Glyc* means "sugar.") Hyperglycemia is usually caused by a decrease in insulin, which leaves sugar in the bloodstream rather than helping it to enter the cells. The insulin deficiency may be due to the body's inability to produce insulin or may exist because insulin injections were forgotten or not given in sufficient quantity. Infection, stress, or increasing dietary intake can also be a factor in hyperglycemia.

Hyperglycemia typically develops over days and even weeks—in contrast to the typically rapid onset of hypoglycemia. Glucose levels in the blood creep up while the cells of the body begin to starve for sugar. As blood sugar levels increase, the patient may complain of chronic thirst and hunger. In an attempt to rid the blood of excess sugar, the body will increase urination. Nausea is also a frequent complaint.

Extremely high levels of sugar in the blood begin to draw water away from the body's cells, potentially resulting in profound dehydration. Starving body cells begin to burn fats and proteins in a manner that results in excessive waste products being released into the system. These waste products build up and combine with dehydration to cause a condition called *diabetic ketoacidosis (DKA)*.

A person who has diabetic ketoacidosis will commonly have a profoundly altered mental status. He will also have the signs and symptoms of shock, caused by dehydration. A waste product of diabetic ketoacidosis is ketones. A person having this complication will breathe rapidly and often emit a fruity, acetone odor on his breath as the body works to breathe off these byproducts.

Remember that it is not part of the scope of practice for an EMT to determine exactly which condition has caused a diabetic emergency. However, a later section of this chapter, "Hypoglycemia and Hyperglycemia Compared," provides more information on these conditions.

hyperglycemia
(HI-per-gli-SEE-me-ah)
high blood sugar.

diabetic ketoacidosis
(di-ah BET-ic KEY-to-as-id-DO-sis) **(DKA)**
a condition that occurs as the result of high blood sugar (hyperglycemia), characterized by dehydration, altered mental status, and shock.

Inside/Outside

HYPOGLYCEMIA

Inside the body of a hypoglycemic patient, the cells are starving for sugar (even if the cause was too much insulin). Brain cells, and particularly the cells of the reticular activating system, are at a loss for glucose and, therefore, energy. As the body attempts to compensate, the fight-or-flight mechanism of the autonomic nervous system engages. Blood vessels constrict, the heart pumps faster and harder, and breathing accelerates.

Outside of the body we see these changes in the form of signs and symptoms. Starving brain cells result in altered mental status. Confusion, stupor, unconsciousness, and seizures are common. Constricted blood vessels give the patient pale and sweaty skin. The fight-or-flight response increases the pulse rate and the respiratory rate.

Inside/Outside

HYPERGLYCEMIA

In a hyperglycemic patient's body, particularly if he has progressed to diabetic ketoacidosis, major changes are occurring. As sugar levels in the blood skyrocket, water is pulled away from cells, causing a systemic dehydration and potentially hypovolemic shock. Brain cells are damaged as a result. In a last resort measure, cells begin to breakdown fats and proteins, giving off ketones and other waste products.

Outside the body, we see a profound mental status change resulting from dehydration of brain cells. The overall dehydration results in the signs and symptoms of shock, including tachycardia, rapid respirations, and dropping blood pressure. The production of ketones can result in a fruity smell, similar to nail polish remover, on the breath.

PATIENT ASSESSMENT

Diabetic Emergencies

Prehospital treatment of the diabetic depends on rapid identification of the patient with an altered mental status and a history of diabetes (see Scan 21-1). To assess the patient:

1. Ensure a safe scene. People with diabetic emergencies can be agitated and sometimes violent. Always ensure the safety of yourself and your crew before approaching a patient with altered mental status.
2. Perform a primary assessment. Identify altered mental status.
3. Perform a secondary assessment. Gather the history from the patient or bystanders:
   - Gather a history of the present episode. Ask about how the episode occurred, time of onset, duration, associated symptoms, any mechanism of injury or other evidence of trauma, whether there have been any interruptions to the episode, seizures, or a fever.
   - During the SAMPLE history, determine if the patient has a history of diabetes. Question the patient or bystanders about such a history. Look for a medical identification bracelet, wallet card, or other identification of a diabetic condition such as a home-use blood glucose meter. Look in the refrigerator or elsewhere at the scene for medications such as insulin, a medication with a trade name for insulin (such as Humulin), or an oral medication used to treat diabetes (such as metformin, Glucotrol, Glucophage, Micronase) (Figure 21-2). Some diabetic patients use an implanted insulin pump. These small pumps are about the size of an MP3 player and are usually found worn on the belt. The pump will have small catheters that enter

FIGURE 21-2 Look for indications that the patient may have a history of diabetes.

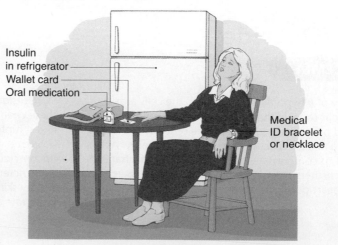

Insulin in refrigerator
Wallet card
Oral medication
Medical ID bracelet or necklace

into the abdomen (Figure 21-3). Also ask about the patient's last meal, last medication dose, and any related illnesses.

- Perform blood glucose monitoring if local protocols permit you to do so. (See the information in the next section.)

4. Determine if the patient is alert enough to be able to swallow.
5. Take baseline vital signs. (In some jurisdictions, oral glucose will be administered before the vital signs are taken.)

The following signs and symptoms are associated with a diabetic emergency:

- Rapid onset of altered mental status:
  - After missing a meal on a day the patient took prescribed insulin
  - After vomiting a meal on a day the patient took prescribed insulin
  - After an unusual amount of physical exercise or work
  - May occur with no identifiable predisposing factor
- Intoxicated appearance, staggering, slurred speech, to unconsciousness
- Cold, clammy skin
- Elevated heart rate
- Hunger
- Uncharacteristic behavior
- Anxiety
- Combativeness
- Seizures

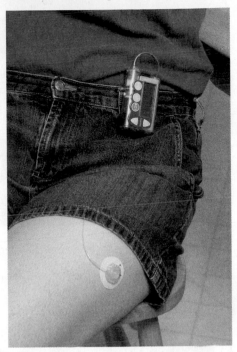

FIGURE 21-3 Some diabetics use an implanted insulin pump.

Decision Point

Is My Patient Hypoglycemic?

This is important because there is an effective field treatment for the patient who is hypoglycemic and able to safely ingest oral glucose.

PEDIATRIC NOTE

Diabetic children are more at risk for medical emergencies than diabetic adults. Children are more active and may exhaust blood sugar levels by playing hard—especially if they have taken their prescribed insulin. Children are also less likely to be disciplined about eating correctly and on time. As a consequence, children are more at risk of hypoglycemia.

Blood Glucose Meters

One of the many advances in managing diabetes has been the development of portable, reliable blood glucose meters (Figure 21-4). People with diabetes now routinely test the level of glucose in their blood at least once a day, and sometimes as often as five or six times a day. By

FIGURE 21-4 Many diabetics use home glucose meters to test their blood glucose levels.

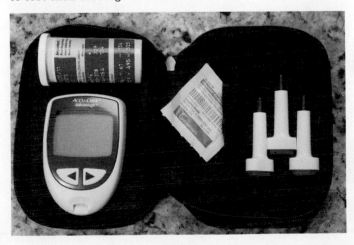

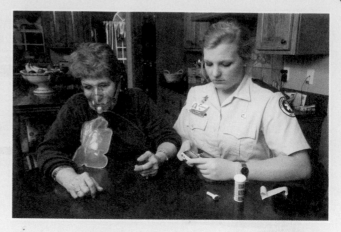

1 Perform a primary assessment. Determine if the patient's mental status is altered.

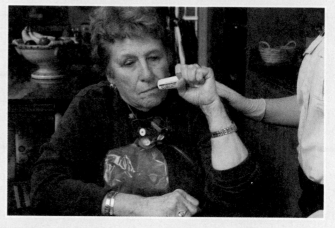

2 Perform a secondary assessment and take the patient's vital signs. Be sure to find out if she has a history of diabetes. Observe for a medical identification device. If your protocols allow, check the patient's blood glucose level (see Chapter 12, "Vital Signs and Monitoring Devices").

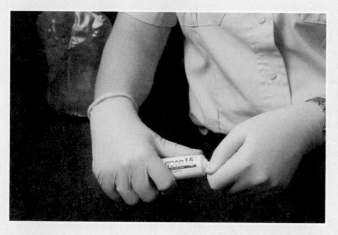

3 If the patient has a history of diabetes, has an altered mental status, and is alert enough to swallow, prepare to administer oral glucose.

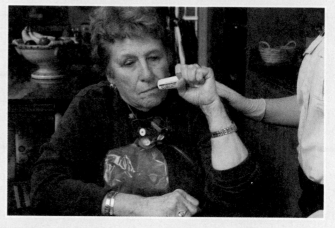

4 Assist the patient in accepting oral glucose.

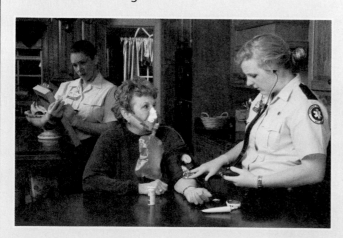

5 Reassess the patient.

determining the amount of glucose in their blood, they can determine very precisely how much insulin they should take and how much and how often they should eat. Keeping blood glucose levels as close to normal as possible leads to significantly fewer diabetes-related complications (heart disease, blindness, and kidney failure, to name a few), so a person with diabetes has a strong motivation to keep his blood glucose level within the normal range. Chapter 12, "Vital Signs and Monitoring Devices" discussed blood glucose meters and the steps for their use.

NOTE: *EMTs must have permission from medical direction or by local protocol to perform blood glucose monitoring using a blood glucose meter.*

If the patient has a glucose meter, the patient or a family member can use it to determine the patient's blood glucose level. Generally, EMTs should not use a patient's glucose meter. There are many different types of these devices on the market, each with its own instructions for use, which may be very different from device to device. Additionally, there is no way for the EMT to know whether the test strips have been stored properly or when the device was last calibrated. These facts are very important if the reading is to be accurate.

A value less than 60 to 80 mg/dL (milligrams per deciliter) in a symptomatic diabetic (i.e., a patient with a mild alteration in mental status or who is diaphoretic (sweaty)) is typical of hypoglycemia and indicates the need for prompt administration of glucose. Patients with values less than 50 mg/dL will typically have significant alterations in mental status that may include complete unresponsiveness. Patients with a blood glucose level that is this low will often be unable to safely receive oral glucose. A reading over 140 (depending on the manufacturer's instructions) indicates hyperglycemia. Patients with glucose levels in the mid and high 100s are often without acute symptoms, although over time this level of hyperglycemia can cause damage to various body organs. Patients with blood glucose levels over 200–300, especially for a prolonged time, may experience dehydration and other more serious symptoms and should receive medical care.

A reading inconsistent with the patient's symptoms (such as 25 mg/dL in a patient who is alert and oriented) should make the EMT question the result. There are many potential causes of inaccurate results, including insufficient blood on the test strip, a strip past its expiration date or not stored properly, or a meter that needs calibration. Although many people use blood glucose meters appropriately and accurately, it is quite common to get an inaccurate reading, especially when the device is not used properly. It is critical that any health care provider using a blood glucose meter to test a patient's blood have the proper training in use of the device and be thoroughly familiar with its care and maintenance. Calibration and testing on a regularly scheduled basis are essential if the device is to give accurate results.

On occasion, the glucometer will display the word *HIGH* rather than a number. Depending on the manufacturer, a "High" or "HI" reading indicates an extremely high glucose level, usually in excess of 500 mg/dL. The word *LOW* usually indicates blood glucose levels which are extremely low (often less than 15 mg/dL).

Remember that the blood glucose monitor is just one tool used in your assessment of a patient with an altered mental status. Blood glucose monitoring, or any other examinations, should never be done before a thorough primary assessment has been performed. Some areas recommend that the blood glucose measurements be done while en route to the hospital.

PATIENT CARE

Diabetic Emergencies

Emergency care of a patient with a diabetic emergency includes the following (see Scans 21-1 and 21-2):

1. Occasionally a person with only mild hypoglycemia and minor altered mental status can be treated by simply giving him something to eat. In a person who is only slightly confused, it may be more appropriate to ask him to ingest a glass of milk or a piece of toast than a tube of oral glucose. You must understand that this course of treatment will take longer to resolve the hypoglycemia and is certainly not appropriate for a patient who has severe hyperglycemia. Always use good clinical judgment to determine if your patient needs more aggressive care.

2. Determine if all of the following criteria for administration of oral glucose are present: The patient has a history of diabetes, has an altered mental status, and is awake enough to swallow.
3. If the patient meets the criteria for administration of oral glucose and if he is able, let the patient squeeze the glucose from the tube directly into his mouth.
4. Reassess the patient. If the patient's condition does not improve after administration of oral glucose, consult medical direction about whether to administer more. If at any time the patient loses consciousness, remove the tongue depressor from his mouth and take steps to ensure an open airway.

If the patient is not awake enough to swallow, treat him like any other patient with an altered mental status. That is, secure the airway, provide artificial ventilations if necessary, and be prepared to perform CPR if needed. Position the patient appropriately. If the patient does not need to be ventilated, place him in the recovery position (on his side) so that he is less likely to choke on or to aspirate fluids or vomitus into his lungs. Request an ALS intercept if available.

Decision Point

Can I Give Oral Glucose?

The most important decision point in choosing to give oral glucose is the patient's ability to swallow. Although a severely hypoglycemic patient may desperately need sugar, if he is unable to protect his airway, the administration of oral gel may be the worst thing you can do. We only administer oral glucose to those patients we feel can swallow it and protect their airway from aspiration.

Hypoglycemia and Hyperglycemia Compared

Many students find that they confuse hypoglycemia and hyperglycemia. Fortunately, the use of reliable blood glucose monitoring in the field has made this decision much easier. It is also important to note that it is not necessary to distinguish between the two conditions in order to give the proper treatment. There are three typical differences between hypoglycemia and hyperglycemia:

- **Onset.** Hyperglycemia usually has a slower onset, whereas hypoglycemia tends to come on suddenly. This is because some sugar still reaches the brain in hyperglycemic (high blood sugar) states. With hypoglycemia (low blood sugar), it is possible that no sugar is reaching the brain. Seizures may occur.
- **Skin.** Hyperglycemic patients often have warm, red, dry skin. Hypoglycemic patients have cold, pale, moist, or "clammy" skin.
- **Breath.** The hyperglycemic patient often has acetone breath (like nail polish remover), whereas the hypoglycemic patient does not.

Also, patients who are hyperglycemic frequently breathe very deeply and rapidly, as though they have just run a race. Dry mouth, intense thirst, abdominal pain, and vomiting are all common signs and symptoms of this condition. The proper treatment is given under close medical supervision in a hospital.

POINT OF VIEW

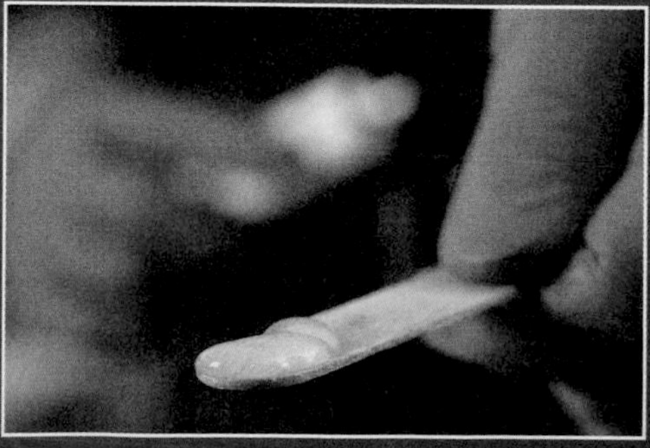

"You'd think after you've been a diabetic most of your life that the needles wouldn't bother you. Actually they've gotten better, smaller. And need less blood.

"Despite how much I try to keep my blood sugar regulated, no matter how much I see my doctor, I end up needing an ambulance a couple of times a year. It is almost embarrassing. I see the same people time after time, and they are always so nice to me.

"I remember the days before we could check my blood sugar. I'd just have to get some sugar. If it wasn't low, it would take days to get me back regulated again after all that sugar. When the EMTs came today they were right on the ball. They checked my sugar and it was the lowest I have ever seen it. They put a blob of that goop on a tongue depressor and put it in my mouth, and I was better pretty quickly.

"But I still get sick of the needles sometimes."

SCAN 21-2 Oral Glucose

MEDICATION NAME
1. Generic: Glucose, oral
2. Trade: Glutose, Insta-glucose

INDICATIONS
Patients with altered mental status and a known history of diabetes mellitus

CONTRAINDICATIONS
1. Unconsciousness
2. Known diabetic who has not taken insulin for days
3. Unable to swallow

MEDICATION FORM
Gel, in toothpaste-type tubes

DOSAGE
One tube

ADMINISTRATION
1. Ensure signs and symptoms of altered mental status with a known history of diabetes.
2. Ensure patient is conscious.
3. Administer glucose.
   a. Place on tongue depressor between cheek and gum, or
   b. Have patient self-administer between cheek and gum.
4. Perform reassessment.

ACTIONS
Increases blood sugar

SIDE EFFECTS
None when given properly. May be aspirated by the patient without a gag reflex.

REASSESSMENT STRATEGIES
If patient loses consciousness or seizes, remove tongue depressor from mouth.

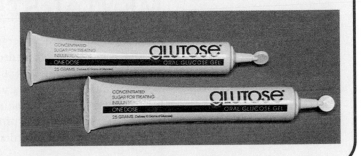

CRITICAL DECISION MAKING

The Taste of Sweet Success

For each of the following patients, determine if the general criteria are met for you to administer glucose to the patient. Oral glucose is carried on your ambulance. For the purposes of this exercise, assume that your blood glucose monitor isn't available. (It is sometimes important to make decisions independent of devices.)

1. Your patient is confused. She doesn't know what day it is and is talking but not making any sense. Her nurse's aide tells you the patient is diabetic and has been having trouble with managing her blood sugar levels. She will occasionally take insulin but not eat and vice versa.

2. At a facility for disabled youth, a 19-year-old man recovering from a head injury was seizing prior to your arrival, but the seizure has stopped. He responds to loud verbal stimulus. He has a history of diabetes.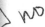

3. You respond to a motor-vehicle collision and find one patient sitting behind the wheel of his car, rocking back and forth, muttering incoherently. The accident was low-speed with a very minor impact. You observe a medical identification bracelet that indicates the patient is diabetic.

There appear to be clear-cut differences between the signs and symptoms of hyperglycemia and hypoglycemia, but distinguishing between them in the field can be difficult and is not necessary. If your system allows the use of blood glucose monitoring, it may provide the patient's actual blood glucose level. This can be used to identify someone with hypo- or hyperglycemia. Remember that this is just one tool in your assessment which, when combined with the patient's history (e.g., food intake and medications taken) and your protocols, will aid in your decision-making process. Always consult medical direction if questions or concerns arise.

Giving glucose will help the hypoglycemic patient by getting needed sugar into his bloodstream and to the brain. Although the hyperglycemic patient already has too much sugar in his blood, the extra dose of glucose will not have time to cause damage in the short time before he reaches the hospital and can be diagnosed and treated. This is why "sugar (glucose) for everyone" is the rule of thumb for diabetic emergencies, whether the patient is hypo- or hyperglycemic, and why you do not need to distinguish between the two conditions.

NOTE: *Some hyperglycemic and hypoglycemic patients will appear to be intoxicated. Always suspect a diabetic problem in cases that seem to involve no more than intoxication. Remember that the patient intoxicated on alcohol may also be a diabetic, with the alcohol breath covering the acetone odor of diabetic ketoacidosis. The alcoholic diabetic is a good candidate for a diabetic emergency, because he tends to neglect eating and taking insulin during prolonged drinking.*

OTHER CAUSES OF ALTERED MENTAL STATUS

In addition to diabetic emergencies, there are many other causes of altered mental status. Examples include hypoxia; drug and alcohol use; brain injuries, both traumatic and medical; metabolic abnormalities; brain tumors; and infectious diseases such as meningitis. In all cases, use a thorough primary assessment to identify immediate life threats. Gather a careful history; then calm the patient and transport him to the hospital.

The following sections provide additional information on three other causes of altered mental status: seizure disorders, stroke, and dizziness or syncope.

Seizure Disorders

● **CORE CONCEPT**
Understanding the causes, assessment, and care of seizure disorders

seizure (SEE-zher)
a sudden change in sensation, behavior, or movement. The most severe form of seizure produces violent muscle contractions called convulsions.

partial seizure
a seizure that affects only one part or one side of the brain.

generalized seizure
a seizure that affects both sides of the brain.

tonic-clonic (TON ik KLON-ik) **seizure**
a generalized seizure in which the patient loses consciousness and has jerking movements of paired muscle groups.

postictal (post-IK-tul) **phase**
the period of time immediately following a tonic-clonic seizure in which the patient goes from full loss of consciousness to full mental status.

aura
a sensation experienced by a seizure patient right before the seizure, which might be a smell, sound, or general feeling.

If the normal functions of the brain are upset by injury, infection, or disease, the brain's electrical activity can become irregular. This irregularity can bring about a sudden change in sensation, behavior, or movement, called a **seizure** (also called a *fit*, *spell*, or *attack* by nonmedical people). A seizure is not a disease in itself but rather a sign of some underlying defect, injury, or disease.

There are two types of seizures: partial and generalized. **Partial seizures** affect only one part, or one side, of the brain. Often these seizures affect only one area of the body and the patient may or may not lose consciousness. **Generalized seizures** affect the entire brain and as a result affect the consciousness of the patient. The seizure EMS is most likely to be called for, a type of generalized seizure characterized by unconsciousness and major motor activity, is called a **tonic-clonic seizure**. A tonic-clonic seizure often comes without warning, although a person may cry out before it begins. The patient will thrash about wildly, using his entire body. The convulsion usually lasts only a few minutes and has three distinct phases:

- **Tonic phase.** The body becomes rigid, stiffening for no more than 30 seconds. Breathing may stop, the patient may bite his tongue (rare), and bowel and bladder control could be lost.

- **Clonic phase.** The body jerks about violently, usually for no more than 1 or 2 minutes (some can last 5 minutes). The patient may foam at the mouth and drool. His face and lips often become cyanotic.

- **Postictal phase.** The *postictal phase* begins when convulsions stop. The patient may regain consciousness immediately and enter a state of drowsiness and confusion, or he may remain unconscious for several hours. Headache is common.

The length of the postictal phase may vary greatly from patient to patient. Some patients come around immediately, whereas others take much longer. It is important to remember that some patients may become combative and even violent toward rescuers during this phase. Safety should always be a priority.

Some seizures are preceded by an **aura**. An aura is a sensation the patient has when a seizure is about to happen. Often the patient notes a smell, a sound, or even just a general feeling right before the seizure begins. It can be important to document this finding when it exists.

Inside/Outside

A tonic-clonic seizure originates in the brain. For any number of possible reasons, neurons in both sides of the brain begin to fire simultaneously in a very disorganized fashion. Think of it as ventricular fibrillation of the brain. This irregular activity significantly disturbs brain activity and, in turn, disrupts any number of bodily functions.

Outside the body, this activity will be seen first as a loss of consciousness. Uncoordinated neurologic function then causes a body-wide contraction of muscles (the tonic phase). During this brief phase, breathing is typically stopped, and you may note that the patient has lost control of his bladder and/or bowels. You may also find blood in the patient's mouth and airway if he has bitten his tongue. Cyanosis is also a common finding in this phase. In the next phase, the clonic phase, the patient typically begins to breathe again, and paired muscle groups begin jerking movements. Often this is seen as flexion and extension of the arms and legs. This typically lasts for only a few minutes. As the seizure concludes, the patient begins the postictal phase. At this point, the patient is unconscious and will slowly regain mental status over a variable period of time. The patient may not know he has had a seizure (amnesia of the event) and confusion and repetetive questions are common.

Not all seizures you will see are generalized tonic-clonic seizures. Although infrequent, partial seizures may require your assistance. In these types of seizures you may see uncontrolled muscle spasm or convulsion in a patient with a fully alert mental status. You may also see a patient who has only a brief loss of consciousness without muscle convulsions. These seizures may be very difficult to distinguish from other disorders. Always use a thorough patient assessment to guide your care.

Causes of Seizures

The most common cause of seizures in adults is failure to take prescribed antiseizure medication. The most common cause of seizures in infants and children 6 months to 3 years of age is high fever (febrile seizures). Other causes include:

- **Hypoxia.** A lack of oxygen frequently causes seizures. These seizures often immediately precede respiratory and/or cardiac arrest.
- **Stroke.** Clots and bleeding in the brain are frequent causes of seizure. We will discuss this topic in greater detail later in this chapter.
- **Traumatic brain injury.** Brain injuries can cause seizures. So can scars formed at the site of previous brain trauma.
- **Toxins.** Drug or alcohol use, abuse, or withdrawal can cause seizures. Other poisons can also alter brain function to cause a seizure.
- **Hypoglycemia.** As we discussed earlier in this chapter, hypoglycemia (low blood sugar) is a frequent cause of seizures.
- **Brain tumor.** A brain tumor may occasionally cause seizures.
- **Congenital brain defects.** Seizures due to congenital defects of the brain (defects one is born with) are most often seen in infants and young children.
- **Infection.** Swelling or inflammation of the brain caused by an infection can cause seizures.
- **Metabolic.** Seizures can be caused by irregularities in the patient's body chemistry (metabolism).
- **Idiopathic.** This means occurring spontaneously, with an unknown cause. This is often the case with seizures that start in childhood.

In addition, seizures may also be seen with:

- Epilepsy
- Measles, mumps, and other childhood diseases
- Eclampsia (a severe complication of pregnancy)
- Heat stroke (resulting from exposure to high temperatures)

epilepsy (EP-uh-lep-see) a medical condition that causes seizures.

Epilepsy is perhaps the best-known of the conditions that result in seizures. Epilepsy is not a disease itself, but rather an umbrella term used when a person has multiple seizures from an unknown cause. Some people are born with epilepsy, whereas others develop epilepsy after a head injury or surgery. Conscientious use of medications allows most epileptics to live normal lives without seizures of any type. However, it is common for an epileptic patient to seize if he fails to take his medications properly or if an illness interferes with the normal medication routine. Remember that, although a patient with seizures may be an epileptic, epilepsy is only one condition that causes seizures.

PATIENT ASSESSMENT

Seizure Disorders

It is very important to be able to describe the seizure to emergency department personnel. If you have not observed the seizure (usually EMS is called after the seizure has taken place), always try to find out what it was like by asking the following questions of bystanders. Be sure to record and report your findings.

- What was the person doing before the seizure started? Was there an aura?
- Exactly what did the person do during the seizure—movement by movement—especially at the beginning? Was there loss of bladder or bowel control?
- How long did the seizure last?
- What did the person do after the seizure? Was he asleep (and for how long)? Was he awake? Was he able to answer questions? (If you are present during the seizure, use the AVPU scale to assess mental status.)

NOTE: *Multiple patients seizing at the same time is a major scene safety red flag. If this occurs, consider the possibility of a chemical weapon or similar weapon of mass destruction and take appropriate precautions.*

PATIENT CARE

Seizure Disorders

Emergency care of a patient with a seizure disorder includes the following.

If You Are Present When a Convulsive Seizure Occurs:

- Place the patient on the floor or ground. If there is no possibility of spine injury, position the patient on his side for drainage from the mouth.
- Loosen restrictive clothing.
- Remove objects that may harm the patient.
- Protect the patient from injury, but do not try to hold the patient still during convulsions (Figure 21-5).

FIGURE 21-5 Protect the seizure patient from injury.

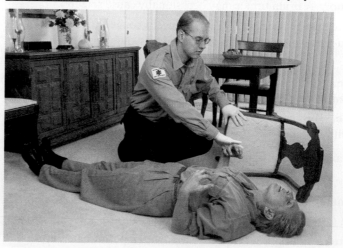

After Convulsions Have Ended:

■ Protect the airway. A patient who has just had a generalized seizure will sometimes drool and will usually be very drowsy for a little while, so you may need to suction the airway. If there is no possibility of spine injury, position the patient on his side for drainage from the mouth.

■ If the patient is cyanotic (blue), ensure an open airway and provide artificial ventilations with supplemental oxygen. Patients who are breathing adequately may be given oxygen by nasal cannula or nonrebreather based on pulse oximetry readings. Hypoxia is common after long periods of seizure activity.

■ Treat any injuries the patient may have sustained during the convulsions, or rule out trauma. Head injury can cause seizures, or the patient may have injured himself during the seizure. Immobilize the neck and spine if trauma is suspected.

■ Transport to a medical facility, monitoring vital signs and respirations closely.

NOTE: *Never place anything in the mouth of a seizing patient. Many objects can be broken and obstruct the patient's airway.*

PEDIATRIC NOTE

Remember that seizures caused by high fevers and idiopathic seizures (with no known cause) are common in children. Seizures in children who frequently have them are rarely life threatening. However, as an EMT, you should treat any seizure in an infant or child as if it is life threatening.

The epileptic is often knowledgeable about his condition, medications, and history. Since seizures may be common for the patient, he may refuse transportation. The patient should be encouraged to accept transportation to a hospital for examination. Should the patient continue to refuse, he should not be left alone after the seizure, and he must not drive. A competent person must remain with the patient.

NOTE: *Seizures usually last no more than 1 to 3 minutes. When the patient has two or more convulsive seizures lasting 5 to 10 minutes or more without regaining full consciousness, it is known as* **status epilepticus***. Some systems consider all patients who are still seizing when EMS arrives on the scene to be in status epilepticus. This is a high-priority emergency requiring immediate transport to the hospital and possible ALS intercept (having an advanced life support team meet your ambulance en route). The paramedics must open and suction the airway and administer a high concentration of oxygen at the scene and while en route.*

status epilepticus (STAT-us or STAT-us ep-i-LEP-ti-kus) a prolonged seizure or situation when a person suffers two or more convulsive seizures without regaining full consciousness.

Types of Seizures

It is beyond the EMT's scope of practice to identify the type of seizure the patient is having. The EMT's job is to treat immediate life threats, gather a history, and provide other normal assessment and care as previously described. However, some additional background information about types of seizures can provide perspective.

Partial Seizures In a simple partial seizure (also called focal motor, focal sensory, or Jacksonian) there is tingling, stiffening, or jerking in just one part of the body. There may also be an aura, which is a sensation such as a smell, bright lights, a burst of colors, or a rising sensation in the stomach. There is no loss of consciousness. However, in some cases the jerking may spread and develop into a tonic-clonic seizure.

A complex partial seizure (also called psychomotor or temporal lobe) is often preceded by an aura. This type of seizure is characterized by abnormal behavior that varies widely from person to person. It may involve confusion, a glassy stare, aimless moving about, lip smacking or chewing, or fidgeting with clothing. The person may appear to be drunk or on drugs. He is not violent but may struggle or fight if restrained. Very rarely, such extreme behavior as screaming, running, disrobing, or showing great fear may occur. There is no loss of consciousness, but there may be confusion and no memory of the episode afterward. In some cases, the seizure may develop into a tonic-clonic seizure.

Generalized Seizures When we think of generalized seizures, we think of the tonic-clonic seizure. However, there are other types of generalized seizures we should know about.

An absence seizure (also called petit mal) is brief, usually only 1 to 10 seconds. There is no dramatic motor activity and the person usually does not slump or fall. Instead, there is a temporary loss of concentration or awareness. An absence seizure may go unnoticed by everyone except the person and knowledgeable members of his family. A child may suffer several hundred absence seizures a day, severely interfering with his ability to pay attention and do well in school. Absence seizures often stop before adulthood but sometimes worsen and become tonic-clonic seizures.

Patient care for the generalized tonic-clonic seizure was described earlier. For a simple or complex partial seizure, do not restrain the person; simply remove objects from his path and gently guide him away from danger. For an absence seizure, if you are aware that it has occurred, simply provide the patient with any information he may have missed.

Stroke

CORE CONCEPT

Understanding the causes, assessment, and care of stroke

stroke

a condition of altered function caused when an artery in the brain is blocked or ruptured, disrupting the supply of oxygenated blood or causing bleeding into the brain. Formerly called a *cerebrovascular accident (CVA)*.

One of the many causes of altered mental status may be a **stroke**. Formerly called a *cerebral vascular accident (CVA)*, the term *stroke* refers to the death or injury of brain tissue that is deprived of oxygen. This can be caused by blockage of an artery that supplies blood to part of the brain or bleeding from a ruptured blood vessel in the brain. A stroke caused by a blockage, called an *ischemic stroke*, can occur when a clot or embolism occludes an artery. This mechanism is responsible for most strokes.

A stroke caused by bleeding into the brain, called a *hemorrhagic stroke*, frequently is the result of longstanding high blood pressure (hypertension). It also can occur when a weak area of an artery (an aneurysm) bulges out and eventually ruptures, forcing the brain into a smaller than usual space within the skull.

Different patients experiencing a stroke may have very different signs and symptoms, depending on the size and location of the arteries involved. One of the most common signs is one-sided weakness (hemiparesis). Because the left side of the brain controls movement on the right side of the body (and vice versa), someone with right-sided weakness from a stroke actually has a problem on the left side of his brain. However, the nerves that control the face muscles do not necessarily cross over in the same way, so sagging or drooping on one side of the face is not a reliable sign of injury to the opposite side.

A less common, but very important, sign of stroke is a headache caused by bleeding from a ruptured vessel. If you find in gathering a history that the patient cried out in pain, clutched his head, and collapsed, this is very important information to relay to the hospital staff. This patient may have had a particular kind of bleeding from an artery under the arachnoid layer of the meninges (the meninges are several layers of tissue that surround the brain and spinal cord). This is called a subarachnoid hemorrhage. Fortunately, most stroke patients are not hemorrhaging and do not experience headaches.

In many cases, you will find it difficult to communicate with the stroke patient. The damage to the brain sometimes causes a partial or complete loss of the ability to use words. The patient may be able to understand you but will not be able to talk or will have great difficulty with speech. Sometimes, the patient will understand you and know what he wants to say, but he will say the wrong words. This difficulty in using words is known as expressive aphasia. *Aphasia* is a general term that refers to difficulty in communication. Another form of it is receptive aphasia. In this case, the patient can speak clearly, but cannot understand what you are saying, so he will clearly say things that do not make much sense or are inappropriate for the situation.

Transient Ischemic Attack

A common occurrence is for an EMT to respond to a patient described as being confused, weak on one side, and having difficulty speaking. The EMT arrives, only to find an elderly patient who is alert, oriented, and perfectly normal without any evident weakness or speech difficulties. This patient may have had a transient ischemic attack (TIA), sometimes called a mini-stroke by laypeople. When this condition occurs, a patient looks as though he is having a stroke because he has the typical signs and symptoms of the condition. However, unlike stroke, a patient with a TIA has complete resolution of his symptoms without treatment within 24 hours (usually much sooner).

With TIA, small clots may be temporarily blocking circulation to part of the brain. When the clot breaks up, the patient's symptoms resolve because the affected brain tissue had only a short period of hypoxia and did not sustain permanent damage. However, this patient is at significant risk of having a full-blown stroke. If the patient refuses transport, you have a responsibility to attempt to persuade the patient to be evaluated as soon as possible so that a subsequent stroke can be prevented.

Always remember that if symptoms are present, it is impossible to distinguish between a stroke and a TIA in the field. Always assume the worst and treat as if it is a stroke.

PATIENT ASSESSMENT

Stroke

A very good way to assess conscious patients for stroke is to evaluate three items that constitute the Cincinnati Prehospital Stroke Scale (Figure 21-6 and Scan 21-3):

■ Ask the patient to grimace or smile. (Demonstrate to the patient what you want him to do, making sure that you show your teeth. This allows you to test control of the facial muscles.) A normal response is for the patient to move both sides of his face equally and to show you his teeth. An abnormal response is unequal movement or no movement at all.

FIGURE 21-6 The Cincinnati Prehospital Stroke Scale.

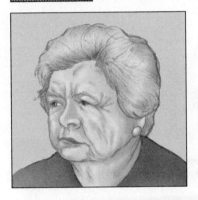

Facial Droop
Normal: Both sides of face move equally
Abnormal: One side of face does not move at all

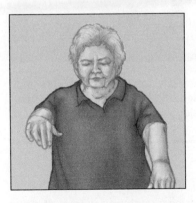

Arm Drift
Normal: Both arms move equally or not at all
Abnormal: One arm drifts compared to the other

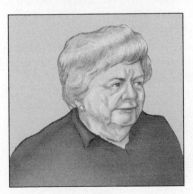

Speech
Normal: Patient uses correct words with no slurring
Abnormal: Slurred or inappropriate words or mute

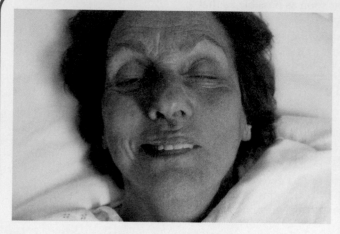

1 Assess for facial droop. The face of a stroke patient often has an abnormal drooped appearance on one side.
(© Edward T. Dickinson, MD)

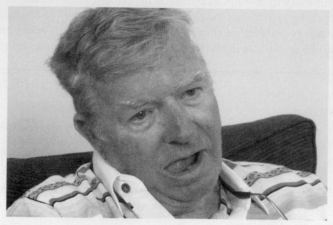

3 Assess for speech difficulties. A stroke patient will often have slurred speech, use the wrong words, or be unable to speak at all.

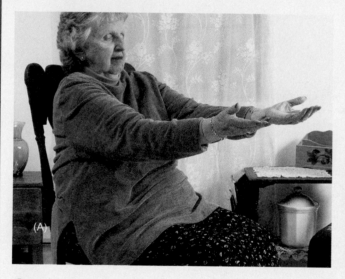

(A)

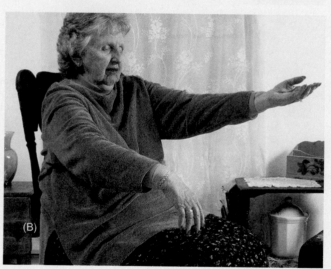

(B)

2 Assess for arm drift by asking the patient to close her eyes and extend her arms for 10 seconds. (A) A patient who has not suffered a stroke can usually hold her arms in an extended position with eyes closed. (B) A stroke patient will often display arm drift. That is, one arm will remain extended but the arm on the affected side will drift downward.

- Ask the patient to close his eyes and extend his arms straight out in front of him for 10 seconds. A normal response is for the patient to move both arms at the same time. An abnormal response is for one arm to drift down or not move at all.

- Ask the patient to say something like, "The sky is blue in Cincinnati." An uninjured person's speech is usually clear. A stroke patient is more likely to show an abnormal response to the test, like slurred speech, the wrong words, or no speech at all.

Other signs and symptoms of stroke, which will often fluctuate in severity while you observe the patient, include:

- Confusion
- Dizziness
- Numbness, weakness, or paralysis (usually on one side of the body)
- Loss of bowel or bladder control

- Impaired vision
- High blood pressure
- Difficult respiration or snoring
- Nausea or vomiting
- Seizures
- Unequal pupils
- Headache
- Loss of vision in one eye
- Unconsciousness (uncommon)

Decision Point

Is My Patient Having a Stroke?

Identify patients who appear to be having a stroke. These patients should be transported promptly to an appropriate facility.

> **NOTE:** *A patient who demonstrates any one of the three findings of the Cincinnati Prehospital Stroke Scale has a 70 percent chance of having an acute stroke.*

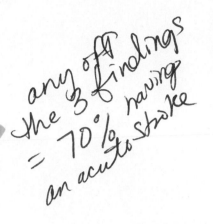

any off the 3 findings = 70% having an acute stroke

PATIENT CARE

Stroke

It is not necessary to determine that a stroke has taken place, although you may suspect it. There are many problems that can mimic strokes, including tumor or infection in the brain, head injury, seizures, hypoglycemia, and bacterial or viral infections that cause weakness or paralysis of facial nerves (Figure 21-7). Treat the patient as you would any patient with similar symptoms:

- For a conscious patient who can maintain his airway, calm and reassure him; monitor the airway; and administer high-concentration oxygen. Transport the patient in a semi-sitting position.

- For an unconscious patient, or a patient who cannot maintain his airway, maintain an open airway; provide high-concentration oxygen, and transport with the patient lying on the affected side.

FIGURE 21-7 Some infections, such as Lyme disease, may cause a temporary facial paralysis known as Bell's palsy.

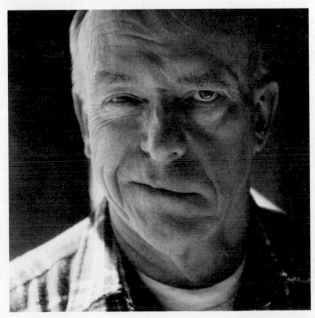

- Transport to a hospital with the capabilities to manage a stroke patient (CT scan at a minimum). Your destination choice may be guided by a local stroke care protocol, so follow local guidelines.

Because of recent research and advances in the treatment of stroke, you may have special protocols for management and transport of patients with signs and symptoms of stroke. New treatments are being used and tried in many hospitals, but time is of the essence if any of these treatments is to be effective. There appears to be a very narrow window within which assessment must be completed and treatment must be started.

The most widespread advance in stroke care is the use of clot-busting (thrombolytic) drugs in cases of ischemic stroke. This therapy can potentially reverse the symptoms of stroke, but patients must meet very specific criteria:

- Definite onset of stroke symptoms less than 3 hours prior to the administration of the thrombolytic drug
- An emergency CT scan of the brain confirming that there is no evidence of a hemorrhagic stroke
- Blood pressure that is not excessively hypertensive at the time the drug is administered

One of the most important things the EMT can do to optimize the care of stroke patients who are potential candidates for thrombolytics is to determine and document the exact time of onset of symptoms. If the person who provides you with the patient's time of onset is someone other than the patient, it is a good idea to document who that person is and how he can be contacted (e.g., cell phone number) if the physician in the emergency department should have to verify any information. In cases where the exact time of onset is not known, the patient will not be able to receive thrombolytics. For example, the patient who awakens at 7 a.m. and is immediately noted by the family to have new stroke symptoms but who was last seen in a normal condition at 11:30 p.m. the night before cannot get thrombolytic therapy, because it is not known when the stroke occurred during the night.

NOTE: *If you suspect the patient has had a stroke, it is important to transport him promptly and notify the hospital of symptoms you see and the results of the Cincinnati Prehospital Stroke Scale. If you have a choice of hospitals, your protocols may direct you to a hospital capable of providing the most recent stroke treatments.*

Dizziness and Syncope

● **CORE CONCEPT**
Understanding the causes, assessment, and care of dizziness and syncope

syncope (SIN-ko-pee)
fainting.

Dizziness and *syncope* (another term for fainting) are common reasons EMS is called. Although this is especially true for the elderly population, these problems can occur to patients of any age. Although these complaints might seem to be harmless, in fact they can be indicators of serious or even life-threatening problems. In many cases you will not be able to diagnose the true cause of the syncope. However, you should use your assessment to rapidly identify and treat life threats and to gather important information that will assist in the overall treatment of the patient.

Dizziness and syncope are separate problems that are sometimes related. It is not uncommon for someone to complain of dizziness before fainting. Because these two conditions are often caused by the same problems, we will consider them together in this chapter.

Dizziness is a common term that means different things to different people. It is important in your assessment to find out what the patient means by "dizziness." Does he mean weakness, as in a sensation of loss of strength? Does he feel vertigo? Vertigo is the sensation of your surroundings spinning around you. Is it lightheadedness, the sensation that he is about to pass out (sometimes called *presyncope* or *near syncope*)? Is it something else?

Syncope is a brief loss of consciousness with spontaneous recovery. Typically, it is very short, from a few seconds to at most a few minutes. The patient usually regains consciousness very soon after being allowed to lie flat (Figure 21-8).

Patients will often have some warning that a syncopal episode or fainting spell is about to occur. This may include such symptoms as lightheadedness, dizziness, nausea, weakness, vision changes, sudden pallor (loss of normal skin color), or sweating. Occasionally incontinence of bladder or bowel occurs as part of the episode, but this is more common with seizures.

Patients may be able to describe specific signs or symptoms that indicate certain causes of the episode are more likely than others. This may include fluttering in the chest (palpitations), a sensation of a racing heart (tachycardia), a slow heart rate (bradycardia), or headache.

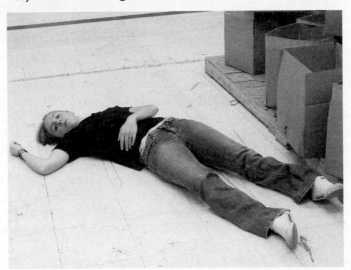

FIGURE 21-8 Loss of consciousness with syncope is usually brief. The patient usually regains consciousness very soon after being allowed to lie flat.

Causes of Dizziness and Syncope

The factors that cause dizziness and syncope are generally related to the brain. Problems like hypoxia, hypoglycemia, and hypovolemia all interfere with normal brain function. These events may happen rapidly, like blood flow to the brain being reduced by a cardiac dysrhythmia; or they may happen slowly, like slow gastrointestinal bleeding that finally reaches the point where the patient is unable to stand without losing consciousness.

There are many causes of dizziness and syncope. The more common ones can be grouped into four categories: hypovolemic, metabolic, environmental/toxicological, and cardiovascular.

Hypovolemic Causes Hypovolemia, or low fluid/blood volume, can cause dizziness or syncope when the patient attempts to sit up or stand. In this case, there is enough blood to perfuse the brain when the patient is lying down. However, when the patient tries to get up, the body is unable to quickly divert enough blood from the legs to the brain. There are several common causes of hypovolemia, including dehydration, internal bleeding, and trauma. The most serious cause of hypovolemia is bleeding.

In a patient with dizziness or syncope, the source of the bleeding may not be obvious. A woman of childbearing age can have a ruptured ectopic pregnancy that results in significant blood loss. (See Chapter 34, "Obstetrics and Gynecology," for more information about ectopic pregnancy.) This is usually accompanied by lower abdominal pain. A slowly bleeding ("leaking") abdominal aortic aneurysm can also lead to life-threatening blood loss. Such an aneurysm often causes the patient to experience abdominal pain radiating to the back. Gastrointestinal bleeding, with or without associated abdominal pain, is fairly common, especially among the older population.

There are other ways to become hypovolemic besides bleeding. Dehydration results from losing more fluid than the patient takes in. This is very common in hot weather, when the patient sweats a great deal but does not drink enough liquid to keep up with this fluid loss (heat exhaustion). It can also happen when someone becomes ill with diarrhea. Because eating or drinking anything is followed by a painful, watery bowel movement, the patient is reluctant to drink any fluids at all and becomes dehydrated. Sometimes, with severe diarrhea, this happens despite the patient's efforts to drink liquids.

Metabolic and Structural Causes When the cause of dizziness or syncope is metabolic, something is wrong with the brain or the structures near it. Because a properly functioning brain is necessary to maintain consciousness, alterations in the brain chemistry or structure can lead to a diminished level of consciousness. Similarly, because the inner and middle ear must be properly functioning for a person to maintain a sense of balance, a problem in this region can lead to dizziness. Inflammation of this area is a very common cause of dizziness. A patient who has been diagnosed with such a problem may be taking the drug meclizine.

Vertigo?

Hypoglycemia deprives the brain of glucose, which it needs all the time to function properly. An interruption in this supply can lead to both dizziness and syncope. If the patient remains unconscious more than a few minutes, however, it is not considered syncope, or fainting. There is likely to be a more serious cause of the episode. Occasionally, a stroke will present with either dizziness or syncope. In this case, there may be other neurological signs and symptoms present, like one-sided weakness, drooping of one side of the face, or slurred speech. A seizure can cause a temporary loss of consciousness, too. You learned about managing a patient having a seizure earlier in this chapter.

Environmental/Toxicological Causes Environmental and toxicological imbalances can lead to alterations in consciousness. Alcohol is the most commonly used drug and, when a patient drinks too much, it can lead to an altered level of consciousness. Many people who are intoxicated display a fluctuating level of consciousness that can appear to be syncope. Other drugs that are central nervous system depressants can cause similar effects. Syncope and near-syncope also commonly occur with carbon monoxide poisoning.

Panic attacks and anxiety attacks can lead a patient to become so anxious that the patient hyperventilates by breathing faster and deeper. When a patient breathes this hard, it can change the blood chemistry in a way that constricts the blood vessels supplying the brain with oxygen. Fortunately, when the patient loses consciousness, the hyperventilation ceases and things return at least partly to normal.

Cardiovascular Causes Cardiovascular causes of dizziness and syncope also deserve mention. A dysrhythmia that results in the heart beating extremely fast (a *tachycardia*) can lead to either dizziness or syncope. This is often the result of a problem with the electrical system in the heart. Ordinarily, increases in the heart rate result in increased blood being pumped out of the heart (greater cardiac output). However, when the heart beats extremely fast, the ventricles do not have time to fill before they pump blood out again. So, even though the heart is beating much faster than normal, it is actually pumping out less blood than usual. A very slow heart rate (a *bradycardia*) may also lead to dizziness or syncope through reduced cardiac output, in this case because the heart is not beating fast enough to pump out sufficient blood. This may not be noticeable to the patient when he is lying flat. When the patient tries to sit or stand, though, dizziness and syncope can occur when blood goes to the legs and the brain does not get sufficient blood.

A cardiovascular cause of syncope that is not the result of a problem with the heart's electrical system is stimulation of the carotid sinus. This area is located in the carotid artery under the mandible. When stimulated, it sends signals to the heart to slow down. Some people have a very sensitive carotid sinus. All that may be needed to stimulate it in some sensitive individuals is turning the head while wearing a shirt with a tight collar.

One of the most common types of syncope is *vasovagal syncope* or simple fainting. This is thought to be the result of stimulation of the vagus nerve, which in turn signals the heart to slow down. When someone is suddenly frightened or put under significant emotional stress, this nerve can be stimulated, leading to reduced cardiac output, which in the upright individual can quickly result in syncope. When the patient reaches a horizontal position, the brain regains perfusion and the patient regains consciousness.

Other Causes The causes previously discussed are just a few of the causes of dizziness and syncope. There are many others. In some cases, you will gather information that suggests one of them is the culprit. In many cases, you will not. Determining the cause can be extremely difficult. In half of the cases of dizziness or syncope, no cause is ever found despite thorough evaluation by emergency physicians and other specialists.

PATIENT ASSESSMENT

Dizziness and Syncope

Dizziness or syncope is usually easily recognized by the patient's complaint of a brief loss of consciousness. The secondary assessment for a patient with dizziness or syncope includes an appropriate history and vital signs. Questions to ask include:

- *Describe what you mean by "dizziness." Let the patient use his own words.*
- *Did you have any warning? If so, what was it like?*
- *When did it start?*

 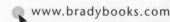

- How long did it last?
- What position were you in when the episode occurred?
- Have you had any similar episodes in the past? If so, what cause was found?
- Are you on medication for this kind of problem?
- Did you have any other signs or symptoms? Nausea? Vomiting (is there blood or material resembling coffee grounds)? Black tarry stools (digested blood)?
- Did you witness any unpleasant sight or experience a strong emotion?
- Did you hurt yourself?
- Did anyone witness involuntary movements of the extremities (like seizures)?

PATIENT CARE

Dizziness and Syncope

When a patient has experienced dizziness or syncope, provide the following care after attending to any threats to life:

1. Administer high-concentration oxygen.
2. Call for ALS if the patient has signs of instability and it is available in your area.
3. Loosen any tight clothing around the neck.
4. Lay the patient flat.
5. Treat any associated injuries the patient may have incurred from the fall.

Decision Point

Is My Patient Stable? Is My Patient Likely to Remain Stable?
The urgency of your treatment and transport will depend on these decisions.

CHAPTER REVIEW

Key Facts and Concepts

- Diabetic emergencies are usually caused by poor management of the patient's diabetes.
- Diabetic emergencies are often brought about by hypoglycemia, or low blood sugar.
- The chief sign of this hypoglycemia is altered mental status.
- Whenever a patient has an altered mental status, a history of diabetes, and can swallow, administer oral glucose.
- Seizures may have a number of causes. Assess and treat for possible spinal injury, protect the patient's airway, and provide oxygen as needed.
- You should gather information about the seizure to give to hospital personnel.

- A stroke is caused when an artery in the brain is blocked or ruptures.
- Signs and symptoms of a stroke commonly include an altered mental status, numbness or paralysis on one side, and difficulty with speech, among other symptoms.
- For stroke patients, ensure an open airway and provide supplemental oxygen. Determine the exact time of onset of symptoms and transport promptly.
- Dizziness and syncope (fainting) may have a variety of causes.
- In the case of syncope, administer oxygen, loosen clothing around the neck, and place the patient flat with raised legs if there is no reason not to. Treat any injuries and transport.

Key Decisions

- Is this patient's altered mental status being caused by hypoxia?
- In a patient with a hypoglycemic emergency, does he have a mental status that would allow the administration of oral glucose?
- Does the seizure patient need artificial ventilation?
- When did the symptoms of the stroke begin?

Chapter Glossary

aura a sensation experienced by a seizure patient right before the seizure, which might be a smell, sound, or general feeling.

diabetes mellitus (di-ah-BEE-tez MEL-i-tus) also called "sugar diabetes" or just "diabetes," the condition brought about by decreased insulin production or the inability of the body cells to use insulin properly. The person with this condition is a diabetic.

diabetic ketoacidosis (di-ah BET-ic KEY-to-as-id-DO-sis) *(DKA)* a condition that occurs as the result of high blood sugar (hyperglycemia), characterized by dehydration, altered mental status, and shock.

epilepsy (EP-uh-lep-see) a medical condition that causes seizures.

generalized seizure a seizure that affects both sides of the brain.

glucose (GLU-kos) a form of sugar, the body's basic source of energy.

hyperglycemia (HI-per-gli-SEE-me-ah) high blood sugar.

hypoglycemia (HI-po-gli-SEE-me-ah) low blood sugar.

insulin (IN-suh-lin) a hormone produced by the pancreas or taken as a medication by many diabetics.

partial seizure a seizure that affects only one part or one side of the brain.

postictal (post-IK-tul) *phase* the period of time immediately following a tonic-clonic seizure in which the patient goes from full loss of consciousness to full mental status.

reticular (ruh-TIK-yuh-ler) *activating system (RAS)* series of neurologic circuits in the brain that control the functions of staying awake, paying attention, and sleeping.

seizure (SEE-zher) a sudden change in sensation, behavior, or movement. The most severe form of seizure produces violent muscle contractions called convulsions.

status epilepticus (STAY-tus or STAT-us ep-i-LEP-ti-kus) a prolonged seizure or situation when a person suffers two or more convulsive seizures without regaining full consciousness.

stroke a condition of altered function caused when an artery in the brain is blocked or ruptured, disrupting the supply of oxygenated blood or causing bleeding into the brain. Formerly called a *cerebrovascular accident (CVA)*.

syncope (SIN-ko-pee) fainting.

tonic-clonic (TON-ik-KLON-ik) *seizure* a generalized seizure in which the patient loses consciousness and has jerking movements of paired muscle groups.

Preparation for Your Examination and Practice

Short Answer

1. List the chief signs and symptoms of a diabetic emergency.
2. Explain how you can determine a medical history of diabetes.
3. Explain what treatment may be given by an EMT for a diabetic emergency and the criteria for giving it.
4. Tell whether treatment for a diabetic emergency should be given before or after baseline vital signs are taken. (Answer according to your local protocol.)
5. Explain the care that should be given to a patient who has had a seizure.
6. Explain the care that should be given to a conscious and to an unconscious patient with suspected stroke.
7. Explain the care that should be given to a patient who has experienced dizziness or syncope.

Thinking and Linking

Think back to Chapter 14, "Assessment of the Medical Patient," and link information from that chapter with information from this chapter as you consider the following question:

1. What parts of the patient's SAMPLE history will provide clues to the cause of the patient's altered mental status?

Think back to Chapter 4, "Medical, Legal, and Ethical Issues," as well as to Chapter 17, "Communication and Documentation," as you consider the following situation:

2. You have given a diabetic patient glucose. The patient is now oriented and does not want to be transported to the hospital. After you have made diligent efforts to persuade the patient to go, the patient still refuses transportation. What do you tell the patient? What do you document in relation to the refusal and your interaction with the patient?

Critical Thinking Exercises

Patients suffering a diabetic emergency are sometimes thought to be drunk. The purpose of this exercise will be to consider how to treat such a patient.

- You are dispatched to a "man behaving oddly" at a train station. When you arrive, you find that the man is unconscious. "He's drunk," a bystander tells you. "He was staggering and slurring his words." As you assess the patient, you find a medical identification bracelet that tells you he is a diabetic. Do you administer oral glucose? How do you proceed?

Pathophysiology to Practice

The following questions are designed to assist you in gathering relevant clinical information and making accurate decisions in the field.

1. How might you differentiate a patient who had a seizure associated with hypoxia from a patient who had a seizure associated with epilepsy?
2. What assessment elements would be important in making this decision?

Street Scenes

While on your day off, you receive a telephone call about working a shift at the county fair. It sounds like fun, so you agree. That Friday night, you and your partner are on stand-by with an ambulance at the first-aid tent. It is 10 p.m. and the evening has been quiet. Just when you think that it will also remain uneventful, you receive a call on the radio that security has an intoxicated person they want you to examine on the midway. Upon arrival, you find a male patient in his 20s, sitting and talking in slurred speech to a deputy sheriff. A security guard tells you that the patient was wandering down the midway and talking incoherently. "I'm sure he's drunk," he tells you, "but the rules say you have to take a look before we transport to the security office."

Street Scene Questions

1. Does this patient need a thorough assessment?
2. What is the first concern when starting to assess this patient?
3. What types of underlying medical problems might make a patient appear to be drunk?

As your partner approaches the patient, he is met with what appears to be an angry patient, who says, "That's all I need—another cop." The patient then pushes the deputy sheriff away, and he turns to you. "This guy is just another drunk," your partner says, "and we are out of here." You almost buy into your partner's hasty evaluation, but you notice a bracelet on the patient's wrist. You approach, introduce yourself, and ask the patient if you can check him out. He reluctantly agrees, and as you take a pulse, which is rapid, you see that his bracelet indicates he has diabetes.

Street Scene Questions

4. Does your assessment plan change at this point?
5. How will you get a SAMPLE history if the patient is alone?
6. What is the priority level of this patient? Is there a need to call for ALS assistance?

After primary and secondary assessments, you find the patient's airway is open with no mucus or other secretions noted, his breathing is at 24 breaths per minute, and his pulse rate is 110.

Just as you finish taking vital signs, a person approaches who says he is a friend of the patient. He confirms that your patient is a diabetic and that he took his insulin before they left for the fair. "He expected to eat here," the friend tells you, "but he was trying to win at the midway games and must have forgotten." You and your partner agree that he could tolerate oral glucose. You explain to your patient what you are doing and apply some to the inside of his cheek. In a few minutes he starts to become more alert, and soon he says he feels fine.

The ALS unit is now on the scene and has checked his sugar level. It is in a normal range. The patient does not want to be transported and, after you talk to medical direction, he is allowed to leave with his friend, who promises to take him directly to a diner for something starchy to eat.

You call back in service and, as you walk to the ambulance, you remind your partner that you can never assume anything. Every patient needs an assessment.

22

Allergic Reaction

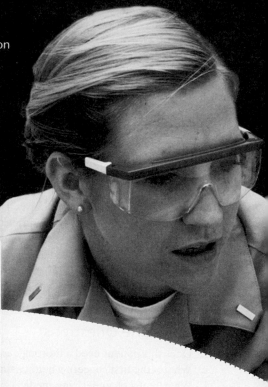

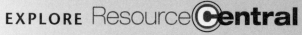

OBJECTIVES

After reading this chapter you should be able to:

22.1 Define key terms introduced in this chapter.

22.2 Differentiate between the signs and symptoms of an allergic reaction and an anaphylactic reaction. (pp. 536, 539)

22.3 Describe the relationship between allergens and antibodies necessary for an allergic reaction to occur. (pp. 531–532)

22.4 Describe the effects of histamine and other chemicals in producing the signs and symptoms of anaphylaxis. (p. 533)

22.5 List common allergens. (pp. 531–532)

22.6 Prioritize the steps in assessment and management of patients with allergic and anaphylactic reactions. (pp. 535–538)

22.7 Recognize the indications for administering and assisting a patient in the use of an epinephrine auto-injector. (pp. 539–541)

22.8 Describe the desired effects and side effects associated with the administration of epinephrine. (pp. 539–541)

22.9 Demonstrate administration of epinephrine by auto-injector. (pp. 537–538)

22.10 Describe the considerations in reassessment of patients with allergic and anaphylactic reactions. (p. 540)

KEY TERMS

allergen, *p. 531*   anaphylaxis, *p. 531*   epinephrine, *p. 539*
allergic reaction, *p. 531*   auto-injector, *p. 536*   hives, *p. 534*

A llergic reactions can be mild or extremely severe. A mild allergic reaction can rapidly develop into a severe reaction. A severe allergic reaction can quickly become life threatening. For these reasons, prompt recognition and appropriate assessment and treatment of allergic reactions can be critical.

ALLERGIC REACTIONS

A natural response of the human body's immune system is to react to any foreign substance—in other words, to defend the body by neutralizing or getting rid of the foreign material. Sometimes the immune response is exaggerated; this exaggerated reaction is called an *allergic reaction*. Almost any of a wide variety of substances can be an *allergen*, something that causes an allergic reaction. For example, cat dander can be an allergen. A person who is allergic to cat dander will itch and sneeze whenever a cat is nearby. The reaction is unpleasant but harmless.

In some people, however, contact with certain foreign substances triggers an immune response that gets out of hand. Consider bee stings. Most people have no reaction to a bee sting other than pain and some swelling at the sting site. However, a few people have very severe, life threatening reactions to bee stings. This kind of severe allergic reaction is called *anaphylaxis*, or *anaphylactic shock*. In anaphylaxis, exposure to the allergen will cause blood vessels to rapidly dilate, which causes a drop in blood pressure (hypotension). Many tissues may swell, including those that line the respiratory system. This swelling can obstruct the airway, leading to respiratory failure.

There are many causes of allergic reactions (in some individuals), such as (Figure 22-1):

- **Insects.** The stings of bees, yellow jackets, wasps, and hornets can cause rapid and severe reactions.

- **Foods.** Foods such as nuts, eggs, milk, and shellfish can cause reactions. In most cases, the effect is slower than that seen with insect stings. An exception is peanuts. Peanut allergies are frequently very severe and very rapid in onset. Many people with allergies to one food will have allergies to related foods (for example, someone who is allergic to almonds is more likely to be allergic to walnuts). Again, peanuts are an exception. People who are allergic to peanuts do not necessarily have any other allergies, including nuts (in part because peanuts are legumes, not nuts).

- **Plants.** Contact with certain plants such as poison ivy, poison sumac, and poison oak (Figure 22-2) can cause a rash that is sometimes severe. The rash associated with poison ivy is actually an allergic reaction. Approximately two-thirds of the population is allergic to the oil on poison ivy leaves. Plant pollen also causes allergic reactions in many people, but rarely anaphylaxis.

- **Medications.** Antitoxins and drugs, especially antibiotics such as penicillin, may cause severe reactions. Just as with foods, people who are allergic to one kind of antibiotic can be allergic to related antibiotics. In the course of evaluating patients, you will hear many of them say they are allergic to penicillin or other antibiotics. Many of them

allergic reaction
an exaggerated immune response.

allergen
something that causes an allergic reaction.

anaphylaxis (an-ah-fi-LAK-sis)
a severe or life-threatening allergic reaction in which the blood vessels dilate, causing a drop in blood pressure, and the tissues lining the respiratory system swell, interfering with the airway. Also called *anaphylactic shock*.

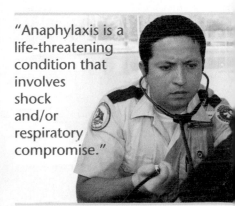

"Anaphylaxis is a life-threatening condition that involves shock and/or respiratory compromise."

FIGURE 22-1 Substances that may cause allergic reactions.

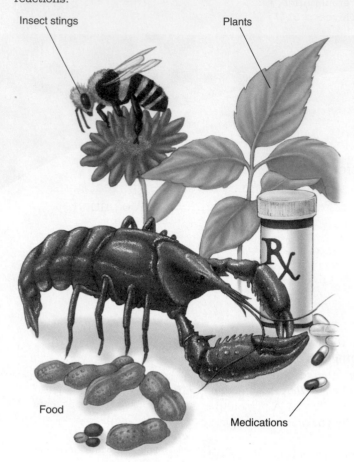

Insect stings

Plants

Food

Medications

FIGURE 22-2 (A) Poison ivy, (B) poison sumac, and (C) poison oak.

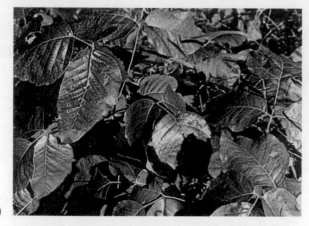

(A)

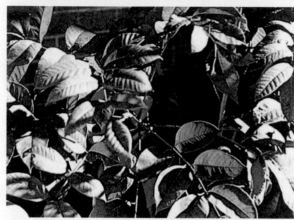

(B)

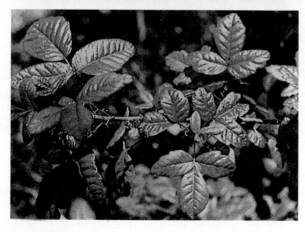

(C)

are wrong, because they confuse side effects, such as nausea or diarrhea, with an allergic reaction.

- **Others.** Dust, chemicals, soaps, makeup, and a variety of other substances can cause allergic reactions—which are occasionally severe—in some people.

One particular product EMTs should be aware of as a possible allergen is latex. Two groups of people are especially likely to be allergic to latex. One of these groups is patients with conditions that require multiple surgeries. The repeated exposure to the latex in doctors' and nurses' gloves is probably the reason many such patients develop a severe allergy to latex. This is very important to understand, because if you wear latex gloves when treating a patient with a latex allergy, you may actually cause an allergic or anaphylactic reaction in the patient.

Inside/Outside

■ Inside

Something that all allergic reactions share is that people do not have them the first time they are exposed to an allergen. This is because the body's immune system has not "learned" to recognize the allergen yet. The first time someone is exposed to an allergen, the immune system forms antibodies in response. These antibodies are the body's attempt to attack the foreign substances. A particular antibody will combine with only the allergen it was formed in response to (or another allergen very similar to the original one).

The second time the person is exposed to the allergen, the antibodies already exist in the person's body. This time, the antibody combines with the allergen, leading to the release of histamine and other chemicals into the bloodstream. Together, these substances have several effects that may lead to a spectrum of allergic reactions including, at times, the life-threatening condition known as anaphylaxis: They dilate blood vessels, decrease the ability of capillaries to contain fluid, cause bronchoconstriction, and promote the production of thick mucus in the lungs.

■ Outside

The dilation of blood vessels reduces the amount of blood returning to the heart, leading to decreased cardiac output and an increased risk of shock. Skin also becomes flushed as blood vessels near the surface open up. When capillaries become leaky, fluid moves into the tissue and appears as swelling, especially around the site of an injection (or sting) (Figure 22-3A) and the face (Figure 22-3B), including the eyes, lips, ears, tongue, and airway. If the area around the vocal cords becomes swollen, the patient may have a muffled voice or display stridor on inspiration. Urticaria, also called hives—red, itchy, possibly raised blotches on the skin (Figure 22-3C)—is another result of the release of histamines and related substances in response to allergens. Bronchoconstriction causes decreased movement of air in the lungs, leading to wheezing and difficulty breathing. Thick mucus worsens this effect. Irritation of nerve endings results in itching.

FIGURE 22-3 Signs of an allergic reaction may include (A) local swelling, (B) facial swelling, and (C) hives. *(Photo A: © Daniel Limmer; Photo B: © Edward T. Dickinson, MD; Photo C: © Charles Stewart, MD and Associates)*

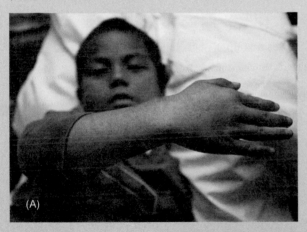

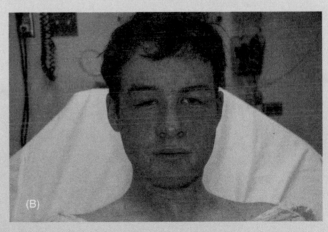

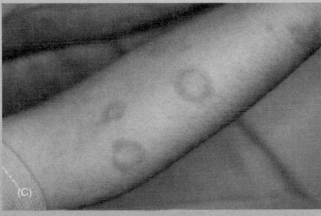

The other group that is becoming more sensitive to latex is health care professionals, including EMTs. Again, this increased sensitivity is probably because of more frequent exposure to latex as a result of practicing Standard Precautions. Fortunately, it is now possible to find virtually all medical equipment and supplies in forms that do not contain latex. Many hospitals and EMS agencies maintain latex-free environments to avoid causing reactions in latex-sensitive individuals.

NOTE: *If you wear latex gloves and notice that your hands seem to be red and itchy after a call, you may be developing an allergy to latex. If you are allergic to latex, it is very important that you protect yourself from further exposure to this allergen. If you do not, the signs will get worse as you continue to wear latex gloves. Some people become extremely sensitive to latex, so it is important that you tell this to any health care provider who is caring for you as a patient. Also discuss this with your own physician so that you become as informed as possible about this topic and learn how to protect yourself.*

There is no way to predict the exact course of an allergic reaction. Severe reactions most often take place immediately, but they are occasionally delayed 30 minutes or more. A mild allergic reaction may turn into more serious anaphylactic shock in a matter of minutes. When a patient with an exposure to a known allergen is displaying only minor signs and symptoms, you must closely monitor the patient for signs of the condition becoming more serious. This patient's airway may swell and close off in just a few minutes. Be prepared to manage the airway and to administer epinephrine if so advised by medical direction.

The signs and symptoms of an allergic reaction or anaphylactic shock can include:

- - - - - - - - - - ● **CORE CONCEPT**

How to identify a patient
experiencing an allergic reaction

hives
red, itchy, possibly raised blotches on
the skin that often result from allergic
reactions.

Skin:

- Itching
- *Hives* (may be localized—especially around an insect sting—or generalized over wide areas of the body)
- Flushing (red skin)
- Swelling of the face (especially the eyes and lips), neck, hands, feet, or tongue
- Warm, tingling feeling in the face, mouth, chest, feet, and hands

Respiratory:

- Patient may report a feeling of tightness in the throat or chest
- Cough
- Rapid breathing
- Labored, noisy breathing
- Hoarseness, muffled voice, or loss of voice entirely
- Stridor (harsh, high-pitched sound during inspiration)
- Wheezing (audible without a stethoscope)

Cardiac:

- Increased heart rate
- Decreased blood pressure

Generalized Findings:

- Itchy, watery eyes
- Headache
- Runny nose
- Patient expresses a sense of impending doom

Signs and Symptoms of Shock:

- Altered mental status
- Flushed, dry skin or pale, cool, clammy skin

- Nausea or vomiting
- Changes in vital signs: increased pulse, increased respirations, decreased blood pressure

Distinguishing Anaphylaxis from Mild Allergic Reaction

Any of the signs and symptoms discussed previously can be associated with an allergic reaction. *To be considered a severe allergic reaction, or anaphylaxis, the patient must have either respiratory distress or signs and symptoms of shock.*

CORE CONCEPT
Differences between a mild allergic reaction and anaphylaxis

PATIENT ASSESSMENT

Allergic Reaction or Anaphylaxis

Conduct the usual assessment sequence, as follows:

1. Perform the primary assessment and care for any immediately life-threatening problems with the patient's airway, breathing, or circulation.
2. Perform a secondary assessment. Inquire about:
   - History of allergies
   - What patient was exposed to
   - How patient was exposed (contact, ingestion, and so on)
   - What signs and symptoms the patient is having
   - Progression (What happened first, next? How rapidly?)
   - Interventions (Has any care been provided? Has the patient taken any medication?)
3. Assess baseline vital signs and get the remainder of the past medical history.

Suspect an allergic reaction whenever the patient has come in contact with a substance that has caused an allergic reaction in the past; whenever the patient complains of itching, hives, or difficulty breathing (respiratory distress); or when the patient shows signs or symptoms of shock (hypoperfusion).

Table 22-1 lists specific signs and symptoms and their likely association with either a non-life-threatening allergic reaction or a life-threatening anaphylactic reaction.

Table 22-1 Distinguishing Allergic from Anaphylactic Reactions

Signs and symptoms in the "Allergic" column are more likely to be associated with allergic reactions that are not life threatening. Signs and symptoms in the "Anaphylactic" column are more likely to be associated with anaphylactic reactions that are life threatening.

SYSTEM	ALLERGIC	ANAPHYLACTIC
Respiratory complaints	Sneezing, cough, mild dyspnea	Moderate to severe dyspnea, tightness in chest
Respiratory sounds	Wheezing	Wheezing, muffled voice, stridor
Skin texture	Local hives	Generalized hives
Skin color	Possible pallor, little or no flushing of skin	Generalized pallor or flushed skin
Swelling	Local swelling	Swelling of face, lips, eyes, tongue, mouth, injection site
Vital signs	Normal or nearly normal vital signs	Tachycardia, hypotension, tachypnea, decreased oxygen saturation
Mental status	Mild, moderate, or severe anxiety	Feeling of impending doom

Decision Points

- Is this an allergic reaction or anaphylaxis?
- Does it have the potential to become anaphylaxis?
- Do I need to administer an epinephrine auto-injector?

PATIENT CARE

Allergic Reaction or Anaphylaxis

------------ ● **CORE CONCEPT**

How to treat a patient
experiencing an allergic reaction

auto-injector

a syringe preloaded with medication
that has a spring-loaded device that
pushes the needle through the skin
when the tip of the device is pressed
firmly against the body.

1. Manage the patient's airway and breathing. Apply high-concentration oxygen through a nonrebreather mask, if you have not already done so during the primary assessment. If the patient has or develops an altered mental status, open and maintain the patient's airway. If the patient is not breathing adequately, provide artificial ventilations.

2. You may be able to assist the patient in administering an epinephrine **auto-injector**, or you may be allowed to carry auto-injectors on your ambulance. To find out if use of an auto-injector is appropriate, consider each of the following:

   • *If* the patient has come in contact with a substance that caused an allergic reaction in the past, *and if* the patient has respiratory distress or exhibits signs and symptoms of shock, *and if* the patient has a prescribed epinephrine auto-injector (*or if* your protocols allow you to carry and use epinephrine auto-injectors), then contact medical direction and, if so ordered, assist the patient with his prescribed auto-injector or administer epinephrine from an auto-injector you carry on the ambulance (Scan 22-1). Record the administration of the epinephrine auto-injector. Transport. Reassess 2 minutes after epinephrine administration and record reassessment findings.

   • *If* the patient has come in contact with a substance that caused an allergic reaction in the past, *but* the patient is *not* wheezing or showing signs of respiratory distress or shock (hypoperfusion), then continue with the assessment. Consult medical direction; if the patient has an epinephrine auto-injector *and if* medical direction so orders, administer epinephrine. Some patients have histories of very rapid onset of severe symptoms, so the physician may wish you to give the medication even though the patient does not appear to need it.

   • *If* the patient has come in contact with a substance that caused an allergic reaction in the past, *and if* the patient complains of respiratory distress or exhibits signs and symptoms of shock, *but* the patient *does not* have a prescribed epinephrine auto-injector available or has never had one prescribed, and your protocols *do not* allow you to carry and use epinephrine auto-injectors, then perform care for shock and transport the patient immediately.

If the patient meets the criteria just listed but does not have an epinephrine auto-injector and your protocols do not allow you to carry and use one, consider requesting an ALS intercept. Paramedics carry and can administer epinephrine.

You probably will not see many patients with allergic reactions. However, most of those you do see will be able to give you a history of their allergies. Once in a while, you will see a patient who has no history and is having his first allergic reaction. In this case, the patient will not be carrying an epinephrine auto-injector because his physician has not prescribed one. Treat the patient for shock and transport immediately. Consider requesting ALS intercept.

Table 22-2 provides a summary of assessment and care of patients with allergic or anaphylactic reactions.

Table 22-2 Summary of Assessment and Care of Patients with Allergic or Anaphylactic Reactions

• Epinephrine prescription • History of exposure • Signs and symptoms of anaphylaxis	• Epinephrine prescription • History of exposure • <u>NO</u> signs and symptoms of anaphylaxis	→	1. Standard treatment 2. Consult physician for order to give epinephrine
• NO epinephrine prescription*	• Epinephrine prescription • NO epinephrine available	→	1. Standard treatment 2. Transport

* In some areas, EMTs carry and administer epinephrine. If this is the case, a prescription for epinephrine is not necessary.

FIRST TAKE STANDARD PRECAUTIONS.

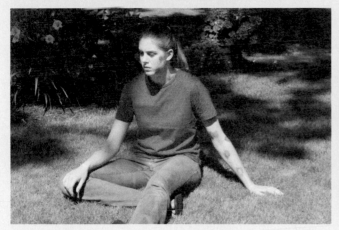

If a patient suffers a severe allergic reaction:

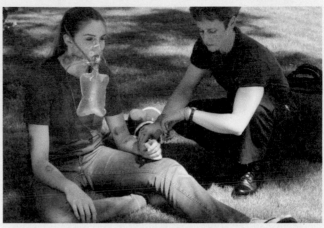

❶ Perform a primary assessment. Provide high-concentration oxygen by nonrebreather mask.

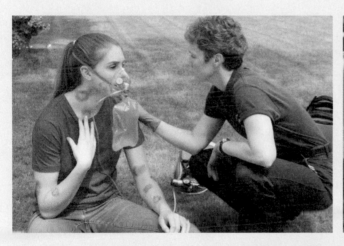

❷ Perform a secondary assessment. Obtain a SAMPLE history.

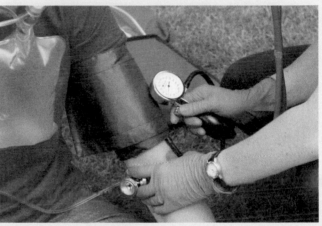

❸ Take the patient's vital signs.

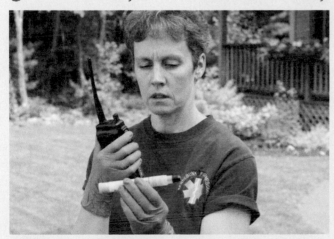

❹ Find out if the patient has a prescribed epinephrine auto-injector and if it is prescribed for this patient or ensure that your protocols allow administering an epinephrine auto-injector you carry on the ambulance. Then check the expiration date and check for cloudiness or discoloration if liquid is visible. Contact medical direction.

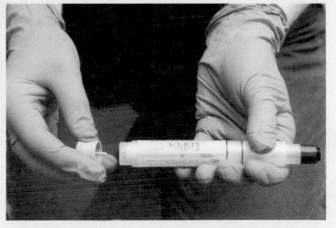

❺ If medical direction orders use of the epinephrine auto-injector, prepare it for use by removing the safety cap. (Photo shows the EpiPen®.)

(continued)

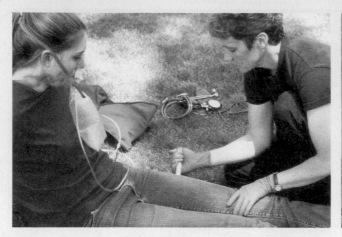

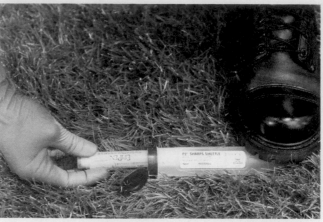

6 Press the injector against the patient's thigh to trigger release of the spring-loaded needle and inject the dose of epinephrine into the patient.

7 Dispose of the used single-dose injector in a portable biohazard container.

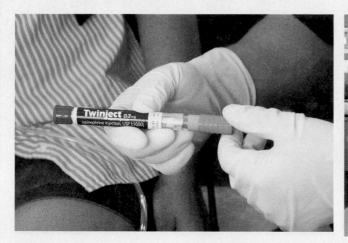

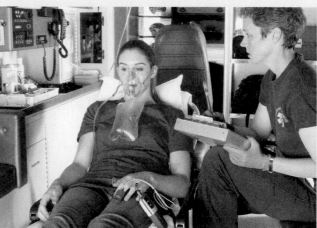

8 If using the Twinject®, follow the manufacturer's directions to remove color-coded caps and administer the first dose. Save the device and transport it with the patient in case the second dose it contains is needed later. (If needed, again follow the manufacturer's directions to remove the color-coded cap and tab to administer the second dose.)

9 Document the patient's response to the medication.

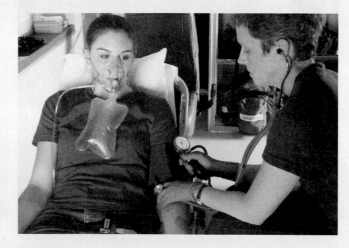

10 Perform a reassessment, paying special attention to the patient's ABCs and vital signs en route to the hospital.

Allergic Reaction or Anaphylaxis?

For each of the following patients, decide whether the presentation is an allergic reaction or anaphylaxis:

1. A patient who has a history of allergy to bee stings and feels her throat "closing up" after a bee sting

2. A patient who reports an unknown allergy and feels like his skin is "just itching all over"

3. A patient who has an "allergy" to dairy products and reports an upset stomach and diarrhea

4. A patient who is allergic to peanuts and has swelling of the face and neck, difficulty breathing, and a rapid pulse

5. A patient who is allergic to penicillin but accidentally took a medication containing penicillin; patient is dizzy but has stable vital signs

SELF-ADMINISTERED EPINEPHRINE

Physicians have long prescribed *epinephrine* in bee sting kits, AnaKits, or EpiPens® for patients who are susceptible to severe allergic reactions. Epinephrine is a hormone produced by the body. When administered as a medication, it will constrict blood vessels (helping to raise the blood pressure and improve perfusion) and dilate the bronchioles (helping to open the airway and improve respiration).

Many people who are subject to severe allergic reactions are prescribed an epinephrine auto-injector by their physician to carry with them and use when such a reaction occurs. An auto-injector is a spring-loaded needle and syringe with a single dose of epinephrine that will automatically release and inject the medication. The reason it is important for a patient with severe allergic reactions to carry an epinephrine auto-injector is that an allergic reaction can become life threatening so quickly that there is not enough time to transport the patient to a hospital to receive the medication.

When authorized by medical direction, you may administer or help the patient administer a dose of epinephrine from an auto-injector that has been prescribed for the patient by a physician. Some states allow EMTs to carry epinephrine auto-injectors on the ambulance to administer with approval from medical direction. After you make sure that the liquid is clear (if you can see it), remove the cap and press the injector firmly against the patient's thigh. Hold it there until the entire dose is injected. (Injection on the outside of the thigh midway between the waist and knee is recommended.) On reassessment 2 minutes after the epinephrine is administered, in addition to some relief of symptoms, expect the patient's pulse to have increased.

The procedure for administering an epinephrine auto-injector is shown in Scan 22-1. Information about epinephrine auto-injectors is summarized in Scan 22-2.

Epinephrine is a very powerful medication. It not only saves lives, it can also occasionally take lives. One of the good things epinephrine does for patients is make the heart beat more strongly. This is beneficial when the patient is hypoperfusing (that is, when the patient is in shock), because one reason for the hypoperfusion is that the patient's blood vessels are dilated and blood is not returning to the heart as quickly. Unfortunately, once you give a drug, you cannot take it back. If the dose of epinephrine in the auto-injector is more than the patient needs, the patient's heart will be working harder than it needs to. This can be dangerous in a patient with a heart condition or who is hypertensive (has high blood pressure).

The power of epinephrine and its possible adverse effects are among the reasons why EMTs have been taught to *give epinephrine only to patients who have been prescribed auto-injectors by their physicians*. They have been evaluated by physicians who have considered the patient's history and physical condition, were satisfied that the patient is a good candidate for epinephrine, and wrote a prescription.

epinephrine (EP-uh-NEF-rin) a hormone produced by the body. As a medication, it constricts blood vessels and dilates respiratory passages and is used to relieve severe allergic reactions.

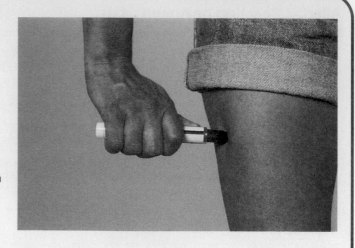

MEDICATION NAME
1. Generic: epinephrine
2. Trade: Adrenalin™
3. Delivery system: EpiPen® or EpiPen Jr.® or Twinject® (adult or child size)

INDICATIONS
Must meet the following three criteria:
1. Patient exhibits signs of a severe allergic reaction, including either respiratory distress or shock (hypoperfusion).
2. Medication is prescribed for this patient by a physician or is carried on the ambulance.
3. Medical direction authorizes use for this patient.

CONTRAINDICATIONS
No contraindications when used in a life-threatening situation.

MEDICATION FORM
Liquid is administered by an auto-injector—an automatically injectable needle-and-syringe system.

DOSAGE
1. Adult: one adult auto-injector (0.3 mg)
2. Infant and child: one infant/child auto-injector (0.15 mg)

ADMINISTRATION
1. Obtain patient's prescribed auto-injector. Ensure:
   a. Prescription is written for the patient who is experiencing the severe allergic reaction or your protocols permit carrying the auto-injector on the ambulance.
   b. Medication is not discolored (if visible).
   c. Medication has not expired.
2. Obtain an order from medical direction, either on-line or off-line.
3. Remove the safety cap(s) from the auto-injector.
4. Grasp the center of the auto-injector (to avoid accidentally injecting yourself).
5. Place the tip of the auto-injector against the patient's thigh.
   a. Lateral portion of the thigh
   b. Midway between waist and knee
6. Push the injector firmly against the thigh until the injector activates.
7. Hold the injector in place until the medication is injected (at least 10 seconds).
8. Record the administration and time.
9. Dispose of a single-dose injector, such as the EpiPen®, in a biohazard container; save a two-dose injector,

such as the Twinject®, and transport it with the patient in case the second dose is later required.

ACTIONS
1. Dilates the bronchioles
2. Constricts blood vessels
3. Makes the capillaries less permeable (leaky)

SIDE EFFECTS
1. Increased heart rate
2. Pallor
3. Dizziness
4. Chest pain
5. Headache
6. Nausea
7. Vomiting
8. Excitability, anxiety

REASSESSMENT STRATEGIES
1. Transport.
2. Continue secondary assessment of airway, breathing, and circulatory status.

If the patient's condition continues to worsen (decreasing mental status, increasing breathing difficulty, decreasing blood pressure):
   a. Obtain medical direction for an additional dose of epinephrine
   b. Treat for shock (hypoperfusion)
   c. Prepare to initiate basic life support procedures (CPR, AED)

If the patient's condition improves, provide supportive care:
   a. Continue oxygen
   b. Treat for shock (hypoperfusion)

Although some patients receive instruction from their physicians in how to use the auto-injector, others will be uncomfortable or afraid to use one because of their unfamiliarity with the device and will prefer to have you help them with it. Ordinarily, when a health care provider gives an injection, the clothing over the injection site is rolled up or down and the area is cleansed with an alcohol pad. These steps are not necessary with an epinephrine auto-injector. The risk of giving a patient an infection because you did not take those steps is so small, in fact, that the manufacturer's instructions for auto-injectors do not advise patients to take those steps. However, your protocols may direct you to act differently. Follow your local protocols.

One of the most difficult things you may have to do is distinguish between the patient with a (localized) allergic reaction, who should not receive epinephrine, and the patient with a (generalized) anaphylactic reaction, who should be given epinephrine. Patients can and do present in many different ways. One patient in anaphylaxis may have severe difficulty breathing with no hives or decreased blood pressure, whereas another patient may have a rapid heartbeat and decreased blood pressure with no difficulty breathing. The important thing to recognize in any patient is the presence of *either* respiratory distress *or signs and symptoms of shock (hypoperfusion)*. Very often, both of these—indications of respiratory distress and indications of shock—are present. However, only *one* of these needs to be present for the patient to be in anaphylaxis.

CORE CONCEPT ●
Who should be assisted with an epinephrine auto-injector

Additional Doses of Epinephrine

A patient with an allergic reaction may have a compromised airway or respiratory function, or these conditions may develop as the allergic reaction progresses. Carefully monitor the patient's airway and breathing throughout your care and transport.

In your reassessment, you will frequently find that the patient's condition improves, although sometimes it will deteriorate. You may need to give additional doses of epinephrine in this case. You will be able to do this only if the patient has one or more extra auto-injectors *and* you have remembered to ask the patient to bring them in the ambulance *and* you obtain permission for the second dose from medical direction. Don't forget: If a patient has an extra epinephrine auto-injector, bring it along.

Most auto-injectors on the market today, such as the EpiPen® and EpiPen Jr®, can give only one dose of epinephrine (Figure 22-4A). Recently, an auto-injector became available that can provide two doses of epinephrine, the Twinject®, which also comes in adult and child sizes (Figure 22-4B). Because administering the second dose from the Twinject® requires you to disassemble part of the apparatus, you should become familiar with the auto-injector before you need to use it.

FIGURE 22-4 Epinephrine auto-injectors: (A) EpiPen® and EpiPen Jr®; (B) the Twinject®, which also comes in child and adult sizes.

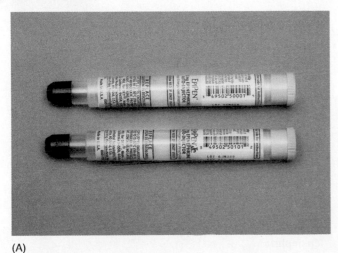

(A)

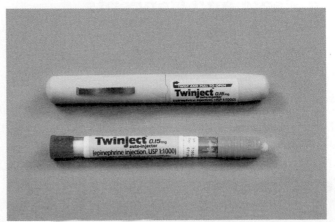

(B)

POINT OF VIEW

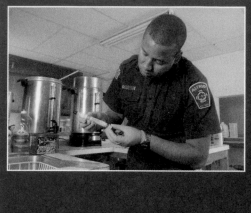

"I was at the lodge the other day. We were preparing for the holiday festival, our biggest fundraiser of the year. It is held during tourist season. We have a dinner and bake sale. I've worked it for the past 20 years, since I was a kid.

"Most people there know I have an allergy to nuts. It seems like all I have to do is look at them sometimes and I blow up and can't breathe. Someone brought some in, and the next thing I know it started. It seemed like seconds and I was wheezing and swelling up.

"My friends knew right away something was wrong. Mikey called 911 while Drew went out to my car to get my EpiPen®. The ambulance must have been right around the corner. They walked in with Drew. They took one look at me and I could see the concern in their eyes. I've seen it before.

"Fortunately, they didn't waste time. They were putting me on oxygen and getting the stretcher while the EMT in charge got the EpiPen®. It saved my life before. It did again today. They actually had to use my second EpiPen® in the ambulance because it was such a bad reaction.

"The guys joked with me when I got out of the hospital. They were going to name the lodge after me if I died. They like to joke. But I'm not sure they know just how close it was."

CHAPTER REVIEW

Key Facts and Concepts

- Allergic reactions are common. Anaphylaxis, a true life-threatening allergic reaction, is rare.

- The most common symptom in all of these cases is itching. Patients with anaphylaxis, though, will also display life-threatening difficulty breathing and/or signs and symptoms of shock (hypoperfusion). These patients will also be extremely anxious. Their bodies are in trouble and are letting the patients know it.

- The signs and symptoms of anaphylaxis are a result of physiological changes: vasodilation, bronchoconstriction, leaky capillaries, and thick mucus.

- By quickly recognizing the condition, consulting medical direction, and administering the appropriate treatment, you can literally make the difference between life and death for these patients.

Key Decisions

- Is the patient's breathing adequate, inadequate, or absent?

- Is the patient having an allergic reaction or is he having a life-threatening anaphylactic reaction? Does the patient have respiratory difficulty or shock?

- Should I assist the patient with or administer epinephrine?

Chapter Glossary

allergen something that causes an allergic reaction.

allergic reaction an exaggerated immune response.

anaphylaxis (an-ah-fi-LAK-sis) a severe or life-threatening allergic reaction in which the blood vessels dilate, causing a drop in blood pressure, and the tissues lining the respiratory system swell, interfering with the airway. Also called *anaphylactic shock*.

auto-injector a syringe preloaded with medication that has a spring-loaded device that pushes the needle through the skin when the tip of the device is pressed firmly against the body.

epinephrine (EP-uh-NEF-rin) a hormone produced by the body. As a medication, it constricts blood vessels and dilates respiratory passages and is used to relieve severe allergic reactions.

hives red, itchy, possibly raised blotches on the skin that often result from allergic reactions.

Preparation for Your Examination and Practice

Short Answer

1. What are the indications for administration of an epinephrine auto-injector?

2. List some of the more common causes of allergic reactions.

3. List signs or symptoms of an anaphylactic reaction associated with each of the following:
   - Skin
   - Respiratory system
   - Cardiovascular system

Thinking and Linking

Think back to Chapter 20, "Cardiac Emergencies," and link information from that chapter with information from this chapter as you consider the following situation:

- Your patient is a 60-year-old who used his friend's EpiPen® and is now complaining of chest pain. He thought he might have been stung and, although he wasn't sure, his friend had said: "Here, I can help you with that," handed him the EpiPen®, and helped him inject himself with epinephrine. You know that one action of epinephrine is making the heart beat more strongly. Could this be causing the patient's chest pain? How? And how should you proceed at this point to assess and care for this patient?

Critical Thinking Exercises

Anaphylactic reactions are truly life threatening. Fortunately, many patients carry their own epinephrine auto-injectors. Many ambulances also carry these lifesaving devices. Yet not all patients who have allergic reactions have anaphylaxis. The purpose of this exercise will be to determine the difference between an allergic reaction and anaphylaxis and to determine whether epinephrine should be administered.

1. Your 24-year-old patient ate a meal that he believes contained shellfish. He is allergic to shrimp. While the kitchen staff rushes to determine if shrimp was used in or near the preparation of the patient's meal, you perform an examination. The patient is sweating and nervous. He appears to be breathing adequately. You do not note any wheezing or stridor. His face is slightly red. His pulse is 88, strong and regular; respirations 24; blood pressure 108/74; and skin warm and moist.

2. You are called to a 50-year-old woman who received a narcotic pain reliever after minor dental surgery. She believes she is allergic to some pain medication but can't remember which one. She has vomited twice. One time she believes she saw blood in her vomit. Her vital signs are pulse 92, strong and regular; respirations 22 and adequate, without wheezes or stridor; blood pressure 148/86; skin warm and dry; pupils equal and reactive to light.

3. Your patient is a parent who came into his daughter's kindergarten class as a helper. After eating a cookie, he developed a funny feeling in his tongue that progressed to swelling. He is anxious and sweaty when you see him. His pulse is 126 and regular, respirations 32 and slightly labored, blood pressure 96/58, skin cool and moist, pupils equal and reactive to light.

Pathophysiology to Practice

The following question is designed to assist you in gathering relevant clinical information and making accurate decisions in the field.

- Anxiety is a common symptom in anaphylactic reactions, but anxiety alone can produce symptoms that resemble an anaphylactic reaction. What would be the effect of epinephrine on a person who appears to be having an anaphylactic reaction but is really having an anxiety attack with no anaphylaxis?

As you respond to a remote neighborhood in your district for an unknown problem, your dispatcher gives you further information about the call. She states that an elderly male has been stung several times by hornets but has not developed difficulty breathing. The dispatcher also tells you there is an ALS unit responding from the other side of town.

As you arrive on-scene, you see an older woman coming out to greet you. She appears upset as she tells you that her 68-year-old husband was doing some work in their storage shed. "I was working in the kitchen when I heard him yelling my name. As I ran outside, I could see him waving his arms around, trying to scare away the hornets."

You find Mr. Meeker sitting forward on a lawn chair at the rear of the house. You notice immediately he is using accessory muscles to breathe and that his face and neck appear flushed. He attempts to explain what has happened but is unable to speak in complete sentences.

Street Scene Questions

1. What is your impression of Mr. Meeker's condition?
2. What do you think might be happening to him?

As you apply a nonrebreather mask to the patient, Mrs. Meeker tells you that he has an allergy to hornet stings and the last time he was stung was shortly after he returned from the war in southeast Asia in the 1960s. You ask, "Does your husband carry an EpiPen®?" She tells you no. He has no other allergies, takes an aspirin daily, and had a heart attack 9 years ago.

You suspect the patient might be experiencing an allergic reaction to the insect stings and that this could be a life-threatening reaction.

As you place Mr. Meeker in the ambulance, your partner reassures the patient's wife and advises her to be careful as she follows the ambulance to the hospital. En route, you assess vital signs and find that the patient's pulse is 136 and thready, his respirations are 28 and shallow, oxygen saturation (his SpO_2) is 93 percent on 15 liters per minute O_2, and he has a blood pressure of 92/60. You notice the patient's respiratory count is falling and that he has become extremely fatigued by breathing.

Street Scene Questions

3. What do you suspect is beginning to happen to your patient?
4. What further treatment should you render?

When you reassess the patient's breathing more closely, you notice his respiratory rate has dropped significantly to about 12. Although that number is in the normal range for an adult, you realize that the depth of the patient's respirations is so shallow that he is not breathing adequately. You connect the bag-valve mask (BVM) to the oxygen tank and ventilate Mr. Meeker about 12 times a minute, making sure you ventilate him deeply enough to make his chest rise. After a few breaths, you are able to match your ventilations to the patient's so that he is not fighting against the BVM.

As it happens, the ALS intercept is delayed in a traffic snarl, and you reach the hospital before the intercept can happen. You advise the emergency department staff that you have a 68-year-old male who has been stung by several hornets and you suspect a severe allergic reaction. The staff relieves you of patient care and thanks you for the report.

Poisoning and Overdose Emergencies

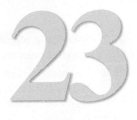

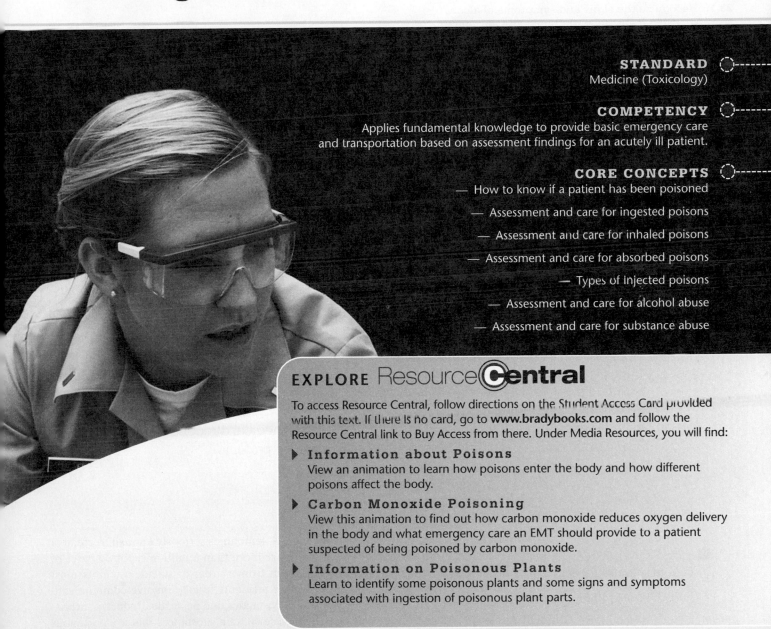

STANDARD ○--------
Medicine (Toxicology)

COMPETENCY ○--------
Applies fundamental knowledge to provide basic emergency care and transportation based on assessment findings for an acutely ill patient.

CORE CONCEPTS ○--------
— How to know if a patient has been poisoned

— Assessment and care for ingested poisons

— Assessment and care for inhaled poisons

— Assessment and care for absorbed poisons

— Types of injected poisons

— Assessment and care for alcohol abuse

— Assessment and care for substance abuse

EXPLORE Resource Central

To access Resource Central, follow directions on the Student Access Card provided with this text. If there is no card, go to **www.bradybooks.com** and follow the Resource Central link to Buy Access from there. Under Media Resources, you will find:

▶ **Information about Poisons**
View an animation to learn how poisons enter the body and how different poisons affect the body.

▶ **Carbon Monoxide Poisoning**
View this animation to find out how carbon monoxide reduces oxygen delivery in the body and what emergency care an EMT should provide to a patient suspected of being poisoned by carbon monoxide.

▶ **Information on Poisonous Plants**
Learn to identify some poisonous plants and some signs and symptoms associated with ingestion of poisonous plant parts.

OBJECTIVES

After reading this chapter you should be able to:

23.1 Define key terms introduced in this chapter.

23.2 Describe the ways in which poisons can enter the body. (pp. 547–548)

23.3 Identify potential dangers to EMS providers and others at scenes where poisoning, alcohol abuse, or substance abuse is involved. (pp. 546–567)

23.4 Collect key elements in the history of a patient who has been poisoned. (pp. 549, 554, 558)

23.5 Describe the use of activated charcoal in the management of ingested poisons. (pp. 550–553)

23.6 Explain the management of patients who have ingested a poison. (p. 553)

23.7 Develop a plan for managing patients who have inhaled poisons. (pp. 554–558)

23.8 Develop a plan for managing patients who have absorbed poisons through the skin. (pp. 558–559, 560)

23.9 Describe the health risks associated with alcohol abuse. (p. 561)

23.10 Recognize the signs and symptoms of alcohol abuse and alcohol withdrawal. (pp. 561–562)

23.11 Recognize signs, symptoms, and health risks associated with abuse of substances, including stimulants, depressants, narcotics, volatile chemicals, and hallucinogens. (pp. 563–566)

23.12 Given a variety of scenarios, develop a treatment plan for patients with emergencies related to alcohol and substance abuse. (pp. 562–563, 566–567)

KEY TERMS

absorbed poisons, *p. 548*
activated charcoal, *p. 551*
antidote, *p. 553*
delirium tremens (DTs), *p. 562*

dilution, *p. 552*
downers, *p. 564*
hallucinogens, *p. 565*
ingested poisons, *p. 547*

inhaled poisons, *p. 547*
injected poisons, *p. 548*
narcotics, *p. 564*
poison, *p. 546*

toxin, *p. 546*
uppers, *p. 563*
volatile chemicals, *p. 565*
withdrawal, *p. 562*

Hard can you, as an EMT, know that the patient you encounter at the scene of an emergency call has been poisoned? Family members or bystanders may report this fact when they call for help. There may be clues at the scene, such as empty pill bottles or containers of toxic substances, and the patient's signs and symptoms may indicate poisoning or overdose. After you identify and treat immediately life-threatening problems, such as airway or breathing difficulties, your main assessment task will be to gather information for medical direction. They will guide your care and management of the poisoning or overdose patient.

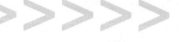

POISONING

CORE CONCEPT
How to know if a patient has been poisoned

poison
any substance that can harm the body by altering cell structure or functions.

toxin
a poisonous substance secreted by bacteria, plants, or animals.

A *poison* is any substance that can harm the body, sometimes seriously enough to create a medical emergency. In the United States, there are more than a million reported cases of poisoning annually. Although some of these result from murder or suicide attempts, most are accidental and involve young children. These incidents usually involve common substances such as medications, petroleum products, cosmetics, and pesticides. In fact, a surprisingly large percentage of chemicals in everyday use contain substances that are poisonous if misused.

We usually think of a poison as some kind of liquid or solid chemical that has been ingested by the poisoning victim. Although this is often the case, many living organisms are capable of producing a *toxin*, a substance that is poisonous to humans. For example, some mushrooms and other common plants can be poisonous if eaten. These include some varieties of house plants, including the rubber plant and certain parts of holiday plants such as mistletoe and holly berries. In addition, bacterial contaminants in food may produce toxins, some of which can cause deadly diseases (such as botulism).

A great number of substances can be considered poisonous, with different people reacting differently to various poisons (Table 23-1). As odd as it may seem, what may be a dangerous poison for one person may have little effect on another. For most poisonous substances, the reaction is far more serious in the ill, the very young, and the elderly.

Table 23-1 Common Ingested Poisons

SUBSTANCE	SIGNS AND SYMPTOMS
Acetaminophen	Nausea and vomiting. Jaundice is a delayed sign. There may be no signs or symptoms.
Acids and alkalis	Burns on or around the lips. Burning in mouth, throat, and abdomen. Vomiting.
Antiarrhythmics (drugs to regulate electrical impulses and the speed of the heart)	Bradycardia, hypotension, decreased consciousness, respiratory depression
Antidepressants (selective serotonin reuptake inhibitors)	Tachycardia, hypertension, nausea, tremors
Antihistamines and cough or cold preparations	Hyperactivity or drowsiness. Rapid pulse, flushed skin, dilated pupils.
Antipsychotics	Drowsiness, coma, tachycardia
Aspirin	Delayed signs and symptoms, including ringing in the ears, deep and rapid breathing, bruising.
Food poisoning	Different types of food poisoning have different signs and symptoms of varying onset. Most include abdominal pain, nausea, vomiting, and diarrhea, sometimes with fever.
Ibuprofen and other nonsteroidal anti-inflammatory drugs (NSAIDs)	Upset stomach, nausea, vomiting, drowsiness, abdominal pain, gastrointestinal bleeding.
Insecticides	Slow pulse, excessive salivation and sweating, nausea, vomiting, diarrhea, difficulty breathing, constricted pupils.
Petroleum products	Characteristic odor of breath, clothing, vomitus. If aspiration has occurred, coughing and difficulty breathing.
Plants	Wide range of signs and symptoms, ranging from none to nausea and vomiting to cardiac arrest.

Once on or in the body, poisons can do damage in a variety of ways. A poison may act as a corrosive or irritant, destroying skin and other body tissues. A poisonous gas can act as a suffocating agent, displacing oxygen in the air. Some poisons are systemic poisons, causing harm to the entire body or to an entire body system. These poisons can critically depress or overstimulate the central nervous system, cause vomiting and diarrhea, prevent red blood cells from carrying oxygen, or interfere with the normal biochemical processes in the body at the level of the cell. The actual effect and extent of damage is dependent on the nature of the poison, on its concentration, and sometimes on how it enters the body. These factors vary in importance depending on the patient's age, weight, and general health.

Poisons can be classified into four types, according to how they enter the body: ingested, inhaled, absorbed, and injected (Figure 23-1).

- **Ingested poisons** (poisons that are swallowed) can include many common household and industrial chemicals, medications, improperly prepared or stored foods, plant materials, petroleum products, and agricultural products made specifically to control rodents, weeds, insects, and crop diseases.
- **Inhaled poisons** (poisons that are breathed in) take the form of gases, vapors, and sprays. Again, many of these substances are in common use in the home, industry, and agriculture. Such poisons include carbon monoxide (from car exhaust, wood-burning stoves, and furnaces), ammonia, chlorine, insect sprays, and the gases produced from volatile liquid chemicals (volatile means "able to change very easily from a liquid into a gas"; many industrial solvents are volatile).

"Poisoning and overdose calls are like detective cases. Get a great history and examine the scene for clues."

ingested poisons
poisons that are swallowed.

inhaled poisons
poisons that are breathed in.

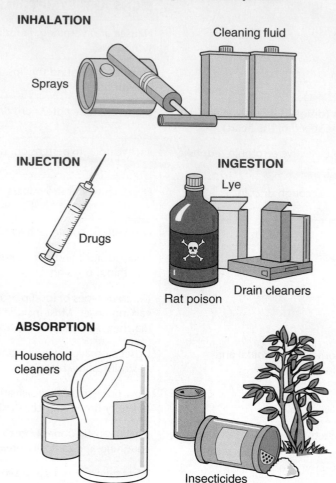

FIGURE 23-1 Poisons enter the body by way of ingestion, inhalation, absorption, and injection.

INHALATION

Sprays

Cleaning fluid

INJECTION

Drugs

INGESTION

Lye

Rat poison

Drain cleaners

ABSORPTION

Household cleaners

Insecticides

absorbed poisons

poisons that are taken into the body through unbroken skin.

injected poisons

poisons that are inserted through the skin; for example, by needle, snake fangs, or insect stinger.

- *Absorbed poisons* (poisons taken into the body through unbroken skin) may or may not damage the skin. Many are corrosives or irritants that will injure the skin and then be slowly absorbed into body tissues and the bloodstream, possibly causing widespread damage. Others are absorbed into the bloodstream without injuring the skin. Examples of these poisons include insecticides and agricultural chemicals. Contact with a variety of plant materials and certain forms of marine life can lead to skin damage and possible absorption into tissues under the skin.

- *Injected poisons* (poisons inserted through the skin) enter the body through a means that penetrates the skin. The most common injected poisons include illicit drugs injected with a needle and venoms injected by snake fangs or insect stingers. These will be discussed under "Substance Abuse," later in this chapter, and in Chapter 33, "Environmental Emergencies."

NOTE: *If you suspect intentional poisoning or attempted suicide, approach the scene with caution and have police backup if indicated.*

PEDIATRIC NOTE

Preventing poisoning is, of course, preferable to treating it. The EMT's own home and the squad building should be "childproofed" against poisoning by keeping medications and other dangerous substances out of children's reach. The EMT can also share poisoning prevention information with members of the public during school visits and community outreach activities.

Ingested Poisons

Ingested poisons are those poisons that have been swallowed. An ingested poison is often a toxic substance that a curious child eats or drinks. In adults, an ingested poison is often a medication on which the patient has accidentally or deliberately overdosed.

CORE CONCEPT ●---------

Assessment and care for ingested poisons

PATIENT ASSESSMENT

Ingested Poison

You must gather information quickly in cases of possible ingested poisoning. In order to determine if activated charcoal is appropriate, on-line medical direction will need certain information:

- **What substance was involved?** Many products have similar names. It is important to get the exact spelling of the substance. If it is possible and safe, bring the container to the hospital with the patient.

- **When did the exposure occur?** Some poisons act very quickly and will require immediate treatment. Others may take longer to affect the body, which may allow for other treatments to be used. It is important for emergency department personnel to know as closely as possible the time of ingestion so that appropriate testing and treatment can be done.

  It is sometimes difficult to determine the time of the exposure from the reports of family members or witnesses. If you cannot get an exact time, determine the earliest and latest possible times of exposure.

- **How much was ingested?** This may be determined by simply counting the number of tablets left in a brand new prescription. However, it can also be difficult to determine, such as when estimating the amount of gasoline spilled on a garage floor. When the amount cannot be reliably estimated, determine the maximum amount that might have been ingested.

- **Over how long a period did the ingestion occur?** Someone who takes a certain medication chronically and then overdoses on it may require very different hospital treatment from the patient who has the same overdose but has never taken that medication before.

- **What interventions has the patient, family, or well-meaning bystanders taken?** Many traditional home remedies for medical problems are harmful, particularly when someone has been exposed to enough of a substance to suffer ill effects. Product labels have been improved over the last few years, but some still contain inaccurate or even dangerous instructions for management of potentially toxic exposures.

- **What is the patient's estimated weight?** This estimate, in combination with the amount of substance ingested, may be critical in determining the appropriate treatment.

- **What effects is the patient experiencing from the ingestion?** Nausea and vomiting are two of the most common results of poison ingestion, but you may also find altered mental status, abdominal pain, diarrhea, chemical burns around the mouth, and unusual breath odors.

Decision Points

- Is the scene safe from whatever poisoned my patient?
- Is my patient at risk for vomiting or other airway complications?
- Do I need to consult another source, such as poison control, medical direction, ALS, or the *DOT Emergency Response Guidebook?*

Food Poisoning

Another way someone can be poisoned is through food that has been improperly handled or cooked. Food poisoning can be caused by several different bacteria that grow when exposed to the right conditions. This frequently happens when raw meat, poultry, or fish is left at room temperature before being cooked or the food does not reach a high enough temperature to kill the bacteria. Some food poisonings are the result of bacteria causing an infection in the patient

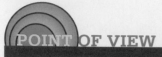

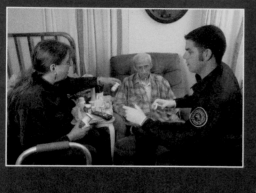

"We were sent to a call for an older patient with an altered mental status. We have a considerable older population in our community and a lot of assisted living places.

"You read in the news that people are getting older and living longer. Medicine has helped people do this. I was on a call the other day. I looked at this nice older man. You wouldn't believe how many medications he had. It was crazy.

"I'm not saying he didn't need them. That's not my place. But with just a little confusion or disorganization he could double up on powerful cardiac meds or change his blood sugar or blood pressure or thyroid levels. His daughter thought that is what happened.

"I guess, on the good side, the medications helped us figure out his medical history. We rarely get the full story from the patient and family.

"I know in this case it took 5 minutes just to get his history list of meds. It actually is an issue we see a lot."

(symptoms may occur a day or so after ingestion); other times it may be the result of toxins formed by the bacteria that contaminate the food, and it is these toxins that result in symptoms (usually within hours of ingestion). Signs and symptoms vary somewhat, depending on the bacteria involved, but frequently include nausea, vomiting, abdominal cramps, diarrhea, and fever.

You can prevent food poisoning at home and at the station by washing your hands, utensils, cutting boards, and any surface the food touches before—and especially after—any contact with raw meat, fish, or poultry (the bacteria can easily be spread to other foods from hands or surfaces); by storing and cooking foods at appropriate temperatures; and by not leaving raw or cooked foods at room temperature for long periods of time.

Activated Charcoal

To provide the proper emergency care for ingested poisons (Scan 23-1), follow the instructions given to you by medical direction or your regional poison control center. In some cases of ingested poisoning, medical direction will order administration of ***activated charcoal*** (Scan 23-2).

Activated charcoal works through adsorption, the process of one substance becoming attached to the surface of another. In contrast to ordinary charcoal, which adsorbs some substances, activated charcoal has been manufactured to have many cracks and crevices. As a result, activated charcoal has an increased amount of surface available for poisons to bind to (similar to corrugated cardboard which, if you cut it open, has many more surfaces than you would expect by looking at the smooth outer surface). Activated charcoal is not an antidote; however, through the adsorption or binding process, in many cases it will prevent or reduce the amount of poison available for the body to absorb.

Many poisons are adsorbed by activated charcoal, but not all. Since there are millions of potential poisons available and the number is always increasing, it makes little sense to memorize lists of poisons where activated charcoal should not be used. Instead, medical direction (possibly in consultation with a poison control center) will determine whether the use of activated charcoal is appropriate.

There are, however, a few instances you should know about where the use of activated charcoal is contraindicated:

- Patients who cannot swallow obviously cannot swallow activated charcoal.
- Patients with altered mental status might choke on activated charcoal and aspirate it into the lungs.
- Patients who have ingested acids or alkalis should not take activated charcoal because the caustic material may have severely damaged the mouth, throat, and esophagus. Activated charcoal cannot help the damage that has already been done, and swallowing it may cause further damage. Examples of such caustic substances are oven cleaners, drain cleaners, toilet bowl cleaners, and lye.

FIRST TAKE STANDARD PRECAUTIONS.

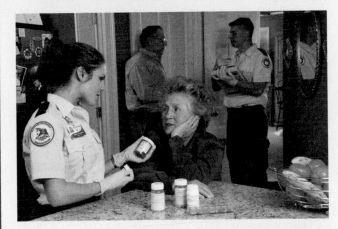

1 Quickly gather information.

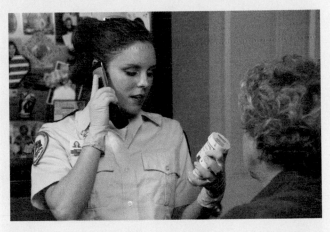

2 Call medical direction on the scene or en route to the hospital.

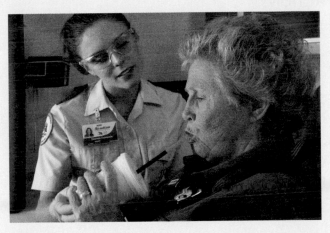

3 If directed, administer activated charcoal. You may wish to administer the medication in an opaque cup that has a lid with a hole for a straw.

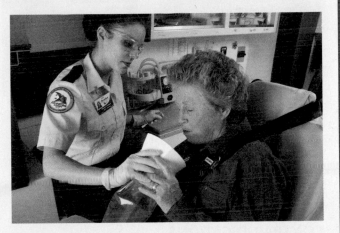

4 Position the patient for vomiting and save all vomitus. Have suction equipment ready.

NOTE: *When a patient has ingested a poison, it provides another reason to avoid mouth-to-mouth contact. Provide ventilations through a pocket face mask or other barrier device.*

- Patients who have accidentally swallowed while siphoning gasoline should not be given activated charcoal. The patient will be coughing violently and possibly aspirating the gasoline. This patient will be unable to swallow activated charcoal.

In addition, activated charcoal is not indicated in cases of food poisoning.

Many brands of activated charcoal are on the market, but some have greater surface area than others. Medical direction can guide you in the selection of an appropriate brand.

Some patients, especially those who have taken an intentional overdose, may refuse to take activated charcoal. Never attempt to force a patient to swallow activated charcoal. If the patient refuses, notify medical direction and continue reassessment and care.

Activated Charcoal vs. Syrup of Ipecac A traditional treatment for poisoning used to be syrup of ipecac. This orally administered drug causes vomiting in most people with just

activated charcoal
a substance that adsorbs many poisons and prevents them from being absorbed by the body.

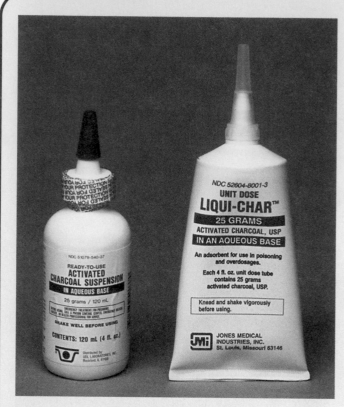

DOSAGE

1. Adults and children: 1 gram activated charcoal/kg of body weight
2. Usual adult dose: 25 to 50 grams
3. Usual pediatric dose: 12.5 to 25 grams

ADMINISTRATION

1. Consult medical direction.
2. Shake container thoroughly.
3. Since medication looks like mud, the patient may need to be persuaded to drink it. Providing a covered container and a straw will prevent the patient from seeing the medication and so may improve patient compliance.
4. If the patient does not drink the medication right away, the charcoal will settle. Shake or stir it again before administering.
5. Record the name, dose, route, and time of administration of the medication.

ACTIONS

1. Activated charcoal adsorbs (binds) certain poisons and prevents them from being absorbed into the body.
2. Not all brands of activated charcoal are the same. Some adsorb much more than others, so consult medical direction about the brand to use.

SIDE EFFECTS

1. Some patients have black stools.
2. Some patients may vomit, particularly those who have ingested poisons that cause nausea. If the patient vomits, repeat the dose once.

REASSESSMENT STRATEGIES

1. Be prepared for the patient to vomit or further deteriorate.

MEDICATION NAME

1. Generic: activated charcoal
2. Trade: SuperChar, InstaChar, Actidose, Liqui-Char, and others

INDICATIONS

Poisoning by mouth

CONTRAINDICATIONS

1. Altered mental status
2. Ingestion of acids or alkalis
3. Inability to swallow

MEDICATION FORM

1. Premixed in water, frequently available in a plastic bottle containing 12.5 grams of activated charcoal
2. Powder—should be avoided in the field

one dose. When vomiting occurs, it results, on the average, in removal of less than one-third of the stomach contents. Because ipecac is slow, is relatively ineffective, and has the potential to make a patient aspirate vomitus, it is rarely used today.

Although poison control centers on rare occasions instruct parents of young children in the proper use of syrup of ipecac, activated charcoal is the medication of first choice for health care providers in most poisoning and overdose cases.

dilution (di-LU-shun)
thinning down or weakening by mixing with something else. Ingested poisons are sometimes diluted by drinking water or milk.

Dilution

Occasionally, medical direction will give an order for **dilution** of a poisonous substance. This means an adult patient should drink one to two glasses of water or milk, whichever is ordered. A child should typically be given one-half to one full glass. Dilution with water may slow absorption slightly, whereas milk may soothe stomach upset. This treatment is frequently advised for patients who, as determined by medical direction or poison control, do not need transport to a hospital.

PATIENT CARE

Ingested Poison

Emergency care of a patient who has ingested poison includes the following steps:

1. Detect and treat immediately life-threatening problems in the primary assessment. Evaluate the need for prompt transport for critical patients.
2. Perform a secondary assessment. Use gloved hands to carefully remove any pills, tablets, or fragments from the patient's mouth; package the material and transport it with the patient.
3. Assess baseline vital signs.
4. Consult medical direction. As directed, administer activated charcoal to adsorb the poison, or water or milk to dilute it. This can usually be done en route.
5. Transport the patient with all containers, bottles, and labels from the substance.
6. Perform reassessment en route.

NOTE: *Sometimes patients who have ingested poisons will require assisted ventilations. Direct mouth-to-mouth ventilation in such a case is dangerous, not only because of the danger of contracting an infectious disease but also because of possible contact with poisonous substances remaining on the patient's lips, in the airway, or in his vomitus. Use a pocket face mask with a one-way valve, a bag-valve-mask unit with supplemental oxygen, or positive pressure ventilation when providing ventilations to a patient who is suspected of ingesting a poison.*

Antidotes

Many laypeople think that every poison has an *antidote*, a substance that will neutralize the poison or its effects. This is not true. There are only a few genuine antidotes, and they can be used only with a very small number of poisons. Modern treatment of poisonings and overdoses consists primarily of prevention of absorption when possible (such as by administration of activated charcoal) and good supportive treatment (such as airway maintenance, administration of oxygen, treatment for shock). In a small number of poisonings, advanced treatments are administered in a hospital (administration of antidotes and kidney dialysis).

antidote
a substance that will neutralize the poison or its effects.

PEDIATRIC NOTE

It is the nature of infants and children to explore their world—and to get into and often taste whatever they find. Children will swallow substances adults cannot imagine swallowing, including horrible-tasting poisonous substances like bleach or lye. The natural curiosity of children makes them the most frequent victims of accidental poisoning.

It is important to find out an infant's or child's weight, which—in combination with the estimated amount of the poisonous substance that was ingested—will help medical direction determine appropriate treatment.

As an EMT, always assume that the infant or child has ingested a lethal amount of the poison. Because it is usually extremely difficult or impossible to be sure exactly how much the child has taken in, always treat for the worst. Call medical direction, administer the recommended treatments, and transport the child to the hospital.

Inhaled Poisons

Inhaled poisons are those that are present in the atmosphere and that you, as well as the patient, are at risk of breathing in. Carbon monoxide poisoning is a common problem. Other possible inhaled poisons include chlorine gas (often from swimming pool chemicals), ammonia (often released from household cleaners), sprayed agricultural chemicals and pesticides, and carbon dioxide (from industrial sources).

CORE CONCEPT
Assessment and care for inhaled poisons

Inside/Outside

Acetaminophen overdose is the most common cause of hospitalization of overdose patients. This is not surprising, given its effectiveness as an analgesic and its presence as an ingredient in many medications. It is very safe in recommended doses for healthy people who do not abuse alcohol or have liver problems, but acetaminophen is very dangerous in overdose. Fortunately, the toxic effects of acetaminophen do not appear right away. After someone takes too much of the drug, the liver becomes overwhelmed and unable to detoxify the substance. Over the next several hours, the liver sustains irreparable damage if nothing is done. If the antidote is given within the first 4 to 12 hours after an overdose, however, the patient should recover with a functioning liver.

Unfortunately, the signs and symptoms of acetaminophen overdose are delayed and not very specific. During the first 4 to 12 hours, the most the patient may experience is loss of appetite, nausea, and vomiting. It isn't until a day or two later that the patient typically experiences right upper quadrant pain and jaundice, when it is too late for the antidote to work.

This points out the importance of several aspects of prehospital assessment and management:

- Suspect acetaminophen poisoning in conjunction with any other overdose.
- It may be appropriate to search medicine cabinets and garbage cans for empty pill bottles, depending on the circumstances.
- Deal with apparent threats to life first. Because the effects of acetaminophen poisoning are delayed, there is time to institute treatment in the hospital.

NOTE: *If you suspect that a patient has inhaled a poison, approach the scene with care. Some EMS systems provide training in the use of protective clothing and self-contained breathing apparatus (SCBA) to be used in a hostile environment (such as chlorine gas, ammonia, or smoke). Remember that many inhaled poisons can also be absorbed through the skin. Go only where your protective equipment and clothing will allow you to go safely to perform your mission, and only after you have been trained in the use of this equipment. Do only what you have been trained to do and go only where your protective equipment will allow you to go safely. If you do not have the necessary equipment or training, get someone there who is properly equipped and trained.*

PATIENT ASSESSMENT

Inhaled Poison

Gather the following information as quickly as possible:

- **What substance was involved?** Get its exact name.
- **When did the exposure occur?** Estimate as well as you can when the patient was exposed to the poisonous gas by finding out the earliest and latest possible times of exposure.
- **Over how long a period did the exposure occur?** The longer someone is exposed to a poisonous gas, the more poison that will probably be absorbed.
- **What interventions has anyone taken?** Did someone remove the patient or ventilate the area right away? When did this happen?
- **What effects is the patient experiencing from the exposure?** Nausea and vomiting are very common in poisoning of all types. With inhaled poisons, find out if the patient is having difficulty breathing, chest pain, coughing, hoarseness, dizziness, headache, confusion, seizures, or altered mental status.

PATIENT CARE

Inhaled Poison

The principal prehospital treatment of inhaled poisoning consists of maintaining the airway and supporting respiration (Scan 23-3). In the case of inhaled poisoning, oxygen is a very important drug. Some inhaled poisons prevent the blood from transporting oxygen in the normal manner. Some prevent oxygen from getting into the bloodstream in the first

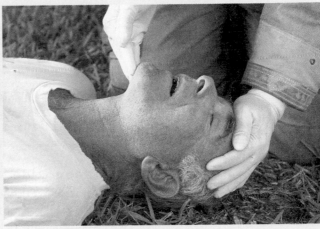

1 Remove the patient from the source of the poison.

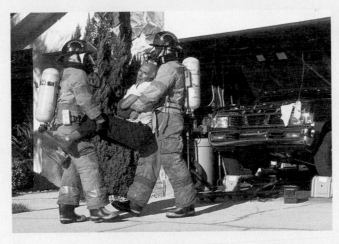

2 Establish an open airway.

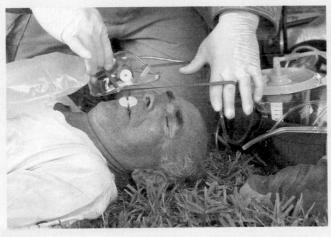

3 Insert an oropharyngeal or nasopharyngeal airway and administer high-concentration oxygen by

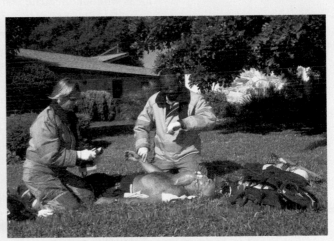

4 Gather the patient's history, take baseline vital signs, and expose the chest for auscultation.

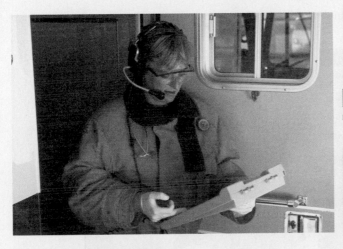

5 Contact medical direction.

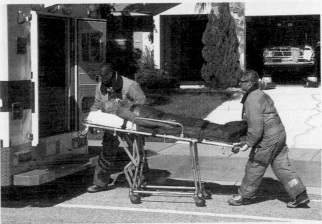

6 Transport the patient.

NOTE: *In the presence of hazardous fumes or gases, wear protective clothing and self-contained breathing apparatus or wait for those who are properly trained and equipped to enter the scene and bring the patient out.*

place. In either case, your ability to keep the airway open, ventilate as needed, and give high-concentration oxygen may make the difference in the patient's survival and quality of life.

Emergency care steps include the following:

1. If the patient is in an unsafe environment, have trained rescuers remove the patient to a safe area. Detect and treat immediately life-threatening problems in the primary assessment. Evaluate the need to promptly transport critical patients.
2. Perform a secondary assessment; obtain vital signs.
3. Administer high-concentration oxygen. This is the single most important treatment for inhaled poisoning after the patient's airway is opened.
4. Transport the patient with all containers, bottles, and labels from the substance.
5. Perform reassessment en route.

Carbon Monoxide

Carbon monoxide (CO), one of the most commonly inhaled poisons, is usually associated with motor-vehicle exhaust and fire suppression. The number of carbon monoxide cases has increased recently because of the carbon monoxide that can accumulate from the use of improperly vented wood-burning stoves and the use of charcoal for heating and indoor cooking in areas without adequate ventilation. Malfunctioning oil-, gas-, and coal-burning furnaces and stoves can also be sources of carbon monoxide. The indoor use of gasoline-powered small engines such as electrical generators or pumps is another common cause of CO poisoning.

Since carbon monoxide is an odorless, colorless, and tasteless gas, you will not be able to directly detect its presence without special equipment (Figure 23-2). Look for indications of possible carbon monoxide poisoning like wood-burning stoves, doors that lead to a garage, bedrooms above a garage where motor repair work is in progress, and evidence that suggests the patient has spent a long period of time sitting in an idling motor vehicle. When inhaled, carbon monoxide prevents the normal carrying of oxygen by the red blood cells. Long exposure, even to low levels of the gas, can cause dramatic effects. Death may occur as hypoxia becomes more severe.

The signs and symptoms of carbon monoxide poisoning are deceptive, because they can resemble those of the flu. Specifically, you may see:

- Headache, especially "a band around the head"
- Dizziness
- Breathing difficulty
- Nausea
- Cyanosis
- Altered mental status; in severe cases, unconsciousness may result

FIGURE 23-2 Special monitors are needed to detect the presence of carbon monoxide in the environment.

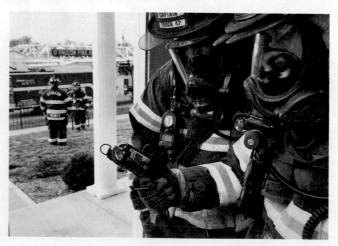

You should suspect carbon monoxide poisoning whenever you are treating a patient with vague, flu-like symptoms who has been in an enclosed area. This is especially true when a group of people in the same area have similar symptoms. A patient with carbon monoxide poisoning may begin to feel better shortly after being removed from the dangerous environment. However, it is still very important to continue to administer oxygen and to transport these patients to a hospital. Oxygen is an antidote for carbon monoxide poisoning, but it takes time to "wash out" the carbon monoxide from the patient's bloodstream. These patients need medical evaluation because they can have serious consequences, including neurological deficits, from their exposure.

NOTE: *There is a commonly accepted idea that a patient exposed to carbon monoxide will have cherry red lips. In fact, cherry red skin is NOT typically seen in patients with carbon monoxide poisoning.*

Smoke Inhalation

Smoke inhalation is a serious problem associated with fire scenes. Smoke inhalation is often associated with thermal burns as well as with the effects of chemical poisons within the smoke. The smoke from any fire source contains many poisonous substances. Modern building materials and furnishings often contain plastics and other synthetics that release toxic fumes when they burn or are overheated. It is possible for the substances found in smoke to burn the skin, irritate the eyes, injure the airway, cause respiratory arrest, and, in some cases, cause cardiac arrest.

As an EMT, you will most likely find irritated (reddened, watering) eyes and, of far greater concern, injury to the airway associated with smoke.

The following signs indicate an airway injured by smoke inhalation:

- Difficulty breathing
- Coughing
- Breath that has a "smoky" smell or the odor of chemicals involved at the scene
- Black (carbon) residue in the patient's mouth and nose
- Black residue in any sputum coughed up by the patient
- Nose hairs singed from superheated air

Move the patient suffering from smoke inhalation to a safe area and provide the same care you would provide for any inhaled poison: assess the patient, administer high-concentration oxygen, and transport.

NOTE: *The body's reaction to toxic gases and foreign matter in the airway can often be delayed. Convince all smoke inhalation patients that they must be seen by a physician, even if they are not yet feeling serious effects.*

"Detergent Suicides"

A method of suicide that is popular in Japan has started to make inroads in the United States. By mixing two easily obtained chemicals, a person can cause the release of toxic hydrogen sulfide gas. In Japan, the chemicals involved are frequently toilet cleaner and bath salts, leading to the name "detergent suicide." The same kind of bath salts are not available in the United States, but other chemicals that are available in the United States can lead to the same result. Typically, a source of acid, such as a strong household cleaner, and a source of sulfur, often a pesticide, will quickly release significant amounts of toxic hydrogen sulfide gas when mixed together.

Hydrogen sulfide is best known for its rotten egg odor, but less well known is that, even at moderate concentrations, it can be quite dangerous. Hydrogen sulfide not only takes the place of oxygen but also bonds with iron in cells, preventing oxygen from binding to those cells and getting to where it is needed. Mild exposure can result in coughing, eye irritation, and sore throat. More severe exposures can lead to dizziness, nausea, shortness of breath, headache, and vomiting. In severe cases, fluid will collect in the lungs (pulmonary edema), resulting in death.

The typical method of committing suicide in Japan with this toxic gas includes combining the chemicals in a small enclosed space and posting warning signs advising people not to try to gain access to the patient but to call a hazardous materials team. Although this warning is common in Japan, it is not clear how often others attempting suicide in this manner will be so courteous toward rescuers.

Although this method of suicide has not yet become common in the United States, EMTs must be extremely careful when approaching a scene where a "detergent suicide" may have taken place. Warning signs to look for include a small enclosed space, such as a car, with tape sealing the windows and doors. Any kind of sign or note warning people not to approach should be taken very seriously. Call the appropriate agency to open the space and remove the body. Do not become another casualty.

Absorbed Poisons

CORE CONCEPT

Assessment and care for absorbed poisons

Absorbed poisons frequently irritate or damage the skin. However, some poisons can be absorbed with little or no damage to the skin.

> **NOTE:** *Just as poisonous substances can be absorbed by patients, they can also be absorbed by EMTs. It is critical that the EMT take protective measures to prevent exposure to these substances. It may be necessary for firefighters to decontaminate a patient before the EMT touches him.*

PATIENT ASSESSMENT

Absorbed Poison

When treating a patient with absorbed poisoning, gather the following information as quickly as possible:

- **What substance was involved?** Get its exact name. (If the exposure occurs at a commercial site, then by law material safety data sheets (MSDS) should be available on-site that will help identify the substance.)
- **When did the exposure occur?**
- **How much of the substance was the patient exposed to?** How large an area of skin was the substance on?
- **Over how long a period did the exposure occur?** The longer someone's skin is exposed to a poison, the more likely it is to be well absorbed.
- **What interventions has anyone taken?** Did someone attempt to wash the substance off the patient? If so, with what? Did anyone attempt to use a chemical to "neutralize" the substance?
- **What effects is the patient experiencing from the exposure?** Common signs and symptoms include a liquid or powder on the patient's skin, burns, itching, irritation, and redness.

PATIENT CARE

Absorbed Poison

Emergency care of a patient with absorbed poisons includes the following steps:

1. Detect and treat immediately life-threatening problems in the primary assessment. Evaluate the need for prompt transport of critical patients.
2. Perform a secondary assessment; obtain vital signs. This includes removing contaminated clothing while protecting oneself from contamination.
3. Remove the poison by doing one of the following:
   - **Powders.** Brush powder off the patient, then continue as for other absorbed poisons.
   - **Liquids.** Irrigate with clean water for at least 20 minutes and continue en route if possible.
   - **Eyes.** Irrigate with clean water for at least 20 minutes and continue en route if possible.
4. Transport the patient with all containers, bottles, MSDS sheets, and labels from the substance.
5. Perform reassessment en route.

 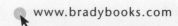

The most important part of the treatment of a patient with an absorbed poison is to get the poison off the skin or out of the eye (Scan 23-4). The best way to do this is by irrigating the skin or the eye with large amounts of clean water. A garden hose or fire hose can be used to irrigate the patient's skin, but care must be taken not to injure the skin further with high pressure.

"Neutralizing" acids or alkalis with solutions such as dilute vinegar or baking soda in water should *not* be done. When incidents like these occur, such substances are almost never readily available. Even if they were, they would not be appropriate. They have never been shown to help, and there is good reason to believe they would make matters worse. When an acid is mixed with an alkali, it is true that the two may be neutralized. It is also true, though, that this reaction produces heat. Skin that has been injured already by an acid or alkali may be further damaged by attempts to neutralize the chemical.

Injected Poisons

As mentioned earlier, the most common injected poisons are illicit drugs injected with a needle (which will be discussed later in this chapter) and the venom of snakes and insects (which will be covered in Chapter 33, "Environmental Emergencies").

CORE CONCEPT ●--------------
Types of injected poisons

Poison Control Centers

Emergency care in poisoning cases presents special problems for the EMT. Signs and symptoms can vary greatly. Some poisons produce a characteristic set of signs and symptoms very quickly, whereas others are subtle and slow to appear. Poisons that act almost immediately usually produce obvious signs, and the particular poison or its container is often still nearby. Slow-acting poisons can produce effects that mimic an infectious disease or some other medical emergency.

There will be times when you will not know the substance that caused the poisoning. In some of these cases, an expert may be able to tell, based on the combination of signs and symptoms. Even when you know the source of the poison, correct emergency care procedures may still be in question. Ideas about proper care keep changing as more research is done on poisoning. This constant change makes it impossible to print guides and charts for poison control and care that will be up-to-date when you use them. Although manufacturers have improved the instructions on many container labels, some still have inaccurate or even dangerous advice.

Fortunately, a network of poison control centers exists to provide information and advice to both laypeople and health care providers. Throughout the United States, it is possible to reach a poison control center 24 hours a day. Dialing 1-800-222-1222 connects you with the poison center covering the area the call is coming from. Your EMS agency may also have a local number for your regional poison center. Either number will work.

An EMT should consult a poison control center only when directed by local protocol. In most cases, EMTs get medical direction from physicians or nurses who are in hospital emergency departments. Unless special arrangements have been made, the poison control center staff does not have the authority to provide on-line medical direction. If the poison control center staff does have the authority to do so, they can tell you what should be done for most cases of poisoning.

If you are permitted to communicate directly with the poison control center in your area, do so by telephone. Even if you have radio contact with your local poison control center, the telephone is the preferred way to communicate. The staff member may need to talk to you for several minutes, far too long a period to monopolize the air waves. The telephone will also allow you to maintain patient confidentiality. Make certain you have memorized the number and/or carry the poison control center number with you into the residence—perhaps pasted inside your kit—so that you do not have to return to the rig to get it.

To help the poison control center staff, gather all of the information you need before you call.

Many people have the impression that the poison control center should be called only for cases of ingested poisonings. However, the center's staff can provide valuable care information for all types of poisoning.

Your community may have special poisoning problems. For example, not every community is exposed to rattlesnakes, jellyfish, or powerful agricultural chemicals. Many EMS systems have compiled lists of poisoning problems specific for their areas. Check to see if this has been done for the area in which you will be an EMT.

FIRST TAKE STANDARD PRECAUTIONS.

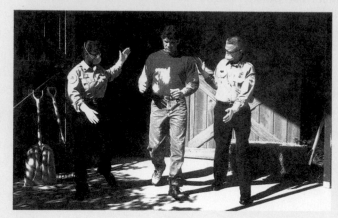

① Remove the patient from the source or the source from the patient. Avoid contaminating yourself with the poison.

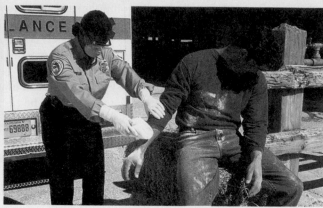

② Brush powders from the patient. Be careful not to abrade the patient's skin.

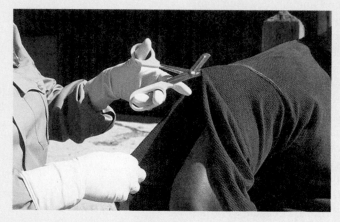

③ Remove contaminated clothing and other articles.

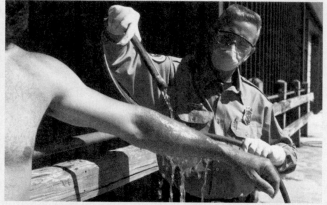

④ Irrigate with clear water for at least 20 minutes. Catch contaminated runoff and dispose of it safely.

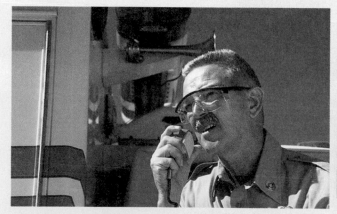

⑤ Contact medical direction.

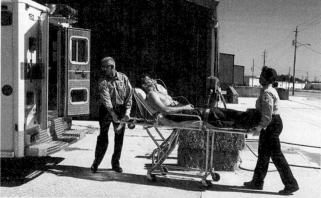

⑥ Transport the patient.

NOTE: *Take care to protect your skin from contact with poisonous substances. Wear protective clothing. If necessary, have firefighters or others who are properly protected hose off the patient before you touch him.*

ALCOHOL AND SUBSTANCE ABUSE

Many patients' conditions are caused directly or indirectly by alcohol or drug abuse—problems that cross all geographic and economic boundaries.

Alcohol Abuse

Many persons consume alcohol without having any problems. However, others occasionally or chronically abuse alcohol. Even though adults can legally drink alcohol, it is still a drug that can have a potent effect on a person's central nervous system. Emergencies arising from the use of alcohol may be due to the effect of alcohol that has just been consumed, or it may be the result of the cumulative effects of years of alcohol abuse.

EMTs often do not take alcohol abuse patients seriously. This may be due to some such patients' belligerent or unusual behavior, frequent calls to EMS when intoxicated, or less than desirable hygiene. Nevertheless, you should provide care for the patient suffering from alcohol abuse the same as you would for any other patient. Patients who appear intoxicated must be treated with the same respect and dignity as those who are "sober."

Above all, you must not neglect your duty to provide medical care. Not only do alcohol-abuse patients often have injuries from accidents and falls but they are also candidates for many medical emergencies. Chronic drinkers (alcoholics) often have derangements in blood sugar levels, poor nutrition, the potential for considerable gastrointestinal bleeding, and other problems. A person can be both intoxicated and having a heart attack or hypoglycemia. If the patient has ingested alcohol and other drugs, this can produce a serious medical emergency. When alcohol is combined with other depressants such as antihistamines and tranquilizers, the effects of alcohol can be more pronounced and, in some cases, lethal.

Since EMT safety is a critical part of all calls, do not hesitate to ask for police assistance with any patient who appears intoxicated or irrational or exhibits potentially dangerous behavior. The nature of intoxication is such that a passive person may suddenly become aggressive. Always be prepared for this event.

CORE CONCEPT
Assessment and care for alcohol abuse

CRITICAL DECISION MAKING

Find the Clues

Poisoning and overdose emergencies are challenging in that you will need to figure out what toxin caused the patient's current signs and symptoms. Your ability to examine the scene and report accurate findings to poison control are vital to the patient's well-being. In each of the following scenarios, decide what information you will need to gather—and where to obtain it—to ensure proper treatment for the patient.

1. Your patient states he has taken an overdose of prescription medications.
2. Your patient is found in a closed garage with the car running.
3. Your patient is found in the garden, confused and drooling.

PATIENT ASSESSMENT

Alcohol Abuse

Keep in mind that, although alcohol abuse may be the patient's only problem, there may be another problem present. Conduct a complete assessment to identify any medical emergencies. Remember that diabetes, epilepsy, head injuries, high fevers, hypoxia, and other medical problems may make the patient appear to be intoxicated when he is not. Also look for injuries. Do not allow the presence of alcohol or the signs and symptoms of alcohol abuse to override your suspicions of other medical problems or injuries.

Since getting a history from any patient who appears intoxicated will be difficult and perhaps unreliable, your powers of observation and resourcefulness will be tested. Family members and bystanders may provide important information.

The following list contains signs and symptoms of alcohol abuse:

- Odor of alcohol on the patient's breath or clothing. By itself, however, this is not enough to conclude alcohol abuse. Be certain that the odor is not "acetone breath," as with some diabetic emergencies.
- Swaying and unsteadiness of movement
- Slurred speech, rambling thought patterns, incoherent words or phrases
- A flushed appearance to the face, often with the patient sweating and complaining of being warm
- Nausea or vomiting
- Poor coordination
- Slowed reaction time
- Blurred vision
- Confusion
- Hallucinations, visual or auditory ("seeing things" or "hearing things")
- Lack of memory (blackout)
- Altered mental status

withdrawal

referring to alcohol or drug withdrawal in which the patient's body reacts severely when deprived of the abused substance.

delirium tremens (duh-LEER-e-um TREM-uns) **(DTs)**

a severe reaction that can be part of alcohol withdrawal, characterized by sweating, trembling, anxiety, and hallucinations. Severe alcohol withdrawal with the DTs can lead to death if untreated.

The alcoholic patient may not be under the influence of alcohol but, instead, may be suffering from alcohol **withdrawal**. This can be a severe condition occurring when the alcoholic patient cannot obtain alcohol, is too sick to drink alcohol, or has decided to quit drinking suddenly. The alcohol-withdrawal patient may experience seizures or **delirium tremens (DTs)**, a condition characterized by sweating, trembling, anxiety, and hallucinations. In some cases, alcohol withdrawal can be fatal. Signs of alcohol withdrawal include:

- Confusion and restlessness
- Unusual behavior, to the point of demonstrating "insane" behavior
- Hallucinations
- Gross tremor (obvious shaking) of the hands
- Profuse sweating
- Seizures (common and often very serious)
- Hypertension
- Tachycardia

Be on the alert for signals—such as depressed vital signs—that the patient has mixed alcohol and drugs. Also, when interviewing the intoxicated patient or the patient suffering from alcohol withdrawal, do not begin by asking the patient if he is taking drugs. He may react to this question as if you are gathering evidence of a crime. Ask if any medications have been taken while drinking. If necessary, when you are certain that the patient knows you are concerned about his well-being, you can repeat the question using the word *drugs*.

NOTE: *All patients with seizures or DTs must be transported to a medical facility as soon as possible.*

PATIENT CARE

Alcohol Abuse

Since alcohol abuse patients often vomit, take Standard Precautions, including gloves, mask, and protective eyewear as necessary. To provide basic care for the intoxicated patient and the patient suffering alcohol withdrawal, follow these steps:

1. Stay alert for airway and respiratory problems. Be prepared to perform airway maintenance, suctioning, and positioning of the patient should the patient lose consciousness, seize, or vomit. Help the patient so that vomitus will not be aspirated. Have a rigid-tip suction device ready. Provide oxygen and assist respirations as needed.
2. Assess for trauma the patient may be unaware of because of his intoxication.

3. Be alert for changes in mental status as alcohol is absorbed into the bloodstream. Talk to the patient in an effort to keep him as alert as possible.
4. Monitor vital signs.
5. Treat for shock.
6. Protect the patient from self-injury. Use restraint as authorized by your EMS system. Request assistance from law enforcement if needed. Protect yourself and your crew.
7. Stay alert for seizures.
8. Transport the patient to a medical facility.

Note that, in some systems, patients under the influence of alcohol who are not suffering from a medical emergency or apparent injury are not transported. They are given over to the police. This may not be wise since some patients having an alcohol-related emergency may die if they don't receive additional care. In addition, EMS personnel may have missed a medical problem or injury. Remember that the patient's condition may worsen as the alcohol continues to be absorbed by his system. Be especially careful of patients with even minor head injuries, since subdural hematoma (see Chapter 31, "Trauma to the Head, Neck, and Spine") is common in alcoholics.

NOTE: *A PATIENT UNDER THE INFLUENCE OF ALCOHOL CANNOT MAKE AN INFORMED REFUSAL OF TREATMENT OR TRANSPORT. If the patient refuses treatment or transport, you should nevertheless treat and arrange for transport of the patient as necessary on the basis of implied consent. Always contact medical direction before transporting a patient against his will. Document this in your prehospital care report.*

Substance Abuse

Substance abuse is a term that indicates a chemical substance is being taken for other than therapeutic (medical) reasons. Many substances have legitimate purposes when used properly. When these same substances are abused, however, the results can be devastating. Not only are substance abuse patients at risk for dangerous effects of the substances they abuse, they are also at increased risk of trauma as a result of their impaired judgment when under the influence and the inherent risks of violence related to "drug deals."

Individuals who abuse drugs and other chemical substances should be considered to have an illness. Therefore, they have the right to the same professional emergency care as any other patient.

The most common drugs and chemical substances that are abused and can lead to problems requiring an EMS response (Figure 23-3) can be classified as uppers, downers, narcotics, hallucinogens, and volatile chemicals.

- ***Uppers*** are stimulants that affect the nervous system and excite the user. Many abusers use these drugs in an attempt to relieve fatigue or to create feelings of well-being. Examples are caffeine, amphetamines, and cocaine. Cocaine may be "snorted," smoked, or injected. Other stimulants are frequently taken in pill form.

CORE CONCEPT

Assessment and care for substance abuse

uppers

stimulants such as amphetamines that affect the central nervous system to excite the user.

FIGURE 23-3 These substances are often abused.

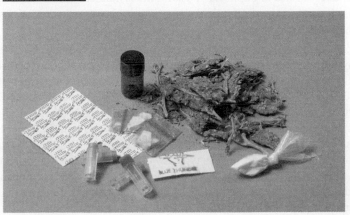

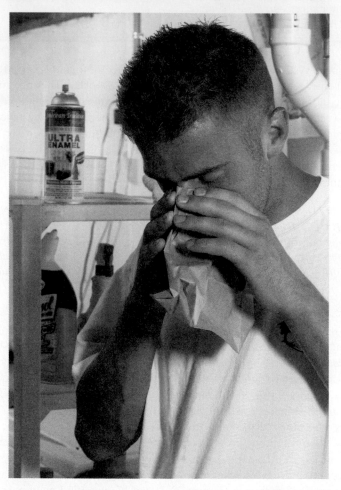

FIGURE 23-4 Volatile chemicals produce vapors that can be inhaled. Methods of inhaling substances include "huffing" (breathing fumes directly or from a substance-impregnated fabric) and "bagging" (breathing fumes from a substance sprayed into a bag).

downers

depressants, such as barbiturates, that depress the central nervous system, which are often used to bring on a more relaxed state of mind.

narcotics

a class of drugs that affect the nervous system and change many normal body activities. Their legal use is for the relief of pain. Illicit use is to produce an intense state of relaxation.

- **Downers** have a depressant effect on the central nervous system. This type of drug may be used as a relaxing agent, sleeping pill, or tranquilizer. Barbiturates are an example, usually in pill or capsule form. One example of a downer that you may encounter on an EMS call is Rohypnol (flunitrazepam), also known as Roofies. Because it is colorless, odorless, tasteless, and has been put into unsuspecting people's drinks, it has become known as a "date rape" drug. Another downer you may see is GHB (gamma-Hydroxybutyrate), also known as Georgia Home Boy or goop. In addition to depressing the central nervous system, it produces a sense of euphoria and sometimes hallucinations. It has caused respiratory depression so severe that patients have required assisted ventilations even though some of them were still breathing.

- **Narcotics** are drugs capable of producing stupor or sleep. They are often used to relieve pain. Many drugs legitimately used for these purposes (such as codeine) are also abused, affecting the nervous system and changing many of the normal activities of the body, often producing an intense state of relaxation or feeling of well-being. A relatively new narcotic, OxyContin (oxycodone), has become a common drug of abuse. This is unfortunate, because it has done an excellent job of controlling chronic pain in patients with certain conditions. Illegal narcotics such as heroin are also commonly abused. Heroin is often injected into a vein. Other narcotics are typically in pill form. Narcotic overdoses are generally characterized by three signs: coma (or depressed level of consciousness), pinpoint pupils, and respiratory depression (slow, shallow respirations). Together, these are sometimes referred to as the opiate triad.

- *Hallucinogens* such as LSD, PCP, and certain types of mushrooms are mind-affecting drugs that act on the nervous system to produce an intense state of excitement or a distortion of the user's perceptions. This class of drugs has few legal uses. They are often eaten or dissolved in the mouth and absorbed through the mucous membranes. A newer hallucinogen is ecstasy, also known as XTC, X, or MDMA (because it is methylenedioxymethamphetamine). Often taken at "rave" parties with other drugs, this hallucinogen also has the stimulant properties of uppers.

- *Volatile chemicals* produce vapors that can be inhaled (Figure 23-4). They can give an initial "rush" and then act as a depressant on the central nervous system. Cleaning fluid, glue, model cement, and solutions used to correct typing mistakes are commonly abused volatile chemicals.

hallucinogens (huh-LOO-sin-uh-jens)
mind-affecting or mind-altering drugs that act on the central nervous system to produce excitement and distortion of perceptions.

volatile chemicals
vaporizing compounds, such as cleaning fluid, that are breathed in by the abuser to produce a "high."

PATIENT ASSESSMENT

Substance Abuse

As an EMT, you will not need to know the names of the many abused drugs or their specific reactions. It is far more important for you to be able to detect possible drug abuse at the overdose level and to relate certain signs to certain types of drugs and drug withdrawal. Table 23-2 provides some of the names of commonly abused drugs. Do not worry about memorizing this list. Read it through so that you can place some of the more familiar drugs into categories in terms of drug type.

The signs and symptoms of substance abuse, dependency, and overdose can vary from patient to patient, even for the same drug or chemical. The problem is made more complex by the fact that many substance abusers take more than one drug or chemical at a time. Often, you will have to carefully combine the information gained from the signs and symptoms, the scene, the bystanders, and the patient in order to determine if you may be

Table 23-2 Commonly Abused Drugs

UPPERS	DOWNERS	NARCOTICS	MIND-ALTERING DRUGS	VOLATILE CHEMICALS
AMPHETAMINE (Benzedrine, bennies, pep pills, ups, uppers, cartwheels) BIPHETAMINE (bam) COCAINE (coke, snow, crack) DESOXYN (black beauties) DEXTROAMPHETAMINE (dexies, Dexedrine) METHAMPHETAMINE (speed, crank, meth, crystal, diet pills, methedrine) METHYLPHENIDATE (Ritalin) PRELUDIN	BARBITURATES (downers, dolls, barbs, rainbows) *Note: Barbiturates include amobarbital, pentobarbital, phenobarbital, and secobarbital:* AMOBARBITAL (blue devils, downers, barbs, Amytal) PENTOBARBITAL (yellow jackets, barbs, Nembutal) PHENOBARBITAL (goofballs, phennies, barbs) SECOBARBITAL (red devils, barbs, Seconal) **OTHER DOWNERS:** CHLORAL HYDRATE (knockout drops, Noctec) METHAQUALONE (Quaalude, ludes, Sopor, sopors) NONBARBITURATE SEDATIVES (various tranquilizers and sleeping pills: Valium or diazepam, Miltown, Equanil, meprobamate, Thorazine, Compazine, Librium or chlordiazepoxide, reserpine, Tranxene or clorazepate, and other benzodiazepines) PARALDEHYDE	CODEINE (often in cough syrup) DEMEROL (meperidine) DILAUDID FENTANYL (Sublimaze) HEROIN ("H," horse, junk, smack, stuff) METHADONE (dolly) MORPHINE OPIUM (op, poppy) PAREGORIC (contains opium) ACETOMINOPHEN WITH CODEINE (1, 2, 3, 4)	*HALLUCINOGENIC:* DMT LSD (acid, sunshine) MESCALINE (peyote, mesc) MORNING GLORY SEEDS PCP (angel dust, hog, peace pills) PSILOCYBIN (magic mushrooms) STP (serenity, tranquility, peace) *NONHALLUCINOGENIC:* HASH, MARIJUANA (grass, pot, tea, wood, dope) THC	AMYL NITRATE (snappers, poppers) BUTYL NITRATE (Locker Room, Rush) CLEANING FLUID (carbon tetrachloride) FURNITURE POLISH GASOLINE GLUE HAIR SPRAY NAIL POLISH REMOVER PAINT THINNER TYPEWRITING CORRECTION FLUIDS

dealing with substance abuse. In many cases, you will not be able to identify the substance involved.

When questioning the patient and bystanders, you will get better results if you begin by asking if the patient has been taking any medications. Then, if necessary, ask if the patient has been taking drugs.

Some significant signs and symptoms related to specific types of drugs include those listed in the following text. These are offered to help you recognize possible drug abuse in general. Your patient care may not change as a result of this knowledge, but information you can gather about what kind of drug the patient may have been taking will be useful to hospital personnel.

The following list features signs and symptoms of drug abuse for various types of drugs:

- **Uppers.** People who abuse these drugs display excitement, increased pulse and breathing rates, rapid speech, dry mouth, dilated pupils, sweating, and the complaint of having gone without sleep for long periods. Repeated high doses can produce a "speed run." The patient will be restless, hyperactive, and usually very apprehensive and uncooperative.

- **Downers.** People who abuse these drugs are sluggish, sleepy patients lacking typical coordination of body and speech. Pulse and breathing rates are low, often to the point of a true emergency.

- **Narcotics.** People who abuse these drugs have a reduced rate of pulse and rate and depth of breathing, which is often seen with a lowering of skin temperature. The pupils are constricted, often pinpoint in size. The muscles are relaxed and sweating is profuse. The patient is very sleepy and does not wish to do anything. In overdoses, coma is common. Respiratory arrest or cardiac arrest may rapidly develop.

- **Hallucinogens.** People who abuse these drugs have a fast pulse rate, dilated pupils, and a flushed face. The patient often "sees" or "hears" things, has little concept of real time, and may not be aware of the true environment. Often what he says makes no sense to the listener. The user may become aggressive or be very timid.

- **Volatile chemicals.** People who abuse these drugs appear dazed or show temporary loss of contact with reality. The patient may develop a coma. The linings of the nose and mouth may show swollen membranes. The patient may complain of a "funny numb feeling" or "tingling" inside the head. Changes in heart rhythm can occur. This can lead to death.

When reading the just-listed signs and symptoms of drug abuse, you will have noticed that many of the indications are similar to those for quite a few other medical emergencies. As an EMT, you must never assume drug abuse is occurring by itself. You must be on the alert for medical emergencies, injuries, and combinations of drug abuse problems with other emergencies.

In addition to the effects of long-term drug use and overdose, you may encounter cases of severe drug withdrawal. Withdrawal occurs when the long-term user of certain drugs such as narcotics suddenly stops taking the drug. As in reactions to the use of various drugs, withdrawal varies from patient to patient and from drug to drug.

In cases of drug withdrawal, you may see:

- Shaking
- Anxiety
- Nausea
- Confusion and irritability
- Hallucinations (both visual and auditory—"seeing things" or "hearing things")
- Profuse sweating
- Increased pulse and breathing rates

PATIENT CARE

Substance Abuse

Your care for the drug-abuse patient will be basically the same for all drugs and will not change unless you are so ordered by medical direction. When providing care for substance-abuse patients, make certain that you are safe and identify yourself as an EMT

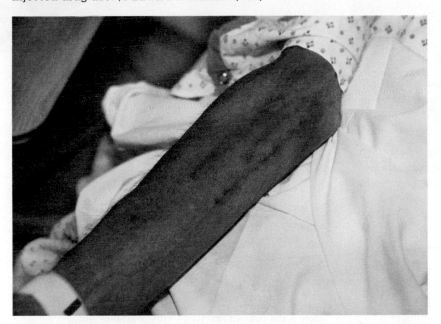

to the patient and bystanders. Since these patients often vomit, take Standard Precautions, including gloves, mask, and protective eyewear as necessary. Be aware of loose hypodermic needles or weapons on the scene that can pose significant risks to you as an EMT.

Emergency care includes the following:

1. Perform a primary assessment. Provide basic life support measures if required.
2. Be alert for airway problems and inadequate respirations or respiratory arrest. Provide oxygen and assist ventilations if needed.
3. Treat for shock. (Treatment for shock will be discussed in Chapter 27, "Bleeding and Shock".)
4. Talk to the patient to gain his confidence and to help maintain his level of responsiveness. Use his name often, maintain eye contact, and speak directly to the patient.
5. Perform a physical exam to assess for signs of injury to all parts of the body. Assess carefully for signs of head injury.
6. Look for gross soft-tissue damage on the extremities resulting from the injection of drugs ("tracks"). Tracks usually appear as darkened or red areas of scar tissue or scabs over veins (Figure 23-5).
7. Protect the patient from self-injury and his attempts to hurt others. Use restraint as authorized by your EMS system. Request assistance from law enforcement if needed.
8. Transport the patient as soon as possible.
9. Contact medical direction according to local protocols.
10. Perform reassessment with monitoring of vital signs. Stay alert for seizures, and be on guard for vomiting that could obstruct the airway.
11. Continue to reassure the patient throughout all phases of care.

NOTE: *Many drug abusers may appear calm at first and then become violent as time passes. Always be on the alert and ready to protect yourself. If the patient creates an unsafe scene and you are not a trained law enforcement officer, GET OUT and find a safe place until the police arrive.*

When dealing with drug abuse, you must also protect yourself from the substance itself. Many hallucinogens can be absorbed through the skin and mucous membranes. Intravenous drug users may possess hypodermic syringes, which pose a hazard of infectious disease transmission through accidental punctures. Take Standard Precautions and follow all infection exposure control procedures. Never touch or taste any suspected illicit substance.

Key Facts and Concepts

- In a poisoned patient, perform a primary assessment and immediately treat life-threatening problems. Ensure an open airway. Administer high-concentration oxygen if the poison was inhaled or injected.

- Next, perform a secondary assessment, including baseline vital signs. Find out if the poison was ingested, inhaled, absorbed, or injected; what substance was involved; how much poison was taken in; when and over how long a period exposure took place; what interventions others have already done; and what effects the patient experienced.

- Consult medical direction. As directed, administer activated charcoal or water or milk for ingested poisons.

- Remove the patient who has inhaled a poison from the environment and administer high-concentration oxygen; remove poisons from the skin by brushing them off or diluting them.

- Transport the patient with all containers, bottles, and labels from the substance.

- Reassess the patient en route.

- Carefully document all information about the poisoning, interventions, and the patient's responses.

Key Decisions

- Is it safe for me to approach the scene and the patient?
- Is the patient breathing adequately?
- How much exposure did the patient have to the poison or drug?
- How is the patient reacting to the poison or drug?
- Are there any specific actions I need to take based on the identity of the poison or drug?

Chapter Glossary

absorbed poisons poisons that are taken into the body through unbroken skin.

activated charcoal a substance that adsorbs many poisons and prevents them from being absorbed by the body.

antidote a substance that will neutralize the poison or its effects.

delirium tremens (duh-LEER-e-um TREM-uns) ***(DTs)*** a severe reaction that can be part of alcohol withdrawal, characterized by sweating, trembling, anxiety, and hallucinations. Severe alcohol withdrawal with the DTs can lead to death if untreated.

dilution (di-LU-shun) thinning down or weakening by mixing with something else. Ingested poisons are sometimes diluted by drinking water or milk.

downers depressants, such as barbiturates, that depress the central nervous system, which are often used to bring on a more relaxed state of mind.

hallucinogens (huh-LOO-sin-uh-jens) mind-affecting or mind-altering drugs that act on the central nervous system to produce excitement and distortion of perceptions.

ingested poisons poisons that are swallowed.

inhaled poisons poisons that are breathed in.

injected poisons poisons that are inserted through the skin; for example, by needle, snake fangs, or insect stinger.

narcotics a class of drugs that affect the nervous system and change many normal body activities. Their legal use is for the relief of pain. Illicit use is to produce an intense state of relaxation.

poison any substance that can harm the body by altering cell structure or functions.

toxin a poisonous substance secreted by bacteria, plants, or animals.

uppers stimulants such as amphetamines that affect the central nervous system to excite the user.

volatile chemicals vaporizing compounds, such as cleaning fluid, which are breathed in by the abuser to produce a "high."

withdrawal referring to alcohol or drug withdrawal in which the patient's body reacts severely when deprived of the abused substance.

Preparation for Your Examination and Practice

Short Answer

1. Name four ways in which a poison can be taken into the body.

2. What is the sequence of assessment steps in cases of poisoning?

3. What information must you gather in a case of poisoning before contacting medical direction?

4. What are the emergency care steps for ingested poisoning?

5. What are the emergency care steps for inhaled poisoning? For absorbed poisoning?

Thinking and Linking

Patients who are exposed to poisons and drugs sometimes have preexisting medical problems. As you work on this exercise, combine what you have learned in this chapter with material from the assessment chapters and Chapter 20, "Cardiac Emergencies."

- A middle-aged woman who was in a house fire is out of the house and coughing quite a bit. She was exposed to smoke for up to 10 minutes because she was asleep when the fire started. How should you interpret her pulse oximeter reading? How should it affect your treatment?

- A despondent older man took his recently deceased wife's medications. Medical direction advises you that one of the medications causes tachycardia. The patient has had a myocardial infarction and has congestive heart failure. He takes nitroglycerin as needed. What should you anticipate may happen to this patient? How should you manage it?

Critical Thinking Exercises

Many pesticides are highly toxic, yet many people who use them refuse to recognize the dangers. The purpose of this exercise will be to consider how you might manage a pesticide poisoning patient who is in denial.

- A local farmer calls 911, concerned because one of his farm hands has tried to clean up some spilled pesticide powder with his hands. On arrival, you find that the patient insists he has brushed all the powder off, feels fine, and doesn't need to go to the hospital. As he talks, he continues to make brushing motions at his jeans on which you can see the marks of a powdery residue. How do you manage the situation?

Pathophysiology to Practice

The following questions are designed to assist you in gathering relevant clinical information and making accurate decisions in the field.

- A young man who kept a rattlesnake was handling it when it bit him on the hand. The area is swollen and discolored. When you call the poison center, the poison information specialist tells you that rattlesnake venom affects primarily the cardiovascular system. What signs and symptoms should you anticipate?

- What if the snake was a coral snake and the poison information specialist told you the venom affects primarily the nervous system? What signs and symptoms should you anticipate?

Street Scenes ━ ━ ━ ━ ━ ━ ━ ━ ━ ━ ━ ━ ━ ━ ━ ━ ━

You and your partner are assigned to the night shift when you are dispatched out for a "possible poisoning." You arrive on-scene within 4 minutes to find a 20-year-old female sitting on the couch with a small child in her arms. The female, Anna Prince, states that she is the child's mother and she believes the child has ingested some lamp oil. The child's name is Maria, and she is 8 months old. Anna states, "I was doing the dishes when I turned around and saw Maria with the oil candle in her hands. I don't know how much she drank or how much she spilled." Maria is crying and coughing excessively, but she is alert and responds to her mother. Her skin is warm, dry, and pink. You also notice that there is some lamp oil on the front of Maria's shirt.

Street Scene Questions

1. What questions would you ask the patient's mother next?
2. What signs or symptoms should you inquire about?

You continue to gather information about the situation and discover that the time of exposure occurred approximately 3 to 4 minutes before 911 was activated. Anna also reports that she neither has the original container that the lamp oil was purchased in, nor does she remember how much oil was left in the candle. You estimate the total container size to be 100 cc and determine that half of the oil is missing. Anna also reports that she gave Maria some water, but Maria vomited after drinking a small amount.

As you continue with your assessment, you find that Maria has a clear upper airway. Her mucous membranes are pink and moist, and her pupils are equal and reactive to light. Anna states that Maria has been sick lately and that she weighed 20 pounds at her last doctor's visit. Maria is currently taking Children's Tylenol for fever reduction and has no known medical allergies. The only medical history that her mother reports is a recent fever and mild cough. Maria's current vital signs include a strong pulse of 140 and regular; respirations are 36 with crying and coughing; and an oxygen saturation of 97 percent.

Street Scene Questions

3. What treatments would you initiate?
4. Should you contact someone for advice? If yes, then who?

You provide the patient with blow-by oxygen, setting the flow rate at 10 liters per minute. You place the child in a car seat that is securely anchored to the ambulance stretcher for transport. The mother also is secured in a seat inside the ambulance. You take the lamp oil candle with you.

You contact poison control, and they advise you that the main concern for Maria is related to aspiration of the oil into the lungs. They advise you that the oil may be a petroleum product with a hydrocarbon base and that activated charcoal and syrup of ipecac are contraindicated. You also contact medical direction; they agree with the recommendations from poison control and order only supportive care.

During transport, you continually monitor your patient's airway and ventilatory status. When you repeat vital signs, respirations are 32 and slightly labored and pulse is 128, regular, and strong. As you arrive at the emergency department, Maria has stopped crying but continues to cough. No other changes occur during the transport.

24 Abdominal Emergencies

○ **STANDARD**
Medicine (Toxicology)

○ **COMPETENCY**
Applies fundamental knowledge to provide basic emergency care and transportation based on assessment findings for an acutely ill patient.

○ **CORE CONCEPTS**
— Understanding the nature of abdominal pain or discomfort

— Becoming familiar with abdominal conditions that may cause pain or discomfort

— How to assess and care for patients with abdominal pain or discomfort

EXPLORE Resource Central

To access Resource Central, follow directions on the Student Access Card provided with this text. If there is no card, go to **www.bradybooks.com** and follow the Resource Central link to Buy Access from there. Under Media Resources, you will find:

▶ **Abdominal Aortic Aneurysm**
View an animation to learn what happens during an abdominal aortic aneurysm.

▶ **Information about STDs**
Learn about sexually transmitted diseases, what health problems can be caused by these diseases, and what an EMT should do to treat a patient suspected of having an STD.

▶ **Information about Hepatitis from the CDC**
Read about hepatitis, what populations are most at risk for contracting viral hepatitis, and why it is important for an EMT to be vaccinated against Hepatitis B.

OBJECTIVES

After reading this chapter you should be able to:

24.1 Define key terms introduced in this chapter.

24.2 Describe the location, structure, and function of the organs in the abdominal cavity. (pp. 571–573)

24.3 Explain the origins and characteristics of visceral, parietal, and tearing pain. (pp. 573–574)

24.4 Associate areas of referred pain with the likely origins of the pain. (p. 574)

24.5 Recognize the common signs and symptoms of abdominal conditions, including appendicitis, peritonitis, cholecystitis, pancreatitis, ulcers,

abdominal aortic aneurysm, hernia, and renal colic. (pp. 574–577)

24.6 Discuss the type of abdominal pain that may indicate cardiac involvement. (p. 577)

24.7 Discuss appropriate assessment and management of patients complaining of abdominal pain. (pp. 577–584)

24.8 Elicit key information in the history of patients complaining of abdominal pain, including history specific to female patients. (pp. 578, 580)

A bdominal emergencies are challenging for EMTs because the cause of the patient's pain is not visible. Further complicating these challenges, many organs within the abdomen will cause pain if affected. This can cause confusion in determining the priority and stability of the patient with abdominal pain.

Fortunately, these challenges can be overcome. The patient assessment process will help you determine the patient's priority. Although there are various potential causes for abdominal pain, the treatment for most conditions is the same and will not require a specific diagnosis. This chapter will detail information about assessing and treating abdominal emergencies.

ABDOMINAL ANATOMY AND PHYSIOLOGY

The abdomen—the area below the diaphragm and above the pelvis—contains a variety of organs that perform digestive, reproductive, endocrine, and regulatory functions. Although we may think the abdomen only handles the digestion of food, in reality organs and structures within the abdomen do much more, including secreting insulin to regulate blood sugar (the islets of Langerhans of the pancreas), filtering blood and assisting with immune response (the spleen), and removing toxins from the body (the liver). Figure 24-1 shows the structures and organs of the abdomen. Table 24-1 lists the structures and organs of the abdomen with their functions.

FIGURE 24-1 The structures and organs of the abdomen.

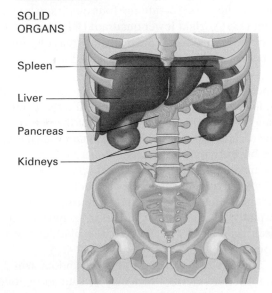

SOLID ORGANS

Spleen
Liver
Pancreas
Kidneys

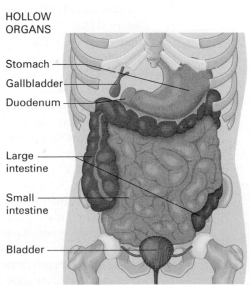

HOLLOW ORGANS

Stomach
Gallbladder
Duodenum

Large intestine

Small intestine

Bladder

Table 24-1 Structures and Organs of the Abdomen

STRUCTURE OR ORGAN	TYPE OF STRUCTURE OR ORGAN	PURPOSE
Esophagus	Hollow digestive	This structure carries food from the mouth and pharynx to the stomach.
Stomach	Hollow digestive	This expandable organ, located below the diaphragm and connected to the esophagus and small intestine, begins the breakdown of foods.
Small intestine	Hollow digestive	The small intestine, consisting of the duodenum, jejunum, and ileum, takes stomach contents and removes nutrients as it passes its contents to the large intestine.
Large intestine (colon)	Hollow digestive	The large intestine absorbs fluid from its contents, creating fecal waste for excretion through the rectum and anus.
Appendix	Hollow lymphatic	This dead-ended sac of bowel rich in lymphatic tissue has no function in digestion. It may become infected (appendicitis), causing pain and requiring surgery.
Liver	Solid digestive Other functions with regulation of the blood and detoxification	This organ is involved in regulating levels of carbohydrate and other substances in the blood. It is involved in bile secretion for digestion of fats, and has many other functions including detoxification of the blood.
Gallbladder	Hollow digestive	This organ stores bile before its release into the intestine.
Spleen	Solid lymphatic tissue	This organ removes abnormal blood cells and is involved in the immune response.
Pancreas	Solid digestive	This organ releases enzymes that assist in breaking down food in the small intestine into absorbable molecules. It also secretes hormones into the blood that regulate blood sugar levels.
Kidneys	Solid urinary	These organs filter and excrete waste. They also regulate water, blood, and electrolyte levels and assist the liver with detoxification.
Bladder	Hollow urinary	This organ collects urine from the kidneys prior to excretion (urination).

The abdomen can be divided into quadrants. Imaginary lines drawn both vertically and horizontally through the umbilicus (the navel) create the four quadrants: right upper quadrant (RUQ), left upper quadrant (LUQ), right lower quadrant (RLQ), and left lower quadrant (LLQ). These quadrants are used to identify and describe areas of pain, tenderness, discomfort, injury, or other abnormalities. The abdominal quadrants are shown in Figure 24-2A.

peritoneum
the membrane that lines the abdominal cavity (the *parietal peritoneum*) and covers the organs within it (the *visceral peritoneum*).

Most of the organs of the abdomen are enclosed within the **peritoneum** (Figure 24-2B). These organs include the stomach, liver, spleen, appendix, small and large colon, and in women the uterus, fallopian tubes, and ovaries. There are two layers of the peritoneum: the *visceral peritoneum*, which covers the organs, and the *parietal peritoneum*, which is attached to the abdominal wall. A slight space between the two layers contains a lubricant fluid.

retroperitoneal space
the area posterior to the peritoneum, between the peritoneum and the back.

The area outside the peritoneum is called *extraperitoneal space* (refer again to Figure 24-2B), which includes the **retroperitoneal space**, the area between the abdomen and the back. The organs in the retroperitoneal area, which is technically not part of the abdomen, include the kidneys, the pancreas, and the aorta. This information will be important when types of pain are discussed later in the chapter. The bladder and most of the rectum is inferior to the peritoneum.

The female reproductive organs and structures also lie within the abdomen and pelvis. These include the ovaries, fallopian tubes, and uterus, which may be sources of abdominal

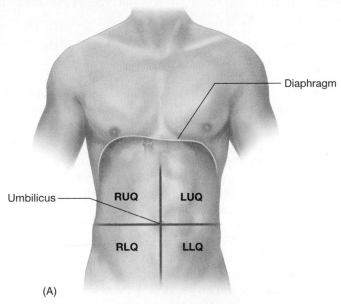

Diaphragm

Umbilicus

| RUQ | LUQ |
| RLQ | LLQ |

(A)

Cross Section of Torso Viewed from the Right

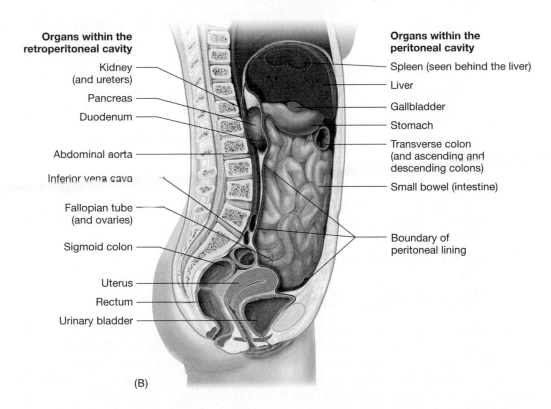

Organs within the retroperitoneal cavity

Kidney (and ureters)

Pancreas

Duodenum

Abdominal aorta

Inferior vena cava

Fallopian tube (and ovaries)

Sigmoid colon

Uterus

Rectum

Urinary bladder

Organs within the peritoneal cavity

Spleen (seen behind the liver)

Liver

Gallbladder

Stomach

Transverse colon (and ascending and descending colons)

Small bowel (intestine)

Boundary of peritoneal lining

(B)

pain. The anatomy of the female reproductive system and the assessment and care for related emergencies are discussed in detail in Chapter 34, "Obstetric and Gynecologic Emergencies."

ABDOMINAL PAIN OR DISCOMFORT

The potential exists for both medical and traumatic emergencies to the abdomen. The traumatic emergencies are covered in Chapter 28, "Soft-Tissue Trauma." This chapter covers the most common acute (sudden or emergent) medical abdominal emergencies.

CORE CONCEPT •

Understanding the nature of abdominal pain or discomfort

[handwritten: Colicks intermittent pain Hollow Organs]

[handwritten: appendix = hollow]

As noted earlier in this chapter, there are many organs within the peritoneal and retroperitoneal cavities. These organs can be sources of a wide range of problems or complaints in patients of all ages. Some classic patterns and types of pain involving the abdomen include the following:

- ***Visceral pain*** originates from the organs (the *viscera*) within the abdomen. The organs themselves do not have a large number of nerve endings to detect pain. Therefore, visceral pain is often described as dull, achy, or intermittent and may be diffuse, or difficult to locate. (The patient may say he has abdominal pain but cannot point to a specific location.) Pain that may be described as *intermittent*, *crampy*, or *colicky* often comes from hollow organs of the abdomen. Pain that is *dull* and *persistent* often originates from solid organs.

- ***Parietal pain***, as the name implies, arises from the parietal peritoneum, the lining of the abdominal cavity—thus, it is often referred to as *peritoneal tenderness*. Because of its more widespread and efficient nerve endings, pain originating from the parietal peritoneum can be more easily located and described than pain from the visceral organs.

  Parietal pain is the direct result of local irritation of the peritoneum. Such irritation may be caused by internal bleeding (as from blood leaking into the peritoneum from an injured spleen) or infection/inflammation (such as pain in the RLQ from an infected appendix). Parietal pain may be sharp or constant and localized to a particular area. When obtaining the history, you may find the patient will describe this type of pain as worsening when he moves and getting better when he remains still or lies with the knees drawn up.

- ***Tearing pain*** is not the most common type of abdominal pain. Most abdominal structures or organs do not have the ability to detect tearing sensations. The exception is the aorta. In cases of an expanding abdominal aortic aneurysm (AAA), the inner layer of the aorta is damaged and blood leaks from the inner portions of the vessel to the outer layers. This causes a tearing of the vessel lining and pockets of blood resting in a weak area of the vessel. Much like a balloon, the area of collected blood creates an expanding pouch in the blood vessel wall. This is often sensed as a "tearing" pain in the back. (Remember that parts of the aorta are in the retroperitoneal space. This is why the pain is felt in the back.)

- ***Referred pain*** is pain felt in a place other than where the pain originates. For example, when a gallbladder is diseased, pain is often felt not in the area of the gallbladder but, instead, in the area of the right shoulder blade. This is because nerve pathways from the gallbladder return to the spinal cord by way of shared pathways with nerves that sense pain in the shoulder area.

[handwritten: Pain felt in another location]

ABDOMINAL CONDITIONS

Many types of abdominal conditions lead to abdominal complaints. Remember that, as an EMT, it is more important to provide proper assessment and management (including transport) than it is to field diagnose specific conditions. Although many conditions have "classic" signs and symptoms, there are many patients who do not display them. Some patients may be pain-free with a raging infection inside the abdomen, whereas others may be in agony from a minor irritant.

Appendicitis

Appendicitis, an infection of the appendix, is the most common cause of a person needing surgery. About 1 in 15 people will develop appendicitis at some time in their lives. Signs and symptoms include nausea and sometimes vomiting, pain in the area of the umbilicus (initially), followed by persistent pain in the right lower quadrant (RLQ). If the appendix ruptures, the patient will typically experience a sudden severe increase in pain. This is a result of the bowel contents being let loose into the peritoneal cavity, leading to peritonitis.

Peritonitis

The peritoneum, the lining of the abdomen, is very sensitive to foreign substances. This is especially true with irritating substances such as gastric juices, bowel contents, and blood. The result of such an insult is peritonitis. Peritonitis may be the result of a medical condition (such as the inflammation of a ruptured appendix) or the result of trauma (such as bleeding from a ruptured spleen). The abdomen typically becomes extremely painful and rigid. This is not a voluntary response like guarding (discussed later in the chapter). Rather, the rigidity of peritonitis is an involuntary response of the muscles over the peritoneum. Peritonitis represents a potentially life-threatening emergency. The patient needs prompt evaluation by a physician to determine the appropriate treatment, which is often surgery.

Cholecystitis/Gallstones

Cholecystitis is an inflammation of the gallbladder, often caused by gallstones. The patient with this condition will experience severe and sometimes sudden right upper quadrant (RUQ) and/or epigastric (upper central abdomen just below the xiphoid process) pain, which may radiate to the shoulder. The pain may be caused or worsened by ingestion of foods high in fat.

Pancreatitis

Pancreatitis, an inflammation of the pancreas, is common in patients with chronic alcohol problems. The pain from pancreatitis is found in the epigastric area. Because of the retroperitoneal location of the pancreas, behind the stomach, the pain may radiate to the back and/or shoulders. This is a serious condition which, in advanced cases, can present with signs of shock.

Gastrointestinal (GI) Bleeding

Bleeding can occur from within the GI system anywhere from the esophagus to the rectum. Depending on the size of the source blood vessel, GI bleeding may be gradual or sudden and massive. Because this type of bleeding occurs inside the lumen of the esophagus, stomach, or intestines, blood eventually has to pass out through the rectum and/or through the mouth. Patients may report the passage of abnormal stools that are dark black or maroon in color and tarry in appearance, or they may simply pass frank blood without stool from the rectum. If the patient is bleeding from an upper GI source (the esophagus, stomach, or first portion of the small bowel), he also may exhibit vomiting of frank blood or "coffee-ground" vomit. The coffee-ground appearance is due to the partial breakdown of blood by digestive enzymes.

Patients most commonly have no significant or constant pain associated with GI bleeding. An exception to this rule is patients with perforated ulcers in the stomach (gastric ulcers). These lesions are the result of acidic gastric juices wearing a hole in the upper gastrointestinal system. If the erosion eats into a blood vessel, GI bleeding will result. If the acid causes erosion all the way through the stomach or proximal small bowel wall, then this very acidic liquid leaks into the peritoneum, resulting in significant abdominal pain from chemical irritation and peritonitis.

Patients with GI bleeding may present in different ways. If the source vessel of the bleed is a small one, the patient may experience a slow loss of blood, referred to as chronic gastrointestinal hemorrhage. This results in the patient becoming pale and weak over a period of days to weeks, unaware that he is bleeding inside. The body can compensate for most of this blood loss over a period of time, but eventually the patient develops signs and symptoms of shock. If the source of bleeding is from a larger blood vessel, the patient may present with brisk bleeding from the rectum or vomiting of either bright red blood or material that resembles coffee grounds. This type of bleeding is associated with the sudden onset of signs and symptoms of hypoperfusion.

Abdominal Aortic Aneurysm

Abdominal aortic aneurysm (AAA) is a ballooning or weakening in the wall of the aorta as it passes through the abdomen. The weakening results in tearing of the internal layer of the blood vessel, which allows blood to escape into the weaker, outer layers. The affected area

Inside/Outside

When the aorta is weakened, it can rupture quite suddenly or leak relatively slowly. It can also dissect, which means that an inner layer of the aorta tears, allowing the high pressures in the aorta to dissect (spread apart) the layers of the vessel. As the pressure continues to exert force on the aorta, the area of dissection can spread. In some cases, the dissection spreads so far that it interferes with or even eliminates the blood flow to an artery that branches off the aorta. In this case, you may see decreased perfusion of an extremity with a decreased or absent pulse.

can gradually grow and rupture. Ruptured aneurysms are associated with an extremely high rate of death if they are discovered after they rupture.

You may encounter a patient who is aware he has an aneurysm. These conditions are sometimes found when a test for another condition, such as an abdominal ultrasound or CT scan, reveals the presence of a small aneurysm. Not all are surgically repaired immediately. If you have a patient who tells you that he has an aneurysm and he has abdominal pain, it is a serious emergency requiring prompt transportation to an appropriate hospital.

Patients with a slowly leaking AAA usually present with gradually developing abdominal pain, which can be described as sharp pain or tearing pain and may radiate to the back. The association of back pain with ruptured AAA is why back pain in older adults is considered a highest-priority dispatch in medical priority dispatch systems. A sudden rupture of the aorta typically causes sudden onset of excruciating abdominal and back pain. Signs of shock are usually present. Depending on the location of the AAA, there may be inequality between the femoral or pedal pulses.

Hernia

A hernia is a hole in the muscle layers of the abdominal wall, allowing tissue—usually intestine—to protrude up against the skin. This can be aggravated by heavy lifting or straining that causes the intestine to push through the weakened area in the abdominal wall. Such a hernia will cause a sudden onset of pain, usually after lifting. A hernia may be palpated as a mass or lump on the abdominal wall or in the creases of the groin (Figure 24-3).

FIGURE 24-3 An inguinal hernia, a protrusion of abdominal-cavity contents through the inguinal canal in the anterior abdominal wall.
(© Edward T. Dickinson, MD)

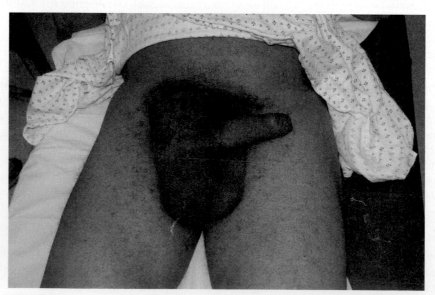

Although it may be very painful, it is a life-threatening condition only if the hernia causes an obstruction or twisting of the intestine.

Because pain at the site of a hernia may indicate obstruction or strangulation of the intestine, all patients with a painful hernia should be transported for further evaluation at the hospital.

Renal Colic

Under certain conditions the kidneys may form small, hard stones. If one of these stones begins to descend down the ureter on the way to the bladder, it can cause severe flank pain that often radiates anteriorly to the groin area. The visceral pain from such a "kidney stone" is often severe and may be associated with nausea and vomiting. These patients are typically described as "writhing," because they move around, trying unsuccessfully to find a position of comfort.

Cardiac Involvement

Pain from a heart attack (myocardial infarction) may be felt as abdominal discomfort. This pain, often described as indigestion or disgestive discomfort, is commonly felt in the epigastric region (the area below the xiphoid, in the upper center of the abdomen). If the patient complains of this type of pain, consider the possibility of cardiac involvement, as described in Chapter 20, "Cardiac Emergencies."

ASSESSMENT AND CARE OF ABDOMINAL PAIN OR DISCOMFORT

CORE CONCEPTS

How to assess and care for patients with abdominal pain or discomfort

There are so many potential causes of abdominal pain that the EMT should not be concerned with field diagnosing a particular cause. Diagnosing can be difficult even in a hospital, where advanced diagnostic tests are available. The focus of your assessment process (Scan 24-1) will be to accurately perform a secondary assessment to describe the condition and identify potentially serious conditions such as shock.

For each of the steps in the assessment process, you may observe specific concerns and points of interest in the abdominal pain patient.

Scene Size-Up

As you approach and take the important scene size-up steps, be prepared to protect your face and clothes in case vomiting occurs. Odors can be clinically important. For example, blood in vomit or feces creates a distinctly strong odor. Identifying this odor early will help you identify potential shock. Your search for a mechanism of injury may help you determine if this is a traumatic versus a medical condition.

Primary Assessment

The general impression you obtain as you approach the patient will be valuable in determining the seriousness of the patient's condition and the urgency of your care. First, the patient's level of consciousness will help you determine the required airway care. If the patient is conscious, you will be able to begin talking to him to gain information, and if the patient is talking, you will know he has an open airway. Unconscious patients require airway care, and any history will be obtained from family or bystanders.

At this stage of assessment, you will be able to notice the early signs of shock. An altered mental status; anxiety; pale, cool, or moist skin; and rapid pulse and respirations will alert you to shock—long before you would take a blood pressure or see trends in the blood pressure.

The position of the patient also provides important clues. Does the patient appear to be in pain? Is he guarding the abdomen (Figure 24-4)? Is he in the fetal position?

Apply oxygen to all patients with abdominal pain or distress at 15 lpm via nonrebreather mask.

NOTE: *Abdominal pain or discomfort should always be considered an emergency—even if signs of shock are not present.*

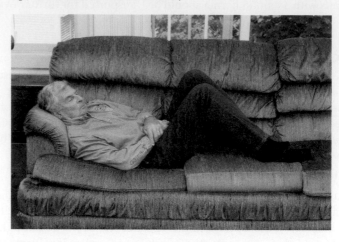

FIGURE 24-4 The patient with abdominal pain will often be found in a position of guarding (knees drawn up, arms across the abdomen).

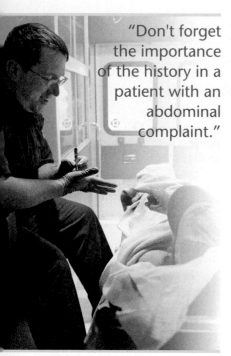

"Don't forget the importance of the history in a patient with an abdominal complaint."

History

The history is vital in the assessment of the patient with an abdominal emergency. Be systematic in your interviewing of the patient.

History of the Present Illness

Have the patient describe the pain in his own words by answering your open-ended questions.

While gathering information about the patient's signs and symptoms, use the OPQRST mnemonic (onset, provocation/palliation, quality, region/radiation, severity, time) as a mental checklist to help you elicit information from the patient about his pain or discomfort.

- **Onset.** *When did the pain or discomfort begin? Did it begin while at rest or during activity? How did the pain begin? Did it begin as steady and severe, or did it gradually build to this point?*

- **Provocation/palliation.** *What makes the pain better or worse? Does any position make the pain better or worse? Does movement affect the pain?*

- **Quality.** *Describe the sensation in your abdomen to me.*

- **Region/Radiation.** *Point to or show me where the pain or discomfort is.* (Remember that the patient's pain or discomfort may span more than one region or quadrant or may be difficult for the patient to localize.) *Do you have pain anywhere else? Does the pain radiate or shoot to other parts of your abdomen, back, or body?*

- **Severity.** *How severe is the pain or discomfort?* Ask the patient to report the pain on a 1-to-10 scale.

- **Time.** *How long have you had the pain or discomfort? Has it changed over time? Is it better or worse?*

Keep in mind that using only the word *pain* in talking to the patient about his symptoms may cause your history to be inaccurate. If you ask the patient if he has "pain" in his abdomen, he may reply, "No." The patient may have discomfort, pressure, bloating, cramping, or another sensation that he would not call "pain." This response will reduce the effectiveness of your exam, care for the patient, and subsequent reporting. The initial use of open-ended questions will help you to get accurate information in the patient's own words.

History Specific to Female Patients

When female patients, especially those within childbearing years, have abdominal pain, you must ask additional questions as part of the history.

Emergencies such as ectopic pregnancy (a pregnancy developing outside of the uterus) can be life-threatening conditions and must be considered in the history. Other conditions, such as ruptured ovarian cysts, pelvic inflammatory disease, and menstrual irregularities, can also cause significant pain.

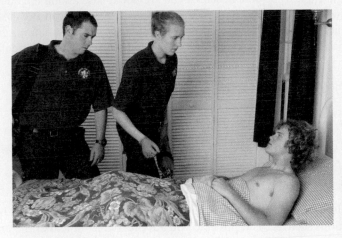

1 Perform a scene size-up.

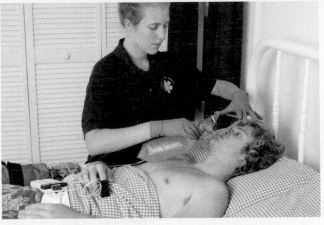

2 Perform a primary assessment and apply oxygen.

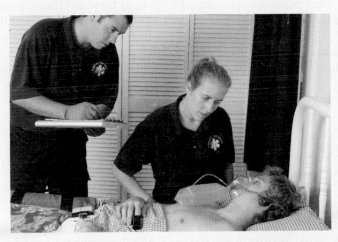

3 Take a patient history.

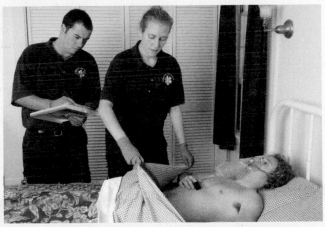

4 Expose the site.

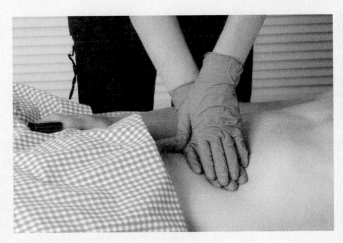

5 Palpate the abdominal quadrants.

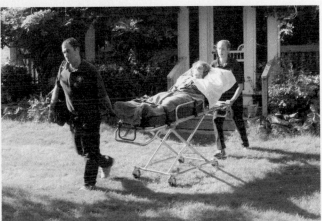

6 Transport the patient.

The questions you will need to ask of a female in childbearing years who is suffering abdominal pain are highly personal but important to include in the history. Ask the questions directly, with the terminology taught in class. If the patient senses you are not at ease asking the questions, she will be uneasy answering them. Assuring privacy for the patient while you ask these questions may help communication. Remember, this is important assessment information.

The following list includes important questions to ask when gathering a female patient's history:

Where are you in your menstrual cycle?

Is your period late?

Do you have bleeding from the vagina now that is not menstrual bleeding?

If you are menstruating, is the flow normal?

Have you had this pain before?

If so, when did it happen and what was it like?

If the patient is within childbearing years, ask if she believes she is pregnant or could be pregnant. If you ask a questions such as, "Is it possible you are pregnant?" it leaves the answer to the patient's judgment.

Some patients may not even be fully aware of how one becomes pregnant. Some may not realize that, even if they have used birth control devices or techniques, they could be pregnant.

If the answer is "Yes" to any of these questions, suspect ectopic pregnancy. (Even if the answers are "No," pregnancy—with ectopic pregnancy being the potential cause of the patient's pain—is still a possibility.) An ectopic pregnancy is a serious emergency, requiring *immediate* transport to the hospital.

NOTE: *Ectopic pregnancy occurs at the beginning of pregnancy. A patient with an ectopic pregnancy will not "look pregnant"—that is, she will not have an abdomen that appears outwardly pregnant.*

Detailed information on emergencies related to the female reproductive system can be found in Chapter 34, "Obstetric and Gynecologic Emergencies."

Past Medical History

After you have elicited information about the patient's signs and symptoms (the OPQRST questions) already discussed under "History of the Present Illness," continue with questions pertaining to the patient's allergies, medications, pertinent past history, last oral intake, and events leading to the present emergency.

Allergies   Inquire if the patient has any allergies and, if so, what he is allergic to.

Medications   Ask if the patient takes any medications. This includes over-the-counter, herbal, and illegal medications or drugs. For example, aspirin used to prevent heart attack and stroke can cause bleeding in the stomach. Some illegal substances can cause abdominal distress in use and withdrawal. Diabetics can experience abdominal pain as a symptom of blood sugar abnormalities for which they may be taking prescribed medications.

Pertinent Past History   The patient's medical history may provide information about past problems that may be related to the current problem. If the patient has a history of past abdominal problems, ask what these conditions are, if the pain resembles past experiences with the condition, and what happened last time. (Was it serious? Was the patient in shock? Was surgery necessary?) A patient's cardiac history with epigastric discomfort may lead you to be concerned for heart attack.

Last Oral Intake   This is very important in patients with abdominal complaints. Determine the patient's last oral intake (liquids, meals, snacks). Additionally, determine if this intake and the intake over the past hours-to-days has been normal for this patient.

Events Leading to the Emergency   The events leading up to the call for EMS (similar to the onset question in the OPQRST questions) can help you determine a timeline and progression of signs and symptoms. Ask again specifically about activity (even over the past few days) which seems related to the problem. Vomiting, nausea, diarrhea, and/or constipation are also important history items. Ask specifically if any dark red, bright red, or coffee-ground-like substances were noted in the vomit or feces, indicating internal bleeding.

Geriatric patients may present some dilemmas when you are assessing abdominal pain. Older people may have a decreased ability to perceive pain. This will, of course, make obtaining a history and description of the pain or discomfort more difficult. It is also important to remember that older patients are likely to have a more serious cause of their abdominal pain than younger patients. Research has demonstrated that elderly patients with abdominal pain are up to nine times more likely to die than younger patients with the same cause of the abdominal pain.

Many geriatric patients also take medications (e.g., beta blockers such as atenolol or metoprolol) for high blood pressure or heart conditions, which will reduce the heart rate. These medications may prevent the patient's pulse from rising during shock. An EMT could find a pulse of 72 and think that shock isn't present when in fact it is.

Physical Examination of the Abdomen

Assessment of the abdomen involves two procedures for EMS personnel: inspection and palpation. You may see some health care providers in the hospital auscultating (listening to) bowel sounds. This can be a long process (listening 3 minutes per quadrant) which will not change prehospital care and is not recommended as part of prehospital assessment.

Before you physically assess the abdomen, you will have asked the patient where it hurts. The patient may have pointed to a spot or may have moved his hand around an area indicating diffuse pain or discomfort. This will be important for your physical exam.

First, inspect the patient's abdomen. Look for distention, bloating, discoloration, abnormal protrusions, or other signs that appear abnormal or unusual. You may have to ask the patient or family members if the current appearance of the abdomen is normal or changed, since body types and shapes vary widely.

Then palpate the abdominal quadrants. Always palpate the area that has pain or discomfort *last*. If this area is palpated first and causes additional pain, it will mask or alter the patient's response to palpation of the other quadrants.

To palpate the abdomen, use the fingertips of several fingers and gently press into the abdomen in each quadrant. While palpating, feel for rigidity or hardening and ask or observe whether this causes pain for the patient. If the initial gentle palpation does not cause pain or discomfort, you may palpate a bit deeper. Once you have found pain, discomfort, or abnormality, there is no need to palpate further in that area.

You may observe that the patient is guarding the abdomen. The term *guarding* is used to describe two possible presentations: the patient drawing his arms down across the abdomen (review Figure 24-5) or the patient tensing the muscles before you touch the abdomen. Guarding is a voluntary or involuntary attempt to protect the abdomen and prevent further pain.

In cases of abdominal aortic aneurysm, you may palpate a pulsating mass (abnormal bulge or lump). This mass may be found in conjunction with tearing or sharp pain in the

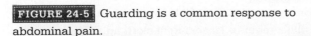

FIGURE 24-5 Guarding is a common response to abdominal pain.

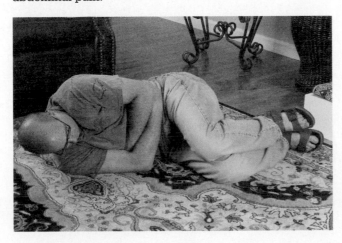

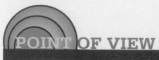

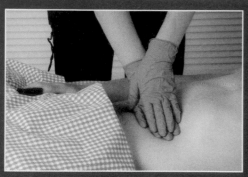

"I went to bed feeling like I had a stomachache. But I woke up with some really bad pain. It was so bad I could barely roll over and call 911 for the ambulance.

"The EMTs came and started to take care of me. They asked me questions and took my blood pressure. Then they pressed on my belly. Whoa! Did that hurt like a. . . . Well, I won't use those words here. Trust me. It hurt a lot. I yelled and almost startled the EMT. I know he had to do it to check me out.

"I found out the reason I was in so much pain. It was my appendix. They said if I hadn't gotten to surgery when I did it may have burst. I'm thankful for what the EMTs did—even if it did almost send me through the roof."

back. This indicates an advanced aneurysm. If you gently palpate this mass, do not palpate it again. Instead, report this mass to the receiving hospital. Some patients may have knowledge of an aneurysm which, when first found, was not serious and has worsened, or it was inoperable. This history is important.

Remember that the aorta normally creates a slight sensation of pulsing on deeper palpation of the abdomen, especially in very thin patients. The presence of the pulsating *mass* indicates an aneurysm. In larger patients, you will not be able to palpate a mass, even though an aneurysm is present. In this case, the patient's report of tearing pain may be the only indication of a possible aortic aneurysm.

NOTE: *A common assessment error is not assessing the lower quadrants properly. The lower quadrants extend from the umbilicus downward to the pelvis. In most people, this extends well below the belt- or waistline and requires loosening of clothing to actually assess the lower quadrants (Figure 24-6).*

Vital Signs

Vital signs should be taken initially and then every 5 minutes for a patient complaining of abdominal pain. These vital signs are pulse, respiration, blood pressure, and skin color, temperature, and condition. Mental status is also important to observe. Remember that shock will appear initially with increased pulse and respirations; pale, moist skin; and anxiety. Falling blood pressure will be a late sign. Shock will be discussed in detail in Chapter 27, "Bleeding and Shock."

Since patients with abdominal pain may have an increased pulse simply as a result of the pain, serial vitals taken over time will help identify potentially dangerous trends. Calming,

FIGURE 24-6 Adequate examination of the lower abdominal quadrants, well below the beltline or waistline, requires loosening of clothing.

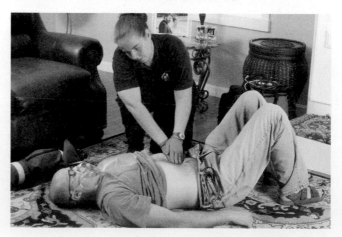

placing the patient in a position of comfort, and administering oxygen may actually reduce the pulse, which is a good sign.

Respirations may also be affected by abdominal pain. If breathing worsens the abdominal pain, the patient may be breathing shallowly and sometimes more rapidly.

General Abdominal Distress

You may be called to evaluate patients who have complaints that appear nonspecific but involve the digestive system. Nausea, vomiting, and diarrhea are examples. Some of these complaints will result from digestive system disorders, whereas other causes could be cardiac issues, diabetic issues, food poisoning, or the flu.

Your assessment and care for these patients, like any others discussed in this chapter, will involve providing a proper scene size-up and primary assessment with appropriate airway care. Your history, physical exam, and vital signs assessments will be critical for determining the patient's priority and condition (stable vs. unstable).

The assessment techniques discussed previously in the chapter will apply in the same manner to these patients. Determining if there is pain, tenderness, discomfort, or any associated complaints; the time of onset (sudden vs. over a period of time); fever and malaise; and abdominal inspection and palpation are all appropriate.

Patient care will involve monitoring for airway problems if the patient is vomiting. Place the responsive patient in a position of comfort. Place the unresponsive patient or the patient who is having difficulty maintaining an airway in a left lateral recumbent position for drainage from the mouth.

PATIENT ASSESSMENT

Abdominal Distress

To assess a patient suffering from abdominal pain or distress:

1. Perform a scene size-up, looking for clues to a possible mechanism of injury while taking Standard Precautions as well as safety precautions.
2. Perform a primary assessment including the general impression of the patient's level of distress, mental status, airway, breathing, and circulation. Apply oxygen. Make a transport/priority decision. Vomiting may cause airway compromise, so be prepared to suction.
3. Assist the patient to a position of comfort. Calm and reassure the patient. This will help the patient and, by relaxing him, also help complete your next assessment steps.
4. Perform a history, physical examination, and vital signs.
5. Perform a reassessment every 5 minutes en route.

NOTE: *Vomiting and diarrhea will require both strict attention to Standard Precautions during patient care and careful cleaning and disinfection of the equipment and ambulance after the call.*

Decision Point

• Is my patient in shock or developing shock?

PATIENT CARE

Abdominal Distress

Although there are many types of abdominal emergencies, the care you will provide for all abdominal conditions is the same. You may find patients who appear unstable and obviously have a serious condition as well as those who are in pain, yet appear stable. In every case, despite the differences in patient presentation, you should follow these steps when treating a patient with an abdominal emergency.

1. While performing the primary assessment, maintain the patient's airway. If the patient has an altered level of responsiveness, this will compromise the airway. Keep in mind that patients with abdominal emergencies may vomit. Suction whenever necessary.
2. Administer 15 lpm of oxygen to the patient by nonrebreather mask.

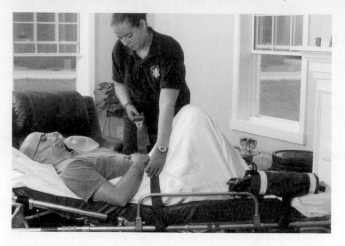

FIGURE 24-7 Place the responsive patient without airway problems or signs of shock in a position of comfort and transport the patient to an appropriate facility.

3. Place the patient in a position of comfort (Figure 24-7). However, if shock and/or airway problems are present, position the patient to treat these conditions. The left laterally recumbent position will help maintain the airway.
4. Transport the patient promptly to an appropriate facility.

You should always work to calm the patient and reduce his anxiety. Patients who are in pain will require calming and reassurance.

Never give a patient with a complaint of abdominal pain or discomfort anything by mouth.

NOTE: *This chapter has talked in great detail about assessment of the abdomen, searching for abnormal findings. Keep in mind, however, that the absence of abnormal findings does not mean the patient's condition is not serious. PATIENTS WITH ABDOMINAL PAIN SHOULD ALWAYS BE CONSIDERED AT LEAST POTENTIALLY UNSTABLE AND TRANSPORTED PROMPTLY.*

CRITICAL DECISION MAKING

Assessing a Patient with Abdominal Pain

Each patient with abdominal pain will receive a history and physical examination. In the following patient presentations, determine what part or parts of the history or physical examination are missing.

1. A 26-year-old female patient complains of pain in her lower left abdominal quadrant. The pain radiates from the left to the right lower quadrant. She denies allergies or medications. The pain came on while she was sitting at her desk earlier in the day. Her vital signs are pulse 104 and slightly irregular, respirations 22, blood pressure 128/90, skin warm and dry.

2. A 14-year-old boy complains of abdominal pain. It began slowly over a day or two and has gradually become more severe. His parents are present. The patient denies medical history, allergies, or meds. He hasn't eaten since yesterday because of the pain. His vital signs are pulse 96, strong and regular; respirations 20 and adequate; blood pressure 104/72; skin warm and dry.

3. A 56-year-old man complains of severe pain in both lower quadrants of his abdomen which developed suddenly and without apparent provocation. The pain is intermittent and comes in waves. He has a history of high blood pressure and high cholesterol and takes medications for both. His pulse is 88, strong and regular; respirations 18 and adequate; blood pressure 158/104; skin cool and moist.

Key Facts and Concepts

- All complaints of abdominal pain or distress must be treated as serious emergencies requiring transport.

- As an EMT, your responsibility is primarily to assess the patient and report your findings. Field diagnosing the cause of an abdominal complaint is often more difficult and time-consuming than diagnosing in the emergency department, where there are many more resources available than in the field.

- Your assessment should include a thorough patient history, physical exam, and vital signs.

- Look for signs and symptoms that can signal serious trouble. This includes the sudden onset of tearing pain radiating to the back; vomiting blood or coffee-ground material; the presence of black, tarry stools; or signs and symptoms of shock.

- Emergency care will consist of protecting the patient's airway, administering high-concentration oxygen by nonrebreather mask, placing the responsive patient in a position of comfort, placing the unresponsive patient or patient with difficulty maintaining an airway in the left lateral recumbent position, and transporting the patient to the hospital.

- Take all appropriate Standard Precautions and carefully clean and disinfect equipment and the ambulance, especially if the patient has vomited or had diarrhea.

Key Decisions

- Is the patient's airway at risk because of vomiting?
- Is the patient displaying signs and symptoms of shock?
- Does the patient's presentation suggest any critical problems (e.g., tearing abdominal pain radiating to the back)?
- Do I need to transport this patient immediately for definitive care in a hospital?

Chapter Glossary

parietal pain a localized, intense pain that arises from the parietal peritoneum, the lining of the abdominal cavity.

peritoneum the membrane that lines the abdominal cavity (the *parietal peritoneum*) and covers the organs within it (the *visceral peritoneum*).

referred pain pain that is felt in a location other than where the pain originates.

retroperitoneal space the area posterior to the peritoneum, between the peritoneum and the back.

tearing pain sharp pain that feels as if body tissues are being torn apart.

visceral pain a poorly localized, dull, or diffuse pain that arises from the abdominal organs, or viscera.

Preparation for Your Examination and Practice

Short Answer

1. List five signs and symptoms of abdominal distress.
2. Describe the difference between visceral and parietal pain and describe a condition that may be responsible for each.
3. Describe the emergency care for a patient experiencing abdominal pain or distress.
4. Name the four abdominal quadrants and explain how the quadrants are determined.

Thinking and Linking

Think back to Chapter 20, "Cardiac Emergencies," and link information from that chapter with information from this chapter as you consider the following situation:

- Your patient is an elderly male with a history of cardiac problems. He is complaining of central chest pressure without radiation. En route to the hospital, he says, "I'm going to be sick." He then vomits approximately a cup of material that looks like coffee grounds. How could the patient's bleeding be connected to his chest pain? What treatment available in an ambulance might help this patient?

Critical Thinking Exercises

Abdominal pain can have many causes and can vary significantly in severity. The purpose of this exercise will be to consider some elements of the history and management for such a patient.

- You are called to a patient with abdominal pain. You arrive to find him sitting on the couch, doubled over with pain. He describes the pain as severe and says it began as "on and off" over the past several days. It became severe within the hour. What additional questions would you ask the patient? What position would he likely be most comfortable in?

Pathophysiology to Practice

The following question is designed to assist you in gathering relevant clinical information and making accurate decisions in the field.

- Although it is sometimes difficult to determine the cause of abdominal pain in young and middle-aged patients, it is even more difficult for elderly patients. They often have vague symptoms of abdominal problems rather than the traditional presentations of particular diseases. Describe two of the more likely causes for an elderly patient with generalized abdominal pain to have sustained life-threatening internal bleeding.

Street Scenes

You are dispatched to the Shop-Till-You-Drop supermarket for a "sick woman." You arrive at a scene that appears safe and observe store workers around an approximately 75-year-old woman who appears sweaty and somewhat pale. She is sitting in a chair brought over by a store employee. The employee tells you that the woman was standing in the checkout line and told the cashier that her stomach hurt and she felt ill. She vomited into the trash can the employee provided and then began to feel a bit weak and dizzy. She was placed in the chair to await EMS.

You introduce yourself and find the woman oriented but looking tired, breathing adequately but a bit rapidly, and having a slightly increased radial pulse. You ask the clerk to bring you the trash can the patient vomited into. She thinks your request is kind of weird, but she complies.

Street Scene Questions

1. What is your initial impression of this patient?
2. What is the significance of the patient's initial presentation?
3. Why would you want to see the trash can?

You ask your partner to administer oxygen and get a set of vitals while you get a history. The trash can contains a considerable amount of a reddish-brown substance you believe may be partially digested blood. You radio for advanced life support before you begin the history, and realize the patient must be promptly transported.

Street Scene Questions

4. Why would you request advanced life support?
5. Do you agree with the transport priority? Why or why not?

The patient reports diffuse pain across the upper abdominal quadrants that has been increasing slightly over the past few days. It is not worsened or made better by anything in particular and is slightly tender to palpation. No rigidity is noted. She has eaten and drunk normally over the past several days and has no history of abdominal problems. She has had one "mini-stroke" a few months ago. She takes an unknown blood pressure medication and an aspirin a day to prevent further strokes. Her pulse is 104, respirations 26, blood pressure 102/68, skin pale and moist.

You promptly move the patient to the stretcher and into the ambulance. An ALS engine arrives and a paramedic jumps in with her equipment. You explain that you are concerned about a potentially serious condition and shock. The paramedic agrees.

Street Scene Questions

6. Do you believe this patient is in shock? Explain your reasoning.
7. What effect might her history have on her current condition?
8. What position should the patient be placed in?

Because of the patient's apparent history of high blood pressure, you think that the blood pressure of 102/68, which would usually not be considered low, may actually indicate shock for this patient. The paramedic thinks that the aspirin taken for stroke prevention may have caused bleeding in her stomach.

The paramedic begins advanced care, including an IV and electrocardiogram. As a precaution, he checks the patient's blood sugar level and finds it is within normal limits. The paramedic obtains a second set of vital signs: pulse 112, respirations 28, blood pressure 100/64, skin unchanged. The patient insists on sitting up because she feels she may vomit again.

You arrive at the hospital a short time later and make a report to the physician. The patient is, in fact, bleeding internally and will be admitted for further care.

Behavioral and Psychiatric Emergencies and Suicide

STANDARD ⊙------
Medicine (Psychiatric)

COMPETENCY ⊙------
Applies fundamental knowledge to provide basic emergency care and transportation based on assessment findings for an acutely ill patient.

CORE CONCEPTS ⊙------
— The nature and causes of behavioral and psychiatric emergencies
— Emergency care for behavioral and psychiatric emergencies
— Emergency care for potential or attempted suicide
— Emergency care for aggressive or hostile patients
— When and how to restrain a patient safely and effectively
— Medical/legal considerations in behavioral and psychiatric emergencies

EXPLORE Resource Central

To access Resource Central, follow directions on the Student Access Card provided with this text. If there is no card, go to **www.bradybooks.com** and follow the Resource Central link to Buy Access from there. Under Media Resources, you will find:

▶ **How to Apply Soft Restraints**
Learn how to properly apply soft restraints in this video and discuss when and why you would restrain a patient.

▶ **Eating Disorders**
Watch a video on eating disorders to learn how to differentiate between common types of disorders and identify some complications associated with eating disorders.

▶ **Fact Sheet on Suicide**
Read facts on suicide, such as who is at risk, some warning signs, and how an EMT should assess and manage a suicidal patient.

OBJECTIVES

After reading this chapter you should be able to:

25.1 Define key terms introduced in this chapter.

25.2 Recognize behaviors that are abnormal in a given context. (p. 588)

25.3 Discuss medical and traumatic conditions that can cause unusual behavior. (p. 589)

25.4 For a patient whose abnormal behavior appears to be caused by stress, discuss techniques to calm the patient and gain his cooperation. (p. 590)

25.5 Discuss assessment of a patient who appears to be suffering from a behavioral or psychiatric emergency. (p. 591)

(continued)

KEY TERMS

behavior, *p. 588*   behavioral emergency, *p. 588*   excited delirium, *p. 595*   positional asphyxia, *p. 597*

A s an EMT, you will respond to many emergencies in which the patient is behaving in unexpected and sometimes dangerous ways. The unusual behavior may be the result of stress, physical trauma or illness, drug or alcohol abuse, or a psychiatric condition (mental disorder).

>>>>>>
BEHAVIORAL AND PSYCHIATRIC EMERGENCIES

What Is a Behavioral Emergency?

● CORE CONCEPT
The nature and causes of behavioral and psychiatric emergencies

behavior
the manner in which a person acts.

behavioral emergency
when a patient's behavior is not typical for the situation; when the patient's behavior is unacceptable or intolerable to the patient, his family, or the community; or when the patient may harm himself or others.

We all exhibit *behavior*. Behavior is defined as the manner in which a person acts or performs. It involves any or all activities of a person, including physical and mental activity. Of course, behavior differs from person to person and from situation to situation.

A *behavioral emergency* exists when a person exhibits abnormal behavior—that is, behavior within a given situation that is unacceptable or intolerable to the patient, the family, or the community.

A key part of that definition is "within a given situation." You may have observed that, in your own life or in that of friends or family, behavior varies, depending on the situation at hand. For example, if a person is notified unexpectedly of the death of a loved one, a common reaction is screaming, crying, throwing things, or other emotional outbursts. In the context of the situation, this behavior would not be unusual. If the same behaviors were exhibited for no apparent reason in the middle of a shopping center, they might indicate a behavioral emergency.

Remember that you will be exposed to persons from other cultures and with different lifestyles. Some behaviors may seem unusual to you but might be quite normal to the person performing them. Behavioral conditions require full patient assessment, including primary and secondary assessments, just like any other emergency. Remain objective. Do not judge patients hastily or solely on the way they look or act.

Psychiatric Conditions

Some, but not all, behavioral emergencies are caused by psychiatric conditions, which may also be called mental disorders.

The National Institute of Mental Health (NIMH), in its document *The Numbers Count: Mental Disorders in America (2008)*, notes that in any given year 26.2 percent of adult Americans suffer from a diagnosable mental disorder. Almost 10 percent of the population has a mood disorder (e.g., depression) and just over 20 percent have anxiety or panic issues. Much smaller percentages are involved for conditions such as schizophrenia (1.1 percent) and bipolar disorder (2.6 percent). Some have more than one condition simultaneously. Based on these statistics, it is clear you will be called to deal with people experiencing psychiatric crisis. This chapter will help you understand and care for this significant patient population.

Physical Causes of Altered Mental Status

It is helpful to consider patients who are exhibiting crisis or unusual behavior to be having an altered mental status from a *non*psychiatric cause until proven otherwise. Many medical and traumatic conditions are likely to alter a patient's behavior. These problems may include:

- Low blood sugar, which may be the cause of rapid onset of erratic or hostile behavior (similar to alcohol intoxication), dizziness and headache, fainting, seizures, sometimes coma, profuse perspiration, hunger, drooling, and rapid pulse but normal blood pressure. (See Chapter 21, "Diabetic Emergencies and Altered Mental Status.")

- Lack of oxygen, which may cause restlessness and confusion, cyanosis (blue or gray skin), and altered mental status.

- Stroke or inadequate blood to the brain, which may cause confusion or dizziness, impaired speech, headache, loss of function or paralysis of extremities on one side of the body, nausea and vomiting, and rapid full pulse.

- Head trauma, which can cause personality changes ranging from irritability to irrational behavior, altered mental status, amnesia or confusion, irregular respirations, elevated blood pressure, and decreasing pulse.

- Mind-altering substances, which can cause highly variable signs and symptoms depending on the substance ingested. (See Chapter 23, "Poisoning and Overdose Emergencies.")

- Excessive cold, which may cause shivering, feelings of numbness, altered mental status, drowsiness, staggering walk, slow breathing, and slow pulse.

- Excessive heat, which may cause decreased or complete loss of consciousness. (See Chapter 33, "Environmental Emergencies.")

When dealing with someone who appears to be having a behavioral emergency, always consider the possibility that his unusual behavior is caused by something other than a psychological problem (Figure 25-1). Chapter 21, "Diabetic Emergencies and Altered Mental Status," discussed many of the common causes of altered mental status.

CRITICAL DECISION MAKING

Psych Condition . . . or Hidden Medical Condition?

You will respond to many behavioral emergencies during your EMS experience. Sometimes patients with medical problems appear to be psychiatric patients, but they actually aren't. Other times, patients with a psychiatric history have medical problems that aren't related to their psychiatric condition. For each of these patients, describe how your assessment would determine if the patient was suffering from a medical problem or a psychiatric problem.

1. Your patient is a 56-year-old man who was found to be "talking to God" and generally mumbling at the grocery store.

2. Your patient is a 21-year-old student who was found on the outskirts of his campus, acting strangely, with a slight smell of alcohol on his breath.

3. Your patient is an 84-year-old woman who is in a nursing home. She has a history of depression and cardiac problems. This morning she became agitated and angry with the staff.

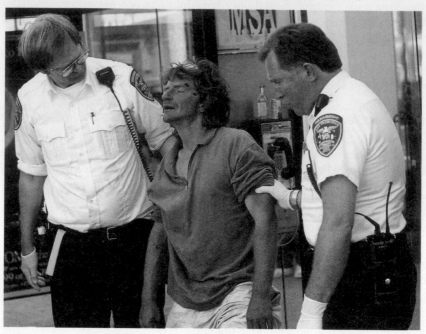

Situational Stress Reactions

When faced with severe, unexpected stress, most patients will display emotions such as fear, grief, and anger. These are typical stress reactions at the accident scene and common reactions to serious illness and death. In the vast majority of cases, as you begin to take control of the situation and treat the patient as an individual, your personal interaction will inspire confidence in your ability to help. The patient will begin to calm down and may even begin to feel able to cope with the emergency.

Be as unhurried as you can. If you rush your patient assessment and interview, the patient may feel as if the situation is out of control. The patient also may believe that you are concerned about the problem but not about him. Let the patient know that you are there to help.

Whenever you care for a patient who is displaying typical stress reactions, act in a calm manner, giving the patient time to gain control of his emotions. Quietly and carefully evaluate the situation, keeping your own emotions under control. Let the patient know that you are listening to what he is saying, and honestly explain things to the patient. Stay alert for sudden changes in behavior.

By acting in this manner, you are applying crisis management techniques to help the patient deal with stress. If the patient does not begin to interact with you or calm down, and if there are no apparent physical causes for the behavior, you must assume that there is a problem of a more serious nature, such as a psychiatric problem. Proceed according to the recommendations in the following segments of this chapter.

EMERGENCY CARE FOR BEHAVIORAL OR PSYCHIATRIC EMERGENCIES

CORE CONCEPT

Emergency care for behavioral and psychiatric emergencies

Behavioral and Psychiatric Emergencies

Behavioral and psychiatric problems have a wide variety of manifestations and presentations. One patient may be withdrawn and not wish to communicate, whereas another may be agitated, talkative, or exhibiting bizarre or threatening behavior. Some patients may act as if they wish to harm themselves or others.

Follow these general rules when dealing with a patient who is experiencing a behavioral or psychiatric emergency:

- Identify yourself and your role.
- Speak slowly and clearly. Use a calm and reassuring tone.
- Make eye contact with the patient.
- Listen to the patient. You can show you are listening by repeating part of what the patient says back to him.
- Do not be judgmental. Show compassion, not pity.
- Use positive body language. Avoid crossing your arms or looking uninterested.
- Acknowledge the patient's feelings.
- Do not enter the patient's personal space. Stay at least 3 feet from the patient. Making the patient feel closed in can cause an emotional outburst.
- Be alert for changes in the patient's emotional status. Watch for increasingly aggressive behavior and take appropriate safety precautions.

PATIENT ASSESSMENT

Behavioral or Psychiatric Emergency

To assess a patient who appears to be suffering a behavioral or psychiatric emergency:

- Perform a careful scene size-up. If there are indications at the time of dispatch that the call may involve a potentially violent or agitated patient, then police should be requested to respond to the scene, arriving ahead of EMS units to assure the scene is safe ("secure") for EMS to enter.
- Identify yourself and your role. It may not be obvious to the patient who you are and what you intend to do.
- Complete a primary assessment, including assessment of the patient's mental status (level of responsiveness; orientation to person, place, and time).
- Perform as much of the detailed examination as possible. Be alert for medical and traumatic conditions that could be causing the patient's behavior.
- Gather a thorough patient history. This will alert you to past psychiatric problems, or psychiatric medications the patient may be taking (or not taking—causing the outburst). This may also alert you to conditions such as diabetes that can closely mimic a psychiatric condition.

The following are common presentations, or signs and symptoms, of patients experiencing psychiatric emergencies:

- Panic or anxiety
- Unusual appearance, disordered clothing, or poor hygiene
- Agitated or unusual activity, such as repetitive motions, threatening movements, or withdrawn stance
- Unusual speech patterns, such as too rapid or pressured-sounding speech (as if being forced out), or an inability to carry on a coherent conversation
- Bizarre behavior or thought patterns
- Suicidal or self-destructive behavior
- Violent or aggressive behavior with threats or intent to harm others

Decision Points

- Is the scene safe?
- Is my patient having a behavioral/psychiatric crisis, or is this an altered mental status from a physical cause?

Inside/Outside

The nervous system works through the use of neurotransmitters. Electrical impulses travel along neurons until they reach a synapse—a space between nerve cells. Neurotransmitters are chemicals within the body that transmit the message from the distal end of one neuron (the presynaptic neuron) to the proximal end of the next neuron (postsynaptic neuron). Although it sounds like a complicated process, it actually takes only milliseconds.

Neurotransmitters are released from a neuron, then travel across the synapse to the next neuron. The receptors on the postsynaptic neuron receive the neurotransmitter. This is the mechanism by which the impulse is moved along the nervous system. After the impulse is transmitted, the neurotransmitter goes through a process called reuptake, in which the neurotransmitter is returned to the presynaptic neuron.

Neurotransmitters—or the lack of neurotransmitters—have been implicated in depression and other mental disorders. Medications prescribed for these conditions are designed to affect the relevant neurotransmitters. One commonly prescribed class of drugs is the selective serotonin reuptake inhibitor (SSRI). This medication is believed to elevate mood by preventing the reuptake of the neurotransmitter serotonin in the synapse. Prozac, Paxil, and Zoloft are trade names of commonly prescribed SSRI medications.

Newer medications offer reuptake inhibition of more than one neurotransmitter. In addition to serotonin, neurotransmitters include norepinephrine, epinephrine, and dopamine.

PATIENT CARE

Behavioral or Psychiatric Emergency

Emergency care of a patient having a behavioral or psychiatric emergency involves these steps:

- Be alert for personal or scene safety problems throughout the call.

- Treat any life-threatening problems during the primary assessment.

- Be alert for medical or traumatic conditions that could mimic a behavioral emergency. Treat conditions you identify (e.g., low blood sugar level).

- Be prepared to spend time talking to the patient. Use the skills listed earlier in dealing with the patient. Remember to talk in a calm, reassuring voice. Use positive body language and good eye contact. Avoid unnecessary physical contact and quick movements.

- Encourage the patient to discuss what is troubling him.

- Never play along with any visual or auditory hallucinations that a patient may be experiencing. Do not lie to the patient.

- If it appears it will help, involve family members or friends in the conversation. Evaluate the patient's response to the presence of others. If it agitates the patient, ask the others to leave.

Suicide

CORE CONCEPT

Emergency care for potential or attempted suicide

Each year in this country, thousands of people commit suicide. Suicide is the eighth leading cause of death, but the third leading cause of death in the 15- to 24-year-old age group. Depression and suicide have also reached alarming levels in the senior citizen population. Many more suffer both physical and emotional injuries in suicide attempts. Anyone may become suicidal if emotional distress is severe, regardless of gender, age, or ethnic, social, or economic background.

People attempt suicide for many reasons, including depression caused by chemical imbalance, the death of a loved one, financial problems, the end to a love affair, poor health, loss of esteem, divorce, fear of failure, and alcohol and drug abuse. People attempt to end their lives by any one of a variety of methods. You may observe suicides or attempted suicides by drug overdose, hanging, jumping from high places, ingesting poisons, inhaling gas, wrist-cutting, self-mutilation, stabbing, or shooting.

PATIENT ASSESSMENT

Potential or Attempted Suicide

Factors often associated with a risk for suicide appear in the following list. Although some or even all of them may be present in a patient, it is not possible to use these characteristics to predict who will or who will not commit suicide:

- **Depression.** Take seriously a patient's feelings and expressions of despair or suicidal thoughts.
- **High current or recent stress levels.** If these are present, take the threat of suicide seriously.
- **Recent emotional trauma.** This could be job loss, loss of a significant relationship, serious illness, arrest, or imprisonment.
- **Age.** High suicide rates occur at ages 15 to 25 and over age 40. The elderly are a population where suicide rates are increasing.
- **Alcohol and drug abuse.**
- **Threats of suicide.** The patient may have told others that he is considering suicide. Take all threats of suicide seriously.
- **Suicide plan.** A patient who has a detailed suicide plan is more likely to commit suicide. Look for a plan that includes a method to carry out the suicide, notes, giving away personal possessions, or getting affairs in order.
- **Previous attempts or suicide threats.** These could include a history of self-destructive behavior. Often patients who have attempted suicide on a previous occasion are considered to be "looking for attention" and are not taken seriously on subsequent attempts. However, statistics reveal that a person who has attempted suicide in the past is more likely to commit suicide than one who has not.
- **Sudden improvement from depression.** A patient who has made the decision to commit suicide may actually appear to be coming out of a depression. The fact that the decision has been made and an end is in sight can cause this apparent "improvement." You may find family members and friends of suicidal patients who will report that the patient had seemed "better" in the past few days.

NOTE: *Whenever you are called to care for a patient who has attempted or may be about to attempt suicide, your first concern must be your own safety. Not all patients will wish to harm you, but the mechanism used to attempt suicide will be capable of causing death. It could intentionally or accidentally be turned on you.*

PATIENT CARE

Potential or Attempted Suicide

Patients who are in an emotional, psychiatric, or attempted-suicide emergency are cared for in similar ways. In all cases, your personal interaction with the patient is key. Try to establish visual and verbal contact as soon as possible. Avoid arguing. Make no threats, and show no indication of using force.

Remember that you are the first professional to begin both the physical and mental health care of the patient. The more reassurance you can provide for the patient, the easier it will be for the hospital emergency department staff to continue care.

Emergency care includes the following steps:

1. Treatment must begin with scene size-up. Make sure it is safe to approach the patient. If the scene is not safe, request assistance from the police and wait until they have secured the scene. Do not leave the patient alone unless you are at risk of physical harm. Try to talk with the patient from a safe distance until the police arrive. Take Standard Precautions.
2. When the scene is secure, look for and treat life-threatening problems to the extent that the patient will permit it. Seek police assistance in restraining the patient if necessary for care of life-threatening problems.
3. As possible, perform a secondary assessment and provide emergency care.
4. Perform a detailed physical exam only if it is safe and you suspect the patient may have an injury.

5. Perform a reassessment. Watch for sudden changes in the patient's behavior and physical condition.
6. Contact the receiving hospital and report on the patient's current mental status and other essential information.

Note that a physical exam may be difficult with the emotional or psychiatric patient. Because of this, you may not be able to proceed beyond the primary assessment.

Throughout your interaction with the patient, speak slowly and patiently await answers to your questions. As you gain the patient's confidence, explain what questions must be answered and what must be done as part of the physical exam and taking vital signs. Let the patient know that you think it would be best if he goes to the hospital and that you need his cooperation and help. Back off if necessary. If the patient's fear or aggression increases, do not push the issues of the examination or transport. Instead, try to reestablish the conversation and give the patient more time before you again suggest that going to the hospital is a good idea.

Transport all suicidal patients. Seek police assistance, if necessary. Report any attempted suicide or expression of suicidal thoughts to the medical facility, police, or government agency designated by your state law and local protocols.

Aggressive or Hostile Patients

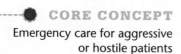

CORE CONCEPT

Emergency care for aggressive or hostile patients

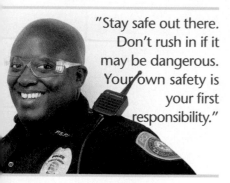

"Stay safe out there. Don't rush in if it may be dangerous. Your own safety is your first responsibility."

Aggressive or disruptive behavior may be caused by trauma to the brain and nervous system, metabolic disorders, stress, alcohol, other drugs, or psychological disorders. Sometimes you will know that your patient is aggressive from the information you receive from dispatch. Other times the scene may provide quick clues (such as drugs, yelling, unclean conditions, broken furniture). Neighbors, family members, or bystanders may tell you that the patient is dangerous or angry or has a history of aggression or combativeness. The patient's stance (tense muscles, fists clenched, or quick irregular movements, for example) or his position in the room may give you an early warning of possible violence. On rare occasions, you may start with an apparently calm patient who suddenly turns aggressive.

As already noted, when a patient acts as if he may hurt himself or others, your first concern must be your own safety. Take the following precautions:

- Do not isolate yourself from your partner or other sources of help. Make certain that you have an escape route. Do not let the patient come between you and the door. If a patient should become violent, retreat and wait for police assistance.

- Do not take any action that may be considered threatening by the patient. To do so may bring about hostile behavior directed against you or others.

- Always be on the watch for weapons. Stay out of kitchens, as they are filled with dangerous weapons. Stay in a safe area until the police can control the scene.

PATIENT ASSESSMENT

Aggressive or Hostile Patient

Your assessment of the aggressive or hostile patient may not go beyond the primary assessment phase until the patient is appropriately calmed or restrained. Most of your time may be spent trying to calm the patient and ensuring everyone's safety. However, aggression or hostility in a patient should never be used as an excuse for not assessing the patient as thoroughly as possible. An aggressive or hostile patient:

- Responds to people inappropriately
- Tries to hurt himself or others
- May have a rapid pulse and breathing
- Usually displays rapid speech and rapid physical movements
- May appear anxious, nervous, or "panicky"

PATIENT CARE

Aggressive or Hostile Patient

Follow these steps for the emergency care of an aggressive or hostile patient:

1. Treatment begins with scene size-up. Make sure it is safe to approach the patient. If needed, request assistance from law enforcement before making your approach. Practice Standard Precautions.
2. Seek advice from medical direction if the patient's behavior prevents normal assessment and care procedures.
3. As part of reassessment, watch for sudden changes in the patient's behavior. An agitated patient who suddenly becomes silent may be experiencing a serious medical emergency. Complete reassessments involve rechecking the primary assessment frequently and upon any change in mental status.
4. Seek assistance from law enforcement, as well as from medical direction, if restraint seems necessary.

Reasonable Force and Restraint

CORE CONCEPT
When and how to restrain a patient safely and effectively

Reasonable force is the force necessary to keep a patient from injuring himself or others. Reasonableness is determined by looking at all circumstances involved, including the patient's strength and size, type of abnormal behavior, mental status, and available methods of restraint. Understand that you may protect yourself from attack, but otherwise you must avoid actions that can cause injury to the patient.

In addition, in most localities an EMT cannot legally restrain a behavioral emergency patient, move such a patient against his will, or force such a patient to accept emergency care—even at the family's request. The restraint and forcible moving of patients is usually within the jurisdiction of law enforcement. The police (and, in some areas, a physician) can order you to restrain and transport a patient to the appropriate medical facility. However, the physician is not empowered to order you to take action that could place you in danger. If the police order restraint and transport for the patient, they must perform or assist with these procedures as necessary. Remember to follow local protocol.

At times, a patient with a medical or traumatic emergency may display violent behavior to the extent that restraint is necessary before the patient can receive the medical treatment he needs. For example, a diabetic patient with hypoglycemia may be acting abnormally and even aggressively. If the patient's behavior interferes with or prevents treatment and the EMT can safely restrain the patient, he should do so in order to initiate treatment. Similarly, a patient with a head injury may be hypoxic and acting abnormally. Again, if it can be done safely, the EMT should institute the needed treatment which, in this case, includes restraint so the patient can be safely transported to a facility where his head injury can be treated.

Determining whether a particular patient has a medical or traumatic emergency that is causing his abnormal behavior can be difficult. Consider whether the patient is capable of giving or refusing informed consent, consult medical direction, and administer the care that is in the patient's best interest without endangering yourself.

Never try to assist in restraining a patient unless there are sufficient personnel to do the job. You must be able to ensure your safety as well as the patient's safety. If you help the police or a physician to restrain a patient, make certain that the restraints are humane. For example, handcuffs and plastic "throwaway" criminal restraints should not be used because of the soft-tissue damage they can inflict. Initially, the police may have to use such restraints. However, in some states they can be replaced with soft restraints such as leather cuffs and belts. If authorized in your state and by local protocol, an ambulance should carry leather cuffs, a waist-size belt, and at least three short belts. Restraints for the wrists and ankles can be made from gauze roller bandages.

excited delirium
bizarre and/or aggressive behavior, shouting, paranoia, panic, violence toward others, insensitivity to pain, unexpected physical strength, and hyperthermia, usually associated with cocaine or amphetamine use. Also called agitated delirium.

NOTE: *The medical literature refers to a condition called **excited delirium** (also called agitated delirium). In this situation, a patient begins to act extremely agitated or psychotic. It is believed that a patient with this condition has an elevated temperature and sometimes alcohol or drug intoxication. The patient will cease struggling, and often*

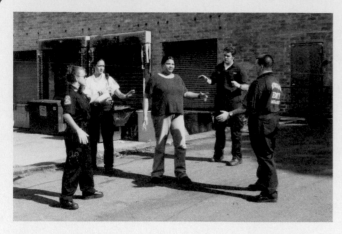

1 Plan your approach to the patient in advance and remain outside the range of the patient's arms and legs until you are ready to act.

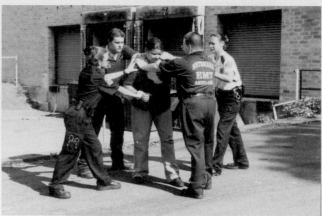

2 Assign one EMT to each limb, and have all the EMTs approach the patient at the same time.

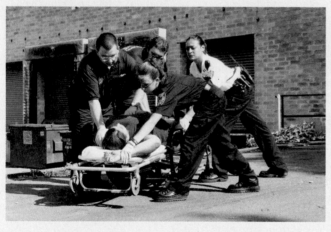

3 Place the patient on the stretcher as his/her condition and local protocols indicate. Do not let go until the patient is properly secured.

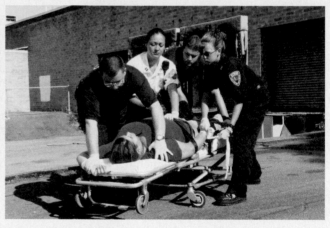

4 Use multiple straps or other soft restraints to secure the patient to the stretcher.

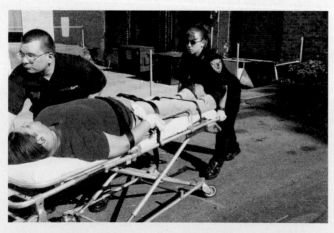

5 When the patient is secure, assess distal circulation and continually monitor airway and breathing. *(Photos 1–5 © Craig Jackson/In the Dark Photography)*

NOTE: *A fifth rescuer, if available, can control the patient's head—taking special care, however, not to be bitten.*

within minutes the patient is found to have inadequate or absent respirations and subsequently dies. It is important for the EMT to be alert for this sequence of events if patients exhibit this behavior and monitor the patient constantly throughout the call.

Do not remove police restraints until you and the police are certain that soft restraints will hold the patient. To ensure everyone's safety once they are on, do not remove soft restraints, even if the patient appears to be acting rationally.

Follow these guidelines when a patient must be restrained (Scan 25-1):

- Be sure to have adequate help.
- Plan your activities; have a well-delineated plan of action before initiating the restraint.
- Estimate the range of motion of the patient's arms and legs and stay beyond that range until ready.
- Once the decision to restrain the patient has been reached, act quickly.
- Have one EMT talk to and reassure the patient throughout the restraining procedure.
- Approach with a minimum of four persons, one assigned to each limb, all to act at the same time. (Five rescuers would allow an extra person to control the head. However, the rescuer at the head should use caution to prevent being bitten.)
- Secure all four limbs with restraints approved by medical direction.
- Position the patient face up. The position will be dictated by what the restraining process itself permits, the patient's condition (e.g., injuries, breathing problems), and local protocols. Monitor the patient's airway. Never "hog tie" the patient or restrain the patient in any manner that will impair breathing. Patients who have been improperly restrained have died as a result of a condition often referred to as ***positional asphyxia***. Carefully monitor all restrained patients. Many times a patient will become quiet and stop fighting, leading EMTs and police officers to relax because the patient appears to have calmed down. In some cases, the patient has stopped breathing and dies. It can't be repeated enough: *Monitor your restrained patient constantly throughout the call.*
- Use multiple straps or other restraints to ensure that the patient is adequately secured. Anticipate that the patient's behavior may turn more violent and be sure that restraint is adequate for this possibility.
- If the patient is spitting on rescuers, place a surgical mask on the patient if he has no breathing difficulty or likelihood of vomiting and if local protocols permit, or have rescuers wear protective masks, eyewear, and clothing.
- Reassess the patient's distal circulation frequently and adjust restraints as safe and necessary if distal circulation is diminished.
- Use sufficient force, but avoid unnecessary force.
- Document the reasons why the patient was restrained and the technique of restraint.

positional asphyxia
inadequate breathing or respiratory arrest caused by a body position that restricts breathing.

Transport to an Appropriate Facility

Your medical protocols or procedures should direct you to the most appropriate medical facility within your service area. Not all hospitals are prepared to treat behavioral emergencies.

Medical/Legal Considerations

A patient who refuses emergency care or transport is a significant medical/legal risk for EMS agencies and EMTs. What should you do when a behavioral emergency patient refuses or resists your efforts to provide care?

Most states have a provision in law that will allow a patient to be transported against his will if he is a danger to himself or others. This is an exception to the rule that patients must provide consent for their care and transportation. Know your state laws on treating patients without consent. Many states give this authority to law enforcement personnel. It will always be beneficial to have the police present if the patient must be restrained as a matter of safety.

CORE CONCEPT
Medical/legal considerations in behavioral and psychiatric emergencies

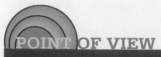

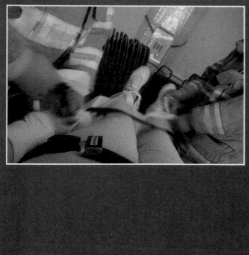

"I was at a group therapy session when I started noticing people were watching me. They did that for awhile. When I would talk they would whisper and giggle and point. I heard voices. They whispered, too. I couldn't see the people, but I heard the voices very clearly. They were talking about me.

"I stood up and yelled. "'Don't say those things! Oh yes, you. Stop it right now!'" They kept going. The voices got louder. I started pushing people and throwing chairs. They had no right to do this to me. The voices just laughed. People pointed and whispered. I knew what they were thinking.

"The ambulance came. The police came. I got tied down and taken to the hospital.

"Some of what I tell you is based on what my counselor told me. I don't remember it all. You see, I am schizophrenic. I guess you could say reality isn't my strong point sometimes. I can joke about it now. What I experienced are called paranoid delusions. I get them a lot. I can usually control them. But sometimes when I can't afford my pills or I get fed up with the fact that I feel groggy all the time or when I can't have sex I stop taking them.

"That's when I hear voices and get restrained and taken to the hospital. Man, there has got to be a better way."

You may also be required to contact medical direction about the psychiatric patient who refuses care. Many communities have mental health teams that will respond to the scene to help with the care of a patient with behavioral problems. This team will also help evaluate the need for transporting the patient against his will.

Emotionally disturbed patients sometimes accuse EMS personnel of sexual misconduct. If possible, EMTs of the same sex as the patient should attend to the emergency care of disturbed patients. For the aggressive or violent patient, make sure law enforcement officers accompany you to the hospital to protect you and the patient. In the event of a legal problem, they can serve as third-party witnesses.

For more information on this topic, review Chapter 4, "Medical, Legal, and Ethical Issues."

CHAPTER REVIEW

Key Facts and Concepts

- As an EMT, you will respond to many behavioral emergencies. Be sure to ensure your own safety before entering a scene or caring for a violent or potentially violent patient.

- A considerable portion of the population has a diagnosable psychiatric condition. However, not all patients are violent. It is important to remember that patients in crisis are patients—and people—who need your compassion as well as your care.

- Always consider patients acting in an unusual or bizarre fashion to be experiencing an altered mental status; this will help

you to avoid overlooking a medical or traumatic cause for the patient's problem.

- Because the treatment for these patients usually requires long-term management, little medical intervention can be done in the acute psychiatric situation. However, the way you interact with the patient during the emergency and assess your patient throughout the call is crucial for their continued well-being.

Key Decisions

- Is the patient a danger to me, my crew, or bystanders?
- Is the patient a threat to himself?
- Is the patient experiencing a medical or traumatic condition (e.g., diabetic emergency, head injury) that may explain his behavior?
- Does the patient require restraint?
- Have I assessed my patient thoroughly and frequently?
- Could my patient be experiencing a worsening of his condition because of the restraints?

Chapter Glossary

behavior the manner in which a person acts.

behavioral emergency when a patient's behavior is not typical for the situation; when the patient's behavior is unacceptable or intolerable to the patient, his family, or the community; or when the patient may harm himself or others.

excited delirium bizarre and/or aggressive behavior, shouting, paranoia, panic, violence toward others, insensitivity to pain, un-

expected physical strength, and hyperthermia, usually associated with cocaine or amphetamine use. Also called *agitated delirium*.

positional asphyxia inadequate breathing or respiratory arrest caused by a body position that restricts breathing.

Preparation for Your Examination and Practice

Short Answer

1. Name several conditions that can alter a person's mental status and behavior.
2. List several methods that can help calm the patient who is suffering a behavioral or psychiatric emergency.
3. Describe the signs and symptoms of a behavioral or psychiatric emergency.
4. Describe what you can do when scene size-up reveals that it is too dangerous to approach the patient.
5. List several factors that can help you assess the patient's risk for suicide.
6. Research your state law. Then describe the circumstances that must exist for you to treat and transport a behavioral emergency patient without consent.

Thinking and Linking

Think back to Chapter 21, "Diabetic Emergencies and Altered Mental Status," as well as Chapter 23, "Poisoning and Overdose Emergencies," and link information from those chapters with information from this chapter as you consider the following situation:

- You are called to a patient who is acting bizarrely. List some indications (clues at the scene, signs and symptoms) that might indicate the abnormal behavior was actually due to a diabetic condition or overdose emergency.

Think back to Chapter 3, "Lifting and Moving Patients," and link information from that chapter with information from this chapter as you consider the following situation:

- The police have subdued a violent psychiatric patient. They ask you to transport the patient to the hospital. What would you use to restrain the patient's extremities? What transport device would you use? How would you secure the patient's extremities to that device?

Critical Thinking Exercises

Behavioral and psychiatric emergencies come in a wide variety of presentations. The purpose of this exercise will be to consider an assessment issue, a management issue, and a transport issue association with such behavioral and psychiatric patients.

1. You are transporting a psychiatric patient who was restrained by the police. The patient was highly agitated but now begins to act sleepy. Should you reassess the patient? If so, how?
2. You are called to respond to an intoxicated minor who is physically aggressive, threatens suicide, and whose parents permit you to treat but not transport. How would you manage this patient?
3. You are treating a patient who has attempted suicide but appears stable. It is the patient's fourth attempt. Your part-

ner says "He's just looking for attention—we shouldn't even take him to the hospital." What do you think? What should you say to your partner?

Pathophysiology to Practice

The following questions are designed to assist you in gathering relevant clinical information and making accurate decisions in the field.

1. Why could a diabetic patient appear to be having a psychiatric emergency?
2. Why could a head injury patient appear to be having a psychiatric emergency?
3. Why does hypoxia cause unusual behavior?

It's a sunny and relatively quiet summer afternoon when you are dispatched to a small manufacturing company for an individual "acting in a bizarre manner." The dispatcher is trying to get additional information, but it is difficult. Your response time is 5 minutes, and you are met outside by the manager. He tells you that about 15 minutes ago a worker kicked a table and disrupted some of the equipment. When he was approached by coworkers, he said, "Stay away, or I will hurt myself." The manager says the patient has a knife, but no one has seen it.

Street Scene Questions

1. What is your first and most important concern?
2. How should you handle the matter of scene safety?
3. When should you approach the patient?

You contact the dispatcher who informs you that two police officers are responding and should be on-scene in 3 minutes. You make sure that your crew and bystanders are in a safe position in the event the patient exits the building. When the officers pull up, you tell them what you know. The police tell you to wait outside. They enter the building and find the patient still very agitated. While you wait outside, a coworker of the patient approaches and says that she might have some information that could help. Supposedly, the patient is on antidepressant drugs and his wife recently left him. She believes that he could hurt himself but she doubts he will hurt anyone else. At this point, one of the police officers tells you that the patient is calm and they have frisked him.

Street Scene Questions

4. How should the patient be approached?
5. What are the safety concerns when working with an agitated patient?
6. Does this patient need a medical assessment?

You decide that only you should approach the patient so as not to overwhelm him. There is already a police officer standing next to him. As you approach, you introduce yourself and tell the patient that you need to ask some questions and get some medical information. You listen to him and, during the medical history, you ask if he has taken more medication than he should. He says that he took his morning dose but that is all. You take a set of vital signs and continue to listen. After a few minutes, the patient agrees to go to the hospital with you.

You ask your partner to move the ambulance to a back door so the patient doesn't have to pass coworkers on the way out. You have discussed the situation with the police officers and you feel confident that there is no longer a safety issue and that they won't be needed for the transport. The police searched the patient for weapons and found none. The patient is placed on the stretcher with all safety straps applied. You listen to the patient all the way to the hospital, being compassionate and acknowledging the patient's feelings as well as you can. Your partner calls the hospital on the radio and gives an ETA of 5 minutes.

Later, as you walk away from the patient in the emergency department, he smiles and thanks you for listening.

Hematologic and Renal Emergencies

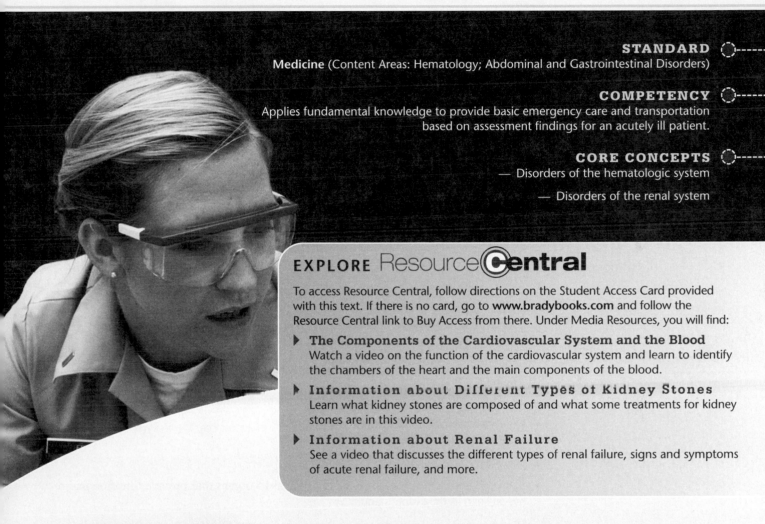

STANDARD ○------

Medicine (Content Areas: Hematology; Abdominal and Gastrointestinal Disorders)

COMPETENCY ○------

Applies fundamental knowledge to provide basic emergency care and transportation based on assessment findings for an acutely ill patient.

CORE CONCEPTS ○------

— Disorders of the hematologic system

— Disorders of the renal system

EXPLORE Resource Central

To access Resource Central, follow directions on the Student Access Card provided with this text. If there is no card, go to **www.bradybooks.com** and follow the Resource Central link to Buy Access from there. Under Media Resources, you will find:

▶ **The Components of the Cardiovascular System and the Blood**
Watch a video on the function of the cardiovascular system and learn to identify the chambers of the heart and the main components of the blood.

▶ **Information about Different Types of Kidney Stones**
Learn what kidney stones are composed of and what some treatments for kidney stones are in this video.

▶ **Information about Renal Failure**
See a video that discusses the different types of renal failure, signs and symptoms of acute renal failure, and more.

OBJECTIVES

After reading this chapter you should be able to:

26.1 Define key terms introduced in this chapter.

26.2 Describe the structure and function of the hematologic system. (pp. 602–603)

26.3 Identify medications that can interfere with blood clotting. (p. 603)

26.4 Explain the pathophysiology and complications of sickle cell anemia. (pp. 603–604)

26.5 Discuss assessment and management for patients with emergencies related to sickle cell anemia. (pp. 604–605)

26.6 Describe the structure and function of the renal system. (pp. 605–606)

26.7 Describe the causes and consequences of acute and chronic renal failure. (p. 607)

26.8 Explain the purpose of hemodialysis and peritoneal dialysis. (pp. 607–609)

26.9 Recognize patients with complications of end-stage renal disease, dialysis, and missed dialysis. (p. 610)

26.10 Provide treatment for patients with complications of end-stage renal disease, dialysis, and missed dialysis. (pp. 610–611)

26.11 Describe special considerations for patients who have received a kidney transplant. (p. 611)

Our good health depends on the human body's multiple organ systems working seamlessly together. As an EMT, you will focus much of your medical attention on acute emergencies that can be attributed to the cardiovascular and respiratory systems. In this chapter, we will discuss patients who have diseases or problems with their *hematologic system* (pertaining to blood) or *renal system* (pertaining to the kidneys). (*Hematology* is the medical specialty concerned with blood disorders. *Nephrology* is the medical specialty concerned with renal/kidney diseases.) Dozens of medical conditions can arise from diseases involving these two body systems. However, certain patients with certain diseases in this group are most likely to require EMS services as a result of their illnesses.

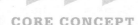

THE HEMATOLOGIC SYSTEM

CORE CONCEPT

Disorders of the
hematologic system

Our blood—although central to the function of our cardiovascular system—actually represents its own organ system. As you learned in Chapter 5, "Medical Terminology and Anatomy and Physiology," each component of the blood has specific functions that, when all are working properly, are critical to a patient's health and survival, such as:

- Control of bleeding by clotting

- Delivery of oxygen to the cells

- Removal of carbon dioxide from the cells

- Removal and delivery of other waste products to organs that provide filtration and removal such as the kidneys and liver

Blood is made up of solid components (including red blood cells, white blood cells, and platelets) suspended in a liquid called plasma. The solid components of blood are created in the bone marrow that forms the specialized core of many of the body's bones. Red blood cells, white blood cells, and platelets survive in the circulation for only a finite period of time—and are then removed from the circulation by means such as the filtration by the spleen.

Each component of the blood has specialized functions.

- **Red blood cells (RBCs).** RBCs make up the majority of the cells in the circulation and give blood its characteristic red color. These cells contain specialized molecules called *hemoglobin* that bind to oxygen and are responsible for oxygen delivery to the cells.

- **White blood cells (WBCs).** WBCs are critical blood cells that respond to infection and are mediators of the body's immune response. (See Chapter 22, "Allergic Reaction.")

- **Platelets.** Platelets are actually fragments of larger cells that are crucial to the formation of clots. Clumping (called aggregation) of platelets is the body's most rapid response to stop bleeding from an injured site. However, in some situations the clumping of platelets is not desirable, such as when plaque in a coronary artery ruptures. In this situation, the rapid clumping of platelets can cause a clot that then completely blocks the coronary artery and results in a heart attack (myocardial infarction). One of the

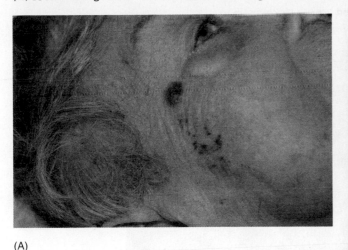

(A)

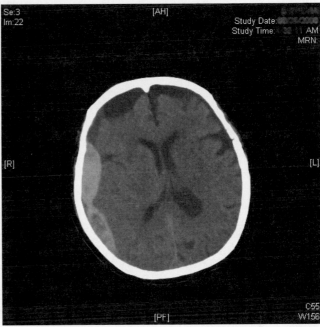

(B)

most effective and widely available drugs to prevent the aggregation of platelets is aspirin. That is why patients who are having an acute heart attack, or a potential heart attack, are routinely given an aspirin.

- **Plasma.** Plasma is the liquid in which the blood cells and platelets are suspended. Plasma contains dissolved nutrients and also carries certain crucial proteins such as the clotting factors. These clotting factors form the most stable clots, replacing the initial efforts of the platelets to stop bleeding.

NOTE: *There are certain medical conditions in which the normal ability to form clots can worsen the patient's disease; for example, in those at risk for heart attacks or strokes, or those with abnormal cardiac rhythms such as atrial fibrillation. For this reason, thousands of patients are on prescription drugs commonly referred to as "blood thinners." Drugs such as Coumadin (warfarin) and Lovenox® (enoxaparin) inhibit certain clotting factors. Other drugs, such as aspirin and Plavix® (clopidogrel), inhibit platelet aggregation. Patients on these medications are more prone to have life-threatening bleeding when they are injured than patients who are not on these medications. In some EMS systems, injured patients taking these medications are frequently upgraded to trauma center transport, even with apparently minor injuries, because of their increased risk of uncontrolled bleeding. Follow your local protocols (Figure 26-1).*

Anemia

Lack of a normal number of red blood cells in the circulation is called *anemia*. There are many reasons why a patient becomes anemic. *Acute anemia* may be the result of trauma or of sudden massive bleeding from the gastrointestinal tract. *Chronic anemia* occurs over time and can be caused by conditions such as recurrent heavy menstrual periods, slow gastrointestinal blood loss, or diseases that affect the bone marrow or the structure of the hemoglobin molecule itself. Patients with chronic anemia will often appear more pale than normal (from a lack of circulating red blood cells) and often complain of fatigue and shortness of breath with exertion (because of a lack of adequate oxygen being delivered to the body's cells).

anemia
lack of a normal number of red blood cells in the circulation.

Sickle Cell Anemia

Sickle cell anemia (SCA) is an inherited disease in which patients have a genetic defect in their hemoglobin that results in an abnormal structure of the red blood cells. Sickle cell anemia can occur in patients of African, Middle Eastern, or Indian descent but is most common in patients of African descent.

sickle cell anemia (SCA)
an inherited disease in which a genetic defect in the hemoglobin results in abnormal structure of the red blood cells.

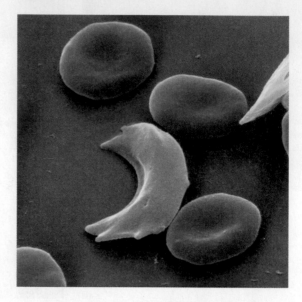

FIGURE 26-2 Scanning electron photomicrograph of normal red blood cells contrasted with a sickle cell.

(©Photo Researchers, Inc.)

A normal red blood cell is donut-shaped with a depression rather than a hole in the center. Normal red blood cells are able to be compressed as they move and squeeze through small capillaries to deliver oxygen to the cells of the body's organs. Patients with sickle cell disease have red blood cells composed of defective hemoglobin that causes them to lose their ability to have a normal shape and compressibility. These abnormal RBCs resemble the shape of a sickle when observed under a microscope (Figure 26-2). Because of their abnormal shapes, these RBCs do not survive in the circulation as long as normal RBCs. This results in chronic anemia.

The complications of SCA are generally attributed to the sludging of the abnormally shaped red blood cells, which causes blockages within the body's small blood vessels. The complications of sickle cell anemia include:

- **Destruction of the spleen.** The spleen, as it filters the blood, becomes blocked by the abnormal RBCs. Because the spleen is important in fighting infections, its loss places patients with SCA at higher risk for severe, life-threatening infections.

- **Sickle cell pain crisis.** Sickle cell crisis is caused by the sludging of sickled RBCs in capillaries, which results in severe pain in the arms, legs, chest, and/or abdomen.

- **Acute chest syndrome.** Chest syndrome is characterized by shortness of breath and chest pain associated with hypoxia (low oxygen saturation) when blood vessels in the lungs become blocked.

- **Priapism.** Painful prolonged erections in males occur because sludging RBCs prevent normal blood drainage from the erect penis.

- **Stroke.** Stroke can occur when sludging RBCs block blood vessels that supply the brain.

- **Jaundice.** The liver becomes overwhelmed by the breakdown in red blood cells, resulting in yellowish pigmentation of body tissues.

Despite advances in modern medical care, patients with SCA still have an abnormally short life span.

NOTE: *Some patients may tell you that they have "sickle cell trait" as part of their past medical history. These patients carry the gene for sickle cell disease but do not have the disease. Therefore, these patients do not suffer the complications of sickle cell anemia and have normal life spans. It is estimated that 1 in 12 African Americans have sickle cell trait.*

Inside/Outside

We have just listed some common complications of sickle cell anemia. As you assess your patient, what outside signs and symptoms are associated with which inside complications? The following chart makes the connections.

OUTSIDE	INSIDE
Infection	The spleen may be so damaged from the sickled red blood cells that it no longer functions. This means that the spleen's normal role in immune function is lost, predisposing the sickle cell patient to more frequent and severe infections.
Pain in bones, joints, abdomen, soft tissues	A vaso-occlusive crisis is a condition where sickled red blood cells block microcirculation. This causes hypoxia and severe pain in the affected organs. This often occurs in bones and joints but can also involve the abdomen and soft tissues.
Difficulty breathing, chest pain, cough, fever	When vaso-occlusive crisis occurs in the lungs it can result in acute chest syndrome. Patients will complain of difficulty breathing (often severe), chest pain, cough, and sometimes fever.
Prolonged penile erection	Sickled red blood cells are believed to block blood that is trying to exit the corpus spongiosum, causing the prolonged, painful erection of the penis called priapism.
Stroke symptoms	Sickle cell patients (adults and children) are more likely to experience ischemic stroke. The exact mechanism for this isn't known. While sickled cells may affect the microcirculation of the brain and cause stroke, many strokes involve larger vessels in the arterial circulation.
Yellowed skin, yellowed eye whites	The liver is overwhelmed with the massive breakdown of red blood cells. This lack of normal liver function causes jaundice (a yellowish pigmentation of the skin, whites of the eyes, and other body tissues and fluids).

PATIENT CARE

Sickle Cell Anemia

Emergency treatment of a patient with sickle cell anemia is as follows:

1. Administer high-concentration supplemental oxygen.
2. Monitor patients with acute chest syndrome for signs of inadequate respiration and provide bag-valve-mask ventilation as necessary.
3. Monitor patients with high fever for signs of hypoperfusion, and treat for shock as necessary.
4. Transport patients with acute stroke symptoms to a designated stroke center, if available. Follow local protocols.

Decision Point

- Should I request ALS to provide pain control for my SCA patient?

THE RENAL SYSTEM

The renal system is made up of two kidneys, two ureters (to carry urine from each kidney to the bladder), and a single urethra (to carry urine from the bladder to the outside of the body) (Figure 26-3).

As you learned in Chapter 5, "Medical Terminology and Anatomy and Physiology," the kidneys are responsible for the filtration of the blood and the removal of certain waste products, excessive salts, and excessive fluid from the body. In addition, in times of dehydration the kidneys also help the body retain needed fluid. Because they perform these critical functions, the kidneys are essential to life.

CORE CONCEPT
Disorders of the renal system

FIGURE 26-3 The renal system.

Renal System

kidney

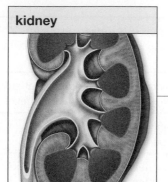

Filters blood and
produces urine

ureter

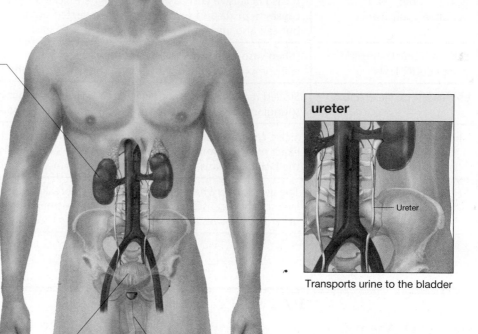

Ureter

Transports urine to the bladder

urinary bladder

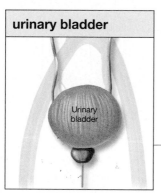

Urinary
bladder

Stores urine

male urethra

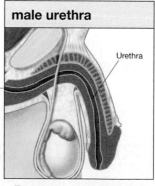

Urethra

Transports urine to exterior

female urethra

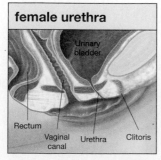

Urinary
bladder

Rectum

Vaginal
canal

Urethra

Clitoris

Transports urine to exterior

Many diseases involve the renal system. Urinary tract infections are perhaps the most common disease process that afflicts the renal and urinary system. Similarly, stones that form in the kidneys can cause severe flank pain when the stone becomes lodged in the ureter and is unable to pass into the bladder.

This chapter, however, will focus not on the most common or most painful disease of the renal system. Instead, it will discuss the challenges of patients whose kidneys no longer function properly—or at all—and the emergencies that arise as a result of this organ system failure.

Renal Failure

The most serious disease of the kidneys is called **renal failure**. Renal failure occurs when the kidneys lose their ability to adequately filter the blood and remove toxins and excess fluid from the body.

There are many reasons why patients develop renal failure. Some causes for renal failure are sudden (acute) and some develop gradually over time (chronic). *Acute renal failure* can occur as a result of shock, toxic ingestions, and other causes. Some patients who experience acute renal failure can recover normal kidney function if the underlying cause of the insult to the kidneys is rapidly identified and corrected. An example of this would be severe dehydration in a patient trapped in a building collapse for several days who, with aggressive treatment with intravenous fluids, can recover normal renal function over time. However, others who suffer acute renal failure never recover normal kidney function. Causes of *chronic renal failure* can include inherited diseases such as polycystic kidney disease. More commonly, however, the long-term damage is caused by poorly controlled diabetes and/or high blood pressure that results in the loss of normal renal function.

Patients who go on to develop irreversible renal failure—to the extent that their kidneys can no longer provide adequate filtration and fluid balance to sustain life—are defined as patients with **end-stage renal disease (ESRD)**. Patients with ESRD usually require **dialysis** to survive. More than half a million Americans have ESRD, and more than 350,000 of these patients are on chronic dialysis.

Dialysis is the process by which an external medical system independent of the kidneys is used to remove toxins and excess fluid from the body. There are two general types of dialysis: *hemodialysis* and *peritoneal dialysis*. Over 90 percent of ESRD patients who require dialysis get hemodialysis in specialized outpatient dialysis centers rather than peritoneal dialysis. Only 8 percent of U.S. dialysis patients treat themselves at home with home hemodialysis or peritoneal dialysis. The vast majority of the more than 350,000 Americans on dialysis who are treated in dialysis centers undergo three treatments a week, each lasting 3 or 4 hours. Although some patients get to their dialysis appointments by their own means, many others utilize medical transport to get to and from dialysis. This need for medical transport has created a frequent interface between EMTs and patients with ESRD.

Hemodialysis

In hemodialysis (HD), the most common form of dialysis, a patient is connected to a dialysis machine that pumps his blood through specialized filters to remove toxins and excess fluid (Figure 26-4). A patient is connected to a dialysis machine by two large catheters. One catheter allows blood to flow out of the body into the dialysis machine and the other catheter returns blood to the body after filtration. This creates a circuit by which the blood

renal failure
loss of the kidneys' ability to filter the blood and remove toxins and excess fluid from the body.

end-stage renal disease (ESRD)
irreversible renal failure to the extent that the kidneys can no longer provide adequate filtration and fluid balance to sustain life; survival with ESRD usually requires dialysis.

dialysis
the process by which toxins and excess fluid are removed from the body by a medical system independent of the kidneys.

machine @ clinic

POINT OF VIEW

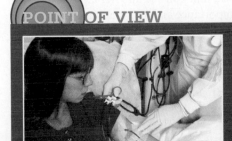

"I have a friend who is on dialysis. She is young—not someone you would think of as sick. Three times a week she goes for her treatments. Sometimes I go to keep her company—or I stop by when we are on a call at the hospital next door. It sure has made me more aware of dialysis and the people who get it. It seems like a miracle sometimes that dialysis is even possible. She has told me how it keeps her alive—and what happens when she misses her appointment."

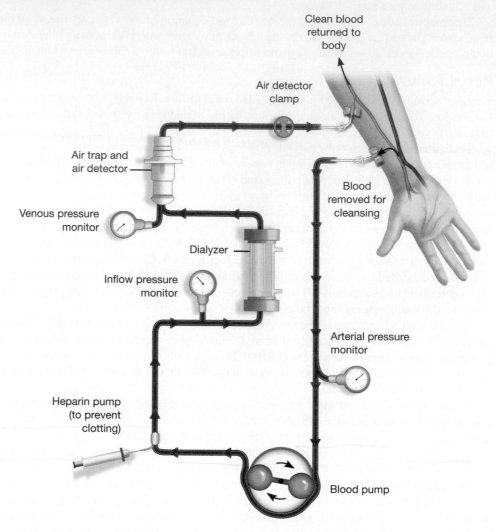

is removed from the body, filtered, and returned to the body continuously over several hours while the patient is connected to the machine.

Because HD requires a large blood flow from the body, ESRD patients on this type of chronic dialysis have specialized means of access to the body's blood circulation. Hemodialysis patients will have either a specialized two-port catheter that is inserted in one of the major veins of the torso (Figure 26-5) or have a special surgically created fistula in one of their extremities that connects arterial and venous blood flow (Figure 26-6). Because a fistula contains turbulent flow between a surgically connected artery and vein (A-V), a properly functioning A-V fistula will have a characteristic vibration, called a *thrill*, when gently palpated. ESRD patients are very protective of their fistulas and will insist that you use another extremity to obtain a blood pressure. This is appropriate, given the importance and vulnerability of the fistula.

thrill
a vibration felt on gentle palpation, such as that which typically occurs within an arterial-venous fistula.

Peritoneal Dialysis

Patients who manage their ESRD with peritoneal dialysis (PD) usually do so in their own home. PD is a slower process than HD and requires multiple treatments every day for most patients. Despite requiring more frequent treatments, many patients prefer PD over HD because it allows them to be treated at home. Outside the United States and Canada, PD is the most common form of dialysis.

Peritoneal dialysis works by utilizing the large surface area inside the peritoneal cavity that surrounds the abdominal organs as a means of removing toxins and excess fluid from the body. ESRD patients on PD have a permanent catheter that is implanted

FIGURE 26-5 A two-port catheter for hemodialysis inserted into a major vein of the torso. *(© Edward T. Dickinson, MD)*

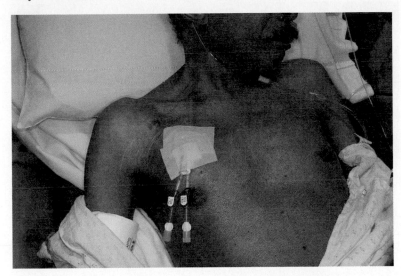

through their abdominal wall and into the peritoneal cavity (Figure 26-7). Several liters of a specially formulated dialysis solution are run into the abdominal cavity and left in place for several hours, where it absorbs waste material and excess fluid; then the fluid is drained back out into the bag and is discarded. The PD fluid setup looks much like a large IV bag and tubing. Each cycle of filling and draining the peritoneal cavity is called an ***exchange***.

There are two types of peritoneal dialysis: ***continuous ambulatory peritoneal dialysis (CAPD)*** and ***continuous cycler-assisted peritoneal dialysis (CCPD)***. In CAPD, the most common type of PD, the fluid is left in the peritoneal cavity by clamping the catheter for 4 to 6 hours. The patient then repeats the exchange several times a day. This is a simple gravity exchange process where the bag is elevated above the abdominal catheter in order to run dialysis fluid in, and then lowered below the level of the abdomen to drain the fluid out.

Continuous cycler-assisted peritoneal dialysis (CCPD) uses the same type of peritoneal catheter as CAPD. However, rather than using a gravity exchange, a machine is used to fill and empty the abdominal cavity with dialysis fluid three to five times during the night while the person sleeps. In the morning, the last fill remains in the abdomen with a dwell time that lasts the entire day.

exchange
one cycle of filling and draining the peritoneal cavity in peritoneal dialysis.

continuous ambulatory peritoneal dialysis (CAPD)
a gravity exchange process for peritoneal dialysis in which a bag of dialysis fluid is raised above the level of an abdominal catheter to fill the abdominal cavity and then lowered below the level of the abdominal catheter to drain the fluid out.

continuous cycler-assisted peritoneal dialysis (CCPD)
a mechanical process for peritoneal dialysis in which a machine fills and empties the abdominal cavity of dialysis solution.

FIGURE 26-6 A fistula surgically connects an artery and a vein in an extremity. *(© Edward T. Dickinson, MD)*

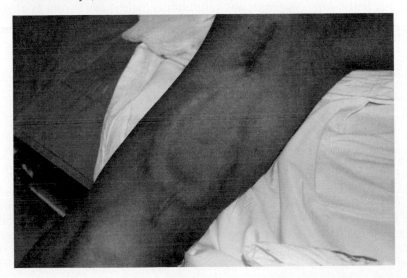

FIGURE 26-7 Peritoneal dialysis. *(© Edward T. Dickinson, MD)*

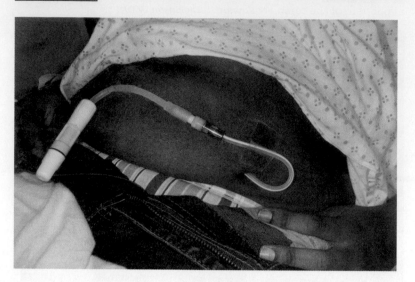

Medical Emergencies with End-Stage Renal Disease

Medical emergencies encountered in patients with ESRD can be broadly divided into two groups: those that arise from the loss of normal kidney function and those that are complications of their dialysis treatments. In addition, never forget that the vast majority of dialysis patients have other underlying diseases such as diabetes and high blood pressure, so these patients are at risk for medical emergencies related to those diseases as well, independent of their renal failure.

Complications of ESRD

The most serious complications of ESRD seen by the EMT occur when patients fail to be dialyzed. Bad weather, illness, and poor compliance are all common reasons why patients with ESRD miss their dialysis appointments.

Because these patients lack the ability to rid the body of excess fluid, patients who have missed dialysis will often present with signs and symptoms similar to those seen in congestive heart failure (see Chapter 20, "Cardiac Emergencies"). These include shortness of breath, because of fluid buildup in the lungs, and the accumulation of fluids elsewhere, such as the ankles, hands, and face. In addition, because patients with ESRD can no longer balance and clear excess electrolytes as well as other toxins, patients who have missed dialysis may suffer from electrical disturbances of the heart (dysrhythmias). This is because the proper functioning of the heart's electrical system requires that the balance of electrolytes in the bloodstream be kept within a certain tight range. Elevated levels of the electrolyte potassium are particularly dangerous, and can result in patient death from dysrhythmias.

PATIENT CARE

ESRD Patient Who Has Missed Dialysis

When encountering an ESRD patient who has missed dialysis and is experiencing problems, follow these steps:

1. Assess the ABCs.
2. When you obtain vital signs, obtain a blood pressure on an arm that does not have a fistula.
3. Place the patient in a position of comfort; this is usually sitting upright on the stretcher.
4. Administer oxygen at 15 lpm by nonrebreather mask.
5. Monitor the patient's vital signs carefully and be prepared to attach and use the automatic external defibrillator (AED) if the patient becomes unresponsive and pulseless. Be aware that ESRD patients who suffer cardiac arrest may not respond to defibrillation. Paramedics carry certain drugs that can be administered in the field to help stabilize ESRD-induced dysrhythmias. Consider ALS backup, but do not delay transport to the hospital.
6. Transport the patient to a hospital with renal dialysis capabilities.

• Should I request ALS for management of this patient's side effects of missed dialysis?

Complications of Dialysis

The major complications for patients on hemodialysis have to do with the fact that they must frequently have large blood vessels accessed multiple times each week for their dialysis. Other complications include:

• Bleeding from the site of the A-V fistula when the dialysis needles are removed while being disconnected from the machine.

• Clotting and loss of function of the A-V fistula. This results in the fistula feeling hard to the touch and in loss of the normal thrill felt on palpation.

• Bacterial infection of the blood due to contamination at the A-V fistula or dialysis catheter site during machine connection and disconnection.

The most common serious complication of ESRD patients on peritoneal dialysis is acute *peritonitis*, a bacterial infection within the peritoneal cavity. Patients on PD who develop peritonitis may develop abdominal pain, fever, and the tell-tale sign that their dialysis fluid appears cloudy when it is drained from the peritoneal cavity rather than its normal clear appearance. Infected peritoneal dialysis fluid is much like chicken broth in color and turbidity.

peritonitis
bacterial infection within the peritoneal cavity.

PATIENT CARE

ESRD Patient with Complications of Dialysis

When encountering an ESRD patient who is experiencing complications of dialysis, follow these steps:

1. Assess the ABCs.
2. Immediately control any serious bleeding from the site of the A-V fistula. Use direct pressure, elevation, and hemostatic dressings as needed. Generally, a tourniquet should be avoided in this situation as it may damage the A-V fistula. Contact medical direction if bleeding remains uncontrolled and you are considering tourniquet use.
3. Administer oxygen at 15 lpm by nonrebreather mask.
4. Be aware that ESRD patients with peritonitis or a bacterial infection in their blood may present in shock with signs of hypoperfusion. Treat for shock by keeping the patient supine and warm.
5. If peritonitis is suspected in a patient on peritoneal dialysis, transport the bag of exchanged dialysis fluid with the patient so it may be tested for bacteria at the hospital to confirm the diagnosis.

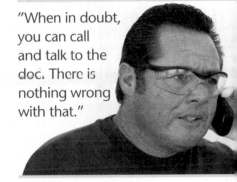

"When in doubt, you can call and talk to the doc. There is nothing wrong with that."

Finally, never forget that the vast majority of dialysis patients have other underlying diseases such as diabetes and high blood pressure, so they are at increased risk for medical emergencies related to those diseases as well, independent of their renal failure.

Kidney Transplant Patients

Kidneys are the most commonly transplanted organs. Patients with end-stage renal disease may be candidates for renal transplant which, if successful, can provide the patient with a normally functioning kidney and end his need for dialysis.

There are approximately 16,000 kidney transplants performed by specialized surgeons in the United States each year. Thanks to the kindness of organ donors, a renal transplant places a single healthy kidney in the lower abdomen of the patient with ESRD. The surgeon then connects a blood supply and a ureter to the transplanted kidney, allowing the patient the opportunity to regain normal renal function.

Patients with kidney transplants spend the rest of their lives on a special class of drugs that prevent organ rejection by suppressing the body's immune system. However, these same drugs that help protect the transplanted kidney also make these patients more susceptible to serious infections.

CRITICAL DECISION MAKING

Should You Request Advanced Life Support?

Determine if you would request advanced life support for the following patients and, if so, why.

1. A 29-year-old patient with sickle cell anemia who has severe pain in his arms and chest

2. A 42-year-old patient who recently completed his peritoneal dialysis and complains of severe abdominal pain that is worsened by movement

3. A 55-year-old female who refused to leave her house to go to her hemodialysis appointments and now complains of severe difficulty breathing, has a rapid pulse, and is anxious

4. A 37-year-old sickle cell anemia patient who complains of extreme fatigue

CHAPTER REVIEW

Key Facts and Concepts

- Blood delivers oxygen to the cells, removes carbon dioxide from the cells, and controls bleeding by clotting.

- Blood consists of red blood cells, white blood cells, and plasma.

- Anemia is a lack of red blood cells in circulation.

- Sickle cell anemia is an inherited disease in which a defect in the hemoglobin results in a "sickle" shape to red blood cells. This mis-shaping inhibits movement of the red blood cells through capillaries, causing "sludging" and blockages in smaller blood vessels.

- The renal system is comprised of the kidneys, the ureters, the bladder, and the urethra.

- The kidneys perform a vital filtering of the blood to remove waste products. They also help maintain a water balance within the body.

- Problems with the renal system include infection, kidney stones, and renal failure.

- Renal failure is a condition in which the kidneys are unable to filter waste and provide a balance of fluids in the body.

- In dialysis, an external system filters the blood and removes excess fluid from the body. Dialysis may be performed in either of two ways: hemodialysis or peritoneal dialysis. Dialysis at dialysis centers is generally performed three times per week.

- The main complications with patients in end-stage renal disease generally occur after the patient has missed a dialysis appointment.

Key Decisions

- Does my patient have a history of sickle cell disease or end-stage renal disease?

- Does my patient have an A-V fistula?

- Will I need to make an early request for advanced life support because of complications from a missed dialysis appointment?

Chapter Glossary

anemia lack of a normal number of red blood cells in the circulation.

continuous ambulatory peritoneal dialysis (CAPD) a gravity exchange process for peritoneal dialysis in which a bag of dialysis fluid is raised above the level of an abdominal catheter to fill the abdominal cavity and lowered below the level of the abdominal catheter to drain the fluid out.

continuous cycler-assisted peritoneal dialysis (CCPD) a mechanical process for peritoneal dialysis in which a machine fills and empties the abdominal cavity of dialysis solution.

dialysis the process by which toxins and excess fluid are removed from the body by a medical system independent of the kidneys.

end-stage renal disease (ESRD) irreversible renal failure to the extent that the kidneys can no longer provide adequate filtration and fluid balance to sustain life; survival with ESRD usually requires dialysis.

exchange one cycle of filling and draining the peritoneal cavity in peritoneal dialysis.

peritonitis bacterial infection within the peritoneal cavity.

renal failure loss of the kidneys' ability to filter the blood and remove toxins and excess fluid from the body.

sickle cell anemia (SCA) an inherited disease in which a genetic defect in the hemoglobin results in abnormal structure of the red blood cells.

thrill a vibration felt on gentle palpation, such as that which typically occurs within an arterial-venous fistula.

Preparation for Your Examination and Practice

Short Answer

1. What is sickle cell anemia?
2. What is sludging in a patient with sickle cell anemia?
3. What is a thrill?
4. What is the difference between hemodialysis and peritoneal dialysis?
5. What are the complications that may be seen if a patient misses a dialysis appointment?

Thinking And Linking

Think back to Chapter 20, "Cardiac Emergencies," and link information from that chapter with information from the section on end-stage renal disease in this chapter as you consider the following situations:

1. You are treating a patient who has missed dialysis. Because of a fluid buildup, the patient has signs and symptoms similar to congestive heart failure. What are these signs and symptoms?
2. Your patient, who has missed dialysis, says he is having palpitations. Why?

Critical Thinking Exercises

Renal diseases and sickle cell anemia can result in life-threatening emergencies. The purpose of this exercise is to analyze the complaints of two such patients.

- You have a patient who is transported routinely for dialysis three times per week. She was sick and cancelled the trip yesterday. Now she calls saying she can't breathe and feels like she is going to die. Is it possible that she has a legitimate complaint after missing dialysis by only one day?

- You have a patient with a history of sickle cell crisis who is complaining of severe pain in his legs. The patient refuses to move because it hurts so much. Your partner thinks the patient is being overdramatic and falsely complaining of pain to

get drugs from the hospital. Do you agree with your partner? Why or why not? What should you do for the patient?

Pathophysiology to Practice

The following questions are designed to assist you in gathering relevant clinical information and making accurate decisions in the field.

- You are treating a patient who is complaining of stroke symptoms. He has a history of sickle cell disease. Does sickle cell disease make the diagnosis of a stroke more likely or less likely in this patient? Why?

- A patient with sickle cell anemia tells you of severe, recurring infections. Why would an SCA patient have this problem?

Street Scenes -

You are sent to a "routine transfer" nonemergency call to transport a 64-year-old patient from a long-term care facility to a dialysis appointment. You arrive to find the patient with an altered mental status and "not feeling well."

You note the patient has poor color, which the staff tells you is normal for the patient. The patient is somewhat anxious and her skin is warm to the touch.

Street Scene Questions

1. What are your initial steps in assessing this patient?
2. How does the dialysis history fit into the patient picture at this point?

You complete a primary assessment and find the patient is breathing somewhat rapidly but adequately at 28/minute. The patient has peripheral pulses and no obvious external bleeding. Pulse oximetry reveals a saturation of 94 percent. The patient will respond to questions but is sleepy and a little confused. The staff says this is a new development in the patient, who is usually quite oriented.

Street Scene Questions

3. What assessments should you perform next?
4. Do you believe the patient's condition is related to her dialysis?

The patient's pulse and respirations are slightly elevated. Her blood pressure is 108/58, her skin is warm and dry, and her pupils are equal and reactive to light. The patient has a slight difficulty breathing and some fluid is noticeable around her ankles. Her lungs show some mild crackles (also known as rales) in the bases. Blood glucose is 102. Even though the patient cannot follow instructions for the stroke scale, she does not have facial droop or slurred speech. The staff says she seemed fine when she went to bed last night.

Street Scene Question

5. The staff asks you to take the patient to her dialysis appointment and says they think "she'll be fine by the time she gets back." Should you transport her to dialysis or to a hospital?

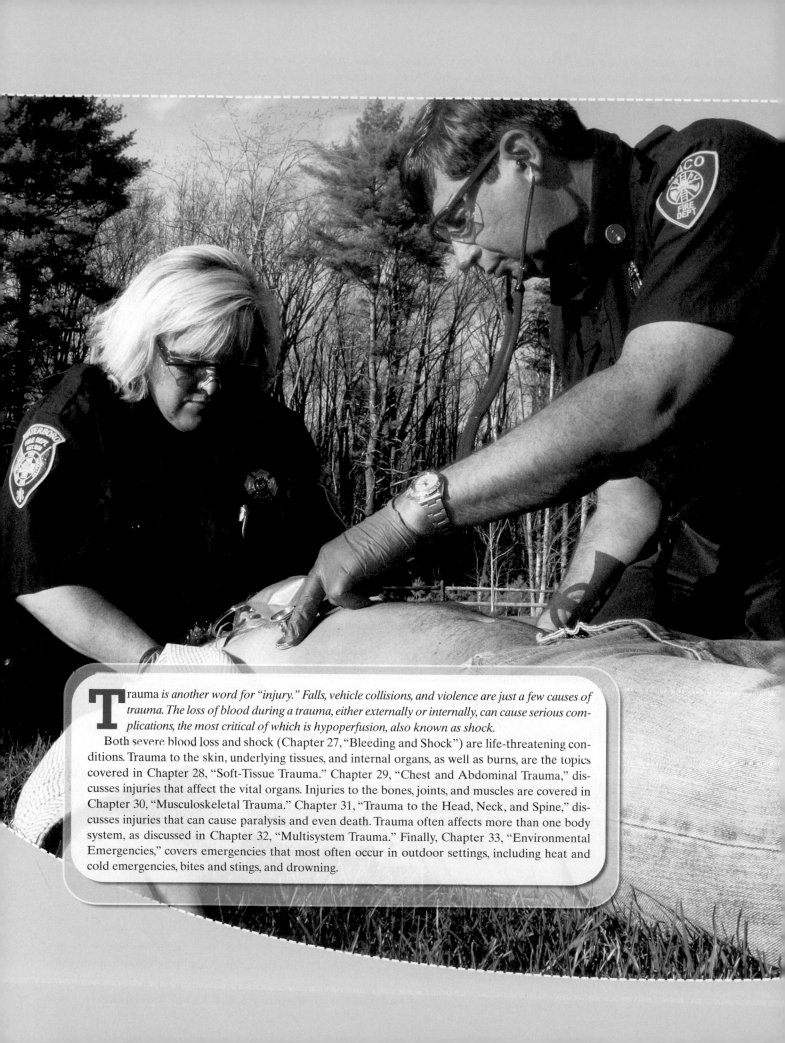

Trauma *is another word for "injury." Falls, vehicle collisions, and violence are just a few causes of trauma. The loss of blood during a trauma, either externally or internally, can cause serious complications, the most critical of which is hypoperfusion, also known as shock.*

Both severe blood loss and shock (Chapter 27, "Bleeding and Shock") are life-threatening conditions. Trauma to the skin, underlying tissues, and internal organs, as well as burns, are the topics covered in Chapter 28, "Soft-Tissue Trauma." Chapter 29, "Chest and Abdominal Trauma," discusses injuries that affect the vital organs. Injuries to the bones, joints, and muscles are covered in Chapter 30, "Musculoskeletal Trauma." Chapter 31, "Trauma to the Head, Neck, and Spine," discusses injuries that can cause paralysis and even death. Trauma often affects more than one body system, as discussed in Chapter 32, "Multisystem Trauma." Finally, Chapter 33, "Environmental Emergencies," covers emergencies that most often occur in outdoor settings, including heat and cold emergencies, bites and stings, and drowning.

Trauma Emergencies

Bleeding and Shock

CORE CONCEPTS
— How to recognize arterial, venous, and capillary bleeding

— How to evaluate the severity of external bleeding

— How to control external bleeding

— Signs, symptoms, and care of a patient with internal bleeding

— Signs, symptoms, and care of a patient with shock

EXPLORE Resource Central

To access Resource Central, follow directions on the Student Access Card provided with this text. If there is no card, go to **www.bradybooks.com** and follow the Resource Central link to Buy Access from there. Under Media Resources, you will find:

▶ **Types of Shock**
View an animation and learn some of the most common causes of shock.

▶ **Some Ways to Control Bleeding**
Watch a video to learn about different types of external bleeding and what materials you can use to control bleeding.

▶ **Dressing Selection and Bandaging**
See a video that discusses the types and purposes of wound dressings.

OBJECTIVES

After reading this chapter you should be able to:

27.1 Define key terms introduced in this chapter.

27.2 Describe the structure and function of the circulatory system, including the functions of the blood. (pp. 617–619)

27.3 Explain the concept of perfusion. (p. 619)

27.4 Compare and contrast arterial, venous, and capillary bleeding. (pp. 620–621)

27.5 Discuss causes and effects of severe external bleeding. (pp. 621–622, 629)

27.6 Discuss assessment and management of external bleeding, including methods of controlling external bleeding. (pp. 622–629)

27.7 Identify patients at risk for internal bleeding. (pp. 630–631)

27.8 Recognize signs of internal bleeding and discuss patient care for internal bleeding. (pp. 630–632)

27.9 Discuss the causes of shock and its effects on the body. (p. 632)

27.10 Explain the concepts of compensated, decompensated, and irreversible shock. (p. 633)

27.11 Discuss the types of shock. (p. 633)

27.12 Relate the signs and symptoms of shock to the body's attempts to compensate for blood loss. (pp. 632–634)

27.13 Discuss the management of patients in shock. (pp. 634–638)

KEY TERMS

arterial bleeding, *p. 620*

capillary bleeding, *p. 621*

cardiogenic shock, *p. 633*

compensated shock, *p. 633*

decompensated shock, *p. 633*

hemorrhage, *p. 619*

hemorrhagic shock, *p. 633*

hemostatic agents, *p. 626*

hypoperfusion, *p. 619*

hypovolemic shock, *p. 633*

irreversible shock, *p. 633*

neurogenic shock, *p. 633*

perfusion, *p. 619*

pressure dressing, *p. 625*

shock, *p. 619*

tourniquet, *p. 627*

venous bleeding, *p. 621*

The leading cause of death in the United States for persons between the ages of 1 and 44 is trauma. As an EMT, you will be called upon to provide emergency care to victims of traumatic injuries varying in severity from minor to life threatening. It is vital that you learn to recognize the signs and symptoms of serious trauma and shock. Early identification, appropriate care, and expeditious transport to an appropriate medical facility contribute greatly to the patient's chance of survival. Understanding the signs, symptoms, and management of bleeding and shock is a vital part of good prehospital care.

THE CIRCULATORY SYSTEM

Main Components

The circulatory (or cardiovascular) system is responsible for the distribution of blood to all parts of the body. This system has three main components: the heart, blood vessels, and the blood that flows through them. All components must function properly for the system to remain intact (Figure 27-1). (You may wish to review the information about the heart and the circulatory system in Chapter 5, "Medical Terminology and Anatomy and Physiology.")

The heart is a muscular organ that lies within the chest, behind the sternum. Its job is to pump blood, which supplies oxygen and nutrients to the body's cells. To provide a sufficient supply of oxygen and nutrients to all parts of the body, the heart must pump at an adequate rate and rhythm.

The blood is circulated throughout the body through three major types of blood vessels (Figure 27-2):

- **Arteries.** The arteries carry oxygen-rich blood away from the heart. They are under a great deal of pressure during the heart's contractions. (Taking the patient's blood pressure is a means of measuring arterial pressure.) An artery has a thick, muscular wall that enables it to dilate or constrict, depending on the amount of oxygen and nutrients needed by the cells or organs it feeds.

- **Capillaries.** Oxygen-rich blood is emptied from the arteries into microscopically small capillaries, which supply every cell of the body. In areas where capillaries and body cells

FIGURE 27-1 The circulatory system.

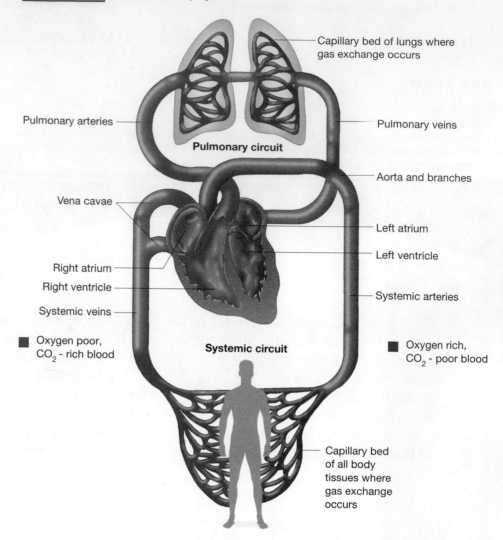

Capillary bed of lungs where gas exchange occurs

Pulmonary arteries

Pulmonary veins

Pulmonary circuit

Aorta and branches

Vena cavae

Left atrium

Left ventricle

Right atrium

Right ventricle

Systemic arteries

Systemic veins

Oxygen poor, CO_2 - rich blood

Systemic circuit

Oxygen rich, CO_2 - poor blood

Capillary bed of all body tissues where gas exchange occurs

are in contact, a vital "exchange" takes place. Oxygen and nutrients are given up by the blood and pass through the extremely thin capillary walls into the cells. At the same time, carbon dioxide and other waste products given up by the cells pass through the capillary walls and are taken up by the blood.

- **Veins.** Blood that has been depleted of oxygen and loaded with carbon dioxide and other wastes in the capillaries empties into the veins, which carry it back to the heart. Veins have one-way valves that prevent the blood from flowing in the wrong direction. Blood in a vein is under much less pressure than blood in an artery.

The blood has several functions.

- **Transportation of gases.** Blood carries inhaled oxygen from the lungs to the body's cells, and it carries carbon dioxide from the body's cells back to the lungs where it is then exhaled.

- **Nutrition.** Blood circulates nutrients from the intestines or storage tissues (such as fatty tissue, the liver, and muscle cells) to the other body cells.

- **Excretion.** Blood carries waste products from the cells to organs, such as the kidneys, that excrete (eliminate) them from the body.

- **Protection.** Blood carries antibodies and white blood cells, which help fight disease and infection. Blood also contains platelets and clotting factors that work to control bleeding from damaged blood vessels by forming blood clots.

FIGURE 27-2 Comparative structure of arteries, capillaries, and veins.

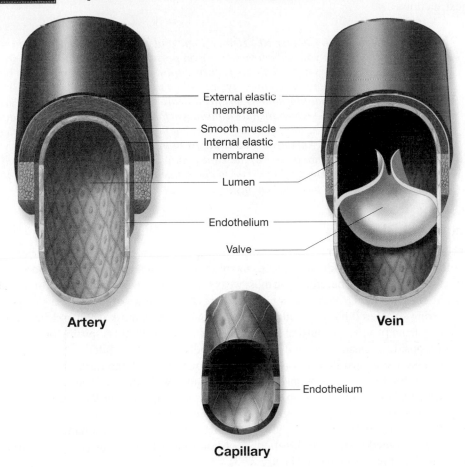

Artery

Vein

Capillary

- External elastic membrane
- Smooth muscle
- Internal elastic membrane
- Lumen
- Endothelium
- Valve
- Endothelium

- **Regulation.** Blood carries substances that control the body's functions, such as hormones, water, salt, enzymes, and chemicals. Blood also helps regulate body temperature by carrying body heat to the lungs and skin surface where it is dissipated.

The adequate circulation of blood throughout the body, which fills the capillaries and supplies the cells and tissues with oxygen and nutrients, is called **perfusion**. If, for some reason, blood is not adequately circulated, some of the body's cells and organs do not receive adequate supplies of oxygen, and dangerous waste products build up. Inadequate perfusion of the body's tissues and organs is called **hypoperfusion**, which is also known as **shock**. (*Hypo-* means "low," so *hypoperfusion* means "low perfusion.")

Recall that the heart, blood vessels, and blood are the three main components of the circulatory system. These components may be likened to a pump, pipes, and fluid in the pipes. For the circulatory system to function properly, all three components must function properly. If any component fails, or "leaks," the body will try in various ways to compensate and maintain adequate perfusion. However, if the problem is not corrected and the condition quickly reverses, adequate perfusion cannot be maintained and shock (hypoperfusion) will result.

perfusion
the supply of oxygen to, and removal of wastes from, the body's cells and tissues as a result of the flow of blood through the capillaries.

hypoperfusion
(HI-po-per-FEW-zhun)
the body's inability to adequately circulate blood to the body's cells to supply them with oxygen and nutrients. *See also* shock.

shock
the body's inability to adequately circulate blood to the body's cells to supply them with oxygen and nutrients, which is a life-threatening condition. Also known as *hypoperfusion*.

BLEEDING

Severe bleeding, or **hemorrhage**, is the major cause of shock (hypoperfusion) in trauma. The body contains a certain amount of blood to circulate through the blood vessels. If enough blood volume is lost, perfusion will not occur in all cells. Inadequate perfusion of the body's cells will eventually lead to the death of tissues and organs. The cells and tissues of the brain, the spinal cord, and the kidneys are the most sensitive to inadequate perfusion.

hemorrhage (HEM-o-rej)
bleeding, especially severe bleeding.

Bleeding, or hemorrhage, is classified as either external or internal, as explained in the next sections.

NOTE: *As discussed in Chapter 26, "Hematologic and Renal Emergencies," a growing number of patients that you will encounter are on prescription medications that are designed to limit the body's natural ability to form blood clots. Often referred to as* blood thinners, *these medications are commonly prescribed to patients with a history of stroke, irregular heartbeat (atrial fibrillation), artificial heart valves, or a history of a heart attack. These medications—which include aspirin, warfarin (Coumadin), and clopidogrel (Plavix)—act to prevent strokes or heart attacks, but in the setting of external or internal bleeding can result in life-threatening bleeding from injuries that might be relatively minor for a patient who is not on one of these medications. When treating patients with external or internal bleeding, it is important to determine whether or not they are on blood thinners as part of your past medical history.*

External Bleeding

Whenever bleeding is anticipated or discovered, you must use Standard Precautions to avoid exposure of your skin and mucous membranes. Blood and open wounds pose a risk of infection to the EMT. Therefore, you must wear protective gloves when caring for any bleeding patient. You should also wear a mask and protective eyewear if there is a chance of encountering splattered blood. In addition, you should wear a mask when assisting a patient suffering from profuse or spurting (arterial) bleeding, or one who is spitting or coughing up blood. Consider wearing a gown if clothing may become contaminated.

Although Standard Precautions decrease the possibility of exposure to blood and body fluids, you should nevertheless *always* wash your hands with soap and water immediately after each call. Gloves may develop tears or small holes without your knowledge. Always remove the gloves carefully, turning them inside out as you take them off. This reduces the possibility of blood or fluid on the gloves coming in contact with your hands.

External bleeding may be classified according to which of the three types of blood vessels is injured and losing blood (Figure 27-3):

- Arterial bleeding
- Venous bleeding
- Capillary bleeding

Arterial bleeding is usually bright red in color, because it is still rich in oxygen. It is often rapid and profuse, spurting with each heartbeat; however, as the patient's systolic blood pressure drops, the strength of the spurting may decrease. As explained earlier, blood in an artery is under high pressure, and arteries have thick, muscular walls that maintain the pres-

- - - - - - - - - ● **CORE CONCEPT**

How to recognize arterial, venous, and capillary bleeding

arterial bleeding
bleeding from an artery, which is characterized by bright red blood that is rapid, profuse, and difficult to control.

FIGURE 27-3 Three types of external bleeding.

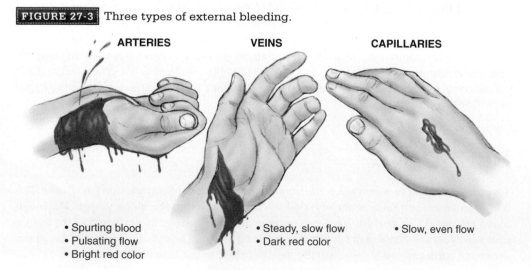

ARTERIES   **VEINS**   **CAPILLARIES**

- Spurting blood
- Pulsating flow
- Bright red color

- Steady, slow flow
- Dark red color

- Slow, even flow

sure. For this reason, arterial bleeding is the most difficult bleeding to control. Control measures may need to continue throughout transport to the hospital.

Venous bleeding is usually dark red or maroon in color, because it has already passed its oxygen to the cells and picked up carbon dioxide and wastes. Bleeding from the veins has a steady flow. It is usually easy to control (although it can be profuse), because veins return blood to the heart under low pressure. Because venous pressure may be lower than atmospheric pressure, large veins may actually suck in debris or air bubbles in the presence of an open wound. Bleeding from the large veins in the neck is an especially serious problem. An air bubble, or embolism, may be carried directly to the heart, interfering with the regular heart rhythm or even completely stopping it. An air embolism also can cause damage to the brain or lungs if lodged there.

Capillary bleeding is usually slow and "oozing" due to the capillaries' small size and low pressure. Most capillary bleeding is considered minor and is easily controlled. It often clots spontaneously, or with minimal treatment. As you would expect, the color of capillary blood is usually somewhere between the bright red of arterial blood and the darker red of venous blood. Capillary bleeding usually results from a minor injury such as a scrape. However, these wounds can easily become contaminated, leading to infection. You may also see capillary bleeding from the edges of more serious wounds.

Severity of External Bleeding

The severity of a patient's bleeding depends on the speed and amount of blood lost in relation to the patient's physical size. Whereas a sudden loss of 1 liter (1,000 cc) of blood is considered serious in the average adult, losing half that amount (500 cc) is considered serious in a child. In a 1-year-old infant, with a total blood volume of only about 800 cc, a loss of even 150 cc is considered serious. If the bleeding is slow and occurs over a long time, the body can adjust better to this loss and maintain adequate oxygenation to the tissues, particularly in a healthy person. However, an elderly or chronically ill patient will have more difficulty maintaining normal oxygenation. If, at any time, the patient begins to exhibit signs and symptoms of shock (hypoperfusion), the bleeding is immediately considered serious.

The body's natural response to bleeding is constriction of the injured blood vessel and clotting. However, a serious injury may prevent effective clotting, thereby allowing continued bleeding. Wounds that are large or deep may not clot well. Uncontrolled bleeding or significant blood loss can eventually lead to death.

venous bleeding
bleeding from a vein, which is characterized by dark red or maroon blood and a steady, easy-to-control flow.

capillary bleeding
bleeding from capillaries, which is characterized by a slow, oozing flow of blood.

CORE CONCEPT

How to evaluate the severity of external bleeding

PATIENT ASSESSMENT

External Bleeding

It is important for you to learn to estimate the amount of external blood loss in order to predict potential shock (hypoperfusion), properly triage (prioritize) patients, and identify bleeding that must be treated during the primary assessment.

It is sometimes difficult to estimate blood loss when the blood has flowed onto the floor or when carpeting or clothing has absorbed it. An exercise that may help you better estimate external blood loss is pouring a pint of liquid on the floor to note its appearance, and soaking an article of clothing in a pint of fluid to note how wet it feels and looks. Since estimating external blood loss is difficult, it is important for you to watch for signs and symptoms of shock (hypoperfusion), which are listed in Table 27-1.

No matter how small blood loss appears to be, if the patient shows any signs or symptoms of shock (hypoperfusion), the bleeding is considered serious. However, do not wait for signs and symptoms to appear before beginning treatment. Any patient with a significant amount of blood loss should be treated to prevent the development of shock. Many of the signs and symptoms of shock appear late in the process. By the time they develop, it may be too late for the patient to recover.

Decision Points

• Does my patient have severe bleeding that must be controlled during the primary assessment?

• Is my patient in shock or developing shock?

Table 27-1 Signs of Shock

SIGNS (IN ORDER OF APPEARANCE)	DESCRIPTION
Altered mental status	Altered mental status occurs because the brain is not receiving enough oxygen. The brain is very sensitive to oxygen deficiencies. When it is deprived of oxygen, even slightly, behavioral changes may be noted. These changes may begin as anxiety and progress to restlessness and sometimes combativeness.
Pale, cool, and clammy skin	When the body senses low blood volume, natural mechanisms take over in an attempt to correct the problem. One of these mechanisms is to divert blood from nonvital areas to vital organs. Blood is quickly directed away from the skin to such organs as the brain and heart. This results in the loss of color and temperature in the skin. Infants and children may exhibit capillary refill times of greater than 2 seconds. *Note: In anaphylactic and neurogenic shock (rare) the skin is typically warm, flushed, and dry because the circulatory system has lost the ability to constrict blood vessels in the skin.*
Nausea and vomiting	In the body's continuing effort to keep blood perfusing the vital organs, blood is diverted from the digestive system. This causes feelings of nausea and occasionally vomiting.
Vital sign changes	The first vital signs to change are the pulse and respirations: • The pulse will increase in an attempt to pump more blood. As the pulse gradually increases, it becomes weak and thready. Most patients will become tachycardic with significant blood loss; however, a significant number do not, so you cannot rely solely on this sign. • Respirations also increase in an attempt to increase the amount of oxygen in the blood. The respirations will become shallower and labored as shock progresses. • Blood pressure is one of the last signs to change. When blood pressure drops, the patient is clearly in a state of serious, life-threatening shock. • A narrowing of the pulse pressure may also occur. This means that the difference between the systolic and diastolic pressures will decrease (become closer together).
	Late signs of shock that you may encounter include thirst, dilated pupils, and in some cases cyanosis around the lips and nail beds.

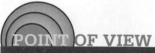

POINT OF VIEW

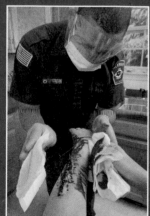

"I remember waiting to see if it would hurt.

"It wasn't the blood. That didn't bother me. I just sat there and waited for the pain. Things were in slow motion. The knife had gone into my forearm. Everyone stopped what they were doing and stared. I grabbed my arm and felt the warm blood drip down over my fingers. But it still didn't seem real.

"I heard someone scream. Someone else called 911. It took me a minute to get my head around what happened. It seemed like only a few seconds had gone by when the EMS people showed up. They put a bandage on my arm and made sure the bleeding had stopped.

"As I look back on it now, I am amazed at how detached I was from the whole thing. I guess some would call that shock.

"And for the record, once I got composed again, it hurt. Oh yes, trust me. It hurt."

Controlling External Bleeding

CORE CONCEPT

How to control external bleeding

The control of external bleeding is one of the most important elements in the prevention and management of shock (hypoperfusion). If bleeding is not controlled, shock will continue to develop and worsen, leading to the patient's death.

External Bleeding

Patient assessment and care always begin with the ABCs. After taking Standard Precautions, maintain the patient's airway, monitor respirations, and ventilate, if necessary. Assess circulation by taking a radial pulse; assessing skin color, temperature, and condition; and controlling external bleeding. Severe external bleeding must be identified and controlled during the primary assessment. The major methods of controlling external bleeding are (Scan 27-1):

- Direct pressure
- Elevation
- Hemostatic agent
- Tourniquet

Other methods include splinting, cold application, and use of the pneumatic anti-shock garment (PASG). Each of these methods will be more thoroughly discussed later in this chapter.

In addition to controlling external bleeding, an important treatment for any trauma patient is administration of oxygen. Blood loss decreases perfusion. This means that less oxygen is delivered to the tissues. The administration of supplemental oxygen will increase the oxygen saturation of the blood that is still in the patient's circulatory system, improving oxygenation of the tissues.

Standard Precautions and infection control are mandatory when attempting to control external bleeding. Always wear disposable gloves when caring for the patient and cleaning up after the call. Follow your local infection exposure control plan regarding cleaning and disposal of contaminated bandages, sheets, and other materials and supplies.

Direct Pressure The most common and effective way to control external bleeding is by applying direct pressure to the wound. This can be done with your gloved hand, a dressing and your gloved hand, or by a pressure dressing and bandage.

1. Apply pressure to the wound until the bleeding is controlled. If the bleeding is mild, use a sterile dressing. If the bleeding is severe or spurting, immediately place your gloved hand directly on the wound. Do not waste time trying to find a dressing (Figure 27-4).

2. Hold the pressure firmly until the bleeding is controlled. Remember, your goal is limiting additional blood loss.

FIGURE 27-4 In cases of profuse bleeding, do not waste time finding a dressing. Instead, use your gloved hand to apply direct pressure.

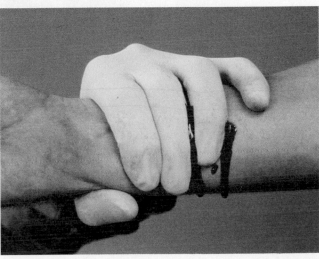

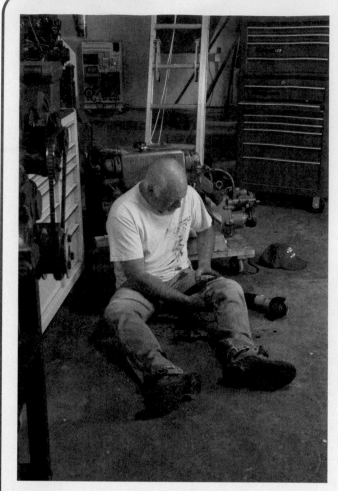

1 Perform a scene size-up, look for hazards, and determine the necessity of Standard Precautions.

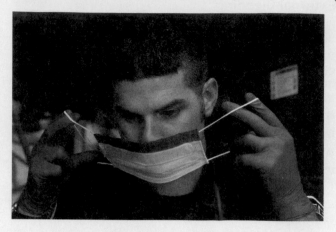

2 Take Standard Precautions.

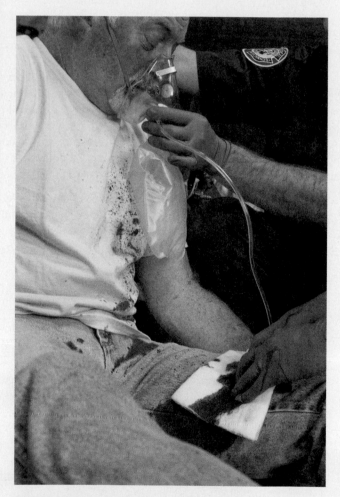

3 Apply direct pressure. If another EMT is available, administer oxygen.

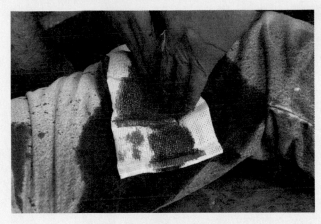

④ Hemostatic dressings may be used to stop bleeding if pressure alone doesn't work. Use your gloved hand to push the dressing into the wound.

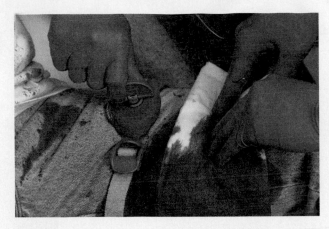

⑤ If pressure and hemostatic dressings do not stop the bleeding, apply and tighten a tourniquet until the bleeding stops.

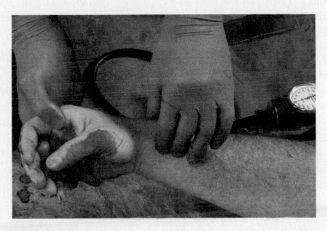

⑥ Assess and treat the patient for shock.

3. Once the bleeding has been controlled, bandage a dressing firmly in place to form a pressure dressing (see the following explanation).

4. Do not remove a dressing once it has been placed on the wound. Removal of a dressing may destroy clots or cause further injury to the site. If a dressing becomes blood soaked, apply additional dressings on top of it and hold them firmly in place. You may need to continue holding direct pressure on the wound until you and the patient arrive at the hospital.

Application of a ***pressure dressing*** will control most external bleeding. Place several gauze pads on the wound. Hold the dressings in place with a self-adhering roller bandage wrapped tightly over the dressings and above and below the wound site. You must create enough pressure to control the bleeding.

As previously noted, dressings should not be removed from the wound. If bleeding continues, place additional dressings over the existing one and apply pressure by hand. You may also apply a tighter bandage (which does not hinder circulation). Several types of dressings may be used to control external bleeding (Figure 27-5).

You may be unable to apply an effective pressure dressing to some areas of the body. For example, bleeding from the armpit may require you to apply continuous direct pressure with your gloved hand and a dressing. Remember that direct pressure is usually the quickest and most effective method of controlling external bleeding.

pressure dressing
a bulky dressing held in position with a tightly wrapped bandage, which applies pressure to help control bleeding.

FIGURE 27-5 Various types of dressings.

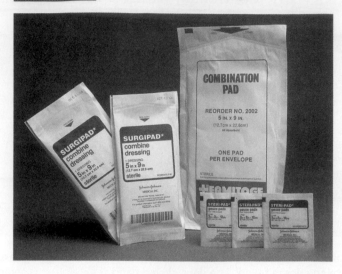

NOTE: *After controlling bleeding from an extremity using a pressure dressing, always check for a distal pulse to make sure that the dressing has not been applied too tightly. If you do not feel a pulse, adjust the pressure applied by the dressing to reestablish circulation. Check distal pulses frequently while the patient is in your care.*

Elevation Elevation of an injured extremity has never been proven to decrease bleeding, but if it can be done quickly and easily, it makes sense to employ this method at the same time you apply direct pressure. When you elevate an injury above the level of the heart, gravity helps reduce the blood pressure in the extremity, slowing bleeding. However, do not use this method if you suspect possible musculoskeletal injuries, impaled objects in the extremity, or spine injury.

To use elevation in controlling external bleeding, apply direct pressure to the injury site. Elevate the injured extremity, keeping the injury site above the level of the heart.

hemostatic (HEM-o-STAT-IK) **agents**
substances applied as powders, dressings, gauze, or bandages to open wounds to stop bleeding.

Hemostatic Agents ***Hemostatic agents*** are relatively new to civilian EMS but have been used extensively in the military. They are frequently carried on ambulances and may also be purchased at pharmacies and sporting goods stores.

Most hemostatic agents seen in the field today are either hemostatic dressings (Figure 27-6) or specially formulated hemostatic gauze wraps (bandages) (Figure 27-7). The advantage of hemostatic gauze is that a length of the leading edge of the gauze can be wadded up and inserted into the wound as a dressing, then secured in position, using the remaining wrap as a bandage. (The original hemostatic agents were formulated as loose powders or granules to be poured into the wound and packed in with a gloved hand, but these formulations are now used only rarely by EMS providers as hemostatic dressings and hemostatic gauze have gained favor.)

FIGURE 27-6 Hemostatic sponge/dressing.
(©Edward T. Dickinson, MD)

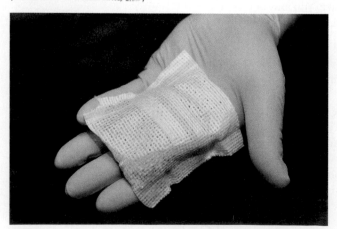

FIGURE 27-7 Hemostatic bandage.
(©Edward T. Dickinson, MD)

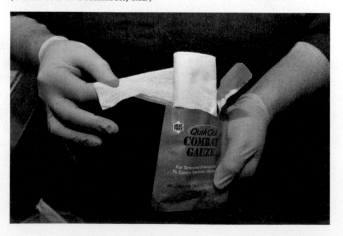

Hemostatic dressings that are placed directly into wounds contain an absorbent substance that traps red blood cells. When the dressings are placed deep into the bleeding wounds, it is believed that they speed or assist clotting and stop bleeding.

To use these dressings, open the package and follow the manufacturer's directions. Some dressings must be placed into a wound in a specific orientation. Maintain pressure on the wound over the dressing.

Regardless of the type of agent used, continue manual pressure and monitor the patient's bleeding. Hemostatic agents are frequently successful in stopping bleeding. If they do not work, you should use a tourniquet. Always follow local protocols.

Tourniquet A *tourniquet* (Figure 27-8) is a device that closes off all blood flow to and from an extremity. Previously believed to be an extreme last resort, tourniquets have moved into mainstream care for patients with severe bleeding that can't be controlled by direct pressure. At one point it was believed that the use of a tourniquet was a "life or limb" decision; that is, although use of a tourniquet will stop blood flow, it will likely result in amputation of the limb.

tourniquet (TURN-i-ket)
a device used for bleeding control that constricts all blood flow to and from an extremity.

Testing in battle has shown that the risks of using a tourniquet, while present, are believed to be justified in the presence of bleeding that cannot otherwise be controlled. In civilian use, with the exception of wilderness applications or prolonged entrapment, it is extremely rare for transport time to take longer than an hour. In these cases, it appears that the risk of permanent damage to an extremity is considerably less than the risk of death from uncontrolled bleeding (Figure 27-9).

Remember that patients who have severe bleeding may also have other injuries or conditions such as airway compromise, inadequate breathing, or chest injury, which will also require your urgent attention. In these cases, the use of a tourniquet offers the additional benefit of allowing you to treat these conditions.

The decision to use a tourniquet is an important one. You must recognize the situation as one in which you will be unable to stop the bleeding with direct and fingertip pressure. In this case, you will apply and then tighten a tourniquet.

NOTE: *Some systems may also authorize the use of hemostatic agents in this situation as an alternative. See the discussion of hemostatic agents next.*

Tourniquets are used only on extremity injuries. In addition, do not apply the tourniquet over a joint (elbow or knee). Place the tourniquet approximately 2 inches above the bleeding wound. There are several brands of commercial tourniquets available (such as the MAT shown in Figure 27-9). These devices fasten around the extremity and are tightened by a turning or twisting mechanism.

Tourniquets can also be made from ambulance equipment such as a cravat. Improvised tourniquets should be at least 2 to 4 inches wide and several layers thick. Never use narrow

FIGURE 27-8 The Mechanical Advantage Tourniquet (MAT).

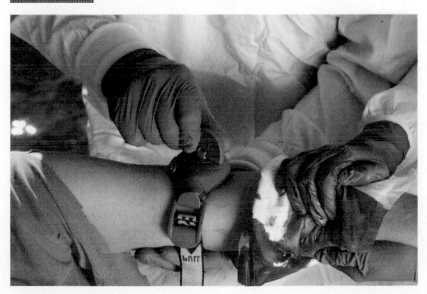

FIGURE 27-9
A commercial tourniquet in place to control bleeding from a gunshot wound. *(©Edward T. Dickinson, MD)*

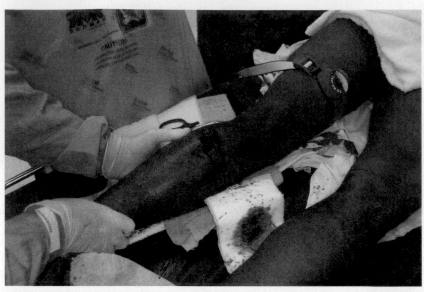

material such as a rope or wire that could cut into the skin. A blood pressure cuff may also be used as a tourniquet (Figure 27-10). If so, monitor the cuff pressure to be sure the cuff does not gradually deflate.

Once a tourniquet has been applied, do not remove or loosen it unless ordered by medical direction. Loosening a tourniquet may dislodge clots that have formed, resulting in further bleeding. If you must use a tourniquet, keep it in place.

While you are applying a tourniquet, have another rescuer apply direct pressure. This may slow the bleeding until the tourniquet is applied. To properly apply a tourniquet, follow these steps:

1. Select a site no farther than 2 inches from the wound. If the wound is on a joint, or just distal to the joint, apply the tourniquet above the joint. The tourniquet should be between the wound and the heart.

2. If using a commercial tourniquet, place the strap around the limb, pull the free end through the buckle or catch, and tighten this end over the pad. Tighten to the point where bleeding is controlled. Do not tighten beyond that point.

   If you are using cravats, or triangular bandages, wrap the material around the injured limb and tie a knot over the pad. Slip a pen, stick, or similar device into the knot and ro-

FIGURE 27-10 A blood pressure cuff used as a tourniquet.

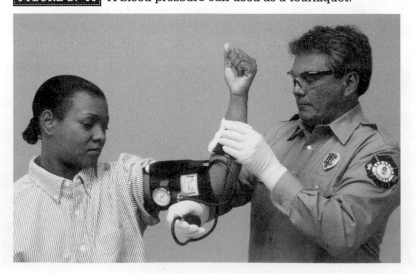

tate to tighten the tourniquet. Tighten to the point that bleeding is controlled, but no more than this point. Secure the device in place with tape or by tying with the ends of the cravat.

3. Attach a notation to the patient to alert other rescuers and hospital staff that a tourniquet has been applied and indicate the time of the application. Note this on your prehospital care report as well. Do not cover the extremity. You must visually monitor the wound site and the effectiveness of the tourniquet. Leave the tourniquet in open view. Advise hospital staff of the application of a tourniquet during your radio report and in person upon your arrival at the emergency department.

You may arrive at a scene to find that well-meaning bystanders have already applied a tourniquet to an injury, which may or may not have been necessary. If the EMT determines that the bleeding is not severe, and other means would control it, medical direction may be contacted about removing the tourniquet. Always follow your local protocols for this situation. If you are directed to remove the tourniquet, have another rescuer apply direct pressure to the wound while you release the tourniquet. If you find that the "tourniquet" applied by a layperson has not stopped the bleeding, immediately apply direct pressure and remove it. Proceed as you normally would.

Other Methods of Bleeding Control

Although the methods of bleeding control listed previously in the chapter are the ones that most experts agree are the most effective, a variety of other techniques may have a benefit in limited or specific applications or may still be a part of the protocols in some areas. These methods include using splints, cold applications, and the pneumatic anti-shock garment (PASG).

Splinting   Bleeding associated with a musculoskeletal injury may be controlled by proper splinting of the injury. Since the sharp ends of broken bones may cause tissue and vessel injury, stabilizing them and preventing further movement of the bone ends prevents additional damage. There are several types of splints used for stabilizing injured extremities. (Splinting musculoskeletal injuries will be discussed in detail in Chapter 30, "Musculoskeletal Trauma.")

Inflatable splints, also called air splints, may be used to control internal and external bleeding from an extremity. This type of splint may be used to control bleeding even if there is no suspected bone injury. The splint produces a form of direct pressure. Air splints are useful if there are several wounds to the extremity or one that extends over the length of the extremity. Air splints are most effective for venous and capillary bleeding. However, they are not usually effective for the high-pressure bleeding caused by an injured artery—at least not until the arterial pressure has decreased below that of the splint. However, you may use an air splint to maintain pressure on a bleeding wound after other manual methods, such as a pressure dressing, have already controlled the bleeding.

Cold Application   A traditional method of controlling bleeding is the application of ice or a cold pack to the injury. The cold minimizes swelling and reduces the bleeding by constricting the blood vessels. Application of cold should not be used alone but rather in conjunction with other manual techniques. Application of cold will also reduce pain at the injury site.

NOTE: *Never apply ice or cold packs directly to the skin. This can cause frostbite and further damage to the tissue. Always wrap ice or a cold pack in a cloth or towel before applying it to the skin. Do not leave it in place for longer than 20 minutes at a time.*

Pneumatic Anti-Shock Garment   Although the use of the PASG is controversial, some experts still believe that it is useful in controlling bleeding from the areas the garment covers. The PASG controls external bleeding from the lower extremities by direct pressure, similarly to the air splint. It is also useful in providing indirect pressure to help control internal bleeding in the pelvic and abdominal cavities. *Never* inflate only the abdominal section of the PASG. Use of the PASG when there is shock present with a chest wound is generally not advised. Follow your local protocols regarding the use of the PASG or contact medical direction for advice.

If your local protocols call for PASG use, remove the patient's lower outer garments to improve application of the garment and to allow for easier insertion of a urinary catheter later. If clothing cannot be removed, remove the patient's belt and any sharp objects from the pockets. Since transport will be required, place the PASG on the spine board before placing the patient on the PASG. An inflated anti-shock garment should be removed only when a physician is present or directing someone to remove it. Removal should only take place when vital signs have just been monitored and indicate that the patient is stable, and when an operating room is immediately available.

Use of the PASG in the treatment of shock (hypoperfusion) will be discussed later in this chapter.

Special Situations Involving Bleeding

Bleeding most often occurs from a wound caused by direct trauma (striking or being struck or cut by something, such as in a collision, a fall, a stabbing, or a shooting). However, you may also find external bleeding from other causes, such as bleeding from the ears caused indirectly by a head injury or a nosebleed caused by high blood pressure.

Head Injury   Traumatic injuries resulting in a fractured skull may cause bleeding or loss of cerebrospinal fluid (CSF) from the ears or nose. However, this fluid loss is not due to direct trauma to the ears or nose. Instead, the head injury results in increased pressure within the skull, which forces fluid out of the cranial cavity. You should not attempt to stop this bleeding or fluid loss, as doing so may increase the pressure in the skull. Do not apply pressure to the ears or nose. Allow the drainage to flow freely, using a gauze pad to collect it.

Nosebleed   Nosebleeds, also called *epistaxis*, may be caused by direct trauma to the nose. However, bleeding from the nose may also be caused by medical problems such as high blood pressure (hypertension). Tiny capillaries in the nose may burst because of increased blood pressure, sinus infection, or digital trauma (nose picking). Controlling bleeding from the nose is sometimes more difficult if the patient is taking certain medications, such as an anticoagulant like Coumadin. To stop a nosebleed, follow these steps:

1. Have the patient sit down and lean forward.

2. Apply or instruct the patient to apply direct pressure to the fleshy portion around the nostrils.

3. Keep the patient calm and quiet.

4. Do not let the patient lean back. This can allow blood to flow down the esophagus to the stomach as the patient swallows, resulting in nausea and vomiting.

5. If the patient becomes unconscious or is unable to control his own airway, place the patient in the recovery position (on his side) and be prepared to provide suction and aggressive airway management.

Internal Bleeding

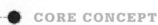
CORE CONCEPT

Signs, symptoms, and care of a patient with internal bleeding

Internal bleeding is bleeding that occurs inside the body. The bleeding itself is not visible, but many of the signs and symptoms are very apparent. There are several reasons why internal bleeding can be very serious:

- Damage to the internal organs and large blood vessels can result in loss of a large quantity of blood in a short period of time.

- Blood loss cannot be seen. Whereas external bleeding is easy to identify, internal bleeding is hidden. Patients may die of blood loss without having any external bleeding.

- Severe internal blood loss may even occur from injuries to the extremities. Sharp bone ends of a fractured femur can cause enough tissue and blood vessel damage to cause shock (hypoperfusion).

PATIENT ASSESSMENT

Internal Bleeding

Since internal bleeding is not visible, and may not be obvious, you must identify patients who may have internal bleeding by performing a thorough history and physical exam. Suspicion of internal bleeding and estimates of its severity should be based on the mechanism of injury as well as clinical signs and symptoms. If a patient has a mechanism of injury that suggests the possibility of internal bleeding, treat as though the patient has internal bleeding.

Blunt trauma is the leading cause of internal injuries and bleeding. Mechanisms of blunt trauma that may cause internal bleeding are:

- Falls
- Motor-vehicle or motorcycle crashes
- Auto-pedestrian collisions
- Blast injuries

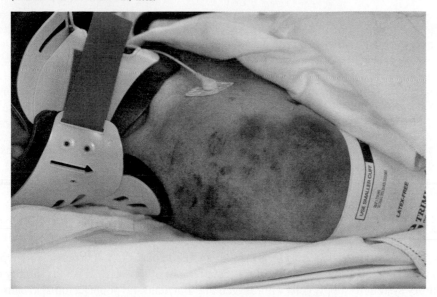

FIGURE 27-11 Bruising is one sign of internal bleeding.
(© Edward T. Dickinson, MD)

Penetrating trauma is also a common cause of internal injuries and bleeding. It is often difficult to judge the severity of the wound even when the size and length of the penetrating object are known. Always assess your patient for exit wounds. Mechanisms of penetrating trauma are:

- Gunshot wounds
- Stab wounds from a knife, ice pick, screwdriver, or similar object
- Impaled objects

Signs of Internal Bleeding

Many of the signs of internal bleeding that you will see are also signs of shock (hypoperfusion). These signs have developed as a result of uncontrolled internal bleeding. They are late signs, indicating that a life-threatening condition has already developed. If you wait until signs of internal bleeding or shock develop before beginning treatment, you have waited too long. Signs of internal bleeding are:

- Injuries to the surface of the body, which could indicate underlying injuries.
- Bruising, swelling (Figure 27-11), or pain over vital organs (especially in the chest and abdomen). Basic knowledge of anatomy is important for this reason.
- Painful, swollen, or deformed extremities.
- Bleeding from the mouth, rectum, vagina, or other body orifice.
- A tender, rigid, or distended abdomen.
- Vomiting a coffee-ground-like substance or bright red vomitus, indicating the presence of blood. (Red blood is usually "new." Dark blood is usually "old.")
- Dark, tarry stools or bright red blood in the stool.
- Signs and symptoms of shock. Remember that the signs listed in Table 27-1 are late signs. They will appear only after internal bleeding has already resulted in significant blood loss.

Remember, your best clue indicating the possibility of internal bleeding may be the presence of a mechanism of injury that could have caused internal bleeding.

PATIENT CARE

Internal Bleeding

Care for the patient with internal bleeding centers on the prevention and treatment of shock (hypoperfusion). Definitive treatment for internal bleeding can only take place in the hospital. Patients with suspected internal bleeding must be considered serious and warrant immediate transport to the hospital.

NOTE: *Unnecessary treatment for internal injuries will not harm the patient; however, death may result from not treating a patient who needs it.*

As with all patients, your first priority is the standard ABCs; that is, ensure an open airway, adequate breathing, and circulation. Patients with internal bleeding may deteriorate quickly. Monitor the ABCs and vital signs often. Be prepared to maintain the patient's airway, to provide or assist ventilations, or to administer CPR as needed.

1. Maintain the ABCs and provide support as needed.
2. Administer high-concentration oxygen by nonrebreather mask, if oxygen administration has not already begun.
3. Control any external bleeding. If you suspect internal bleeding in an injured extremity, apply an appropriate splint.
4. Provide prompt transport to an appropriate medical facility. Internal bleeding must often be controlled in the operating room.

SHOCK (HYPOPERFUSION)

● CORE CONCEPT

Signs, symptoms, and care of a patient with shock

Shock, also known as hypoperfusion, is inadequate tissue perfusion. (Perfusion and hypoperfusion were defined at the beginning of this chapter.) In other words, it is the inability of the circulatory system to supply cells with oxygen and nutrients. Hypoperfusion also causes the inadequate removal of waste products from the cells. The result of untreated shock is death.

Causes of Shock

As discussed previously, the circulatory system consists of three components: the heart, blood vessels, and blood. Failure of any of these components—the pumping of the heart, the supply of blood, the integrity of the blood vessels, or the ability of the vessels to dilate and constrict—means that perfusion of the brain, lungs, and other body organs will not be adequate.

Blood vessels can play an important role in the development of shock (if they are *not* functioning properly) or in the body's ability to compensate for shock (if they are functioning properly). Blood vessels can change their diameter, either by dilating or constricting. These changes in size are governed by the need for blood in various areas of the body. In an area of the body that is doing more work, blood vessels dilate to allow more blood to flow to that area. At the same time, in another area of the body that is not working as hard, vessels will constrict. For example, if you are running, blood flow to the muscles in the legs increases through dilated arteries. At the same time, blood flow to the digestive system lessens because vessels supplying these organs have been constricted to compensate for the dilation of the arteries in the legs.

Since the amount of blood in the body does not change, this balance between dilation of some vessels and constriction of others is necessary to keep the system full. The same amount of blood is in the body, but it is distributed differently. If all the blood vessels in the body dilated at one time, there would not be enough blood to fill the entire circulatory system. Circulation would fail, tissues would not be adequately perfused, and the patient would develop shock.

As shock develops, the failure of one component of the system may cause adverse effects on another. If blood is being lost through external bleeding, the heart rate will increase in an effort to circulate the remaining blood to all the tissues. However, the increased heart rate causes increased bleeding. As more blood is lost, the heart tries to compensate by increasing its rate even more. If left untreated, the process continues until the patient dies.

In early shock, the body attempts to compensate for blood loss. Most of the signs and symptoms of shock are caused by the body's compensating mechanisms attempting to adequately perfuse the tissues. Shock may develop if (1) the heart fails as a pump, (2) blood volume is lost, or (3) blood vessels dilate, creating a vascular container capacity that is too great to be filled by the available blood.

Severity of Shock

Shock (hypoperfusion) is the body's reaction to decreased blood circulation to the organ systems. It is the result of the inadequate perfusion of tissues with oxygen and nutrients and the inadequate removal of metabolic waste products. If untreated, shock will cause cell and

Inside/Outside

When pressure receptors in the aorta and carotid artery sense decreased flow, they stimulate the release of epinephrine and norepinephrine into the bloodstream. This causes blood vessels to constrict, especially in the skin, kidneys, and gastrointestinal tract. When blood vessels in the skin constrict, the skin becomes cool and pale. Sweat glands empty their contents, causing the sweaty skin so commonly seen in this situation. When blood vessels in the kidneys constrict, the kidneys produce less urine, thereby preventing the loss of more fluid. Constriction of blood vessels in the GI tract causes the stomach to try to empty its contents, leading to nausea and vomiting. All of these reactions are part of the "fight-or-flight" response the body experiences when under extreme stress.

organ malfunction and, ultimately, death. Prompt recognition of this condition and aggressive treatment are vital to ensure patient survival.

Shock is classified into three categories of severity: compensated shock, decompensated shock, and irreversible shock.

- In **compensated shock**, the body senses the decrease in perfusion and attempts to compensate for it. For a time, the body's compensating mechanisms work, and the patient maintains his blood pressure. Some early signs of shock are actually caused by the body's compensating mechanisms at work. You will note an increased heart rate (to increase blood flow) and increased respirations (to increase oxygenation of the blood). Constriction of the peripheral circulation (to redirect blood to the vital core organs) results in pale, cool skin and, in infants and children, increased capillary refill time.

- **Decompensated shock** begins at the point when the body can no longer compensate for the low blood volume or lack of perfusion. Late signs of shock, such as falling blood pressure, develop.

- **Irreversible shock** exists when the body has lost the battle to maintain perfusion to the organ systems. Cell damage occurs, especially in the liver and kidneys. Even if adequate vital signs can be restored, the patient may die days later due to the failure of irreparably damaged organs.

Types of Shock

Regardless of the cause, shock is the circulatory system's failure to provide sufficient blood and oxygen to all the body's vital tissues. The three major types of shock are hypovolemic shock, cardiogenic shock, and neurogenic shock.

- **Hypovolemic shock** is most commonly seen by EMTs. When it is caused by uncontrolled bleeding, or hemorrhage, it can be called **hemorrhagic shock**. The bleeding can be internal, external, or a combination of both. Hypovolemic shock may also be caused by burns or crush injuries, where plasma is lost, or by severe dehydration.

- **Cardiogenic shock** may develop in patients suffering a myocardial infarction, or heart attack. It develops from the inadequate pumping of blood by the heart. The strength of the heart's contractions may be decreased because of the damage to the heart muscle. Alternatively, the heart's electrical system may be malfunctioning, causing a heartbeat that is too slow, too fast, or irregular. Other cardiac problems, such as congestive heart failure, may also cause shock. You must watch for low blood pressure, edema in the feet and ankles, and other signs of heart failure. (Review Chapter 20, "Cardiac Emergencies.")

- **Neurogenic shock** may result from the uncontrolled dilation of blood vessels due to nerve paralysis caused by spinal cord injuries. Although there is no actual blood loss, the dilation of the blood vessels increases the circulatory system's capacity to the point where the available blood can no longer adequately fill it. With sepsis (massive infection) or an anaphylactic (severe allergic) reaction, vasodilation may also cause shock. Neurogenic shock is rarely seen in the field.

compensated shock
when the patient is developing shock but the body is still able to maintain perfusion. *See* shock.

decompensated shock
when the body can no longer compensate for low blood volume or lack of perfusion. Late signs such as decreasing blood pressure become evident. *See* shock.

irreversible shock
when the body has lost the battle to maintain perfusion to vital organs. Even if adequate vital signs return, the patient may die days later due to organ failure.

hypovolemic (HI-po-vo-LE-mik) shock
shock resulting from blood or fluid loss.

hemorrhagic (HEM-or-AJ-ik) shock
shock resulting from blood loss.

cardiogenic shock
shock, or lack of perfusion, brought on not by blood loss, but by inadequate pumping action of the heart. It is often the result of a heart attack or congestive heart failure.

neurogenic shock
hypoperfusion due to nerve paralysis (sometimes caused by spinal cord injuries) resulting in the dilation of blood vessels that increases the volume of the circulatory system beyond the point where it can be filled.

Infants and children present a special problem when assessing for shock. They have such efficient compensating mechanisms that they can maintain a normal blood pressure until half of their blood volume is gone. By the time their blood pressure drops, they are already near death. The potential for shock must be considered and cared for early. Do not wait for signs of shock to appear.

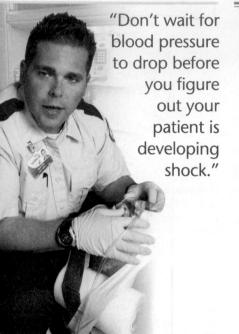

"Don't wait for blood pressure to drop before you figure out your patient is developing shock."

PATIENT ASSESSMENT

Shock (Hypoperfusion)

Many of the signs and symptoms of shock are the same no matter what the cause (hypovolemic, cardiogenic, or neurogenic). The symptoms follow a logical progression as shock develops and worsens. The signs and symptoms, in the order they appear, are as follows (Figure 27-12 and Table 27-1):

- **Altered mental status.** The brain is very sensitive to any decrease in oxygen supply. When the brain is deprived of oxygen, even slightly, mental and behavioral changes may be seen. These may include anxiety, restlessness, and combativeness.

- **Pale, cool, and clammy skin.** When the body senses inadequate tissue perfusion, it attempts to correct the problem by diverting, or shunting, blood from nonvital areas to the vital organs. Blood is quickly directed away from the skin and sent to organs such as the heart and brain. This results in loss of skin color and temperature. Infants and young children may have a capillary refill time of greater than 2 seconds. (Delayed capillary refill time is considered an unreliable sign of shock in patients over the age of 5 when capillary refill time can more readily be influenced by other factors.) Note that in neurogenic shock (rare) the skin is typically warm, flushed, and dry because the circulatory system has lost the ability to constrict blood vessels in the skin.

- **Nausea and vomiting.** In the body's efforts to direct blood to the vital organs, blood is diverted from the digestive system, resulting in nausea and sometimes vomiting.

- **Vital sign changes.** The first vital signs to change are the respiratory and pulse rates:
  - The pulse will increase in an attempt to pump more blood. As it continues to increase and blood loss worsens, the pulse becomes weak and thready.
  - Respirations increase in an attempt to raise the oxygen saturation of the blood left in the system. As shock progresses, respirations become more rapid, labored, shallow, and sometimes irregular.
  - Blood pressure drops because the body's compensating mechanisms can no longer keep up with the decrease in perfusion or blood loss. Decreased blood pressure is a *late* sign of shock. By the time the blood pressure drops, the patient is in a truly life-threatening condition.
  - Pulse oximetry might not be accurate in patients with shock. Oximeters rely on adequate perfusion to get an accurate reading. Patients with shock may not be adequately perfusing their extremities.

- **Other signs.** Late signs of shock include thirst, dilated pupils, and sometimes cyanosis around the lips and nail beds.

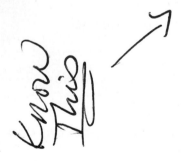

Emergency Care for Shock

Emergency care for the patient in shock includes airway maintenance and the administration of high-concentration oxygen. Increasing the blood's oxygen saturation will improve oxygen supply to the tissues. You must also attempt to stop what is causing the shock, such as external bleeding, and attempt to maintain perfusion.

Remember that *transportation is an intervention.* Your most significant treatment for the shock patient may be early recognition of the problem and prompt transportation to a hospital where the patient will receive definitive care.

The term *golden hour* has been used to describe the optimal time from the infliction of a traumatic injury until the patient receives definitive treatment in a hospital—usually surgery. However, trauma programs and experts have ceased using the term *golden hour* because there is no research that clearly identifies the optimal time between injury and definitive care.

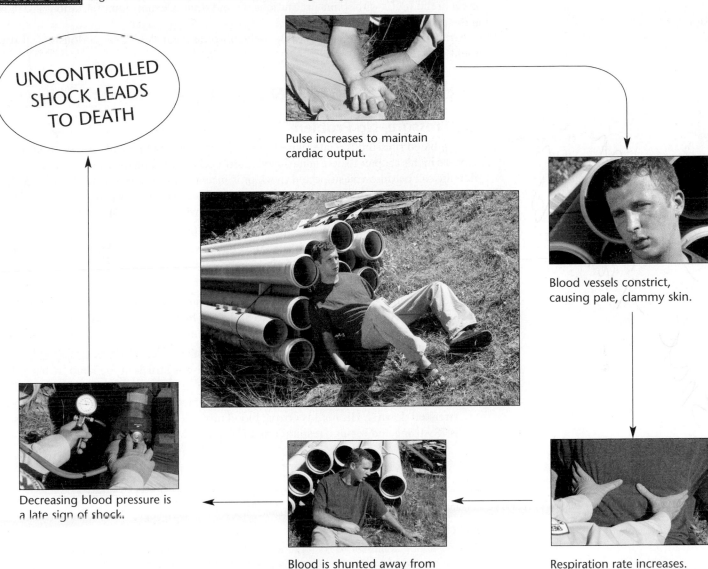

UNCONTROLLED SHOCK LEADS TO DEATH

Pulse increases to maintain cardiac output.

Blood vessels constrict, causing pale, clammy skin.

Decreasing blood pressure is a late sign of shock.

Blood is shunted away from the gastrointestinal organs, causing nausea.

Respiration rate increases.

Furthermore, EMTs should never consider an hour the ideal time if less time can be taken. Perhaps a better statement is that *every minute between the time of injury and the patient getting to an operating suite is, in fact, like gold to the patient—and to his chances of survival.*

Note that the clock begins running at the time of injury, not the time of your arrival on-scene. If the patient is not quickly found, or you have a long response time to the scene, much of this critical time, formerly called the golden hour, may have already ticked away. Therefore, your goal in caring for trauma and shock patients is to limit on-scene time and provide immediate transportation to the hospital. Be sure to alert the receiving hospital as soon as possible, as they may need to call in a surgeon or activate a trauma team. The clock does not stop with the patient's arrival at the hospital. It stops in the operating room.

For the reasons just discussed, limiting the time spent at the scene is vital. The goal for on-scene time when caring for a trauma or shock patient has been stated as a maximum of 10 minutes (unless lengthy extrication is required). This time limit is often called the *platinum 10 minutes.* Like the golden hour, there is no research that proves 10 minutes is the ideal on-scene time. The best rule is simply to take as little time as possible at the scene.

In order to keep scene time as short as possible, keep procedures done at the scene to a minimum. In patients showing signs of shock, or a mechanism of injury that suggests that possibility, some elements of patient assessment, such as detailed exams and treatments, are best done in the ambulance en route to the hospital. On-scene assessment and care should consist of the ABCs with spinal precautions, a rapid trauma exam, immobilization, and moving the patient to the ambulance.

Always drive safely and responsibly to the hospital regardless of the seriousness of your patient's condition.

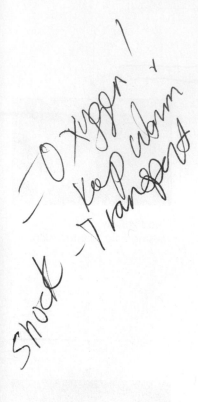

CRITICAL DECISION MAKING

No Pressure, No Problem

Falling blood pressure is a late sign of shock. In the following patients, use material you learned in this chapter to determine if your early decision making would lead you to expedite the call because you suspected shock or if, instead, you believe the patient will likely be stable. You will not be provided a blood pressure—but in each patient you will find enough information to make a proper early decision without a blood pressure reading.

1. Your patient was working on scaffolding that collapsed, causing him to fall one story (about 10 feet). He is conscious, is alert but anxious, and complains of pain to the right side of his chest. His pulse is 102 and regular, respirations 26, skin cool and moist, and pupils equal and reactive to light.

2. Your patient is found sitting in a bathroom stall at an upscale restaurant. He is pale, sweaty, and leaning against the wall. He tells you he has recently had a problem with bleeding hemorrhoids. There is bright red blood in the toilet bowl. When you stand the patient up to move him to the stretcher, he feels like he is going to pass out.

3. You are called to an assault. A 27-year-old man was struck in the head by his girlfriend. She used a telephone to strike him once in the nose and again in the forehead. The police called you to evaluate his nosebleed. The patient's shirt has blood streaked down it. His nose is oozing blood now. He is alert and oriented. His pulse is 78, strong and regular; respirations 14; and skin warm and dry.

PATIENT CARE

Shock (Hypoperfusion)

Care for shock is similar to the care for bleeding described earlier. Remember Standard Precautions when caring for any patient who is bleeding externally. The emergency care steps for shock (Scan 27-2) are as follows:

1. Maintain an open airway and assess the respiratory rate. If the patient is breathing adequately, apply high-concentration oxygen by nonrebreather mask. Assist ventilations or perform CPR, if necessary.

2. Control any external bleeding.

3. Apply and inflate the PASG if approved or ordered by your local medical direction (Scan 27-3). The PASG is usually indicated for bleeding in areas covered by the garment, pelvic injury, and some abdominal trauma. Always follow your local protocols for use of the PASG. Alternative treatments for pelvic injuries, which also help treat for shock, are discussed in Chapter 30, "Musculoskeletal Trauma."

   Use of the PASG is usually contraindicated in cardiogenic shock, or if there are abnormal lung sounds. Special consideration should be taken if your patient has bleeding in areas not covered by the garment.

   Use of the PASG when there is shock in the presence of a chest wound is generally not advised. If your female patient is pregnant, inflate only the leg sections. If your patient is a child, it is recommended that only the leg sections be inflated. This is because the top of the abdominal section of the pediatric-size garment often covers the lower portion of a child's chest, which can interfere with the child's respirations.

4. Splint any suspected bone injuries or joint injuries. However, if your patient is in shock, do not use your valuable on-scene time for this. Splints should be applied en route to the hospital. Do not take time to individually splint multiple injuries. You can splint the entire body by securing the patient to a long spine board. This will adequately stabilize the injuries until further care can be given.

FIRST TAKE STANDARD PRECAUTIONS.

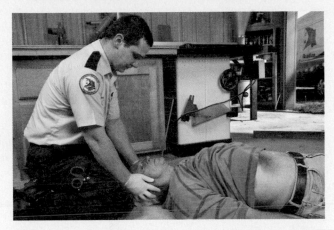

1 Perform manual stabilization of the head and neck. Maintain an open airway.

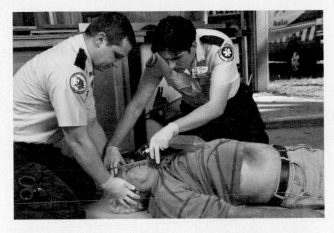

2 Administer oxygen by nonrebreather mask.

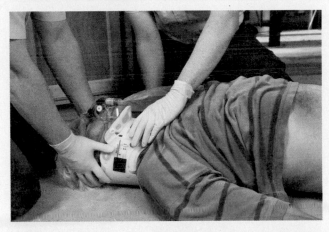

3 If the patient may have a spine injury, apply a cervical collar.

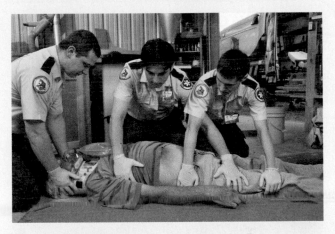

4 Log roll the patient onto a spine board.

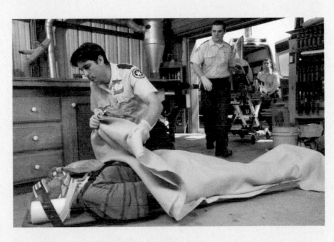

5 Prepare the patient for prompt transport. Maintain warmth.

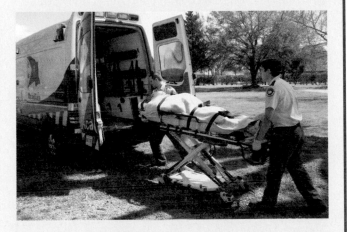

6 Transport the patient.

5. Prevent loss of body heat by covering the patient with a blanket.
6. Transport the patient immediately. Detailed exams and care procedures should be done en route to the hospital. Notify the receiving hospital as soon as possible. Give them information on the patient's injuries and condition. Contact medical direction, if necessary. If your on-scene time is extended due to extrication, or your transport time to the hospital is lengthy, request an ALS intercept, if available. This may be a ground ambulance or a helicopter service. If you have the patient loaded in your ambulance, begin transport and ask that the ALS unit intercept your unit en route. Time is of the essence.
7. If the patient is conscious, speak calmly and reassuringly throughout your assessment, care, and transport. Fear increases the body's work and worsens developing shock.

NOTE: *The traditional practice of elevating the legs as a treatment for shock is no longer recommended. However, if elevating the legs is part of your local protocols, it will do no harm if there is no possibility of spine injury. In any case, elevation would be unnecessary if you are applying and inflating the PASG.*

SCAN 27-3 Applying the Pneumatic Anti-Shock Garment (PASG)

FOLLOW LOCAL PROTOCOLS REGARDING APPLICATION AND INFLATION.

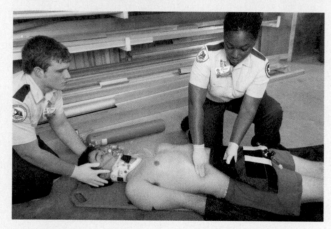

❶ Place PASG on spine board, then patient on PASG. Position so the top of the garment is three finger-widths below the bottom of the rib cage.

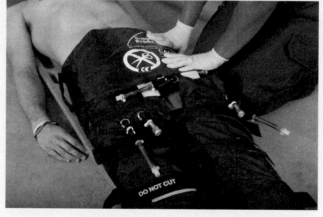

❷ Apply the garment.

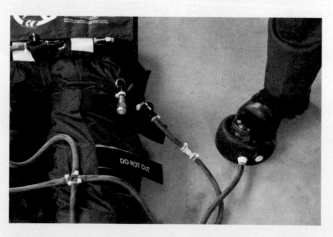

❸ Inflate the garment.

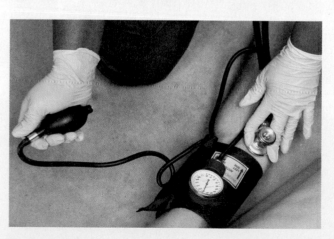

❹ Monitor and record vital signs every 5 minutes. If the garment loses pressure, add air as needed.

CHAPTER REVIEW

Key Facts and Concepts

- Almost all external bleeding can be controlled by direct pressure and elevation. When these don't work, apply a tourniquet if the bleeding is on an extremity.

- Emergency care for internal bleeding is based on the prevention and treatment of shock.

- Early signs of shock are often restlessness, anxiety, pale skin, and rapid pulse and respirations.

- If shock remains uncontrolled, the patient's blood pressure falls, a late sign of shock.

- Signs and symptoms of shock may not be evident early in the call, so treatment based on the mechanism of injury may be lifesaving.

- Treat shock by maintaining the airway; administering high-concentration oxygen; controlling bleeding; and keeping the patient warm. One of the most important treatments is early recognition of shock and immediate transport to a hospital.

Key Decisions

- Has direct pressure controlled the patient's bleeding or do I need to apply a tourniquet?

- What can I use for a tourniquet that will control bleeding but not damage tissue?

- Is a patient with pale, cool skin; tachycardia; and rapid, shallow respirations in shock or just under stress? How will continuing assessment help in making that decision?

- When treating a patient with shock, what should I do at the scene and what should I do en route to the hospital?

Chapter Glossary

arterial bleeding bleeding from an artery, which is characterized by bright red blood that is rapid, profuse, and difficult to control.

capillary bleeding bleeding from capillaries, which is characterized by a slow, oozing flow of blood.

cardiogenic shock shock, or lack of perfusion, brought on not by blood loss, but by the heart's inadequate pumping action. It is often the result of a heart attack or congestive heart failure.

compensated shock when the patient is developing shock but the body is still able to maintain perfusion. *See* shock.

decompensated shock when the body can no longer compensate for low blood volume or lack of perfusion. Late signs such as decreasing blood pressure become evident. *See* shock.

hemorrhage (HEM-o-rej) bleeding, especially severe bleeding.

hemorrhagic (HEM-or-AJ-ik) *shock* shock resulting from blood loss.

hemostatic (HEM-o-STAT-IK) *agents* substances applied as powders, dressings, gauze, or bandages to open wounds to stop bleeding.

hypoperfusion (HI-po-per-FEW-zhun) the body's inability to adequately circulate blood to the body's cells to supply them with oxygen and nutrients. *See also* shock.

hypovolemic (HI-po-vo-LE-mik) *shock* shock resulting from blood or fluid loss.

irreversible shock when the body has lost the battle to maintain perfusion to vital organs. Even if adequate vital signs return, the patient may die days later due to organ failure.

neurogenic shock hypoperfusion due to nerve paralysis (sometimes caused by spinal cord injuries) resulting in the dilation of blood vessels that increases the volume of the circulatory system beyond the point where it can be filled.

perfusion the supply of oxygen to, and removal of wastes from, the body's cells and tissues as a result of the flow of blood through the capillaries.

pressure dressing a bulky dressing held in position with a tightly wrapped bandage, which applies pressure to help control bleeding.

shock the body's inability to adequately circulate blood to the body's cells to supply them with oxygen and nutrients, which is a life-threatening condition. Also known as *hypoperfusion*.

tourniquet (TURN-i-ket) a device used for bleeding control that constricts all blood flow to and from an extremity.

venous bleeding bleeding from a vein, which is characterized by dark red or maroon blood and a steady, easy-to-control flow.

Preparation for Your Examination and Practice

Short Answer

1. Name the three main types of blood vessels, and describe the type of bleeding you would expect to see from each one.

2. List the patient care steps for external bleeding control.

3. Define perfusion and hypoperfusion.

4. List the signs and symptoms of shock. Which would you expect to see early? Which are late signs? Explain what causes each of them.
5. List the three major types of shock and what causes each one.
6. List the emergency care steps for treating a patient in shock.

Thinking And Linking

Think back to Chapters 10–15 on scene size-up and patient assessment as well as Chapters 18–26 on medical emergencies. Link information from those chapters with information from this chapter as you consider the following questions:

1. You respond to a shopping center parking lot for a motor-vehicle collision. You find an older male patient unresponsive in his vehicle. What facts could you gather at the scene that would help you determine whether the patient's unresponsiveness was caused by trauma and shock or a medical condition?
2. What medical conditions can cause shock or present with signs and symptoms similar to shock?

Critical Thinking Exercises

Assessing and treating a patient at the scene of a collision is a challenge. The purpose of this exercise will be to consider assessment and care for such a patient.

- A patient has been involved in a motor-vehicle collision. There is considerable damage to his vehicle. The steering column and wheel are badly deformed. The patient complains of a "sore chest." You note no external bleeding. The patient's vital signs are pulse 116, respirations 20, blood pressure 106/70. How would you proceed to assess and care for this patient?

Pathophysiology to Practice

The following question is designed to assist you in gathering relevant clinical information and making accurate decisions in the field.

- A patient who was found unresponsive is in severe shock. She has no signs of trauma and has no medical history. How could an overdose of medication have caused her condition?

Street Scenes -

Your ambulance is dispatched with an EMR unit from the fire department, Squad 31, to a 46-year-old male with injuries from a fall. Squad 31 is on-scene first, gathering a history and taking a set of vital signs. You arrive about 3 minutes later. Arnold Johnson, your patient, is sitting in a chair and looking anxious.

Mr. Johnson likes to do odd jobs around the house. Today's project was to fix a loose shelf in the kitchen. He got out his ladder and tools and started to work. As he reached to hammer his first nail, he lost his footing and fell a few feet, hitting his left side on the corner of the kitchen table. It hurt, but he went back to finish the shelf. After a few minutes, he realized he was in considerable discomfort. As the pain increased and Arnold started to feel worse, he knew something was wrong and called 911.

Street Scene Questions

1. What is the priority for this patient? Does a primary assessment still need to be done?
2. What assessment information do you want to receive from Squad 31?
3. Is the mechanism of injury important information for this patient?

You approach the patient as your partner gets the EMR information. You notice that Mr. Johnson is pale and seems to have an increased respiratory rate. Your partner gives you the patient history from Squad 31, including their impression that the patient may have broken some ribs. The EMR staff report the following vital signs: a thready pulse of 110, respiratory rate of 24 and labored, and a blood pressure of 130/85. As you move on to the secondary assessment, your partner prepares the stretcher. You are becoming more concerned. You ask Arnold's wife if this is his normal color and she tells you he is very pale. At that point, the patient tells you he feels nauseated and thinks he might throw up.

Street Scene Questions

4. What is the treatment priority for this patient?
5. How often should you get a new set of vital signs?

You load the patient on the stretcher, ask him how he feels, and notice he is not as alert as when you arrived on the scene about 10 minutes ago. You administer oxygen by way of nonrebreather mask and move toward the ambulance, concerned that this patient may be bleeding internally. Once en route to the hospital, you get another set of vital signs and realize the pulse is weak and has increased by 10 beats per minute. The respiratory rate is now 28 and seems more labored. The blood pressure is 124/80. You do a detailed assessment of the abdomen, and the patient reacts with tenderness in the left upper quadrant. The closest hospital is a trauma center, and you tell your partner this is a high priority. You continue patient care with 15 lpm of oxygen by nonrebreather mask and keep the patient warm. You take another set of vital signs, followed by a radio report to the hospital. You end the transmission by advising ETA in 7 minutes.

A short time after you give your prehospital care report to ED personnel, you overhear a surgeon turn to a nurse and quietly say, "Get an operating room set up. This patient likely has a severe spleen injury."

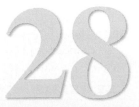

Soft-Tissue Trauma

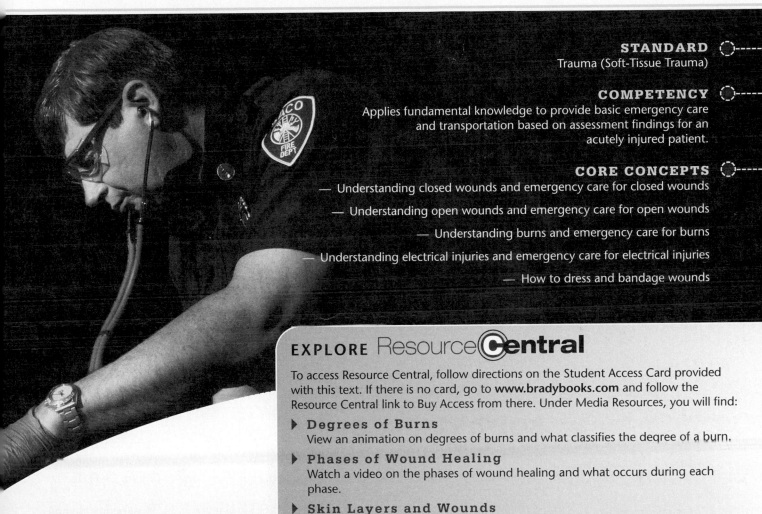

STANDARD ⟡----
Trauma (Soft-Tissue Trauma)

COMPETENCY ⟡----
Applies fundamental knowledge to provide basic emergency care and transportation based on assessment findings for an acutely injured patient.

CORE CONCEPTS ⟡----
— Understanding closed wounds and emergency care for closed wounds
— Understanding open wounds and emergency care for open wounds
— Understanding burns and emergency care for burns
— Understanding electrical injuries and emergency care for electrical injuries
— How to dress and bandage wounds

EXPLORE Resource Central

To access Resource Central, follow directions on the Student Access Card provided with this text. If there is no card, go to **www.bradybooks.com** and follow the Resource Central link to Buy Access from there. Under Media Resources, you will find:

▶ **Degrees of Burns**
View an animation on degrees of burns and what classifies the degree of a burn.

▶ **Phases of Wound Healing**
Watch a video on the phases of wound healing and what occurs during each phase.

▶ **Skin Layers and Wounds**
See a video on skin layers and their purposes and why you should know how deep a wound may be.

OBJECTIVES

After reading this chapter you should be able to:

28.1 Define key terms introduced in this chapter.

28.2 Describe the structure and function of the skin. (pp. 642–644)

28.3 Describe types of closed soft-tissue wounds and the assessment and management of closed soft-tissue wounds. (pp. 644–646)

28.4 Predict injuries that may be indicated by various contusion (bruise) types and locations. (p. 646)

28.5 Describe types of open soft-tissue wounds and general assessment and care for open soft-tissue wounds. (pp. 646–652)

28.6 Describe specific treatment for abrasions and lacerations, puncture wounds, impaled objects, avulsions, amputations, and genital injuries. (pp. 652–659)

28.7 Discuss complications associated with burns. (p. 659)

28.8 Classify burns by agent, source, depth, and severity. (pp. 660–665)

28.9 Describe specific treatment for thermal burns and chemical burns. (pp. 666–670)

28.10 Describe assessment and management for electrical burns. (pp. 670–671)

(continued)

KEY TERMS

abrasion, *p. 646*	crush injury, *p. 645*	laceration, *p. 647*	rule of palm, *p. 663*
amputation, *p. 648*	dermis, *p. 643*	open wound, *p. 646*	subcutaneous layers, *p. 644*
avulsion, *p. 648*	epidermis, *p. 642*	partial thickness burn, *p. 660*	superficial burn, *p. 660*
closed wound, *p. 644*	full thickness burn, *p. 661*	puncture wound, *p. 647*	
contusion, *p. 645*	hematoma, *p. 645*	rule of nines, *p. 662*	

E MTs are frequently called to deal with injuries to the soft tissues of the body. These injuries may range from minor scrapes and bruises to life-threatening bleeding or amputations. Although serious external bleeding is uncommon, this is an opportunity for the EMT to make a significant difference in a patient's life. Many soft-tissue injuries are open wounds, which can be very upsetting to the patient. Your emotional care and demeanor will mean a great deal. Overall, the assessment and care of the patient with a soft-tissue injury will be a challenging part of your responsibilities as an EMT.

>>>>>> ## SOFT TISSUES

The soft tissues of the body include the skin, fatty tissues, muscles, blood vessels, fibrous tissues, membranes (tissues that line or cover organs), glands, and nerves (Figure 28-1). Teeth, bones, and cartilage are considered hard tissues.

The most obvious soft-tissue injuries involve the skin (Figure 28-2). Most people do not think of the skin as a body organ, but it is. In fact, it is the largest organ of the human body. The skin's total surface area is over 20 square feet. Its major functions are:

- **Protection.** The skin is a barrier that keeps out microorganisms (germs), debris, and unwanted chemicals. Underlying tissues and organs are protected from environmental contact.

- **Water balance.** The skin helps prevent water loss and stops environmental water from entering the body. This helps preserve the chemical balance of body fluids and tissues.

- **Temperature regulation.** Blood vessels in the skin can dilate (increase in diameter) to carry more blood to the skin, allowing heat to radiate away from the body. When the body needs to conserve heat, these vessels constrict (decrease in diameter) to prevent heat loss. The sweat glands found in the skin produce perspiration, which will evaporate and help cool the body. The fat that is part of the skin serves as a thermal insulator.

- **Excretion.** Salts, carbon dioxide, and excess water can be released through the skin.

- **Shock (impact) absorption.** The skin and its layers of fat help protect the underlying organs from minor impacts and pressures.

epidermis (ep-i-DER-mis) the outer layer of the skin.

The skin has three major layers: the epidermis, the dermis, and the subcutaneous layer. The outer layer of the skin is the *epidermis*. The outermost epidermis is composed of dead cells, which are rubbed off or sloughed off and are replaced. The pigment granules of the skin and living cells are found deeper in the epidermis. The cells of the innermost portion are actively dividing, replacing the dead cells of the outer layers. The epidermis contains no blood

FIGURE 28-1 Soft tissues.

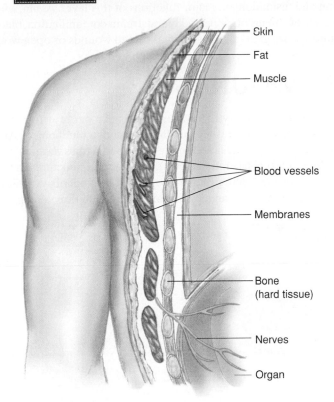

FIGURE 28-2 The skin.

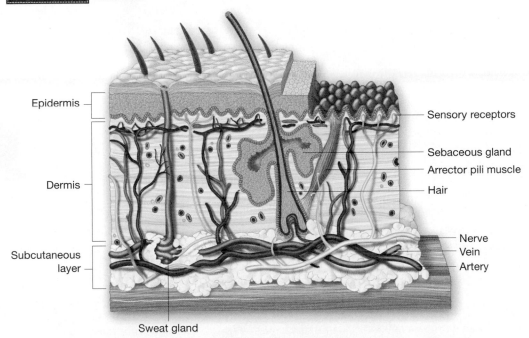

vessels or nerves. Except for certain types of burns and injuries due to cold, injuries of the epidermis present few problems in EMT-level care.

The layer of skin below the epidermis is the **dermis**. This layer is rich with blood vessels, nerves, and specialized structures such as sweat glands, sebaceous (oil) glands, and hair follicles. Specialized nerve endings in the dermis are involved with the senses of touch, cold, heat, and pain. Once the dermis is opened to the outside world, contamination and infection become major problems. Such wounds can be serious, especially when accompanied by profuse bleeding and intense pain.

dermis (DER-mis)
the inner (second) layer of the skin found beneath the epidermis. It is rich in blood vessels and nerves.

subcutaneous (SUB-ku-TAY-ne-us) **layers**
the layers of fat and soft tissues found below the dermis.

The layers of fat and soft tissue below the dermis are called the **subcutaneous layers**. Shock absorption and insulation are major functions of this layer. Again, when these layers are injured there are problems of tissue and bloodstream contamination, bleeding, and pain.

Soft-tissue injuries are generally classified as closed wounds or open wounds.

CLOSED WOUNDS

● CORE CONCEPT
Understanding closed wounds and emergency care for closed wounds

closed wound
an internal injury with no open pathway from the outside.

A **closed wound** is an internal injury; that is, there is no open pathway from the outside to the injured site. These wounds usually result from the impact of a blunt object. Although the skin itself may not be broken, there may be extensively crushed tissues beneath it. Closed wounds can be simple bruises, internal lacerations (cuts), and internal punctures caused by fractured bones, crushing forces, or the rupture (bursting open) of internal organs (Figure 28-3). Internal bleeding from a closed wound can range from minor to life threatening.

FIGURE 28-3 Closed wounds.

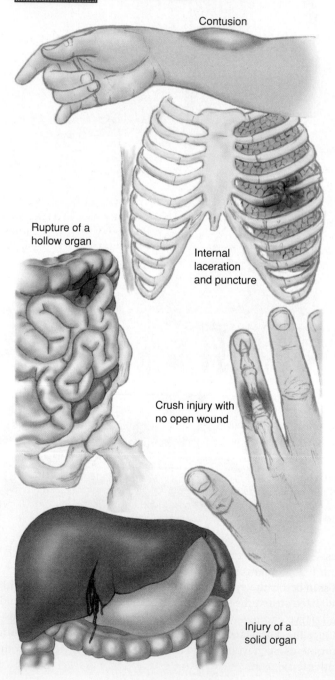

Contusion

Rupture of a hollow organ

Internal laceration and puncture

Crush injury with no open wound

Injury of a solid organ

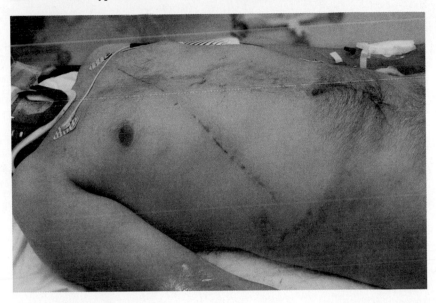

FIGURE 28-4 Contusions, such as these created by a seat belt, are the most common type of closed wound. *(© Edward T. Dickinson, MD)*

Types of Closed Wounds

There are three types of closed wounds: contusions, hematomas, and crush injuries.

Contusions

A ***contusion*** is a bruise, the most frequently encountered type of closed wound (Figure 28-4). In a contusion, the epidermis remains intact, but cells and blood vessels in the dermis are damaged. A variable amount of internal bleeding occurs at the time of injury and may continue for a few hours. There is pain, swelling, and discoloration at the wound site. Swelling and discoloration may occur immediately or may be delayed as much as 24 to 48 hours. The swelling is caused by a collection of blood under the skin or within the damaged tissues. Other organs such as the kidneys or brain may also be contused.

contusion (kun-TU-zhun)
a bruise.

Hematomas

Blood almost always collects at the injury site. This results in a ***hematoma***. A hematoma differs from a contusion in that hematomas involve a larger amount of tissue damage, including damage to larger blood vessels with greater internal blood loss. As much as a liter of blood may accumulate in a hematoma.

hematoma (hem-ah-TO-mah)
a swelling caused by the collection of blood under the skin or in damaged tissues as a result of an injured or broken blood vessel.

Closed Crush Injuries

Force can be transmitted from the body's exterior to its internal structures, even when the skin remains intact and the only indication of injury is a simple bruise. This force can cause the internal organs to be crushed or ruptured, causing internal bleeding. This is called a ***crush injury***. Solid organs such as the liver and spleen normally contain considerable amounts of blood. When crushed, they bleed severely and cause shock. Contents of hollow organs, such as digested food or urine, can leak into the body cavities, causing severe inflammation and tissue damage.

crush injury
an injury caused when force is transmitted from the body's exterior to its internal structures. Bones can be broken; muscles, nerves, and tissues damaged; and internal organs ruptured, causing internal bleeding.

Emergency Care for Closed Wounds

Closed wounds require strict attention to Standard Precautions, even though the patient's skin is not broken.

PATIENT ASSESSMENT

Closed Wounds

Bruising may be an indication of internal injuries and related internal bleeding (Table 28-1). In addition, consider the possibility of closed soft-tissue injuries whenever there is swelling, pain, or deformity, as well as a mechanism of blunt trauma. Always consider the mechanism

Table 28-1   Contusions (Bruises) as Signs of Soft-Tissue Injury

SIGN	INDICATES
Large bruise or bruised areas directly over the body	Possible injury to underlying organs such as the spleen, liver, or kidneys.
Swelling or deformity at the site of the bruise	Possible underlying fracture.
Bruise on the head or neck	Possible injury to the cervical spine or brain. Search for blood in the mouth, nose, and ears.
Bruise on the trunk or signs of damage to the ribs or sternum	Possible chest injury. Determine if the patient is coughing up frothy red blood, which may indicate a punctured lung, and assess for difficult breathing. Use your stethoscope to listen for equal air entry and any unusual breath sounds.
Bruise on the abdomen	Possible injury to the abdominal organs. Look to see if the patient has vomited. If so, is there any substance in the vomitus that looks like coffee grounds (partially digested blood)? Palpate to detect if the patient's abdomen is rigid or tender.

Note: Treatment for internal bleeding is discussed in Chapter 27, "Bleeding and Shock"; treatment of head injury is discussed in Chapter 31, "Trauma to the Head, Neck, and Spine"; and treatment of chest and abdominal injuries is discussed in this chapter.

---

of injury (MOI) when you examine a patient with a closed wound. Crush injuries may be difficult or impossible to identify during assessment, so you must rely on the MOI. Patients with a significant MOI should be considered to have internal bleeding and shock until they are ruled out in the emergency department.

PATIENT CARE

Closed Wounds

Take the appropriate Standard Precautions and follow these steps for emergency care of a patient with closed wounds:

1. Manage the patient's airway, breathing, and circulation. Apply high-concentration oxygen by nonrebreather mask.
2. *Manage as if there is internal bleeding* and *provide care for shock* if you believe that there is any possibility of internal injuries.
3. Splint extremities that are painful, swollen, or deformed.
4. Stay alert in case the patient vomits.
5. Continue to monitor the patient for the development of shock and transport as soon as possible.

OPEN WOUNDS

- - - - - - - ● CORE CONCEPT
Understanding open wounds and emergency care for open wounds

open wound
an injury in which the skin is interrupted, exposing the tissue beneath.

abrasion (ab-RAY-zhun)
a scratch or scrape.

An ***open wound*** is an injury in which the skin is interrupted, or broken, exposing the tissues underneath. The interruption can come from the outside, as a laceration, or from the inside when a fractured bone end breaks the skin.

Types of Open Wounds

There are numerous types of open wounds, including abrasions, lacerations, punctures, avulsions, amputations, crush injuries, blast injuries, and high pressure injection injuries.

Abrasions

The classification of ***abrasion*** includes simple scrapes and scratches in which the outer layer of the skin is damaged but not all the layers are penetrated. Abrasions can range in severity (Figure 28-5). Skinned elbows and knees, *road rash*, *mat burns*, *rug burns*, and *brush burns*

 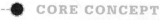

FIGURE 28-5 (A)Abrasions are usually the least serious type of open wound. (B) Some abrasions are more severe.
(Photos A and B: © Edward T. Dickinson, MD)

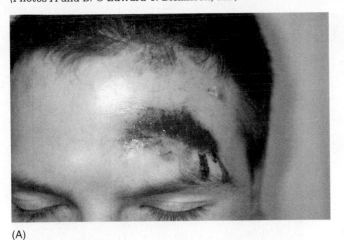

(A)

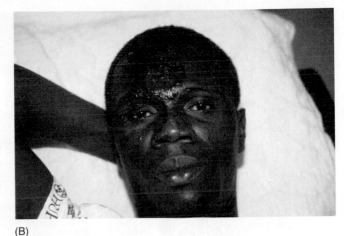

(B)

are examples of abrasions. With abrasions, there may be no detectable bleeding or only the minor ooze of blood from the capillary beds. The patient may be experiencing great pain, even if the injury is minor. Because of dirt or other substances ground into the skin, the opportunity for infection is great.

Lacerations

A *laceration* is a cut. It may be smooth or jagged (Figure 28-6). This type of wound is often caused by an object with a sharp edge, such as a razor blade, broken glass, or a jagged piece of metal. However, a laceration can also result from a severe blow or impact with a blunt object. If the laceration has rough edges, it may tend to fall together and obstruct the view as you try to determine the wound depth. It is usually impossible to look at the outside of a laceration and determine the extent of the damage to underlying tissues. If significant blood vessels have been torn, bleeding will be considerable. Sometimes the bleeding is partially controlled when blood vessels are stretched and torn. This is due to the natural retraction and constriction of the cut ends that aid in rapid clot formation.

laceration (las-er-AY-shun)
a cut.

Punctures

When a sharp, pointed object passes through the skin or other tissue, a *puncture wound* has occurred. Typically, puncture wounds are caused by objects such as nails, ice picks, splinters, or knives (Figure 28-7). Often, there is no severe external bleeding, although internal bleeding may be profuse. The threat of contamination must always be seriously considered.

puncture wound
an open wound that tears through the skin and destroys underlying tissues. A *penetrating puncture wound* can be shallow or deep. A *perforating puncture wound* has both an entrance and an exit wound.

FIGURE 28-6 (A) Some lacerations have smooth edges, and (B) some have jagged edges.
(Photo A: © Edward T. Dickinson, MD; Photo B: © Dr. Paula Moynahan, Moynahan Medical Center)

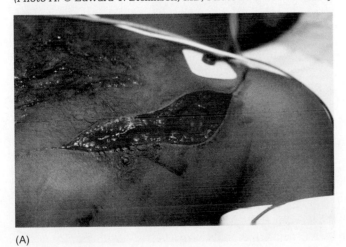

(A)

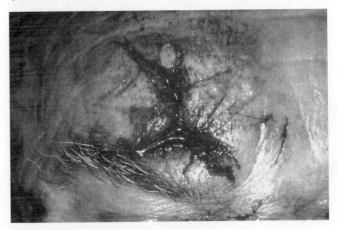

(B)

FIGURE 28-7 (A) The knife penetrating this patient's back constitutes a serious puncture wound. (B) An X-ray of the same wound. *(Photos A and B: © Edward T. Dickinson, MD)*

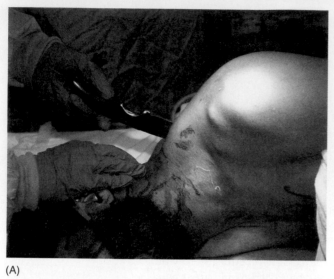
(A)

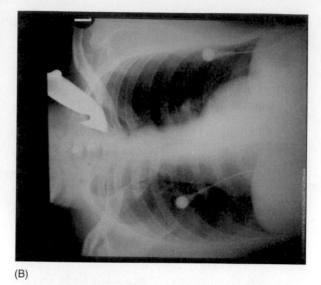
(B)

A puncture wound can be shallow or deep. In either case, tissues and blood vessels are injured. If the object causing the injury passes through the body and out again, the exit wound may be more serious than the entrance wound, as in a gunshot wound.

Avulsions

avulsion (ah-VUL-shun)
the tearing away or tearing off of a piece or flap of skin or other soft tissue. This term also may be used for an eye pulled from its socket or a tooth dislodged from its socket.

In an ***avulsion***, flaps of skin and tissues are torn loose or pulled off completely. When the tip of the nose is cut or torn off, this is an example of an avulsion. The same applies to the external ear (Figure 28-8A). A degloving avulsion occurs when the hand is caught in a roller. In this type of incident, the skin is stripped off like a glove (Figure 28-8B). An eye pulled from its socket (extruded) is also a form of avulsion. The term *avulsed* is used in reporting the wound, as in "an avulsed eye" or "an avulsed ear." When tissue is avulsed, it is cut off from its oxygen supply and will soon die.

Amputations

amputation (am-pyu-TAY-shun)
the surgical removal or traumatic severing of a body part, usually an extremity.

The extremities are sometimes subject to ***amputation***. Amputated fingers, toes, hands, feet, or limbs are completely cut through or torn off (Figure 28-9). Jagged skin and bone edges can sometimes be observed. There may be massive bleeding; or the force that amputates a

FIGURE 28-8 (A) An avulsion of the ear lobe. (B) An avulsion injury that caused a degloving.
(Photos A and B: © Edward T. Dickinson, MD)

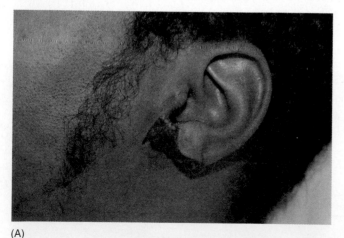
(A)

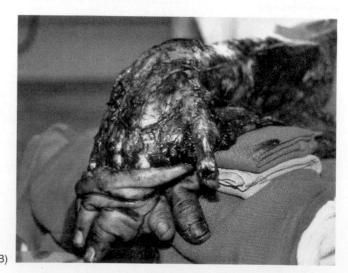
(B)

FIGURE 28-9 (A) Amputated leg. (B) Hand with thumb amputated. *(Photos A and B: © Edward T. Dickinson, MD)*

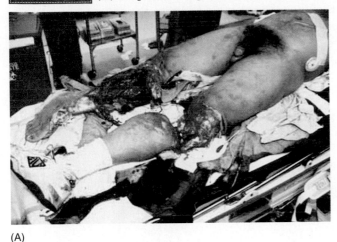

(A)

(B)

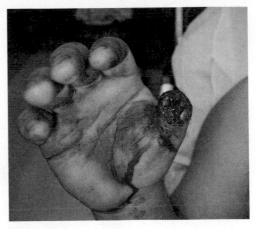

limb may close off torn blood vessels, limiting the amount of bleeding. Often, blood vessels collapse, or they retract and constrict, which limits bleeding from the wound site.

Open Crush Injuries

Although crush injuries were discussed earlier in this chapter as closed wounds, crush injuries also can be open wounds. An open crush injury can result when an extremity is caught between heavy items, such as pieces of machinery. Blood vessels, nerves, and muscles are involved, and swelling may be a major problem with resulting loss of blood supply distally. Bones are fractured and may protrude through the wound site. Soft tissues and internal organs can be crushed to produce profuse bleeding, both externally and internally (Figure 28-10).

Blast Injuries

When a patient is injured from a blast or explosion, he may sustain a combination of all of the injuries just described. The unusual characteristics of a blast mean that a mixture of open and closed injuries can be the result (Figure 28-11). Primary injuries occur because of the intense high pressure (pressure wave) that hits the patient. Injuries can include damage to any air- or fluid-filled body organ or cavity, especially pressure injury to the lungs. Secondary injury is the result of projectiles such as debris hitting the patient (blast wave), leading to open wounds such as shrapnel wounds. Tertiary (third level) injuries occur if the patient is picked up and moved to a different location. Tertiary injuries can include not just soft-tissue injuries but also fractures, avulsions, and amputations. Finally, the patient may sustain additional

"Don't get distracted by wounds that are obvious and gross and miss the big things—the things (like airway or breathing problems or shock) that can kill your patient."

FIGURE 28-10 An open crush injury.
(© Edward T. Dickinson, MD)

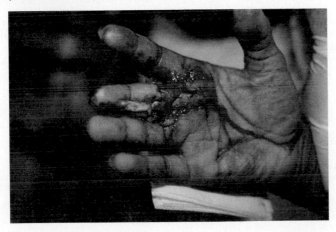

FIGURE 28-11 Blasts can cause injury with the initial blast, when the patient is struck by debris, or when the patient is thrown by the blast. In addition, the patient may sustain additional injuries such as from exposure to chemicals or toxins or be injured by structural collapse.

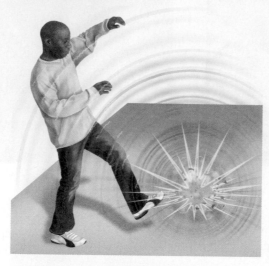

(A) Pressure Wave/Primary Injury
Air molecules slam into one another, creating a pressure wave moving outward from the blast center, causing pressure injuries.

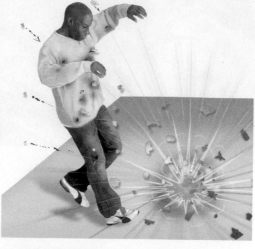

(B) Blast Wave/Secondary Injury
Instantaneous combustion of the explosive agent creates superheated gases. The resulting pressure blows the bomb casing apart. Pieces of the bomb projectiles that cause injuries by impacting the patient.

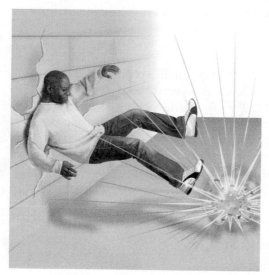

(C) Patient Displacement/Tertiary Injury
The blast wind may propel the patient to the ground or against objects, causing further injuries.

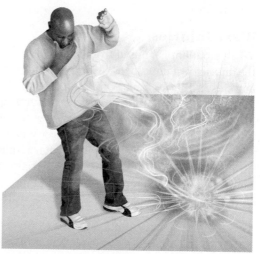

(D) Patient Exposed to Hazardous Material or Structural Collapse/Quaternary Injury
The patient may also be exposed to harmful chemicals or toxins or may be injured by structural collapse.

injuries such as exposure to chemicals or toxins, burns, and crush injuries. These are sometimes referred to as quaternary (fourth level) injuries.

High Pressure Injection Injuries

An uncommon but important injury can occur when a patient is working with a machine that injects grease, paint, air, or some other substance under high pressure. If the nozzle injects the substance into the patient, typically the finger, rather than the object it was intended for, this can lead to significant injury. These machines may use pressures of thousands of pounds per square inch, which results in a wound that is much worse than it looks. There is typically very little (or even no) injury apparent on inspection. The real damage is not visible because it is under the skin. When the high pressure device injects its solution, it can travel a significant distance; for example, moving through most or all of a limb. The injected solution causes extensive tissue damage, both from the force of the pressure and from the toxic nature of some solutions. Over the course of the next few hours, tissue begins to die. If the patient does not get the appropriate treatment early enough, there is a high probability that at least part, and perhaps all, of the patient's limb will have to be amputated.

EMT treatment for high pressure injection includes elevating and splinting the limb. Although the patient may complain of severe pain, do *not* apply cold. This causes vasoconstriction and can lead to further tissue damage and death from lack of perfusion. If the incident occurred just before your arrival, the patient may not have any pain and may not wish to go to an emergency department. It is nonetheless vital that you persuade the patient to be evaluated in an ED as soon as possible. If the patient delays treatment, he may end up losing his hand or forearm.

Emergency Care for Open Wounds

Open wounds require strict attention to Standard Precautions. In addition to wearing gloves, a gown and protective eyewear may also be required. Remember to properly dispose of all soiled materials and wash your hands after each call.

PATIENT ASSESSMENT

Open Wounds

Airway, breathing, circulation, and severe bleeding are identified and treated in the primary assessment. Once the primary assessment and the appropriate physical examination have been completed, care for the individual wounds begins.

Decision Point

- Does this injury affect my patient's airway, breathing, or circulation?

PATIENT CARE

Open Wounds

The following steps are general guidelines for emergency care of open wounds. Steps for specific kinds of open wounds appear on the following pages. Be sure to take appropriate Standard Precautions when performing these steps.

1. Expose the wound. Clothing that covers a soft-tissue injury must be lifted, cut, or split away. For some articles of clothing, this is best done with scissors or a seam cutter. Do not attempt to remove clothing in the usual manner, which can aggravate existing injuries and cause additional damage and pain.
2. Clean the wound surface. Do not try to pick embedded particles and debris from the wound. Simply remove large pieces of foreign matter from the surface. When possible, use a piece of sterile dressing to brush away large debris while protecting the wound from contact with your soiled gloves. Do not spend much time cleaning the wound. Control of bleeding is the priority.
3. Control bleeding. Start with direct pressure, or direct pressure and elevation. When necessary, apply a tourniquet (see Chapter 27, "Bleeding and Shock").
4. For all serious wounds, provide care for shock, including administration of high-concentration oxygen (see Chapter 27, "Bleeding and Shock").
5. Prevent further contamination. Use a sterile dressing. When none is available, use the cleanest cloth material at the scene.
6. Bandage the dressing in place after you have controlled the bleeding. If an extremity is involved, check for a distal pulse to make certain that circulation has not been interrupted by the application of a tight bandage. With the exception of a pressure dressing, bleeding must be controlled before bandaging is started. Periodically recheck the bandage to make certain that bleeding has not restarted.

7. Keep the patient lying still. Any movement will increase circulation and could restart bleeding.
8. Reassure the patient. This will help ease the patient's emotional response and perhaps lower his pulse rate and blood pressure. In some cases, this may help to reduce the bleeding rate. Also, a patient who feels reassured will usually be more willing to lie still, reducing the chances of restarting bleeding.

TREATING SPECIFIC TYPES OF OPEN WOUNDS

Treating Abrasions and Lacerations

In treating abrasions, take care to reduce wound contamination. Although bleeding from a long, deep laceration may be difficult to control, direct pressure over a dressing usually works well. The air-inflated splint can be useful in the management of this type of wound when it is applied over a dressing. Do not pull apart the edges of a laceration in an effort to see into the wound.

Most lacerations can be cared for by bandaging a dressing in place. Some EMS systems recommend using special wound-closure strips for minor lacerations. (A butterfly bandage is made up of thin strips of adhesive bandaging and is designed to bring the sides of a laceration together.) Bandage a gauze dressing over the butterfly strip.

NOTE: *Do not underestimate the effects of a laceration. When evaluating a laceration, check the pulse, as well as motor and sensory function, distal to the injury. The patient may need stitches, plastic surgery, antibiotics, or a tetanus shot at the hospital, so do not put on bandages and leave the patient at the scene. Serious infection or scarring could result.*

Treating Puncture Wounds

Use caution when caring for puncture wounds. An object that appears to be embedded only in the skin may actually go all the way to the bone. In such cases, it is possible that the patient may not have any serious pain. Even an apparently moderate puncture wound may cause extensive internal injury with serious internal bleeding. What appears at first to be a simple, shallow puncture wound may be only part of the problem. There also could be a severe exit wound that requires immediate care, so be sure to search for one.

Gunshot wounds are puncture wounds that can fracture bones and cause extensive soft-tissue and organ injury. The seriousness of the wound cannot be determined by the caliber of the bullet or the point of entry and exit. The bullet may have tumbled through tissues, deflected off a bone, fragmented, or exploded inside the body (Figure 28-12A, 28-12B, and 28-12C). All bullet wounds are considered serious. If the bullet has penetrated the body, you must assume that there is considerable internal injury. Close-range shootings often have burns around the entry wound (Figure 28-12D). Remember that any gunshot wound to the face, no matter how minor, can create airway problems. Air guns fired at close range can cause serious damage by injecting air into the tissues.

All stab wounds should be considered serious, especially when they involve the head, neck, chest, abdomen, groin, or are inflicted proximal to the knee or elbow.

Care for a patient with a moderate or serious puncture wound includes these steps:

1. Reassure the alert patient. Such wounds can be frightening.
2. Search for an exit wound, especially when there is a gunshot wound. Control bleeding and provide adequate wound treatment to both the entry and exit wounds.
3. Assess the need for basic life support whenever there is a gunshot wound. Care for shock, administering high-concentration oxygen.
4. Follow your local protocols with regard to immobilizing the spine when the patient's head, neck, or torso is involved. Many EMS systems have included this step in their protocols, but the wisdom of doing so is in question. There is some evidence to suggest that immobilizing a patient with a penetrating injury may extend prehospital time and lead

FIGURE 28-12 (A)Bullets travel in an unpredictable path once they are inside the patient's body and can therefore cause damage to multiple organs and bones. (B) A gunshot wound to the right flank. (C) X-ray of the same wound showing tumbling of the bullet within the body. (D) A close-range gunshot with burns around the entry wound. *(Photos B, C, and D: © Edward T. Dickinson, MD)*

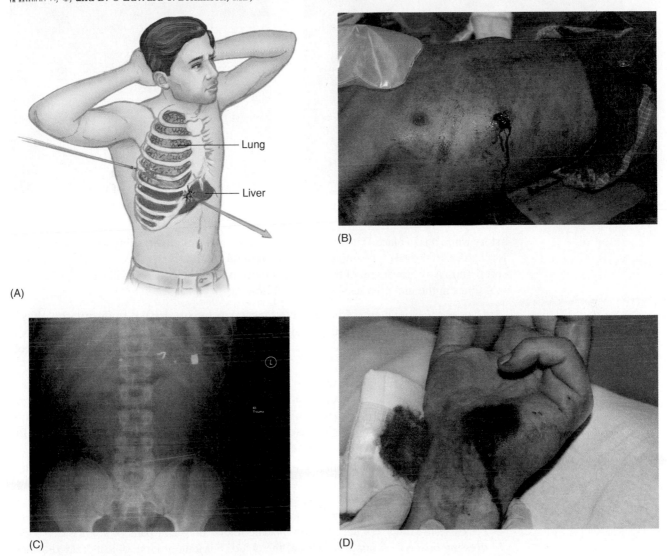

(A)

Lung

Liver

(B)

(C)

(D)

to worse outcomes for patients, yet there is disagreement in the trauma community about how to treat these patients. Again, follow your local protocols.

5. Transport the patient. If the object that caused the puncture wound is available, and if the scene of the emergency is not a crime scene, take the object to the emergency department for examination as well.

Treating Impaled Objects

A puncture wound may contain an impaled object. The object may be a knife, a fence post or guard rail, a shard of glass, or even a wooden stick—or part of any of these that has broken off in the wound (Figure 28-13), piercing any part of the body. Even though it is rare, you may be confronted with an impaled object that is long enough to make transport impossible unless the object is shortened. In such cases, contact the emergency department physician for specific directions. Usually, someone must hold the object, keeping it very stable, while you gently cut through it at the desired length. A fine-toothed saw with rigid blade support (e.g., a hack saw or reciprocating saw) should be used. In some cases, you may need to leave the object in place as found. The challenge in these cases is stabilization of the object.

In general, when caring for a patient with a puncture wound involving an impaled object, *do not remove the impaled object.* The object may be plugging bleeding from a major

FIGURE 28-13 (A) Part of a knife impaled in a wound near the clavicle. (B) X-ray of the same impaled knife fragment. *(Photos A and B: © Edward T. Dickinson, MD)*

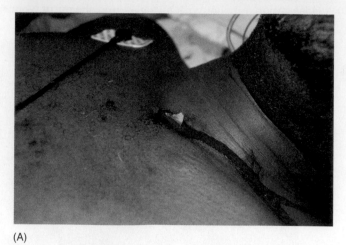

(A)

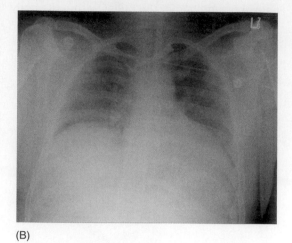

(B)

artery while it is in place. If you remove it, you may cause severe bleeding when the pressure is released. Removal of the object also may cause further injury to nerves, muscles, and other soft tissues. Any movement of the impaled object at the skin's surface will be magnified several times in the inner tissues. Proceed as follows:

1. Expose the wound area. Cut away clothing, taking great care not to disturb the object. Do not attempt to lift clothing over the object, as you may accidentally move it. Long impaled objects may have to be stabilized by hand during exposure, bleeding control, and dressing.

2. Control profuse bleeding by direct pressure, if possible. Be careful to position your gloved hands on either side of the object and exert pressure downward. *Do not put pressure on the object.* Apply pressure with great care if the object has a cutting edge, such as a knife or a shard of glass; otherwise, you may cause additional injury to the patient. Be careful not to injure your hands or damage your gloves.

3. While you continue to stabilize the object and control bleeding, have another trained rescuer place several layers of bulky dressing around the injury site so that the dressings surround the object on all sides (Figure 28-14). Manual stabilization must continue until the stabilizing dressings are secured in place.

   Have the other rescuer begin by placing folded universal pads or some other bulky dressing material on opposite sides of the object. For long or large objects, folded towels, blankets, or pillows may have to be used in place of dressing pads. Remove your hands from under the pads. Place them on top and apply pressure as each layer is placed in position. The next layer of pads should be placed on opposite sides of the object, perpendicular to the first layer. Continue this process until as much of the object as possible has been stabilized.

FIGURE 28-14 Stabilize an impaled object with a bulky dressing.

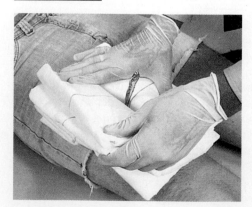

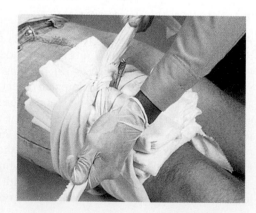

Once bandaged in place, the dressings will stabilize the object and exert downward pressure on bleeding vessels. Keep in mind that there is a limited amount of time that can be given to stabilizing an impaled object. Stay in contact with the Medical Director for directions and recommendations.

4. Secure the dressings in place. Although adhesive strips may hold the dressings in place, blood around the wound site, sweat, and body movements may not allow you to use tape. Triangular bandages folded into strips (cravats) can be applied by tying one above and one below the impaled object. The cravats should be wide (no less than 4 inches in width once folded). A thin rigid splint can be used to push the cravats under the patient's back when they are needed to care for objects impaled in the trunk of the body.

5. Care for shock. Provide oxygen at the highest possible flow and concentration. When appropriate, oxygen administration and heat conservation measures should be accomplished as soon as possible. When working by yourself, these may have to be delayed while you attempt to control bleeding.

6. Keep the patient at rest. Position the patient for minimum stress. If possible, immobilize the affected area—for example, with a splint or a spine board. Provide emotional support.

7. Transport the patient carefully and as soon as possible. Avoid any movement that may jar, loosen, or dislodge the object. If the object was removed by bystanders before you arrived, bring it to the hospital for examination.

8. Reassure the patient throughout all aspects of care. An alert patient who is afflicted with an impaled object is usually very frightened.

Object Impaled in the Cheek

A dangerous situation exists when the cheek has been penetrated by a foreign object. First, the object may go into the oral cavity and create an airway obstruction, or it may stay impaled in the cheek wall but work its way free and enter the oral cavity later. Second, when the cheek wall is perforated, bleeding into the mouth and throat can be profuse and interfere with breathing, or it may make the patient nauseated and induce vomiting. External wound care will not stop the flow of blood into the mouth.

If you find a patient with an object impaled in the cheek, you should (Figure 28-15):

1. Examine the wound site. Gently inspect both the external cheek and the inside of the mouth. Use your penlight and look into the patient's mouth. If need be, carefully use your gloved fingers to probe the inside cheek to determine if the object has passed through the cheek wall. This is best done with a dressing pad used to protect your fingers and any wound you touch.

2. Remove the object, *if* you find perforation and *you can see both ends* of the object. Pull it out in the direction that it entered the cheek. If this cannot be easily done, leave the object

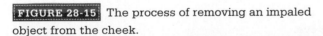 **FIGURE 28-15** The process of removing an impaled object from the cheek.

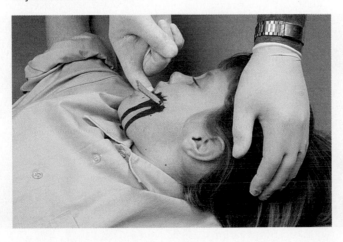

in place. Do not twist the object. *If you find perforation but the tip of the object is also impaled into a deeper structure* (e.g., the palate), *stabilize the object*. Do not try to remove it.

3. Position the patient. Make certain that you allow for drainage (the possibility of spine injuries may require you to immobilize the head, neck, and spine first, then tilt the patient and the spine board as a unit).

4. Monitor the patient's airway, once the object is removed or stabilized. *Be prepared to suction as necessary.* Keep in mind that an object penetrating the cheek wall also may have caused teeth or dentures to break, creating potential airway obstruction. Pay close attention, especially if the patient is not alert. Blood in the patient's mouth can compromise the airway.

5. Dress the outside of the wound using a pressure dressing and bandage or apply a sterile dressing and use direct hand pressure to control the bleeding. You may be able to place gauze on the inside of the cheek to help control bleeding into the mouth, but only if the patient is alert and cooperative. Monitor the patient's mental status closely, and make sure the dressing does not work its way into the airway.

6. Provide oxygen and care for shock. You may have to use a nasal cannula if constant suctioning is required. If any dressing materials are placed in the patient's mouth, use of standard face masks can be dangerous unless you leave 3 to 4 inches of the dressing outside of the patient's mouth.

Puncture Wound or Object Impaled in the Eye

Use loose dressings for a puncture wound to the eye with no impaled object. If you find an object impaled in the eye, you should (Figure 28-16):

1. Stabilize the object. Place a roll of 3-inch gauze bandage or folded 4 × 4s on either side of the object, along the vertical axis of the head, in a manner that will stabilize the object.

2. Apply rigid protection. Fit a disposable paper drinking cup or paper cone over the impaled object and allow it to come to rest on the dressing rolls. Do not allow it to touch the object. Do not use a Styrofoam cup, which can flake.

3. Have another rescuer stabilize the dressings and cup while you secure them in place with a self-adherent roller bandage or with a wrapping of gauze. Do not secure the bandage on top of the cup.

4. Dress and bandage the uninjured eye. This will help to reduce sympathetic eye movements.

5. Provide oxygen and care for shock.

6. Reassure the patient and provide emotional support.

This method can also be used as a pressure dressing to control bleeding in the area of the eye.

FIGURE 28-16 Managing an object impaled in the eye.

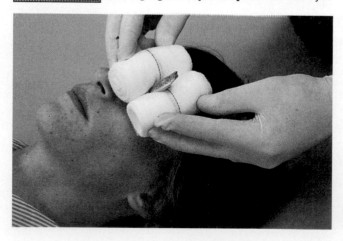
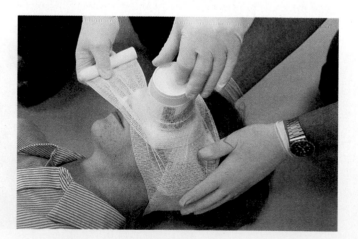

NOTE: *In some EMS systems, step 4 is not part of the recommended treatment for an injured eye. Covering both eyes often makes a patient anxious. Furthermore, covering the uninjured eye seems to make little, if any, difference in patient outcome. However, you should follow your local protocols.*

An alternative to the previous method calls for the rescuer to make a thick dressing with several layers of sterile gauze pads or universal dressings. A hole approximately the size of the impaled object is cut in the center of this pad. The rescuer then carefully passes this dressing over the impaled object and positions the pad so that the impaled object is centered in the opening. The rest of the procedure remains the same as previously described. If your EMS system instructs you to use this technique, remember that you must take great care not to touch the object as the dressing is set in place.

Treating Avulsions

Emergency care for avulsions requires the application of large, bulky pressure dressings. In addition, you should make every effort to preserve any avulsed parts and transport them to the medical facility along with the patient. It may be possible to surgically restore the part or to use it for skin grafts.

In cases in which flaps of skin have been torn loose but not off, follow these steps:

1. Clean the wound surface.
2. Fold the skin back to its normal position as gently as possible.
3. Control bleeding and dress the wound using bulky pressure dressings.

If skin or another body part is torn from the body, control bleeding and dress the wound using a bulky pressure dressing. Save the avulsed part and wrap it in a sterile dressing kept moist with sterile saline. Make certain that you label the avulsed part with what it is, the patient's name and date, and the time the part was wrapped and bagged. Your records should show the approximate time of the avulsion. Be sure to keep the part as cool as possible, without freezing it, by placing it in a cooler or any other available container so that it is on top of a cold pack or a *sealed* bag of ice. Do not use dry ice. Do not immerse the avulsed part in ice, cooled water, or saline. Label the container the same as the label used for the saved part.

NOTE: *The care of avulsed tissues is directed by local protocols, which are often written to match the reimplantation procedures of the hospitals in your EMS system. Some EMS systems prefer that the dressing used to wrap the avulsed part be moistened with sterile normal saline (sterile distilled water is not recommended). This saline must be from a fresh sterile source. Keep in mind that once a sterile source of saline has been opened, it is no longer considered sterile. Take great care if you use this method, since the saline may carry microorganisms from your gloved hand through the dressing to the avulsed part. During your care, remember that avulsions appear grotesque and will be frightening to your patient. Provide reassurance to your patient throughout the call.*

Treating Amputations

Never complete an amputation. As in other external bleeding situations, the most effective method to control bleeding is a snug pressure dressing.

1. Apply the pressure dressing. Place it over the stump.
2. Use pressure points to control bleeding. A tourniquet should not be applied unless other methods used to control bleeding have failed.
3. Care for the amputated part (Figure 28-17). When possible, wrap it in a sterile dressing and secure the dressing with a self-adhesive gauze bandage. Wrap or bag the amputated part in a plastic bag and keep cool by cold packs. Do not immerse the amputated part directly in water or saline. In addition, do not let the part come in direct contact with ice or it may freeze.

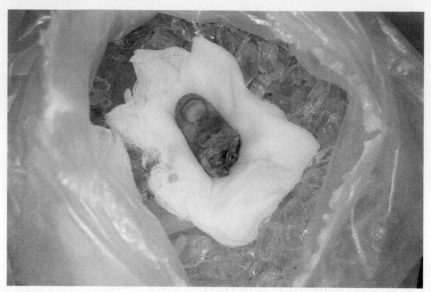

FIGURE 28-17 Care for an amputated part. The amputated digit sits upon sterile saline soaked gauze, awaiting replantation. *(© Edward T. Dickinson, MD)*
NOTE: This is the thumb that was amputated from the hand shown in Figure 28-9B.

Treating Genital Injuries

Injuries to the genitals are not very common, but they often bleed heavily and cause significant anxiety in patients. The genitals are very vascular (contain lots of blood vessels), so when they are injured they bleed heavily. Because they are also part of the reproductive system, injuries in this area can affect a patient's ability to have children. Males tend to sustain trauma to the genitals more frequently than females because of the less-protected position of male genitalia, but anyone can sustain a genital injury.

Specific injuries that occur to the genitals are:

- Lacerations, contusions, and abrasions, which can result from either blunt or penetrating trauma (Figure 28-18A).

- Avulsions, including a degloving injury of the penis (Figure 28-18B), in which the skin and tissue are pulled off and torn in the same way as a degloving injury to the hand, as described earlier.

- Blunt trauma, including straddle injuries in which the patient injures the perineum by landing heavily on a narrow structure.

- Zipper injuries, which are especially common in uncircumcised boys. The foreskin may get caught in the zipper of the patient's pants.

- Foreign bodies and impaled objects in the vagina or penis.

- Blood at the meatus (Figure 28-18C), which is often an indication of a disruption of the urethra. In patients who have sustained blunt trauma, the cause of the urethral injury may be a fracture of the pelvis, which will be further discussed in Chapter 30, "Musculoskeletal Trauma."

Care for a patient with a genital injury includes these steps:

1. Control bleeding as you would for other soft-tissue injuries.
2. Preserve any avulsed parts as described in your local protocols.
3. Consider whether the injury you see suggests another, possibly more serious, injury (e.g., blood at the meatus suggesting pelvic trauma).
4. Display a calm, professional manner to maintain the patient's dignity. Although treatment is usually the same as for other soft-tissue injuries, the modest patient may need more reassurance.

FIGURE 28-18 Genital trauma can present in various ways. (A) Gunshot wound to the scrotum. (B) Avulsion of the penis. (C) Blood at the meatus, indicating disruption of the urethra that is likely associated with pelvic trauma.
(Photos A and C: © Edward T. Dickinson, MD; Photo D: © Dr. Paula Moynahan, Moynahan Medical Center)

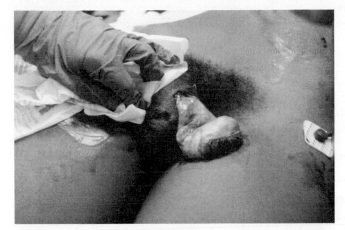

(A)

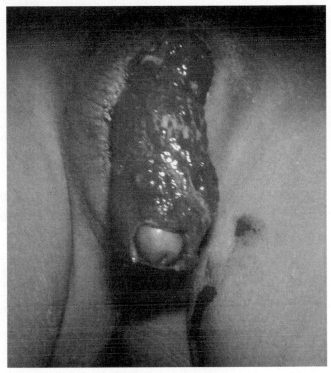

(C)

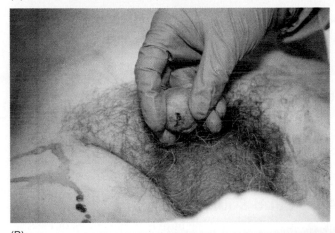

(B)

5. If the patient is a child or other possibly vulnerable person, inquire in a nonthreatening way whether sexual abuse was involved.

6. Dress and bandage the wound in accordance with the principles of bandaging (covered later in this chapter).

BURNS

Most people think of burns as injuries to the skin, but burns can affect much more. Burn injuries often involve structures below the skin, including muscles, bones, nerves, and blood vessels. Burns can injure the eyes beyond repair. Respiratory system structures can be damaged, producing airway obstruction due to tissue swelling, and even cause respiratory failure and respiratory arrest. In addition to the physical damage caused by burns, patients often suffer emotional and psychological problems that begin at the emergency scene and may last a lifetime.

When caring for a burn patient, always think beyond the burn. For example, a medical emergency or accident may have led to the burn. The patient may have had a heart attack while smoking a cigarette and the unattended cigarette caused a fire. During the patient assessment, you should detect the heart problem even though the burn may be the most obvious injury. Conversely, a fire or burn may cause or aggravate another injury or medical condition. For example, someone trying to escape a fire may fall and suffer spinal damage and fractures. As an EMT, you should not only detect the burn but detect the spinal damage and fractures as well.

CORE CONCEPT

Understanding burns and emergency care for burns

Burns

When your patient has been burned, patient assessment involves classifying, then evaluating, the burns. Burns can be classified and evaluated in three ways:

- By agent and source
- By depth
- By severity

All three are important in deciding the urgency and the kind of emergency care the burn requires. These classifications are discussed in detail in the following text.

NOTE: *Patient assessment should not be neglected in order to begin immediate burn care.*

Table 28-2 Agents and Sources of Burns	
AGENTS	**SOURCES**
Thermal	Flame; radiation; excessive heat from fire, steam, hot liquids, and hot objects
Chemicals	Various acids, bases, and caustics
Electricity	Alternating current, direct current, and lightning
Light (typically involving the eyes)	Intense light sources; ultraviolet light can also be considered a source of radiation burns
Radiation	Usually from nuclear sources; ultraviolet light can also be considered a source of radiation burns

Classifying Burns by Agent and Source

Burns can be classified according to the agent causing the burn (e.g., chemicals or electricity). Noting the source of the burn (e.g., dry lime or alternating current) can make the classification more specific. You should report the agent and also, when practical, the source of the agent (Table 28-2). For example, a burn can be reported as "chemical burns from contact with dry lime."

Never assume the agent or source of the burn. What may appear to be a thermal burn could in fact be caused by radiation. You may find minor thermal burns on the patient's face and forget to consider light burns to the eyes. Always gather information from your observations of the scene, bystanders' reports, and the patient interview.

Classifying Burns by Depth

Burns involving the skin are classified as superficial, partial thickness, and full thickness burns (Figure 28-19). These classifications are also sometimes called first-degree, second-degree, and third-degree burns, with first-degree burns corresponding to superficial burns, and so on, as described next.

- A ***superficial burn*** (Figure 28-20) involves only the epidermis (the outer layer of the skin). It is characterized by reddening of the skin and perhaps some swelling. An example is a sunburn. The patient will usually complain about pain (sometimes severe) at the site. The burn will heal of its own accord, without scarring. Superficial burns are also called first-degree burns.

- In a ***partial thickness burn*** (Figure 28-21), the epidermis is burned through and the dermis (the second layer of the skin) is damaged, but the burn does not pass through to underlying tissues. There will be deep intense pain, noticeable reddening, blisters, and a mottled (spotted) appearance to the skin. Burns of this type cause swelling and blistering for 48 hours after the injury, as plasma and tissue fluids are released and rise to the

superficial burn
a burn that involves only the epidermis, the outer layer of the skin. It is characterized by reddening of the skin and perhaps some swelling. A common example is a sunburn. Also called a first-degree burn.

partial thickness burn
a burn in which the epidermis (first layer of skin) is burned through and the dermis (second layer) is damaged. Burns of this type cause reddening, blistering, and a mottled appearance. Also called a *second-degree burn*.

FIGURE 28-19 Burns are classified by depth.

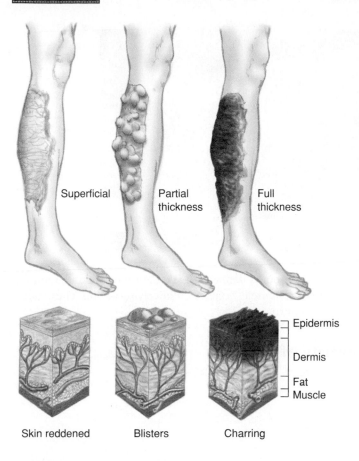

Superficial   Partial   Full
thickness   thickness

Epidermis

Dermis

Fat
Muscle

Skin reddened   Blisters   Charring

FIGURE 28-20 A superficial burn.
(Charles Stewart, MD, and Associates)

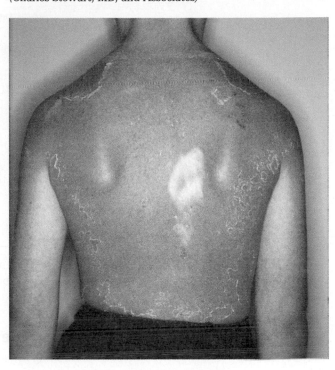

FIGURE 28-21 (A and B) Partial thickness burns.
(Photos A and B: © Edward T. Dickinson, MD)

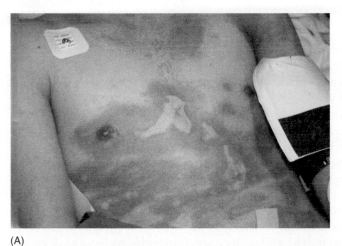

(A)

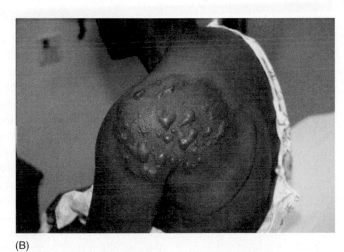

(B)

top layer of skin. When treated with reasonable care, partial thickness burns will heal themselves, producing very little or no scarring. Partial thickness burns are also called second-degree burns.

- In a ***full thickness burn*** (Figure 28-22), all the layers of the skin are damaged. Some full thickness burns are difficult to tell apart from partial thickness burns; however, there are usually areas that are charred black or brown or areas that are dry and white. The patient may complain of severe pain or, if enough nerves have been damaged, he may not feel any pain at all (except at the periphery of the burn where adjoining partial thickness burns may be causing pain). This type of burn may require skin grafting. As these burns

full thickness burn
a burn in which all the layers of the skin are damaged. There are usually areas that are charred black or areas that are dry and white. Also called a *third-degree burn*.

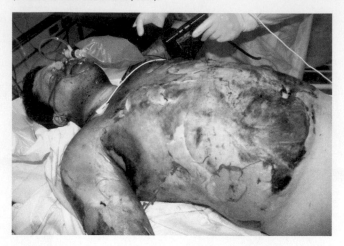

FIGURE 28-22 A full thickness burn.
(© Edward T. Dickinson, MD)

heal, dense scars form. Full thickness burns damage all layers of the skin and additionally may damage subcutaneous tissue, muscle, bone, and underlying organs. These burns are sometimes called third-degree burns.

Determining the Severity of Burns

When determining the severity of a burn, consider the following factors:

- Agent or source of the burn
- Body regions burned
- Depth of the burn
- Extent of the burn
- Age of the patient
- Other illnesses and injuries

The agent or source of the burn can be significant in terms of patient assessment. A burn caused by electrical current may cause only small areas of skin injury but pose a great risk of severe internal injuries. Chemical burns are of special concern since the chemical may remain on the skin and continue to burn for hours or even days, eventually entering the bloodstream. This is sometimes the case with certain alkaline chemicals.

When you are considering the body regions burned, keep in mind that any burn to the face is of special concern since it may involve injury to the airway or the eyes (Figure 28-23). The hands and feet also are areas of concern because scarring may cause loss of movement of fingers or toes. Special care is required to avoid aggravation to these injury sites when moving the patient and to prevent the damaged tissues from sticking to one another. When the groin, genitalia, buttocks, or medial thighs are burned, potential bacterial contamination can be far more serious than the initial damage to the tissues. Note that circumferential burns (burns that encircle the body or a body part) can be very serious because they constrict the skin. When they occur to an extremity, they can interrupt circulation to the distal tissues. When they occur around the chest, they can restrict breathing by limiting chest wall movement. In addition, the burn healing process can be very complicated. This is particularly true when circumferential burns occur to joints, the chest, and the abdomen where the encircling scarring tends to limit normal functions.

The depth of the burn is important to determine its severity. In partial thickness and full thickness burns, the outer layer of the skin is penetrated. This can lead to contamination of exposed tissues and the invasion of harmful chemicals and microorganisms into the circulatory system.

You also will need to roughly estimate the extent of the burn area. The amount of skin surface involved can be calculated quickly by using the ***rule of nines*** (Figure 28-24). For an adult, each of the following areas represents 9 percent of the body surface: head and neck,

rule of nines
a method for estimating the extent of a burn. For an adult, each of the following areas represents 9 percent of the body surface: the head and neck, each upper extremity, the chest, the abdomen, the upper back, the lower back and buttocks, the front of each lower extremity, and the back of each lower extremity. The remaining 1 percent is assigned to the genital region. For an infant or child, the percentages are modified so that 18 percent is assigned to the head, 14 percent to each lower extremity.

FIGURE 28-23 A singed face signals danger of airway burns or burns to
the eyes. (© *Edward T. Dickinson, MD*)

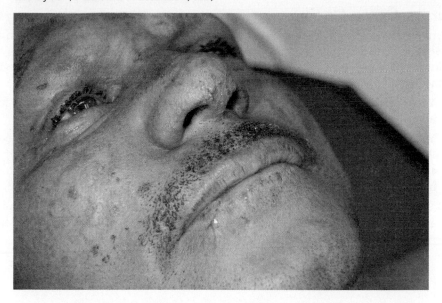

each upper extremity, chest, abdomen, upper back, lower back and buttocks, the front of
each lower extremity, and the back of each lower extremity. These make up 99 percent of the
body's surface. The remaining 1 percent is assigned to the genital region.

In the rule of nines, the percentages are modified for infants and young children, whose
heads are much larger in relationship to the rest of the body. An infant's or young child's
head and neck are counted as 18 percent; each upper extremity as 9 percent; chest and abdomen as 18 percent; the entire back as 18 percent; each lower extremity as 14 percent; and
the genital region as 1 percent. (This adds up to 101 percent, but it is only used to give a
rough determination. Some systems count each lower limb as 13.5 percent to achieve an
even 100 percent.)

An alternative way to estimate the extent of a burn is the ***rule of palm***, which uses the
patient's own hand to approximate the surface area. The rule of palm can be applied to any
patient—infant, child, or adult. Since the palm of the hand equals about 1 percent of the
body's surface area, mentally compare the patient's palm with the size of the burn to estimate its extent. (For example, a burn the size of five palms = 5 percent of the body.) The rule

rule of palm
a method for estimating the extent of
a burn. The palm of the patient's own
hand, which equals about 1 percent of
the body's surface area, is compared
with the patient's burn to estimate its
size.

FIGURE 28-24 Rule of nines.

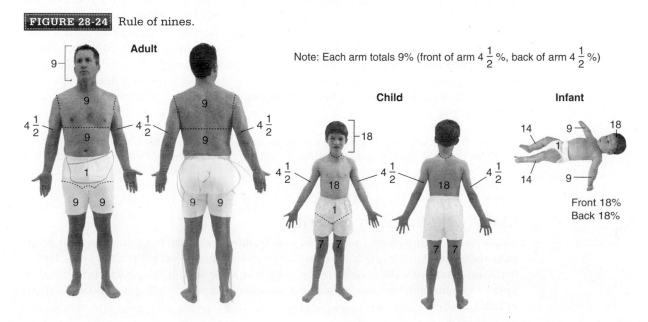

Note: Each arm totals 9% (front of arm $4\frac{1}{2}$ %, back of arm $4\frac{1}{2}$ %)

Adult

Child

Infant

Front 18%
Back 18%

CRITICAL DECISION MAKING

Burns—by the Numbers

Burns are a type of soft-tissue injury. Decisions about burn care and transportation are often determined by an approximation of body surface area affected. For each of the following patients, determine the approximate body surface area burned and the degree of the burn.

1. Your patient fell asleep by the pool and was sunburned over the backs of both legs, his back, and the backs of both arms. The skin is bright red.

2. Your patient works at a fast food restaurant. She was by the fryer when someone threw in an ice cube as a joke to scare her. Hot grease splashed up and covered the anterior portion of her left forearm and her entire right hand. The skin is red and blistered.

3. Your patient fell asleep while smoking. He has circumferential burns on both legs and has burned the entire right arm. The legs are red and blistered. The patient's right arm is severely charred and peeling.

---

of palm may be easier to apply to smaller or localized burns, whereas the rule of nines may be easier for larger or more widespread burns.

The patient's age is a major factor in considering the severity of burns. Infants, children under age 5, and adults over age 55, because of their anatomy and physiology, have the most severe responses to burns and the greatest risk of death. They also have different healing patterns than other age groups.

GERIATRIC NOTE

Burn intensity and body-area involvement that would be minor to moderate in a young adult could be fatal for an aged person. In late adulthood, the body's ability to cope with injury is reduced by aging tissues and failing body systems. The ability of tissues to heal from any injury is lessened and the time of healing is increased.

When determining the severity of a burn, you also must consider the other illnesses and injuries a patient may have. Obviously, a patient with an existing respiratory illness will be especially vulnerable to exposure to heated air or chemical vapors. Likewise, the stress of a fire or other environmental emergency will be of particular concern for patients with heart disease. Patients with respiratory ailments, heart disease, or diabetes will react more severely to burn damage. What may be a minor burn for a healthy adult could be of major significance to a patient with a pre-existing medical condition. Similarly, the stress of a burn added to other injuries sustained during the emergency may lead to shock or other life-threatening problems that would not have resulted from the nonburn injuries or the burn alone.

NOTE: *All burns are to be treated as more serious if accompanied by other injuries or medical problems. If you discover that the patient has a decreased blood pressure, always assume that he has other serious injuries. Attempt to determine the patient's problem through standard assessment techniques.*

Classifying Burns by Severity

The severity of burns must be classified to determine the order and type of care, to determine the order of transport, and to provide maximum information to the emergency department. In some cases, the severity of the burn may determine if the patient is to be taken directly to a hospital with special burn-care facilities. For most adults, use the classifications in Table 28-3.

Table 28-3 Classifications of Burn Severity: Adults

CLASSIFICATIONS BY THICKNESS, PERCENT OF BODY SURFACE AREA, AND COMPLICATING FACTORS

Minor Burns

- Full thickness burns of less than 2 percent of the body surface, excluding the face, hands, feet, genitalia, or respiratory tract
- Partial thickness burns of less than 15 percent of the body surface
- Superficial burns of 50 percent of the body surface or less

Moderate Burns

- Full thickness burns of 2 to 10 percent of the body surface, excluding the face, hands, feet, genitalia, or respiratory tract
- Partial thickness burns of 15 to 30 percent of the body surface
- Superficial burns that involve more than 50 percent of the body surface

Critical Burns

- All burns complicated by injuries of the respiratory tract, other soft-tissue injuries, and injuries of the bones
- Partial thickness or full thickness burns involving the face, hands, feet, genitalia, or respiratory tract
- Full thickness burns of more than 10 percent
- Partial thickness burns of more than 30 percent
- Burns complicated by musculoskeletal injuries
- Circumferential burns

Note: Burns which, by the prior classification, are moderate should be considered critical in a person less than 5 or greater than 55 years of age. See Table 28-4 for classifications for children less than 5 years of age.

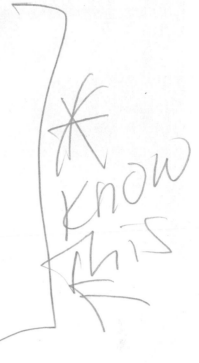

GERIATRIC NOTE

Note that burns usually classified as moderate are considered critical in adults over 55 years of age.

PEDIATRIC NOTE

Burns pose greater risks to infants and children than adults. This is because their body surface area is greater in relation to their total body size. This results in greater fluid and heat loss than would occur in an adult patient. Infants have a higher risk of shock, airway problems, and hypothermia from burns. Additionally, the classification of burn severity differs in patients less than 5 years of age, as shown in Table 28-4. When a child has been burned, consider the possibility of child abuse.

Table 28-4 Classifications of Burn Severity: Children Less than 5 Years of Age

CLASSIFICATIONS BY THICKNESS AND PERCENT OF BODY SURFACE AREA

Minor Burns

- Partial thickness burns of less than 10 percent of the body surface

Moderate Burns

- Partial thickness burns of 10 to 20 percent of the body surface

Critical Burns

- Full thickness burns of any extent or partial thickness burns of more than 20 percent of the body surface

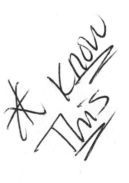

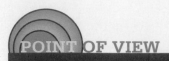

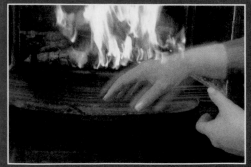

(© Edward T. Dickinson)

"I was tending the fire. I do it all the time. We were about to put in a movie, so I may have gotten a bit greedy and wanted to load the fireplace up so it would burn long and hot.

"The wood was nice and dry and a small fire had been going for awhile. But like I said, I decided it would be a good idea to build up the fire, and I put too much wood in. The wood shifted. I moved to catch some of the pieces, and then I heard a whoosh. The shift must've created an air flow that fed the fire. Well, that fire certainly caught. And so did my hand.

"I didn't think my hand was in the fire for that long, but it must've been. I felt the heat first. I'm not sure why, but I noticed hairs burning on my wrist before I even noticed the pain . . . and redness . . . and blistering. It got most of my hand and up my wrist a little.

"The EMTs came and put a dressing on my hand. I knew it was bad by looking at it. They were even more concerned, because they knew a burn to the hand can be really serious. They called the doctor on the radio who said to go to a hospital different than my normal one. They took me to a hospital with a specialty in treating burns.

"I'll tell you this: I'll never try to overfeed a fire again. Burns hurt a lot—and for a long time."

FIGURE 28-25 Chemical burns to the eyes. *(© Western Ophthalmic Hospital/Science Photo Library/Photo Researchers, Inc.)*

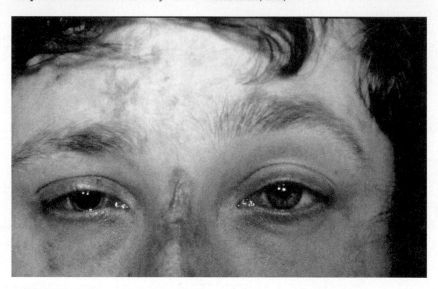

Treating Specific Types of Burns

There are special approaches to the care of thermal burns, general chemical burns, and chemical burns to the eyes (Figure 28-25).

PATIENT CARE

Thermal Burns

As an EMT, you will have to care for thermal burns caused by scalding liquids, steam, contact with hot objects, flames, flaming liquids, and gases. Sunburn can also be severe in infants and young children, who may have other heat-related injuries.

The steps for basic care of thermal burns are given in Table 28-5. Currently, dry sterile dressings are recommended by the national EMT curriculum for all burns. The standing orders for burn care are determined by your EMS Medical Director and the regional EMS system. Some EMS systems state that all partial thickness and full thickness burns are to be wrapped with dry sterile dressing or a burn sheet, whereas other burn centers recommend moist dressings for partial thickness burns to less than 10 percent of the body and dry dressings for more severe cases. The latter protocol is now being adopted by most EMS systems.

Table 28-5 Care for Thermal Burns

1. *Stop the burning process!*
   - Flame—Wet down, smother, then remove any affected clothing.
   - Semi-solid (grease, tar, wax)—Cool with water. Do not remove the substance.
2. Ensure an open airway. Assess breathing.
3. Look for signs of airway injury: soot deposits, burnt nasal hair, facial burns.
4. Complete the primary assessment.
5. Treat for shock. Provide high-concentration oxygen. Treat serious injuries.
6. Evaluate burns by depth (see below), extent (rule of nines or rule of palm), and severity.

DEPTH OF BURN	OUTER SKIN LAYER IS BURNED	SECOND SKIN LAYER IS BURNED	TISSUE BELOW SKIN IS BURNED	COLOR CHANGES	PAIN	BLISTERS
Superficial	Yes	No	No	Red	Yes	No
Partial thickness	Yes	Yes	No	Deep red	Yes	Yes
Full thickness	Yes	Yes	Yes	Charred black or white	Yes/no	Yes/no

7. *Do not* clear debris. Remove clothing and jewelry.
8. Wrap with dry sterile dressing.
9. *Burns to hands or feet*—Remove the patient's rings or jewelry that may constrict blood flow with swelling. Separate fingers or toes with sterile gauze pads.

Burns to the eyes—Do not open the patient's eyelids if burned. Be certain the burn is thermal, not chemical. Apply sterile gauze pads to *both* eyes to prevent sympathetic movement. (Some local protocols recommend covering only the injured eye. Follow your local protocols.) If the burn is chemical, flush the eyes for 20 minutes en route to the hospital.
FOLLOW LOCAL BURN CENTER PROTOCOLS, AND TRANSPORT ALL BURN PATIENTS AS SOON AS POSSIBLE.

Note that EMTs must manage burns correctly until the patient can be transferred to the care of a medical facility's staff. Never apply ointments, sprays, or butter (which would trap the heat against the burn site and have to be scraped off by the hospital staff). Do not break blisters. Do not apply ice to any burn (as it can cause tissue damage). Keep the burn site clean to prevent infection. Keep the patient warm, as the temperature regulation function of the skin may be affected by the burn.

NOTE: *Do not attempt to rescue persons trapped by fire unless you are trained to do so and have the equipment and personnel required. The simple act of opening a door might cost you your life. In some fires, opening a door or window may greatly intensify the fire or even cause an explosion.*

PATIENT CARE

Chemical Burns

Chemical burns require immediate care, and in an ideal situation people at the scene will begin this care before you arrive. At many industrial sites, workers and Emergency Medical Responders are trained to provide initial care for incidents involving the chemicals in use at that facility. Most major industries have emergency deluge-type safety showers to wash dangerous chemicals from the body. However, this will not always be the case. Be prepared for situations in which nothing has been done and there is no running water near the scene.

Emergency care for a patient with chemical burns includes the following:

1. The primary care procedure is to *wash* away the chemical with flowing water. If a dry chemical is involved, *brush* away as much of the chemical as possible and then flush the skin (Figure 28-26). Simply wetting the burn site is not enough. Continuous flooding of the affected area is required, using a copious but gentle flow of water. Avoid hard sprays that may damage badly burned tissues. Continue to wash the area for at least 20 minutes, and continue the process en route to the hospital. Take steps as needed to avoid

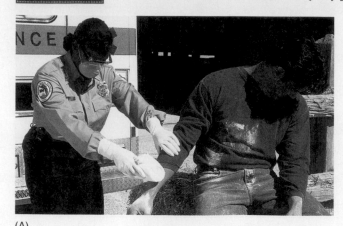

(A)

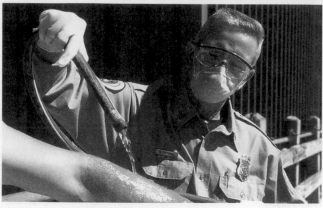

(B)

contaminating yourself with the chemical agent. Remove the patient's contaminated clothing, shoes, socks, and jewelry as you apply the wash. *Do not contaminate skin that has not been in contact with the chemical.*

2. Apply a sterile dressing or burn sheet.
3. Treat for shock.
4. Transport.

Continue to be on the alert for delayed reactions that may cause renewed pain or interfere with the patient's ability to breathe. If the patient complains of increased burning or irritation, wash the burned areas again with flowing water for several minutes.

Treating Specific Chemical Burns

When possible, find out the exact chemical or mixture of chemicals that were involved in the incident. Most industrial sites will have a material safety data sheet (MSDS) that provides specific emergency information about the chemical agents being used. Some special chemical burns require specific care procedures.

- **Mixed or strong acids or unidentified substances.** Many of the chemicals used in industrial processes are mixed acids, whose combined action can be immediate and severe. The pain produced from the initial chemical burn may mask any pain being caused by renewed burning due to small concentrations left on the skin.

  When the chemical is a strong acid (e.g., hydrochloric acid or sulfuric acid), a combination of acids, or an unknown, play it safe and continue washing even after the patient claims he is no longer experiencing pain.

- **Dry lime.** If dry lime is the burn agent, do not wash the burn site with water. To do so will create a corrosive liquid. Brush the dry lime from the patient's skin, hair, and clothing. Make certain that you do not contaminate the patient's eyes or airway.

  Use water only after the lime has been brushed from the body, contaminated clothing and jewelry have been removed, and the process of washing can be done quickly and continuously with running water.

- **Carbolic acid (phenol).** Carbolic acid does not mix with water. When available, use alcohol for the initial wash of unbroken skin, followed by a long steady wash with water. (Follow local protocols.)

- **Sulfuric acid.** Heat is produced when water is added to concentrated sulfuric acid, but it is still preferable to wash rather than leave the contaminant on the skin.

- **Hydrofluoric acid.** This acid is used for etching glass as well as many other manufacturing processes. Burns from it may be delayed, so treat all patients who may have come into contact with the chemical, even if burns are not in evidence. Flood the affected area with water. Do not delay care and transport to find neutralizing agents. (Follow local protocols.)

- **Inhaled vapors.** Whenever a patient is exposed to a caustic chemical and may have inhaled the vapors, provide high-concentration oxygen (humidified, if available) and transport as soon as possible. This is very important when the chemical is an acid that is known to vaporize at standard environmental temperatures. (Examples include hydrochloric acid and sulfuric acid.)

Inside/Outside

Although part of the treatment for both acid and alkali burns is irrigation, alkali burns should be irrigated longer because of the different ways in which these chemicals react with the human body.

When acids encounter tissue, they break down proteins. This results in coagulated tissue that limits further progression of the acid. Alkalis, on the other hand, break down protein, but they also liquefy the damaged tissue. In fact, this process, called saponification, is how soap has been made for centuries. A strong alkali like lye is mixed with fat or oil. The chemical reaction that occurs changes the two substances into soap.

Because a strong alkali liquefies dead tissue, the alkali is able to eat into the tissue much farther than an acid can. Continued irrigation is the best method of diluting and removing the alkali and limiting the damage it causes.

There is a well-known exception to the principle of acids causing limited damage. Hydrofluoric acid not only causes burns like any other acid, but it also penetrates much more deeply. The fluoride released from the acid combines with calcium and magnesium in the tissue until the fluoride is used up. This typically results in significant tissue damage, since there isn't that much calcium or magnesium outside of bone. Much of the damage is internal and not visible, especially with low concentrations. Higher concentrations will cause both internal damage and external damage. Hydrofluoric acid is used in industrial applications such as glass etching and electronics manufacturing, but it is also available in some rust removers intended for use around the home.

If you encounter a patient with a hydrofluoric acid exposure, you must irrigate copiously and for as long as you can or until medical direction tells you to stop. Hydrofluoric acid burns can cause great tissue damage with few external signs, so do your best to persuade a reluctant patient to go to the emergency department for further treatment.

PATIENT CARE

Chemical Burns to the Eyes

A corrosive chemical can burn the globe of a person's eye before he can react and close the eyelid. Even with the lid shut, chemicals can seep through onto the globe.

To care for chemical burns to the eye, you should take the following steps:

1. *Immediately* flood the eyes with water. Often the burn will involve areas of the face as well as the eye. When this is the case, flood the entire area. Avoid washing chemicals back into the eye or into an unaffected eye (Figure 28-27).
2. Keep running water from a faucet, low-pressure hose, bucket, cup, bottle, rubber bulb syringe, IV setup, or other such source flowing into the burned eye. The flow should be from the medial (nasal) corner of the eye to the lateral corner. Since the patient's natural reaction will be to keep the eyes tightly shut, you may have to hold the eyelids open.
3. Start transport and continue washing the eye for at least 20 minutes or until the patient's arrival at the medical facility.
4. After washing the eye, cover both eyes with moistened pads.

FIGURE 28-27 Emergency care of chemical burns to the eye.

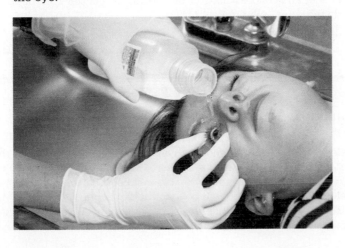

5. Wash the patient's eyes for 5 more minutes if he begins to complain about renewed burning sensations or irritation.

> **NOTE:** *Protect yourself during the washing process for a chemical burn. Wear protective gloves and eyewear and control the wash to avoid splashing.*

> **NOTE:** *Do not use neutralizers such as vinegar or baking soda in a patient's eyes.*

> **NOTE:** *Some scenes where chemical burns have taken place can be very hazardous. Always evaluate the scene. There may be large pools of dangerous chemicals around the patient. Acids could be spurting from containers. Toxic fumes may be present. If the scene will place you in danger, do not attempt a rescue unless you have been trained for such a situation and have the needed equipment and personnel at the scene.*

ELECTRICAL INJURIES

● **CORE CONCEPT**

Understanding electrical injuries
and emergency care for
electrical injuries

Electric current, including lightning, can cause severe damage to the body. In these cases, the skin is burned where the energy enters the body and where it flows into a ground. Along the path of this flow, tissues are damaged due to heat. In addition, significant chemical changes take place in the nerves, heart, and muscles, and body processes are disrupted or may completely shut down.

> **NOTE:** *The scenes of injuries due to electricity are often very hazardous. Assume that the source of electricity is still active unless a qualified person tells you that the power has been turned off. Do not attempt a rescue unless you have been trained to do this kind of rescue and have the necessary equipment and personnel. For information about electrical hazards at the scene of a vehicle collision, see Chapter 10, "The Scene Size-Up," and Chapter 40, "Highway Safety and Vehicle Extrication."*

PATIENT ASSESSMENT

Electrical Injuries

The victim of an electrical accident may have any or all of the following signs and symptoms (Figure 28-28):

- Burns where the energy enters and exits the body
- Disrupted nerve pathways displayed as paralysis
- Muscle tenderness, with or without muscular twitching
- Respiratory difficulties or respiratory arrest
- Irregular heartbeat or cardiac arrest
- Elevated blood pressure or low blood pressure with the signs and symptoms of shock
- Restlessness or irritability if conscious, or loss of consciousness
- Visual difficulties
- Fractured bones and dislocations from severe muscle contractions or from falling (This can include the spinal column.)
- Seizures (in severe cases)

PATIENT CARE

Electrical Injuries

Follow these steps to provide emergency care to a patient with electrical injuries:

1. Provide airway care. Electrical shock may cause severe swelling along the airway.
2. Provide basic cardiac life support as required. Since cardiac rhythm disturbances are common, be prepared to perform defibrillation if necessary.
3. Care for shock and administer high-concentration oxygen.
4. Care for spine injuries, head injuries, and severe fractures. All serious electrical shock patients should be fully immobilized because electrical current can cause severe muscular

FIGURE 28-28 (A) Injuries due to electrical shock and (B) entrance wound (right hand) and exit wound (left forearm) from an electrical shock. *(Photo B: © Edward T. Dickinson, MD)*

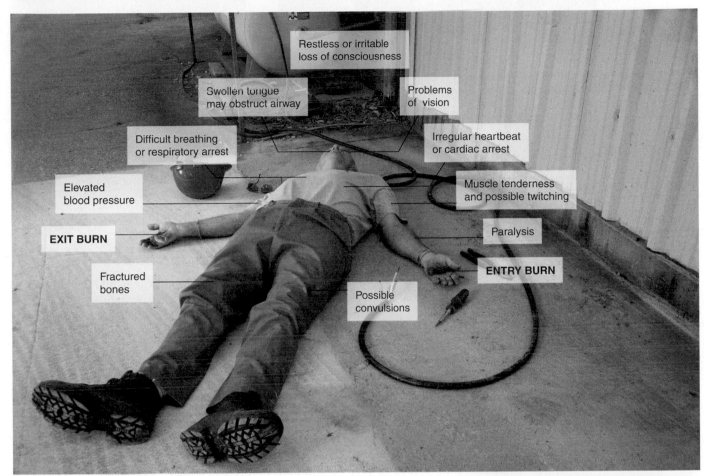

Restless or irritable loss of consciousness

Swollen tongue may obstruct airway

Problems of vision

Difficult breathing or respiratory arrest

Irregular heartbeat or cardiac arrest

Elevated blood pressure

Muscle tenderness and possible twitching

EXIT BURN

Paralysis

Fractured bones

ENTRY BURN

Possible convulsions

(A)

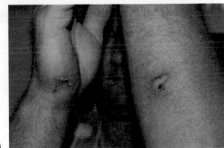

(B)

contraction. Also, the patient may have been thrown by a high-voltage current. In either case, there is the possibility of a spinal injury that requires immobilization.

5. Evaluate electrical burns, looking for at least two external burn sites: contact with the energy source and contact with a ground.
6. Cool the burn areas and smoldering clothing the same as you would for a flame burn.
7. Apply dry sterile dressings to the burn sites.
8. Transport as soon as possible. Some problems have a slow onset. If there are burns, there also may be more serious hidden problems. In any case of electrical shock, heart problems may develop.

Remember that the major problem caused by electrical shock is usually not the burn. Respiratory and cardiac arrest are real possibilities. Be prepared to provide basic cardiac life support measures with automated defibrillation.

NOTE: *Make certain that you and the patient are in a safe zone (not in contact with any electrical source and outside the area where downed or broken wires or other sources of electricity can reach you).*

FIGURE 28-29 (A) Dressings cover wounds and (B) bandages hold dressings in place.

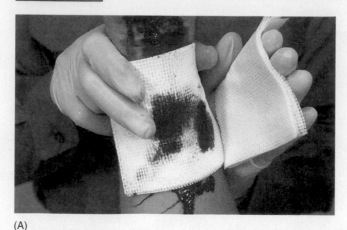

(A)

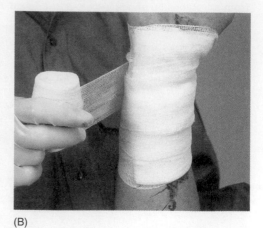

(B)

DRESSING AND BANDAGING

● **CORE CONCEPT**

How to dress and bandage
wounds

dressing

any material (preferably sterile) used
to cover a wound that will help control
bleeding and prevent additional
contamination.

bandage

any material used to hold a dressing
in place.

universal dressing

a bulky dressing.

Most cases of open wound care require the application of a dressing and a bandage (Figure 28-29 and Scan 28-1). A ***dressing*** is any material applied to a wound in an effort to control bleeding and prevent further contamination. Dressings should be sterile. A ***bandage*** is any material used to hold a dressing in place. Bandages need not be sterile.

NOTE: *Be certain to wear disposable gloves and other barrier devices to avoid contact with the patient's blood and body fluids. Follow infection control procedures.*

Various dressings are carried in emergency care kits. These dressings should be sterile, meaning that all microorganisms and spores that can grow into active organisms have been killed. Dressings also should be aseptic, meaning that all dirt and foreign debris have been removed. Many EMS systems now also carry hemostatic dressings used to stop bleeding (Figure 28-30). In emergency situations, when commercially prepared dressings are not available, clean cloth, towels, sheets, handkerchiefs, and other similar materials may be suitable alternatives.

The most popular dressings are individually wrapped sterile gauze pads, typically 4 inches square. A variety of sizes are available, referred to according to size in inches, such as $2 \times 2s$, $4 \times 4s$, $5 \times 9s$, and $8 \times 10s$.

Large bulky dressings, such as the multitrauma or ***universal dressing***, are available when bulk is required for profuse bleeding or when a large wound must be covered. These dressings are especially useful for stabilizing impaled objects. Sanitary napkins can sometimes be used in place of the standard bulky dressings. Although not sterile, they are separately wrapped and have very clean surfaces. (Do not apply any adhesive surface of the

FIGURE 28-30 (A and B) Application and bandaging of a hemostatic dressing.

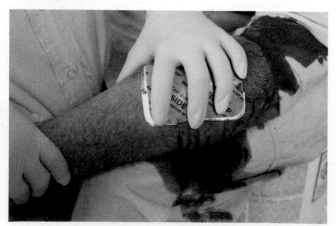

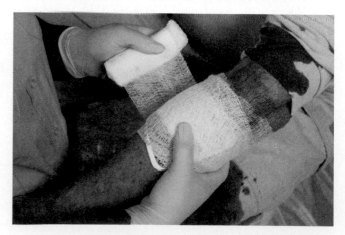

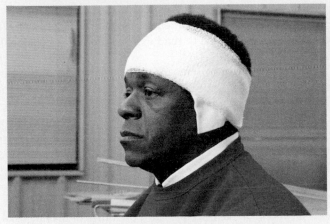

FOREHEAD OR EAR (NO SKULL INJURY). Place the dressing and secure it with a self-adherent roller bandage.

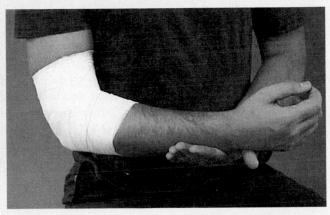

ELBOW OR KNEE. Place the dressing and secure it with a cravat or roller bandage. Apply the roller bandage in a figure-eight pattern.

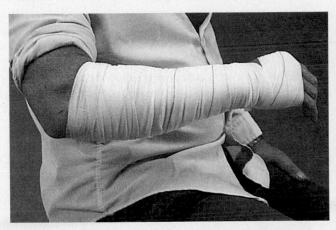

HAND. Place the dressing, wrap it with roller bandages, and secure it at the wrist. When possible, bandage it in the position of function.

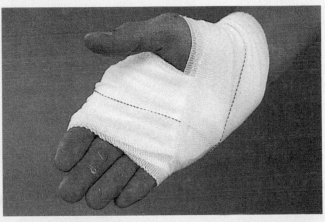

FOREARM OR LEG. Place the dressing and secure it with a roller bandage, distal to proximal. Better protection is offered if the palm or sole is wrapped.

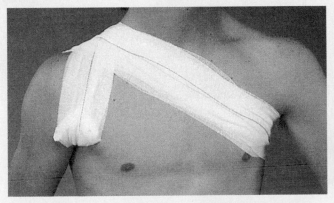

SHOULDER. Place the dressing and secure it with a figure-eight of cravat or roller dressing. Pad under the knot if a cravat is used.

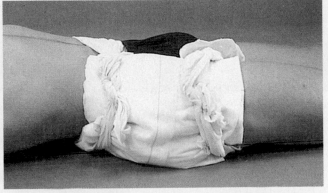

HIP. Place the bandage and use a large dressing to cover the hip. Secure it with the first cravat around the waist and second cravat around the thigh on the injured side.

napkin directly to the wound.) Of course, bulky dressings can be made by building up layers of gauze pads.

A ***pressure dressing*** is used to control bleeding. Gauze pads are placed on the wound and a bulky dressing is placed over the pads. A self-adherent roller bandage is then wrapped tightly over the dressing and above and below the wound. You must check and frequently recheck the distal pulse, and you may need to readjust the pressure to ensure distal circulation.

An ***occlusive dressing*** is used when it is necessary to form an airtight seal. This is done when caring for open wounds to the abdomen, for external bleeding from large neck veins, and for open wounds to the chest. Sterile, commercially prepared occlusive dressings are available in two different forms: plastic wrap and petroleum-gel-impregnated gauze occlusive dressings. Local protocols vary as to which form to use. Nonsterile wrap also can be used in emergency situations. In emergencies, EMTs have been known to fashion occlusive dressings from plastic credit cards, plastic bags, sterile medical equipment wrappers, and defibrillator pads.

Large dressings are sometimes needed in emergency care. Sterile, disposable burn sheets are commercially available. Bed sheets can also be sterilized and kept in plastic wrappers to be used later as dressings. These sheets can make effective burn dressings or may be used in some cases to cover exposed abdominal organs.

Bandages are provided in a wide variety of types. The preferred bandage is the self-adhering, form-fitting roller bandage (Figure 28-31). It eliminates the need to know many specialized bandaging techniques developed for use with ordinary gauze roller bandages.

Dressings can be secured using adhering or nonadhering gauze roller bandages, triangular bandages, strips of adhesive tape, or an air splint. In a situation where one of these is not available, you can use strips of cloth, handkerchiefs, and other such materials. Elastic bandages that are used in the general care of strains and sprains should not be used to hold dressings in place. They can become constricting bands, interfering with circulation. This is very likely to occur as the tissues around the wound site begin to swell after the elastic bandage is in place.

pressure dressing
a dressing applied tightly to control bleeding.

occlusive dressing
any dressing that forms an airtight seal.

FIGURE 28-31 To apply a self-adhering roller bandage, (A) secure it with several overlapping wraps, (B) keep it snug, and (C) cut and tape or tie it in place.

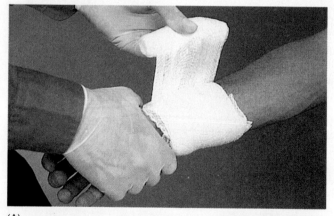

(A)

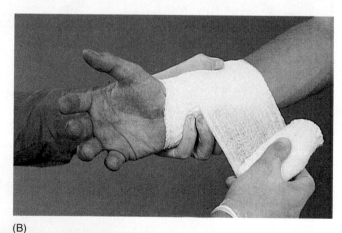

(B)

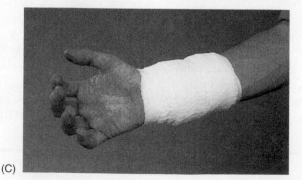

(C)

PATIENT CARE

Dressing Open Wounds

The following rules apply to the general dressing of wounds (Figure 28-32):

1. Take Standard Precautions.
2. Expose the wound. Cut away any clothing necessary so the entire wound is exposed.
3. Use sterile or very clean materials. Avoid touching the dressing in the area that will come into contact with the wound. Grasp the dressing by the corner, taking it directly from its protective pack, and place it on the wound.
4. Cover the entire wound. The entire surface of the wound and the immediate surrounding areas should be covered.
5. Control the bleeding. Use direct pressure and/or hemostatic agents or dressings to stop or slow the bleeding. With the exception of the pressure dressing, a dressing should not be bandaged in place if it has not controlled the bleeding. You should continue to apply dressings and pressure as needed for the proper control of bleeding.
6. Do not remove dressings. Once a dressing has been applied to a wound, it must remain in place. Bleeding may restart and tissues at the wound site may be injured if the dressing is removed. If the bleeding continues, reapply pressure, apply additional hemostatic agent, and put new dressings over the blood-soaked ones.

There is an exception to the rule prohibiting the removal of dressings. If a bulky dressing has become soaked with blood, it may be necessary to remove the dressing so that direct pressure can be reestablished or a new bulky dressing can be added and a pressure dressing created. Protection for the wound site is better maintained if one or more gauze pads are placed over the injured tissues before placing the bulky dressing. This will allow for the removal of a bulky dressing without disturbing the wound.

FIGURE 28-32 To dress an open wound, (A) expose the wound site, (B) control the bleeding, (C) dress and bandage the wound, and (D) keep the patient at rest.

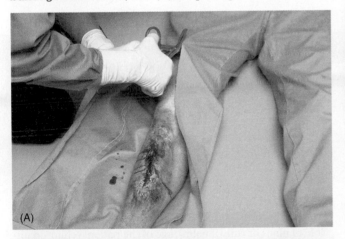
(A)

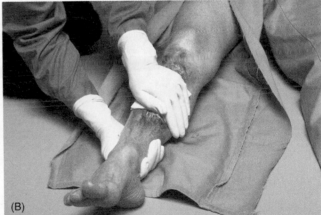
(B)

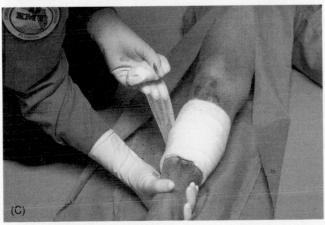
(C)

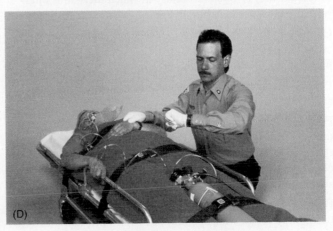
(D)

Bandaging Open Wounds

The following rules apply to general bandaging:

1. Do not bandage too tightly. All dressings should be held snugly in place, but they must not restrict the blood supply to the affected part.
2. Do not bandage too loosely. Hold the dressing by bandaging snugly, so the dressing does not move around or slip from the wound. Loose bandaging is a common error in emergency care.
3. Do not leave loose ends. Any loose ends of gauze, tape, or cloth may get caught on objects when the patient is moved.
4. Do not cover the tips of fingers and toes. When bandaging the extremities, leave the fingers and toes exposed whenever possible to observe skin color changes that indicate a change in circulation and to allow for easier neurologic reassessment. Pain, pale or cyanotic skin, cold skin, numbness, and tingling are all indications that a bandage may be too tight. The exception is burned fingers or toes, which have to be covered.
5. Cover all edges of the dressing. This will help to reduce additional contamination. The flutter-valve dressing for an open chest wound is an exception (see Chapter 29, "Chest and Abdominal Trauma").

Two special problems occur when bandaging an extremity. First, point pressure can occur if you bandage around a very small area. It is best to wrap a large area, ensuring a steady, uniform pressure. Apply the bandage from the smaller diameter of the limb to the larger diameter (distal to proximal) to help ensure proper pressure and contact. Second, the joints have to be considered. You can bandage across a joint, but do not bend the limb once the bandage is in place. Doing so may restrict circulation, loosen the dressing and bandage, or do both. In some cases, it may be necessary to apply an inflatable or rigid splint, or to use a sling and swathe to prevent the joint's movement.

CHAPTER REVIEW

Key Facts and Concepts

- Soft-tissue injuries may be closed (internal, with no pathway to the outside) or open (an injury in which the skin is interrupted, exposing the tissues below).
- Closed injuries include contusions (bruises), hematomas, and crush injuries. Open wounds include abrasions, lacerations, punctures, avulsions, amputations, and crush injuries.
- For open wounds, expose the wound, control bleeding, and prevent further contamination.
- For both open and closed injuries, take appropriate Standard Precautions; note the mechanism of injury; protect the patient's airway and breathing; administer high-concentration oxygen by nonrebreather mask; treat for shock; and transport.
- Burn severity is determined by considering the source of the burn, body regions burned, depth of the burn (superficial,

partial thickness, and full thickness), extent of the burn (by rule of nines or rule of palm), age of the patient (children under 5 and adults over 55 react most severely), and other patient illnesses or injuries.

- Care for burns includes stopping the burning process (using water for a thermal burn, brushing away chemicals), covering a thermal burn with a dry sterile dressing, flushing a chemical burn with sterile water, protecting the airway, administering oxygen, treating for shock, and transporting the patient to a medical facility.
- For treatment of electrical injuries, be sure that you and the patient are in a safe zone away from possible contact with electrical sources. Protect the airway, breathing, and circulation. Be prepared to care for respiratory or cardiac arrest. Treat for shock, care for burns, and transport the patient.

Key Decisions

- Does our patient have an adequate airway?
- Is the patient's breathing adequate, inadequate, or absent?
- If the wound is penetrating, is there an exit wound?
- What is the best way to immobilize an impaled object?
- Do we need to cool the burn area to stop the burning?

- Does our burn patient need to go to a special destination?
- Is there respiratory involvement with the burn?
- Have we sufficiently irrigated the chemical burn?
- Does our patient's electrical burn have an exit wound?
- Is the bandage on our patient's extremity snug enough without limiting circulation?

Chapter Glossary

abrasion (ab-RAY-zhun) a scratch or scrape.

amputation (am-pyu-TAY-shun) the surgical removal or traumatic severing of a body part, usually an extremity.

avulsion (ah-VUL-shun) the tearing away or tearing off of a piece or flap of skin or other soft tissue. This term also may be used for an eye pulled from its socket or a tooth dislodged from its socket.

bandage any material used to hold a dressing in place.

closed wound an internal injury with no open pathway from the outside.

contusion (kun-TU-zhun) a bruise.

crush injury an injury caused when force is transmitted from the body's exterior to its internal structures. Bones can be broken; muscles, nerves, and tissues damaged; and internal organs ruptured, causing internal bleeding.

dermis (DER-mis) the inner (second) layer of the skin found beneath the epidermis. It is rich in blood vessels and nerves.

dressing any material (preferably sterile) used to cover a wound that will help control bleeding and prevent additional contamination.

epidermis (ep-i-DER-mis) the outer layer of the skin.

full thickness burn a burn in which all the layers of the skin are damaged. There are usually areas that are charred black or areas that are dry and white. Also called a *third-degree burn*.

hematoma (hem-ah-TO-mah) a swelling caused by the collection of blood under the skin or in damaged tissues as a result of an injured or broken blood vessel.

laceration (las-er-AY-shun) a cut.

occlusive dressing any dressing that forms an airtight seal.

open wound an injury in which the skin is interrupted, exposing the tissue beneath.

partial thickness burn a burn in which the epidermis (first layer of skin) is burned through and the dermis (second layer) is damaged. Burns of this type cause reddening, blistering, and a mottled appearance. Also called a *second-degree burn*.

pressure dressing a dressing applied tightly to control bleeding.

puncture wound an open wound that tears through the skin and destroys underlying tissues. A *penetrating puncture wound* can be shallow or deep. A *perforating puncture wound* has both an entrance and an exit wound.

rule of nines a method for estimating the extent of a burn. For an adult, each of the following areas represents 9 percent of the body surface: the head and neck, each upper extremity, the chest, the abdomen, the upper back, the lower back and buttocks, the front of each lower extremity, and the back of each lower extremity. The remaining 1 percent is assigned to the genital region. For an infant or child, the percentages are modified so that 18 percent is assigned to the head, 14 percent to each lower extremity.

rule of palm a method for estimating the extent of a burn. The palm of the patient's own hand, which equals about 1 percent of the body's surface area, is compared with the patient's burn to estimate its size.

subcutaneous (SUB-ku-TAY-ne-us) *layers* the layers of fat and soft tissues found below the dermis.

superficial burn a burn that involves only the epidermis, the outer layer of the skin. It is characterized by reddening of the skin and perhaps some swelling. A common example is a sunburn. Also called a first-degree burn.

universal dressing a bulky dressing.

Preparation for Your Examination and Practice

Short Answer

1. List three types of closed soft-tissue injuries.
2. List four types of open soft-tissue injuries.
3. Explain when you would remove an object impaled in the cheek and when you would, instead, stabilize an object impaled in the cheek.
4. Describe the three classifications (depths) of burns.
5. Differentiate between a dressing and a bandage.
6. List the qualities and purpose of an effective bandage. How can you tell if a bandage is improperly applied?

Thinking and Linking

Think back to Chapter 2, "The Well-Being of the EMT," as you consider the following question:

- What Standard Precautions are required for the following calls?
    a. An agitated person with a lip laceration and missing teeth

b. A small cut to the left hand, which is oozing blood

c. A laceration to the right forearm with bright red spurting blood

Think back to Chapter 1, "Introduction to Emergency Medical Services and the Health Care System," and the discussion of specialized trauma and other treatment centers under "Components of the EMS System" as you consider the following question:

- Which specialty centers should the following patients be transported to (if the center is available in your region)?

  a. A patient with partial thickness burns on 35 percent of his body

  b. A patient with suspected internal bleeding and trauma

  c. A patient with an amputated hand

Critical Thinking Exercises

Assessing a wound that is covered can be tricky. The purpose of this exercise will be to consider one such situation.

- A 21-year-old male lacerated his anterior elbow when he fell through a window. There is a lot of blood around the patient. Bystanders have applied numerous towels and washcloths over the wound (at least 3 inches thick). There are so many dressings on the wound, in fact, that you can't tell if it is still bleeding. The patient is alert, but pale and anxious. The radial pulse on his uninjured arm is weak and rapid. How much assessment of the wound should you do and how do you do it without making things worse?

Pathophysiology to Practice

The following question is designed to assist you in gathering relevant clinical information and making accurate decisions in the field.

- Patients with extensive burns lose large amounts of fluid internally because of damage to the cell membranes. If you find a patient with a recent burn (less than 1 hour old) who is tachycardic, pale, and hypotensive, why should you look for a source of bleeding?

Street Scenes

Late Sunday evening, you respond to #4 Mountain View Apartments. You and your partner are met by the manager and a security guard, who lead you to Mary, a 42-year-old female sitting in a chair in the manager's office with a thick towel wrapped around her right forearm. Standard Precautions are in place. You greet the patient and identify yourself, then ask, "What happened?" You note the trail of blood spots on the floor leading to an outside door.

"I locked myself out of my apartment," she tells you. "So, I wrapped my coat around my arm and broke the glass window above my kitchen sink. I thought the coat would protect me, but I was wrong."

Street Scene Questions

1. What is your general impression of this patient?
2. What priority would you assign to her?
3. What interventions are appropriate at this time?

Your general impression is of an alert female patient holding a blood-soaked towel to her right forearm. Primary assessment shows her airway open and clear, respirations normal, and a regular pulse in her right wrist. You assign her a low transport priority.

You ask Norma, your partner, to go to Mary's apartment accompanied by the security guard to see if she can learn anything more about the mechanism of injury. Meanwhile, you observe that the bleeding is being controlled and begin a secondary assessment. You gently remove the towel and note there is no active bleeding from a smooth and deep laceration with muscle and tendons visible. You dress and bandage the wound.

There are no other injuries or medical problems present. You do, however, detect an odor of alcohol on Mary's breath. "Have you had any alcohol today?" you ask.

"Yes, I drank two beers about 3 hours ago. That's all!" she exclaims. However, with the odor on her breath, you figure she must have had more than two beers. Focusing on her right arm, you find pulses still present in that extremity. She is also able to feel your finger touch her palm. However, when you ask her to wiggle her fingers, her ring and little fingers remain motionless. She also tells you it hurts to move her fingers. Norma returns and tells you there is a pool of blood on Mary's patio.

Street Scene Questions

4. Would you change the priority of transport of this patient based on what you now know? Why or why not?
5. What interventions are appropriate for this patient?

While you continue with the patient history, Norma obtains baseline vital signs. You learn Mary is taking thyroid medication and a blood thinner for a medical condition. You ask when she received her last tetanus shot, and she tells you she cannot remember.

Norma informs you that Mary's pulse is equal in both extremities at a rate of 128 and regular; her blood pressure is 156/94, her respirations are 24 and unlabored; pupils are equal and reactive to light; and her skin is warm, dry, and a normal color.

You contact medical direction, concerned about the loss of movement in Mary's affected extremity. The doctor tells you that you should stabilize Mary's arm with a sling.

You apply a sling, reassess Mary's vitals, and find no significant changes. Reassessing her pulse, motor function, and sensation, you find Mary still unable to move her fourth and fifth digits on her right hand. You place her on your cot, load her into the ambulance, and transport her to the closest facility, monitoring her condition throughout the 15-minute ride. You find no other significant changes occurring.

Chest and Abdominal Trauma

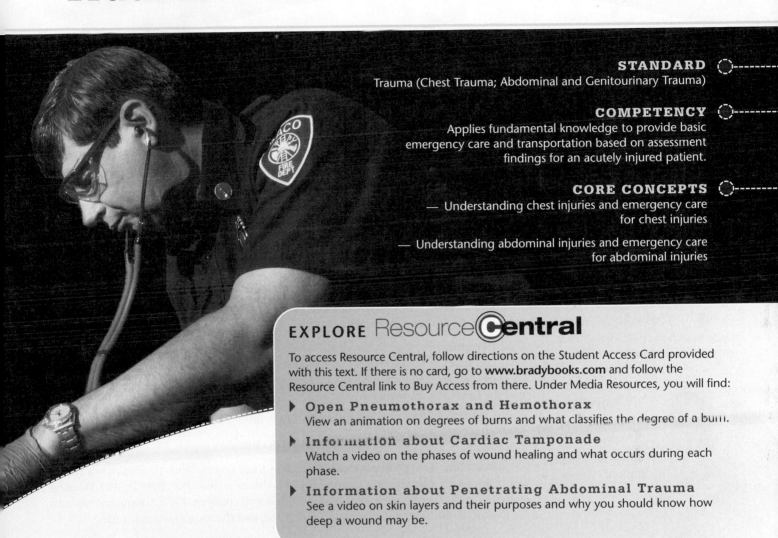

29

STANDARD ⚪------

Trauma (Chest Trauma; Abdominal and Genitourinary Trauma)

COMPETENCY ⚪------

Applies fundamental knowledge to provide basic emergency care and transportation based on assessment findings for an acutely injured patient.

CORE CONCEPTS ⚪------

— Understanding chest injuries and emergency care for chest injuries

— Understanding abdominal injuries and emergency care for abdominal injuries

EXPLORE Resource Central

To access Resource Central, follow directions on the Student Access Card provided with this text. If there is no card, go to **www.bradybooks.com** and follow the Resource Central link to Buy Access from there. Under Media Resources, you will find:

▶ **Open Pneumothorax and Hemothorax**
View an animation on degrees of burns and what classifies the degree of a burn.

▶ **Information about Cardiac Tamponade**
Watch a video on the phases of wound healing and what occurs during each phase.

▶ **Information about Penetrating Abdominal Trauma**
See a video on skin layers and their purposes and why you should know how deep a wound may be.

OBJECTIVES

After reading this chapter you should be able to:

29.1 Define key terms introduced in this chapter.

29.2 Describe mechanisms of injury commonly associated with chest injuries. (p. 680)

29.3 Describe specific chest injuries, including flail chest, open chest wounds, pneumothorax, tension pneumothorax, hemothorax, hemopneumothorax, traumatic asphyxia, cardiac tamponade, aortic injury, and *commotio cordis* and the assessment and management for each of these specific injuries. (pp. 680–688)

29.4 Discuss mechanisms and types of abdominal injuries. (pp. 688–689)

29.5 Demonstrate the assessment and management of patients with blunt and penetrating abdominal injuries, including management of evisceration. (pp. 690–692)

Although serious injuries to the chest, abdomen, and genitalia are not that common, they are injuries that EMTs must be comfortable with and able to expeditiously handle. Many of these injuries can be life threatening. The EMT must be able to recognize injuries that require prompt prehospital treatment and those that require prompt transport to a facility capable of dealing with them. Even injuries that do not appear life threatening at first can develop into much more serious problems en route to the hospital. The EMT's assessment and reassessment skills will be important to the ultimate outcome of these patients.

>>>>>>

● CORE CONCEPT

Understanding chest injuries and emergency care for chest injuries

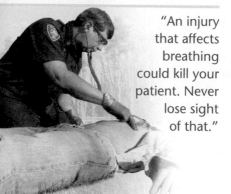

"An injury that affects breathing could kill your patient. Never lose sight of that."

CHEST INJURIES

The chest can be injured in a number of ways:

- **Blunt trauma.** A blow to the chest can fracture the ribs, the sternum, and the costal (rib) cartilages. Whole sections of the chest can collapse. With severe blunt trauma, the lungs and airway can be damaged. In addition, the great vessels (aorta and venae cavae) and the heart may be seriously injured.

- **Penetrating objects.** Bullets, knives, pieces of metal or glass, steel rods, pipes, and various other objects can penetrate the chest wall, damaging internal organs and impairing respiration.

- **Compression.** Compression injuries develop from severe blunt trauma in which the chest is rapidly compressed, such as when a driver strikes his chest on the steering column or when a person is trapped in a trench-wall collapse. The sternum and ribs can be fractured, the heart can be severely squeezed, and the lung(s) can rupture.

Closed Chest Injuries

Chest injuries are classified as either closed or open. In a closed chest injury, the skin is not broken, leading many people to think that the damage done is not serious. However, such injuries, sustained through blunt trauma and compression injuries, can cause contusions and lacerations of the heart, lungs, and great vessels.

Closed chest injuries may cause a condition known as *flail chest* (Figure 29-1). This condition is defined as a fracture of two or more consecutive ribs in two or more places. (Some sources say three or more ribs in two or more places.) The most important factor to remember—even more than the number of broken ribs—is that flail chest leaves a portion of the chest wall unstable, which affects breathing and reduces lung expansion. This can lead to inadequate breathing and hypoventilation.

Because the flail segment is not attached, it is free to independently move. When the patient's chest expands to inhale, negative pressure draws air into the lungs. This negative pressure also draws the flail segment inward. When the patient's chest moves inward, positive pressure is created that pushes air out of the lungs, and this positive pressure also pushes the flail segment outward. Thus, the movement of the flail segment is opposite to the movement of the remainder of the chest cavity. This is called *paradoxical motion* (Figure 29-2).

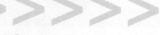

flail chest
fracture of two or more adjacent ribs in two or more places that allows for free movement of the fractured segment.

paradoxical motion
movement of ribs in a flail segment that is opposite to the direction of movement of the rest of the chest cavity.

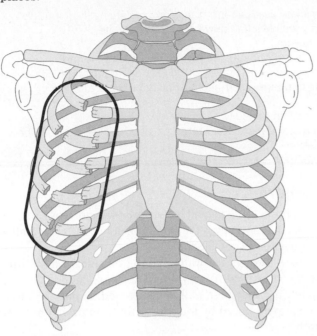

FIGURE 29-1 Flail chest occurs when blunt trauma creates a fracture of two or more ribs in two or more places.

FIGURE 29-2 Paradoxical motion.

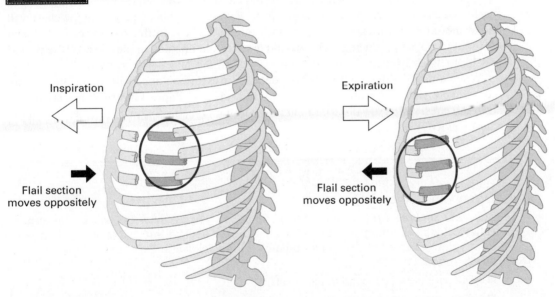

Inspiration

Flail section
moves oppositely

Expiration

Flail section
moves oppositely

PATIENT ASSESSMENT

Flail Chest

The patient with flail chest will have a mechanism of injury capable of causing it, difficulty breathing, pain at the injury site, and likely signs of shock and hypoxia.

The characteristic paradoxical motion may be difficult to observe in early stages since the chest wall muscles will tighten and naturally splint the area. This muscle tightening, combined with efforts necessary to breathe, will eventually cause the patient to become fatigued. In turn, this will cause the flail segment to become more visible—and will also make assisting ventilations necessary. When a flail segment is visible, it may be a late sign that appears once the patient becomes tired and weak.

Passitive Pressure Ventialations

Flail Chest

1. Perform a primary assessment. Flail segments should be identified as early in the assessment as possible since they pose a threat to life.
2. Administer oxygen.
3. If the patient is breathing inadequately, assist ventilations.
4. Use a bulky dressing to stabilize the flail segment. Tape the dressing into place. The tape or bandage used should not encircle the chest or interfere with chest expansion.
5. Monitor the patient carefully.
6. Watch the patient's respiratory rate and depth. If respirations become too shallow, assist ventilations.

Open Chest Injuries

Whenever the skin is broken, the patient has an open wound. However, the term *open chest wound* usually means that not only is the skin broken but the chest wall is also penetrated (for example, by a bullet or a knife blade).

An object can pass through the wall from the outside, or a fractured and displaced rib can penetrate the chest wall from within. The heart, lungs, and great vessels can be injured at the same time the chest wall is penetrated. It may be difficult to tell if the chest cavity has been penetrated by looking at the wound. Do not open the wound to determine its depth.

Specific signs (as noted in the following Patient Assessment section) will indicate possible open chest injury.

You must consider all open wounds to the chest to be life-threatening wounds. Open chest wounds are usually penetrating puncture wounds, which may penetrate the chest wall one or more times (for example, a gunshot wound may have both an entrance and an exit wound). An object producing such a wound may remain impaled in the chest, or the wound may be completely open.

When air enters the chest cavity, the delicate pressure balance within the chest cavity is destroyed. This causes the lung on the injured side to collapse. (Injuries associated with air in the chest cavity are discussed in more detail under the heading "Injuries within the Chest Cavity.")

Open Chest Wound

sucking chest wound
an open chest wound in which air is "sucked" into the chest cavity.

The term **sucking chest wound** is used when the chest cavity is open to the atmosphere. Each time the patient breathes, air can be sucked into the opening. This patient will develop severe difficulty breathing. The following signs indicate a sucking chest wound:

- The patient has a wound to the chest.
- There may or may not be the characteristic sucking sound associated with an open chest wound.
- The patient may be gasping for air.

Keep in mind that the object penetrating the chest wall may have seriously damaged a lung, major blood vessel, or the heart itself.

Decision Points

- Does my patient have a chest injury that must be treated during the primary assessment?
- Does my patient have an open chest injury that requires an occlusive dressing?
- Does my patient have an injury or injuries that require minimal scene time and prompt transport to a trauma center?

PATIENT CARE

Open Chest Wound

An open chest wound is a *true emergency* that requires rapid initial care and immediate transport to a medical facility. Follow these steps:

1. Maintain an open airway. Provide basic life support, if necessary.
2. Seal the open chest wound as quickly as possible. If need be, use your gloved hand. Do not delay sealing the wound in order to find an occlusive dressing.
3. Apply an occlusive dressing to seal the wound. When possible, the dressing should be at least 2 inches wider than the wound. If there is an exit wound in the chest, apply an occlusive dressing over this wound, too. Create a flutter-valve dressing with one corner or side unsealed. These dressings will be discussed in detail later under the heading "Occlusive and Flutter-Valve Dressings."
4. Administer high-concentration oxygen.
5. Care for shock.
6. Transport as soon as possible. Unless other injuries prevent you from doing so, keep the patient positioned on the injured side. This allows the uninjured lung to expand without restriction.
7. Consider advanced life support intercept if it will not delay the patient's arrival at the hospital.

Occlusive and Flutter-Valve Dressings

Care for an open chest wound involves application of a dressing that will allow air to escape the chest cavity while preventing air from entering. These dressings—called occlusive, one-way, or flutter-valve dressings—usually involve taping the dressing in place and leaving a side or corner of the dressing unsealed (Figures 29-3 and 29-4). As the patient inhales, the dressing will seal the wound. As the patient exhales, the free corner or edge will act as a flutter valve to release air that is trapped in the chest cavity.

The danger of a *pneumothorax* developing into a *tension pneumothorax* (see the description of pneumothorax and tension pneumothorax under the heading "Injuries within the Chest Cavity") is the reason why medical authorities recommend the flutter-valve (three-sided) occlusive dressing instead of an occlusive dressing sealed on all four sides. If you find that blood or tissue begins to accumulate under the dressing and prevents air escape, you may need to briefly remove the dressing, wipe away the accumulated material, and reseal the dressing on three sides. Commercial devices, such as the Asherman Chest Seal, seal all the wound edges and have a valve that allows pressure relief.

You may have to maintain hand pressure over the occlusive dressing en route to the hospital. The tape also may not stick well to bloody skin or to skin that is sweaty from shock.

pneumothorax
air in the chest cavity.

tension pneumothorax
a type of pneumothorax in which air that enters the chest cavity is prevented from escaping.

FIGURE 29-3 Creating a flutter valve to allow air to escape from the chest cavity.

On inspiration, dressing seals wound, preventing air entry

Expiration allows trapped air to escape through untaped section of dressing

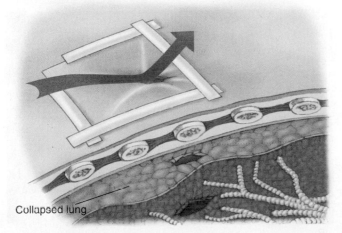

Collapsed lung

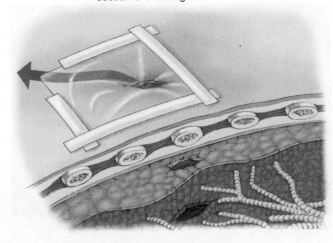

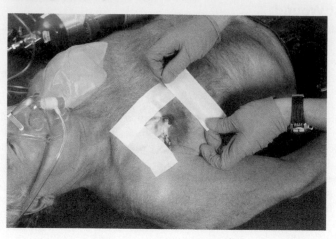

FIGURE 29-4 Seal three edges of an occlusive dressing for an open chest wound.

Note that if a commercial occlusive dressing is not available, you may have to improvise. Most ambulances carry sterile disposable items that are wrapped in plastic. The inside surface of the plastic is sterile. If you do not have an occlusive dressing, use one of these wrappers or the wrapper from an IV bag. Keep in mind that household plastic wrap is not thick enough to make an effective occlusive dressing for an open chest wound. If nothing else is available, household plastic or saran wrap can be used, but it must be folded several times to be of the proper thickness. Even then, it may fail. If there is no other choice, aluminum foil may be used to make the seal. Be careful, however, as foil edges may lacerate the patient's skin and may tear when lifted to release pressure.

A commercial alternative to taping an occlusive material over a sucking chest wound is the Asherman Chest Seal (Figure 29-5). Because it includes a one-way valve in its design, there is no need to leave an edge unsealed. To use it, quickly dry the skin around the wound and apply the seal's adhesive surface to the wound, being careful to center the device (and the one-way valve) over the wound. Once the valve is placed directly over the wound, air will be able to escape from the thoracic cavity but not enter it.

NOTE: *Once a chest wound is sealed, you must continue to monitor the patient and stay alert for complications. Even if you use a flutter valve or a commercial chest seal device, you still must monitor the patient for a buildup of pressure. The free corner or edge of the dressing may stick to the chest, blood may accumulate under the dressing, or the dressing may be drawn into the wound, causing the valve to fail.*

FIGURE 29-5 (A) An open chest wound from a gun shot. (B) An Asherman Chest Seal applied to the wound. *(Photos A and B: © Edward T. Dickinson, MD)*

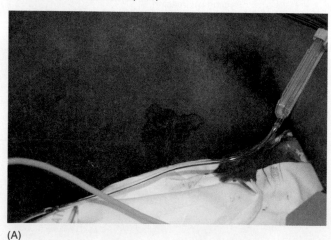

(A)

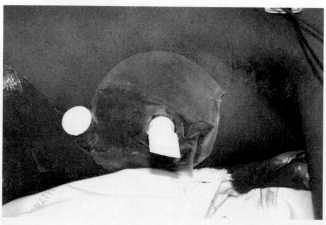

(B)

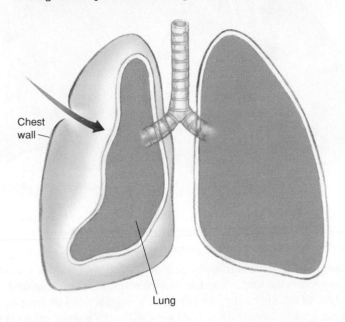

Chest wall

Lung

Injuries within the Chest Cavity

Because each of the organs inside the chest cavity is vital to life, any chest injury has the potential to be serious. Since, the blood vessels that run through the chest are the largest in the body, injury to these vessels is often fatal. In fact, the chest can hold over 3 liters of blood. It is possible to bleed to death within the chest cavity and never spill a drop outside the body.

Since chest injuries have the potential to be serious—even fatal—it is important to describe some of the specific injuries that may occur within the chest cavity. The signs and symptoms of different chest injuries often overlap, so you may only be able to narrow the possibilities instead of determining the patient's exact problem. This is sufficient for you to assess and care for them effectively as described at the end of this section.

- **Pneumothorax and tension pneumothorax.** Pneumothorax occurs when air enters the chest cavity, possibly causing collapse of a lung. The air can enter through an external wound (Figure 29-6), the air may enter the cavity through a punctured lung, or both events may occur. Tension pneumothorax, which is most often found with a closed chest injury or after a sealed occlusive dressing has been applied to an open chest wound, is especially critical. The lung may be punctured by a broken rib or other cause. If there is no opening to the outside of the chest, air that leaks from the lung has no avenue of escape. It builds up in the chest cavity and puts pressure on the heart, great blood vessels, and the unaffected lung, reducing cardiac output and the lungs' ability to oxygenate the blood.

  Patients with pneumothorax will have diminished or absent lung sounds on the affected side. As the pneumothorax progresses to a tension pneumothorax, the jugular veins in the neck may become distended (unless blood volume is low). Signs of shock will also be present. The trachea may shift to the opposite side but this is a very late sign and one which is difficult to detect.

- **Hemothorax and hemopneumothorax** (Figure 29-7). Hemothorax is a condition in which the chest cavity fills with blood. With hemopneumothorax, the chest cavity fills with both blood and air. It is easy to compare these two complications with pneumothorax if you remember that *pneumo* means "air" and *hemo* means "blood." In pneumothorax, there is a buildup of air in the thorax. In hemothorax and hemopneumothorax, blood creates or adds to the pressure.

  Hemothorax can be caused when lacerations within the chest cavity are produced by penetrating objects or fractured ribs. Blood will flow into the space around the lung, the lung may collapse, and the patient will experience a loss of blood, leading to shock.

FIGURE 29-7 Pneumothorax, hemothorax, and hemopneumothorax.

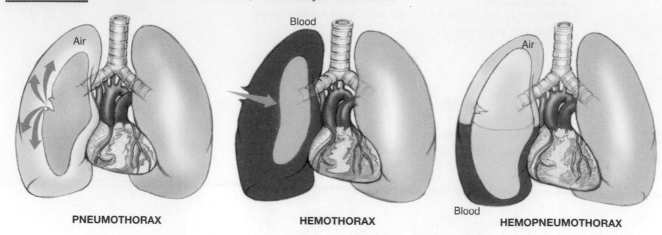

Air

Blood

Air

Blood

PNEUMOTHORAX   **HEMOTHORAX**   **HEMOPNEUMOTHORAX**

Hemopneumothorax involves a combination of blood and air that usually produces the same results: a collapsed lung and loss of blood leading to shock.

Patients with hemothorax usually present with signs of shock.

- **Traumatic asphyxia.** Traumatic asphyxia is associated with sudden compression of the chest. When this occurs, the sternum and the ribs exert severe pressure on the heart and lungs, forcing blood out of the right atrium and up into the jugular veins in the neck. The pressure of the blood being forced into the head and neck will usually result in blood vessels in and near the skin rupturing, causing extensive bruising of the face and neck (Figure 29-8).

  Patients with traumatic asphyxia present with a mechanism of injury that can cause compression of the chest. The patient's neck and face will be a darker color than the rest of the body (red, purple, or blue). Depending on the amount of pressure and how long the pressure was exerted on the torso, the patient may also have bulging eyes, distended neck veins, and broken blood vessels in the face.

- **Cardiac tamponade.** When an injury to the heart causes blood to flow into the surrounding pericardial sac, the condition produced is cardiac tamponade. The heart's unyielding sac fills with blood and compresses the chambers of the heart to a point where they will no longer adequately fill, backing up blood into the veins. This is usually the result of penetrating trauma like a stab wound. The pericardium is very tough, with limited ability to quickly stretch. It is also "self-sealing," in that little or no blood will be able to escape when the heart is lacerated.

  Patients who experience cardiac tamponade will usually have distended neck veins. The patient will exhibit signs of shock and a narrowed pulse pressure.

FIGURE 29-8 A patient suffering traumatic asphyxia.
(© Edward T. Dickinson, MD)

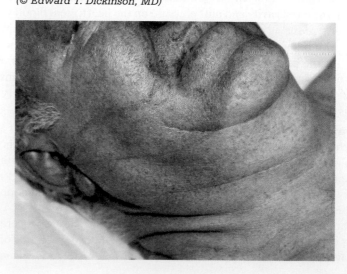

- **Aortic injury and dissection.** Trauma can also cause injury to the aorta, the largest artery in the body. Damage to this large, high-pressure vessel causes massive, often fatal bleeding. Penetrating trauma can cause direct damage to the aorta. Blunt trauma, such as deceleration from a severe motor-vehicle collision (e.g., head-on), can sever or tear the aorta.

  The aorta can also be damaged without trauma. Degeneration of the aorta, often worsened by high blood pressure or other diseases, causes weakening of this large vessel. Aortic dissection is a condition where the inner layer of the wall of the aorta begins to tear. Blood from the interior of the vessel leaks into the outer layers and eventually causes a balloon-like protrusion, called an *aneurysm*. As pressure builds in the aneurysm, there is an increased risk of rupture, leading to the patient's death. The aorta runs from the left ventricle through the chest and abdomen, and these injuries can occur anywhere along its path.

  The patient with an aortic injury may complain of pain in the chest, abdomen, or back—depending on the injury's location. The patient will often exhibit signs of shock. The patient may have differences in pulse or blood pressure between the right and left arms (in proximal aortic injury) or differences in pulses between the arms and the legs or the legs themselves (in abdominal aortic injury). In thin patients or those with a large aneurysm in the abdomen, the aneurysm may occasionally be palpated. Other than routine abdominal palpation, however, you should not probe the abdomen specifically for aneurysms, as it may cause injury to the patient, such as rupture of the aorta.

  Commotio cordis is an uncommon condition that is easy to recognize and treat. When someone gets hit in the center of the chest, the result is usually a bruise or even perhaps a fracture. In *commotio cordis* (Latin for commotion or disturbance of the heart), however, the impact occurs just when the heart is vulnerable. There are several hundredths of a second during each heartbeat when the heart, if sufficiently stimulated, will go into ventricular fibrillation (VF). A patient in *commotio cordis* experiences this condition. An example of this is the young athlete who tries to catch a baseball, but misses. The ball strikes him in the center of the chest and the patient collapses in cardiac arrest.

  If you obtain a history like this with a young patient, treat the patient like any other patient in ventricular fibrillation. Do *not* treat the patient as a trauma patient, delaying defibrillation because of the concern about internal blood loss. If the patient receives defibrillation and CPR quickly enough, the patient has a very good chance of survival. He usually has a very healthy heart that will respond well to CPR and defibrillation.

PATIENT ASSESSMENT

Injuries within the Chest Cavity

The following are common signs of pneumothorax:

- Respiratory difficulty
- Uneven chest wall movement
- Reduction of breath sounds on the affected side of the chest (listen with stethoscope)

Signs of tension pneumothorax include those items in the previous list plus:

- Increasing respiratory difficulty
- Indications of developing shock, including rapid, weak pulse; cyanosis; and low blood pressure due to decreased cardiac output
- Distended neck veins
- Tracheal deviation to the uninjured side (which is a late sign and difficult to observe)
- Reduced or absent breath sounds on the affected side of the chest

The following signs may commonly indicate a hemothorax:

- Signs of pneumothorax plus coughed-up frothy red blood

The following are common potential signs of traumatic asphyxia:

- Distended neck veins
- Head, neck, and shoulders appearing dark blue or purple
- Bloodshot and bulging eyes
- Swollen and blue tongue and lips
- Chest deformity

The following are common signs of cardiac tamponade:

- Distended neck veins
- Very weak pulse
- Low blood pressure
- Steadily decreasing pulse pressure (Pulse pressure is the difference between systolic and diastolic readings.)

The following are common signs of aortic injury or dissection:

- Tearing chest pain radiating to the back
- Differences in pulse or blood pressure between the right and left extremities or between the arms and legs
- Palpable pulsating mass (if the abdominal aorta is involved)
- Cardiac arrest

PATIENT CARE

Injuries within the Chest Cavity

The treatment is the same for all of the previously noted types of injuries within the chest cavity:

1. Maintain an open airway. Be prepared to apply suction.
2. Administer high-concentration oxygen.
3. Follow local protocols as to the preferred type of dressing for any open wound.
4. Care for shock.
5. Transport as soon as possible.
6. Consider ALS intercept if it will not delay the patient's arrival at the hospital. ALS personnel can perform procedures such as chest decompression that can greatly benefit a patient suffering from certain chest injury complications.

CRITICAL DECISION MAKING

What's the Likely Cause?

For each of the following patient presentations, determine what you believe is the likely cause:

1. You are called to a man who was jogging when he suddenly had a sharp pain in his right chest. He has difficulty breathing but is oriented, and he is in pain that changes when he breathes. He has diminished lung sounds in the upper right chest.

2. Your patient was stabbed in the right side of his chest. He is hypotensive, has distended neck veins, has no lung sounds on the right side of his chest, and has diminished sounds on the left side of his chest.

3. Your patient was shot in the chest near the 4th intercostal space on the left side. He has hypotension, distended neck veins, narrowing pulse pressure, and adequate lung sounds on both sides of the chest.

● CORE CONCEPT

Understanding abdominal injuries and emergency care for abdominal injuries

evisceration (e-vis-er-AY-shun)

an intestine or other internal organ protruding through a wound in the abdomen.

ABDOMINAL INJURIES

Abdominal injuries can be open or closed, with a closed injury usually caused by blunt trauma. Internal bleeding can be severe if organs and major blood vessels are lacerated or ruptured. Very serious and painful reactions can occur when the hollow organs are ruptured and their contents leak into the abdominal cavity. Penetrating wounds to the abdomen can be caused by objects such as knives, ice picks, arrows, and the broken glass and twisted metal of vehicular collisions and structural accidents. Very serious penetrating wounds can be caused by bullets, even when the bullet is small caliber. Open wounds of the abdomen may be so large and deep that organs protrude through the wound opening. This is known as an *evisceration* (Figure 29-9).

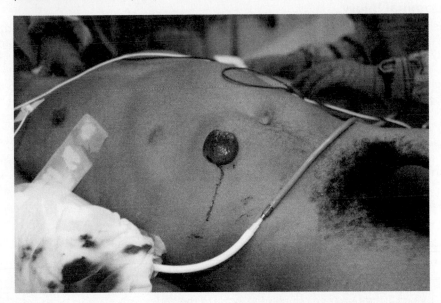

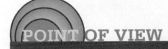
POINT OF VIEW

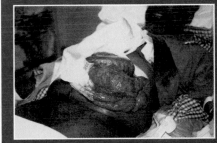

"I was bringing in a patient with an altered mental status from a nursing home when our Medical Director called me over to one of the big trauma bays. She asked me if I had ever seen an evisceration. I said 'You mean . . . ,' and she smiled and motioned me inside. I am a pretty new EMT. I'm glad I saw it there at the hospital before I saw it on the street. It was like amazing and gross at the same time. She showed me how delicate the tissue is and why we handle the exposed organs gently. You certainly don't see that all the time."

(© Edward T. Dickinson)

A more common condition than an evisceration is blunt trauma to one or more abdominal organs. The liver is the most commonly injured organ because of its relatively large size and position in the upper right quadrant and under the lowermost ribs on the right side. The liver is very vascular; therefore, when it is injured, it can bleed profusely, often to the point of life-threatening blood loss. Another very vascular organ is the spleen, located in the left upper quadrant and under the lowermost ribs on the left. Like the liver, the spleen can produce life-threatening blood loss.

The diaphragm is occasionally injured, from either blunt trauma or penetrating trauma. If there is a sudden severe force applied to the abdomen, that pressure can be posteriorly and superiorly transmitted. This can be so great that the diaphragm partially detaches, allowing abdominal contents to enter the thoracic cavity. A penetrating injury like a stab wound can also injure the diaphragm. If the resulting wound is significant, abdominal contents can enter the thoracic cavity in this manner, too.

Hollow organs in the abdomen include the stomach, small and large bowel, gallbladder, and urinary bladder. If these organs are injured, they often spill their contents into the abdominal cavity, leading to severe irritation and often peritonitis. This can cause the abdominal muscles to involuntarily contract, leading to rigidity of the abdominal wall.

Retroperitoneal organs, located in the posterior abdomen, are less commonly injured than the organs inside the peritoneal cavity. The pancreas, for instance, lies across the spine. Unless a knife or bullet hits it or there is significant force to the center of the abdomen, this organ is rarely injured. The kidneys are also retroperitoneal, with protection from the muscles of the back and the lower ribs that cover their superior portion. If a kidney is injured, it is usually from a direct blow.

Information on abdominal emergencies from medical causes may be found in Chapter 24, "Abdominal Emergencies."

Abdominal Injury

Gunshot wounds without exit wounds can cause serious abdominal damage, just as those with exit wounds do. A misconception about bullet wounds is that internal damage can be easily assessed. On the contrary, any projectile entering the body can be deflected, or it can explode and send out pieces in many directions (Figure 29-10). Do not believe that only the structures directly under the entrance wound have been injured. Also, keep in mind that the bullet's pathway between the entrance wound and exit wound is seldom a straight line.

Further complicating the problem, penetrating abdominal wounds can be associated with wounds in adjacent areas of the body. For example, a bullet can enter the chest cavity, pierce the diaphragm, and cause widespread damage in the abdomen. A complete patient assessment is essential in determining the probable extent of injuries. Always assess for an exit wound.

The following are some common signs and symptoms of abdominal injury:

- Pain, often starting as mild pain then rapidly becoming intolerable
- Cramps
- Nausea
- Weakness
- Thirst
- Obvious lacerations and puncture wounds to the abdomen
- Lacerations and puncture wounds to the pelvis and middle and lower back or chest wounds near the diaphragm
- Indications of blunt trauma, such as a large bruised area or an intense bruise on the abdomen
- Indications of developing shock, including restlessness; pale, cool, and clammy skin; rapid shallow breathing; a rapid pulse; and low blood pressure (Sometimes patients with abdominal injury who are in extreme pain show an initial elevated blood pressure.)
- Coughing up or vomiting blood; the vomitus may contain a substance that looks like coffee grounds (partially digested blood)
- Rigid and/or tender abdomen, which the patient tries to protect (guarded abdomen)
- Distended abdomen

FIGURE 29-10 X-ray showing two bullets that entered the patient's abdomen on the right side (at the paper clips), and then fragmented throughout the abdomen. *(© Edward T. Dickinson, MD)*

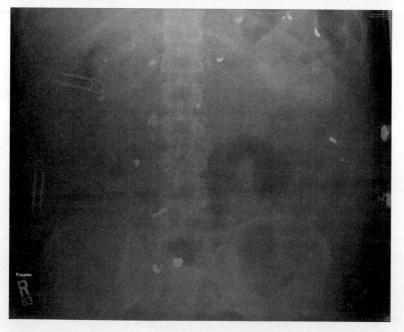

- Patient who tries to lie very still, with the legs drawn up, in an effort to reduce the tension on the abdominal muscles

Decision Points

- Does my patient have an abdominal injury that must be treated during the primary assessment?
- Does my patient have an open abdominal injury that requires an occlusive dressing?
- Does my patient have an injury or injuries that require minimal scene time and prompt transport to a trauma center?

Inside/Outside

THE PATH OF THE BULLET

A patient who has gunshot wounds in the lower ribs and at the same level in the back may appear to have a chest wound. In reality, you need to treat him for both a chest wound and an abdominal wound. It is obvious that the bullet may have penetrated the lung, but since the spleen and liver are posterior to the lowermost left and right ribs, you must assume they may have been injured at the same time. If the patient was inhaling deeply when he was shot (resulting in the abdominal organs taking up less space in the chest), the spleen and liver may not have been in the direct path of the bullet. But bullets often take paths that are not straight. If the bullet tumbled or produced cavitation, the spleen or liver may very well have sustained serious injury. You will need to be alert to the possibility of both a chest and an abdominal injury.

PATIENT CARE

Abdominal Injury

Some emergency care steps apply to both closed and open abdominal injuries. However, other additional care steps are necessary for open abdominal injuries.

For both closed and open abdominal injuries:

1. Stay alert for vomiting and keep the airway open
2. Place the patient on his back, legs flexed at the knees, to reduce pain by relaxing abdominal muscles.
3. Administer high-concentration oxygen.
4. Care for shock.
5. Apply the PASG, if protocols allow. Many EMS systems do not use the pneumatic anti-shock garment (PASG), but if you work in one that does, and if the garment is indicated according to local protocols, you should apply the anti-shock garment.
6. Give nothing to the patient by mouth. This could induce vomiting or pass through open wounds in the esophagus, stomach, or intestine and enter the abdominal cavity.
7. Constantly monitor vital signs.
8. Transport as soon as possible.

Additional steps for open abdominal injuries:

9. Control external bleeding and dress all open wounds.
10. Do not touch or try to replace any eviscerated, or exposed, organs. Apply a sterile dressing moistened with sterile saline over the wound site. Some EMS systems may recommend that you apply an occlusive dressing as well. It may be necessary to re-moisten the dressings with additional saline in order to ensure that the eviscerated organ or organs do not dry out. In cases of large eviscerations, maintain warmth by placing layers of bulky dressing over the moistened dressing (Scan 29-1).
11. Do not remove any impaled objects. Stabilize impaled objects with bulky dressings that are bandaged in place. Leave the patient's legs in the position in which you found them to avoid muscular movement that may move the impaled object.

NOTE: *Do not use aluminum foil as an occlusive dressing. Foil has been known to cut eviscerated organs.*

FIRST TAKE STANDARD PRECAUTIONS.
Cover the dressed wound to maintain warmth. Secure the covering with tape or cravats tied above and below the position of the exposed organ.

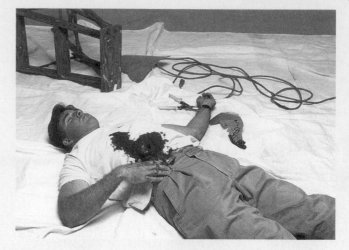

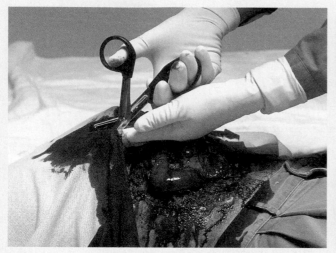

Open abdominal wound with evisceration.

1 Cut away clothing from the wound.

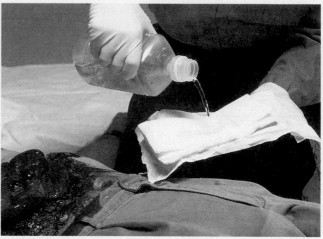

2 Soak a sterile dressing with sterile saline.

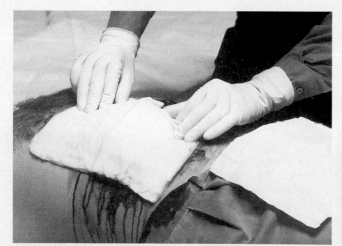

3 Place the moist dressing over the wound. It may be necessary to remoisten the dressing with additional sterile saline to keep the eviscerated organ or organs from drying out.

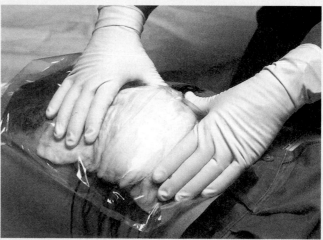

4 Apply an occlusive dressing over the moist dressing if your local protocols recommend taking this action.

CHAPTER REVIEW

Key Facts and Concepts

- An open chest or abdominal wound is considered to be one that penetrates not only the skin but also the chest or abdominal wall to expose internal organs. Open chest and abdominal wounds are life threatening. For an open chest or abdominal wound, apply an occlusive dressing. For both open and closed injuries, take appropriate Standard Precautions; note the mechanism of injury; protect the patient's airway and breathing; administer high-concentration oxygen by nonrebreather mask; treat for shock; and transport.

- A flail chest is characterized by paradoxical motion. If the patient is unable to adequately breathe, assist the patient's ventilations.

- Seal an open chest wound with an occlusive dressing taped on three sides or in some other manner so that it acts as a one-way valve, allowing air out of the chest, but not in. Alternatively, use a commercial device such as the Asherman Chest Seal with a one-way valve to relieve pressure. Monitor the patient for changes and be prepared to manually relieve any pressure in the chest.

- Closed chest wounds are sometimes difficult to distinguish or may occur together. Assess the patient, including breath sounds, and maintain ventilation, oxygenation, and perfusion.

- A patient who collapses in cardiac arrest after a force is applied to the center of his chest should receive CPR and defibrillation like any other arrest from a cardiac cause.

- If a patient develops signs of a tension pneumothorax, arrange immediately for an ALS intercept or transport promptly to a facility that can treat this injury.

- When solid abdominal organs are injured, life-threatening amounts of blood loss can occur.

- When hollow abdominal organs are injured, their contents spill into the abdominal cavity and cause irritation and peritonitis.

Key Decisions

- Is the patient's breathing adequate, inadequate, or absent?
- Is the patient displaying signs of shock?
- Is there an open wound in the chest that needs to be sealed?
- Is the patient displaying signs of a tension pneumothorax?
- Is there an open wound in the abdomen that needs to be dressed and covered?

Chapter Glossary

evisceration (e-vis-er-AY-shun) an intestine or other internal organ protruding through a wound in the abdomen.

flail chest fracture of two or more adjacent ribs in two or more places that allows for free movement of the fractured segment.

paradoxical motion movement of ribs in a flail segment that is opposite to the direction of movement of the rest of the chest cavity.

pneumothorax air in the chest cavity.

sucking chest wound an open chest wound in which air is "sucked" into the chest cavity.

tension pneumothorax a type of pneumothorax in which air that enters the chest cavity is prevented from escaping.

Preparation for Your Examination and Practice

Short Answer

1. What signs and symptoms would alert you that your patient has a flail chest?
2. What are the differences between a pneumothorax and a tension pneumothorax?
3. Describe the care for an open wound to the chest.
4. Describe the care for an open abdominal wound.

Thinking and Linking

Think back to Chapter 2, "The Well-Being of the EMT," as you consider the following question:

- What Standard Precautions are required for the following calls?

1. An open wound in the chest that makes a sucking noise when the patient breathes
2. A patient with paradoxical motion in the lower left ribs
3. An evisceration of the abdomen with bowel visible

Think back to Chapter 1, "Introduction to Emergency Medical Services and the Health Care System," and the discussion of specialized trauma and other treatment centers under the heading "Components of the EMS System," as you consider the following question:

- Which specialty centers should the following patients be transported to (if the center is available in your region)?

1. A patient with a collapsed lung
2. A patient with suspected internal bleeding and trauma

Critical Thinking Exercises

Chest trauma can be difficult to assess and treat in the emergency setting. The purpose of this exercise will be to consider assessment and care for one severe chest injury.

- You have been caring for a patient who was shot in the chest with a nail gun, and have applied an occlusive dressing around the wound. The patient is now suddenly beginning to deteriorate. He is having extreme difficulty breathing and his color has worsened. Breath sounds have become almost totally absent on the side with the impaled nail. What complication might you suspect is causing his worsening condition? How could this be corrected?

Pathophysiology to Practice

The following questions are designed to assist you in gathering relevant clinical information and making accurate decisions in the field.

1. Your patient, who sustained a blunt injury to the chest, is starting to have more difficulty breathing and his respirations are not as deep as they were originally. What factors should you consider in deciding whether to ventilate him? What condition might you cause if you ventilate him?

2. A 64-year-old male is tachycardic, pale, sweaty, and hypotensive. The only injury he has sustained was when he fell 2 days ago and struck his lower left ribs hard on some furniture. He hasn't been feeling well since then, but today he felt much worse. What injured organ is most likely the cause of his condition? Why did it take so long for the patient to develop shock?

Street Scenes

At the scene of a collision between two cars at an intersection, you find a 30-year-old male who was the driver of the car that was hit on the driver's door. He is able to tell you that his chest hurts "very bad" and that he has slight difficulty breathing. His skin is slightly pale and sweaty, he answers questions appropriately, and he is holding his arm across his lower chest.

Street Scene Questions

1. What is your general impression of this patient?
2. What priority would you assign to him?
3. What interventions are appropriate at this time?

Your general impression is of a 30-year-old male who appears to be injured. Your primary assessment reveals normal mental status, an open airway, slightly labored but adequate breathing and a weak, rapid radial pulse, with no external bleeding visible. You assign him a high priority for now, with the understanding that you may change his priority later.

You apply a cervical collar and begin administering oxygen by nonrebreather mask. You also coordinate extrication activities with the fire department on the scene.

Assessment of the patient reveals significant tenderness over the middle ribs on the left side. Breath sounds are difficult to hear because of the noise of the extrication equipment. His upper abdomen on the left side is a little tender but not guarded or rigid.

Street Scene Questions

4. Would you change the priority of transport of this patient based on what you now know? Why or why not?
5. What interventions are appropriate for this patient?

You decide this patient is still a high priority, because he is at high risk for internal bleeding in the chest, the abdomen, or both. You would like to get him out of the car as soon as possible, because one of the most important interventions is prompt transport to a hospital capable of taking care of a serious trauma patient. If advanced life support is available, you will call for it. You continue administration of oxygen by nonrebreather mask and monitor the patient for signs of fatigue that might indicate a need for assisted ventilations.

Your partner obtains a pulse of 116, blood pressure 110/80, and respirations 22 and shallow. His oxygen saturation is 99 percent.

As soon as the patient is free from entanglement in the wreckage, you perform a rapid extrication and get him onto a backboard. En route to the hospital, you reevaluate the patient and find that, although you have found no new injuries, his chest pain is getting worse and he is having more difficulty breathing. As you approach the hospital, you observe that his respirations are becoming shallower. They are still adequate by the time you arrive at the emergency department, but you can see a clear trend in the patient's condition that will require treatment soon.

You advise the trauma team of your observation as you give your report and turn over care of the patient.

Musculoskeletal Trauma

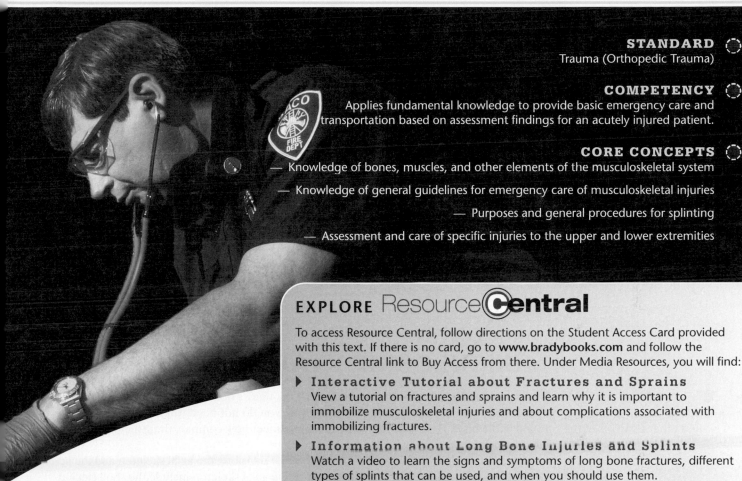

STANDARD
Trauma (Orthopedic Trauma)

COMPETENCY
Applies fundamental knowledge to provide basic emergency care and transportation based on assessment findings for an acutely injured patient.

CORE CONCEPTS
— Knowledge of bones, muscles, and other elements of the musculoskeletal system
— Knowledge of general guidelines for emergency care of musculoskeletal injuries
— Purposes and general procedures for splinting
— Assessment and care of specific injuries to the upper and lower extremities

EXPLORE Resource Central

To access Resource Central, follow directions on the Student Access Card provided with this text. If there is no card, go to **www.bradybooks.com** and follow the Resource Central link to Buy Access from there. Under Media Resources, you will find:

▶ **Interactive Tutorial about Fractures and Sprains**
View a tutorial on fractures and sprains and learn why it is important to immobilize musculoskeletal injuries and about complications associated with immobilizing fractures.

▶ **Information about Long Bone Injuries and Splints**
Watch a video to learn the signs and symptoms of long bone fractures, different types of splints that can be used, and when you should use them.

▶ **Application of a Sager Splint**
Learn how to properly apply a Sager splint and what you should do before applying this splint.

OBJECTIVES

After reading this chapter you should be able to:

30.1 Define key terms introduced in this chapter.

30.2 Describe the anatomy of elements of the musculoskeletal system. (pp. 696–702, 703–704)

30.3 Associate mechanisms of injury with the potential for musculoskeletal injuries. (p. 702)

30.4 Describe the four types of musculoskeletal injury (fracture, dislocation, sprain, and strain) and define open and closed extremity injuries. (p. 706)

30.5 Discuss the assessment of musculoskeletal injuries, including compartment syndrome. (pp. 707–709)

30.6 Discuss the general care of musculoskeletal injuries. (pp. 709–712)

30.7 Describe specific consideraitons for splinting. (pp. 712–716, 728–743)

30.8 Discuss considerations in the assessment and management of specific types of injuries, including:
a. Shoulder girdle injuries (pp. 717–718)
b. Pelvic injuries (pp. 718–720)
c. Hip dislocation (pp. 720–721)
d. Hip fracture (pp. 721–723)
e. Femoral shaft fracture (pp. 723–724)
f. Knee injury (p. 724)
g. Tibia or fibula injury (pp. 725–726)
h. Ankle or foot injury (pp. 726–727)

angulated fracture, *p. 706*
bones, *p. 696*
cartilage, *p. 702*
closed extremity injury,
  p. 706
comminuted fracture, *p. 706*

compartment syndrome,
  p. 708
crepitus, *p. 708*
dislocation, *p. 706*
extremities, *p. 696*
fracture, *p. 706*

greenstick fracture, *p. 706*
joints, *p. 696*
ligaments, *p. 702*
manual traction, *p. 710*
muscles, *p. 702*
open extremity injury, *p. 706*

sprain, *p. 706*
strain, *p. 706*
tendons, *p. 702*
traction splint, *p. 705*

Musculoskeletal injuries are common. As an EMT, you will be called upon to treat injuries to muscles and bones, which range from minor to life threatening. Many musculoskeletal injuries can have a grotesque appearance. When called upon to fully evaluate the patient, do not be distracted from life-threatening conditions by a deformed limb.

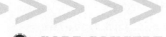

MUSCULOSKELETAL SYSTEM

CORE CONCEPT

Knowledge of bones, muscles, and other elements of the musculoskeletal system

The musculoskeletal system is composed of all the body's bones, joints, and muscles, as well as cartilage, tendons, and ligaments. As an EMT, you do not need to know every structure found in the body. However, you do need to remember how complex the structures are and what kinds of damage may be done in case of injury.

Review the skeleton (Figure 30-1) and its major divisions, the axial skeleton and the appendicular skeleton (Figure 30-2). The bones of the axial skeleton include the skull (including the cranium and face), the sternum, the ribs, and the spine including the cervical, thoracic, and lumbar vertebrae, the sacrum, and the coccyx (Figure 30-3).

In this chapter, we will pay special attention to the appendicular skeleton, particularly the **extremities** —the upper extremities (clavicles, scapulae, arms, wrists, and hands) and the lower extremities (pelvis, thighs, legs, ankles, and feet) (Figure 30-4).

Anatomy of Bone

Bones are formed of dense connective tissue. As components of the skeleton, they provide the body's framework. They need to be strong to provide support and protection for the internal organs, but they also need to be somewhat flexible to withstand stress. The bones store salts and metabolic materials and provide a site for the production of red blood cells. Because of this, bones are very vascular—that is, they contain a rich supply of blood. It is important to know this because, simply stated, bones bleed. Although broken bone ends may cause damage to surrounding tissue and blood vessels, the bones themselves also bleed. This is why a patient with a fractured pelvis, hip, or femur—or multiple fractures—may actually develop shock from blood loss from the bone itself.

Joints are the places where bones articulate, or meet, and are a critical element in the body's ability to move.

Generally, bones are classified according to their appearance—long, short, flat, and irregular (Figure 30-5). The bones found in the arm and thigh are examples of long bones. The

extremities (ex-TREM-i-teez)
the portions of the skeleton that include the clavicles, scapulae, arms, wrists, and hands (upper extremities) and the pelvis, thighs, legs, ankles, and feet (lower extremities).

bones
hard but flexible living structures that provide support for the body and protection to vital organs.

joints
places where bones articulate, or meet.

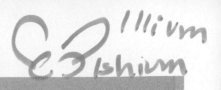

FIGURE 30-1 Human skeleton.

Skeletal System

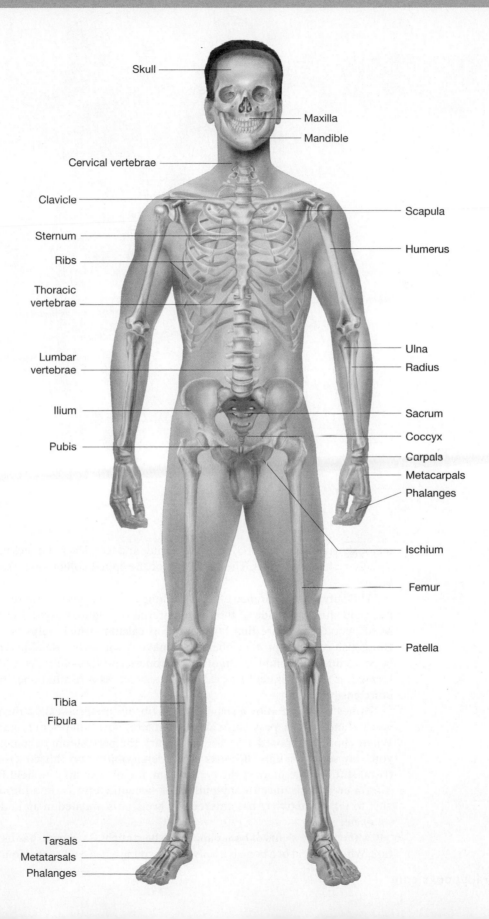

Skull

Maxilla

Mandible

Cervical vertebrae

Clavicle

Scapula

Sternum

Humerus

Ribs

Thoracic vertebrae

Lumbar vertebrae

Ulna

Radius

Ilium

Sacrum

Coccyx

Pubis

Carpals

Metacarpals

Phalanges

Ischium

Femur

Patella

Tibia

Fibula

Tarsals

Metatarsals

Phalanges

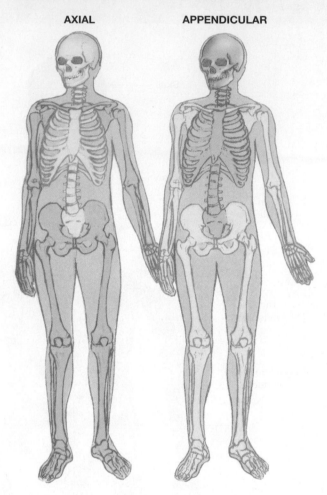

FIGURE 30-2 Highlighted in pink: The axial skeleton comprises the skull, spine, ribs, and sternum. The extremities comprise the appendicular skeleton.

AXIAL   APPENDICULAR

major short bones of the body are in the hands and feet. The flat bones include the sternum, shoulder blades, and ribs. The vertebrae of the spinal column are examples of irregular bones.

The outward appearance of a typical long bone creates the impression that it is a simple, rigid structure made of the same material throughout. Actually, it is quite complex. Most people are aware that bone contains calcium, which helps to make it very hard. Bone also contains protein fibers that make it somewhat flexible. The strength of our bones is due to a combination of this hardness and flexibility. As we age, less protein is formed in the bones, and less calcium is stored. As a result, bones become brittle and more easily break.

Bones are covered by a strong, white, fibrous material called the *periosteum*. Blood vessels and nerves pass through this membrane as they enter and leave the bone. When bone is exposed as a result of injury, the periosteum becomes visible. Although you may see fragments of bones and foreign objects on this covering, do not remove them. If they have pierced the periosteum, the objects may be held firmly in place and offer a great resistance to any pulling or sweeping efforts. In addition, you will not be able to tell if the object has entered the bone or is impaled in an underlying blood vessel or nerve.

Although the shafts of bones appear to be straight, each bone has its own unique curvature. When the end of a bone is involved in forming a ball-and-socket joint, it will be rounded

FIGURE 30-3 Bones of the axial skeleton.

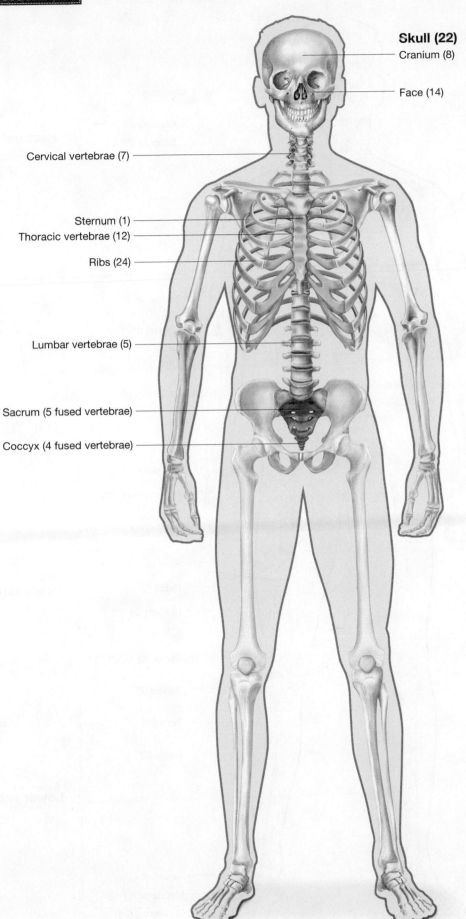

Skull (22)
Cranium (8)

Face (14)

Cervical vertebrae (7)

Sternum (1)
Thoracic vertebrae (12)
Ribs (24)

Lumbar vertebrae (5)

Sacrum (5 fused vertebrae)

Coccyx (4 fused vertebrae)

FIGURE 30-4 Bones of the appendicular skeleton.

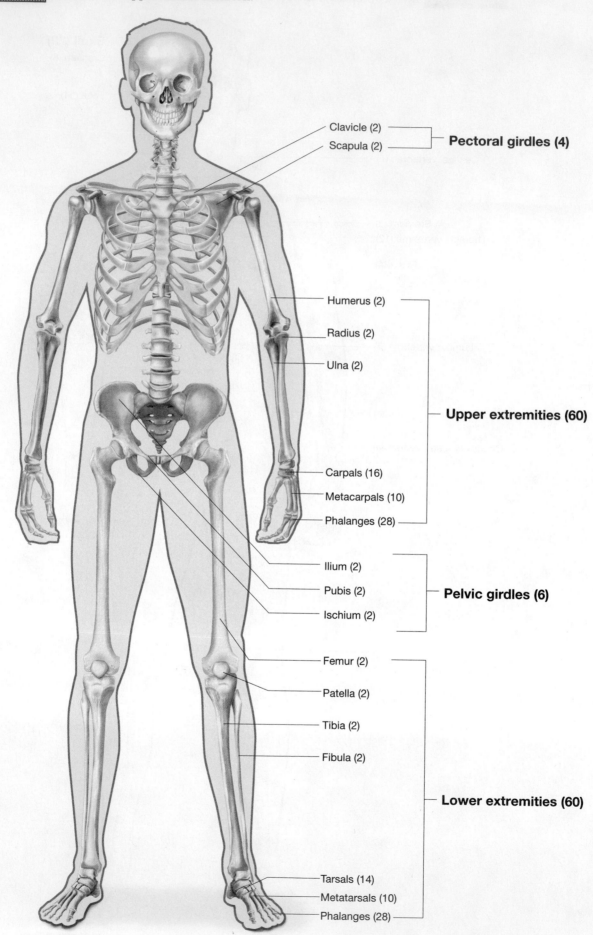

Clavicle (2)
Scapula (2)
Pectoral girdles (4)

Humerus (2)

Radius (2)

Ulna (2)

Upper extremities (60)

Carpals (16)

Metacarpals (10)

Phalanges (28)

Ilium (2)

Pubis (2)
Pelvic girdles (6)

Ischium (2)

Femur (2)

Patella (2)

Tibia (2)

Fibula (2)

Lower extremities (60)

Tarsals (14)

Metatarsals (10)

Phalanges (28)

FIGURE 30-5 Bones are classified by shape.

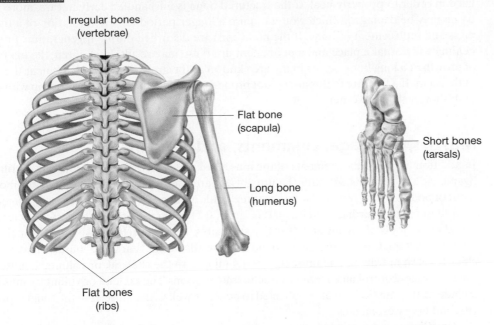

Irregular bones
(vertebrae)

Flat bone
(scapula)

Short bones
(tarsals)

Long bone
(humerus)

Flat bones
(ribs)

to allow for rotational movement. This rounded end, called the head of the bone, is connected to the shaft by the neck. Bone marrow, which is contained in the center of bones, is the site of red blood cell production.

Self-Healing Nature of Bone

The most common bone injury is a break, or fracture (Figure 30-6). The first effects of a bone injury are swelling of soft tissue and the formation of a blood clot in the area of the fracture. Both the swelling and the clotting are due to the destruction of blood vessels in the periosteum and the bone as well as to loss of blood from adjacent damaged vessels.

Interruption of the blood supply causes death to the cells at the injury site. Cells a little farther from the fracture remain intact and, within a few hours, begin to more rapidly divide. They soon grow together to form a mass of tissue that completely surrounds the fracture site. New bone is generated from this mass to eventually heal the damaged bone. The whole process can take weeks or months, depending on the bone that has been fractured, the type of fracture, and the patient's health and age.

FIGURE 30-6 (A) Open fracture and dislocation to the ankle. (B) X-ray of same injury. *(Photos A and B: © Edward T. Dickinson, MD)*

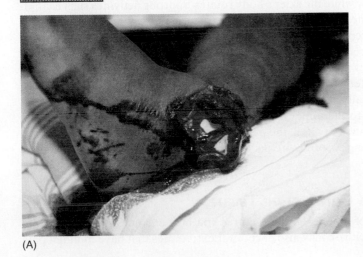

(A)

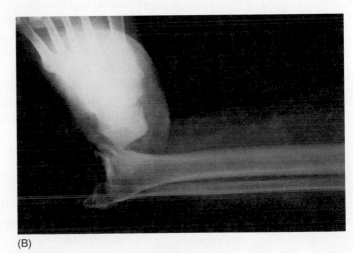

(B)

It is very important for a broken bone to be immobilized quickly and remain immobilized in order to properly heal. If the fractured bone is mishandled early in care, more soft tissue may be damaged, which would require a longer period for the formation of a tissue mass and replacement of bone. If the bone ends are disturbed during regeneration, proper healing will not take place and a permanent disability may result. In children, the majority of growth of a long bone occurs in the area known as the growth plate, which is near the end of the shaft. If a fracture in this area is not properly handled, the child may grow up with one limb shorter than the other.

Muscles, Cartilage, Ligaments, and Tendons

In addition to bones, the elements of the musculoskeletal system are the muscles, cartilage, ligaments, and tendons. *Muscles* (Figure 30-7A) are the tissues or fibers that cause movement of body parts or organs. There are three kinds of muscles: skeletal (voluntary), smooth (involuntary), and cardiac (myocardial) (Figure 30-7B). Smooth, or involuntary, muscles are found in the walls of organs and digestive structures. These muscles move food through the digestive system. Cardiac muscle is found in the walls of the heart. The muscles that are of chief concern in trauma and musculoskeletal injury are the skeletal, or voluntary, muscles. These muscles control all conscious or deliberate motions. The skeletal or voluntary muscles include all the muscles that are connected to bones as well as the muscles in the tongue, pharynx, and upper esophagus.

Cartilage is connective tissue that covers the outside of the bone end (epiphysis) and acts as a surface for articulation, allowing for smooth movement at joints. Cartilage, which is less rigid than bone, forms or helps to form some of the more flexible structures of the body, such as the septum of the nose (the wall between the nostrils), the external ear, the trachea, and the connections between the ribs and sternum (breastbone).

Tendons are bands of connective tissue that bind the muscles to bones. The tendons allow for the power of movement across the joints. *Ligaments* are connective tissues that support joints by attaching the bone ends and allowing for a stable range of motion. Two mnemonics can help you distinguish between the connective functions of tendons and ligaments: MTB = muscle-tendon-bone; BLB = bone-ligament-bone (Figure 30-8).

muscles
tissues or fibers that cause movement of body parts and organs.

cartilage
tough tissue that covers the joint ends of bones and helps to form certain body parts such as the ear.

tendons
tissues that connect muscle to bone.

ligaments
connective tissues that connect bone to bone.

GENERAL GUIDELINES FOR EMERGENCY CARE

Mechanisms of Musculoskeletal Injury

CORE CONCEPT
Knowledge of general guidelines for emergency care of musculoskeletal injuries

There are basically three types of mechanisms that cause musculoskeletal injuries: direct force, indirect force, and twisting force. An example of *direct force* is a person being struck by an automobile, causing crushed tissue and fractures. *Twisting or rotational forces* can cause stretching or tearing of muscles and ligaments, as well as broken bones, such as occur when a ski digs into the snow while the skier's body rotates. Sporting activities such as football, basketball, soccer, in-line skating, skiing, snowboarding, and wrestling—in addition to motor-vehicle collisions—account for many musculoskeletal injuries.

It is easy to see how direct forces cause injuries, but an *indirect force* can be just as powerful. For example, a well-known injury pattern occurs when people fall from heights and land on their feet. The direct forces cause injuries to the feet and ankles, whereas indirect forces usually cause injuries to the knees, femurs, pelvis, and spinal column. In fact, most injuries to the upper extremities are caused by forces applied to an outstretched arm. In the course of a fall, the person reaches out with an arm in an effort to break the fall and, in doing so, often breaks the radius, ulna, or clavicle, or dislocates the shoulder.

Injury to Bones and Connective Tissue

A fracture is the breaking of a bone. Some fractures you may encounter are grossly deformed and painful. However, you may also encounter extremities that have minimal pain

FIGURE 30-7 (A) The muscular system.

Muscular System

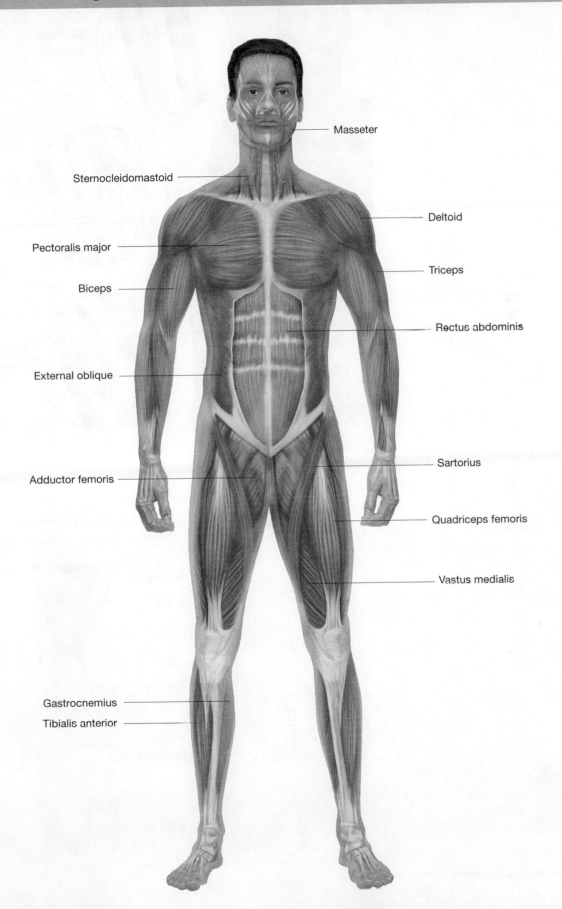

Masseter

Sternocleidomastoid

Deltoid

Pectoralis major

Triceps

Biceps

Rectus abdominis

External oblique

Sartorius

Adductor femoris

Quadriceps femoris

Vastus medialis

Gastrocnemius

Tibialis anterior

FIGURE 30-7 (B) Three types of muscle.

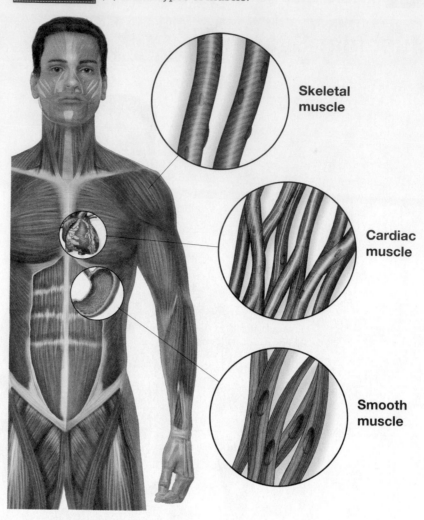

Skeletal muscle

Cardiac muscle

Smooth muscle

FIGURE 30-8 Tendons tie muscle to bone. Ligaments tie bone to bone.

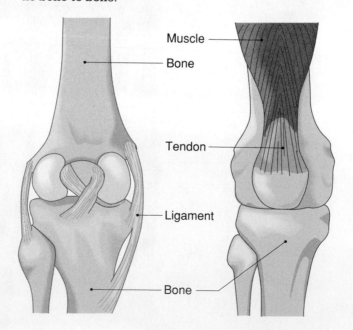

Muscle

Bone

Tendon

Ligament

Bone

and deformity but are, in fact, fractured. Unless there is a very obvious deformity, it is not possible or even important for you to decide if a patient's injury is a fracture, a dislocation, a sprain, or a severe bruise. Most patients simply present with pain, swelling, and—sometimes—deformity. It will take an X-ray or other imaging process to precisely diagnose the injury. In the field, therefore, the worst must be assumed, and a patient with signs and symptoms of a fracture—a painful, swollen, or deformed extremity—should be treated as though he has a fracture. Although most fractures are not life threatening, remember that bones are living tissue. Even in simple uncomplicated fractures, bones bleed. For example, a simple closed tibia-fibula fracture typically causes a 1-pint (500 cc) blood loss. Fractures of the femur typically cause a 2-pint (1,000 cc) blood loss, and pelvic fractures cause a 3- to 4-pint (1,500–2,000 cc) blood loss (Figure 30-9).

In World War I, the battlefield death rate from closed fractures of the femur was about 80 percent, because of complications such as blood loss. Two surgeons noticed that large muscle groups in the thigh go into spasms (contract, or shrink), forcing the broken femoral ends to override each other, injuring the blood vessels. To correct the problem, they invented the ***traction splint***, a splint that applies constant pull along the length of the leg to help stabilize the fractured bone and reduce muscle spasms. With early application of a traction splint, the mortality rate from femur fractures dropped to under 20 percent (and is much lower today).

Remember that splinting an extremity with a suspected fracture can prevent additional blood loss, pain, and complications from nerve and blood vessel injury. Therefore, treat for the worst (a fracture) and immobilize. Physicians in the hospital will diagnose the actual injury with an X-ray.

traction splint

a splint that applies constant pull along the length of a lower extremity to help stabilize the fractured bone and to reduce muscle spasm in the limb. Traction splints are used primarily on femoral shaft fractures.

FIGURE 30-9 Bones bleed. In fact, there may be considerable blood loss, even from an uncomplicated closed fracture.

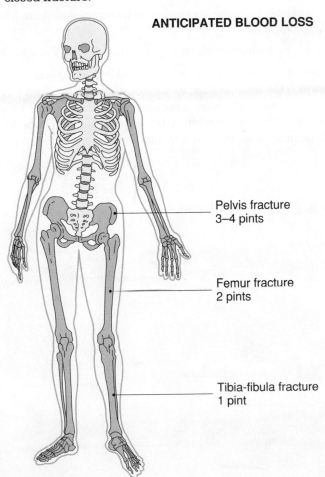

ANTICIPATED BLOOD LOSS

Pelvis fracture
3–4 pints

Femur fracture
2 pints

Tibia-fibula fracture
1 pint

FIGURE 30-10 (A) Open fracture. (B) Closed fracture. *(Photos A and B: © Edward T. Dickinson, MD)*

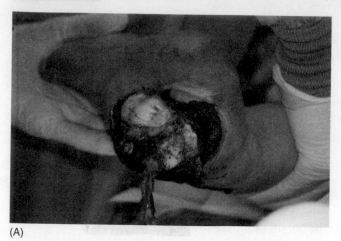
(A)

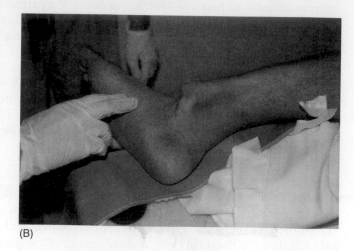
(B)

There are four types of musculoskeletal injury:

- **Fracture.** A fracture is any break in a bone. Fractures can be classified as open or closed (Figure 30-10), and are also classified by the way a bone is broken—***comminuted fractures*** if broken in several places (Figure 30-11), ***greenstick fractures*** if the break is incomplete (Figure 30-12), or ***angulated fractures*** if the broken bone is bent at an angle (Figure 30-13).
- **Dislocation.** The disruption or "coming apart" of a joint is called a dislocation (Figure 30-14). In order for a joint to dislocate, the soft tissue of the joint capsule and ligaments must be stretched beyond the normal range of motion and torn.
- **Sprain.** A sprain is caused by the stretching and tearing of ligaments. It is most commonly associated with joint injuries.
- **Strain.** A strain is a muscle injury caused by overstretching or overexertion of the muscle.

A ***closed extremity injury*** is one in which the skin is not broken. An ***open extremity injury*** is one in which the skin has been broken or torn through from the inside by the injured bone or from the outside by something that has caused a penetrating wound with associated injury to the bone. An open injury is a serious situation because of the increased likelihood of contamination and subsequent infection.

fracture (FRAK-cher)
any break in a bone.

comminuted fracture
a fracture in which the bone is broken in several places.

greenstick fracture
an incomplete fracture.

angulated fracture
fracture in which the broken bone segments are at an angle to each other.

dislocation
the disruption or "coming apart" of a joint.

sprain
the stretching and tearing of ligaments.

strain
muscle injury resulting from overstretching or overexertion of the muscle.

closed extremity injury
an injury to an extremity with no associated opening in the skin.

open extremity injury
an extremity injury in which the skin has been broken or torn through from the inside by an injured bone or from the outside by something that has caused a penetrating wound with associated injury to the bone..

FIGURE 30-11 Comminuted fracture.

FIGURE 30-12 Greenstick fracture.

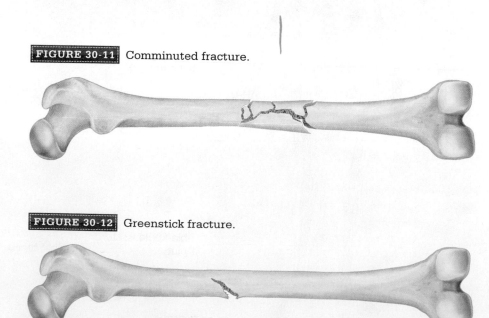

FIGURE 30-13 (A) A closed angulated fracture. (B) An X-ray of the same fracture. *(Photos A and B: © Edward T. Dickinson, MD)*

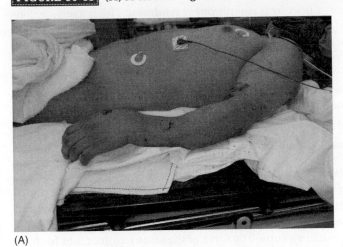

(A)

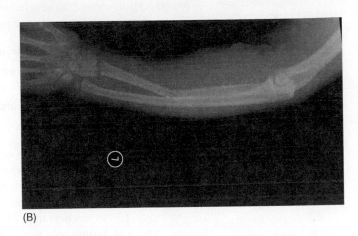

(B)

FIGURE 30-14 A right shoulder dislocation.
(© Edward T. Dickinson, MD)

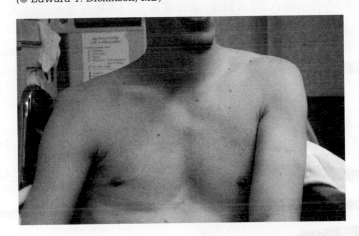

Although many closed injuries can be handled simply in the hospital emergency department, patients with open fractures require surgery. Proper splinting and prehospital care of musculoskeletal injuries help prevent closed injuries from becoming open ones.

Assessment of Musculoskeletal Injuries

Examination involves your senses and the skills of inspection (looking), palpation (feeling), and auscultation (listening). One of the basic principles of assessment is that it is difficult to do a proper examination on patients when they are fully clothed. However, it often is difficult, impractical, or inadvisable to completely disrobe or cut away a patient's clothing due to weather, the patient's modesty, or patient refusal. A good rule of thumb is to cut or remove clothing according to the environment and severity of the situation.

In cases of severe extremity trauma, injuries can be very obvious. However, when treating trauma patients, *your priority must be to rapidly identify and treat life-threatening conditions first.* Do not let a grotesque but relatively minor extremity injury sidetrack you—or the patient. The pain or terrible appearance of an extremity injury may distract the patient from awareness of other injuries or symptoms, such as abdominal pain from internal bleeding. Be sure to assess the patient fully and ask appropriate questions to avoid missing other injuries. Only after your primary assessment and rapid trauma assessment have ruled out obvious life-threatening airway, breathing, or circulation problems and injuries to the head, spine, chest, and abdomen should you focus your attention on musculoskeletal injuries to the extremities.

Compartment Syndrome

compartment syndrome
injury caused when tissues such as blood vessels and nerves are constricted within a space as from swelling or from a tight dressing or cast.

A critical complication of extremity fracture is *compartment syndrome*. This is a serious condition caused by severe swelling in the extremity—in this case, as the result of a fracture. Compartment syndrome progresses as follows:

1. A fracture or crush injury causes bleeding and swelling within the extremity.

2. Pressure and swelling caused by the bleeding within the muscle compartment becomes so great that the body can no longer perfuse the tissues against the pressure.

3. Cellular damage occurs and causes additional swelling.

4. Blood flow to the area is lost. The limb itself may be lost if the pressure is not relieved.

Signs and symptoms of compartment syndrome are similar to those of the injury that caused the condition. Expect to see pain and swelling. The patient may complain of a sensation of pressure. The extremity may feel "hard" on palpation when compared to the uninjured side, and distal circulation, sensation, and motor function (CSM) may be reduced or absent.

EMTs can best treat compartment syndrome by some of the same treatments as for fracture, including cold application and elevation of the extremity (if this can be done safely after splinting). Prompt transport to an appropriate facility is important.

PATIENT ASSESSMENT

Musculoskeletal Injuries

Signs and symptoms of musculoskeletal injuries in a patient include the following:

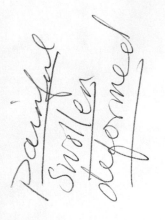

crepitus (KREP-i-tus)
a grating sensation or sound made when fractured bone ends rub together.

- **Pain and tenderness.** The patient with a painful, swollen, or deformed extremity experiences pain when the injured part is touched or moved. Generally, a patient will hold the injured part still, or guard it, in an effort to minimize pain. When examining a conscious patient, ask him to point to the location of the pain, if possible. Then, initially avoiding that location, carefully examine the injured part to assess if there are any other painful or injured areas. With unresponsive patients, suspicion of injury must be based on other physical findings.

- **Deformity or angulation.** The force of trauma causes bones to fracture and become deformed, or angulated, out of the anatomical position. Note that when a patient has joint injuries, the deformity is sometimes subtle. When in doubt, look at the uninjured side and compare it to the injured one.

- **Grating,** or *crepitus*. This is a sound or feeling caused by broken bone ends rubbing together. It can be painful for the patient, so never intentionally cause crepitus. The patient may report grating noises or sensations that occurred prior to your arrival and examination.

- **Swelling.** When bones break and soft tissue is torn, bleeding causes swelling that may increase the proportions of a deformity. Rings, watches, and other jewelry can easily constrict and injure underlying tissue. Therefore, slide or cut them off as soon as possible if swelling is likely to occur.

- **Bruising.** Ecchymosis, or large black-and-blue discoloration of the skin, indicates an underlying injury that may be hours or days old. Obvious bruises indicate the need for splinting.

- **Exposed bone ends.** Bone ends protruding through the skin indicate a fracture that requires splinting. Again, the more gruesome the appearance of the extremity, the greater the temptation is for you to treat that injury first. Remember that you should care for life-threatening injuries first. Extremity injuries rarely kill patients.

- **Joints locked into position.** When joints are dislocated, they may lock into normal or abnormal anatomical positions. Joint injuries usually need to be splinted as found.

- **Nerve and blood-vessel compromise.** Examine for pulses, sensation, and movement distal to the injury site. This must be accomplished before and after splinting. Check for nerve injury by asking the patient if he can sense your touch and can move all his fingers or toes. Any problem of sensation or movement must be noted. Next, feel for pulses in the wrist (radial), ankle (posterior tibial), or foot (dorsalis pedis). Obviously, to accurately examine for sensation, movement, and pulses, the patient's gloves and footwear must be removed.

Another method of assessing compromise to an extremity when a musculoskeletal injury is suspected is to learn and follow the "six Ps":

Pain or tenderness
Pallor (pale skin or poor capillary refill)
Paresthesia, or the sensation of "pins and needles"
Pulses diminished or absent in the injured extremity
Paralysis or the inability to move
Pressure

(6 p's)

Decision Points

- Do my patient's musculoskeletal injuries add up to serious multiple trauma?
- Does my patient have circulation, sensation, and motor function distal to the suspected fracture or dislocation?

PATIENT CARE

Musculoskeletal Injuries

Emergency care of a patient with musculoskeletal injuries includes the following steps:

1. Take and maintain appropriate Standard Precautions.
2. Perform the primary assessment. Remember, do not get distracted from your primary assessment and from determining patient priority by focusing on a dramatic-looking or painful extremity injury. Keep in mind, however, that multiple fractures, especially to the femurs, can cause life-threatening external or internal bleeding.
3. During the secondary assessment, apply a cervical collar if you suspect a spine injury.
4. After life-threatening conditions have been addressed, any suspected extremity fracture must be splinted. For a low-priority (stable) patient, splint individual injuries before transport. For a high-priority (unstable) patient, immobilize the whole body on a long spine board, then "load and go." If time and the patient's condition permit, you may be able to splint a specific injury en route.
5. If appropriate, cover open wounds with sterile dressings, elevate the extremity, and apply a cold pack to the area to help reduce swelling.

NOTE: *If a primary assessment reveals that your patient is unstable, managing extremity injuries becomes a low priority. An unstable patient with "load and go" problems must have the ABCs managed and the entire body splinted or immobilized on a long spine board. Do not take time to individually splint each injury. It is not in the patient's best interest to waste time treating minor injuries and delivering a perfectly packaged but unsavable patient to the hospital.*

Splinting

Emergency care for all suspected extremity fractures starts by splinting. *For any splint to be effective, it must immobilize adjacent joints and bone ends.* Effective splinting minimizes the movement of disrupted joints and broken bone ends, and it decreases the patient's pain. It helps prevent additional injury to soft tissues such as nerves, arteries, veins, and muscles. It can prevent a closed fracture from becoming an open fracture, a much more serious condition, and it can help to minimize blood loss. In the case of the spine, splinting on a backboard prevents injury to the spinal cord and helps to prevent permanent paralysis.

 CORE CONCEPT

Purposes and general procedures for splinting

Realignment of the Deformed Extremity

The object of realignment (straightening) is to assist in restoring effective circulation to the extremity and to fit it to a splint. Some injuries, such as certain wrist fractures, may be easily splintable because they are only slightly deformed. In this case, the only reason to attempt realignment is to restore circulation to the hand if it appears to be cyanotic or lacks a pulse.

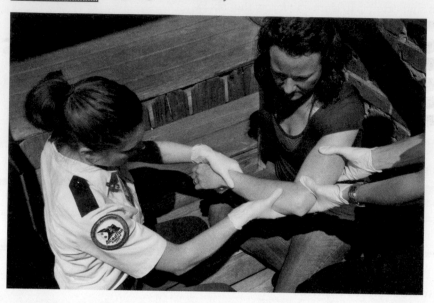

FIGURE 30-15 Aligning an extremity.

The thought of realigning an angulated injury can be a frightening one. However, remember these points:

- If the extremity is not realigned, the splint may be ineffective, causing increased pain and possible further injury (including an open fracture) during transportation.

- If the extremity is not realigned, the chance of nerves, arteries, and veins being compromised increases. When distal circulation is compromised or shut down, tissues beyond the injury become starved for oxygen and die.

- Pain is increased for only a moment during realignment under traction. Pain is reduced by effective splinting.

Due to the size and weight of extremities, attempting to splint one in the deformed position is usually futile and only increases the chance of its becoming an open fracture. When angulated injuries to the tibia or fibula, femur, radius or ulna, or humerus cannot be fit into a rigid splint, realign the bone. Also realign a long bone when the distal extremity is cyanotic or lacks pulses, indicating compromised circulation.

The general guidelines for realigning an extremity are as follows (Figure 30-15):

1. One EMT grasps the distal extremity, while a partner places one hand above and one hand below the injury site.

2. The partner supports the site while the first EMT pulls gentle *manual traction* in the direction of the long axis of the extremity. If you feel resistance or if it appears that bone ends will come through the skin, stop realignment and splint the extremity in the position found.

3. If no resistance is felt, maintain gentle traction until the extremity is properly aligned and splinted.

Generally, injured joints should be splinted in the position found unless the distal extremity is cyanotic or lacks pulses. If these conditions are present, try to align the joint to a neutral anatomical position using gentle traction, provided that no resistance is felt.

Strategies for Splinting

Effective splinting may require some ingenuity. Even though you carry different types of splinting devices, many situations will require you to improvise. In a pinch, you can use pillows or rolled blankets as soft splints. For rigid splints, you can use a piece of lumber, cardboard, a rolled newspaper, an umbrella, a cane, a broom handle, a catcher's shin guard, or a tongue depressor for a finger. A bystander can often rummage through his car trunk and find something suitable.

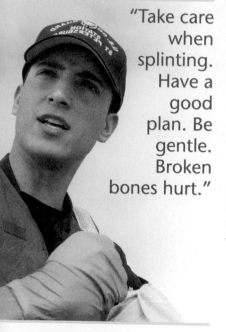

"Take care when splinting. Have a good plan. Be gentle. Broken bones hurt."

manual traction
the process of applying tension to straighten and realign a fractured limb before splinting. Also called *tension*.

FIGURE 30-16 Splints and accessories for musculoskeletal injuries.

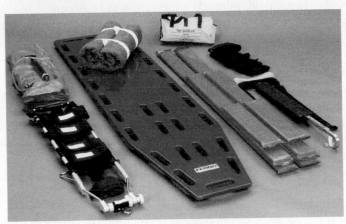

Splints carried on EMS units come in three basic types: rigid splints, formable splints, and traction splints (Figure 30-16). Rigid splints require the limb to be moved to the anatomical position. They tend to provide the greatest support and are ideally used to splint long-bone injuries. Examples are cardboard, wood, Velcro, pneumatic splints such as air splints and vacuum splints, and the pneumatic anti-shock garment. Formable splints are capable of being molded to different angles and generally allow for considerable movement. They are most commonly used to immobilize joint injuries in the position found. Examples are pillow and blanket splints. Traction splints are used specifically for femur fractures.

Regardless of the method of splinting, general rules that apply to all types of immobilization are as follows:

- **Care for life-threatening problems first.** If the patient is unstable, do not waste time with splinting. You can align the injuries in the anatomical position and immobilize the whole body to a long spine board.

- **Expose the injury site.** Before moving the injured extremity, expose the area and control any bleeding.

- **Assess distal CSM.** Because complications of musculoskeletal injury include nerve and blood vessel injury, assess and record distal circulation, sensation, and motor function (CSM) both before and after splinting. (Review Scan 13-4 in Chapter 13, "Assessment of the Trauma Patient," which illustrates how to assess distal function.)

- **Align long-bone injuries to the anatomical position.** Do this under gentle traction, if severe deformity exists or distal circulation is compromised.

- **Do not push protruding bones back into place.** However, when you realign deformed open injuries, they may slip back into position under traction.

- **Immobilize both the injury site and adjacent joints.** In order for splints to be effective, they must keep the injury site and the joints above and below still. (If the joint is injured, splint to immobilize the joint and the adjacent bones.)

- **Choose a method of splinting.** This is always dictated by the severity of the patient's condition and priority decision. If the patient is a high priority for "load and go" transport, choose a fast method of splinting. If the patient is a low priority for transport, choose a slower-but-better splinting method. The methods of splinting from slowest to fastest are:

  Each site is individually splinted (slowest but best).

  The limb is secured to the torso or an uninjured leg (a bit faster, but second choice to individual splints).

  The entire body is secured to a spine board (fastest, but only better than no splint at all).

- **Splint before moving the patient to a stretcher or other location, if possible.** A good rule of thumb is "least handling causes least damage." Sometimes patients must be extricated from where they are before ideal splinting techniques can occur. Attempt to immobilize the extremity as well as you can. (For example, prior to extrication, the injured extremity might be immobilized to the uninjured one.)

- **Pad the voids.** Many rigid splints do not conform to body curves and allow too much movement of the limb. Pad the voids, or spaces between the body part and the splint, to ensure proper immobilization and increase patient comfort.

Hazards of Splinting

By far the most serious hazard of splinting is "splinting someone to death"—splinting before life-threatening conditions are addressed, or spending time splinting a high-priority patient instead of immediately getting the patient into the ambulance and to the hospital. Remember that deformed fractures look painful and grotesque. Do not let that distract you from your priorities.

Always ensure the patient's airway, breathing, and circulation before going on to care for other injuries. Remember, the method of splinting is always dictated by the severity of the patient's condition and by the priority for transportation.

Other hazards include improper or inadequate splinting. If a splint is applied too tightly, it can compress soft tissue and injure nerves, blood vessels, and muscles. If it is applied too loosely or inappropriately, it will allow so much movement that further soft-tissue injury or an open fracture may occur. In addition, because rescue workers may be insecure about realigning a deformed injury, they may attempt to splint it in a deformed position and actually do more harm than good. Remember, it can be very difficult to splint deformed long-bone injuries well enough to prevent excessive movement.

Splinting Long-Bone and Joint Injuries

Before you start the splinting process, select a splint appropriate to the severity of the patient's condition and method of transportation. Be sure to have cravats, padding, and roller bandages immediately at hand.

The splinting of joints usually requires considerable ingenuity. In most cases, formable splints are used to splint the joint in the position it is found. If the distal extremity is pulseless or cyanotic, try to align it to the anatomical position using gentle traction. As with long-bone splinting, get all of your equipment ready before starting the splinting process.

To splint long-bone or joint injuries, follow these guidelines (Scans 30-1 and 30-2):

1. Take appropriate Standard Precautions and, if possible, expose the area to be splinted.
2. Manually stabilize the injury site. This can be done either by you or by a helper.
3. Assess circulation, sensation, and motor function (CSM). Check for pulses and see if the patient can feel your touch distal to the injury. Ask the patient to wiggle his fingers or toes to assess movement. Do not ask the patient to grasp, press, or pull an extremity you believe may be fractured. This will cause unnecessary pain and may aggravate the injury.
4. Realign the injury if deformed or if the distal extremity is cyanotic or pulseless. Be sure to attempt to realign an injured joint only if the distal extremity is pulseless or cyanotic.
5. Measure or adjust the splint and move it into position under or alongside the limb. Maintain manual stabilization or traction during positioning and until the splinting procedure is complete.
6. Apply and secure the splint to immobilize adjacent joints and the injury site.
7. Reassess CSM distal to the injury.

If using a vacuum splint (Scan 30-3), use the previous steps to assess and prepare the extremity for splinting. Move the vacuum splint into position. Place the splint around the extremity, leaving the distal end (fingers or toes) exposed. Using the pump, withdraw the air from the splint until it is firm and then secure the Velcro straps. Monitor the patient.

Traction Splint

Splinting a femur injury is different from splinting other long-bone or joint injuries. The major problem with femur fractures is the tendency for the large muscle groups of the thigh

FIRST TAKE STANDARD PRECAUTIONS.

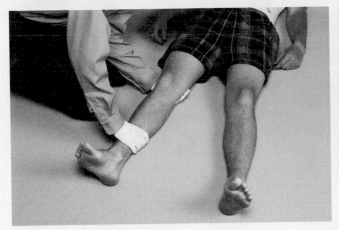

1 Manually stabilize the injured limb.

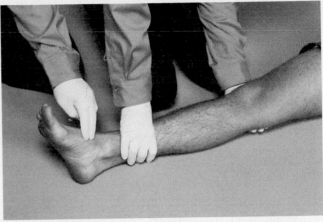

2 Assess distal circulation, sensation, and motor function (CSM).

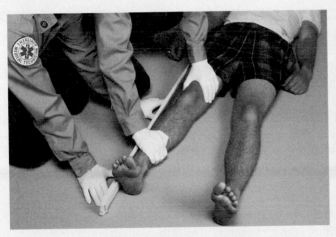

3 Measure the splint. It should extend several inches beyond the joints above and below the injury.

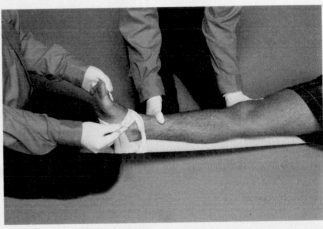

4 Apply the splint and immobilize the joints above and below the injury.

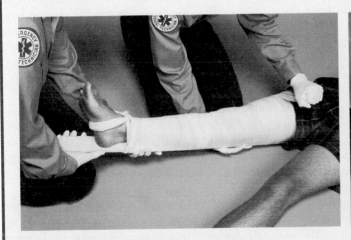

5 Secure the entire injured extremity.

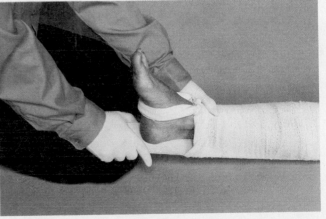

6 Secure the foot in the position of function . . .

(continued)

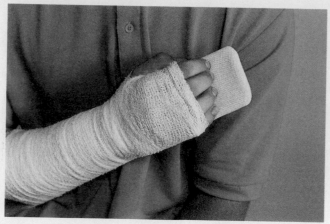

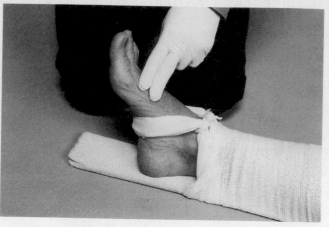

. . . Or, if splinting an arm, secure the hand in the position of function. This is the position the hand would be in if the patient were holding a palm-sized ball. A roll of bandage can be placed in the patient's hand to help maintain the position of function.

7 Reassess distal CSM.

(quadriceps and hamstrings) to go into spasm, forcing the bone ends to override each other, causing pain and further soft-tissue injury. A traction splint counteracts the muscle spasms and greatly reduces the pain.

Traction splints come in two basic varieties: bipolar and unipolar. A bipolar splint cradles the leg between two metal rods; a unipolar splint has a single metal rod that is placed alongside the leg. Examples of the bipolar splint are the half-ring splint, Hare, and Fernotrac. Examples of the unipolar splint are the Sager and the Kendrick traction devices. (Applying a bipolar traction splint will be shown later in Scan 30-9. Applying a unipolar splint will be shown in Scan 30-10.)

One of the most common EMT questions is, "How much traction should I pull?" An answer commonly given is, "Pull enough traction to give the patient some relief from the pain." This answer can be misleading. When the thigh muscles begin to spasm and the bones begin to override, the patient is in real pain. When manual or mechanical traction is applied, you are pulling against a muscle spasm, and that hurts, too. Most patients do not begin to feel relief with the traction splint until it has been applied for several minutes and the muscle spasm begins to subside. With the Sager unipolar splint, traction can be measured. The amount of traction applied should be roughly 10 percent of the patient's body weight and not exceed 15 pounds. With a bipolar splint, firm traction should be applied to align the limb. Exert and maintain a firm pull to prevent bones from continuing to override.

No traction splint applied in the field pulls true traction. Instead, all exert "countertraction." The splint pulls on an ankle hitch and the splint frame is anchored against the pelvis. Once anchored, a pull is felt on the leg. With bipolar splints, any movement of the pelvis off the ground causes a shifting of the splint and loss of traction. Unipolar splints, such as the Sager, are anchored against the pubis between the legs and are less apt to shift and cause a loss of traction during patient movement.

The indications for a traction splint are a painful, swollen, deformed mid-thigh with no joint or lower leg injury. A traction splint is contraindicated if there is a pelvis, hip, or knee injury; if there is an avulsion or partial amputation where traction could separate the extremity; or if there is an injury to the lower third of the leg that would interfere with the ankle hitch.

When possible, use three rescuers to apply a traction splint. One can support the injury site when the limb is lifted to position the traction splint.

FIRST TAKE STANDARD PRECAUTIONS.

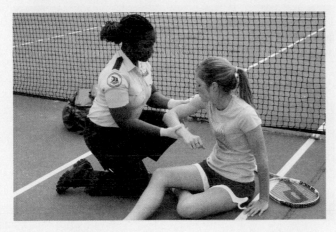

1 Manually stabilize the injured limb, in this case an injured elbow.

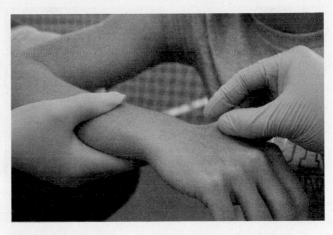

2 Assess distal pulse, motor function, and sensation (CSM).

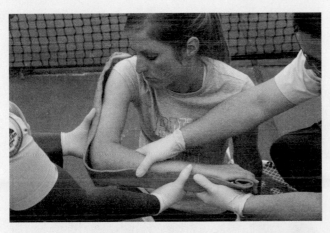

3 Select the proper splint material. Immobilize the site of injury and bones above and below.

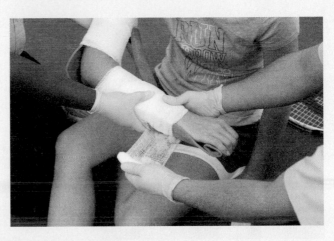

4 Secure the splint.

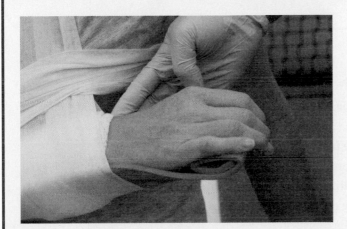

5 Reassess distal CSM.

FIRST TAKE STANDARD PRECAUTIONS.

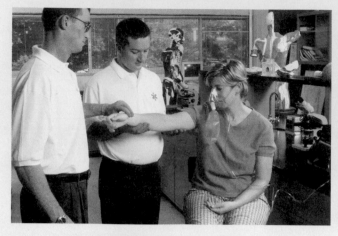

❶ Stabilize the extremity and check distal circulation, sensation, and motor function (CSM).

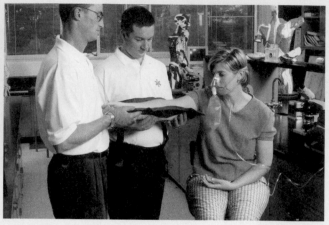

❷ Apply the splint to the extremity and secure it with the straps.

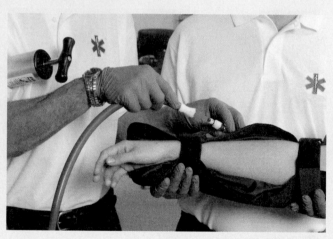

❸ Remove the air from the splint with the pump provided by the manufacturer.

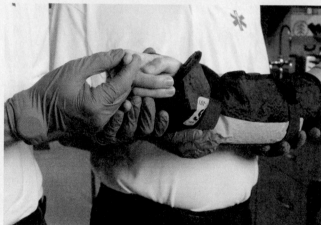

❹ Reassess distal CSM.

General guidelines for the application of a traction splint are as follows:

1. Take Standard Precautions and, if possible, expose the area to be splinted.
2. Manually stabilize the leg and apply manual traction.
3. Assess CSM distal to the injury.
4. Adjust the splint to the proper length, and position it at or under the injured leg.
5. Apply the proximal securing device (ischial strap).
6. Apply the distal securing device (ankle hitch).
7. Apply mechanical traction.
8. Position and secure support straps.
9. Reevaluate the proximal and distal securing devices, and reassess CSM distal to the injury.
10. Secure the patient's torso and the traction splint to a long spine board to immobilize the hip and to prevent movement of the splint.

Inside/Outside

INSIDE	OUTSIDE
Bones are vascular. Bone marrow is involved in the production of red blood cells.	Patients with skeletal injuries—especially those involving long bones and multiple bones—will experience shock.
There are many types of fractures. Greenstick fractures, comminuted fractures, and fractures without displaced bone ends do not appear deformed.	You may see patients who have fractures without obvious deformity. This is why you splint all actual and suspected musculoskeletal fractures.
Swelling and inflammation are the body's natural responses to injury. The body sends blood and cells to the affected area to fight infection. This causes a swollen, often warm extremity around the injury.	Some patients may appear to have a fracture but actually don't. The swelling—especially in areas where the bone is close to the skin—can cause the appearance of fracture.

EMERGENCY CARE OF SPECIFIC INJURIES

The specific injuries described in this section are usually identified as fractures or dislocations. Remember that you do not need to determine the exact nature of an extremity injury. You will simply immobilize any painful, swollen, or deformed extremity. Specific techniques are discussed on the following pages and illustrated later in Scans 30-4 through 30-15.

CORE CONCEPT ●

Assessment and care of specific injuries to the upper and lower extremities

Upper Extremity Injuries

PATIENT ASSESSMENT

Shoulder Girdle Injuries

The following are common signs and symptoms of an injury to the shoulder girdle:

- Pain in the shoulder may indicate several types of injury. Look for specific signs.
- A dropped shoulder, with the patient holding the arm of his injured side against the chest, often indicates a fracture of the clavicle.
- A severe blow to the back over the scapula may cause a fracture of that bone. (All the bones of the shoulder girdle can be felt except the scapula. Only the superior ridge of the scapula, called its spine, can be easily palpated. Injury to the scapula is rare but must be considered if there are indications of a severe blow at the site of this bone.)

Check the entire shoulder girdle. Feel for deformity and tenderness where the clavicle joins the anterior scapula (the acromion). Feel and look along the entire clavicle for deformity from the sternum medially to the shoulder laterally. Note if the head of the humerus can be felt or moves in front of the shoulder. This is a sign of possible anterior dislocation or fracture.

PATIENT CARE

Shoulder Girdle Injuries

Emergency care of a patient with a shoulder girdle injury includes the following steps:

1. Assess distal CSM. If distal CSM is impaired, immobilize and transport as soon as possible, notifying the receiving facility.
2. It is not practical to use a rigid splint for injuries to the clavicle, scapula, or the head of the humerus. Use a sling and swathe (Scan 30-4). If there is a possible cervical-spine injury, do not tie a sling around the patient's neck.

3. If there is evidence of a possible anterior dislocation of the head of the humerus (the bone head is pushed toward the front of the body), place a thin pillow between the patient's arm and chest before applying the sling and swathe.
4. Do not attempt to straighten or reduce any dislocations.
5. Reassess distal CSM.

NOTE: *Sometimes a dislocated shoulder will reduce itself (the displaced head of the humerus "pops back into place"). When this happens, check distal CSM. Apply a sling and swathe and transport the patient. The patient must be seen by a physician.*

Lower Extremity Injuries

PATIENT ASSESSMENT

Pelvic Injuries

Fractures of the pelvis may occur with falls, in motor-vehicle collisions, or when a person is crushed by being squeezed between two objects. Pelvic fractures may be the result of direct or indirect force. The following are common signs and symptoms of a pelvic injury:

■ Complaint of pain in the pelvis, hips, groin, or back. This may be the only indication, but it is significant if the mechanism of injury indicates possible fracture. Usually, obvious deformity is associated with the pain.

■ Painful reaction when pressure is applied to the iliac crests (wings of the pelvis) or to the pubic bones.

■ Complaint that the patient cannot lift his legs when lying on his back. (Do not test for this, but do check for sensation.)

■ Foot on the injured side may turn outward (lateral rotation). This also may indicate a hip fracture.

■ Patient has an unexplained pressure on the urinary bladder and the feeling of having to empty the bladder.

■ Bleeding from the urethra, rectum, or vaginal opening in the setting of a high-impact mechanism of injury. Blood at the meatus of the penis (opening of the urethra) is a finding unique to pelvic trauma/fracture (Figure 30-17A).

NOTE: *Indications of pelvic fractures mean that there may be serious damage to internal organs, blood vessels, and nerves. Internal bleeding may be profus and lead to shock. Any force strong enough to fracture the pelvis also can cause injury to the spine.*

FIGURE 30-17 (A) Blood at the meatus of the penis is a sign of a pelvic fracture. (B) A pelvic wrap can help to stabilize a fractured pelvis. Shown here is a commercial pelvic binding device placed on a severely injured patient with an open pelvic fracture. *(Photos A and B: © Edward T. Dickinson, MD)*

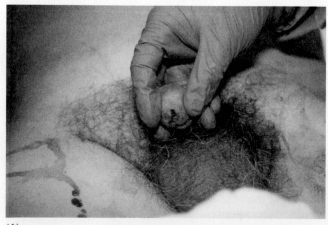

(A)

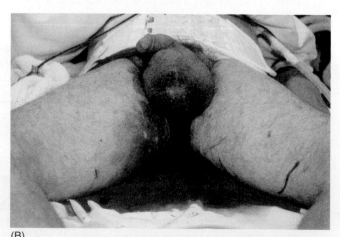

(B)

PATIENT CARE

Pelvic Injuries

Emergency care for pelvic injuries includes the following steps:

1. Move the patient as little as possible. If you must move the patient, move him as a unit. Never lift the patient with the pelvis unsupported. Warning: Use caution when using a log roll to move a patient with a suspected pelvic fracture. Roll the patient gently to the uninjured side, when possible.
2. Determine CSM distal to the injury site.
3. Straighten the patient's lower limbs into the anatomical position if there are no injuries to the hip joints and lower limbs and if it can be done without meeting resistance or causing excessive pain.
4. Prevent additional injury to the pelvis by stabilizing the lower limbs. Place a folded blanket between the patient's legs, from the groin to the feet, and bind them together with wide cravats. Thin rigid splints can be used to push the cravats under the patient. The cravats can then be adjusted for proper placement at the upper thigh, above the knee, below the knee, and above the ankle.
5. If permitted by local protocol, apply a pneumatic anti-shock garment (PASG) to stabilize the pelvis in a patient with hypotension (blood pressure below 90).
6. Assume that there are spinal injuries. Immobilize the patient on a long spine board. When securing the patient, avoid placing the straps or ties over the pelvic area.
7. Reassess distal CSM.
8. Care for shock, providing high-concentration oxygen.
9. Transport the patient as soon as possible.
10. Monitor vital signs.

Once the patient is in the ambulance, some EMTs are allowed to make adjustments to improve patient comfort and reduce muscle spasms of the abdomen and lower limb by gently flexing the legs and placing a pillow under the knees. If you are allowed to follow this protocol, be extremely careful not to move the spine, since the patient may have associated spinal injuries.

NOTE: *It may be very difficult to tell a fractured pelvis from a fracture of the upper femur. When there is doubt, to protect blood vessels and nerves associated with the femur-pelvis (hip) joint, care for the patient as if there is a pelvic fracture. Remember, there may also be spinal injuries.*

Pelvic Wrap

One method of treating pelvic injuries is the pelvic wrap. Performed with commercially available devices (Figure 30-17B) or formed from a sheet (these steps are described in the following text), the wrap reduces internal bleeding and pain while providing stabilization to the pelvis. It may also prevent further injury. Since many systems no longer carry the pneumatic anti-shock garment (PASG), the pelvic wrap provides an alternative treatment for suspected pelvic fracture.

The pelvic wrap should be performed on patients who have pelvic deformity or instability (movement upon palpation) whether or not signs of shock are present. Some systems may also recommend use of the pelvic wrap with a mechanism of injury that would indicate pelvic injury (e.g., motorcycle crashes, auto-pedestrian collisions) even if obvious deformity is not present. A sheet may be placed on the backboard even if the wrap is not immediately secured in the event evidence of instability or shock develops. Always follow your local protocols.

To apply a sheet as a pelvic wrap:

1. Complete a scene size-up and primary assessment.
2. Once you determine the patient is a candidate for a pelvic wrap (unstable pelvis with or without signs of shock or positive MOI), prepare a backboard with a sheet, folded flat, approximately 10 inches wide and lying across the backboard (Figure 30-18A).
3. Carefully roll the patient to the backboard. Center the sheet at the patient's greater trochanter (the bony prominence at the proximal end of the femur). This will position the sheet lower than the iliac "wings." This is the correct position.

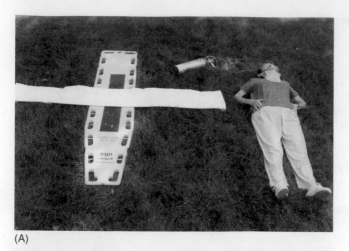
(A)

(B)

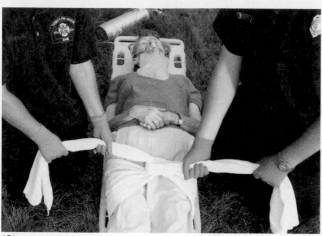
(C)

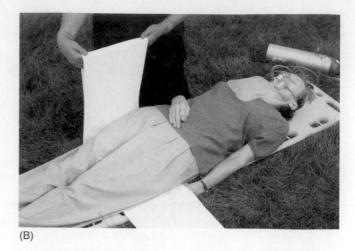

FIGURE 30-18 (A) For a pelvic wrap, lay a sheet, folded flat, approximately 10 inches wide onto the backboard. (B) Bring the sides of the sheet together. (C) Tie the sheet firmly without overcompression to complete the pelvic wrap.

4. Bring the sides of the sheet around to the front of the patient (Figure 30-18B). As you bring the sides of the sheet together and tie them, you will cause compression and stabilization of the pelvis. The sheet should feel firm enough on the pelvis to keep it in normal position without overcompression (Figure 30-18C).

5. Secure the sheet using ties or clamps so that the compression is maintained.

NOTE: *Some EMS services prefer to apply the pelvic wrap to the patient* before *moving the patient to the backboard to reduce the pain of that move.*

Pneumatic Anti-Shock Garment

The pneumatic anti-shock garment (PASG, also known as a MAST garment) may be used (where available) for splinting a suspected pelvic fracture in a patient with hypotension (blood pressure below 90). Some EMS systems also use the anti-shock garment for splinting hip, femoral, and multiple leg fractures. An anti-shock garment is to be applied in accordance with local protocols. In many localities, its application requires an order from a physician. (Review Chapter 27, "Bleeding and Shock," Scan 27-3, "Applying the Pneumatic Anti-Shock Garment (PASG).")

When pelvic fracture is a possibility, always be alert for shock and possible injuries to internal organs. Always take vital signs before applying an anti-shock garment and monitor the vital signs every 5 minutes thereafter.

PATIENT ASSESSMENT

Hip Dislocation

A hip dislocation occurs when the head of the femur is pulled or pushed from its pelvic socket. It is difficult to tell a hip dislocation from a fracture of the proximal (uppermost portion of the) femur. Conscious patients will complain of intense pain with both types of injury. Patients who have had a surgical replacement of the hip joint are at increased risk of hip dislocation. The hip can be either anteriorly or posteriorly dislocated.

FIGURE 30-19 A right posterior hip dislocation from dashboard impact.
(© Edward T. Dickinson, MD)

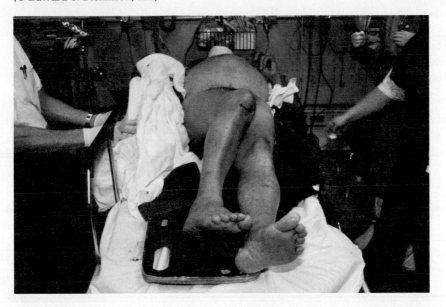

The following are common signs and symptoms of a hip dislocation:

- **Anterior hip dislocation.** The patient's entire lower limb is rotated outward and the hip is usually flexed.

- **Posterior hip dislocation** (most common). The patient's leg is rotated inward, the hip is flexed, and the knee is bent (Figure 30-19). The foot may hang loose (foot drop), and the patient is unable to flex the foot or lift the toes. Often, there is a lack of sensation in the limb. These signs indicate possible damage, caused by the dislocated femoral head, to the sciatic nerve, the major nerve that extends from the lower spine to the posterior thigh. This injury often occurs when a person's knees strike the dashboard during a motor-vehicle collision.

PATIENT CARE

Hip Dislocation

Emergency care of a patient with a hip dislocation includes the following steps:

1. Assess distal CSM.
2. Move the patient onto a long spine board. Some systems use a scoop-style stretcher. When this device is used, the limb should be immobilized.
3. Immobilize the limb with pillows or rolled blankets.
4. Secure the patient to the long spine board with straps or cravats.
5. Reassess distal CSM. If there is a pulse, motor, or sensory problem, notify medical direction and immediately transport.
6. Care for shock by providing high-concentration oxygen.
7. Transport carefully, monitor vital signs, and continue to check for nerve and circulation impairment.

   NOTE: *If you find a painful, swollen, or deformed thigh and the leg is flexed and will not straighten, the patient may also have a fractured femur.*

PATIENT ASSESSMENT

Hip Fracture

As noted earlier, a hip fracture is a fracture of the proximal femur, not the pelvis. The fracture can occur to the femoral head, the femoral neck, or at the portion of the femur just below the neck of the bone.

The following are common signs and symptoms of a hip fracture:

- Pain is localized, although some patients also complain of pain in the knee.
- Sometimes the patient is sensitive to pressure exerted on the lateral prominence of the hip (greater trochanter).
- Surrounding tissues are discolored; however, discoloration may be delayed.
- Swelling may be evident.
- Patient is unable to move his limb while on his back.
- Patient complains about being unable to stand.
- Foot on injured side usually turns outward; however, it may rotate inward (rarely).
- Injured limb may appear shorter.

GERIATRIC NOTE

Direct force (as occurs in a motor-vehicle collision) and twisting forces (as may occur in falls) can cause a hip fracture. Elderly people are more susceptible to this type of injury than others because of their brittle bones or bones weakened by disease.

PATIENT CARE

Hip Fracture

Be certain to assess distal CSM before and after splinting and during transport. The patient should be managed for shock and receive oxygen at a high concentration. You should place the patient on a long spine board or orthopedic stretcher after splinting.

One of the following emergency care methods can be used to stabilize a hip fracture (Figure 30-20):

- **Bind the legs together.** Place a folded blanket between the patient's legs and bind the legs together with wide straps, Velcro-equipped straps, or wide cravats. Carefully place the patient on a long spine board and use pillows to support the lower limbs. Secure the patient to the board. An orthopedic stretcher can be used in place of the long spine board.
- **Padded boards.** Use thin splints to push cravats or straps under the patient at the natural voids (such as the small of the back and back of the knees) and readjust them so that they will pass across the chest, the abdomen just below the belt, below the crotch, above and below the knee, and at the ankle. Splint with two long padded boards. Ideally, one should be long enough to extend from the patient's armpit to beyond the foot. The other should be long enough to extend from the crotch to beyond

FIGURE 30-20 For a patient with a hip or pelvic injury, (A) bind the legs together or (B) splint with a padded long board. Apply an anti-shock garment, if local protocols indicate.

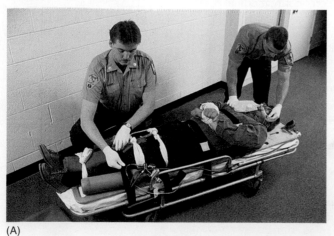

(A)

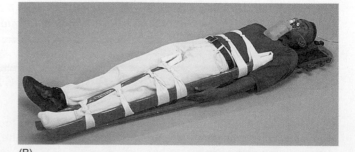

(B)

the foot. Cushion with padding in the armpit and crotch and pad all voids created at the ankle and knee. Secure the boards with the cravats or straps.

- **Apply an anti-shock garment.** Do this if local protocols indicate.

Femoral Shaft Fracture

Because the femur is a large, strong bone, considerable force is necessary to cause a fracture of the femoral shaft. Remember also that muscle contractions can cause bone ends to ride over each other. The bone ends may or may not protrude from an open wound. Never assume that a wound on the thigh is superficial because you do not see bone ends. Always check for signs and symptoms that this wound may be an open fracture.

The following are common signs and symptoms of a femoral shaft fracture:

- The patient may complain of pain, which is often intense.
- Often there will be an open fracture with deformity and sometimes with the end of the bone protruding through the wound. When the injury is a closed fracture, often there will be deformity with possible severe angulation.
- The injured limb may appear to be shortened because the contraction of the thigh muscles caused the bone ends to override each other.

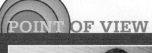

POINT OF VIEW

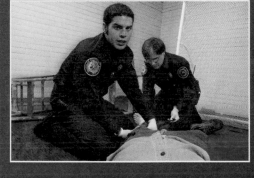

"I was building this really cool indoor driving range in the loft over the barn. I put down green artificial turf. It was going to be great. I was hanging the net when the ladder gave way and I fell.

"It's funny, but on the way down I had time to get a sinking feeling: knowing it was going to hurt when I landed, hoping I didn't break anything, and thinking that probably no one would even hear me. I hit the floor and broke my leg. I knew, because I heard—and felt—the twist, then the break.

"I yelled for about 5 minutes before a neighbor heard me. But then the EMTs came pretty quickly, and they were good guys. They didn't sugar coat the situation. They said it might hurt when they put the splint on and when they carried me down the narrow barn stairs. I hadn't even thought of how they would get me downstairs. I'm not a small guy.

"But they did it. They did it well. They were right, it hurt some, but I appreciate them telling me the truth.

"I guess I've got about 8 weeks before I get to take the first swing in my new driving range."

Femoral Shaft Fracture

Emergency care of a patient with a femoral shaft fracture includes the following steps:

1. Control any bleeding by applying direct pressure (avoiding the possible fracture site) forcefully enough to overcome the barrier of muscle mass. The femoral artery pressure point may be used.
2. As soon as possible, manage the patient for shock (hypoperfusion) and provide high-concentration oxygen.
3. Assess distal CSM.
4. Apply a traction splint. (See Scans 30-9 and 30-10.) If a traction splint is not available, bind the legs together after placing them in the anatomical position.
5. Reassess distal CSM.

NOTE: *The traction splint should not be applied if you suspect that there may be additional injuries or fractures to the area of the knee or tibia/fibula of the same limb. If* *local protocols permit, you may use an anti-shock garment if there are multiple leg fractures. It is not, however, a good splint for the lower leg since it does not immobilize the ankle.*

PEDIATRIC NOTE

When traction-splinting thigh injuries in children, be sure to use appropriately sized splints. Warning: Studies of mechanisms of injury indicate that infants and children with fractured femurs often have injuries to internal organs.

PATIENT ASSESSMENT

Knee Injury

The knee is a joint and not a single bone. Fractures can occur to the distal femur, to the proximal tibia and fibula, and to the patella (kneecap). The following are common signs and symptoms of a knee injury:

- Pain and tenderness
- Swelling
- Deformity with obvious swelling

PATIENT CARE

Knee Injury

There are two general emergency care methods used for immobilizing the knee—one if the knee is bent, the other if it is straight:

- **Knee is bent.** Assess distal CSM. Immobilize the knee in the position in which the leg is found. Tie two padded board splints to the thigh and above the ankle so that the knee is held in position. You can use a pillow to support the leg. Reassess distal CSM. (See Scan 30-11.)
- **Knee is straight or returned to the anatomical position.** Assess distal CSM. Immobilize the knee with two padded board splints or a single padded splint. When using two padded boards, placing one medial and one lateral offers the best support. Remember to pad the voids created at the knee and ankle. Reassess distal CSM. (See Scans 30-12 and 30-13.)

Do not confuse a knee dislocation with a patella dislocation. The patella can become displaced when the lower leg and knee are twisted, as in a skiing or racquetball accident. In a patellar dislocation, the knee will be stuck in flexion and the kneecap will be displaced and laterally palpable. A knee dislocation occurs when the tibia itself is forced either anteriorly or posteriorly in relation to the distal femur. Always check for a distal pulse, since the dislocated knee joint can compress the popliteal artery and stop the major blood supply to the lower leg. If there is no pulse, this is a true emergency. Contact medical direction for permission to gently move the lower leg anteriorly to allow for a pulse, and immediately transport the patient.

What may appear to be a dislocation may prove to be a fracture or a combined fracture and dislocation. Even if you believe that the patient has suffered a dislocated patella and the kneecap has repositioned itself, realize that other damage may be hidden. Whether you suspect a fracture, a dislocation, a sprain, or a strain, always splint the injury and transport the patient.

Once splinting is done, monitor the patient. If there is a loss of distal CSM, or if the foot becomes discolored (white, mottled, or blue) and turns cold, transport the patient without delay. Notify medical direction while en route.

Tibia or Fibula Injury

The following are common signs and symptoms of a tibia or fibula injury:

- Pain and tenderness
- Swelling
- Possible deformity (You might expect to see a deformity of the lower leg when the tibia or fibula is fractured. However, such deformity is often absent.)

PATIENT CARE

Tibia or Fibula Injury

Emergency care of a patient with a tibia or fibula injury includes providing care for shock and administering high-concentration oxygen. Because immobilizing the leg can help to relieve pain and control bleeding, apply a splint using one of the following methods. Remember to assess distal CSM before and after application.

- **Air-inflated splint.** Apply an air-inflated splint (Figure 30-21). Slide the uninflated splint over your hand and gather it in place until the lower edge clears your wrist. Using your free hand, grasp the patient's foot and leg just above the injury site. While maintaining manual traction, have your partner slide the splint over your hand and onto the injured leg. Your partner must make sure that the splint is relatively wrinkle free and that it covers the injury site. Continue to maintain traction while your partner inflates the splint. Test to see if you can cause a slight dent in the plastic with fingertip pressure. Remember to check periodically to see that the pressure in the splint has remained adequate and has not decreased or increased.

FIGURE 30-21 An air splint may be used for a lower leg injury.

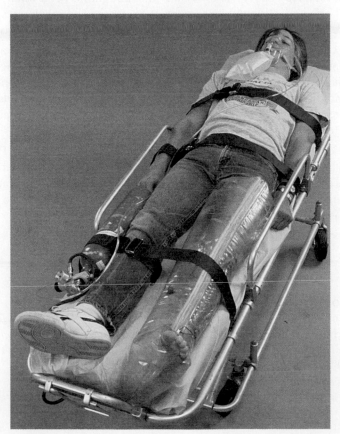

- **Two-splint method.** You can immobilize the fracture using two rigid board splints (Scan 30-14).
- **Single splint with an ankle hitch.** A single splint with an ankle hitch can be applied (Scan 30-15).

PATIENT ASSESSMENT

Ankle or Foot Injury

Sprains (torn ligaments) and fractures are the most common musculoskeletal injuries to the ankle and foot. It is often difficult to distinguish between them, so always treat for a fracture. The following are common signs and symptoms of an ankle or foot injury:

- Pain
- Swelling
- Possible deformity

CRITICAL DECISION MAKING

Sticks and Stones May Break My Bones, but Trauma Centers Save Me

Care for patients with musculoskeletal injuries depends on each patient's overall condition. Patients with isolated fractures may routinely be splinted and transported, whereas those with multiple fractures are at an increased risk of shock and should be treated as multiple-trauma patients. For each of these patients, determine whether you would stay and splint or, as a higher priority, consider transport to a trauma center, using a backboard as the main splinting device.

1. You are called to a patient who tripped and tried to catch himself with an outstretched arm. He believes he broke his wrist and hit his head when he fell. He is alert and oriented. His vital signs are pulse 88, strong and regular; respirations 16; blood pressure 140/84; skin warm and dry; and pupils equal and reactive to light.

2. You are called to an industrial complex where a large spool pinned a man by the legs. The workers are able to move the spool for you to safely access the patient. The patient is in extreme pain. Your physical examination reveals deformity in both thighs and the patient's left lower leg. The patient is agitated. His pulse is 112 and regular, respirations 24 and adequate, blood pressure 108/64, and pupils equal and reactive to light.

3. Your patient was ejected from a vehicle and found about 20 feet away. He complains only of a broken arm. Your physical assessment doesn't reveal any other injuries. The patient is alert and oriented. His pulse is 130 and weak, respirations 28 and adequate, blood pressure 88/56, skin cool and moist, and pupils equal and reactive to light.

PATIENT CARE

Ankle or Foot Injury

Long splints, extending from above the knee to beyond the foot, can be used. However, soft splinting is an effective, rapid method and is recommended for most patients (Figure 30-22). To soft splint, you should follow the emergency care steps described in the following list:

1. Assess distal CSM.
2. Stabilize the limb. Remove the patient's shoe if possible, but only if it removes easily and can be done with no movement to the ankle.
3. Lift the limb, but do not apply manual traction (tension).

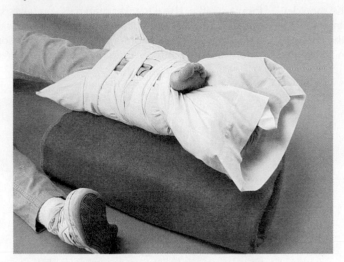

FIGURE 30-22 A pillow splint may be used for an injured ankle.

4. Place three cravats on the floor under the ankle. Then place a pillow lengthwise under the ankle on top of the cravats. The pillow should extend 6 inches beyond the foot.
5. Gently lower the limb onto the pillow, taking care not to change the ankle's position. Stabilize by tying the cravats, and adjust them so they are at the top of the pillow, midway, and at the heel.
6. Tie the pillow to the ankle and foot.
7. Tie a fourth cravat loosely at the arch of the foot.
8. Elevate with a second pillow or blanket. Reassess distal CSM.
9. Care for shock (hypoperfusion) if needed.
10. Apply an ice pack to the injury site to reduce bleeding and swelling, if appropriate. Do not apply the ice pack directly to the skin.

Note that a commercial splint with a foot and leg that extends above the knee may be better than a pillow since it will also immobilize the knee, the joint adjacent to the ankle.

A sling is a triangular bandage used to support the shoulder and arm. Once the patient's arm is placed in a sling, a swathe can be used to hold the arm against the side of the chest. Commercial slings are available. Velcro straps can be used to form a swathe. Use whatever materials you have on hand, provided they will not cut into the patient. Also, remember to assess distal pulse, motor function, and sensation both before and after immobilizing or splinting an extremity.

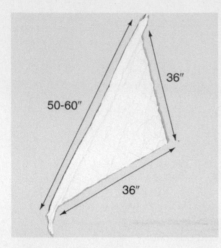

1 Prepare the sling by folding cloth into a triangle.

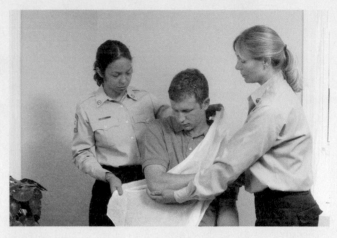

2 Position the sling over the top of the patient's chest as shown. Fold the injured arm across his chest. . . .

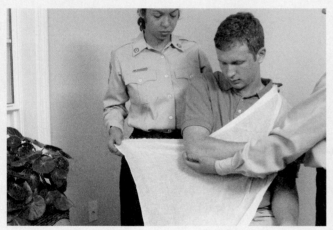

. . . If the patient cannot hold his arm, have someone assist him until you tie the sling.

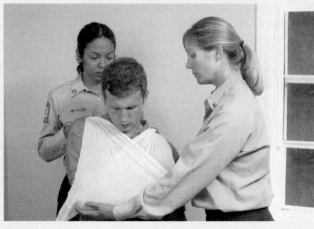

3 Extend one point of the triangle beyond the elbow on the injured side. Take the bottom point and bring it up over the patient's arm. Then take it over the top of the injured shoulder.

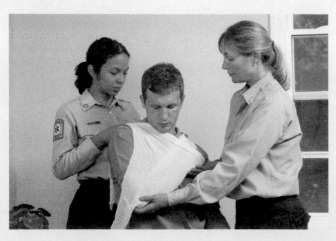

4 If appropriate, draw up the ends of the sling so that the patient's hand is about 4 inches above the elbow.

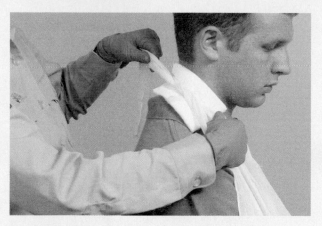

5 Tie the two ends of the sling together, making sure that the knot does not press against the back of the patient's neck. Pad with bulky dressings. (If spine injury is possible, pin the ends to the patient's clothing. Do not tie them around the neck.)

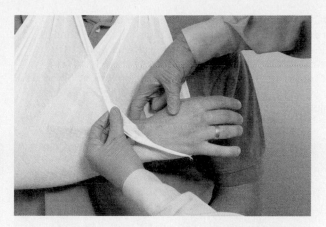

6 Check to be sure you have left the patient's fingertips exposed. Then assess distal circulation, sensation, and motor function (CSM). If the pulse has been lost, take off the sling and repeat the procedure. Then check again.

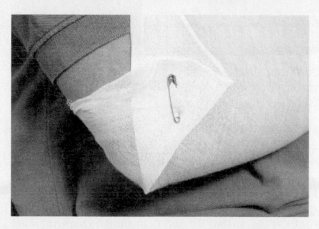

7 To form a pocket for the patient's elbow, take hold of the point of material at the elbow and fold it forward, pinning it to the front of the sling. Or . . .

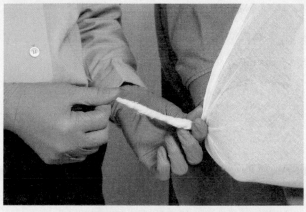

. . . If you do not have a pin, twist the excess material and tie a knot in the point.

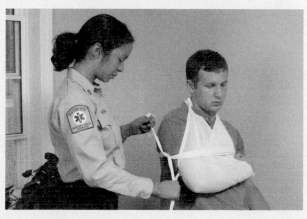

8 Form a swathe from a second piece of material. Tie it around the chest and the injured arm, over the sling. Do not place it over the patient's arm on the uninjured side.

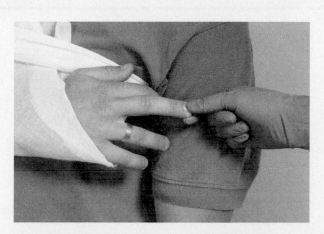

9 Reassess distal circulation, sensation, and motor function (CSM). Treat for shock, and provide high-concentration oxygen. Take vital signs. Perform detailed assessments and reassessments as appropriate.

SIGNS: Injury to the humerus can take place at the proximal end (shoulder), along the shaft of the bone, or at the distal end (elbow). Deformity is the key sign used to detect fractures to this bone in any of these locations; however, assess for all signs of skeletal injury, including pain or swelling. Follow the rules and procedures for care of an injured extremity.

NOTE: *Assess distal circulation, sensation, and motor function both before and after immobilizing or splinting an extremity.*

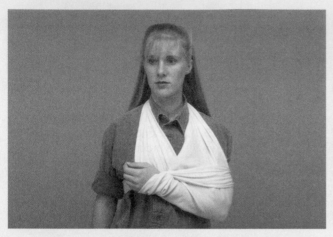

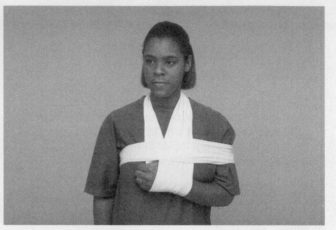

VARIATION ONE: Apply a sling and swathe. If you have only enough material for a swathe, bind the patient's upper arm to her body, taking great care not to cut off circulation to the forearm.

VARIATION TWO: If you have only a narrow or short length of material to use as a sling, apply it so that it supports the wrist only.

NOTE: *Before applying a sling and swathe to care for injuries to the humerus, check the patient's distal circulation, sensation, and motor function (CSM). If you do not feel a pulse, attempt to straighten any slight angulation if the patient has a closed fracture (follow local protocol). Otherwise, prepare for immediate immobilization and transport. If straightening of the angulation fails to restore the pulse or function, splint with a medium board splint, keeping the forearm extended. If there is no sign of circulation or sensory or motor function, you will have to attempt a second splinting. If this fails to restore distal function, immediately transport the patient. Do not try to straighten angulation of the humerus if there are any signs of fracture or dislocation of the shoulder or elbow.*

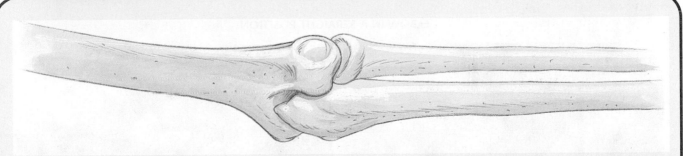

SIGNS: The elbow is a joint and not a bone. It is composed of the distal humerus and the proximal ulna and radius, which form a hinge joint. You will have to decide if the injury is truly to the elbow. The location of deformity and tenderness will direct you to the injury site.

CARE: If there is a distal pulse, the dislocated elbow should be immobilized in the position in which it is found. The joint has too many nerves and blood vessels to risk movement. When a distal pulse is absent, make one attempt to slightly reposition the limb after contacting medical direction. Do not force the limb into the anatomical position.

ELBOW IN OR RETURNED TO THE BENT POSITION

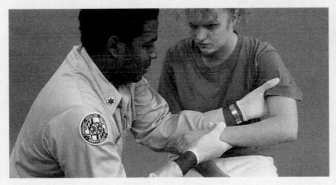

1 Move the limb only if necessary for splinting or if the pulse is absent. *Stop* if you meet resistance or significantly increase the pain.

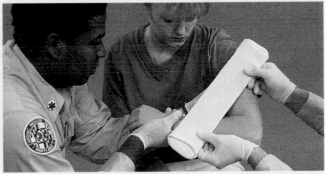

2 Use a padded board splint that will extend 2 to 6 inches beyond the arm and wrist when placed diagonally.

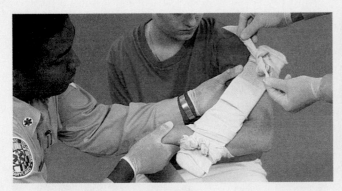

3 Place the splint so it is just proximal to the elbow and wrist. Use cravats to secure it to the forearm, then the arm.

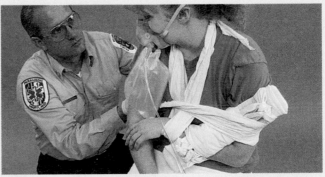

4 A wrist sling can be applied to support the limb. Keep the elbow exposed. Apply a swathe, if possible.

NOTE: *Assess the distal pulse, motor function, and sensation both before and after immobilizing or splinting an extremity.*

(continued)

ELBOW IN A STRAIGHT POSITION

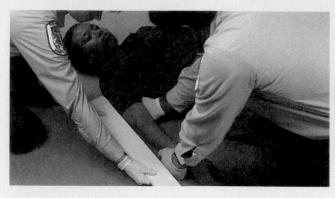

1 Assess distal circulation, sensation, and motor function (CSM).

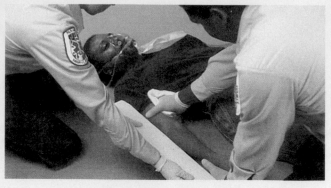

2 Use a padded board splint that extends from under the armpit to a point past the fingertips. Pad the armpit.

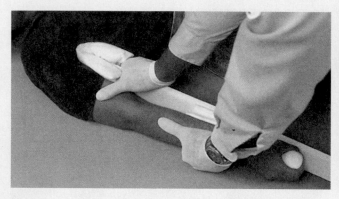

3 Place a roll of bandages in the patient's hand to help maintain the position of function. Place the padded side of the board against the medial side of the limb. Pad all voids.

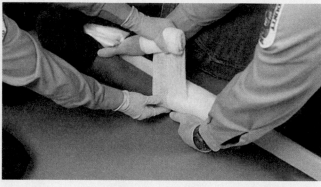

4 Secure the splint. Leave the patient's fingertips exposed.

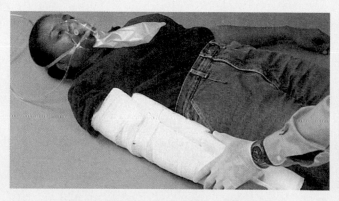

5 Place pads between the patient's side and the splint.

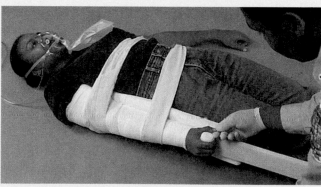

6 Secure the splinted limb to the body with two cravats. Avoid placing the cravats over the suspected injury site. Reassess the distal circulation, sensation, and motor function (CSM).

SIGNS:
- *Forearm.* Deformity and tenderness. If only one bone is broken, deformity may be minor or absent.
- *Wrist.* Deformity and tenderness.
- *Hand.* Deformity and pain. Dislocated fingers are obvious.

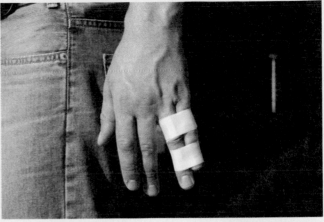

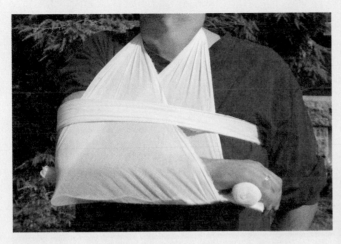

CARE: Injuries occurring to the forearm, wrist, or hand can be splinted using a padded rigid splint that extends from the elbow past the fingertips. The patient's elbow, forearm, wrist, and hand all need the support of the splint. Tension must be provided throughout the splinting. A roll of bandages should be placed in the patient's hand to ensure the position of function. After rigid splinting, apply a sling and swathe.

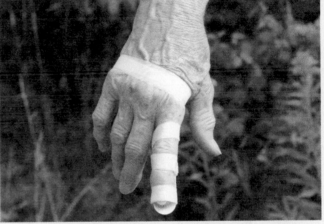

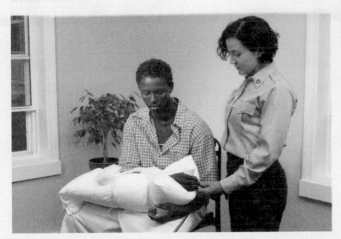

ALTERNATIVE CARE: Injuries to the hand and wrist can be cared for with soft splinting by placing a roll of bandages in the hand to maintain the position of function, then tying the forearm, wrist, and hand into the fold of one pillow or between two pillows. An injured finger can be taped to an adjacent uninjured finger or splinted with a tongue depressor. Some emergency department physicians prefer that care be limited to a wrap of soft bandages. Do not try to "pop" dislocated fingers back into place.

NOTE: *Assess the distal circulation, sensation, and motor function both before and after immobilizing or splinting an extremity.*

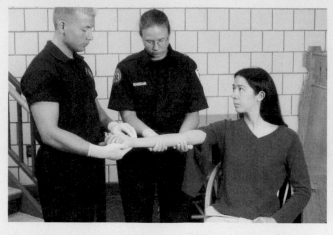

1 Check distal circulation, sensation, and motor function (CSM). Grasp the hand of the patient's injured limb as though you were going to shake hands and apply steady tension.

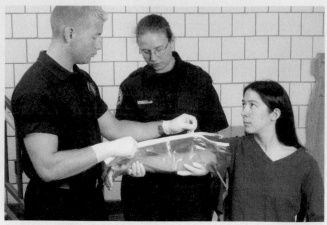

2 While you support her arm, your partner gently slides the splint over your hand and onto the patient's injured limb. The lower edge of the splint should be just above her knuckles. Make sure the splint is free of wrinkles.

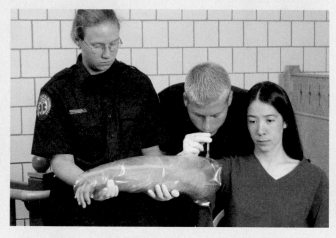

3 Continue to support the arm while your partner inflates the splint by mouth to a point where you can make a slight dent in the plastic when you press it with your thumb.

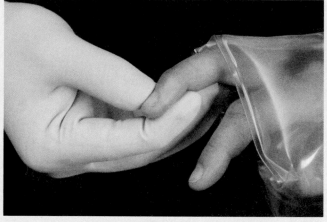

4 Continue to assess distal circulation, sensation, and motor function (CSM).

NOTE: *Air-inflated splints may leak. When applied in cold weather, an inflatable splint will expand when the patient is moved to a warmer place. Variations in pressure also occur if the patient is moved to a different altitude. Frequently monitor the pressure in the splint with your fingertip. Air-inflated splints may stick to the patient's skin in hot weather.*

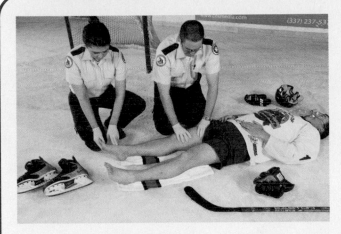

1 Take Standard Precautions.

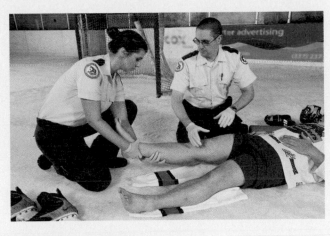

2 Manually stabilize the injured leg.

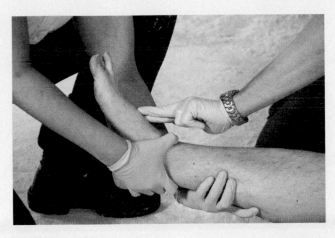

3 Assess circulation, sensation, and motor function (CSM).

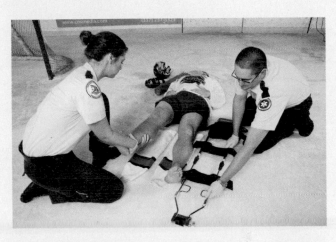

4 Adjust the splint to the proper length and position it next to the injured leg.

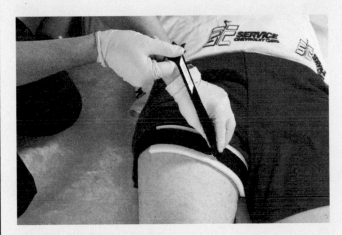

5 Apply the ischial securing device.

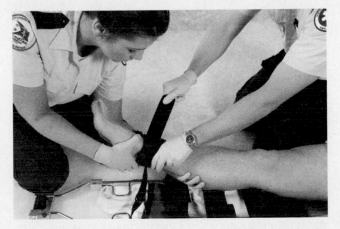

6 Apply an ankle hitch.

NOTE: *Assess the distal circulation, sensation, and motor function both before and after immobilizing or splinting an extremity.*

(continued)

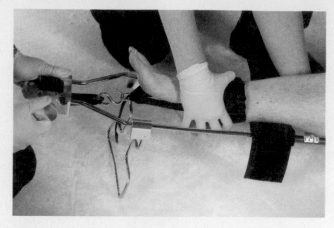

7 Apply manual traction.

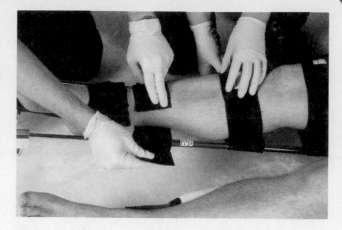

8 Secure support straps, as appropriate.

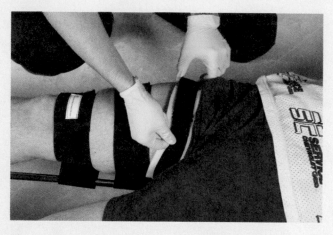

9 Reevaluate the ischial securing device.

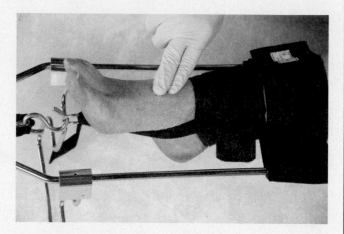

10 Reassess CSM function.

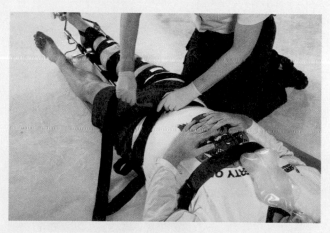

11 Secure the patient's torso to the long board to immobilize the hips.

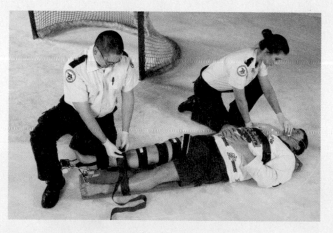

12 Secure the splint to the long board to prevent movement of the splint.

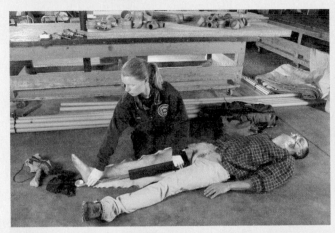

1 Place the splint medially.

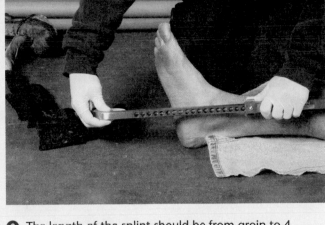

2 The length of the splint should be from groin to 4 inches below the heel. Unlock the clasp to extend the splint.

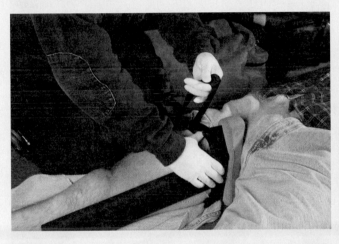

3 Secure the thigh strap.

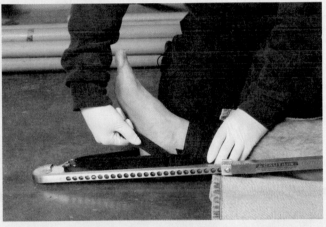

4 Wrap the ankle harness above the ankle (malleoli) and secure it under the heel.

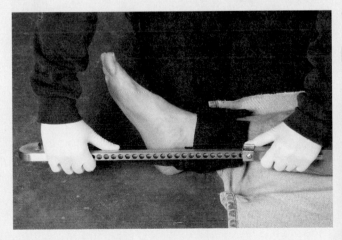

5 Release the lock and extend the splint to achieve the desired traction (in pounds on the pulley wheel).

NOTE: *Assess distal circulation, sensation, and motor function both before and after immobilizing or splinting an extremity.*

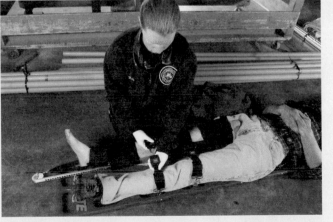

6 Secure the straps at the thigh, lower thigh and knee, and lower leg. Strap the ankles and feet together. Secure the patient to the spine board.

If there is a distal pulse and nerve function, or the limb cannot be straightened without meeting resistance or causing severe pain, knee injuries should be splinted with the knee in the position in which it is found.

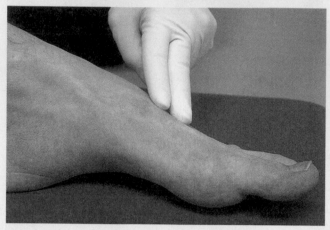

1 Assess distal CSM.

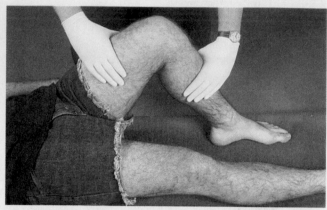

2 Stabilize the knee above and below the injury site.

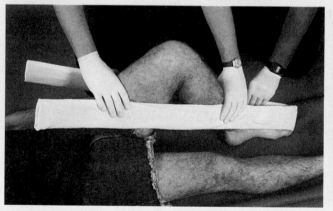

3 Place the padded side of the splints next to the injured extremity. Note that they should be equal in length and extend 6 to 12 inches beyond the mid-thigh and mid-calf.

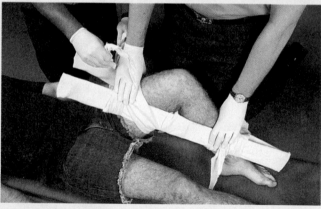

4 Place a cravat through the knee void and tie the boards together.

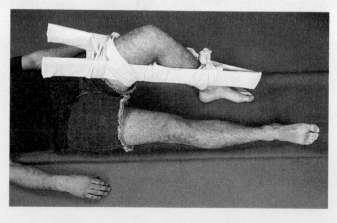

5 Using a figure-eight configuration, secure one cravat to the ankle and the boards, and the second cravat to the thigh and the boards. Reassess distal CSM.

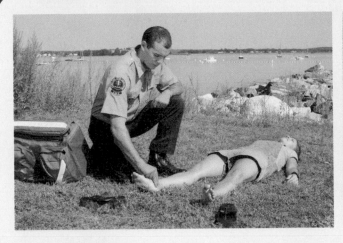

1 Assess distal CSM.

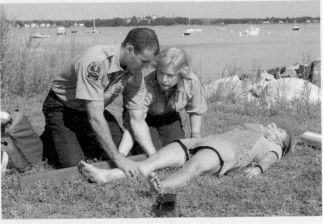

2 Stabilize. The padded board splint should extend from the buttocks to 4 inches beyond the heel.

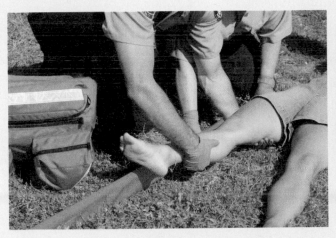

3 Maintain stabilization and lift the limb.

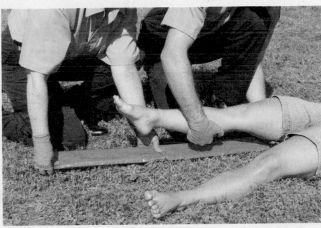

4 Place the splint along the posterior of the limb.

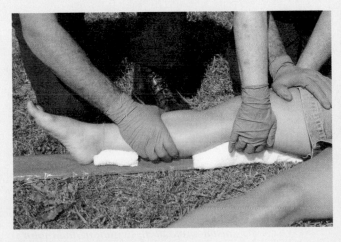

5 Pad the voids.

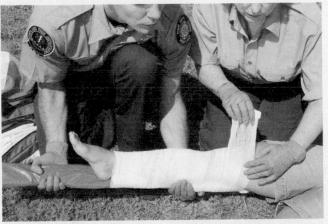

6 Use a 6-inch roller bandage or cravats to secure the injured leg to the splint.

(continued)

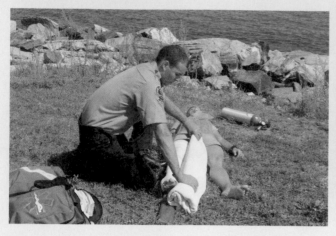

7 Place the folded blanket between the patient's legs, groin to feet.

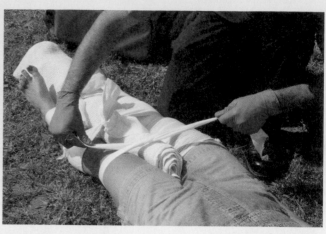

8 Tie the patient's thighs, calves, and ankles together. Do not tie the knot over the injured area.

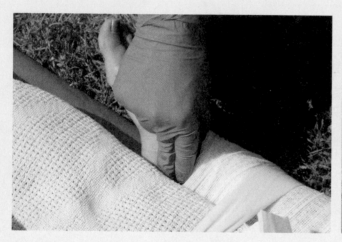

9 Reassess the distal CSM.

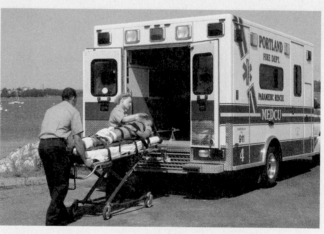

10 Provide emergency care for shock, and continue to administer high-concentration oxygen.

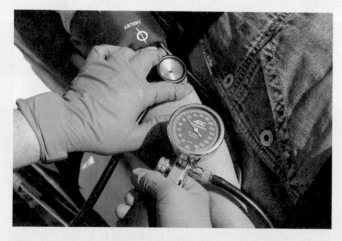

11 Monitor distal pulse and vital signs.

NOTE: *Assess distal circulation, sensation, and motor function both before and after immobilizing or splinting an extremity.*

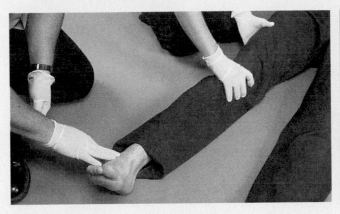

① Stabilize the injured limb, and assess distal CSM.

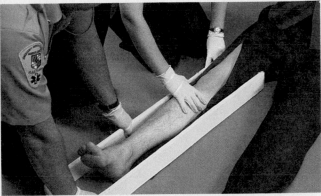

② Measure the padded board splints, medial from groin, lateral from iliac crest, both to 4 inches beyond the foot.

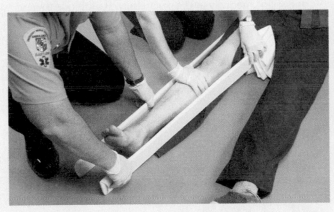

③ Position the splints.

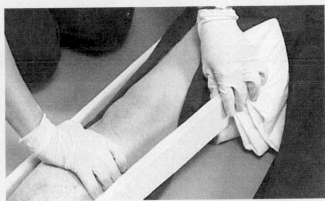

④ Pad the groin.

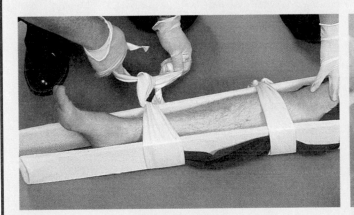

⑤ Secure the splints at the thigh, above and below the knee, and at mid-calf. Pad all voids.

NOTE: *Assess distal circulation, sensation, and motor function both before and after immobilizing or splinting an extremity.*

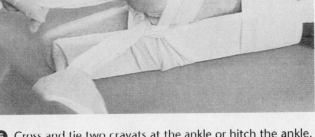

⑥ Cross and tie two cravats at the ankle or hitch the ankle. Reassess distal CSM, care for shock, and provide high-concentration oxygen.

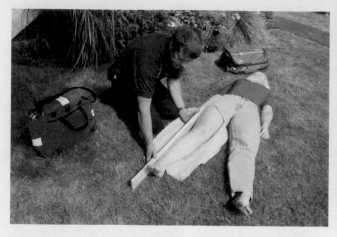

1 Assess the distal CSM. Measure the splints. They should extend above the knee and below the ankle.

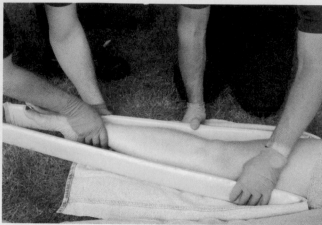

2 Apply manual traction (tension) on the leg, then place one splint medially and one laterally. Padding is toward the leg.

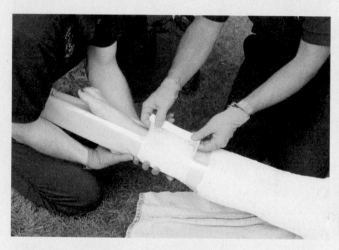

3 Secure the splints, padding the voids.

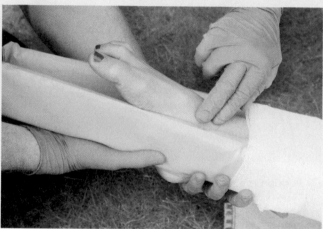

4 Reassess distal CSM.

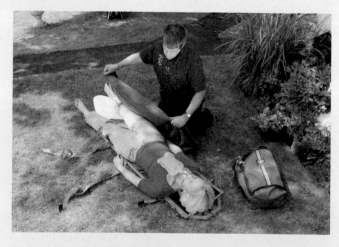

5 Provide emergency care for shock, and administer high-concentration oxygen. Transport on a long spine board.

NOTE: *Assess distal circulation, sensation, and motor function both before and after immobilizing or splinting an extremity.*

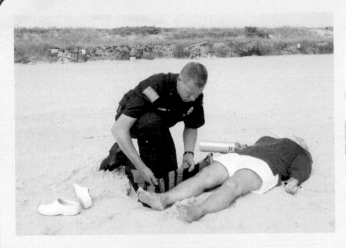

1 Assess distal CSM. Measure the splint.

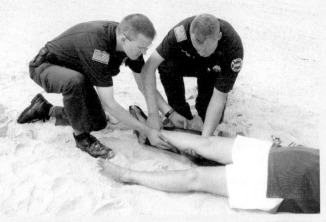

2 Lift the limb off the ground.

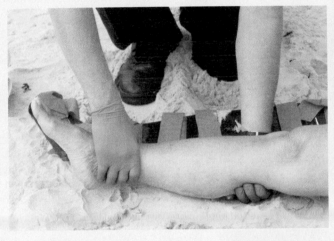

3 Apply manual traction (tension).

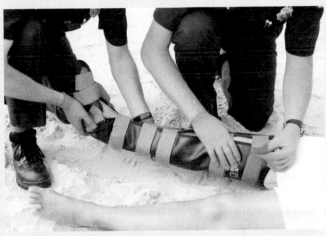

4 Secure the splint to the injured leg.

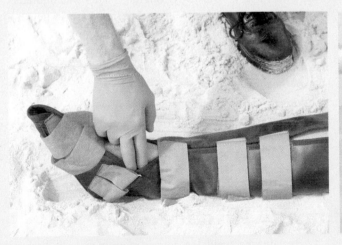

5 Reassess distal CSM.

NOTE: *Assess distal circulation, sensation, and motor function both before and after immobilizing or splinting an extremity.*

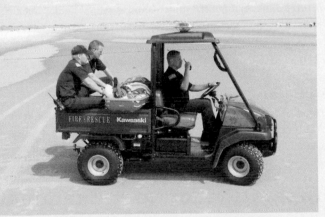

6 Care for shock, and continue to administer high-concentration oxygen. Package the patient and prepare to transport.

CHAPTER REVIEW

Key Facts and Concepts

- Bones bleed. Fractures cause blood loss from within the bone as well as from tissue damage around the bone ends. Serious or multiple fractures can cause shock.

- Splinting of long-bone fractures involves immobilizing the bone ends as well as the adjacent joints.

- Splinting protects the patient from further injury, reduces pain, and helps control bleeding.

- You may need to be creative while splinting. There are many correct ways to splint the same extremity.

- Injuries to bones and joints should be splinted prior to moving the patient.

- If the patient has multiple trauma or appears to have shock (or a significant potential for shock), do not waste time splinting individual fractures. Place the patient on a long spine board and secure the limbs to the board. You can splint individual fractures en route if time and priorities allow.

Key Decisions

- Have I fully addressed life threats and maintained my priorities—even in the presence of a grossly deformed extremity?

- Does the patient have an injury that requires splinting?

- Does the patient have multiple fractures, multiple trauma, or shock?

- Does the patient have adequate CSM distal to the musculoskeletal injury?

- Should I align the angulated extremity fracture?

Chapter Glossary

angulated fracture fracture in which the broken bone segments are at an angle to each other.

bones hard but flexible living structures that provide support for the body and protection to vital organs.

cartilage tough tissue that covers the joint ends of bones and helps to form certain body parts such as the ear.

closed extremity injury an injury to an extremity with no associated opening in the skin.

comminuted fracture a fracture in which the bone is broken in several places.

compartment syndrome injury caused when tissues such as blood vessels and nerves are constricted within a space as from swelling or from a tight dressing or cast.

crepitus (KREP-i-tus) a grating sensation or sound made when fractured bone ends rub together.

dislocation the disruption or "coming apart" of a joint.

extremities (ex-TREM-i-teez) the portions of the skeleton that include the clavicles, scapulae, arms, wrists, and hands (upper extremities) and the pelvis, thighs, legs, ankles, and feet (lower extremities).

fracture (FRAK-cher) any break in a bone.

greenstick fracture an incomplete fracture.

joints places where bones articulate, or meet.

ligaments connective tissues that connect bone to bone.

manual traction the process of applying tension to straighten and realign a fractured limb before splinting. Also called *tension*.

muscles tissues or fibers that cause movement of body parts and organs.

open extremity injury an extremity injury in which the skin has been broken or torn through from the inside by an injured bone or from the outside by something that has caused a penetrating wound with associated injury to the bone.

sprain the stretching and tearing of ligaments.

strain muscle injury resulting from overstretching or overexertion of the muscle.

tendons tissues that connect muscle to bone.

traction splint a splint that applies constant pull along the length of a lower extremity to help stabilize the fractured bone and to reduce muscle spasm in the limb. Traction splints are used primarily on femoral shaft fractures.

Preparation for Your Examination and Practice

Short Answer

1. Describe the basic anatomy of bone and its purposes.

2. Identify the signs and symptoms of musculoskeletal injury.

3. Describe basic emergency care for painful, swollen, or deformed extremities, including general guidelines for splinting long bones and joints.

4. Explain why angulated deformed injuries to the long bones should be realigned to the anatomical position.

5. List the basic principles of splinting.

6. Describe the hazards of splinting.

7. Describe the basic types of splints carried on ambulances.

Thinking and Linking

Think back to Chapter 27, "Bleeding and Shock," and link information from that chapter with information from this chapter as you consider the following situations:

- Blood loss can be significant with a fracture—even with a closed fracture. For each of the following, describe the signs and symptoms of shock you might see and whether you would expect the patient to compensate or eventually decompensate for the blood loss:
  - Fractured tibia and fibula
  - Both tibias and fibulas fractured

- Femur fracture
- Pelvic fracture

Think back to Chapter 3, "Lifting and Moving Patients," and Chapter 10, "Scene Size-Up," and link information from those chapters with information from this chapter as you consider the following situation:

- You have a patient who was thrown from an ATV deep in the woods. He complains of pain to his thigh and hip. What treatment and transportation devices would you use? What assistance would you call for in the scene size-up?

Critical Thinking Exercises

Shock and pain are often associated with musculoskeletal injuries. The purpose of this exercise will be to consider how you might deal with these factors when your patient has a musculoskeletal injury.

1. List three assessment findings that you would use to help determine if your musculoskeletal injury patient is in shock.

2. Patients who suffer fractures can be in extreme pain. Pain can cause anxiety and elevated pulse rates. How could you differentiate between a patient with a rapid pulse and anxiety from pain versus a patient with rapid pulse and anxiety from shock?

Pathophysiology to Practice

The following questions are designed to assist you in gathering relevant clinical information and making accurate decisions in the field.

1. Why do broken bones cause shock?

2. Why would you attempt to straighten an extremity that has no pulses distal to the extremity?

3. Can a patient have a fracture without obvious deformity? Explain your answer.

Street Scenes

You and your crew arrive for duty at the firehouse when you are called out for a "fall injury." A police unit is already on-scene, and they inform you that it is safe. Exiting your engine and taking Standard Precautions, you observe a tall woman in her twenties in jogging clothes leaning on the front hood of a car. She is wincing. The police officer standing next to her approaches and introduces you to your patient. She says her name is Desta.

Your primary assessment reveals that Desta has a good airway and that she is breathing fine. "What happened, Desta, and why did you call EMS this morning?"

"I fell off that wall while trying to climb over it," she answers, simultaneously pointing to a 4-foot rock wall approximately 100 feet away. "When I landed, I heard something crack in my right leg. I hopped on one foot to this car, and called for help." You quickly make a mental note that the surface she landed on is asphalt.

Street Scene Questions

1. What priority would you assign to this patient? Why?
2. How would you continue your assessment?

Desta's mental status seems normal. There are no signs of bleeding anywhere on her body. You assign a low priority to her, and continue your assessment by performing a history and physical exam. Desta tells you that she is taking no medications. You ask if she has any allergies and she smiles as she replies, "Rock walls, apparently." She laughs, then suddenly grimaces in pain as she unintentionally shifts her weight onto her right leg.

You obtain baseline vital signs and learn Desta's pulse is 88 and regular, respirations are 16 and unlabored, and blood pressure is 108/72. Her pupils are equal and reactive. She states she has no pain anywhere but in her lower right leg.

Street Scene Questions

3. What signs might you expect to find with a broken long bone?
4. What are your major concerns with possible broken bones in the extremities?

You assist Desta from her standing position onto your cot, carefully supporting her right leg. Then you expose the extremity. About 2 inches above the ankle, you observe swelling and a noticeable, unnatural curve to her leg. The skin is not broken. You are concerned that she might have nerve and muscle damage below the injury, but she is able to move her toes and feel you touch her foot. You also detect a pulse below the injury site.

Street Scene Question

5. What interventions are appropriate for this patient?

A member of your crew brings an air splint, which provides immobilization to the joint above and below the injury site. You maintain manual traction, being careful not to unnecessarily move the extremity, and apply the splint. After application, the patient states her leg feels more secure. You reassess her vitals as well as pulses, motor function, and sensation below the injury site. Everything appears to be normal. During transport, you continue to check distal pulses, motor function, and sensation on the affected extremity. Transport to the hospital is uneventful.

31 Trauma to the Head, Neck, and Spine

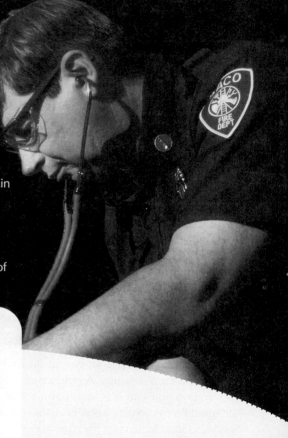

○ **STANDARD**
Trauma (Head, Facial, Neck, and Spine Trauma)

○ **COMPETENCY**
Applies fundamental knowledge to provide basic emergency care and transportation based on assessment findings for an acutely injured patient.

○ **CORE CONCEPTS**
— Understanding the anatomy of the nervous system, head, and spine

— Understanding skull and brain injuries and emergency care for skull and brain injuries

— Understanding wounds to the neck and emergency care for neck wounds

— Understanding spine injuries and emergency care for spine injuries

— Understanding immobilization issues and how to immobilize various types of patients with potential spine injury

EXPLORE Resource Central

To access Resource Central, follow directions on the Student Access Card provided with this text. If there is no card, go to **www.bradybooks.com** and follow the Resource Central link to Buy Access from there. Under Media Resources, you will find:

▶ **Applying a Cervical Collar**
Watch a video on how to properly apply a cervical collar and what you should pay particular attention to prior to applying the collar.

▶ **Traumatic Brain Injury from Neurosurgerytoday.org**
Read about what defines a traumatic brain injury, some signs and symptoms, and treatment and management of these injuries.

▶ **First Aid for Eye Emergencies**
Learn how to assess a patient with a traumatic eye injury and what you should do for particular injuries, such as a chemical burn to the eye.

OBJECTIVES

After reading this chapter you should be able to:

31.1 Define key terms introduced in this chapter.

31.2 Describe the components and function of the nervous system and the anatomy of the head and spine. (pp. 747–750)

31.3 Describe types of injuries to the skull and brain. (pp. 750–759)

31.4 Describe the general assessment and management of skull fractures and brain injuries. (pp. 754–757)

31.5 Describe specific concerns in management of cranial injuries with impaled objects. (p. 757)

31.6 Describe specific concerns in management of injuries to the face and jaw. (pp. 757–759)

31.7 Define nontraumatic brain injuries. (p. 757)

31.8 Explain the purpose and elements of the Glasgow Coma Scale. (pp. 759–760)

31.9 Discuss the assessment and management of open wounds to the next. (pp. 761, 762)

31.10 List types and mechanisms of spine injury. (pp. 761–765)

31.11 Discuss the assessment and management of spine and spinal cord injury. (pp. 765–767, 768)

31.12 Discuss issues in the immobilization of the head, neck, and spine specifically for the following:
a. Applying a cervical collar (pp. 767–769)
b. Immobilizing a seated patient, including rapid extrication for high priority patients (pp. 769–774)

c. Applying a long backboard (pp. 775–778)
d. Rapid extrication from a child safety seat (pp. 778–780)
e. Immobilizing a standing patient (pp. 781–784)
f. Immobilizing a patient wearing a helmet (pp. 732–786)

31.13 Discuss issues in selective spine immobilization. (pp. 787–788)

KEY TERMS

central nervous system, p. 747
concussion, p. 751
contusion, p. 751
cranium, p. 748
dermatome, p. 764

foramen magnum, p. 752
hematoma, p. 752
herniation, p. 753
intracranial pressure (ICP), p. 752
laceration, p. 752

malar, p. 748
mandible, p. 748
maxillae, p. 748
nasal bones, p. 748
neurogenic shock, p. 765
orbits, p. 748

peripheral nervous system, p. 747
spinous process, p. 749
temporomandibular joint, p. 748
vertebrae, p. 749

Y ou have probably noticed that, throughout the earlier chapters of this book, there have been many cautions for patients with possible injuries to the head and spine. This is because injuries to these areas are extremely serious and may result in severe permanent disability or death if improperly treated or missed during your assessment. Second only to proper assessment and care of the ABCs, proper assessment and care for head and spine injuries will be your most important responsibility as an EMT.

NERVOUS AND SKELETAL SYSTEMS

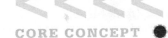

The following segments briefly review the anatomy of the nervous system, head, and spine. For more information on these areas, review Chapter 5, "Medical Terminology and Anatomy and Physiology."

CORE CONCEPT

Understanding the anatomy of the nervous system, head, and spine

Nervous System

The components of the *nervous system* are the brain and the spinal cord as well as the nerves that enter and exit the brain and spinal cord and extend to the various parts of the body. The nervous system provides overall control of thought, sensations, and motor functions, whereas the skeletal system provides support and protection. The skull protects the brain, whereas the bones of the spine protect the spinal cord (Figure 31-1). Whenever the skull or the spine is injured, suspect nervous system damage as well.

The nervous system (Figure 31-2) is divided into two subsystems: the central nervous system and the peripheral nervous system. The *central nervous system* consists of the brain and the spinal cord. The *peripheral nervous system* includes the pairs of nerves that enter and exit the spinal cord between each pair of vertebrae, the 12 pairs of cranial nerves that travel from the brain without passing through the spinal cord, and all of the body's other motor

nervous system

provides overall control of thought, sensation, and the body's voluntary and involuntary motor functions. The components of the nervous system are the brain and the spinal cord as well as the nerves that enter and exit the brain and spinal cord and extend to the various parts of the body.

central nervous system

the brain and the spinal cord.

FIGURE 31-1 Enhanced color spinal cord. *(© Photo Researchers, Inc.)*

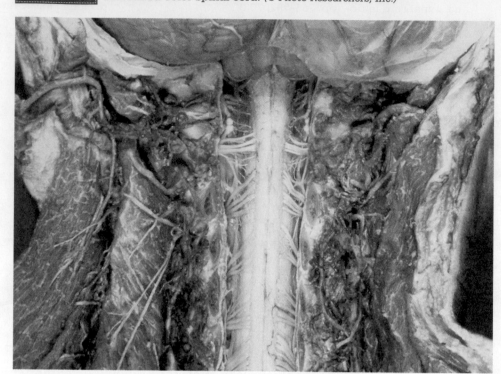

peripheral nervous system
the nerves that enter and exit the spinal cord between the vertebrae; the 12 pairs of cranial nerves that travel between the brain and organs without passing through the spinal cord; and all of the body's other motor and sensory nerves.

autonomic nervous system
controls involuntary functions.

cranium (KRAY-ne-um)
the bony structure making up the forehead, top, back, and upper sides of the skull.

mandible (MAN-di-bl)
the lower jaw bone.

temporal (TEM-po-ral) **bone**
bone that forms part of the side of the skull and floor of the cranial cavity. There is a right and a left temporal bone.

temporomandibular (TEM-po-ro-mand-DIB-yuh-lar) **joint**
the movable joint formed between the mandible and the temporal bone, also called the TMJ.

maxillae (mak-SIL-e)
the two fused bones forming the upper jaw.

nasal (NAY-zul) **bones**
the bones that form the upper third, or bridge, of the nose.

malar (MAY-lar)
the cheek bone, also called the zygomatic bone.

orbits
the bony structures around the eyes; the eye sockets.

cerebrospinal (suh-RE-bro-SPI-nal) **fluid (CSF)**
the fluid that surrounds the brain and spinal cord.

and sensory nerves. *Neurons* are the specialized nerve cells that transmit nervous system impulses throughout the body (Figure 31-3).

Messages from the body to the brain are carried by sensory nerves. Messages from the brain to the muscles are carried by motor nerves. The motor nerves control voluntary movements, or those we consciously control, such as running or grasping. As the nerves exit the brain, prior to traveling down the spinal cord, they cross over to the opposite side of the body. This is why an injury to the left side of the brain may produce effects such as weakness or lack of sensation on the right side of the body.

Some nerves control involuntary functions—those we do not consciously control—including heartbeat, breathing, control of the diameter of your vessels, control of the round sphincter muscles closing your bladder and bowel, and digestion. These nerves are part of the ***autonomic nervous system***. (Autonomic means automatic.)

Anatomy of the Head

The skull is made up of the ***cranium*** and the facial bones (Figure 31-4). The cranium, the portion of the skull that encloses the brain, is formed by the forehead, top, back, and upper sides of the skull. The cranial floor is the inferior wall of the brain case, the bony floor beneath the brain. The cranial bones are fused together to form immovable joints.

There are 14 irregularly shaped bones forming the face. The facial bones are fused into immovable joints, except for the ***mandible***, which joins on each side of the cranium with a ***temporal bone*** to form the ***temporomandibular joint***, sometimes referred to as the TM joint.

The upper jaw is made up of two fused bones called the ***maxillae***. Each is known as a *maxilla*. The upper third, or bridge, of the nose contains two ***nasal bones***. There is a cheek bone on each side of the skull which can be called the ***malar*** or *zygomatic* bone. The malars and the maxillae form a portion of the ***orbits*** (sockets) of the eyes.

The brain is held within the skull. The spinal cord exits the base of the brain and leaves the skull through a large hole where the spinal column is attached. The brain is bathed in a fluid called ***cerebrospinal fluid (CSF)***, which also circulates down the spine around the spinal cord.

FIGURE 31-2 Nervous system.

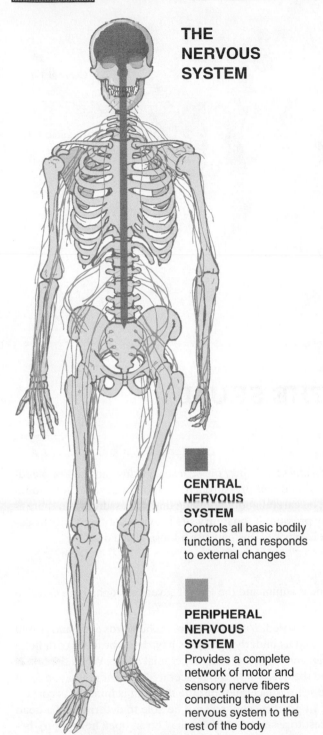

THE
NERVOUS
SYSTEM

CENTRAL NERVOUS SYSTEM
Controls all basic bodily functions, and responds to external changes

PERIPHERAL NERVOUS SYSTEM
Provides a complete network of motor and sensory nerve fibers connecting the central nervous system to the rest of the body

FIGURE 31-3 Neurons are the specialized nerve cells that transmit nervous system impulses throughout the body. (© Photo Researchers, Inc.)

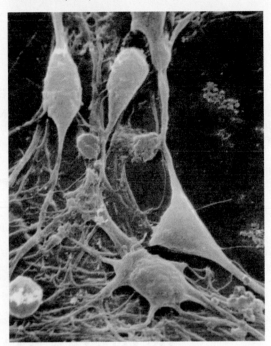

Anatomy of the Spine

The spine is made up of 33 irregularly shaped bones, called ***vertebrae*** (singular *vertebra*), which sit one on top of another to form the spinal column. Each vertebra has a ***spinous process***, a bony bump you can feel along the center of a person's back. Every vertebra has a hollow space like the hole in a donut. These hollow spaces form a channel that runs the length of the spinal column and contains the spinal cord, which is cushioned by the cerebrospinal fluid.

The vertebrae are divided into five areas (shown in Figure 31-5). From top to bottom, they are: 7 cervical (in the neck), 12 thoracic (to which the ribs attach), 5 lumbar (mid-back), 5 sacral (lower back), and 4 coccygeal (in the coccyx, or tailbone). Both the sacral and coccygeal vertebrae are fused together, forming the posterior portion of the pelvis.

vertebrae (VERT-uh-bray)
the bones of the spinal column (singular vertebra).

spinous (SPI-nus) **process**
the bony bump on a vertebra.

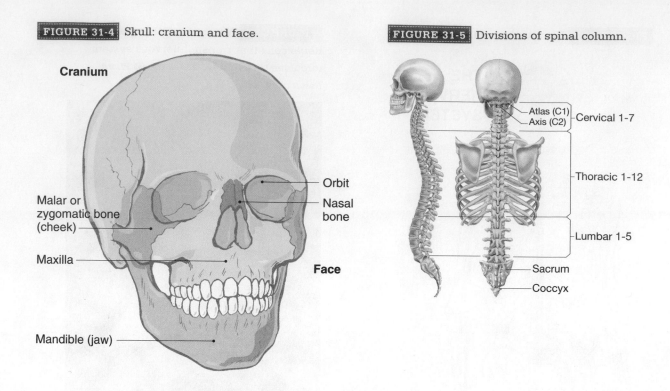

Cranium

Malar or zygomatic bone (cheek)

Maxilla

Mandible (jaw)

Orbit

Nasal bone

Face

Atlas (C1)
Axis (C2)
Cervical 1-7

Thoracic 1-12

Lumbar 1-5

Sacrum

Coccyx

INJURIES TO THE SKULL AND BRAIN

Scalp Injuries

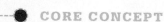

CORE CONCEPT

Understanding skull and brain injuries and emergency care for skull and brain injuries

The scalp has many blood vessels, so any scalp injury may cause a profuse amount of bleeding. Control scalp bleeding by applying direct pressure. Dress and bandage as you would other soft-tissue injuries. However, be careful about applying direct pressure when there is a possible skull injury. Do not apply pressure if the injury site shows bone fragments or depression of the bone or if the brain is exposed. Instead, use a loose gauze dressing.

Skull Injuries

Skull injuries include fractures to the cranium and the face. If severe enough, there can also be injuries to the brain.

Skull injuries can be either open or closed. With most injuries, the words *open* and *closed* refer to whether or not the skin and its underlying tissues have been broken. With head injuries, however, the words *open* and *closed* refer to the cranial bones. When the bones of the cranium are fractured, and the overlying scalp is lacerated, the patient has an *open head injury* (Figure 31-6). If the scalp is lacerated but the cranium is intact, it is considered to be a *closed head injury*. In practice, you may not be able to determine if a head injury is open or closed. It is safest to assume that there may be an open head injury beneath any contusion or laceration of the scalp. You should also be aware that a head injury may be present with *no* external injury.

NOTE: *Whenever you suspect a skull or brain injury, also suspect spine injury.*

Brain Injuries

Brain injuries can be classified as direct or indirect. *Direct injuries* to the brain can occur in open head injuries, with the brain being lacerated, punctured, or bruised by the broken bones or by foreign objects. *Indirect injuries* to the brain may occur with either closed or open head injuries. In an indirect injury, the shock of impact on the skull is transferred to the brain. Indirect injuries to the brain include concussions and contusions.

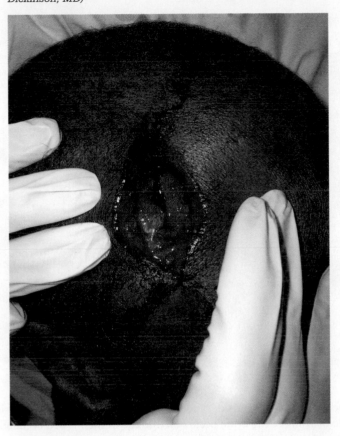

FIGURE 31-6 An open skull fracture. (© *Edward T. Dickinson, MD*)

NOTE: *One of the first and most significant signs of head injury is altered mental status. In some patients, it would be easy to assume the patient was intoxicated or on drugs when the true underlying problem is a head injury. Never assume a patient with an altered mental status is simply intoxicated or on drugs. Use your assessment (palpation) and history.*

Traumatic Brain Injuries

A traumatic brain injury (TBI) is an injury that disrupts the normal functioning of the brain. It may be a brief (e.g., concussion) or long-term condition with permanent damage to the brain. The Centers for Disease Control estimates that 1.7 million people sustain a traumatic brain injury each year in the United States.

The following section describes types of traumatic brain injury. It is not necessary for you as an EMT to diagnose the specific conditions (this is done in the hospital), but knowing the types of injuries and how they present will help you understand these conditions, identify critical patients, and make appropriate transport decisions.

Concussion A *concussion* (Figure 31-7) may be so mild that the patient is unaware of the injury. When a person strikes his head in a fall, or is struck by a blunt object, a certain amount of the force is transferred through the skull to the brain. Usually there is no detectable damage to the brain and the patient may or may not become unconscious. Most patients with a concussion will feel a little "groggy" after receiving a blow to the head, and a headache is also common. If there is a loss of consciousness, it usually lasts only a short time and does not tend to recur. Sometimes, after a head blow, bystanders will say the patient "just sat there staring off into space for a few minutes." Some loss of memory (amnesia) of the events surrounding the incident is fairly common. A common saying is that the fighter did not see the punch that did him in. Actually, he probably did see the punch but then forgot it because of the concussion.

Contusion A bruised brain, or brain *contusion*, can occur with closed head injuries, when the force of the blow is great enough to rupture blood vessels on or within the brain. A contusion is often caused by a collision or blow that causes the brain to hit the inside of

concussion
mild closed head injury without detectable damage to the brain. Complete recovery is usually expected.

contusion
in brain injuries, a bruised brain caused when the force of a blow to the head is great enough to rupture blood vessels.

FIGURE 31-7 Closed head injuries.

CONCUSSION
- Mild injury, usually with no detectable brain damage
- May have brief loss of consciousness
- Headache, grogginess, and short-term memory loss common

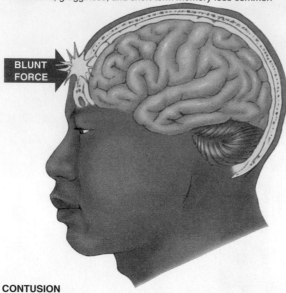

BLUNT FORCE

CONTUSION
- Unconsciousness or decreased level of responsiveness
- Bruising of brain tissue

FIGURE 31-8 Meninges (covering layers) of the brain.

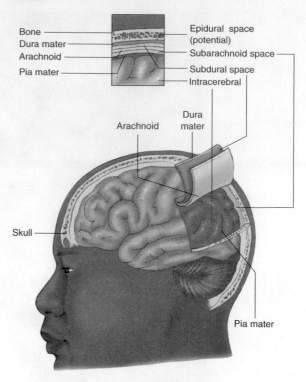

Bone
Dura mater
Arachnoid
Pia mater

Epidural space (potential)
Subarachnoid space
Subdural space
Intracerebral

Arachnoid
Dura mater
Skull
Pia mater

---

laceration (las-uh-RAY-shun)
in brain injuries, a cut to the brain.

the skull, bounce off the opposite side, and then rebound to strike the first side of the skull again. When the bruising of the brain occurs on the side of the blow, it is called a *coup injury*; when it occurs on the side opposite the blow, it is called a *contrecoup injury*.

Laceration A *laceration*, or cut, to the brain can occur from the same forces that might cause a contusion. The inner skull has many sharp, bony ridges that can lacerate a moving brain. A laceration or a puncture wound can also be caused by an object penetrating the cranium.

hematoma (HE-mah-TO-mah)
in a head injury, a collection of blood within the skull or brain.

Hematoma A *hematoma* is a collection of blood within tissue. A hematoma inside the cranium is named according to its location, which may be inside or outside the dura, the brain's protective outer covering (Figure 31-8), or within the brain itself. A *subdural hematoma* is a collection of blood between the brain and the dura. An *epidural hematoma* is blood between the dura and the skull. An *intracerebral hematoma* occurs when blood pools within the brain (Figure 31-9).

Intracranial Pressure

There is limited room for expansion inside the patient's hard skull. When a hematoma develops, pressure increases inside the skull. This is referred to as increasing **intracranial pressure (ICP)**. There is a typical progression that is seen with this condition.

intracranial (IN-truh-KRAY-ne-ul) **pressure (ICP)**
pressure inside the skull.

The hematoma expands and places pressure on the brain, pushing and compressing the brain tissue. Since the cranium is a rigid container, the brain is forced toward the only space available—the opening at the base of the skull called the **foramen magnum**.

foramen magnum (FOR-uh-men MAG-num)
the opening at the base of the skull through which the spinal cord passes from the brain.

The time it takes for symptoms to develop from an increased ICP depends on the rate of bleeding into the skull and the location of the bleed. A small subdural hematoma obtained in an assault or a fall could take from hours up to 2 days before serious symptoms develop, whereas a brisk epidural bleed may almost instantly develop and show symptoms.

The body has mechanisms to deal with increasing pressure within the brain. The body's highest priority is to perfuse the brain with oxygen. When intracranial pressure increases, the body must increase the blood pressure to pump blood into and perfuse the brain. This is why you will see increasing blood pressure in patients with intracranial pressure.

As ICP increases and cerebral perfusion decreases, carbon dioxide levels increase, and this causes brain tissue to swell. This swelling worsens intracranial pressure and creates a vi-

FIGURE 31-9 Hematomas within the cranium.

CRANIAL HEMATOMAS

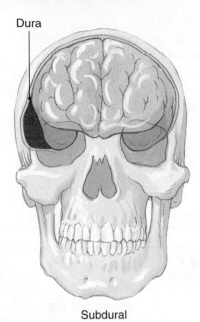
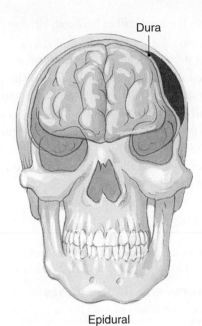
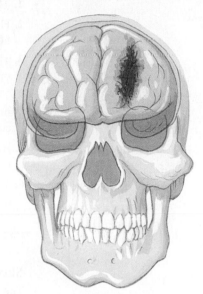

Dura

Dura

Subdural

Epidural

Intracerebral

cious cycle in which the body increases blood pressure in an attempt to perfuse the brain while carbon dioxide builds and increases swelling.

As the hematoma continues to grow, swelling worsens, and the brain is pushed downward toward the foramen magnum, compressing the brainstem. The brainstem regulates our most vital functions, including breathing, heartbeat, and blood pressure. As this area is compressed, in addition to an altered mental status, you may see dilated pupils or sluggish pupil reaction, abnormal respiration patterns, increased systolic blood pressure, and a decreased pulse rate.

As the brain and brainstem become severely compressed and pushed downward (***herniation***), the patient may exhibit decorticate or decerebrate posturing. These may be neurological posturing, such as flexing the arms and wrists and extending the legs and feet (decorticate posture) (Figure 31-10A) or extending the arms with the shoulders rotated inward and wrists flexed and with the legs extended (decerebrate posture) (Figure 31-10B). These postures may be assumed spontaneously or in response to a painful stimulus.

herniation (her-ne-AY-shun)
pushing of a portion of the brain through the foramen magnum as a result of increased intracranial pressure.

FIGURE 31-10 (A) Decorticate posturing. (B) Decerebrate posturing.

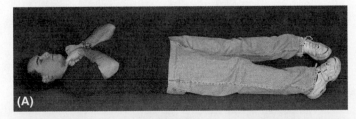

(A)

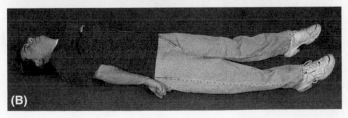

(B)

A patient who has an epidural or subdural hematoma (remembering that there are variables such as the size and location of the bleed as well as concurrent injuries) may present in the following sequence:

1. The patient falls and strikes his head. He appears OK at first.

2. He develops a slight altered mental status after about 10 minutes. This is because the hematoma is beginning to place pressure on one or both cerebral hemispheres.

3. The altered mental status worsens. Soon the patient responds to loud verbal stimulus only by moaning. His blood pressure begins to increase.

4. The patient is now totally unresponsive to any stimuli. His blood pressure is 220/106. You notice his pulse beginning to drop. It had been 88 and now it is 54. His pupils have become unequal or nonreactive.

5. Respirations become slightly irregular. Blood pressure continues to increase. The pulse now drops to 48/minute.

6. The patient begins decerebrate posturing. You may see some seizure activity, followed by decorticate posturing. Death follows if uncorrected by intervention at a trauma center.

PATIENT ASSESSMENT

Skull Fractures and Brain Injuries

The signs of skull fracture and of brain injury are very similar, as noted in the following list (Figure 31-11):

■ Although visible bone fragments and perhaps bits of brain tissue are the most obvious signs of skull fracture, most skull fractures do not produce these signs.

■ The patient may have an altered mental status. Check mental status by using the AVPU scale (alert, verbal stimulus, painful stimulus, unresponsive). If the patient is alert, check for orientation to person, place, and time. Some EMS agencies also use the Glasgow Coma Scale (described later in this chapter).

■ There may be a deep laceration or severe bruise or hematoma to the scalp or forehead. Do not probe or separate the wound opening to determine wound depth.

FIGURE 31-11 Signs of cranial fracture or brain injury.

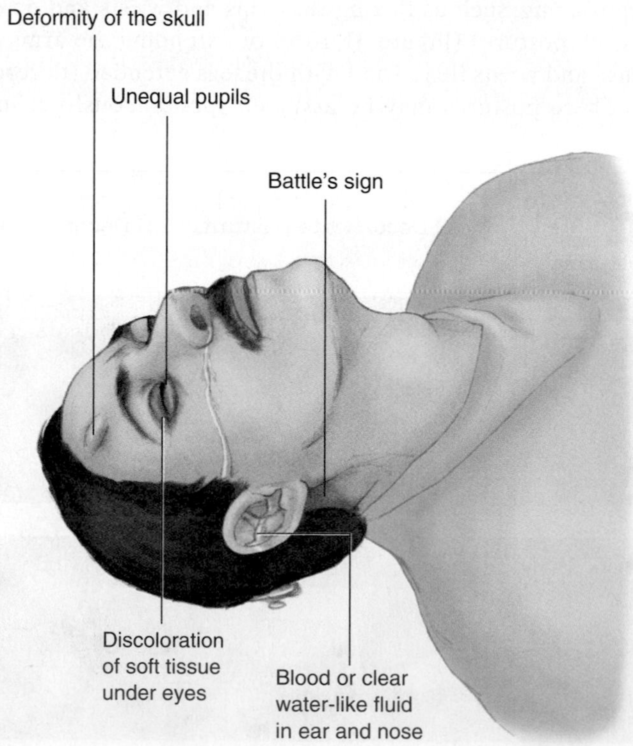

Deformity of the skull

Unequal pupils

Battle's sign

Discoloration of soft tissue under eyes

Blood or clear water-like fluid in ear and nose

FIGURE 31-12 Battle's sign. (© Edward T. Dickinson, MD)

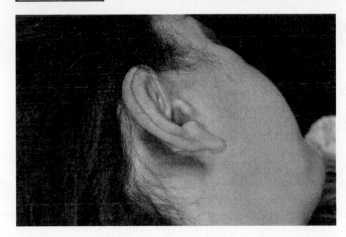

- Depressions or deformity of the skull, large swellings ("goose eggs"), or anything unusual about the shape of the cranium may be visible.
- Severe pain may exist at the site of a head injury. Pain may range from a headache to severe discomfort. Do not palpate the injury site with your fingertips as you may push bone fragments into the injury.
- "Battle's sign," a bruise behind the ear (late sign), may be present (Figure 31-12).
- Pupils are unequal or nonreactive to light (Figure 31-13).
- "Raccoon eyes," black eyes, or discoloration of the soft tissues are present under both eyes (late sign).
- One eye appears to be sunken.
- Bleeding exists from the ears and/or nose.
- Clear fluid flows from the ears and/or nose.
- The patient displays a personality change, ranging from irritable to irrational behavior (a major sign).
- The patient has an increased blood pressure and decreased pulse rate (Cushing's triad, also called Cushing's reflex).
- The patient has irregular breathing patterns.

FIGURE 31-13 Unequal pupils. (© Edward T. Dickinson, MD)

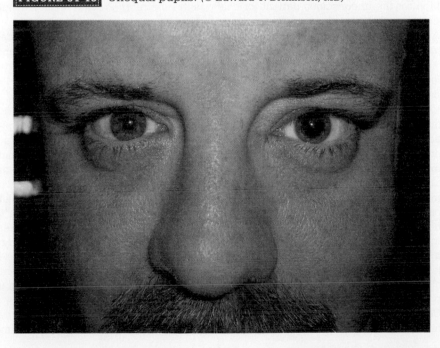

- There is a temperature increase (late sign due to inflammation, infection, or damage to temperature-regulating centers).
- Blurred or multiple-image vision is present in one or both eyes.
- Impaired hearing or ringing occurs in the patient's ears.
- Equilibrium problems exist. The patient may be unable to stand still with his eyes closed or may stumble when attempting to walk. (Do not test for this.)
- Forceful or projectile vomiting may occur.
- The patient may exhibit decorticate or decerebrate posturing.
- The patient may experience paralysis or disability on one side of the body.
- Seizures may be present.
- The patient has deteriorating vital signs.

Note that shock (hypoperfusion) from blood loss is generally not a sign of head injury, except in infants. There simply is not enough room within the adult skull to permit enough bleeding to cause shock. If there is head injury with shock, look for indications of blood loss somewhere else on the body.

With so many factors to consider, possible skull or brain injury can be very difficult to definitively determine. Therefore, assume the patient has a skull or brain injury when the mechanism of injury and the location of the injury indicate a possible head injury.

Decision Points

- Does my patient have a serious or potentially serious head injury? Should he be transported to a trauma center?
- Do my patient's complaint and mechanism of injury indicate spinal stabilization and immobilization are warranted?

PATIENT CARE

Skull Fractures and Brain Injuries

Emergency care of a patient with skull fractures and brain injuries includes the following steps:

1. Take appropriate Standard Precautions.
2. Assume there is a spine injury. Provide manual stabilization of the head on first patient contact, and use the jaw-thrust maneuver to open the airway. For the unconscious patient, insert an oropharyngeal airway without hyperextending the neck. Have suctioning equipment ready, since these patients are prone to vomiting.
3. Monitor the unconscious patient for changes in breathing. Provide artificial ventilations if breathing is inadequate.
4. Apply a rigid cervical collar, immobilize the neck and spine, and, if appropriate, determine the method of extrication, either normal or rapid (discussed later in this chapter).
5. Administer high-concentration oxygen by nonrebreather mask, and evaluate the need for artificial ventilations with supplemental oxygen. This is critical if there is any brain damage.
6. In some EMS systems, if the patient shows signs of increased intracranial pressure (such as decreased mental status associated with dilated pupils or sluggish pupil reaction, abnormal respiration patterns, increased systolic blood pressure, and a decreased pulse rate.), EMTs are instructed to ventilate the patient with supplemental oxygen at the rate of approximately 20 breaths per minute. This *slight* hyperventilation will help reduce brain tissue swelling by lowering carbon dioxide levels and raising oxygen levels. The procedure is not without risk, however. Too much ventilation can decrease blood flow to the brain. This process is reserved for patients with critical head injuries, where the benefit is felt to outweigh the risk. Hyperventilating a breathing patient with a bag-valve mask and oral airway is extremely difficult to do and runs a serious risk of inflating the stomach and causing aspiration of stomach contents. Follow your local protocol. Hyperventilation is not a routine part of the management for all head injury patients—only those who are believed to have increasing intracranial pressure.
7. Control bleeding. Do not apply direct pressure if the injury site shows bone fragments or depression of the bone or if the brain is exposed. Do not attempt to stop the flow of

blood or cerebrospinal fluid from the ears or the nose. If the skull is fractured, you may increase intracranial pressure and the risk of infection. Instead, use a loose gauze dressing.

8. Keep the patient at rest. This can be a critical step.
9. Talk to the conscious patient and provide emotional support. Ask the patient questions so that he will have to concentrate. This procedure also will help you to detect changes in the patient's mental status.
10. Dress and bandage open wounds. Stabilize any penetrating objects. (Do not remove any objects or fragments of bone.)
11. Manage the patient for shock even if signs of shock are not yet present. However, do not elevate the legs unless signs of shock are present and your local protocols permit. Avoid overheating.
12. Be prepared for vomiting. Have a suction unit ready for use.
13. Transport the patient promptly.
14. Monitor vital signs every 5 minutes en route to the hospital.

Decision Point

• Does my patient have increasing intracranial pressure? Should I hyperventilate my patient?

If you are not certain of the severity of the patient's injuries, or if there is evidence of cervical-spine injury, or if the patient with a head injury is unconscious, then the patient must be immobilized to a long spine board. With the entire head, neck, and body rigidly immobilized, the patient may be rotated into a lateral recumbent position so that blood and saliva can freely drain. If the patient vomits, the vomitus is also less likely to cause an airway obstruction or be aspirated (breathed into the lungs) in this position. Some patients with a head injury will vomit without warning. Many vomit without first experiencing nausea. The vomiting is likely to be projectile vomiting (forceful, explosive vomiting). If injuries prevent lateral positioning, constant monitoring and frequent suctioning are required.

Cranial Injuries with Impaled Objects

If there is an object impaled in the cranium, do not remove it. Instead, stabilize the object in place with bulky dressings. (See information on stabilizing impaled objects in Chapter 28, "Soft-Tissue Trauma.") This, with care in handling, will minimize accidental movement of the object.

A lengthy impaled object can make transporting the patient impossible until the object is cut or shortened. Pad around the object with bulky dressings, then carefully (and rigidly) stabilize the object on both sides of where the cut will be made. Cutting should be done with a tool that will not cause the object to move or vibrate when it is finally severed. A hand hacksaw with a fine-tooth blade can be carefully controlled and produces only a small amount of heat. In any case in which you may have to cut an impaled object, seek advice from medical direction or the emergency department physician.

Injuries to the Face and Jaw

Facial fractures are usually caused by an impact, as when a child is struck in the face by a baseball bat or when someone is thrown against a windshield. Bone fragments may lodge in the back of the pharynx and cause airway obstruction. Blood, blood clots, dislodged teeth, or a separated palate may also block the airway. Signs of a facial fracture are shown in Figure 31-14.

NOTE: *The face is part of the skull. Therefore, brain injury may accompany a blow of sufficient force to the face. Treat this patient as you would any patient with a suspected skull or brain injury.*

The mandible is subject to dislocation as well as to fracture. As with any facial injury, there may be pain, discoloration, swelling, and facial distortion. In addition, when the mandible is injured or dislocated, the patient may be unable to move the lower jaw or may have difficulty speaking. There may be an improper alignment of the upper and lower teeth and bleeding around the teeth (Figure 31-15).

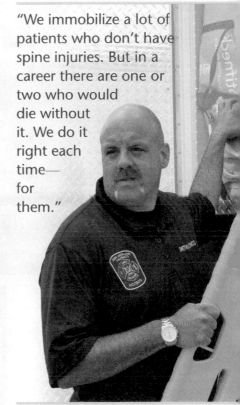

"We immobilize a lot of patients who don't have spine injuries. But in a career there are one or two who would die without it. We do it right each time— for them."

FIGURE 31-14 Signs of facial fracture.

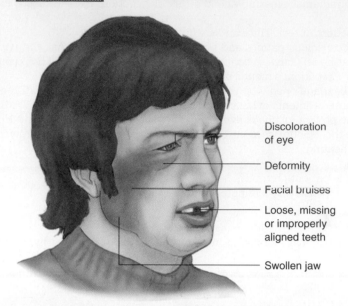

Discoloration of eye

Deformity

Facial bruises

Loose, missing or improperly aligned teeth

Swollen jaw

FIGURE 31-15 Facial injuries: (A) a complex intraoral-facial laceration; (B) an open displaced jaw (mandible) fracture; (C) a CT scan of the injury shown in photo B. *(Photos A, B, and C: © Edward T. Dickinson, MD)*

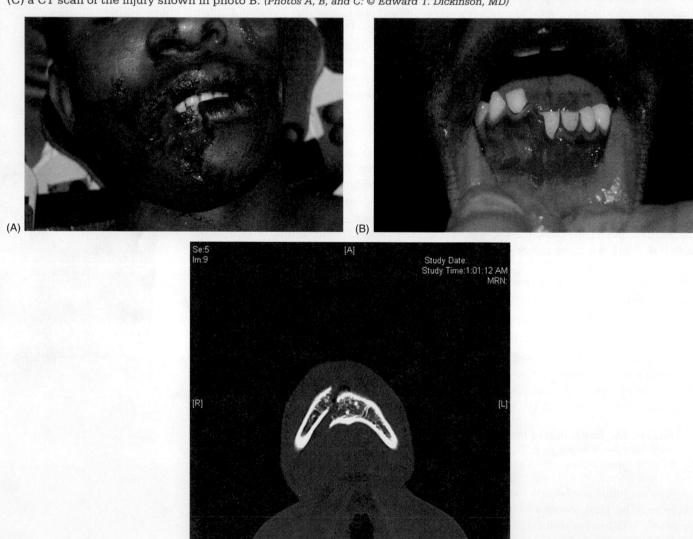

(A)

(B)

(C)

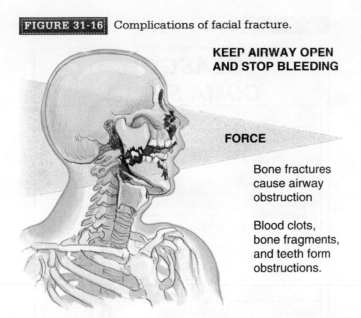

FIGURE 31-16 Complications of facial fracture.

**KEEP AIRWAY OPEN
AND STOP BLEEDING**

FORCE

Bone fractures
cause airway
obstruction

Blood clots,
bone fragments,
and teeth form
obstructions.

The primary concern with facial fractures is the patient's airway (Figure 31-16). Be prepared to suction to remove debris, including loose teeth and blood, from the airway. Because of possible spinal injury, use the jaw-thrust maneuver to open the airway. Control profuse bleeding. (See Chapter 28, "Soft-Tissue Trauma," for care of an object impaled in the cheek.) Apply a rigid collar and immobilize the patient on a spine board. If possible, position the patient to allow drainage from the mouth. Care for shock.

Nontraumatic Brain Injuries

Many of the signs of brain injury may be caused by an internal brain event such as a hemorrhage or blood clot. (See the information on stroke in Chapter 21, "Diabetic Emergencies and Altered Mental Status.") The signs of nontraumatic (not caused by external trauma) brain injury will be the same as those for a traumatic injury, except that there will be no evidence of trauma and no mechanism of injury.

Glasgow Coma Scale

All head-injury patients must be constantly monitored during transport. Be prepared in case the patient vomits or has a seizure. What you observe and report can have a great bearing on the ED staff's initial actions upon your arrival. The early signs of deterioration are subtle changes in mental status that may be overlooked if you are not watching for them.

Some EMS agencies use the Glasgow Coma Scale (GCS) (Figure 31-17), in addition to AVPU, for ongoing neurological assessment. Some systems would immediately transport a patient with a GCS score of less than 14 directly to the trauma center if they are within 30 minutes transport time. When using this score, keep the following considerations in mind:

NOTE: *Do not spend extra time at the scene calculating a GCS score. Calculate the score en route to the hospital to avoid prolonged scene times.*

- **Eye opening.** Spontaneous eye opening means that the patient opens his eyes without your having to do anything. If his eyes are closed, say "Open your eyes" to see if he will obey. Try a normal level of voice. If this fails, shout the command. Should the patient's eyes remain closed, apply an accepted painful stimulus (such as pinching a toe, scratching the palm or sole, or rubbing the sternum). Note any eye injuries or injuries to the face that prevent the patient from opening the eyes. If the injuries are more than minor ones, do not ask the patient to open his eyes.

FIGURE 31-17 Glasgow Coma Scale.

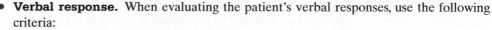

GLASGOW COMA SCALE

Eye Opening	Spontaneous	4	
	To Voice	3	
	To Pain	2	
	None	1	
Verbal Response	Oriented	5	
	Confused	4	
	Inappropriate Words	3	
	Incomprehensible Sounds	2	
	None	1	
Motor Response	Obeys Command	6	
	Localizes Pain	5	
	Withdraws (pain)	4	
	Flexion (pain)	3	
	Extension (pain)	2	
	None	1	
Glasgow Coma Score Total			

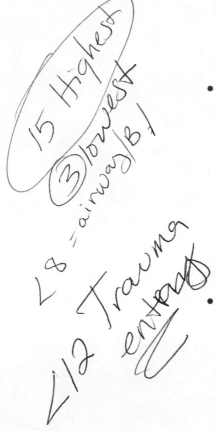

15 Highest
3 lowest
≤8 = airway/BV
≤12 Trauma entry

- **Verbal response.** When evaluating the patient's verbal responses, use the following criteria:
  - *Oriented.* The patient, once aroused, can tell you who he is, where he is, and the day of the week. A person who can answer all three of these questions appropriately is said to be alert on the AVPU scale.
  - *Confused.* The patient cannot answer the previous questions, but he can speak in phrases and sentences.
  - *Inappropriate words.* The patient says or shouts a word or several words at a time. Usually this requires physical stimulation. The words do not fit the situation or a particular question. Often, the patient curses.
  - *Incomprehensible sounds.* The patient responds with mumbling, moans, or groans.
  - *No verbal response.* Repeated stimulation, both verbal and physical, does not cause the patient to speak or make any sounds.
- **Motor response.** The following criteria are used to evaluate motor response:
  - *Obeys command.* The patient must be able to understand your instruction and carry out the request. For example, you may ask the patient (when appropriate) to hold up two fingers.
  - *Localizes pain.* If the patient fails to respond to your commands, apply pressure to one of the nail beds for 5 seconds or firm pressure to the sternum. Note if the patient attempts to remove your hand. Do not apply pressure over an injury site. Do not apply pressure to the sternum if the patient is experiencing difficulty breathing.
  - *Withdraws, after painful stimulation.* Note if the elbow flexes, if the patient moves slowly, if there is the appearance of stiffness, if he holds his forearm and hand against the body, or if the limbs on one side of the body appear to be paralyzed (hemiplegic position).
  - *Posturing, after painful stimulation.* Note if the legs and arms extend, if there is apparent stiffness with these moves, and if there is an internal rotation of the shoulder and forearm.
  - *No motor response to pain.* Repeated painful stimulation does not cause the patient to grimace or make any motions.

WOUNDS TO THE NECK

Because large arteries and veins lie close to the surface of the neck, the potential for serious bleeding from an open wound is great. Since the pressure in a large vein is likely to be lower than atmospheric pressure, the possibility of an *air embolism* (air bubble) being sucked in through a vein is also great. An air embolus can be carried to the heart and interfere with the heart's ability to circulate blood or it may actually cause cardiac arrest. The treatment of wounds to neck veins is aimed at stopping bleeding and preventing an embolus from entering the circulation.

CORE CONCEPT

Understanding wounds to the neck and emergency care for neck wounds

air embolism (air EM-boh-lizm)
a bubble of air in the bloodstream.

PATIENT ASSESSMENT

Open Neck Wound

An injury that has severed a major artery or vein of the neck will produce severe bleeding. Arterial bleeding will be profuse, with bright red blood spurting from the wound. Venous bleeding will also be profuse with dark red to maroon-colored blood flowing steadily from the wound.

PATIENT CARE

Open Neck Wound

Follow these steps for providing emergency care to a patient with an open neck wound (Scan 31-1):

1. Ensure an open airway.
2. Place your gloved hand over the wound.
3. Apply an occlusive dressing to the wound. The dressing should be a thick material that will not be sucked into the wound and must extend 2 inches past the sides of the wound. Seal the dressing on all four sides.
4. Place a dressing over the occlusive dressing.
5. Apply pressure as needed to stop the bleeding. Be careful not to compress both carotid arteries at once.
6. Once bleeding has stopped, bandage the dressing in place. Take care not to restrict the airway or the arteries and veins of the neck.
7. If the mechanism of injury could have caused cervical injury, immobilize the spine.

INJURIES TO THE SPINE

Injuries to the spine must be considered whenever there is serious trauma to any part of the body. Spine injury can be associated with head, neck, and back injuries—and also with chest, abdominal, and pelvic injuries. Even injuries to the upper and lower extremities can be caused by forces intense enough to produce spine injury.

As an EMT, you should "uptriage," or overtreat, patients with potential spine injuries because you cannot rule out a spine injury in the field and because the costs in terms of pain, suffering, disability, and dollars are very high when a spine-injured patient is unintentionally made worse by failure to immobilize the spine.

Injuries to the spinal column include fractures with and without bone displacement, dislocations, muscular strains, and disk injury including compression. The vertebral column may be injured without damage to the spinal cord or spinal nerves. For example, a fractured coccyx is below the level of the spinal cord. Muscular strains are relatively simple injuries. However, when displaced fractures or dislocations occur, the cord, disk, and spinal nerves may be severely injured.

CORE CONCEPT

Understanding spine injuries and emergency care for spine injuries

Mechanisms of Spine Injury

A simple rule of thumb is: If the mechanism of injury exerts great force on the upper body (Figure 31-18) or if there is any soft-tissue damage to the head, face, or neck due to trauma

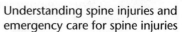

FIRST TAKE STANDARD PRECAUTIONS.

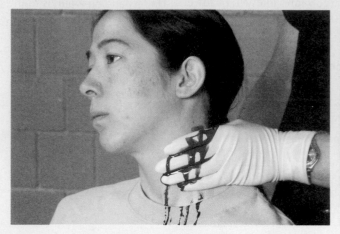

❶ Do not delay! Place your gloved palm over the wound.

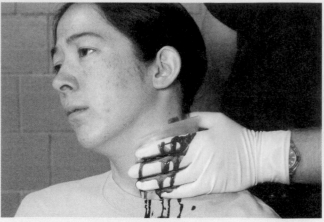

❷ Place an occlusive dressing over the wound. It must be heavy plastic and sized to be 2 inches larger in diameter than the wound site.

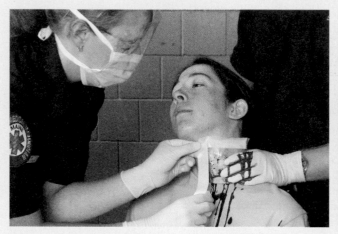

❸ Seal the dressing with tape on all four sides.

NOTE: *For demonstration purposes, the patient is upright.*

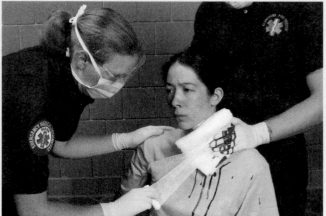

❹ Cover the occlusive dressing with a large gauze dressing. Bring a bandage over the dressing and wrap it in a figure-eight configuration, winding the bandage under the arm opposite the wound. Never wind the bandage around the patient's neck.

(such as from being thrown against a dashboard), assume possible cervical-spine injury. Any blunt trauma above the clavicles may damage the cervical spine.

Some parts of the spine are more susceptible to injury than others. Because it is somewhat splinted by the attached ribs, the thoracic spine is not usually damaged except in the most violent collisions or in gunshot wounds. The pelvic-sacral spine attachment helps to protect the sacrum in the same way. However, the cervical and lumbar vertebrae are susceptible to injury because they are not supported by other bony structures.

The spine is most often injured by compression or excessive flexion, extension, or rotation from falls, diving injuries, and motor-vehicle collisions. Spine injuries in EMS workers often result from not adhering to the proper lifting techniques, causing lateral bending or disk injuries. When the spine is excessively pulled, it can cause a "distraction" injury. This mechanism of spine injury occurs in a hanging. Years ago, rescuers were taught to pull traction on the neck of an injured patient sitting in an automobile. However, this actually had

FIGURE 31-18 Mechanisms of injury to the upper body.

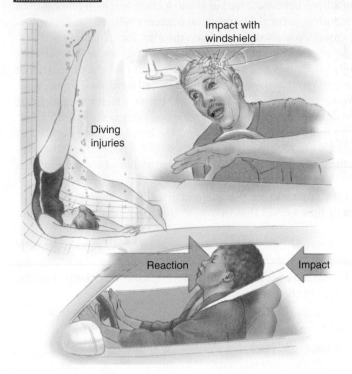

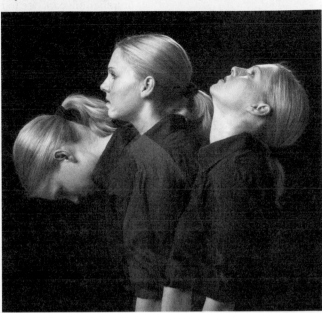

the potential to cause injury, so today EMTs are taught to manually stabilize the head and neck, or hold it still.

Maintain a high degree of suspicion of a potential spine injury when your patient is a victim of a motor-vehicle or motorcycle collision, was struck by a vehicle, received blunt injury to the spine or above the clavicles, was involved in a diving incident, was found hanging by his neck, or was found unconscious due to trauma.

The adult skull weighs more than 17 pounds and rests on a very small area of the cervical spine (like a pumpkin on a broom handle). Motor-vehicle collisions produce violent whiplash injuries because of the speed and sudden deceleration of the vehicle (Figure 31-19). When a vehicle strikes another vehicle or a fixed object head on, the neck can whip quickly back and forth. Although the vehicle decelerates abruptly, the head continues to travel forward at the same speed that the vehicle was traveling, even though the body is held by seat restraints. This neck movement may exceed the normal range of motion. Virtually the same thing occurs when the vehicle is struck from behind.

A fall can generate enough force to fracture or dislocate vertebrae. Assume that any fall three times the patient's height or with enough force to cause open fractures to the ankles will also be accompanied by a spine injury. Needless disability has been caused when head injuries or other injuries resulting from a fall were noted and cared for but spinal injuries were overlooked.

Today, more and more people are participating in sports of all kinds: in-line skating, mountain biking, surfing, rock climbing, and others too numerous to mention. Many sports mishaps can cause spine injury. Sledding or skiing can hurl a person into a tree or other fixed object, twisting or compressing the spinal column. There may be no open wound or fracture of an extremity, or signs of injury may be hidden by bulky clothing. As a result, improper care may be rendered as the patient with a possible spinal injury is placed on a stretcher without adequate examination and immobilization.

Diving incidents often produce injury to the cervical spine. When the diver strikes the diving board, the side or bottom of the pool, or an underwater object, the head can be severely forced beyond its normal limits of motion (flexion, extension, or compression). Cervical vertebrae may be fractured or dislocated, ligaments may be severely sprained, and the spinal cord may be compressed or otherwise traumatized in the cervical region and at other spots along the cord.

Football and other contact sports can generate forces severe enough to produce spinal injury. Spear tackling, using the head, has been outlawed in grade schools and high schools for a number of years due to the incidence of cervical compression fractures. When a game involves player contact or falling to the ground, you should remain on the alert for spinal injury.

The brain is the master organ of life. Messages from all over the body are received by the brain, which determines the body's response. The brain sends messages to the muscles so that we can move, or to a particular organ so that it will carry out a desired function. For example, it may tell the adrenal gland to dump epinephrine into the bloodstream, which increases heart rate. Any major head injury can damage the brain, causing vital body functions to fail.

The spinal cord is a relay between most of the body and the brain. A large number of the messages to and from the brain are sent through the spinal cord. Therefore, damage to the cord can isolate a part of the body from the brain, resulting in loss of function of this region—possibly forever.

A **dermatome** is an area of the body surface that is innervated by a single spinal nerve. (Figure 31-20 provides an idea of how nerves that originate from the spine innervate specific parts of the body.)

The healing power of nerve tissue is limited. This is especially true in certain areas. If nerve tissue in the brain or spinal cord is damaged, to a certain extent function is lost and cannot be restored. As an EMT, your initial care will often prevent additional damage to the brain, spinal cord, and major nerves of the patient's body.

dermatome (DERM-uh-tohm)
an area of the skin that is innervated
by a single spinal nerve.

FIGURE 31-20 Dermatomes are areas of the skin that are innervated by various segments of the spinal cord. Those labeled "C" are innervated by levels of the cervical spine, "T" the thoracic spine, "L" the lumbar spine, and "S" the sacral spine.

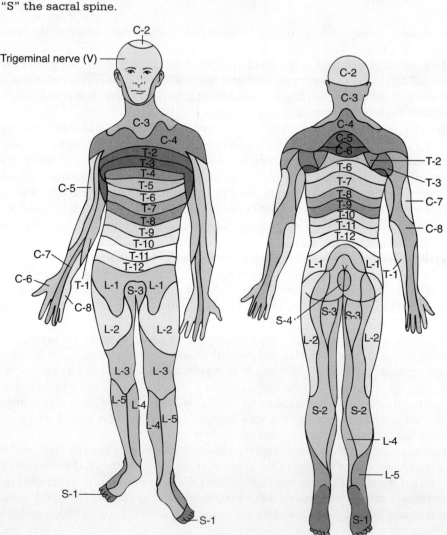

Inside/Outside

THREE EXAMPLES OF DYSFUNCTION FROM SPINAL INJURY

The spinal cord is the conduit through which messages are transmitted from the brain to the body and from the body to the brain. These messages may be as simple as the brain telling your hand to move to pick up something or as vital as directing the diaphragm to contract so that breathing takes place.

Injuries to the spine can cause many problems, including paralysis. The location of injury on the spine dictates how the body is affected. Perhaps the most catastrophic trauma is injury to the cervical spine. Because of its proximal location, the cervical spine affects the entire body; critically, the primary muscles of breathing are innervated by nerves that originate from the third to the fifth cervical vertebrae (C3 to C5).

The phrenic nerve originates primarily from the 4th cervical vertebra (C4), with some innervation also from C3 and C5. The major function of the phrenic nerve is control of the diaphragm. Since the diaphragm is the primary muscle of breathing, if the diaphragm should lose innervation from the phrenic nerve, the patient would no longer be able to breathe effectively and would die. Patients who require a ventilator after a spine injury often have an injury at or above this region of the spine.

Neurogenic shock, as discussed in Chapter 27, "Bleeding and Shock," is a form of shock (hypoperfusion) resulting from nerve paralysis, which can be caused by spinal cord injuries and can, in turn, cause uncontrolled dilation of blood vessels.

The sympathetic nervous system originates from the thoracic and lumbar spine. You will recall that the sympathetic nervous system—the "fight-or-flight" system—is responsible for vital functions such as heart rate, vascular tone, and dilation of bronchiolar smooth muscle.

Now imagine a serious spine injury to this region. You would observe a patient who exhibits low blood pressure and hypoperfusion. This is because the body has lost control over the smooth muscle that regulates the size of blood vessels. The vessels increase in size as they lose tone, but the amount of blood inside the vessels remains the same, so the patient's blood pressure plummets. Since the sympathetic nervous system is no longer functioning and is unable to release epinephrine and norepinephrine, the body cannot increase the heart rate or force of contractions as it normally would to raise blood pressure and combat shock. In most shock states, the skin is pale, cool, and moist. However, neurogenic shock presents differently, with skin that frequently is dry and may even be warm. In most shock states, the pulse is rapid, but in neurogenic shock, the pulse is often low (60–80/minute).

Remember that not all injuries to the spine result in instant paralysis. It may take a period of time for the effects to develop. In some cases, the vertebrae protecting the spinal cord remain in position for awhile but then may lose integrity as the patient moves around or is moved. The patient presentation depends on the location of the spinal injury. The higher the cord injury, the greater the effect it will have on the body. It should also be noted that different spinal tracts are responsible for different functions. For example, a patient who injures the anterior portion of the spinal cord will lose sensation to pain and the ability to move but still may be able to feel light touch (a function of the posterior portion of the spinal cord).

This is why sensation or the ability to move does not rule out spinal injury.

PATIENT ASSESSMENT

Spine and Spinal Cord Injury

The most common causes of spinal cord injury are motor-vehicle collisions, falls, diving incidents, and gunshot wounds. You must do a complete assessment of the patient. Assume that all unconscious trauma patients have a spinal injury.

Whenever in doubt, assume that there are spine injuries and immobilize the patient's torso, head, and neck. The following are common signs and symptoms of spine injury:

- **Paralysis of the extremities.** Paralysis of the extremities may occur. *Paralysis of the extremities is probably the most reliable sign of spinal cord injury in conscious patients.*

- **Pain without movement.** The pain is not always constant and may occur anywhere from the top of the head to the buttocks. Pain in the leg is common for certain types of injury to the lower spine. Other painful injuries can mask this symptom of spinal injury.

- **Pain with movement.** The patient normally tries to lie perfectly still to prevent pain. However, do not ask the patient to move just to determine if it will cause pain. If the patient experiences pain in the neck or back with voluntary movements, including spinal pain with movement in apparently uninjured shoulders and legs, this is a good indicator of possible spinal injury.

- **Tenderness anywhere along the spine.** Gentle palpation of the injury site, when accessible, may reveal point tenderness.

neurogenic shock
a state of shock (hypoperfusion) caused by nerve paralysis that sometimes develops from spinal cord injuries.

These signs and symptoms are reliable indicators of possible spinal injury in the conscious patient. If any one of them is present, you have sufficient reason to immobilize the patient. In the field, it is not possible to rule out spinal injury even when the patient has no pain and is able to move his limbs. The mechanism of injury alone may be the deciding factor. Additional signs of spinal injury may include:

- **Impaired breathing.** Watch the patient breathe. If there is only a slight movement of the abdomen, with little or no movement of the chest, it is safe to assume that the patient is breathing with the diaphragm alone (diaphragmatic breathing). This is also true if there is a reversal of normal breathing patterns with the rib cage collapsing on inspiration and rising on expiration. Damage to the nerves that control the movement of the rib cage can cause this breathing pattern. The nerves that control the diaphragm are located high in the cervical area (the third, fourth, and fifth cervical nerves) and are often unharmed, but the intercostal (between-the-ribs) nerves that control the chest muscles are often damaged in cervical and thoracic injuries. As a result, when the diaphragm moves downward to pull in air, the ribs, instead of expanding, collapse. When the diaphragm relaxes and air is expelled, the rib cage rises—which is the opposite of the normal pattern.

    Impaired breathing is characteristic of spinal cord injury. Check abdominal movement from the side by placing your hand on the patient's abdomen and looking for reversed movements during respiration. Panting due to respiratory insufficiency may develop.

- **Deformity.** Removing a patient's clothing to check for deformity of the spine is not recommended. *Obvious spinal deformities are rare.* However, if you note a gap between the spinous processes (bony extensions) of the vertebrae, or if you can feel a broken spinous process, you must consider the patient to have serious spinal injuries. It is also possible to feel tight muscles in spasm.

- **Priapism.** Persistent erection of the penis is a sign of spinal injury affecting nerves to the external genitalia.

- **Loss of bowel or bladder control.** This may indicate spinal injury.

- **Nerve impairment to the extremities.** The patient may experience loss of use, weakness, numbness, tingling, or loss of feeling in the upper and/or lower extremities—especially below the suspected level of the injury.

- **Neurogenic shock.** This kind of shock can be caused by the failure of the nervous system to control the diameter of blood vessels. The pulse rate may be normal—or even slow in the setting of a low or falling blood pressure—because a message to "speed up" the heart may be prevented from getting to the heart due to the cord injury.

- **Soft-tissue injuries associated with trauma.** Traumatic soft-tissue injuries to the head and neck may signal injury of the cervical spine. Traumatic soft-tissue injuries to the shoulders, back, or abdomen may signal injury of the thoracic or lumbar spine. Traumatic soft-tissue injuries to the lower extremities may signal injury of the lumbar or sacral spine.

Assessment for a responsive patient with suspected spinal injury includes the following strategies:

- Ascertain the mechanism of injury.

- Ask these questions (and tell the patient not to move while answering):
    - What happened?
    - Where does it hurt? Does your neck or back hurt?
    - Can you move your hands and feet?
    - Can you feel me touching (lightly) your fingers? Your toes?
    - Do you feel "pins and needles" (tingling) in your legs? Anywhere?

- Inspect for contusions, deformities, lacerations, punctures, penetrations, and swelling.

- Palpate for tenderness or deformity.

- Assess the patient's equality of strength in the extremities by checking hand grip or pushing against the patient's hands and feet.

Assessment strategies for an unresponsive patient with suspected spinal injury include the following:

- Ascertain from bystanders the mechanism of injury and information about the patient's mental status prior to your arrival.

- Inspect for contusions, deformities, lacerations, punctures, penetrations, and swelling.

- Palpate for areas of tenderness (some unresponsive patients will withdraw from or react to pain) or deformity.

NOTE: *The ability to walk, move the extremities, feel sensation, or experience a lack of pain in the spinal area does not rule out the possibility of spinal column or spinal cord injury.*

Decision Point

- Has a spine injury affected the efficiency or function of the respiratory system or circulatory system? How can I support these vital functions?

PATIENT CARE

Spine and Spinal Cord Injury

Regardless of where the apparent spinal injury is located on the cord, your care is the same. Perform the primary assessment and rapid trauma assessment and determine the patient's priority, since this will be important in deciding how to immobilize him (Figure 31-21).

For all patients with possible spinal injury, and for all trauma victims when there is doubt as to the extent of injury, emergency care includes the following steps:

1. Provide manual in-line stabilization for the head and neck on first patient contact. Place the head in a neutral in-line position unless the patient complains of pain or the head is not easily moved into that position. If that is the case, steady the head in the position found. Maintain manual stabilization until the patient is properly secured to a backboard.
2. Assess the patient's airway, breathing, and circulation. If necessary, open and control the airway with the jaw-thrust maneuver, maintaining in-line stabilization of the head.
3. In your rapid trauma exam, assess the head and neck, then apply a rigid cervical collar. Make sure the collar is properly sized, as a wrong-size collar may do more harm than good by hyperextending the neck if too large or allowing flexion if too small. Also make sure the collar is not applied in a way that will obstruct the airway. Maintain manual stabilization even after the collar is in place until the patient is secured to a backboard, since no collar completely restricts motion.
4. Quickly assess sensory and motor function in all four extremities if the patient is responsive.
5. Based on the patient's priority, apply the appropriate spinal immobilization device at the appropriate speed. (Scans 31-2 through 31-8 are provided in this chapter in order to demonstrate the proper procedure to use based upon the patient's condition and the position in which he is found.)
6. If the patient has paralysis or weakness of the extremities, administer high-concentration oxygen via nonrebreather mask and evaluate the need for artificial ventilations with supplemental oxygen. This is critical should there be any cord damage.
7. Reassess sensory and motor function in all four extremities if the patient is responsive.

NOTE: *Do not spend much time trying to rule out spinal injury in an unresponsive patient. If there is a mechanism of injury associated with spinal injury, immobilize the patient and treat as if there is a spinal injury.*

IMMOBILIZATION ISSUES

Tips for Applying a Cervical Collar

Cervical-spine immobilization devices, or rigid extrication collars, are designed to limit flexion, extension, and lateral movement when combined with an immobilization device such as a long backboard or a vest-style device. Even though there have been marked improvements

CORE CONCEPT ●----------
Understanding immobilization issues and how to immobilize various types of patients with potential spine injury

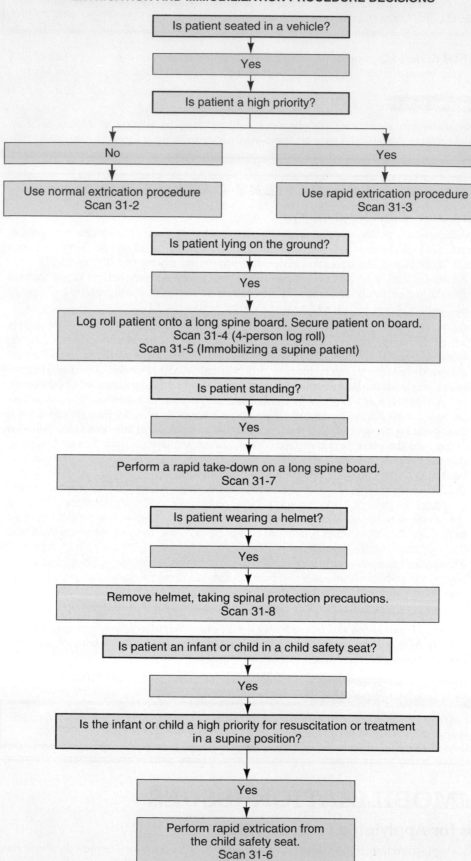

FIGURE 31-21 Choose appropriate extrication and immobilization procedures.

EXTRICATION AND IMMOBILIZATION PROCEDURE DECISIONS

Is patient seated in a vehicle?

Yes

Is patient a high priority?

No | Yes

Use normal extrication procedure
Scan 31-2

Use rapid extrication procedure
Scan 31-3

Is patient lying on the ground?

Yes

Log roll patient onto a long spine board. Secure patient on board.
Scan 31-4 (4-person log roll)
Scan 31-5 (Immobilizing a supine patient)

Is patient standing?

Yes

Perform a rapid take-down on a long spine board.
Scan 31-7

Is patient wearing a helmet?

Yes

Remove helmet, taking spinal protection precautions.
Scan 31-8

Is patient an infant or child in a child safety seat?

Yes

Is the infant or child a high priority for resuscitation or treatment
in a supine position?

Yes

Perform rapid extrication from
the child safety seat.
Scan 31-6

in collars, there is still no collar that completely eliminates movement of the spine. For this reason, when applying a collar, always manually maintain the neck and head in a neutral position in alignment with the rest of the body.

Review the information on manual stabilization in Chapter 11, "The Primary Assessment," and on cervical-collar sizing and application in Chapter 13, "Assessment of the Trauma Patient."

Tips for Immobilizing a Seated Patient

When a patient is found in a sitting position, you will need to decide his priority. If the patient is stable and a low priority, use the normal procedure for spinal immobilization as shown in Scan 31-2. In such situations, where time is not of the essence, the patient must be secured to a short spine board or extrication vest that will immobilize the head, neck, and torso until he can be transferred to a long spine board.

In high-priority situations when there is not enough time to apply a short board or extrication vest—or if the patient must be moved rapidly because of dangers at the scene or to provide access to other, potentially more seriously injured patients—the patient should be immobilized manually while moving him onto the long spine board. This rapid extrication technique is shown in Scan 31-3.

The normal extrication technique is as follows: You manually stabilize the patient's head and neck during primary assessment. After examining the head and neck in the rapid trauma assessment, you apply a rigid collar. Then you secure the patient to a short spine board or extrication vest.

A vest-style extrication device (such as the one shown in Figure 31-22) is a flexible piece of equipment useful for immobilizing patients with possible injury to the cervical spine. It can be used when the patient is found in a bucket seat, in a short compact car seat, in a seat with a contoured back, or in a confined space. It is also useful when the short spine board cannot be inserted into a car because of obstructions. A number of commercial vest-style extrication devices, such as the KED, Kansas Backboard, XP-1, and LSP Halfback Vest, are available. Use the devices approved by your EMS system.

A short spine board (Figure 31-23) is just a shortened version of a long spine board. It is the original extrication device and has been used for many years. It is used less frequently now, however, because today's contoured automobile seat backs do not accommodate a flat board. Also, the short spine board is often too wide and too high to be used effectively in a small car.

A particular sequence must be followed in all applications, whether of a flexible extrication device or a short spine board. That sequence is: secure the torso first and the head last. This ensures greater stability during the strapping process and may help prevent compression of the cervical spine. If the patient has suffered abdominal injuries or displays diaphragmatic breathing that prevents adequate securing of the torso, the torso straps will still be needed but care must be taken so as not to interfere with breathing.

There are a number of special considerations when applying a short board to the patient:

- Assessment of the back, shoulder blades, arms, or collarbones must be done before the device is placed against the patient.

FIGURE 31-22 Ferno KED (Kendrick Extrication Device).

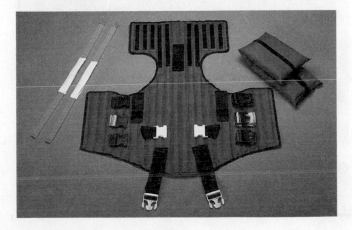

FIGURE 31-23 Short spine board.

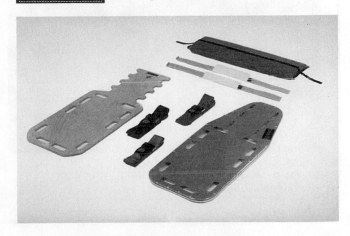

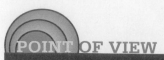
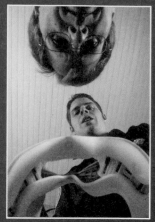

"I was sitting on the sofa at my daughter's house, and when I got up to change the TV, I got dizzy and passed out—passed out good! When I woke up there were these two cute young guys directly over me. Everything around them was white. I was confused. For a minute I thought I was in heaven.

"Then I felt my head. It hurt. I was trying to figure out what was going on. Nothing made sense. The EMTs were so kind. They stopped what they were doing and explained what had happened. They had to explain a couple of times. All I remember was my head hurting and being confused.

"My doctor had just changed my blood pressure medication, and I guess that's why I felt faint when I stood up fast. My daughter said that when I fell I hit my head on the coffee table. Because of that, the EMTs put a collar around my neck and put me on the most uncomfortable board. They said it was necessary, and I believed them. But after the ride to the hospital on that board, my back hurt worse than my head.

"At 75, and with blood pressure problems, I have to learn to take my time. Now I get up slowly. I don't want to have that happen again!"

SCAN 31-2　Spinal Immobilization of a Seated Patient

FIRST TAKE STANDARD PRECAUTIONS.

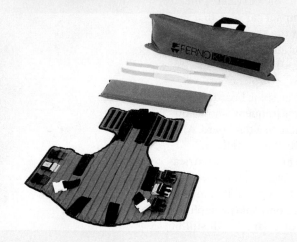

❶ Select an immobilization device.

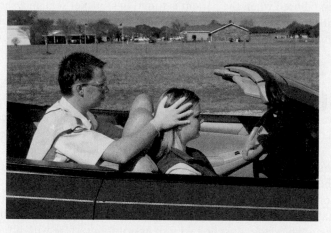

❷ Manually stabilize the patient's head in a neutral, in-line position.

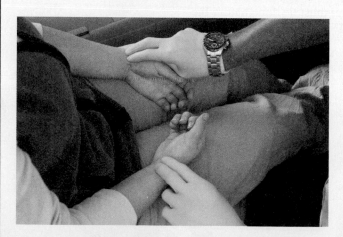

❸ Assess distal circulation, sensation, and motor function (CSM).

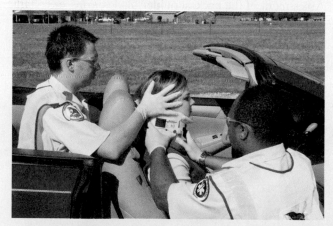

❹ Apply the appropriately sized extrication collar.

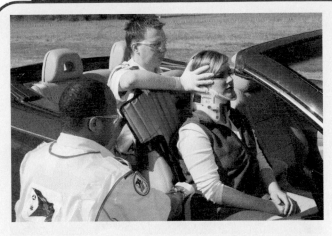

5 Position the immobilization device behind the patient.

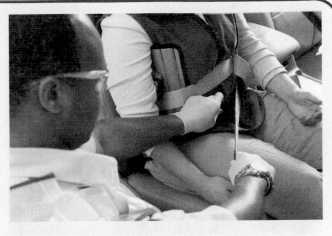

6 Secure the device to the patient's torso.

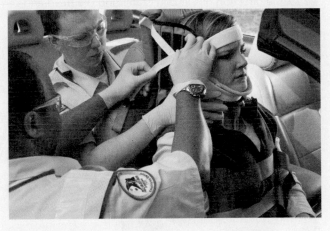

7 Evaluate and pad behind the patient's head as necessary. Secure the patient's head to the device.

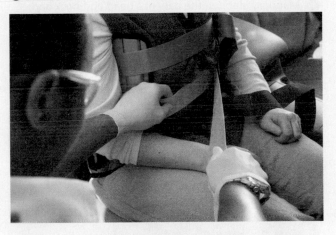

8 Evaluate and adjust the straps. They must be tight enough so the device does not move up, down, left, or right excessively, but not so tight as to restrict the patient's breathing.

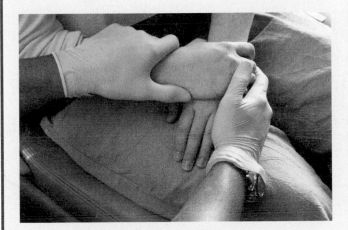

9 As needed, position or secure the patient's wrists and legs.

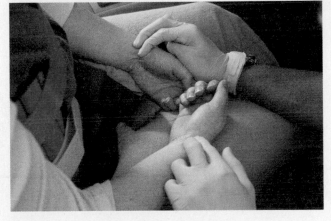

10 Reassess distal circulation, sensation, and motor function (CSM), and transfer the patient to the long board.

NOTE: *In the photos, the roof of the vehicle has been removed to allow for easier illustration of the positions of the EMTs. In most cases, this procedure will be done and should be practiced with the roof intact.*

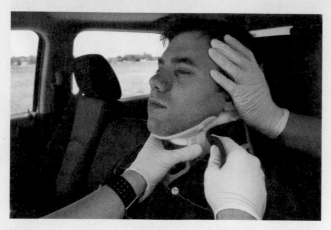

1 Manually stabilize the patient's head and neck and have a second EMT apply a cervical collar.

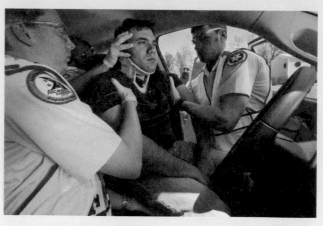

2 At the direction of the EMT stabilizing the head and neck, two EMTs each lift the patient by the armpits and buttocks/thighs just enough for a bystander or additional rescuer to slide a long spine board between the patient and the vehicle seat.

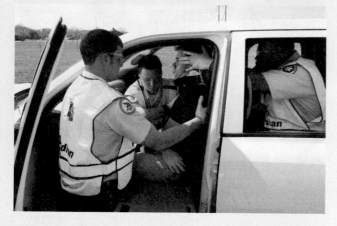

3 The EMTs reposition their hands so the EMT on the front seat inside the vehicle holds the patient's legs and pelvis, while the EMT outside the vehicle holds the upper chest and arms.

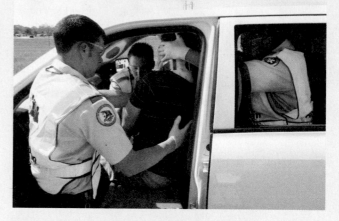

4 At the direction of the EMT holding the head and neck, carefully turn the patient a quarter turn so his back is toward the door of the vehicle.

NOTE: *The rapid extrication procedure is only for critical or unstable high-priority patients who must be moved in less time than would be required to apply a short spine board or extrication vest inside the vehicle before moving the patient to the long spine board (Scan 31-2).*

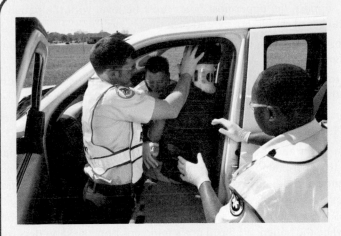

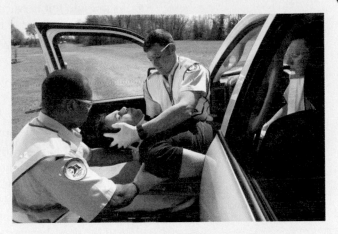

❺ The EMT who was holding the pelvis temporarily holds the chest so the EMT who was holding the chest can take over head and neck stabilization. The EMT in the back seat can then reach over the seat and assist with the chest, and the EMT inside on the front seat can move his hands back to the pelvis.

❻ At the direction of the EMT at the head and neck, gently lower the patient to the spine board. *Note: Sometimes it may be necessary to move the patient inside the vehicle a few inches so there is ample room to lay him down without touching the upper door opening.*

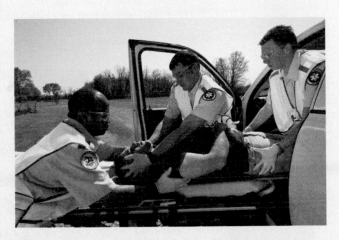

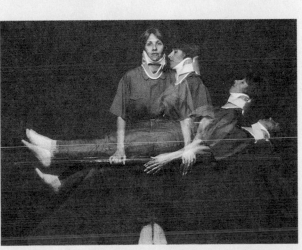

❼ As a bystander or additional rescuer holds the end of the spine board, the EMTs slide the patient to the head end of the board.

❽ Quickly apply straps to the patient's chest, pelvis, and legs and remove the patient to a stretcher or the ground, under the direction of the EMT stabilizing the head and neck. *Note: Since the patient's head is not yet fully immobilized (it is only being manually held stable by the EMT and collar), DO NOT walk more than a few steps with the patient. Once on stable ground or the stretcher, apply a head immobilizer or blanket roll and wide tape.*

As you move the patient from a sitting to a supine position, her spine must not bend, twist, or get jolted. Handle her very gently, and make sure you have enough assistance to perform the move correctly.

- The EMT applying the board must angle it, without striking or jarring, to fit between the arms of the rescuer who is stabilizing the head from behind the patient.

- To provide full cervical support, the uppermost holes must be level with the patient's shoulders. The base of the board should not extend past the coccyx.

- Never place a chin cup or chin strap on the patient, as it can prevent him from opening his mouth if he has to vomit.

- Avoid applying the first torso strap too tightly. This could aggravate an abdominal injury or limit respirations for the diaphragmatic breathing patient.

- Some buckles have quick-release mechanisms. Be careful not to accidentally loosen these buckles when moving the patient.

- Do not pad between the collar and the board. This will create a pivot point that may cause the cervical spine to hyperextend when the head is secured. Instead, pad the occipital region, but only enough to fill any void. This will help keep the head in a neutral position. Sometimes when the shoulders are rolled back to the board, the head will come back to the board far enough so padding is not needed. Never use excessive padding behind the head, because when the patient is placed in a supine position, the shoulders will fall back but the head will not be able to. This will place the patient in an undesirable position of flexion.

- Follow the instructions provided by the manufacturer of the device you are using.

- After applying the short spine board, the packaging of the patient will be completed as shown in Figure 31-24.

FIGURE 31-24 Seated patient, "packaged."

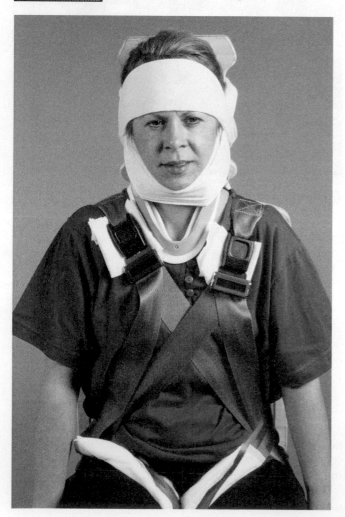 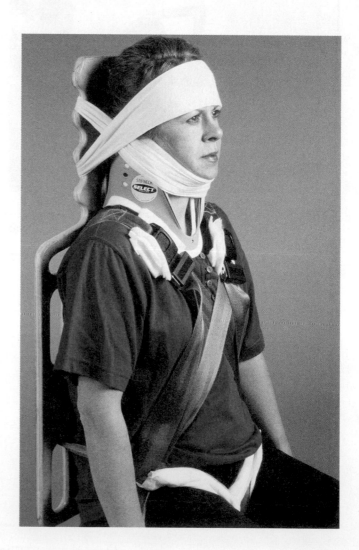

FIGURE 31-25 Long spine board with head immobilizer.

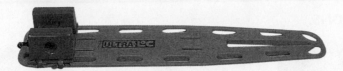

Tips for Applying a Long Backboard

The following tips relate to immobilization of the supine patient:

- You will need to log roll the patient to apply the long backboard (Scans 31-4 and 31-5). This procedure must be done carefully, keeping the patient's spine in alignment. Quickly assess the posterior body before rolling the patient back onto the board. Whenever a move is done involving neck stabilization, the EMT holding the head calls for the move ("We will turn on three: One ... two ... three").

- Pad voids between the patient's head and torso and the board. Be careful not to cause extra movement or to move the patient's spine out of alignment.

- When a patient is secured to a long spine board (Figure 31-25), the head is secured last. Strapping is easier with Velcro or speed-clip straps.

- Additional immobilization for the head and neck can be provided with light foam-filled cushions, a commercial head immobilization device (Figure 31-26) (such as the Ferno Washington head immobilizer, Bashaw CID, or the Laerdal Head Bed), or a blanket roll. If used, these are applied after securing the patient's body to the long backboard. Secure the head with 3-inch hypoallergenic adhesive tape. The tape offers support, especially if the patient and board are to be tilted to allow for drainage. However, blood on the patient's skin and hair may make using tape impractical. You should learn to use cravats or self-adhering roller bandages as a backup method. Do not tape or tie the cravats across the patient's eyes.

- If the patient is a full-term pregnant woman, immobilize her on the backboard. Then tilt the board to the left by propping up the right side to minimize the effect of the uterus compressing the vena cava and causing hypotension and dizziness.

- Unless the spine board has straps specifically intended to criss-cross the shoulders and chest, it is best to strap across the upper chest, the pelvis, and the thighs. If you will need to stand the patient up to carry him out of a tight building, up a basement stairwell, or into a small elevator, make sure the straps are secure under the patient's armpits and tight on the thighs.

FIGURE 31-26 (A) Ferno head immobilizer and (B) disposable head immobilizer. *(Photos A and B: © Ferno, Inc.)*

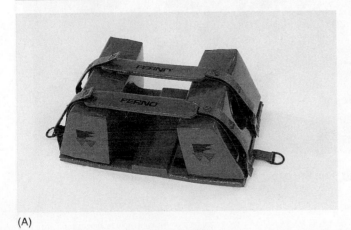

(A)

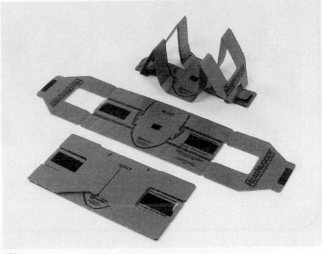

(B)

FIRST TAKE STANDARD PRECAUTIONS.

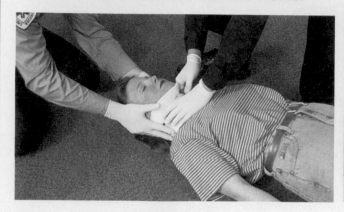

① Stabilize the head and neck. Apply a rigid cervical collar.

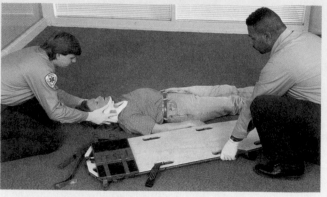

② Place the board parallel to the patient.

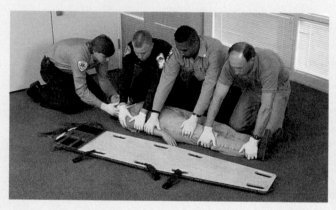

③ Have three rescuers kneel at the patient's side opposite the board, leaving room to roll the patient toward them. Place rescuers at the shoulder, waist, and knee. One EMT will continue to stabilize the head, while the others reach across the patient to properly position their hands.

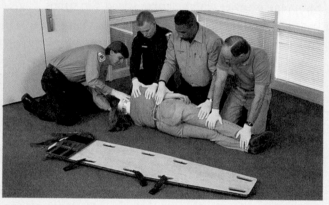

④ The EMT at the head and neck directs the others to roll the patient as a unit.

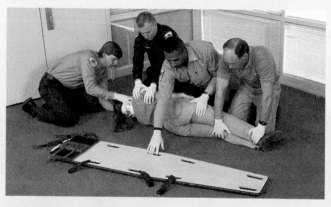

⑤ The EMT at the patient's waist grips the spine board and pulls it into position against the patient. (This can be done by a fifth rescuer.)

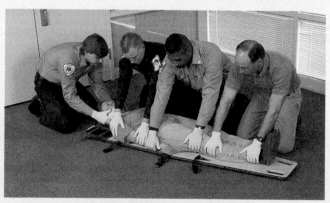

⑥ Roll the patient as a unit onto the board.

FIRST TAKE STANDARD PRECAUTIONS.

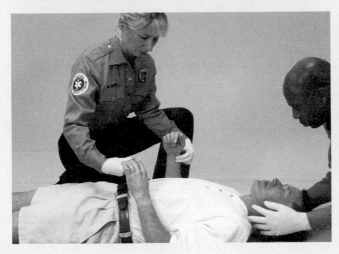

1 Place the patient's head in a neutral, in-line position and maintain manual stabilization of the head and neck. Assess distal circulation, sensation, and motor function (CSM).

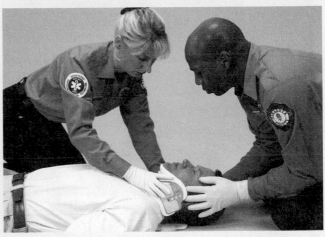

2 Apply an appropriately sized rigid cervical collar.

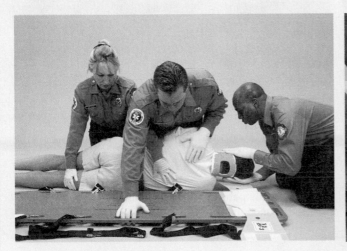

3 Position an immobilization device.

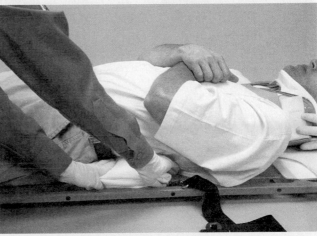

4 Move the patient onto the device without compromising the integrity of the spine. Once the patient is in position, apply padding to voids between the torso and board.

(continued)

- If your service transports to a helicopter, make sure that your backboard fits. There are some restrictions on the size or taper of the long backboard, depending on the helicopter's loading configuration, so find this out ahead of time.

- For a water rescue or diving injury, there are various specialty backboards, such as the Miller board, that are designed to float up beneath the patient and use Velcro closures for ease of application.

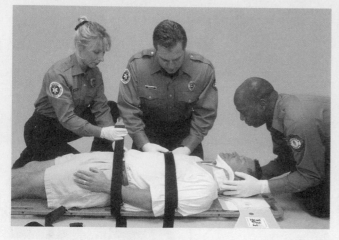

5 Secure the patient's torso to the board first.

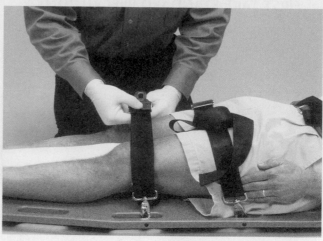

6 Secure the patient's legs (above and below the knee).

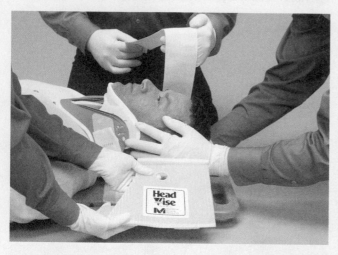

7 Pad and immobilize the patient's head last.

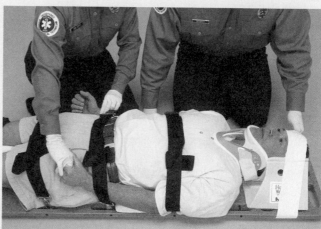

8 Reassess the patient's distal circulation, sensation, and motor function (CSM).

PEDIATRIC NOTE

When immobilizing a 6-year-old or younger child, provide padding beneath the shoulder blades to compensate for the child's large head. Pad from the shoulders to toes as needed to establish a neutral position.

If you do not carry a pediatric long spine immobilization device, then practice immobilizing children using adult equipment and lots of towels or blankets to pad around the child. EMTs are usually very good at improvising. In this case, however, the first time you improvise should be in the classroom so you will work quickly in the field!

PEDIATRIC NOTE

Occasionally, EMTs are confronted at a motor-vehicle collision with an infant or young child who was riding in a child safety seat. At one time, it was recommended that, if the child did not need immediate resuscitation or need to be placed supine for any reason, the child could be immobilized in the child safety seat. *Immobilizing a child in a child safety seat is no longer recommended, because the integrity of a safety seat may have been compromised in the collision.*

The procedure for rapid extrication from the child safety seat is shown in Scan 31-6.

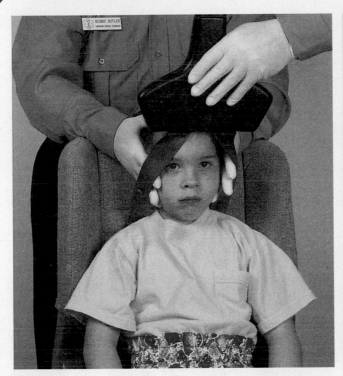

① EMT #1 stabilizes the car seat in the upright position and applies manual stabilization of the patient's head and neck. EMT #2 prepares equipment, and then loosens or cuts the seat straps and raises the front guard.

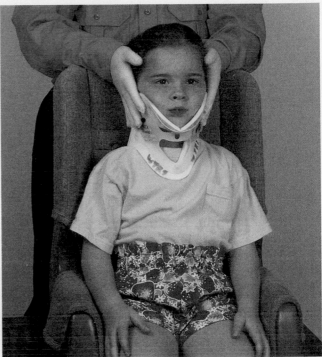

② The cervical collar is applied to the patient as EMT #1 maintains manual stabilization of the head and neck.

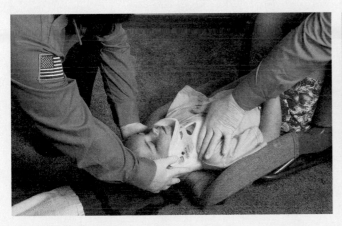

③ As EMT #1 maintains manual stabilization, EMT #2 places the child safety seat on the center of the backboard and slowly tilts it into the supine position. EMTs are careful not to let the child slide out of the chair. For the child with a large head, place a towel under the area where the shoulders will eventually be placed on the board to prevent the head from tilting forward.

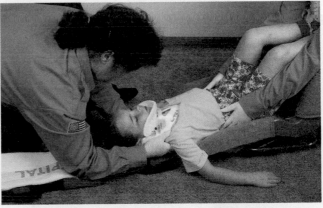

④ EMT #1 maintains manual stabilization and calls for a coordinated long axis move onto the backboard.

(continued)

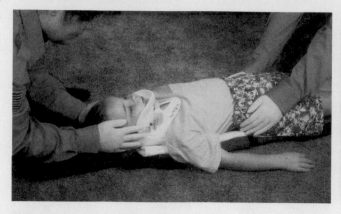

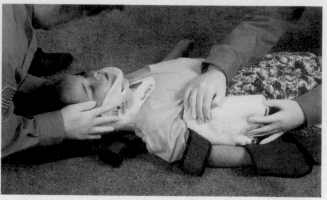

5 EMT #1 maintains manual stabilization, as the move onto the board is completed, with the child's shoulders over the folded towel.

6 EMT #1 maintains manual stabilization, as EMT #2 places rolled towels or blankets on both sides of the patient.

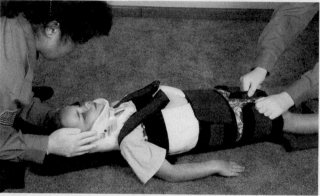

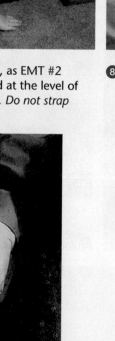

7 EMT #1 maintains manual stabilization, as EMT #2 straps or tapes the patient to the board at the level of the upper chest, pelvis, and lower legs. *Do not strap across the abdomen.*

8 EMT #1 maintains manual stabilization, as EMT #2 places rolled towels on both sides of the head, then tapes the head securely in place across the forehead and cervical collar. *Do not tape across the chin to avoid pressure on the neck.*

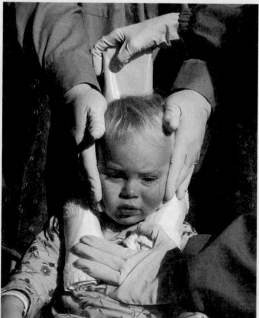

The newborn and infant procedure is exactly the same as for a child, except that an armboard is inserted behind the child in Step 2. If the infant is very small, the armboard may actually be used as the spine board.

CRITICAL DECISION MAKING

More than a Pain in the Neck

You have learned the procedure for immobilizing patients. However, the decision-making process that leads up to the immobilization is equally important. Which patients do you immobilize and which do not require immobilization?

NOTE: *Use the general concepts from this chapter to make your determination. Your protocols in the field may vary.*

1. Your patient was the driver of a vehicle that was struck in the rear end while stopped at a light. The patient denies pain, but you observe her rubbing her neck and looking like she may have some pain.

2. Your patient was in the back seat of a car that was hit broadside (T-bone). She doesn't complain of neck pain, but her head was knocked into the side of the car during the collision. She has a large hematoma on the right side of her head from the impact.

3. Your patient was a passenger in a car that was struck in the driver's side in a minor collision. She denies all injury and isn't sure she wants to go to the hospital.

Tips for Dealing with a Standing Patient

When you approach a vehicle and see the tell-tale spider-web-cracked windshield, you know whoever sat behind that crack needs full spinal immobilization. Even if this patient is up and walking around at the collision scene, he still has the potential for a spine injury. He simply may not yet have dislocated the fracture or ligament injury site. Since it would be dangerous to have him sit down or lie down on your long backboard, you should use a backboard to carefully but rapidly take him down to the supine position without compromising his spine.

Some EMS providers advocate strapping the patient onto the long board while the patient is standing. However, this is often not practical in the field. (It works in the classroom because the simulated patients are not in shock, intoxicated, head injured, combative, or just dizzy!)

The easiest technique is the rapid takedown which, like all skills in this text, should be demonstrated by a qualified instructor and practiced in the classroom prior to use in the field. The procedure takes three EMTs, a set of collars, and a long backboard. (See Figure 31-27 and Scan 31-7.)

FIGURE 31-27 Standing takedown at the scene of an emergency.
(© Howard Paul/Emergency! Stock)

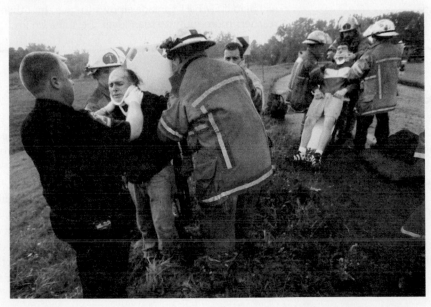

FIRST TAKE STANDARD PRECAUTIONS.

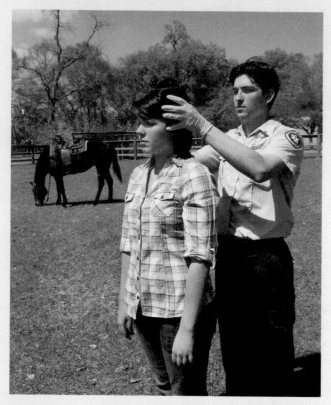

❶ Position your tallest crew member (EMT #1) behind the patient and have him manually stabilize the head and neck. His hands should not leave the patient's head until the entire procedure is complete and the head is secured to the long spine board.

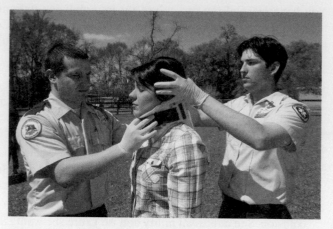

❷ EMT #2 applies a properly sized cervical collar to the patient. EMT #1 continues manual stabilization (the collar aids, but does not replace, manual stabilization).

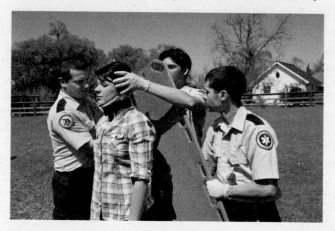

❸ EMT #1 continues manual stabilization, as EMT #2 and another rescuer position a long spine board behind the patient, being careful not to disturb EMT #1's manual stabilization of the patient's head and neck. It will help if EMT #1 spreads elbows to give the other rescuers more room to maneuver the spine board.

Patient Found Wearing a Helmet

Helmets are worn in many sporting events and by many motorcycle riders. Even ski resorts are starting to advocate the use of helmets. Sporting helmets are typically open in the front, making it easier to access the patient's airway than when a patient is wearing a motorcycle helmet, which has a shield and often a full face section that is not removable.

Face, neck, and spine care and airway management or resuscitation may call for the removal of the helmet, especially if the helmet will prevent you from reaching the patient's mouth or nose. If the helmet is left on, shields can be lifted and face guards removed. One EMT must manually steady the patient's head and neck while the other cuts, snaps off, or unscrews the guard. Do not attempt to remove a helmet if doing so causes increased pain, or if the helmet proves difficult to remove, unless there is a possible airway obstruction or ventilatory assistance must be provided. Indications for leaving the helmet in place or for removing the helmet are summarized in the following text.

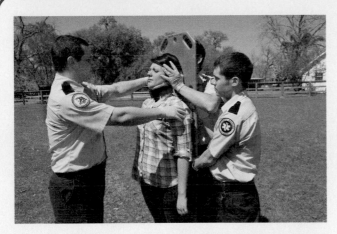

4 EMT #1 continues manual stabilization. EMT #2 looks at the spine board from the front of the patient and does any necessary repositioning to be sure it is centered behind the patient.

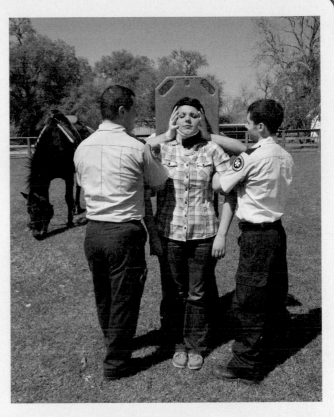

5 EMT #1 continues manual stabilization. EMT #2 and the third rescuer extend the arms that are nearest the patient under the patient's armpits and grasp the spine board. (Once the board is tilted down, the patient will actually be temporarily suspended by the armpits.) To keep the patient's arms secure, they will use the other hand to grasp the patient's arm just above the elbow and hold it against the patient's body.

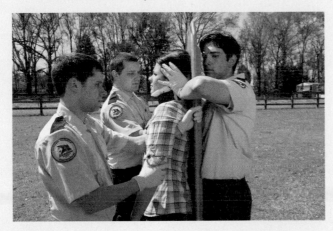

6 EMT #2 and the third rescuer, when reaching under the patient's armpits, must grasp a handhold on the spine board at the patient's armpit level or higher.

(continued)

Indications for leaving the helmet in place:

- Helmet fits snugly, allowing little or no movement of the patient's head within the helmet.
- There are absolutely no impending airway or breathing problems nor any reason to resuscitate or ventilate the patient.
- Removal would cause further injury.
- Proper spinal immobilization can be done with the helmet in place.
- There is no interference with the EMT's ability to assess the airway or breathing.

Indications for removing the helmet:

- The helmet interferes with the EMT's ability to assess and manage airway and breathing.
- The helmet is improperly fitted, allowing excessive head movement.
- The helmet interferes with immobilization.
- Cardiac arrest is present.

Many experienced EMS providers put the controversy of removal versus nonremoval into the following perspective: If your child injured his neck playing football, would you want the

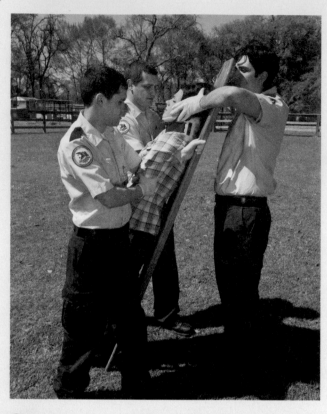

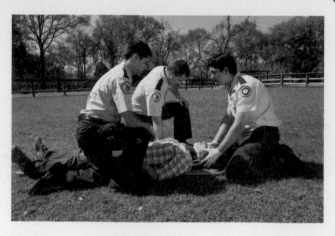

8 EMT #1 maintains manual in-line stabilization throughout the procedure.

7 EMT #1 continues manual stabilization. EMT #2 and the third rescuer maintain their grasp on the spine board and patient. EMT #1 explains to the patient what is going to happen, then gives the signal to begin slowly tilting the board and patient to the ground. As the board is lowered, EMT #1 walks backward and crouches, keeping up with the board as it is lowered and allowing the patient's head to slowly move back to the neutral position against the board. EMT #1 must accomplish all this without interfering with the lowering of the board. EMT #1 may need to rotate somewhat so that, once the board is almost flat, he is holding the head down on the board. Once the patient's head comes in contact with the board, it must not be allowed to leave the board, to avoid flexing the neck. The job of the two rescuers doing the lowering of the board is to control it so that it is slowly lowered and even on both sides. They should also move into a squatting position as they lower the board to avoid injuring their backs.

trainer and the EMT to work together carefully to remove the helmet at the scene, or would you prefer this to be left to emergency department personnel who probably will not have the help of the trainer nor the benefit of lots of practice in the helmet removal technique?

Note that if a football player is wearing shoulder pads and a helmet, you should either remove the pads and the helmet or you should leave them both on. Taking off one, but not the other, will result in hyperflexion or hyperextension because of the space the pads occupy behind the patient's shoulders.

When a helmet must be removed, it is a two-rescuer procedure, as shown in Scan 31-8.

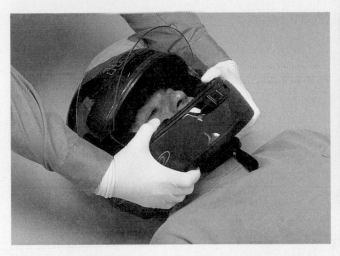

1 EMT #1 is positioned at the top of the patient's head and maintains manual stabilization. Two hands hold the helmet stable while the fingertips hold the lower jaw.

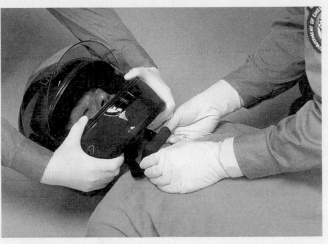

2 EMT #2 opens, cuts, or removes the chin strap.

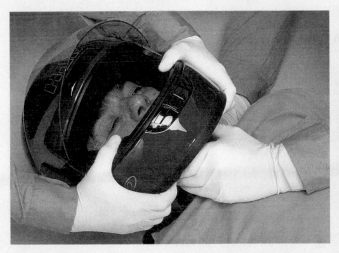

3 EMT #2 then places one hand on the patient's mandible and, using the other hand, reaches in behind the neck and stabilizes the occipital region. Using the combination of the hand in front of the chin and the hand behind the neck, EMT #2 should be able to securely hold the patient's head. If the patient has glasses on, they should be removed now, prior to removal of the helmet.

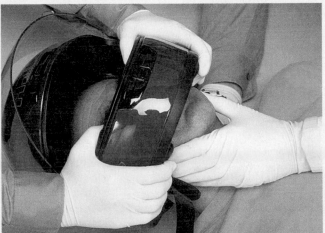

4 EMT #1 can now release manual stabilization and slowly remove the helmet. The lower sides, or ear cups, of the helmet will have to be gently pulled out to clear the ears.

NOTE: *If the patient has shoulder pads and you are removing a football helmet, remember to remove the shoulder pads or pad behind the head to keep it aligned with the padded shoulders. With either helmet-removal method, manual stabilization must be maintained until the patient is secured to a long spine board with full immobilization of the head.*

(continued)

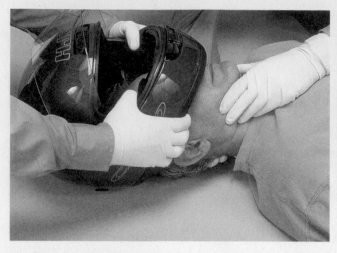

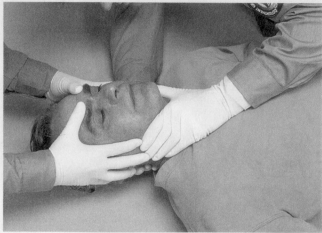

5 The helmet should come off straight with no backward tilting. A full-face helmet may need to be tilted just enough for the chin guard to clear the nose. EMT #2 must support and prevent the head from moving as the helmet is removed.

6 EMT #1, after removing the helmet, reestablishes manual stabilization and maintains an open airway by using the jaw-thrust maneuver.

HELMET REMOVAL—ALTERNATIVE METHOD

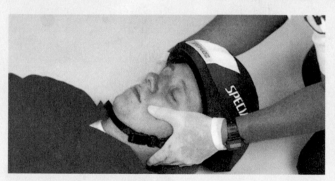

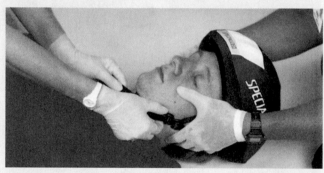

1 EMT #1 applies manual stabilization with the patient's neck in a neutral position.

2 EMT #2 removes the chin strap.

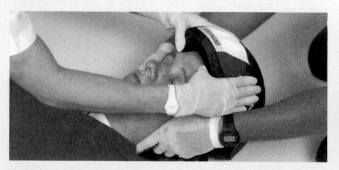

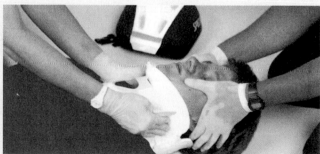

3 EMT #2 removes the helmet, pulling out on each side to clear the ears.

4 EMT #1 maintains manual stabilization as EMT #2 applies a cervical collar.

Selective Spine Immobilization

The traditional approach to spine immobilization in EMS has been to immobilize any patient whose assessment or mechanism of injury suggests the possibility of spine injury. But what exactly does that mean? A serious MOI to one EMT may not seem serious to another EMT. In some EMS systems, providers now have specific indications for spine immobilization. Use of these indications may be limited to advanced level providers in some systems. In others, EMT level providers may be authorized to use them.

This approach is sometimes incorrectly referred to as a "spine clearance protocol." EMTs do not clear spines (i.e., determine there is no spine injury). Instead, in systems that employ this approach, each patient's condition and circumstances are evaluated and compared to a protocol to determine whether spine immobilization is indicated for that patient. In some cases, an EMT may immobilize patients he would not have immobilized before institution of such a protocol.

Typical elements of such a protocol (Table 31-1 and Figure 31-28) include evaluation of both the mechanism of injury and the patient's condition. Patient condition is further broken down into injury-related conditions, such as paralysis, and non-injury-related conditions, such as intoxication, that limit the reliability of the assessment.

These protocols may also differentiate patients by age. Differences in elderly and pediatric patients (as compared to adults) pose special assessment and immobilization challenges.

Most protocols also allow the EMT an "out" by encouraging the provider to immobilize a patient when clinical judgment suggests that it is appropriate, even if none of the other conditions are present.

Although spine immobilization causes pain and discomfort in some patients, that concern is insignificant when compared to the devastating lifelong consequences of failure to immobilize an injured spine. Before you use a selective spine immobilization protocol, be sure you have been trained in the specific indications and contraindications of such a protocol and that your Medical Director has approved it.

When in doubt, immobilize!

Table 31-1   Typical Elements of a Selective Spine Immobilization Protocol

Immobilize the patient's spine if one or more of the following are present.

MECHANISM OF INJURY	PATIENT CHARACTERISTICS THAT ARE INJURY RELATED
• Violent impact to head, neck, torso, or pelvis • Moderate-to-high-speed motor-vehicle incident • Pedestrian struck by a vehicle • Explosion • Ejection from a vehicle • Shallow-water diving incident • Fall: Some protocols include all falls, whereas others include only falls greater than a particular height, commonly three times the patient's height (There may be differences with elderly patients.) • Axial load • Penetrating trauma in or near the spine • Sports injury to the head or neck	• Spine pain, tenderness, or deformity • Neurological deficit or complaint • Pain on movement of the neck or back
PATIENT CHARACTERISTICS THAT ARE NOT DIRECTLY INJURY RELATED	EMT CHARACTERISTICS
• Altered mental status • Intoxication from alcohol or other drugs • Inability to communicate • Distracting injury (e.g., a leg injury so painful the patient might not feel a less obvious injury to the spine) • Stress significant enough to prevent the patient from feeling pain	• The EMT suspects that the patient is not being truthful. • The EMT suspects that there is more to the incident than meets the eye. • The EMT's clinical judgment or suspicions suggest the patient should be immobilized.

FIGURE 31-28 Maine EMS spine assessment protocol.

NOTE: This is an example. Local protocols will determine your ability to make the judgments necessary for selective spine immobilization.

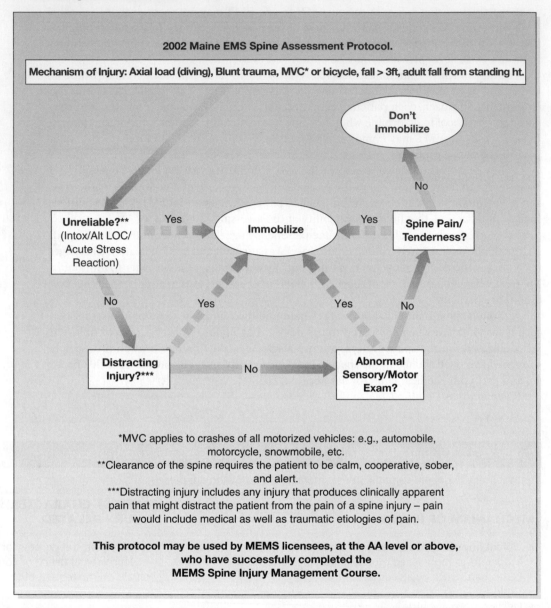

2002 Maine EMS Spine Assessment Protocol.

Mechanism of Injury: Axial load (diving), Blunt trauma, MVC* or bicycle, fall > 3ft, adult fall from standing ht.

*MVC applies to crashes of all motorized vehicles: e.g., automobile, motorcycle, snowmobile, etc.
**Clearance of the spine requires the patient to be calm, cooperative, sober, and alert.
***Distracting injury includes any injury that produces clinically apparent pain that might distract the patient from the pain of a spine injury – pain would include medical as well as traumatic etiologies of pain.

This protocol may be used by MEMS licensees, at the AA level or above, who have successfully completed the MEMS Spine Injury Management Course.

CHAPTER REVIEW

Key Facts and Concepts

- The two main divisions of the nervous system are the central nervous system and the peripheral nervous system.

- You should maintain a high index of suspicion for head or spine injury whenever there is a relevant mechanism of injury.

- You must provide cervical spine stabilization before beginning any other patient care when head or spine injury is suspected.

- Altered mental status is an early and important indicator of head injury. Monitor and document your patient's mental status throughout the call.

- A traumatic brain injury is any injury that disrupts function of the brain and may include anything from a slight concussion to a severe hematoma.

- Always secure the torso to the backboard before the head.

Key Decisions

- Does my patient have a mechanism of injury that would indicate the need for spinal immobilization?

- Does my patient's potential head or spine injury require prompt transport to a trauma center?

Chapter Glossary

air embolism (air EM-boh-lizm) a bubble of air in the bloodstream.

autonomic nervous system controls involuntary functions.

central nervous system the brain and the spinal cord.

cerebrospinal (suh-RE-bro-SPI-nal) ***fluid (CSF)*** the fluid that surrounds the brain and spinal cord.

concussion mild closed head injury without detectable damage to the brain. Complete recovery is usually expected.

contusion in brain injuries, a bruised brain caused when the force of a blow to the head is great enough to rupture blood vessels.

cranium (KRAY-ne-um) the bony structure making up the forehead, top, back, and upper sides of the skull.

dermatome (DERM-uh-tohm) an area of the skin that is innervated by a single spinal nerve.

foramen magnum (FOR-uh-men MAG-num) the opening at the base of the skull through which the spinal cord passes from the brain.

hematoma (HE-mah-TO-mah) in a head injury, a collection of blood within the skull or brain.

herniation (her-ne-AY-shun) pushing of a portion of the brain through the foramen magnum as a result of increased intracranial pressure.

intracranial (IN-truh-KRAY-ne-ul) ***pressure (ICP)*** pressure inside the skull.

laceration (las-uh-RAY-shun) in brain injuries, a cut to the brain.

malar (MAY-lar) the cheek bone, also called the *zygomatic bone*.

mandible (MAN-di-bl) the lower jaw bone.

maxillae (mak-SIL-e) the two fused bones forming the upper jaw.

nasal (NAY-zul) ***bones*** the bones that form the upper third, or bridge, of the nose.

nervous system provides overall control of thought, sensation, and the body's voluntary and involuntary motor functions. The components of the nervous system are the brain and the spinal cord as well as the nerves that enter and exit the brain and spinal cord and extend to the various parts of the body.

neurogenic shock a state of shock (hypoperfusion) caused by nerve paralysis that sometimes develops from spinal cord injuries.

orbits the bony structures around the eyes; the eye sockets.

peripheral nervous system the nerves that enter and exit the spinal cord between the vertebrae; the 12 pairs of cranial nerves that travel between the brain and organs without passing through the spinal cord; and all of the body's other motor and sensory nerves.

spinous (SPI-nus) ***process*** the bony bump on a vertebra.

temporal (TEM-po-ral) ***bone*** bone that forms part of the side of the skull and floor of the cranial cavity. There is a right and a left temporal bone.

temporomandibular (TEM-po-ro-mand-DIB-yuh-lar) ***joint*** the movable joint formed between the mandible and the temporal bone, also called the TMJ.

vertebrae (VERT-uh-bray) the bones of the spinal column (singular vertebra).

Preparation for Your Examination and Practice

Short Answer

1. Name the two components of the central nervous system and discuss their functions.

2. List five signs of a brain injury and explain why mechanism of injury is important in determining possible brain injury.

3. Describe the appropriate emergency treatment of a patient with a possible head or brain injury.

4. List five mechanisms of injury that would support suspicion of a spine injury.

5. Describe the appropriate emergency care for a patient with a possible spine injury.

Thinking and Linking

Think back to Chapter 3, "Lifting and Moving Patients," and link information from that chapter with information from this chapter as you explain how you would immobilize and transport the following patients found at the scene of an automobile collision.

1. A patient seated on the driver's side of a collision car, complaining of neck pain

2. A patient who was thrown from one of the collision cars and is lying on his side in a ditch

3. A patient from one of the collision cars who is found on his feet and is wandering around the scene

Critical Thinking Exercises

Head and spine injuries are among the most dangerous issues to the patient and the most challenging to the EMT. The purpose of this exercise will be to consider how you might manage such patients.

1. Your 24-year-old patient has been involved in a serious motor-vehicle collision. He complains of back pain and presents with significant hypotension but his pulse is normal and his skin is pink, warm, and dry. What condition involving the spine could account for this?
2. You are treating a patient with a head injury. He has an altered mental status and a significant mechanism of injury to the head. Your partner thinks you should hyperventilate. When should you hyperventilate? What are the signs and symptoms that would indicate this is necessary?
3. You are called to the scene of a motor-vehicle collision. After ensuring scene safety and taking Standard Precautions, you approach the car, which has struck a bridge abutment, and note a deformed steering wheel. The driver's side door is open and, out on the middle of the bridge, you see a person you presume to be the driver wandering erratically toward the opposite side of the bridge. How should you proceed?

Pathophysiology to Practice

The following question is designed to assist you in gathering relevant clinical information and making accurate decisions in the field.

- You encounter patients who experience pain in the areas listed below. From the three choices given for each, choose the dermatome associated with it.).
  Nipple level (C-4, T-4, or L-2)
  Navel (T-10, L-1, or S-3)
  Little finger (C-5, C-8, or C-2)
  Big toe (S-1, L-4, or T-12)

Street Scenes

You and your partner are dispatched to the city park for a patient with a head injury. Arriving on-scene, you determine the scene is safe and observe a group of teenage boys huddled around a person who is lying on the ground. Taking Standard Precautions, you grab your equipment and approach the patient. Your partner asks, "What happened?"

"We were jumping ramps on our bicycles when Lee tried to do a flip," states one of the boys. "He hit the ground head first. I told that fool he should be wearing a helmet!" You observe a young male lying supine on the asphalt parking lot, eyes closed, with blood oozing from the top of his head from what appears to be an abrasion.

One of the boys identifies himself as Lee's brother and tells you that Lee is 13 years old. He states he lives just around the corner. You ask if his mother is home and he says she is. You ask him to go tell his mother what happened and to immediately come to the park.

Street Scene Questions

1. What is your general impression of this patient?
2. What immediate treatment should be provided?

Your general impression is of an unconscious male with a head and possible spine injury, so your partner provides manual stabilization of the head and neck. Lee's airway is patent, he is breathing normally, and you observe no other bleeding other than the laceration on the top of his head. You decide this is a high-priority trauma patient.

"Lee," you call out. "Lee, can you hear me?"

Lee opens his eyes and asks, "What happened?" Though the patient responds to verbal stimuli, it is apparent that he does not know what happened. He is able to tell you what day it is (Saturday), but not the date.

"Lee, I am going to give you a number to remember. It's number 51. Can you say that?" you ask.

He replies, "51." About this time, Lee's mother arrives. You briefly recount what you know. She seems concerned, but not overly upset. You apply a rigid collar to further restrict the motion of the patient's neck. You learn that Lee is on no medications, has no allergies, and has no medical history. He ate lunch 2 hours ago. You obtain baseline vitals and find his pulse is 80 and normal; respirations are 24 and unlabored; blood pressure is 108/74, skin is pink, warm, and dry; and pupils are equal and reactive to light.

Street Scene Question

3. How should you monitor changing levels of responsiveness in a patient with a head injury?

"Lee, tell me what day it is today. Then tell me that number I asked you to keep in mind," you say.

"Saturday. But what number?" he responds.

You place Lee on a nonrebreather mask at 15 liters per minute and also apply a loose dressing to the abrasion on his forehead. There is no other sign of injury on his body. Lee denies any neck pain and has good pulses, motor function, and sensation in all extremities.

The fire department rescue squad is now on-scene, and they help you restrict motion of the patient's neck and spine by securing Lee to a rigid board. Lee continues to have good pulses, motor function, and sensation in all extremities. When asked to recall the number again, he states, "I think it was 37." You tell him it is "51" and ask him to repeat it. "51," he says.

On-line medical direction has no other orders for you, but tells you to keep an eye on his airway and mental status. You allow his mother to ride in the ambulance with you. You assess vitals once more en route, noting no significant changes. You once again ask Lee what day and what number and this time he looks at you and says, "Saturday, and I think it's 51." You tell him he's correct. He groans and states he has a headache. The rest of the transport is uneventful.

Multisystem Trauma

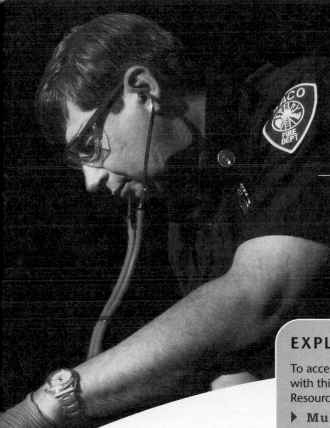

STANDARD ◌--------
Trauma (Multisystem Trauma)

COMPETENCY ◌--------
Applies fundamental knowledge to provide basic emergency care and transportation based on assessment findings for an acutely injured patient.

CORE CONCEPTS ◌--------
— How to balance the critical trauma patient's need for prompt transport against the time needed to treat all of the patient's injuries at the scene

— How to determine the severity of the trauma patient's condition, priority for transport, and appropriate transport destination

— How to select the critical interventions to implement at the scene for a multiple-trauma patient

— How to calculate a trauma score

EXPLORE Resource Central

To access Resource Central, follow directions on the Student Access Card provided with this text. If there is no card, go to **www.bradybooks.com** and follow the Resource Central link to Buy Access from there. Under Media Resources, you will find:

▶ **Multiple System Injuries in Front-End Collisions**
Watch an animation of what happens to the body during a front end collision.

▶ **Information about Entrance and Exit Wounds**
View an animation on entrance and exit wounds and discuss the importance of a complete assessment to identify all wounds.

▶ **Types of Injuries from Motor Vehicle Collisions**
Watch an animation of different types of collisions that occur during an auto crash and discuss types of injuries you can anticipate from different collisions.

OBJECTIVES ------------------------------------

After reading this chapter you should be able to:

32.1 Define key terms introduced in this chapter.

32.2 Describe the considerations for teamwork, timing, and transport decisions in assessing and managing patients with multisystem trauma or multiple trauma. (p. 792)

32.3 Discuss the physiologic, anatomic, and mechanism of injury criteria for determining patient severity with regard to trauma triage and transport decisions. (pp. 793–796)

32.4 Recognize special patient considerations that increase the patient's priority for transport, as age, anticoagulation bleeding disorders, burns, time-sensitive extremity injuries, end-stage renal disorders requiring dialysis, and pregnancy. (p. 796)

32.5 Discuss general principles of multisystem trauma management. (pp. 796–800)

32.6 Describe the purposes of trauma scoring systems. (pp. 800–801)

T here are many differences between trauma patients and medical patients. Medical patients generally call for a single complaint. In contrast, trauma patients often have more than one problem—a head injury and a broken leg, for example. When an emergency concurrently causes damage to more than one area of the body, this is referred to as *multisystem trauma* and is a serious condition.

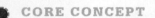

MULTISYSTEM TRAUMA

CORE CONCEPT

How to balance the critical trauma patient's need for prompt transport against the time needed to treat all of the patient's injuries at the scene

multiple trauma
more than one serious injury.

multisystem trauma
one or more injuries that affect more than one body system.

The **multiple trauma** patient has more than one serious injury. The **multisystem trauma** patient has one or more injuries serious enough to affect more than one body system. For example, a patient with a gunshot wound to the chest and a painful, swollen, deformed extremity is a multiple trauma patient, having more than one serious injury. He is also likely to be a multisystem trauma patient. He has a possibility of spinal injury, which will affect the nervous system. Additionally, the gunshot wound to the chest may well affect some or all of the heart and great blood vessels (cardiovascular system), the lungs (respiratory system), and perhaps nearby organs such as the spleen, pancreas, liver, kidneys, stomach, and intestines (endocrine, hepatic, renal, and digestive systems).

When the mechanism of injury suggests that your patient has more than one serious injury, or has an injury or injuries that are likely to affect more than one body system, decisions beyond what are called for on more typical EMS runs become necessary.

For example, consider the patient who has fallen 30 feet from some scaffolding and has an angulated forearm injury. Your primary assessment reveals him to be unresponsive with the airway partially occluded by his tongue. Do you spend time applying a rigid splint to his arm? The answer in this case is no. This patient has life-threatening injuries affecting at least the respiratory system that can only be treated in a hospital emergency department or operating room. Spending additional time at the scene to treat an injury that is not life threatening may reduce the patient's chances of survival.

Now consider an alert patient with no signs or symptoms of shock who has pain and tenderness in the middle of his thigh as well as an angulated forearm. In this case, the patient is stable enough to allow you a few minutes to apply a splint and prevent further injury. In each of these two examples, your actions as an EMT should provide the most benefit to the patient while at the same time reducing risk as much as possible.

These decisions are made easier when your crew works well together and each member knows what to expect from another. This is called *teamwork*. Crew members also must be aware of the importance of moving a multisystem trauma patient to definitive care as soon as possible, since it is rarely possible for EMS providers (even paramedics) to truly stabilize a trauma patient in the field. This is called *timing*. Finally, the appropriate destination must be chosen for the patient. This is a *transport* decision. In areas where some hospitals are designated trauma centers, it is important that protocols specify which patients need to be taken there and when it is (or is not) appropriate for EMS to bypass another hospital.

Determining Patient Severity

When you first approach a trauma scene, you will need to take in as much information as possible in order to make the best decisions. There will be times when you will come upon a horrific crash and see a patient standing there, seemingly uninjured, whereas in a similar crash on a different day you will find a critically injured patient.

Although you have heard much about critical decision making, perhaps the most critical decisions you will make for any trauma patient are determining (1) patient priority/severity, (2) whether to limit scene time or not, and (3) which hospital or transport method is best for your patient.

These decisions are a foundation for the entire call. A wrong decision about patient severity or transport—especially one that delays transport of a patient who needs it—will result in a delay of necessary surgical care at the hospital and create a disorganized, chaotic scene while you try to play catch-up with a crashing patient.

It is also worthwhile to note that there are so many variables at trauma scenes that it is impossible to provide exact guidelines for each situation. The decisions you make will be based on several things, including your patient's condition, the proximity of hospitals, options available for transport (e.g., air medical evacuation), your protocols, and the advice of medical direction.

Consider the following situations. The nature of the area where you provide care may fit one of these situations or be somewhere in between.

- An EMT in a suburban location has a 5-minute transport to a trauma center, so he keeps his scene time short and transports the patient expeditiously to the trauma center.

- Another EMT is 30 minutes from the trauma center and has a patient who is bleeding into his airway. The EMT is having trouble controlling the bleeding. In this case, getting ALS assistance en route or diverting the patient to a closer community hospital is necessary, because it is unlikely the patient will survive the trip to the trauma center without securing the airway.

- A third EMT works in a very rural community. It is 45 minutes to a community hospital and over 2 hours to a trauma center. In this case, a helicopter is summoned to transport this EMT's patient to the trauma center.

You will need to consider many factors when making determinations about patient severity, priority, and transport destination. The next section will cover some of these issues.

The Centers for Disease Control has released guidelines for trauma triage and transport to trauma centers. These take three main factors into consideration: physiological determinants, anatomic criteria, and mechanism of injury.

You will encounter various determinants at different times in the call. You will notice the mechanism of injury as you size-up the scene, observe specific injury patterns as you approach, and notice the patient's mental status and vital signs as you begin to assess the patient. Each of these factors will play into your transport decisions.

Finally, each of the criteria discussed next—physiologic criteria, anatomic criteria, and mechanism of injury—should be considered separately and in sequence, addressing the first of these criteria before the second and addressing the second before the third. For example, if you encounter a patient who is physiologically unstable, he would be transported to a trauma center. However, if your patient is physiologically stable, you would move on to consider the anatomic criteria, and so on.

Determining Severity: Physiologic Criteria

It is believed that the most valuable findings during an assessment are the patient's physiologic conditions (Table 32-1). Any time you have a patient with an altered mental status, hypotension, or an abnormally slow or rapid respiratory rate, you should place this patient at a high priority and transport him promptly to a trauma center when available and following your local protocols.

- Altered mental status (GCS < 14) is a significant indicator of head injury (which may present with unresponsiveness, confusion, or otherwise altered mental status) and hypoxia (which may present with anxiety and/or restlessness).

CORE CONCEPT

How to determine the severity of the trauma patient's condition, priority for transport, and appropriate transport destination

Table 32-1	CDC Trauma Triage Guidelines: Physiologic Criteria
Glasgow Coma Scale	14
Systolic blood pressure	< 90
Respiratory rate	< 10 or > 29 (< 20 in infant less than 1 year)

- Hypotension (systolic blood pressure < 90 mmHg) is a definitive sign for shock and indicates some sort of internal bleeding or other circulatory disturbance.
- Abnormal respiratory rates are also indicative of serious injury. Rapid respiratory rates (> 28) usually indicate shock. Abnormally slow rates (< 10), in contrast, may indicate head injury or later stages of shock. In infants, respiratory rates below 20 are an extremely grave sign.

Determining Severity: Anatomic Criteria

Injuries of certain types or to specific areas of the body require care that is usually available only in a trauma center. For example, it makes sense that injuries to the head and chest could be serious. Other specific injuries require prompt surgical intervention for the patient to recover to the fullest extent possible. This list includes multiple musculoskeletal injuries (more than two long-bone fractures = multiple trauma), amputations, and severely mangled extremities. Pelvic injuries are associated with significant internal bleeding.

These specific anatomic criteria are listed in Table 32-2.

Determining Severity: Mechanism of Injury

A significant mechanism of injury does not guarantee the patient has a serious injury. In the absence of physiologic or anatomic criteria, however, the fact that significant forces have acted on the body causes us as EMTs to act in a more cautious manner.

Some newer vehicles have the ability to transmit data after a crash (telemetry). In addition to notifying police and rescue personnel, the on-board computer in the vehicle may also transmit data such as vehicle speed at the time of the crash, whether the vehicle rolled over or had multiple impacts, which part of the vehicle was struck (e.g., front end), and whether or not the air bag was deployed.

Table 32-3 lists mechanism of injury criteria that may cause you to choose transport to a trauma center over other facilities.

Determining Severity: Special Patients and Considerations

You will read in subsequent chapters that not everyone responds to illness and injury the same way. For example, geriatric patients do not efficiently compensate for shock. Children also respond differently and may benefit by transport to a pediatric specialty facility.

Patients with certain conditions, such as patients on anticoagulants (blood thinners), those with end-stage renal disease, those who are pregnant, and others, may also require transport to a trauma center but are generally decided on a case-by-case basis.

Table 32-2	CDC Trauma Triage Guidelines: Anatomic Criteria

- All penetrating injuries to head, neck, torso, and extremities proximal to elbow and knee
- Flail chest
- Two or more proximal long-bone fractures
- Crushed, degloved, or mangled extremity
- Amputation proximal to wrist and ankle
- Pelvic fractures
- Open or depressed skull fracture
- Paralysis

Table 32-3   CDC Trauma Triage Guidelines: Mechanism of Injury Criteria

FALLS
- Adults: > 20 feet (one story is equal to 10 feet)
- Children: > 10 feet or two to three times the height of the child

HIGH-RISK AUTO CRASH
- Intrusion > 12 in. occupant site; > 18 in. any site
- Ejection (partial or complete) from automobile
- Death in same passenger compartment
- Vehicle telemetry data consistent with high risk of injury.

AUTO V. PEDESTRIAN/BICYCLIST THROWN, RUN OVER, OR WITH SIGNIFICANT (> 20 MPH) IMPACT

MOTORCYCLE CRASH > 20 MPH

One example of a patient who will likely require triage to a higher level of care is a geriatric patient who has had a fall, is on anticoagulant medications, and has a head injury. Even if the patient appears fine after the fall, the risk of intracranial bleeding is high for this patient.

Table 32-4 lists trauma triage guidelines for special patient or system considerations.

Inside/Outside

INTERNAL INJURIES

Multisystem trauma is that which is serious and that often involves internal organs. This inside/outside feature reviews common internal injuries and their outside presentation as a review/summary for serious trauma.

INSIDE	OUTSIDE
Pneumothorax	• Diminished or absent lung sounds on one side • Respiratory distress • Elevated pulse • Possible injury on that side of chest
Tension pneumothorax	• Absent lung sounds on one side • Distended neck veins • Altered mental status • Narrowing pulse pressure • Increased pulse and respirations • Possible injury (penetrating) to the chest • Tracheal deviation (very late sign)
Cardiac tamponade	• Distended neck veins • Narrowing pulse pressure • Increased pulse and respirations • Penetrating injury to the chest
Solid organ damage	• Solid organs are vascular and can bleed profusely causing shock. • A capsule around solid organs such as the liver can mask bleeding and pain, delaying diagnosis. • Injury to these vascular organs is often (although not always) sharp and in predictable patterns/locations (e.g., referred to shoulder)
Hollow organ damage	• Hollow organ damage (e.g., to the small intestine) may cause a spilling of contents into the surrounding abdominal tissue. This frequently causes severe and diffuse pain because of widespread irritation.

Table 32-4 CDC Trauma Triage Guidelines: Special Patient or System Considerations

AGE
- Older adults: Risk of injury or death decreases after age 55 years
- Children: Should be triaged preferentially to pediatric-capable trauma centers

ANTICOAGULATION AND BLEEDING DISORDERS

BURNS
- Without other trauma mechanism: Triage to burn facility
- With trauma mechanism: Triage to trauma center

TIME-SENSITIVE EXTREMITY INJURY

END-STAGE RENAL DISEASE REQUIRING DIALYSIS

PREGNANCY > 20 WEEKS

EMS PROVIDER JUDGMENT

MANAGING THE MULTISYSTEM TRAUMA PATIENT

CORE CONCEPT

How to select the critical interventions to implement at the scene for a multiple-trauma patient

The following scenario describes a typical multiple-trauma call. As you read, ask yourself these questions: When does the EMT recognize that the patient has multiple injuries? What body systems would the EMT suspect have been affected by this patient's injuries? What is the EMT's first decision about managing those injuries, and why do you think he made it? What actions does he take to support the affected body systems? What priorities does he set for his patient?

A Typical Call

You receive a call for a motorcyclist who was hit by a car. The scene is safe, so you approach the patient, an adult male you estimate to be about 25 years old. He appears unresponsive in a pool of blood on the road and is not wearing a helmet (Figure 32-1). Police point to the motorcycle he was riding about 20 feet away.

The patient responds purposefully to a painful stimulus; that is, he tries to push your hand away. He is making gurgling sounds with each breath, so you suction some blood out of his airway. He also is making snoring sounds, so you insert an oropharyngeal airway, which he tolerates and which eliminates the snoring sounds. His breathing is shallow and labored at a rate of about 30, so you have your partner ventilate him with a bag-valve mask and high-concentration oxygen as she simultaneously stabilizes his head with her knees.

There is a pool of blood around the patient's left thigh, which appears angulated. You quickly cut away the left leg of his pants and observe an apparent compound angulated mid-shaft femur fracture with blood flowing heavily from the wound. You apply a tourniquet to stop the bleeding. The patient's radial pulse is rapid and weak, and his skin is pale and sweaty.

You assign this patient a high priority for rapid treatment and transport based on the mechanism of injury, altered mental status, and presence of shock (hypoperfusion). You request ALS intercept en route if it is available and will not delay transport.

You perform a trauma assessment. At the same time, a firefighter with whom you have worked before gets a long backboard and the other equipment necessary to immobilize the patient. By the time he returns, you have finished the rapid trauma assessment and gained the following information: A hematoma (lump) is present on the left side of the patient's head, neck veins are flat, there is no deformity of the cervical spine, breath sounds are decreased on the left side of his chest, his abdomen is soft, his pelvis seems stable, there is an obvious compound angulated midshaft femur fracture on the left side from which the bleeding has been controlled, there are some nonbleeding lacerations on the

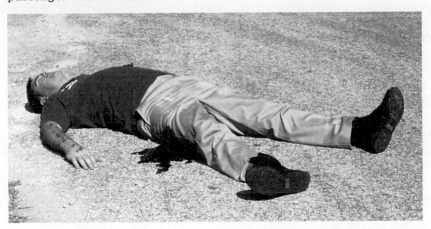

FIGURE 32-1 Unresponsive adult male patient, victim of a motorcycle-passenger vehicle collision.

left forearm and lower leg, and pulses are weak but palpable in all extremities except the leg with the tourniquet.

With a cervical collar in place on the patient, you roll him as a unit and examine his spine and posterior trunk. You find no further injuries. You roll him down on the board, taking care to move the injured leg as little as possible once it is in the anatomical position.

As you quickly immobilize the patient on the board (using the board as a splint for the fractured femur), you make sure the firefighter is available to drive the ambulance so you and your partner can tend to the patient in back. You confirm that the firefighter knows you are to go to the trauma center, not the community hospital that is 5 minutes closer. Your protocols specify that you are to go directly to the trauma center under conditions such as these because of the comprehensive care available there.

You move the patient and board onto the stretcher and into the ambulance, making sure your partner is able to continue ventilating him during the move. Once inside the patient compartment, you repeat the primary assessment. Your general impression is of a young adult male with multiple injuries. His mental status remains unchanged: he again tries to brush your hand away when you apply a painful stimulus. His tongue is prevented from obstructing his airway by an oropharyngeal airway. There is a little bit of gurgling as you carefully listen, so you suction some more blood out of his mouth. There are now no abnormal sounds as your partner ventilates him. Oxygen is flowing, and you see the patient's chest rise with each breath. The bleeding from the thigh remains controlled, and you see no other bleeding wounds. His radial pulse is rapid and weak. The patient is still a high priority.

With a second primary assessment completed, you call the trauma center and notify them of the patient's condition and your estimated time of arrival (10 minutes). You tell them you will give them vital signs as soon as you get them. With the hospital preparing for the patient's arrival, you turn to obtaining vital signs. The patient's pulse is 108, weak and regular; blood pressure 92/56; respirations assisted at 12 per minute; and skin pale and sweaty. You relay this information to the trauma center.

You have a few minutes before you arrive, so you check with your partner to make sure she is still able to ventilate the patient well before you perform a detailed head-to-toe physical exam. You find the patient has equal pupils that are slow to react, a hematoma (lump) on the left side of his head, nothing unusual in or behind the ears, deformity on both sides of his mandible (you conclude this is what is causing the bleeding into his airway), and flat neck veins (you are unable to palpate the cervical spine because the cervical collar is in place). His breath sounds are still decreased on the left side of his chest, his abdomen seems to be firmer than before, his pelvis seems stable, there is an obvious compound midshaft femur fracture on the left side (it is no longer angulated because you straightened it when you put the patient on the board), and there are some nonbleeding lacerations on the left forearm and lower leg. It is more difficult now to palpate peripheral pulses.

You would like to apply a traction splint but realize you do not have enough time or personnel. With just a few minutes before you arrive at the trauma center, you repeat the

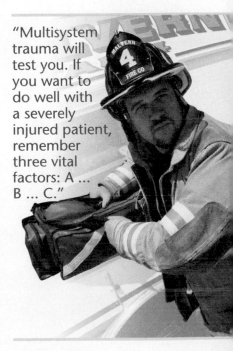

"Multisystem trauma will test you. If you want to do well with a severely injured patient, remember three vital factors: A ... B ... C."

primary assessment one more time. The patient still responds purposefully to painful stimuli, but now he also opens his eyes briefly when you pinch him. You find no other changes. You get another set of vital signs: pulse 120, blood pressure 90 by palpation, respirations assisted at 12 per minute, and skin pale and sweaty.

You arrive at the emergency department and give a report to the trauma team as you transfer your patient to his bed. The patient becomes a bit more responsive in the emergency department, but he is agitated. The staff stabilizes his vital signs for the moment. The emergency department staff asks you and your partner to help apply a traction splint to the patient's fractured femur. You are able to quickly and efficiently do so. The patient goes off for further tests and surgery.

Later you learn that the patient had a cerebral contusion (bruise of the brain), bilateral fracture of the mandible, left hemothorax (blood in the left side of the chest cavity), and a fractured femur.

After a lengthy stay, the patient is able to walk out of the hospital with some temporary assistance from a pair of crutches.

Analysis of the Call

The previous scenario about the injured motorcycle rider shows an example of a patient who has critical injuries. Immediate threats to his life included shock (hypoperfusion) and bleeding into an airway that was partially obstructed by his tongue. Other serious injuries included an apparent head injury, inadequate ventilation, a presumed chest injury, a mandible injury, a compound angulated femur fracture, and a suspected spine injury (based on the mechanism of injury). The EMT in the scenario gave his patient the best possible chance of survival by following the priorities determined by his assessments.

The primary assessment revealed several immediate life threats that the EMT could do something about:

- The airway was partially obstructed by blood, which he suctioned.
- The patient's tongue was partially blocking the airway, causing snoring sounds with breathing, for which he inserted an artificial airway.
- The patient's breathing was shallow and labored at a rate of about 30, which indicated inadequate ventilation, for which the EMT's partner instituted assisted ventilations with high-concentration oxygen.

The EMT then picked up on the seriousness of the patient's condition and made the decision not to treat some injuries the way he ordinarily would. That is, normally he would have applied a traction splint and dressed and bandaged the limb lacerations. Although it was tempting to do so, he realized this would delay transport for a patient who might have very little time to waste. A patient who has bleeding into his airway does not have any time to spare. Accordingly, the EMT used a backboard as a universal splint for the femur and did not bandage the lacerations because they were not bleeding.

Some might say the EMT in the scenario was wrong and should have applied the traction splint in the field. After all, the emergency department staff later asked him to do it, right? In fact, the EMT showed good judgment. The appropriate place to apply a traction splint to this patient was in the emergency department, not in the field. When the emergency department staff asked him to help apply the splint, it was because the patient was stable enough (and because the EMT was more familiar with the device than they were). If the patient's condition had not improved, they would not have asked him to put the splint on. Instead, the patient would have been whisked away for surgery or further tests.

There were two additional ways in which the EMT showed good judgment: he postponed taking vital signs, and he gave the hospital staff time to prepare. That is, the patient was ready to be put in the ambulance before the EMT was able to get vital signs, so he appropriately postponed taking them until they were en route. As tempting as it might be to complete an assessment all at once, the EMT realized that vital signs were not going to change anything he could do and taking them would delay transport. He also called the hospital and gave them an admittedly incomplete report so that they could begin preparations. He made sure to tell them he would get them the patient's vital signs as soon as possible and then he did. This gave the hospital some additional time to notify the trauma team.

Falling for Your Attention

A determination of criticality (whether the patient has a serious condition or not) is one of the most important decisions you can make for the trauma patient. Just identifying when the *potential* for serious injury exists is vital. Your patient priority and transport decisions are based on these determinations. Assume you have a local hospital 15 minutes away and a trauma center 25 minutes away. Determine which of the following patients should be transported to the trauma center and which could be transported to the local hospital—and explain why.

1. Your 30-year-old patient fell 4 feet from a ladder and got his lower leg caught in a rung. He believes he broke his lower left leg. His pulse is 96, strong and regular; respirations 18 and adequate; blood pressure 126/86; pupils equal and reactive to light; and skin warm and dry. He is alert. There are distal pulses in the extremity.

2. Your patient is an 8-year-old male who fell 8–10 feet from a tree to the ground. He is holding his right wrist and says it hurts. As you talk with him and his parents, you note that he appears confused. As you move him to the ambulance, you believe his mental status is decreasing. His vitals are pulse 82, strong and regular; respirations 24; blood pressure 122/86; pupils equal and sluggishly reactive to light; and mental status as previously noted.

3. Your patient is a 32-year-old female who is 30 weeks' pregnant and fell down a flight of stairs. She struck her head and has pain in her left shoulder. Her main concern is the brisk vaginal bleeding that began since the fall.

General Principles of Multisystem Trauma Management

Prepare for a call to a multisystem trauma patient by practicing for it. If you have a regular partner or crew, determine your individual roles beforehand. For example, someone should be designated to manually immobilize the patient's head and, if necessary, ventilate with a bag-valve mask. Depending on the number of people available, you may have to have each person handle several roles. En route to the call, if you have reason to believe you might care for a multisystem trauma patient, review the roles each person will have.

At the scene, follow the assessment steps as you learned them in your EMT course. Follow the priorities you discover in your primary assessment (airway, breathing, and circulation). Then balance the need for scene interventions with the time needed to perform them. As you may recall, the concept of the *golden hour* refers to the need for critical trauma patients to get to surgery within 1 hour of injury (not 1 hour from when you get to the patient). Although the time the patient has to get to surgery has not been scientifically proven to be an hour, the concept is still a useful one in avoiding delays at the scene.

For most critical patients, limit scene treatment to:

- Stabilizing the cervical spine during all interventions
- Suctioning the airway
- Inserting an oral or nasal airway
- Restoring a patent airway by sealing a sucking chest wound
- Ventilating with a bag-valve mask
- Administering high-concentration oxygen
- Controlling bleeding
- Immobilizing the patient with a cervical collar and a long backboard

Principles of multisystem trauma management also include the following:

- **Scene safety is paramount.** Different kinds of trauma tend to have different kinds of dangers. Blunt trauma, which is more common in rural and suburban areas, can be associated with such dangers as bent power poles, leaking fuel, sharp glass and metal edges, and passing traffic. Penetrating trauma, such as stab wounds and gunshot wounds, tend to occur more commonly in urban areas. Risks you will need to consider include the presence of the assailant (especially one who is upset because you are trying to save a person he tried to kill), presence of multiple weapons (on the victim, assailant, and bystanders), absent or delayed police response, and angry crowds.

- **Ensure an open airway.** If you are unable to ventilate your patient without assistance, try other approaches until you find one that works. You might get another person to assist you en route or you might have to switch places with your partner. Other alternatives include using a different device to ventilate, such as a pocket mask with supplemental oxygen, or you and your partner may have to work together to ventilate the patient.

- **Perform urgent or emergency moves as necessary.** For example, if a critical patient is sitting in a vehicle, you will need to perform a rapid extrication.

- **Adapt to the situation.** When a patient is trapped, for example, and part of the patient's body is not accessible, assess as much of him as you can. Keep in mind that when he is extricated you will need to perform a complete examination.

For a multisystem trauma patient, your overall goal is to treat immediate threats to life, which you can treat with prompt transportation to a facility that will provide definitive care (or as close to it as is available). Guard against the temptation in these cases to spend time at the scene treating all of the patient's injuries and immobilizing him perfectly. It is not good patient care to arrive at the hospital with the world's best-packaged corpse.

POINT OF VIEW

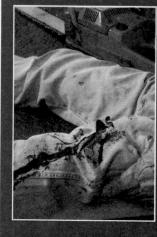

"I pulled the cord on my chainsaw. I really didn't think it would start. It had been in the garage for 2 or 3 years. Imagine my surprise when it fired up—which was nothing compared to my surprise when the saw slipped and cut into my leg.

"I don't remember much else, not even how I got to the ground. I do remember seeing blood and the room getting darker. Then I saw my wife . . . then the EMTs.

"As I came around, I figured it was just a bad cut on my leg. But the EMTs seemed pretty concerned. They were moving quickly. My wife looked worried. I heard the EMTs talking about my vital signs, and then they were moving me to the ambulance.

"On the way, I was a little more coherent. The EMTs told me that they were taking precautions because my pulse was a little high. The leg wound was pretty deep. They took me to a larger hospital close to the city—not my usual hospital. Turns out it was a good thing. I had a lot of muscle and nerve damage, and the hospital where they took me had the staff and equipment to deal with it.

"It was a tough day. My surgeon said the EMTs did a good job by realizing that my leg—and me—were in bad shape and deciding to take me to a hospital that could handle special surgery. They made a good decision—one I am very grateful for."

Trauma Scoring

----------- ● **CORE CONCEPT**

How to calculate a trauma score

trauma score
a system of evaluating trauma patients according to a numerical rating system to determine the severity of the patient's trauma.

In some EMS systems, hospitals ask EMTs and other providers not only to perform the usual assessment of trauma patients but also to evaluate trauma patients according to a numerical rating system. By evaluating certain patient characteristics and assigning a number to each of them, the provider can determine a ***trauma score*** that may do two things.

First, calculating the trauma score may help to determine whether a patient should go to a trauma center. A patient who needs the resources that a trauma center can provide (like 24-hour-a-day availability of trauma surgeons and nurses, operating rooms, special intensive care beds, and so on) should be transported there as expeditiously as possible. In rural areas, this typically means EMS transports to the local hospital where the patient receives enough care to quickly stabilize his condition before he is transferred to a distant trauma center. In more densely populated areas where some local hospitals are trauma centers and some are not, there will be local protocols describing when EMS should transport a patient directly to a trauma center, even if it is necessary to go past a hospital that is not a trauma center. This is where a trauma scoring system can help. By objectively describing the severity of a patient's condition, the score can direct more severely injured patients directly to trauma centers and allow less seriously injured patients to go to local hospitals.

The second major function of a trauma scoring system is to allow trauma centers to evaluate themselves in comparing the outcomes of trauma patients who have similar severity of injuries. In this way, they can improve the quality of care their trauma patients receive and conduct research on trauma care.

Several systems are in use to achieve these purposes. One of the most useful and widely utilized is the Revised Trauma Score (RTS). The RTS evaluates three characteristics of the patient's condition: the Glasgow Coma Scale or GCS (which you learned about in Chapter 31, "Trauma to the Head, Neck, and Spine"), systolic blood pressure, and respiratory rate. The original trauma score included other characteristics that were difficult to evaluate consistently under field conditions and turned out to be unnecessary.

Figure 32-2 shows the values assigned to the EMT's assessment findings in the Revised Trauma Score. Up to four points are assigned for each of the elements of the RTS. The lower the score, the more seriously injured the patient is and the less likely he will survive, even with excellent care.

Follow your local protocols for use of a trauma scoring system, but do not let it interfere with patient care. Manage airway problems and control other immediate threats to life before trying to use a score. In some systems, EMTs are asked to determine the score en route. In others, they may be asked simply to gather all the elements used to calculate the score, but not to assign numerical values. By reporting this information, a physician or nurse at an emergency department can calculate the score and advise you on the appropriate destination for your patient. Follow your local protocol.

FIGURE 32-2 Revised Trauma Score.

REVISED TRAUMA SCORE

Characteristic	Criterion	RTS Points
Glasgow Coma Scale	13–15	4
	9–12	3
	6–8	2
	4–5	1
	3	0
Systolic Blood Pressure	> 89 mmHg	4
	76–89 MmHg	3
	50–75 MmHg	2
	1–49 MmHg	1
	0	0
Respiratory Rate	10–29/min	4
	> 29/min	3
	6–9/min	2
	1–5/min	1
	0	0
Revised Trauma Score (Total)		

Source: Champion H.R., Sacco W.J., Copes W.S., et al. A Revision of the Trauma Score. *J Trauma* 29 (5): 623–9, 1989

Key Facts and Concepts

- Multisystem trauma is a serious condition in which two or more major body systems are injured or affected.

- Recognizing multisystem trauma, triaging properly, transporting promptly, and choosing the correct destination are vital for the survival of your patient.

- The CDC has issued guidelines for trauma triage and transport. These are a guide and should be used in conjunction with your protocols.

- The Revised Trauma Score (RTS) is one method of classifying trauma patients by severity and includes the Glasgow Coma Scale (GCS), systolic blood pressure and respiratory rate.

Key Decisions

- Is my patient seriously injured or potentially seriously injured?

- Should I expedite my scene time?

- Should I transport to a trauma center or assure the patient can be transported to the trauma center (e.g., by contacting air medical evacuation services)?

Chapter Glossary

multiple trauma more than one serious injury.

multisystem trauma one or more injuries that affect more than one body system.

trauma score a system of evaluating trauma patients according to a numerical rating system to determine the severity of the patient's trauma.

Preparation for Your Examination and Practice

Short Answer

1. What considerations must the EMT weigh when considering whether to perform an intervention at the scene?

2. What are the interventions that should generally be performed for a critical trauma patient at the scene?

3. When might it be appropriate for EMTs to bypass a closer hospital for a trauma center?

4. When might it be appropriate not to apply a traction splint in the field to an obviously fractured femur?

Thinking and Linking

Think back to Chapter 20, "Cardiac Emergencies," and link information from that chapter with information from this chapter as you consider the following situation:

- Your patient is a 50-year-old male who has been electrocuted and knocked forcefully to the ground. He's an electrician who thought the power was off when it wasn't. You are taking his vital signs, which seem to be normal, when suddenly he goes into cardiac arrest. Should you use the AED and treat it as a medical arrest . . . or should you transport him immediately without using the AED as for a trauma arrest? Why?

Critical Thinking Exercises

In a patient who has sustained significant trauma, making the correct transport decision is key. The purpose of this exercise will be to determine, and explain, the best transport decision for such a patient.

- You are called to a patient who has been involved in a crash in which the vehicle sustained significant intrusion into the area where the patient was sitting. The patient is alert and complains of pain in his ribs. His vital signs are pulse 96 and regular, respirations 30 and adequate, blood pressure 100/62, pupils equal and reactive, and skin cool and dry. Your partner says the patient is stable and could be easily transported to the community hospital nearby. You think the patient should be transported to the trauma center. How would you justify your decision to your partner?

Pathophysiology to Practice

For each of the following patients, explain why trauma triage guidelines place them at a higher priority:

1. Geriatric patients

2. Penetrating abdominal trauma patients

3. Patients who are on anticoagulants

4. Patients who have an amputated hand

Street Scenes

At 9:15 a.m. your BLS ambulance is dispatched to a busy intersection for a motor-vehicle collision. While responding, you are advised by dispatch that she has had several 911 calls regarding this collision and that there are two vehicles involved. As you arrive on-scene, you observe that a full-size pickup truck apparently struck a smaller compact vehicle head on. Your partner strategically places the ambulance to protect the scene. You notice two occupants slumped over inside the small vehicle, which has fluid draining from under the engine.

Street Scene Questions

1. What is your initial impression of the collision?
2. What additional resources will be necessary on-scene?

The driver of the pickup truck walks over to you and says that he bumped his head but he feels okay. Since he can walk and talk, you move toward the smaller car. As you approach, you note that both air bags have deployed and that the leaking fluid appears to be antifreeze, which does not pose a danger. You call for additional ambulances and make sure the police are en route. The male driver is wearing a full shoulder and lap restraint and appears conscious but "dazed." You notice his unrestrained passenger lying motionless on her left side across the console. Your primary assessment of the passenger reveals an approximately 25-year-old female responding to verbal stimuli, who is verbally abusive and unaware of her surroundings. She is crying and complaining of pain to her right arm. Her airway appears clear as you notice she has sustained severe facial trauma. Her respirations appear slightly labored and shallow. You note a strong and rapid radial pulse and warm and dry skin.

Street Scene Questions

3. Which patient should be transported first?
4. What is your critical decision regarding the female patient?
5. What critical interventions should you perform on-scene?

You realize that the woman is the priority because of her altered mental status and labored respirations. She has a large laceration, which extends from her upper lip up through her hair line,

and you observe angulation to her right humerus. Because of the mechanism of injury and the patient's current status, you decide to perform a rapid extrication. You place a cervical collar on her and spin her onto a board. When she yells, "My baby! Don't hurt my baby!" you note her large abdomen, which is consistent with pregnancy. You place padding under the right side of the backboard, which moves the patient onto her left side. This prevents the baby from compressing the vena cava, which could lower the woman's blood pressure. You move the woman to the ambulance with 15 liters of oxygen by nonrebreather mask in place.

Once in the ambulance, you suction blood that has begun to drain into her mouth from the facial laceration. Her initial vital signs show a pulse rate of 122, slightly labored respirations at a rate of 28, and a blood pressure of 142/94. Her pupils appear equal and reactive, and you notice no fluid exiting the ears. Her neck veins are flat and her trachea appears midline. You expose the patient, auscultate lung sounds, and find the right side sounds diminished, coinciding with tenderness to the right side of her chest. As you assess her large abdomen, she winces and again yells about her baby. You recheck her arm and notice angulation and crepitus. You align it and secure her arm alongside her torso, which acts as a splint. Her remaining extremities appear unremarkable. Your patient's level of responsiveness is not reliable enough for a medical history, but you notice she is wearing a medical identification tag, which states she is allergic to sulfa medication.

Street Scene Questions

6. What further information would you like to obtain about the female patient?
7. To what type of receiving facility should your patient be transported?

While en route to the hospital, you notice the patient's heart rate has increased to 128, her blood pressure has fallen to 122/86, and she is now guarding her abdomen with her left arm. You have contacted medical direction and have been advised to transport the patient to the nearest trauma center. Upon arrival at the trauma center, you update the staff and transfer the patient to their care.

33 Environmental Emergencies

STANDARD
Trauma (Environmental Emergencies)

COMPETENCY
Applies fundamental knowledge to provide basic emergency care and transportation based on assessment findings for an acutely injured patient.

CORE CONCEPTS
— Effects on the body of generalized hypothermia; assessment and care for hypothermia

— Effects on the body of local cold injuries; assessment and care for local cold injuries

— Personal effects on the body of exposure to heat; assessment and care for patients suffering from heat exposure

— Signs, symptoms, and treatment for drowning and other water-related injuries

— Signs, symptoms, and treatment for bites and stings

EXPLORE Resource Central

To access Resource Central, follow directions on the Student Access Card provided with this text. If there is no card, go to **www.bradybooks.com** and follow the Resource Central link to Buy Access from there. Under Media Resources, you will find:

▶ **Snakebites**
Watch this video to learn what types of snakes are poisonous and see how the venom of a snake is injected into a patient.

▶ **Information about Hypothermia**
Read about the different types of hypothermia, learn about the body's reaction to losing heat and find out who is at risk for becoming hypothermic.

▶ **Information about Diving Accidents**
Find out what is the most frequent injury sustained from diving and some ways to prevent diving injuries.

OBJECTIVES

After reading this chapter you should be able to:

33.1 Define key terms introduced in this chapter.

33.2 Describe processes of heat loss and heat production by the body. (pp. 805–806)

33.3 Recognize predisposing factors and exposure factors in relation to hypothermia. (pp. 807–808)

33.4 Recognize signs and symptoms of hypothermia. (pp. 808–809)

33.5 Describe the indications, contraindications, benefits, and risks of passive and active rewarming techniques. (p. 809)

33.6 Prioritize steps in assessment and management of patients with varying degrees of hypothermia. (pp. 808–810)

33.7 Discuss assessment and management for early or superficial local cold injury and for late or deep local cold injury. (pp. 810–813)

33.8 Discuss the effects of heat on the human body. (p. 814)

33.9 Differentiate between assessment and management priorities for heat emergency patients with moist, pale, normal-to-cool skin and those with hot skin that is either dry or moist. (pp. 814–816)

33.10 Anticipate the types of injuries and medical conditions that may be associated with water-related accidents. (pp. 817–818)

33.11 Discuss the assessment and management of the following water-related emergencies:
  a. Drowning (including rescue breathing and care for possible spinal injuries) (pp. 818–822)
  b. Diving accidents (p. 822)
  c. Scuba-diving accidents (pp. 822–824)

33.12 Describe safe techniques for water rescues and ice rescues. (pp. 824–826)

33.13 Discuss the assessment and management of the following types of bites and stings:
  a. Insect bites and stings (pp. 826–828)
  b. Snakebites (pp. 828–830)
  c. Poisoning from marine life (pp. 830–831)

KEY TERMS

active rewarming, *p. 809*
air embolism, *p. 822*
central rewarming, *p. 810*
conduction, *p. 805*
convection, *p. 807*

decompression sickness, *p. 822*
drowning, *p. 818*
evaporation, *p. 807*
hyperthermia, *p. 814*

hypothermia, *p. 807*
local cooling, *p. 811*
passive rewarming, *p. 809*
radiation, *p. 807*
respiration, *p. 807*

toxins, *p. 826*
venom, *p. 826*
water chill, *p. 805*
wind chill, *p. 807*

Environmental emergencies can occur in any setting—wilderness, rural, suburban, and urban areas. They include exposure to both heat and cold; drownings and other water-related injuries; and bites and stings from insects, spiders, snakes, and marine life. The keys to effective management are recognizing the patient's signs and symptoms and providing prompt and proper emergency care. However, as an EMT, you also must recognize that exposure may not be the only danger to the patient. Environmental emergencies can involve preexisting, or cause additional, medical problems and injuries.

EXPOSURE TO COLD

How the Body Loses Heat

If the environment is too cold, body heat can be lost faster than it can be generated. The body attempts to adjust to these temperature differences by reducing perspiration and circulation to the skin—shutting down avenues by which the body usually gets rid of excess heat. Muscular activity in the form of shivering and the rate at which fuel (food) is burned within the body both increase to produce more heat. At a certain point, however, not enough heat is generated to be available to all parts of the body. This may result in damage to exposed tissues and a general reduction or cessation of body functions.

To be able to prevent or compensate for heat loss, the EMT must be aware of the ways in which a body loses heat (Figure 33-1):

- **Conduction.** The transfer of heat from one material to another through direct contact is called **conduction**. Heat will flow from a warmer material to a cooler one. Although body heat transferred directly into cool air is a problem, **water chill** is an even

conduction
the transfer of heat from one material to another through direct contact.

water chill
chilling caused by conduction of heat from the body when the body or clothing is wet.

FIGURE 33-1 Mechanisms of heat loss.

MECHANISMS OF HEAT LOSS

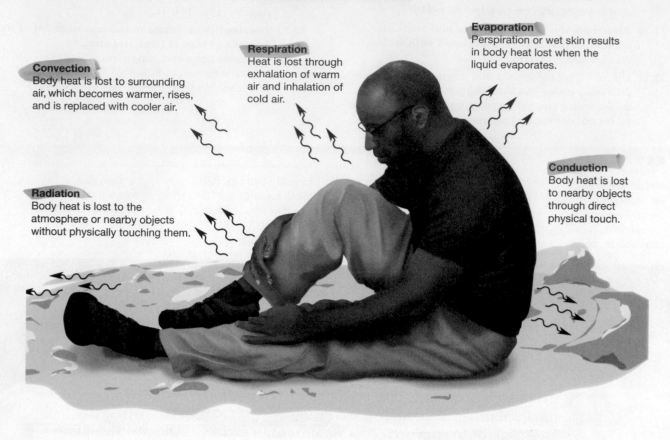

Convection
Body heat is lost to surrounding air, which becomes warmer, rises, and is replaced with cooler air.

Respiration
Heat is lost through exhalation of warm air and inhalation of cold air.

Evaporation
Perspiration or wet skin results in body heat lost when the liquid evaporates.

Conduction
Body heat is lost to nearby objects through direct physical touch.

Radiation
Body heat is lost to the atmosphere or nearby objects without physically touching them.

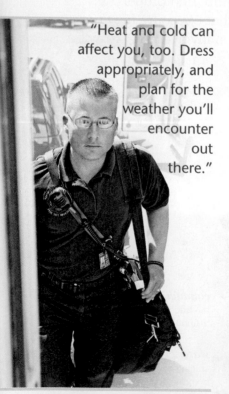

"Heat and cold can affect you, too. Dress appropriately, and plan for the weather you'll encounter out there."

greater problem because water conducts heat away from the body 25 times faster than still air. Patients with wet bodies or clothing are especially susceptible to water chill in cold environments. Heat loss through conduction can be a major problem when a person is lying on a cold floor or another cold surface. However, a person who is standing or walking around in cold weather will lose less heat than a person who is lying on the cold ground.

- **Convection.** When currents of air or water pass over the body, carrying away heat, *convection* occurs. The effects of a cold environment are worsened when moving water or air surround the body. *Wind chill* is a frequent problem. The faster the wind speed, the greater the heat loss. For example, if it is 10°F with no wind, the body will lose heat, but if there is a 20 mph wind, the amount of heat lost by the body is much greater.

- **Radiation.** In conduction and convection, heat is "picked up" by the surrounding (still or moving) air or water. In *radiation*, the body's atoms and molecules send out rays of heat as they move and change. If you were in the vacuum of outer space with no air or water around to pick up heat, you would still lose heat by radiating it out into space. Most radiant heat loss occurs from a person's head and neck.

- **Evaporation.** *Evaporation* occurs when the body perspires or gets wet. As perspiration or water on the skin or clothing vaporizes, the body experiences a generalized cooling effect.

- **Respiration.** *Respiration* causes loss of body heat as a result of exhaled warm air. The amount of heat loss depends on the outside air temperature as well as the rate and depth of respirations.

Generalized Hypothermia

When cooling affects the entire body, a problem known as **_hypothermia_**, or generalized cooling, develops. Exposure to cold reduces body heat. With time, the body is unable to maintain its proper core (internal) temperature. If this cooling is allowed to continue, hypothermia leads to death. (The stages of hypothermia are described in Table 33-1.)

Predisposing Factors

Patients with injuries, chronic illness, or certain other conditions will show the effects of cold much sooner than healthy persons. These conditions include shock (hypoperfusion), burns, head and spinal-cord injuries, generalized infection, and diabetes with hypoglycemia. Those under the influence of alcohol or other drugs also tend to be affected more rapidly and more severely than others. The unconscious patient lying on the cold ground or other cold surface is especially prone to rapid heat loss through conduction and will tend to have greater cold-related problems than one who is conscious and able to walk around.

NOTE: *Be aware that hypothermia can develop in temperatures well above freezing.*

GERIATRIC NOTE

Hypothermia is often an especially serious problem for the aged. The effects of cold temperatures on the elderly are more immediate. During the winter months, many older citizens on small fixed incomes live in unheated rooms or rooms that are kept too cool. Failing body systems, chronic illnesses, poor diets, certain medications, and a lack of exercise may combine with the cold environment to bring about hypothermia.

PEDIATRIC NOTE

Since infants and young children are small with large skin surface areas in relation to their total body mass and have little body fat, they are especially prone to hypothermia. Because of their small muscle mass, infants and children do not shiver very much or at all—another reason the very young are susceptible to the cold. You will learn in Chapter 34, "Obstetric and Gynecologic Emergencies," that a crucial part of the care for newborn infants is to dry them (to prevent heat loss from evaporation) and cover their heads (to prevent heat loss by radiation and convection).

CORE CONCEPT ●

Effects on the body of generalized hypothermia; assessment and care for hypothermia

convection
carrying away of heat by currents of air, water, or other gases or liquids.

wind chill
chilling caused by convection of heat from the body in the presence of air currents.

radiation
sending out energy, such as heat, in waves into space.

evaporation
the change from liquid to gas. When the body perspires or gets wet, evaporation of the perspiration or other liquid into the air has a cooling effect on the body.

respiration
breathing. During respiration, body heat is lost as warm air is exhaled from the body.

hypothermia (HI-po-THURM-e-ah)
generalized cooling that reduces body temperature below normal, which is a life-threatening condition in its extreme.

Table 33-1 Stages of Hypothermia

CORE BODY TEMPERATURE		SYMPTOMS
FAHRENHEIT	**CELSIUS**	
99°F–96°F	37.0°C–35.5°C	Shivering.
95°F–91°F	35.5°C–32.7°C	Intense shivering, difficulty speaking.
90°F–86°F	32.0°C–30.0°C	Shivering decreases and is replaced by strong muscular rigidity. Muscle coordination is affected and erratic or jerky movements are produced. Thinking is less clear, general comprehension is dulled, possible total amnesia exists. Patient generally is able to maintain the appearance of psychological contact with surroundings.
85°F–81°F	29.4°C–27.2°C	Patient becomes irrational, loses contact with the environment, and drifts into a stuporous state. Muscular rigidity continues. Pulse and respirations are slow and cardiac dysrhythmias may develop.
80°F–78°F	26.6°C–20.5°C	Patient loses consciousness and does not respond to spoken words. Most reflexes cease to function. Heartbeat slows further before cardiac arrest occurs.

Obvious and Subtle Exposure

At times, it is obvious that a patient has been exposed to cold and is probably suffering from hypothermia. With other patients, however, exposure is subtle—that is, not so obvious, and not the first thing you may think about. Consider, for example, the elderly patient who has fallen during the night and is not discovered until morning. A broken hip or other injuries may claim your attention, but if your patient has been on the cold floor all night, he is probably also suffering from hypothermia. The patient trapped in a wrecked auto is probably suffering a variety of injuries, but if the weather is cool and extrication from the vehicle takes a while, the patient can easily develop hypothermia as well.

Consider the possibility of hypothermia in the following situations when another condition or injury may be more obvious:

- **Ethanol (alcohol) ingestion.** Has the intoxicated patient passed out on a cold floor or been wandering around outdoors in cool or cold weather?
- **Underlying illness.** Does the patient have a circulatory disorder or other condition that makes him especially susceptible to cold?
- **Overdose or poisoning.** Has the patient been lying in a cold garage or on a cold floor? Is he sweating heavily in a cool environment with evaporation causing excessive heat loss?
- **Major trauma.** Has the patient been lying on the ground or trapped in wreckage during cold weather? Is shock (hypoperfusion, or inadequate circulation of the blood) preventing parts of the body from being warmed by circulating blood?
- **Outdoor resuscitation.** Is your patient getting too cold? If your patient is a drowning patient who has been in the water, has exposure to cool water caused hypothermia?
- **Decreased ambient temperature (for example, room temperature).** Is your patient living in a home or apartment that is too cold?

Remember that the injured patient is more susceptible to the effects of cold than a healthy individual. Protect the patient who is entrapped or for any other reason must remain in a cool or cold environment for a period of time. The major course of action is to prevent additional body heat loss. It may be neither practical nor possible to replace wet clothing, but you can at least create a barrier to the cold with blankets, a salvage cover, an aluminized blanket, a survival blanket, or even articles of clothing. A plastic trash bag can serve as protection from wind and water. Keep in mind that the greatest area of heat loss may be the head, so provide some sort of head covering for the patient.

When the patient's injuries allow, place a blanket between his body and the cold ground or between him and the wreckage he is pinned in. Rotate warm blankets from the heated ambulance to the patient. If the patient will remain trapped for a period of time, plug holes in the wreckage with blankets.

PATIENT ASSESSMENT

Hypothermia

Consider the impact of the following factors when assessing a patient: air temperature, wind chill and/or water chill, the patient's age, the patient's clothing, the patient's health including underlying illness and existing injuries, how active the patient was during exposure, and possible alcohol or drug use.

The following list contains common signs and symptoms of hypothermia. Note that decreasing mental status and decreasing motor function both correlate with the degree of hypothermia:

- Shivering in early stages when the core body temperature is above 90°F. In severe cases, shivering decreases or is absent.
- Numbness, or reduced-to-lost sense of touch.
- Stiff or rigid posture in prolonged cases.
- Drowsiness and/or unwillingness or inability to do even the simplest activities. In prolonged exposures, the patient may become irrational, drift into a stuporous state, or actually remove clothing.
- Rapid breathing and rapid pulse in early stages, and slow to absent breathing and pulse in prolonged cases. (The patient's slow pulse and respirations require that you

spend at least 30 to 45 seconds performing a check for a pulse and respirations.) Blood pressure may be low to undetectable.

■ Loss of motor coordination, such as poor balance, staggering, or inability to hold things.

■ Joint/muscle stiffness, or muscular rigidity.

■ Decreased level of consciousness, or unconsciousness. In extreme cases, the patient has a "glassy stare."

■ Cool abdominal skin temperature. (Place your hand inside the clothing with the back of your hand against the patient's abdomen.)

■ Skin may appear red in early stages. In prolonged cases, skin is pale to cyanotic. In most extreme cases, some body parts are stiff and hard (frozen).

During primary assessment, be sure to check an awake patient's orientation to person, place, and time. (Can he tell you his name? Where he is? What day it is?) Perform a secondary assessment to help you estimate the extent of hypothermia. Assume severe hypothermia if shivering is absent.

Decision Point

● Does my patient have an altered mental status?

Passive and Active Rewarming

Passive rewarming allows the body to rewarm itself. It involves simply covering the patient and taking other steps, including removal of wet clothing, to prevent further heat loss. These actions allow the body to naturally regain its warmth. *Active rewarming* includes application of an external heat source to the body. All EMS systems permit passive rewarming. Although some allow the active rewarming of a hypothermic patient who is alert and responding appropriately, many do not. Follow your local protocols.

Active rewarming can prove to be a dangerous process if the patient's condition is more serious than believed. If you are allowed to rewarm a patient with hypothermia who is alert and responding appropriately, do not delay transport. Rewarm the patient while en route. The emergency care steps that follow assume a protocol that permits active rewarming of a patient who is alert and responding appropriately to your intervention. Follow your local protocols.

passive rewarming
covering a hypothermic patient and taking other steps to prevent further heat loss and help the body rewarm itself.

active rewarming
application of an external heat source to rewarm the body of a hypothermic patient.

PATIENT CARE

Hypothermic Patient Who Is Alert and Responding Appropriately

For the hypothermic patient who is alert and responding appropriately, proceed with active rewarming:

1. Remove all of the patient's wet clothing. Keep the patient dry, dress the patient in dry clothing, or wrap the patient in dry, warm blankets. Keep the patient still and handle him very gently. Do not allow the patient to walk or exert himself. Do not massage his extremities.

2. During transport, actively rewarm the patient. Gently apply heat to the patient's body in the form of heat packs, hot water bottles, electric heating pads, warm air, radiated heat, and even your own body heat. Do not warm the patient too quickly. Rapid warming will circulate peripherally stagnated cold blood and rapidly cool the vital central areas of the body, possibly causing cardiac arrest. If transport is delayed, move the patient to a warm environment if at all possible.

3. Provide care for shock. Provide oxygen, warmed and humidified if possible.

4. Give the alert patient warm liquids at a slow rate. When warm fluids are given too quickly, the patient's circulation patterns change. Blood is sent away from the core and instead routed to the skin and extremities. Do not allow the patient to eat or drink stimulants.

5. Except in the mildest of cases (shivering), transport the patient. Continue to provide high-concentration oxygen and monitor vital signs. Never allow a patient to remain in, or return to, a cold environment.

Take the following precautions when actively rewarming a patient:

■ Rewarm the patient slowly. Handle the patient with great care, just as if there were unstabilized cervical-spine injuries.

central rewarming

application of heat to the lateral chest, neck, armpits, and groin of a hypothermic patient.

- Use *central rewarming*. Heat should be applied to the lateral chest, neck, armpits, and groin. You must avoid rewarming the limbs. If they are warmed first, blood will collect in the extremities due to vasodilation (dilation of blood vessels), possibly causing a fatal form of shock (see Chapter 27, "Bleeding and Shock"). If you rewarm the trunk and leave the lower extremities exposed, you can control the rewarming process and help prevent most of the problems associated with the procedure.

- If transport must be delayed, giving the patient a warm bath is very helpful. However, keep the patient alert enough so that he does not drown. Do not warm the patient too quickly.

- Keep the patient at rest. Do not allow the patient to walk. Since the blood is coldest in the extremities, exercise or unnecessary movement could quickly circulate the cold blood and lower the core body temperature.

- Avoid any rough handling of the hypothermic patient. Such activity may set off fatal dysrhythmias, especially ventricular fibrillation.

POINT OF VIEW

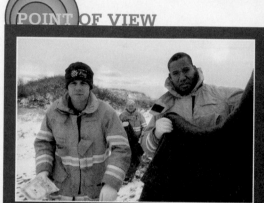

"I was riding my horse on the beach. It is a wonderful feeling. Well, it was until I got thrown. Now, I've been thrown before and you get back up. This time I broke bones.

"To make it worse, it was winter. No one was around.

"I shivered for a while. I yelled and yelled. I tried to move but no luck. Then I stopped shivering and started to get tired. It is funny looking back on that day. I kind of relaxed there at the end. Now I know that means I was on the final glide path. I was heading out.

"Someone finally saw the horse just standing there and came over to figure out why. By that time I was like an ice cube.

"I remember the EMTs coming along and warming me up. Blanket after blanket and the heat in the ambulance was blasting. Those guys must've been boiling. I'm very thankful for them—and for the person that finally called for help. Without them I wouldn't be telling this story."

PATIENT CARE

Hypothermic Patient Who Is Unresponsive or Not Responding Appropriately

A patient who is unresponsive or not responding appropriately has severe hypothermia. For this patient, provide passive rewarming. Do not try to actively rewarm the patient with severe hypothermia. Remove the patient from the environment and protect him from further heat loss. Active rewarming may cause the patient to develop ventricular fibrillation and other complications. Active rewarming can be initiated after arrival at the emergency department in a more monitored setting.

For the patient with severe hypothermia, you should:

1. Ensure an open airway.
2. Provide high-concentration oxygen that has been passed through a warm-water humidifier. If necessary, you can use the oxygen that has been kept warm in the ambulance passenger compartment. If there is no other choice, you can use oxygen from a cold cylinder.
3. Wrap the patient in blankets. If available, use insulating blankets. Handle the patient as gently as possible, as rough handling may cause ventricular fibrillation. Do not allow the patient to eat or drink stimulants. Do not massage his extremities.
4. Transport the patient immediately.

Extreme Hypothermia

In cases of extreme hypothermia, you will find the patient unconscious with no discernible vital signs. The heart rate can slow to less than 10 beats per minute, and the patient will feel very cold to your touch (core body temperature may be below 80°F). Even so, it is possible that a patient in this condition is still alive! Provide emergency care as follows:

- Assess the carotid pulse for 30 to 45 seconds. If there is no pulse, start CPR immediately and prepare to apply the AED.
- If there is a pulse, follow the care steps for a patient who is unresponsive or not responding appropriately as previously listed.

Because the hypothermic patient may not reach biological death for over 30 minutes, the hospital staff will not pronounce a patient dead until after they have rewarmed him and applied resuscitative measures. This means you cannot assume that a severe hypothermia patient is dead on the basis of body temperature and lack of vital signs. As medical personnel point out, "You're not dead until you're warm and dead!"

Localized Cold Injuries

Cold-related emergencies also can result from *local cooling*. Local cooling injuries, those affecting particular (local) parts of the body, are classified as (1) early or superficial and (2) late or deep.

Local cooling most commonly affects the ears, nose, face, hands, and the feet and toes. When a part of the body is exposed to intense cold, blood flow to that part is limited by the constriction of blood vessels. When this happens, tissues freeze. Ice crystals can form in the skin and, in the most severe cases, gangrene (localized tissue death) can set in, which may ultimately lead to the loss of the body part.

As you read the following pages, notice how the signs and symptoms of early or superficial cold injuries are progressive. First, the exposed skin reddens in light-skinned individuals. In dark-skinned individuals, the skin color lightens and approaches a blanched (reduced-color or whitened) condition. As exposure continues, the skin takes on a gray or white blotchy appearance. Exposed skin becomes numb because of reduced circulation. If the freezing process continues, all sensation is lost and the skin becomes dead white.

CORE CONCEPT ●
Effects on the body of local cold injuries; assessment and care for local cold injuries

local cooling
cooling or freezing of particular (local) parts of the body.

PATIENT ASSESSMENT

Early or Superficial Local Cold Injury

Early or superficial local cold injuries (sometimes called frostnip) are brought about by direct contact with a cold object or exposure to cold air. Wind chill and water chill also can be major factors. In this condition, tissue damage is minor and response to care is good. The tip of the nose, tips of the ears, upper cheeks, and fingers (all areas that are usually exposed) are most susceptible to early or superficial local cold injuries. The injury, as its name suggests, is localized with clear demarcation of its limits. Patients are often unaware of the onset of an early local cold injury until someone indicates that there is something unusual about the person's skin color. The following list contains common signs and symptoms:

- The affected area in patients with light skin reddens; in patients with dark skin, it lightens. Both then blanch (whiten). Once blanching begins, the color change can take place very quickly.
- The affected area feels numb to the patient.

PATIENT CARE

Early or Superficial Local Cold Injury

Emergency care for early local cold injury is as follows:

1. Get the patient out of the cold environment.
2. Warm the affected area.
3. If the injury is to an extremity, splint and cover it. Do not rub or massage the area, and do not reexpose it to the cold.

Usually, the patient can apply warmth from his own bare hands, blow warm air on the site, or, if the fingers are involved, hold them in the armpits. During recovery from an early local cold injury, the patient may complain about tingling or burning sensations, which is normal. If the condition does not respond to this simple care, begin to treat for a late or deep local cold injury.

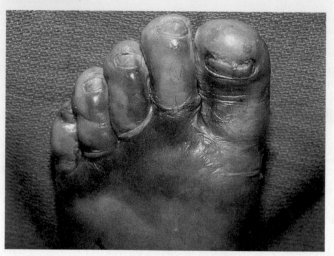

FIGURE 33-2 Local cold injuries. (© *Charles Stewart, MD, and Associates*)

PATIENT ASSESSMENT

Late or Deep Local Cold Injury

Late or deep local cold injury (also known as frostbite) develops if an early or superficial local cold injury goes untreated. In late or deep local cold injury, the skin and subcutaneous layers of the body part are affected. Muscles, bones, deep blood vessels, and organ membranes can become frozen. The following list contains common signs and symptoms of this condition:

- Affected skin appears white and waxy. When the condition progresses to actual freezing, the skin turns mottled or blotchy, and the color turns from white to grayish yellow and finally to grayish blue. Swelling and blistering may also occur (Figure 33-2).

- The affected area feels frozen, but only on the surface. The tissue below the surface is still soft and has its normal resilience, or "bounce." With freezing, the tissues are not resilient and feel frozen to the touch.

  NOTE: *Do not squeeze or poke the tissue. The condition of the deeper tissues can be determined by gently feeling the area. Do the assessment as if the affected area had a fractured bone.*

PATIENT CARE

Late or Deep Local Cold Injury

Initial emergency care for late or deep local cold injury—frostbite and freezing—is as follows:

1. Administer high-concentration oxygen.
2. Transport to a medical facility without delay, protecting the frostbitten or frozen area by covering it and handling it as gently as possible.
3. If transport must be delayed, get the patient indoors and keep him warm. Do not allow the patient to drink alcohol or smoke, because constriction of blood vessels and decreased circulation to the injured tissues may result. Rewarm the frozen part as per local protocol, or request instructions from medical direction.

NOTE: *Never listen to myths and folktales about the care of frostbite. Never rub a frostbitten or frozen area. Never rub snow on a frostbitten or frozen area. There are ice crystals at the capillary level; rubbing the injury site may cause them to seriously damage the already injured tissues. Do not break blisters or massage the injured area. Do not allow the patient to walk on an affected extremity. Do not thaw a frozen limb if there is any chance it will be refrozen.*

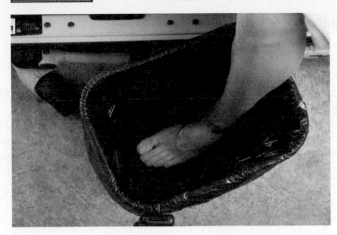

FIGURE 33-3 Rewarming the frozen part.

Active Rapid Rewarming of Frozen Parts

Active rewarming of frozen parts is seldom recommended. The chance of permanently injuring frozen tissues with active rewarming is too great. Consider it only if local protocols recommend it, if you are instructed to do so by medical direction, or if transport will be severely delayed and you cannot reach medical direction for instructions. If you are in a situation where you must attempt rewarming without instructions from a physician, follow the procedure described here.

You will need warm water and a container in which you can immerse the entire site of injury without the limb touching the sides or bottom of the container. If you cannot find a suitable container, fashion one from a plastic bag supported by a cardboard box or wooden crate (Figure 33-3). Proceed as follows:

1. Heat water to between 100°F and 105°F. You should be able to put your finger into the water without experiencing discomfort.

2. Fill the container with the heated water and prepare the injured part by removing clothing, jewelry, bands, or straps. Thawed areas often swell, so you need to remove potentially constricting items beforehand.

3. Fully immerse the injured part. Do not allow the injured area to touch the sides or bottom of the container. Do not place any pressure on the affected part. Continuously stir the water. When the water cools below 100°F, remove the affected part and add more warm water. The patient may complain of moderate pain as the affected area rewarms or he may experience intense pain. Pain is usually a good indicator of successful rewarming.

4. If you complete rewarming of the part (it no longer feels frozen and is turning red or blue), gently dry the affected area and apply a dry sterile dressing. Place dry sterile dressings between the patient's fingers and toes before dressing his hands and feet. Next, cover the site with blankets or whatever is available to keep the area warm. Do not allow these coverings to come in direct contact with the injured area or to put pressure on the site. First try to build some sort of framework on which the coverings can be placed.

5. Keep the patient at rest. Do not allow the patient to walk if a lower extremity has been frostbitten or frozen.

6. Make certain that you keep the entire patient as warm as possible without overheating him. Cover the patient's head with a towel or small blanket to reduce heat loss. Leave the patient's face exposed.

7. Continue to monitor the patient.

8. Assist circulation according to local protocol (some systems recommend rhythmically and carefully raising and lowering the affected limb).

9. Do not allow the limb to refreeze.

10. Transport as soon as possible with the affected limb slightly elevated.

EXPOSURE TO HEAT

Effects of Heat on the Body

CORE CONCEPT

Personal effects on the body of exposure to heat; assessment and care for patients suffering from heat exposure

hyperthermia (HI-per-THURM-e-ah) an increase in body temperature above normal, which is a life-threatening condition in its extreme.

The body generates heat as a result of its constant internal chemical processes. A certain amount of this heat is required to maintain normal body temperature. Any heat that is not needed for temperature maintenance must be lost from the body. If it is not, the result is *hyperthermia*, an abnormally high body temperature. If left unchecked, it will lead to death. Heat and humidity are often associated with hyperthermia.

As you learned earlier, heat is lost through the lungs or the skin. Mechanisms of heat loss include conduction, convection, radiation, evaporation, and respiration. Consider what can happen to the body in a hot environment. Air being inhaled is warm, possibly warmer than the air being exhaled. The skin may absorb more heat than it loses. When high humidity is added, the evaporation of perspiration slows. To make things even more difficult, consider all this in an environment that lacks circulating air or a breeze, which would increase convection and evaporative heat loss.

Since evaporative heat loss is reduced in a humid environment, moist heat can produce dramatic body changes in a short time. Moist heat usually tires people quickly and frequently stops them from harming themselves through overexertion. Dry heat, in contrast, often deceives people. They continue to work or remain exposed to excess heat far beyond what their bodies can tolerate.

The same rules of care apply to heat emergencies as to any other emergency. You will need to perform the appropriate steps of assessment, remaining alert for problems other than those related to heat. Collapse due to heat exhaustion, for example, may result in a fall that can fracture bones. Preexisting conditions such as dehydration, diabetes, fever, fatigue, high blood pressure, heart disease, lung problems, or obesity may hasten or intensify the effects of heat exposure, as will ingestion of alcohol and other drugs.

Age, diseases, and existing injuries all must be considered. The elderly may be affected by poor thermoregulation, prescription medications, and lack of mobility. Newborns and infants also may have poor thermoregulation. Always consider the problem to be greater if the patient is a child or elderly person who is injured or living with a chronic disease.

Patient with Moist, Pale, Normal-to-Cool Skin

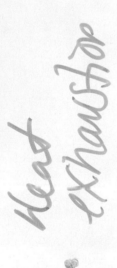

Prolonged exposure to excessive heat can create an emergency in which the patient presents with moist, pale skin that may feel normal or cool to the touch, a condition generally known as *heat exhaustion*. The individual perspires heavily, often drinking large quantities of water. As sweating continues, the body loses salts, bringing on painful muscle cramps (sometimes called *heat cramps*). A person who is actively exercising can lose more than a liter of fluid through perspiration per hour.

Healthy individuals who have been exposed to excessive heat while working or exercising may experience a form of shock brought about by fluid and salt loss. This condition is often seen among firefighters, construction workers, dock workers, and those employed in poorly ventilated warehouses. It is a particular problem during prolonged heat waves early in the summer, before people have become acclimatized to summer heat.

PATIENT ASSESSMENT

Heat Emergency Patient with Moist, Pale, Normal-to-Cool Skin

The following are common signs and symptoms of a heat emergency patient with moist, pale, and normal-to-cool skin:

- Muscular cramps, usually in the legs and abdomen
- Weakness or exhaustion, and sometimes dizziness or periods of faintness
- Rapid, shallow breathing
- Weak pulse

■ Heavy perspiration
■ Loss of consciousness is possible, but is usually brief if it occurs.

Decision Point
● What is the color and condition of my patient's skin?

PATIENT CARE

Heat Emergency Patient with Moist, Pale, Normal-to-Cool Skin

Emergency care of a heat emergency patient with moist, pale, and normal-to-cool skin includes the following steps:

1. Remove the patient from the hot environment and place him in a cool environment (such as in shade or an air-conditioned ambulance).
2. Administer oxygen by nonrebreather mask at 15 liters per minute.
3. Loosen or remove clothing to cool the patient by fanning without chilling him. Watch for shivering.
4. Put the patient in a supine position with legs elevated. Keep him at rest.
5. If the patient is responsive and not nauseated, have him drink small sips of water. If this causes nausea or vomiting, do not give any more water. Be alert for vomiting and airway problems. If the patient is unresponsive or vomiting, do not give water. Transport the patient to the hospital on his left side.
6. If the patient experiences muscular cramps, apply moist towels over cramped muscles.
7. Transport the patient.

Decision Point
● What is the color and condition of my patient's skin?

Patient with Hot Skin, Whether Dry or Moist

When a person's temperature-regulating mechanisms fail and the body cannot rid itself of excessive heat, you will see a patient with hot, dry, or possibly moist skin. When the skin is hot—whether dry or moist—this condition, generally known as *heat stroke,* is a true emergency. The problem is compounded when, in response to loss of fluid and salt, the patient stops sweating, which prevents heat loss through evaporation. Athletes, laborers, and others who exercise or work in hot environments are especially at risk for this condition, as are the elderly who live in poorly ventilated apartments without air conditioning and children left in cars with the windows rolled up.

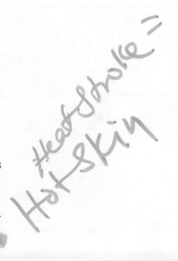

PATIENT ASSESSMENT

Heat Emergency Patient with Hot Skin, Whether Dry or Moist

The following are common signs and symptoms of a heat emergency patient with hot and dry or hot and moist skin:

■ Rapid, shallow breathing
■ Full and rapid pulse
■ Generalized weakness
■ Little or no perspiration
■ Loss of consciousness or altered mental status (Altered mental status is mandatory for a determination of heat stroke.)
■ Dilated pupils
■ Potential seizures; no muscle cramps

Decision Point
● What is the color and condition of my patient's skin?

Heat Emergency Patient with Hot Skin, Whether Dry or Moist

Emergency care of a heat emergency patient with hot and dry or hot and moist skin is as follows (Figure 33-4):

1. Remove the patient from the hot environment and place him in a cool environment (in the ambulance with the air conditioner running on high).
2. Remove the patient's clothing. Apply cool packs to his neck, groin, and armpits. Keep the skin wet by applying water by sponge or wet towels. Aggressively fan the patient.
3. Administer oxygen by nonrebreather mask at 15 liters per minute.
4. Transport immediately. If transport is delayed, continue to attempt to cool the patient with ice packs. Additionally, you can moisten the patient's clothes and fan the body to enhance heat loss by evaporation.

FIGURE 33-4 In heat-emergency cases where the patient's skin is hot (and either dry or moist), aggressively cool.

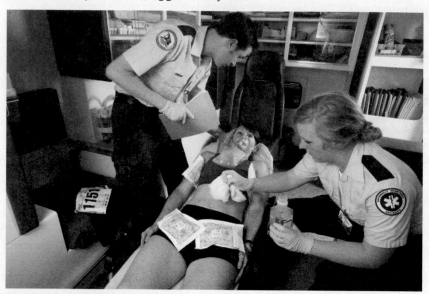

PEDIATRIC NOTE

For infants or young children, cooling is started using tepid (lukewarm) water. This water can then be replaced with cooler water at the recommendation of medical direction.

Beware of what you are told by some patients. They may not believe heat emergencies are serious. Many simply want to return to work. Nevertheless, conduct a thorough primary assessment plus a secondary assessment. If you have any doubts about his condition, tell the patient why he should be transported and seek his permission to do so. You may have to spend a little time with some patients to gain their confidence.

WATER-RELATED EMERGENCIES

Water-Related Accidents

CORE CONCEPT

Signs, symptoms, and treatment for drowning and other water-related injuries

Drowning is the first thing people think of in connection with water-related accidents. However, there are many types of injuries resulting from many types of accidents that can occur on or in the water. Boating, water-skiing, wind surfing, jet-skiing, diving, and scuba-diving accidents can produce fractured bones, bleeding, soft-tissue injuries, and airway obstruction. Even auto collisions can send vehicles or passengers into the water, resulting in any of the

 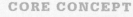

Inside/Outside

Hypothermia and hyperthermia are serious conditions that, when not treated, can lead to death. The following chart explains the pathophysiology behind the main categories of patient presentation.

INSIDE	OUTSIDE
The body undergoes many changes as hypothermia develops. The cardiovascular and central nervous systems are perhaps the most affected by hypothermia. The heart becomes more irritable and prone to dysrhythmias as the body becomes colder. The CNS becomes more sluggish and less responsive.	Hypothermia with normal mental status
At about 91.5°F (33°C) electrical activity in the brain activity becomes abnormal.	Hypothermia with altered mental status
Hyperthermia with cool skin indicates the body is still able to deal with the heat through normal mechanisms (e.g., sweating). Body temperature is a balance of inside and outside temperatures.	Hyperthermia with cool skin
The skin is the major cooling mechanism of the body. When the skin is hot, it indicates that this system is no longer able to dissipate enough heat to maintain a normal body temperature and rapid cooling is necessary. A core temperature that has reached about 105.8°F (41°C) is the critical point.	Hyperthermia with hot skin

injuries usually associated with motor-vehicle collisions as well as the complications caused by the presence of water.

Medical problems such as heart attacks can also cause, or be caused by, water accidents or can simply take place in, on, or near the water. Remember, too, that some water accidents happen far away from pools, lakes, or beaches. For example, bathtub drownings do occur. Adults, as well as children, can drown in only a few inches of water.

> **NOTE:** *Do not attempt a rescue in which you must enter deep water or swim, unless you have been trained to do so and are a very good swimmer. Except for shallow pools and open shallow waters with uniform bottoms, the problems faced in water rescue are too great and too dangerous for the poor swimmer or untrained person. If this bothers you—having to stand by, not being able to help—then take a course in water safety and rescue. (Both the American Red Cross and the YMCA offer water safety and rescue courses.) Otherwise, if you attempt a deep water or swimming rescue, you will probably become a patient yourself.*

PATIENT ASSESSMENT

Water-Related Incidents

Learn to look for the following problems in water-related-incident patients:

- **Airway obstruction.** This may be from water in the lungs, foreign matter in the airway, or swollen airway tissues (which is common if the neck is injured in a dive). Spasms along the airway may be present in some cases of drowning.
- **Cardiac arrest.** This is often related to respiratory arrest or occurs before drowning.
- **Signs of heart attack.** Some untrained rescuers too quickly conclude that chest pains are due to muscle cramps as a result of swimming.
- **Injuries to the head and neck.** These are expected to be found in boating, water-skiing, and diving accidents, but they are also very common in swimming accidents.
- **Internal injuries.** While doing the physical exam, stay on the alert for musculoskeletal injuries, soft-tissue injuries, and internal bleeding.

- **Generalized cooling, or hypothermia.** The water does not have to be very cold and the length of stay in the water does not have to be very long for hypothermia to occur.
- **Substance abuse.** Alcohol and drug use are closely associated with adolescent and adult drownings. Elevated blood alcohol levels have been found in over 30 percent of drowning patients. The screening for drug use has not been as extensive as that done for alcohol, but research indicates that other drugs are a contributory factor in many water-related accidents.
- **Drowning.** The patient may be discovered under or face down in the water. He may be unconscious and without discernible vital signs or may be conscious, breathing, and coughing up water.

Provide assessment and care for any of the previously noted problems as you have learned in other chapters of this text. Drowning is discussed in detail next.

Drowning

drowning

the process of experiencing respiratory impairment from submersion/immersion in liquid, which may result in death, morbidity (illness or other adverse effects), or no morbidity.

In 2002, the World Health Organization (WHO) adopted a definition of *drowning* that is different from the traditional one. According to the WHO, "Drowning is the process of experiencing respiratory impairment from submersion/immersion in liquid. Drowning outcomes are classified as death, morbidity, and no morbidity." Morbidity means the patient experiences illness or other adverse effects, like unconsciousness or pneumonia. The American Heart Association has also adopted this definition of drowning. The WHO definition does not describe near drowning. Hence, the term *near drowning* is no longer used.

The process of drowning often begins as a person struggles to keep afloat in the water. He gulps in large breaths of air as he thrashes about. When he can no longer keep afloat and starts to submerge, he tries to take and hold one more deep breath. As he does, water may enter the airway. There is a series of coughing and swallowing actions, and the patient involuntarily inhales and swallows more water. As water flows past the epiglottis, it triggers a reflex spasm of the larynx. This spasm seals the airway so effectively that no more than a small amount of water reaches the lungs. Unconsciousness soon results from hypoxia (oxygen starvation).

About 10 percent of the people who die from drowning die just from the lack of air. In the remaining patients, the person typically attempts a final respiratory effort and draws water into the lungs, or the spasms subside with the onset of unconsciousness and water freely enters the lungs.

Some patients who drown in cold water can be resuscitated after 30 minutes or more in cardiac arrest. Once the water temperature falls below 70°F, biological death may be delayed. The colder the water, the better the patient's chances for survival, unless generalized hypothermia produces lethal complications.

Rescue Breathing in or out of the Water

Transport for the drowning patient should not be delayed. You may initiate care when the patient is out of the water (already out when you arrive or in the water when you arrive but rescued by others before you initiate care). At other times, you may need to initiate care while the patient is still in the water—especially rescue breathing and immobilization for possible spine injuries. Chest compressions will be effective only after the patient is out of the water.

If needed, rescue breathing should begin without delay. If you can reach the nonbreathing patient in the water, provide ventilations as you support him in a semi-supine position. Continue providing ventilations while the patient is being immobilized and removed from the water. If the patient is already out of the water, begin rescue breathing or CPR on the land.

You may encounter airway resistance as you ventilate the drowning patient. However, you will probably have to ventilate more forcefully than you would other patients. Remember, you must provide air to the patient's lungs as soon as possible.

A patient with water in the lungs usually has water in the stomach, which will add resistance to your efforts to provide rescue breathing or CPR ventilations. Since the patient may have spasms along the airway, or swollen tissues in the larynx or trachea, you may find that some of the air you provide will go into the patient's stomach. Remember, the same problem will occur if you do not properly open the airway or if your ventilations are too forceful.

If gastric distention interferes with artificial ventilation, place the patient on his left side. With suction immediately available, the EMT should place his hand over the epigastric area of the abdomen and apply firm pressure to relieve the distention. This procedure should be done only if the gastric distention interferes with the EMT's efforts to artificially ventilate the patient in an effective manner.

Care for Possible Spinal Injuries in the Water

Injuries to the cervical spine are seen with many water-related accidents. Most often, these injuries are received during a dive or when the patient is struck by a boat, skier or ski, or surfer or surfboard. Even though cervical-spine injuries are the most common of the spine injuries seen in water-related accidents, there can be injury anywhere along the spine.

In water-related accidents, assume that the unconscious patient has neck and spinal injuries. If the patient has head injuries, also assume that there are neck and spinal injuries. Keep in mind that a patient found in respiratory or cardiac arrest will need resuscitation started before you can immobilize the neck and spine. Also, realize that you may not be able to carry out a complete assessment for spinal injuries while the patient is in the water. Take care to avoid aggravating spinal injuries, but do not delay basic life support. Do not delay removing the patient from the water if the scene presents an immediate danger. When possible, keep the patient's neck rigid and in a straight line with the body's midline (Scan 33-1). Use the jaw-thrust maneuver to open the airway.

If the patient with possible spinal injuries is still in the water, you are a good swimmer with proper training, and you are able to aid in the rescue, secure the patient to a long spine board before removing him from the water. This will help prevent permanent neurological damage or paralysis. This type of rescue requires special training in the use of the spine board while in the water. This rigid device can "pop up" very easily from below the water surface. Make certain that you know how to control the board and how to work in the water.

PATIENT CARE

Water-Related Incidents

In all cases of water-related incidents, assume that the unconscious patient has neck and spinal injuries. If the patient is rescued by others while you wait on shore, or if the patient is out of the water when you arrive, you should:

1. Do a primary assessment, protecting the spine as much as possible.
2. Provide rescue breathing. If there is no pulse, begin CPR and prepare to apply the AED. Protect yourself by using a pocket face mask with a one-way valve or bag-valve-mask unit.
3. Look for and control profuse bleeding. Since the patient's heart rate may have slowed down, take a pulse for 60 seconds in all cold-water rescue situations before concluding that the patient is in cardiac arrest.
4. Provide care for shock (as described in Chapter 27, "Bleeding and Shock"), administer high-concentration oxygen, and transport the patient as soon as possible.
5. Continue resuscitative measures throughout transport. Initial and periodic suctioning may be needed.

The drowning patient receiving rescue breathing or CPR should be transported as soon as possible. If resuscitation and immediate transport are not required, cover the patient to conserve his body heat and complete a secondary assessment. Uncover only those areas of the patient's body involved with the stage of the assessment. Care for any problems or injuries detected during the assessment in the order of their priority.

If spinal injury is not suspected, place the patient on his left side to allow water, vomit, and other secretions to drain from the upper airway. Suction as needed. When transport is delayed and you believe that the patient can be moved to a warmer place, do so without aggravating any existing injuries. Do not allow the drowning patient to walk. Transport the patient. A significant number of patients who appear normal after a drowning episode have delayed effects, so persuade the patient to accept transport to a hospital.

Information supplied to the dispatcher or to the hospital from the scene and during transport is critical in cases of drowning. The hospital emergency department staff needs to

HEAD-CHIN SUPPORT

Two Rescuers in Shallow Water

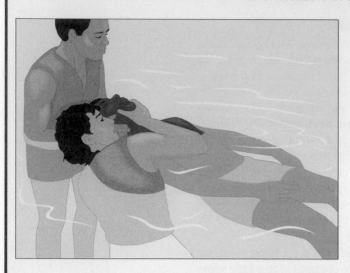

When there are two rescuers present, perform the head-chin support technique to provide in-line stabilization of a patient in shallow water.

HEAD-SPLINT SUPPORT

One Rescuer in Shallow Water

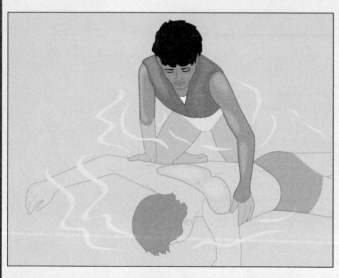

1 When you find a patient face down in shallow water, position yourself alongside the patient.

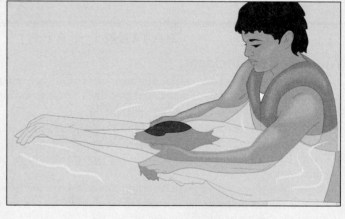

2 Extend the patient's arms straight up alongside his head to create a splint.

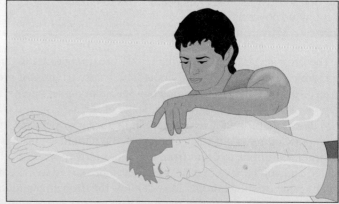

3 Begin to rotate the torso toward you.

NOTE: *Unless you are a very good swimmer and trained in water rescue, do not go into the water to save someone.*

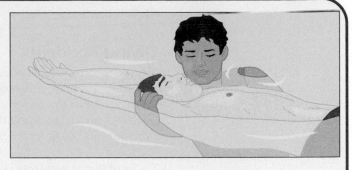

④ As you rotate the patient, lower yourself into the water.

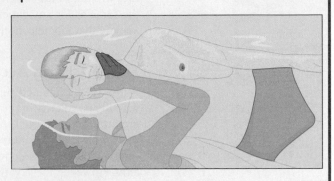

⑤ Maintain manual stabilization by holding the patient's head between his arms.

HEAD-CHIN SUPPORT

One Rescuer in Deep Water

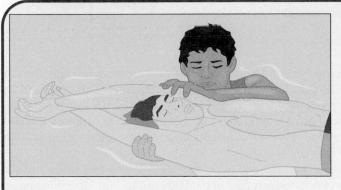

① When you find a patient face down in deep water, position yourself beside him. Support his head with one hand and the mandible with the other.

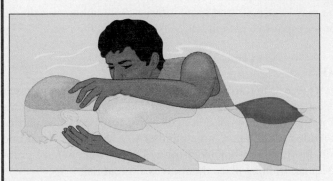

② Rotate the patient by ducking under him.

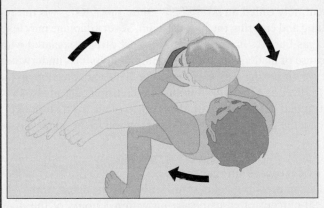

③ Continue to rotate until the patient is face up.

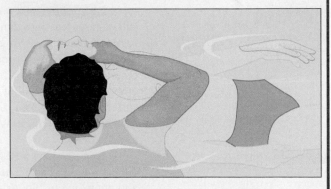

④ Maintain in-line stabilization until a backboard is used to immobilize the patient's spine.

know if this is a fresh- or saltwater drowning, if it took place in cold or warm water, and if it is related to a diving accident. You may be asked to transport the patient to a special facility or to a center having a hyperbaric chamber when decompression therapy is needed.

Diving Accidents

Water-related accidents often involve injuries that occur when individuals attempt dives or enter the water from diving boards. In the majority of these accidents, the patient is a teenager. Basically, the same types of injuries are seen in dives taken from diving boards, poolsides, docks, boats, and the shore. The injury may be due to the diver striking the board or some object on or under the water. From great heights, injury may result from impact with the water.

Most diving accidents involve the head and neck, but you will also find injuries to the spine, hands, feet, and ribs in many cases. Any part of the body can be injured depending on the position that the diver is in when he strikes the water or an object. This means that you must perform a primary assessment. You must also perform a secondary assessment on all diving accident patients. Do not overlook the fact that a medical emergency may have led to the diving accident.

Emergency care for diving accident patients is the same as for any accident patient if they are out of the water. Care provided in the water and during removal from the water is the same as for any patient who may have neck and spine injuries. Remember, you should assume that any unconscious or unresponsive patient has neck and spinal injuries.

Scuba-Diving Accidents

Scuba (self-contained underwater breathing apparatus)-diving accidents have increased with the popularity of the sport, especially since many untrained and inexperienced persons are attempting dives. Today, more than 2 million people scuba dive for sport or as part of their industrial or military job. Added to this are a large number who decide to "try it one time," without the benefits of lessons or supervision. Well-trained divers seldom have problems. However, those with inadequate training place themselves at great risk.

Scuba-diving accidents include all types of body injuries and drownings. In many cases, the scuba-diving accident was brought about by medical problems that existed prior to the dive. There are two special problems seen in scuba-diving accidents: air emboli in the diver's blood and decompression sickness.

An *air embolism*—more accurately called an *arterial gas embolism (AGE)*—is the result of gases leaving a damaged lung and entering the bloodstream. Severe damage may lead to a collapsed lung. Air emboli (gas bubbles in the blood) are most often associated with divers who hold their breath because of inadequate training, equipment failure, underwater emergency, or attempts to conserve air during a dive. However, a diver may develop an air embolism in very shallow water (as little as 4 feet). An automobile-collision patient also may suffer an air embolism if, when trapped below water, he takes gulps of air from air pockets held inside the vehicle. When freed, the patient may develop air emboli in the same way as a scuba diver.

Decompression sickness is usually caused when a diver comes up too quickly from a deep, prolonged dive. The quick ascent causes nitrogen gas to be trapped in the body tissues and then in the bloodstream. Decompression sickness in scuba divers takes from 1 to 48 hours to appear, with about 90 percent of cases occurring within 3 hours of the dive. Divers increase the risk of decompression sickness if they fly within 12 hours of a dive. Because of this delay, carefully consider all information gathered from the patient interview and reports from the patient's family and friends. This information may provide the only clues relating the patient's problems to a scuba dive.

The following are common signs and symptoms of scuba-diving problems:

Air Embolism (Rapid Onset of Signs and Symptoms)

- Blurred vision
- Chest pains
- Numbness and tingling sensations in the extremities

air embolism
gas bubble in the bloodstream. The plural is air emboli. The more accurate term is *arterial gas embolism (AGE)*.

decompression sickness
a condition resulting from nitrogen trapped in the body's tissues, caused by coming up too quickly from a deep, prolonged dive. A symptom of decompression sickness is "the bends," or deep pain in the muscles and joints.

- Generalized or specific weakness, possible paralysis
- Frothy blood in the mouth or nose
- Convulsions
- Rapid lapse into unconsciousness
- Respiratory arrest and cardiac arrest

Decompression Sickness

- Personality changes
- Fatigue
- Deep pain to the muscles and joints (the "bends")
- Itchy blotches or mottling of the skin
- Numbness or paralysis
- Choking
- Coughing
- Labored breathing
- Behavior similar to intoxication (such as staggering)
- Chest pains
- Collapse leading to unconsciousness

For a patient with signs and symptoms of either air embolism or decompression sickness, follow the same emergency care steps:

1. Maintain an open airway.
2. Administer the highest possible concentration of oxygen by nonrebreather mask.
3. Rapidly transport all patients with possible air emboli or decompression sickness.
4. Contact medical direction for specific instructions concerning where to take the patient. You may be sent directly to a hyperbaric trauma care center.
5. Keep the patient warm.
6. Position the patient either supine or on either side (Figure 33-5). Continue to monitor the patient. You may have to reposition the patient to ensure an open airway.

The Diver Alert Network (DAN) was formed to assist rescuers with the care of underwater diving accident patients. The staff, which is available on a 24-hour basis, can be reached by phoning (919) 684-8111. Collect calls will be accepted for actual emergencies. DAN can give you or your dispatcher information on assessment and care and how to transfer the patient to a hyperbaric trauma care center. (A hyperbaric trauma care center is one that has a special pressure chamber for treatment of such conditions.) For nonemergencies, call (919) 684-2948.

FIGURE 33-5 Proper positioning of a scuba-diving accident patient.

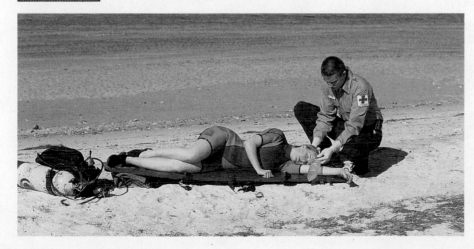

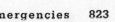

NOTE: *The well-trained scuba diver makes use of a preplanned dive chart. The dive chart, if it is available, may provide you with useful information concerning the nature and duration of the dive. This chart must be transported with the patient.*

Water Rescues

The following is the order of procedures for a water rescue (Figure 33-6), most of which can be performed short of going into the water: reach, throw and tow, row, and go.

- **Reach.** When the patient is responsive and close to shore or poolside, try to reach him by holding out an object for him to grab. Then pull him from the water. Make sure your position is secure. Line (rope) is considered the best choice. If no line is available, use a branch, fishing rod, oar, stick, or other such object—even a towel, blanket, or article of clothing. If no object is available or you have only one opportunity to grab the person (e.g., in strong currents), position yourself flat on your stomach and extend your hand or leg to the patient. (This is not recommended for the nonswimmer.) Again, make certain that you are working from a secure position.

- **Throw and tow.** If the person is conscious and alert but too far away for you to reach and pull from the water, throw an object that will float (Figure 33-7). A personal flotation device (PFD or lifejacket) or ring buoy (life preserver) works best. Other buoyant objects include foam cushions, logs, plastic picnic containers, surfboards, flatboards, large beach balls, and plastic toys. Two empty, capped, plastic milk jugs can keep an adult afloat for hours. Inflatable splints can be used if there is nothing at the scene that will float.

FIGURE 33-6 First try to reach and pull the patient from the water. If that fails, throw him anything that will float and tow him from the water. If that fails, row to the patient.

FIGURE 33-7 Throw the patient any object that will float.

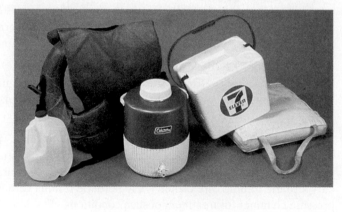

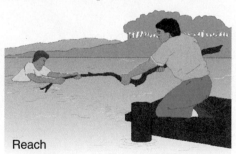

Reach

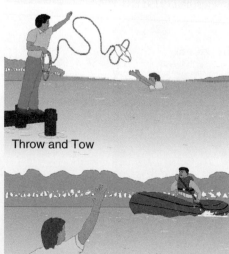

Throw and Tow

Row

Once the conscious patient has a flotation device, try to find a way to tow him to shore. From a safe position, throw the patient a line or another flotation device attached to a line. If you are a good swimmer and you know how to judge the water, wade out no deeper than waist high, wear a personal flotation device, and have a safety line that is secured on shore.

- **Row.** When the patient is too far from shore to allow for throwing and towing, or is unresponsive, you may be able to row a boat to the patient. However, do not attempt to row to the patient if you cannot swim. Even if you are a good swimmer, wearing a personal flotation device is required while you are in the boat.

  If the patient is conscious, tell him to grab an oar or the stern (rear end) of the boat. You must exercise great care when helping the patient into the boat. This is even trickier when you are in a canoe. If the canoe tips over, stay with it and hold onto its bottom and side. Most canoes will stay afloat.

- **Go.** As a last resort, when all other means have failed, you can go into the water and swim to the patient. However, you must be a good swimmer, trained in water rescue and lifesaving. Untrained rescuers can become patients themselves.

Decision Point

- What is the safest way to rescue the patient — considering safety for both the EMT and the patient.

Ice Rescues

Every winter people fall through ice while skating or attempting to cross an ice-covered body of water. Often, the scene becomes a multiple-rescue problem as other individuals fall through the ice while trying to reach the patient. The number-one rule in ice rescue is to protect yourself. Formal ice rescue training is available. In addition, you should wear a cold-water submersion suit and personal flotation device during any ice rescue attempt (Figure 33-8).

FIGURE 33-8 Safe ice rescues require proper equipment.

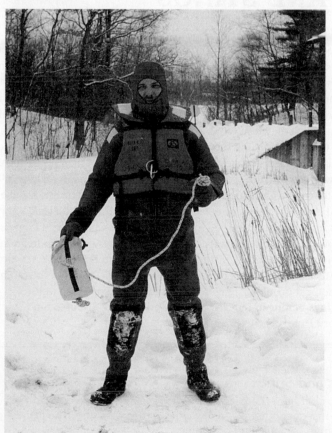

There are several ways in which you can reach a patient who has fallen through ice:

- You can throw a flotation device to the patient.
- You can toss a rope in which a loop has been formed to the patient. The patient can put the loop around his body so that he can be pulled onto the ice and away from the danger area.
- You can use a small, flat-bottomed aluminum boat for an ice rescue. It can be pushed stern (rear end) first by other rescuers and pulled to safety by a rope secured to the bow (front end). The primary rescuer will remain dry and safe if the ice breaks. The patient can be pulled from the water or allowed to grasp the side of the boat, although he may be unable to grasp or to hold on for long.
- A ladder is an effective tool often used in ice rescue. It can be laid flat and pushed to the patient, then pulled back by an attached rope. The ladder also can serve as a surface on which a rescuer can spread out his weight if he must go onto the ice to reach the patient. The ladder should have a line that can be secured by a rescuer in a safe position. Any rescuer on the ladder should have a safety line.

Remember that the patient may not be able to do much to help in the rescue process. In just a matter of minutes, hypothermia may interfere with his mental and physical capabilities.

Whenever possible, do not work alone when trying to perform an ice rescue. If you must work alone, do not walk out onto the ice. Never go onto ice that is rapidly breaking. Never enter the water through a hole in the ice in order to find the patient. Your best course of action will be to work with others, from a safe ice surface or the shore. When there is no other choice, you and your fellow rescuers can elect to form a human chain to reach the patient. However, this is not the safest method to employ, even when all the rescuers are wearing personal flotation devices and using safety lines.

Expect to find injuries to most patients who have fallen through the ice. Treat for hypothermia according to local protocols and treat for any injuries. Transport all patients who have fallen through ice.

BITES AND STINGS

Insect Bites and Stings

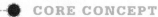

CORE CONCEPT

Signs, symptoms, and treatment for bites and stings

toxins
substances produced by animals or plants that are poisonous to humans.

venom
a toxin (poison) produced by certain animals such as snakes, spiders, and some marine life forms.

Insect stings, spider bites, and scorpion stings are typical sources of injected poisons, or *toxins*—substances produced by animals or plants that are poisonous to humans. (*Venom* is a term for a toxin produced by some animals such as snakes, spiders, and certain marine life forms.) Commonly seen insect stings are those of wasps, hornets, bees, and ants. Insect stings and bites are rarely dangerous. However, 5 percent of the U.S. population will have an allergic reaction to them, which may result in shock. Those who are hypersensitive develop severe anaphylactic shock that is quickly life threatening (see Chapter 22, "Allergic Reaction").

Although all spiders are poisonous, most species cannot get their fangs through human skin. The black widow spider and the brown recluse, or fiddleback, spider (Figure 33-9), are two that can, and their bites can produce medical emergencies. Almost all brown recluse spider bites are painless, and patients seldom recall being bitten. The characteristic lesion appears in only 10 percent of cases, and then only after up to 12 hours (Figure 33-10). EMTs are seldom called to respond to a brown recluse bite. However, black widow bites cause a more immediate reaction.

Scorpion stings are common in the Southwest United States. They do not ordinarily cause deaths, but one rare species (*centruroides exilcauda*) is dangerous to humans and can cause serious medical problems in children, including respiratory failure.

Bites and stings belong in the class of injected poisons discussed in Chapter 23, "Poisoning and Overdose Emergencies."

PATIENT ASSESSMENT

Insect Bites and Stings

Gather information from the patient, bystanders, and the scene. Find out whatever you can about the insect or other possible source of the poisoning. The following are common signs and symptoms of injected poisoning:

- Altered states of awareness
- Noticeable stings or bites on the skin
- Puncture marks (especially note the fingers, forearms, toes, and legs)
- Blotchy skin (mottled skin)
- Localized pain or itching
- Numbness in a limb or body part
- Burning sensations at the site followed by pain spreading throughout the limb
- Redness
- Swelling or blistering at the site
- Weakness or collapse
- Difficult breathing and abnormal pulse rate
- Headache and dizziness
- Chills
- Fever

FIGURE 33-9 (A) Black widow spider. (B) Brown recluse spider. *(Photo A: © Joseph T. Collins/Photo Researchers, Inc.; Photo B: © Breck P. Kent)*

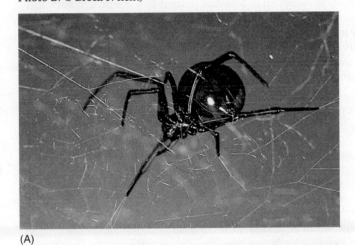

(A)

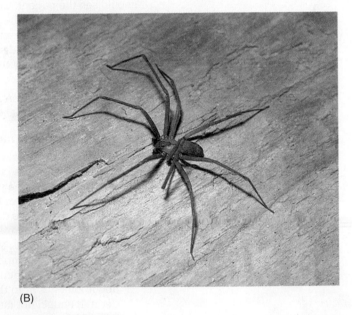

(B)

FIGURE 33-10 Brown recluse spider bite.

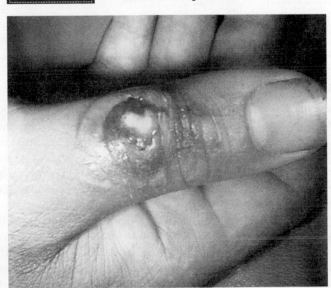

- Nausea and vomiting
- Muscle cramps, chest tightening, joint pains
- Excessive saliva formation, profuse sweating
- Anaphylaxis

NOTE: *Look for medical identification devices that identify persons sensitive to certain stings or bites. Some patients sensitive to stings or bites carry medication to help prevent anaphylactic shock. This situation is described in Chapter 22, "Allergic Reaction."*

PATIENT CARE

Insect Bites and Stings

As an EMT, you are not expected to be able to identify insects and spiders. Proper identification of these organisms is best left to experts. If the patient's problem was caused by a creature that is known locally and is not normally dangerous (such as a bee, wasp, or puss caterpillar), your major concern regarding the patient will be anaphylactic shock. If anaphylactic shock does not develop, care is usually simple.

If the cause of the bite or sting is unknown, or the organism is unknown, a physician should see the patient. Call medical direction or take the patient to a medical facility and let experts decide on the proper treatment for the patient. If possible, transport the stinging object or organism in a sealed container, taking care not to handle it without proper protection, even if it is dead. If you can accomplish this safely, you may save precious minutes needed to identify the toxin.

To provide emergency care for injected toxins:

1. Treat for shock, even if the patient does not present any of the signs of shock.
2. Call medical direction. Skip this only if the organism is known and your EMS system has a specific protocol for care.
3. To remove the stinger or venom sac, the traditional advice was to scrape the site with a blade or a card and to avoid pulling with tweezers (it was thought using tweezers might squeeze more venom into the wound). However, recent research indicates that how you remove the stinger or venom sac is far less important than doing so quickly.
4. Remove jewelry from the patient's affected limb in case the limb swells, which would make removal more difficult later.
5. If local protocol permits and if the wound is on an extremity (not a joint), place constricting bands above and below the sting or bite site. This is done to slow the spread of venom in the lymphatic vessels and superficial veins. The band should be made of 3/4-inch- to 1 1/2-inch-wide soft rubber or other wide soft material. It should be placed about 2 inches from the wound. The band must be loose enough to slide a finger under it. It should not cut off circulation.
6. Keep the limb immobilized and the patient still to prevent distribution of the poison to other parts of the body.

NOTE: *Some EMS systems recommend placing a cold compress on the wound. However, most EMS systems do not use cold for any injected toxin. Follow your local protocols.*

Snakebites

Snakebites require special care but are usually not life threatening. Nearly 50,000 people in the United States are bitten by snakes each year. Although over 8,000 of these cases involve poisonous snakes, on the average fewer than 10 deaths each year are reported from snakebites. (In the United States, more people die each year from bee and wasp stings than from snakebites.) The signs and symptoms of snakebite poisoning may take several hours to appear. If death does result, it is usually not a rapidly occurring event unless anaphylactic shock develops. Most patients who die survive at least 1 to 2 days.

In the United States, there are two types of native poisonous snakes—pit vipers (including rattlesnakes, copperheads, and water moccasins) and coral snakes (Figure 33-11). Up to 25 percent of pit viper bites and 50 percent of coral bites are "dry bites" without venom injection. However, the venomous bite from a diamondback rattler or coral snake is considered very serious. Since each person reacts differently to a snakebite, you should consider

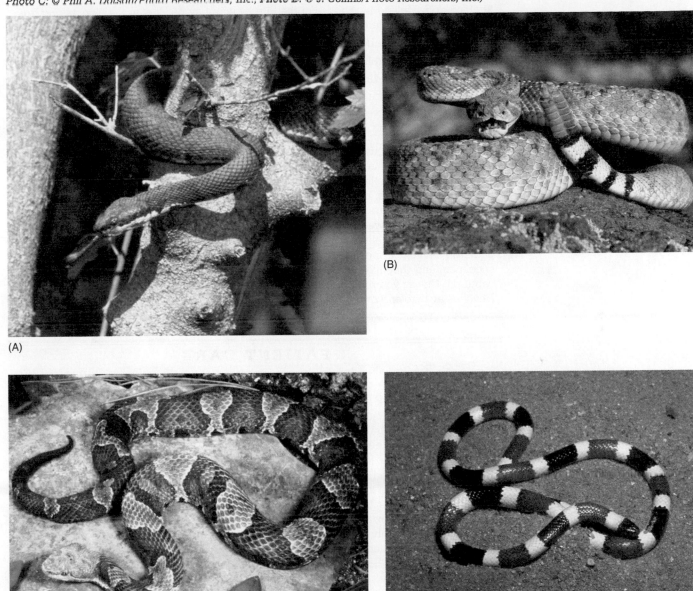

(A)

(B)

(C)

(D)

the bite from any known poisonous snake or any unidentified snake to be a serious emergency. Staying calm and keeping the patient calm and at rest is critical. Since reaction time is slow, there is time to transport the patient without haste.

> **NOTE:** *Native snakes are not the only kind of poisonous animals you may encounter. A number of people have decided to keep poisonous reptiles even though it is illegal to do so in most areas. So, even if you live in an area where there are no poisonous snakes, you may encounter a patient who has sustained a bite from one.*

PATIENT ASSESSMENT

Snakebite

Unless you are dealing with a known species of snake that is not considered poisonous, consider all snakebites to be from poisonous snakes. The patient or bystanders may say that the snake was not poisonous, but they could be mistaken. The signs and symptoms of snakebite may include the following:

- Noticeable bite on the skin, which may appear as nothing more than a discoloration
- Pain and swelling in the area of the bite, which may be slow to develop, taking from 30 minutes to several hours
- Rapid pulse and labored breathing
- Progressive general weakness
- Vision problems (dim or blurred)
- Nausea and vomiting
- Seizures
- Drowsiness or unconsciousness

If the dead or captured snake is at the scene, your role as an EMT is not to identify the snake but to place it in a sealed container and transport it along with the patient. Arrange for separate transport of a live specimen. Do not transport a live snake in the ambulance.

If you see the live, uncaptured snake, take great care or you may be its next victim. When possible, note its size and coloration. Getting close enough to look for details of the eyes or for a pit between the eye and mouth is foolish. The way you classify a snake, whether it is dead or alive, will probably have little to do with your subsequent care of the patient. The medical facility staff will arrange to have an expert classify a captured or dead specimen, and they have protocols to determine patient care if the snake has not been captured. Unless you are an expert in capturing snakes, do not try to catch the snake. *Never delay care and transport in order to capture the snake.*

PATIENT CARE

Snakebite

Emergency care of a patient with snakebite includes:

1. Call medical direction to determine the best receiving facility where antivenom will be most readily available to treat the patient. Rapid transport and the administration of antivenom are the most effective interventions for the treatment of life-threatening snakebite injuries.
2. Treat for shock and conserve body heat. Keep the patient calm.
3. Locate the fang marks. There may be only one fang mark.
4. Remove any rings, bracelets, or other constricting items on the bitten extremity.
5. Keep any bitten extremities immobilized—the application of a splint will help. Do not elevate the limb above the level of the heart.
6. Transport the patient, carefully monitoring vital signs.

NOTE: *Do not place an ice bag or cold pack on the bite unless you are directed to do so by a physician or local protocol. Do not cut into the bite and suction or squeeze the bite site. Never suck the venom from the wound using your mouth. Instead, use a suction cup. However, suctioning is seldom done.*

Research indicates that the use of a *pressure immobilization bandage* may be the most effective technique to slow the spread of venom after a snakebite. This technique involves immediately wrapping the bitten extremity with an elastic (ACE®-type) bandage and then immobilizing the wrapped extremity with a rigid splint or a sling on the upper extremity. The wrap should be only as snug as if you were wrapping a sprained ankle.

The purpose of the pressure immobilization bandage is to restrict the flow of lymph, not of blood. The wrap should be snug but not tight enough to cut off circulation. Monitor for a pulse at the wrist or ankle. Check to be certain that tissue swelling does not cause the constricting bands to become too tight.

Poisoning from Marine Life

Poisoning from marine life forms can occur in a variety of ways—from eating improperly prepared seafood or poisonous organisms to receiving stings and punctures from aquatic life forms. Patients who have ingested spoiled, contaminated, or infested seafood may develop a condition that resembles anaphylactic shock. Therefore, they should receive the same care as any patient in anaphylactic shock. During care, you must be prepared in case the patient vomits. Most patients will show the signs of food poisoning. The care for seafood poisoning is the same as for all other food poisonings.

It is extremely rare for someone in the United States to eat a poisonous variety of marine life, since creatures such as puffer fish and paralytic shellfish are not readily available. For all cases of suspected poisoning due to ingestion, call your on-line medical direction or the poison control center as local protocol directs you. Be prepared for the patient to display vomiting, convulsions, and respiratory arrest.

Venomous marine life forms producing sting injuries include the jellyfish, the sea nettle, the Portuguese man-of-war, coral, the sea anemone, and the hydra. For most victims, the sting produces pain with few complications. Some patients may show allergic reactions and possibly develop anaphylactic shock. These cases require the same care as rendered for any case of anaphylactic shock. Stings to the face, especially those near or on the lip or eye, require a physician's attention. Rinsing the affected area with vinegar will reduce the pain of the sting. However, be careful not to let vinegar get into the patient's mouth or eyes. Once the site has been rinsed with vinegar to inactivate the venom, immersion of the site in hot but non-scalding water (maximum temperature 45°C or 113°F) may further reduce the pain.

Puncture wounds can occur when someone steps on or grabs a stingray, sea urchin, spiny catfish, or other form of spiny marine animal. Although it is true that soaking the wound in non-scalding hot water for 30 to 90 minutes will break down the venom, you should not delay transport. Puncture wounds must be treated by a physician and the patient may need a tetanus inoculation. Remember, the patient could react to the venom by developing anaphylactic shock.

CRITICAL DECISION MAKING

Safety First

Environmental emergencies provide a variety of situations in which an EMT must act. Some patients need to be cooled, others warmed. However, before you even get to treat the patient you must make some safety decisions. Consider the following situations and identify the safety hazards.

1. You are taking a walk while on vacation. You hear a sound from the water and see that several hundred feet out in the water a person is struggling to stay afloat.

2. You are ice skating with the family and hear screaming. Someone has fallen through the ice. A group of people have gathered around the hole, peering downward.

3. You are on a hiking path and hear screaming. A hiker has been bitten by a snake. He is in pain and holding his leg. He is sitting by an outcropping of rocks.

CHAPTER REVIEW

Key Facts and Concepts

- Patients suffering from exposure to heat or cold must be removed from the harmful environment as quickly and as safely as possible.

- Generalized cold injuries involve cooling of the entire body, also referred to as hypothermia. Treatment decisions are based on whether that patient has a normal or altered mental status.

- Patients who have hypothermia with an altered mental status are considered to have severe hypothermia.

- Local cold injury involves an isolated part or parts of the body. It has also been referred to as frostbite. Early local injury sites may be rewarmed gently. Late local injury involves freezing of tissue. You should transport rather than rewarm the patient unless transport is significantly delayed or you are advised by medical direction.

- Hyperthermia is a heat emergency. Its severity is determined by skin temperature. Skin that is normal to cool is considered less severe than skin that is hot to the touch. All heat emergency patients should be removed from the heat and cooled. Altered mental status in the setting of hyperthermia indicates a life-threatening emergency.

- Follow local protocols in reference to rewarming or cooling procedures.
- Immediate resuscitation of the water-related emergency patient may require quick and persistent intervention. Always assure your own safety before attempting any sort of rescue.
- For injection or ingestion of the poisons of insects, spiders, snakes, and marine life, call medical direction and follow your local protocols.

Key Decisions

- Is the scene safe from heat, cold, and venomous creatures?
- How can I safely get the patient from the water?

- Hypothermia: Does the patient have an altered mental status?
- Hyperthermia: Is the patient's skin temperature cool to normal or hot?

Chapter Glossary

active rewarming application of an external heat source to rewarm the body of a hypothermic patient.

air embolism gas bubble in the bloodstream. The plural is air emboli. The more accurate term is *arterial gas embolism (AGE)*.

central rewarming application of heat to the lateral chest, neck, armpits, and groin of a hypothermic patient.

conduction the transfer of heat from one material to another through direct contact.

convection carrying away of heat by currents of air, water, or other gases or liquids.

decompression sickness a condition resulting from nitrogen trapped in the body's tissues, caused by coming up too quickly from a deep, prolonged dive. A symptom of decompression sickness is "the bends," or deep pain in the muscles and joints.

drowning the process of experiencing respiratory impairment from submersion/immersion in liquid, which may result in death, morbidity (illness or other adverse effects), or no morbidity.

evaporation the change from liquid to gas. When the body perspires or gets wet, evaporation of the perspiration or other liquid into the air has a cooling effect on the body.

hyperthermia (HI-per-THURM-e-ah) an increase in body temperature above normal, which is a life-threatening condition in its extreme.

hypothermia (HI-po-THURM-e-ah) generalized cooling that reduces body temperature below normal, which is a life-threatening condition in its extreme.

local cooling cooling or freezing of particular (local) parts of the body.

passive rewarming covering a hypothermic patient and taking other steps to prevent further heat loss and help the body rewarm itself.

radiation sending out energy, such as heat, in waves into space.

respiration breathing. During respiration, body heat is lost as warm air is exhaled from the body.

toxins substances produced by animals or plants that are poisonous to humans.

venom a toxin (poison) produced by certain animals such as snakes, spiders, and some marine life forms.

water chill chilling caused by conduction of heat from the body when the body or clothing is wet.

wind chill chilling caused by convection of heat from the body in the presence of air currents.

Preparation for Your Examination and Practice

Short Answer

1. When is it appropriate to treat a cold emergency with active rewarming and when should you perform passive rewarming?

2. List five situations in which a patient may be suffering from hypothermia along with another, more obvious medical condition or injury.

3. Name the signs and symptoms of a late or deep localized cold injury.

4. Describe the management of a patient suffering from heat emergency who has moist, pale, and cool skin.

5. Describe the management of a patient suffering from a heat emergency who has hot, dry skin.

6. Describe the proper care for a patient suffering from snakebite.

Thinking and Linking

Think back to Chapter 1, "Introduction to Emergency Medical Services and the Health Care System," Chapter 2, "The Well-Being of the EMT," and Chapter 17, "Communication and Documentation." Link information from those chapters to information from this chapter as you consider the following situation:

- You respond to a snakebite. There, you find a patient and witnesses who describe a snake to you in great detail. Where would you find information on what type of snake this was, if it was poisonous, and how to treat the patient? What would you do if the snake was still present?

Think back to Chapter 1, "Introduction to Emergency Medical Services and the Health Care System," Chapter 2, "The Well-Being of the EMT," and Chapter 3, "Lifting and Moving Patients." Link information from those chapters to information from this chapter as you consider the following situation:

- You have a patient who is experiencing hypothermia, is half a mile into the woods, and is not accessible by ambulance. Do you have clothing available that would protect you and your crew/team from hypothermia during the trip in and out? If you will be an EMT in a warm climate, change the situation. It is hot and humid. A hiker has experienced a heat emergency. Can you and your crew/team get the patient out without experiencing a heat emergency yourselves? In either case, what transport device(s) and resources would you use to remove the patient from the woods?

Critical Thinking Exercises

Some environmental emergencies are dangerous for both the patient and the EMT. The purpose of this exercise will be to consider options for patient care in several such circumstances.

1. Your hypothermia patient has an altered mental status. How does this affect your care for the patient? What if you were several hours by snowmobile from the nearest road?

2. What is the underlying pathophysiology that makes hot skin more serious than having cool skin in a heat emergency? What are the implications of hot skin for the care you provide?

3. You are with your family at a local lake. You observe a boat capsize near the middle of the lake and can hear screams from the scene. You are a marginal swimmer. Several civilians begin swimming out to the site. Apply the concepts learned in scene size-up to this scene.

Pathophysiology to Practice

The following questions are designed to assist you in gathering relevant clinical information and making accurate decisions in the field.

1. Why is an altered mental status a major factor in determining whether to actively or passively rewarm a hypothermia patient?

2. Explain why skin temperature (cool or warm *vs.* hot) is a major factor in determining whether to aggressively cool a patient.

Street Scenes

It's very cold out and it's been snowing for hours. Shortly after sundown, you get dispatched for an "unknown man down" call in a downtown area where homeless people often sleep outdoors. As you pull up to the scene, you are met by a police officer who tells you that the man sitting by the heater grate in the sidewalk was going to be taken to the shelter "but something didn't seem right." You get the first-in bag and approach the patient. You ask his name and he says, "Frank." You ask for a last name but he doesn't respond.

"Well, Frank, what's going on?" He just stares. "Do you have any pain?" Again, no response. He just sits with his arms folded over his chest and appears to be shivering. "Frank, we think you need to go to the hospital to get checked out."

"What?" he whispers. You ask the patient if he can stand up but his response is unintelligible. You get the cot and load for transport. The police officer asks you what's wrong and you tell him that you think the patient might be hypothermic.

Street Scene Questions

1. What concerns might you have for this patient?
2. What assessment needs to be performed?
3. Should you rewarm this patient? If so, when should you start?

When you get into the ambulance, you repeat your primary assessment, checking the patient's breathing closely and looking for any external bleeding. Again, you ask the patient if he knows where he is but he responds only with groans. You notice that his clothing is wet, so you turn up the heat in the patient compartment, take off his wet jacket and shirt, and wrap him in more blankets. He is still shivering. You take a set of vital signs and determine his blood

pressure is 90/60, pulse is 120, respiration rate is 28 and shallow, and his skin is flushed. When you feel the abdomen with the back of your hand, it feels cool. You do not smell any alcohol on the patient and when you check distal pulses, motor function, and sensation, you find that he can move all extremities but it is difficult and almost seems painful. His pupils respond to light but appear sluggish. You decide to administer oxygen by nonrebreather mask. You also decide not to actively rewarm the patient but keep him wrapped in blankets, covering his head and keeping the heater turned up.

Street Scene Questions

4. How often should you take vital signs?
5. When moving the patient out of the ambulance and onto the hospital stretcher, what precautions should you take?

You decide to take another set of vital signs after 5 minutes because you think that this patient could be at risk for respiratory arrest or sudden cardiac death. You make sure the AED and the respiratory equipment are close at hand. His vital signs are about the same. You call the hospital, give your report, and advise an ETA of about 5 minutes.

When you get there, you remind your partner that this patient needs to be handled gently. You get another blanket from the emergency department before you make the move. The patient seems to be warming up and you don't want to put him at any additional risk. When you get into the emergency department, you smoothly move the patient to the stretcher and give the prehospital care report. As you are leaving, Frank looks at you and says: "Thanks, you're nice."

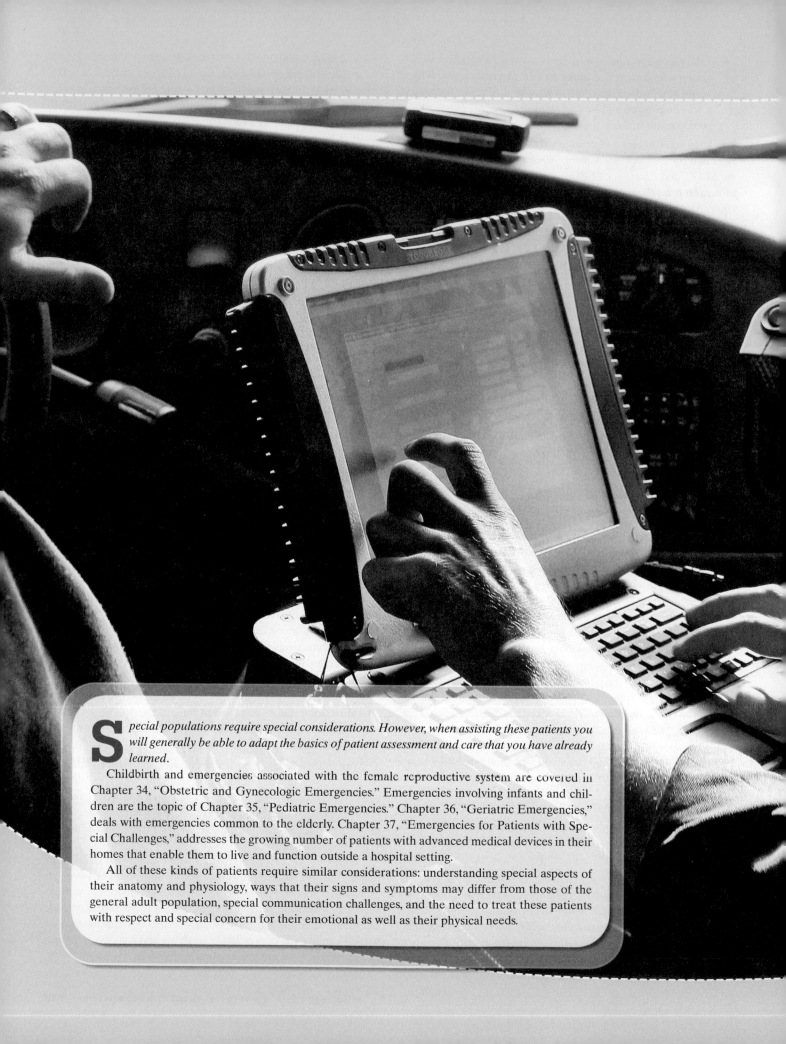

S pecial populations require special considerations. However, when assisting these patients you will generally be able to adapt the basics of patient assessment and care that you have already learned.

Childbirth and emergencies associated with the female reproductive system are covered in Chapter 34, "Obstetric and Gynecologic Emergencies." Emergencies involving infants and children are the topic of Chapter 35, "Pediatric Emergencies." Chapter 36, "Geriatric Emergencies," deals with emergencies common to the elderly. Chapter 37, "Emergencies for Patients with Special Challenges," addresses the growing number of patients with advanced medical devices in their homes that enable them to live and function outside a hospital setting.

All of these kinds of patients require similar considerations: understanding special aspects of their anatomy and physiology, ways that their signs and symptoms may differ from those of the general adult population, special communication challenges, and the need to treat these patients with respect and special concern for their emotional as well as their physical needs.

Special Populations

34 Obstetric and Gynecologic Emergencies

EXPLORE ResourceCentral

To access Resource Central, follow directions on the Student Access Card provided with this text. If there is no card, go to **www.bradybooks.com** and follow the Resource Central link to Buy Access from there. Under Media Resources, you will find:

▶ **Ectopic Pregnancy**
Find out what an ectopic pregnancy is in this animation and learn some of the signs and symptoms a patient might present with.

▶ **Information about Childbirth**
View the stages of labor in this video, learn the signs and symptoms of an imminent birth and find out what equipment you need to prepare for delivery.

▶ **Information about Newborn Resuscitation**
Learn the steps of newborn resuscitation in this video; when you should start chest compressions, and what complications can be caused by meconium aspiration.

OBJECTIVES

After reading this chapter you should be able to:

34.1 Define key terms introduced in this chapter.

34.2 Identify the anatomy of the female reproductive system and fetal development. (pp. 838–840)

34.3 Explain the physiology of pregnancy. (pp. 841–843)

34.4 Explain and describe measures to prevent or correct supine hypotensive syndrome. (p. 843)

34.5 Describe the three stages of labor. (pp. 843–845)

(continued)

34.6 Discuss the assessment of a patient in labor, including history and physical examination. (pp. 845–848)

34.7 Discuss how to decide if delivery is imminent or if the patient in labor should be transported to a medical facility for delivery. (pp. 847–848)

34.8 State findings that may indicate the need for neonatal resuscitation. (p. 848)

34.9 Discuss the role of the EMT in normal childbirth, including preparation and delivery. (pp. 849–853)

34.10 Describe the normal steps in care of the neonate. (pp. 853–856)

34.11 Explain the indications and procedures for neonatal resuscitation, following the inverted pyramid order of priorities. (pp. 857–858)

34.12 Discuss after-delivery care of the mother, including delivery of the placenta, controlling vaginal bleeding, and providing comfort to the mother. (pp. 858–860)

34.13 Describe and discuss the special care required for complications of delivery, including:
a. Breech presentation (p. 861)
b. Limb presentation (p. 862)
c. Prolapsed umbilical cord (pp. 862–863)
d. Multiple birth (pp. 863–864)
e. Premature birth (pp. 864–866)
f. Meconium (p. 866)

34.14 Describe and discuss the special care required for emergencies in pregnancy, including:
a. Excessive prebirth bleeding (pp. 866–867)
b. Ectopic pregnancy (pp. 867–868)
c. Seizures in pregnancy (p. 868)
d. Miscarriage and abortion (pp. 868–869)
e. Trauma in pregnancy (pp. 869–870)
f. Stillbirths (pp. 870–871)
g. Accidental death of a pregnant woman (p. 871)

34.15 Describe and discuss the special care required for gynecological emergencies, including:
a. Vaginal bleeding (p. 871)
b. Trauma to the external genitalia (p. 872)
c. Sexual assault (pp. 872–873)

KEY TERMS

Understanding of the female reproductive system is an important element of your assessment and treatment of any female patient. As an EMT, you should know that the anatomy and physiology of this system can be vastly different from patient to patient. In a nonpregnant female, the organs of reproduction are small and well protected, whereas in a pregnant female these same organs are enlarged and exposed. With pregnancy, a woman's reproductive system will undergo tremendous changes, leading up to the birth of a child.

Childbirth is a natural process that existed long before there were EMTs, and the vast majority of births are uncomplicated. However, you should always remember that, if EMS has been called, something unexpected has occurred and the

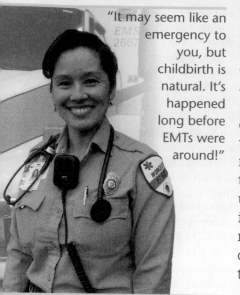

likelihood of a problem has increased. With the potential for complications, the best place to deliver a baby is a hospital. Much of our assessment of the woman in labor will be geared toward making a decision on whether to transport the pregnant woman or prepare for an immediate delivery.

If it does become necessary to assist with an out-of-hospital delivery, one of your main responsibilities in this situation will be to help calm the patient and family members through your unruffled professional manner. However, because childbirth is not a common occurrence in the prehospital setting, it might be easy to get flustered and seem uncertain about the procedures you are performing. Therefore, it is important that you learn about childbirth and practice the procedures required to assist with delivery. If you are ever called upon to assist in a delivery, your skills will contribute to decreased stress and better care of the mother and baby.

>>>>>>

● CORE CONCEPT

Anatomy and physiology of the female reproductive system

ANATOMY AND PHYSIOLOGY

External Genitalia

A woman's external genitalia consist of three major structures: the labia, the perineum, and the mons pubis (Figure 34-1).

FIGURE 34-1 External female genitalia.

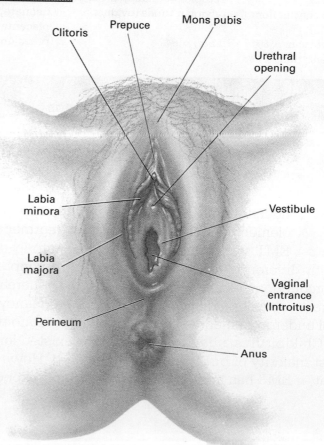

Clitoris
Prepuce
Mons pubis
Urethral opening
Labia minora
Vestibule
Labia majora
Vaginal entrance (Introitus)
Perineum
Anus

The *labia* consist of soft tissues that protect the entrance to the birth canal. The urethral opening and the nerve-rich center of sexual stimulation, called the clitoris, can be found in the anterior aspects of the labia. These tissues are highly vascular and prone to significant bleeding with trauma.

The *perineum* is the soft tissue and muscle found between the vaginal opening and the anus. This tissue is prone to tearing during childbirth. The *mons pubis* is a layer of soft tissue that covers and protects the pubic symphysis. It is the area where hair grows as a woman reaches puberty.

Internal Genitalia

A woman's internal genitalia consist of the vagina, the ovaries, the fallopian tubes (also called the oviducts), and the uterus (Figure 34-2).

The Vagina

The *vagina* is the birth canal. Made up of smooth muscle, it connects the uterus to the outside world and will stretch to accommodate passage of the fetus during delivery. It is also the passageway for menstrual waste products leaving the uterus at the conclusion of the menstrual cycle.

The Ovaries and Fallopian Tubes

The *ovaries* are small, round organs that are located on either side of most women's lower abdominal quadrants. These organs are responsible for producing ova (eggs) for conception. They also produce many of the hormones necessary for the process of reproduction. An ovum produced in the ovaries is transported to the uterus (the place where they will implant and develop) through the *fallopian tubes*, also called the *oviducts*. Each ovary is connected to the uterus by a fallopian tube. If fertilization occurs, it will most likely happen in these tubes. A dangerous condition called *ectopic pregnancy* can occur if the ovum implants in the fallopian tubes. Unlike the uterus, these tubes cannot expand as the fetus develops and are vulnerable to rupture and severe bleeding. (We will discuss ectopic pregnancy in greater detail later in this chapter.)

labia (LAY-be-uh)
soft tissues that protect the entrance to the vagina.

perineum (per-i-NE-um)
the surface area between the vagina and anus.

mons pubis
soft tissue that covers the pubic symphysis; area where hair grows as a woman reaches puberty.

vagina (vah-JI-nah)
the birth canal.

ovary (o-vu-RE)
the female reproductive organ that produces ova.

fallopian (fu-LO-pe-an)
tube the narrow tube that connects the ovary to the uterus. Also called the *oviduct*.

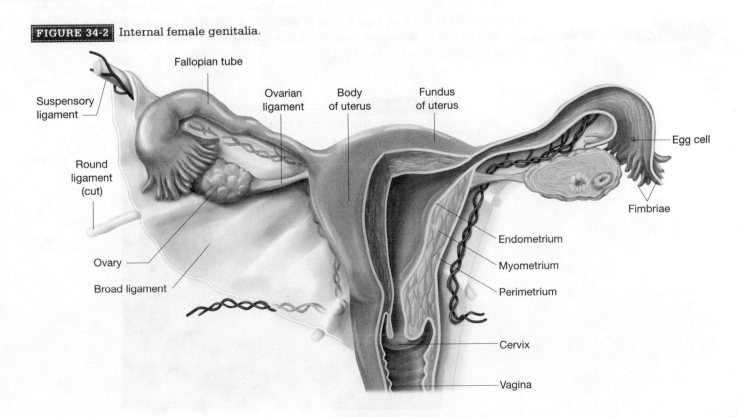

FIGURE 34-2 Internal female genitalia.

Suspensory ligament

Fallopian tube

Ovarian ligament

Body of uterus

Fundus of uterus

Egg cell

Round ligament (cut)

Fimbriae

Ovary

Broad ligament

Endometrium

Myometrium

Perimetrium

Cervix

Vagina

The Uterus

The **uterus** (or womb) is a muscular, hollow organ located along the midline in most women's lower abdominal quadrants. This organ is the intended site for the fertilized egg to implant and develop into a fetus. To accommodate that purpose, the uterus is able to stretch and grow as the fetus gets larger. The top, or fundus, of the uterus can be found as high as the xiphoid process in a late-term pregnant woman. The lower aspect of the uterus is connected to the vagina. A muscular ring called the **cervix** separates these two organs. In a nonpregnant female, the cervix is constricted to close off the uterus. With labor, the cervix thins and dilates to allow the muscular walls of the uterus to contract and push the fetus out through the vagina and into the outside world.

The Female Reproductive Cycle

After a woman reaches the age of puberty, approximately every 28 days her uterus goes through a series of changes to prepare for the potential implantation of a fertilized egg. Hormones such as estrogen and progesterone stimulate these events. In the early phases, the ovaries are stimulated to release an ovum (egg) in a process called **ovulation**. At the same time, the walls of the uterus thicken in preparation for implantation of the egg if fertilization occurs.

The fallopian tubes now move the egg by peristalsis (waves of muscular contraction) toward the uterus. Fertilization typically occurs in the fallopian tubes. If fertilization does not occur, hormone levels once again change and the uterus begins to change as well. Without fertilization, the thickened inner walls of the uterus begin to slough off and are expelled through the vagina. This process is called menstruation and is usually characterized by vaginal bleeding for roughly 3–5 days. If the egg is fertilized and successfully implants, hormones induce other changes that occur with pregnancy.

Fertilization

If the woman has sexual intercourse in the period immediately following ovulation and sperm reaches the ova, fertilization may occur. By combining with the sperm, an ovum becomes an **embryo** and the embryonic stage of pregnancy begins. The embryonic stage occurs roughly from the point of fertilization and lasts 8 weeks. During this stage, the embryo attempts to implant in the lining of the uterus and develop basic connections between itself and the mother

At 8 weeks of development, the fetal stage begins. From this point until delivery, the developing baby is referred to as a **fetus** (Figure 34-3). The fetus will develop over the next 32 weeks (a typical pregnancy lasts about 40 weeks), during which time the woman's body will undergo significant changes.

FIGURE 34-3 Endoscopic photograph of a 5-week-old live fetus in the uterus. A hand and eye are clearly visible. (© Alexander Tsiaras/Science Source/Photo Researchers, Inc.)

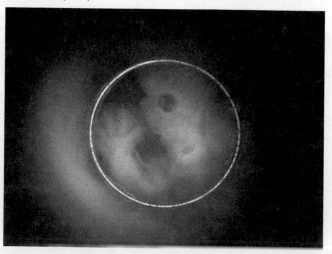

PHYSIOLOGIC CHANGES IN PREGNANCY

Changes in the Reproductive System

Size is the most significant change that pregnancy brings to the reproductive system. As the fetus grows and develops, the uterus simply gets larger. It becomes thinner-walled and less protected by the abdominal cavity. Therefore, it becomes more vulnerable to injury.

The 9 months of pregnancy are divided into three 3-month periods, or trimesters. During the first trimester, the fetus is being formed. Since the fetus remains quite small, there is little uterine growth during this period. After the third month, the uterus grows rapidly, reaching the umbilicus (navel) by the fifth month and the epigastrium (upper abdomen) by the seventh month.

As the fetus develops, other major changes occur in the reproductive system (Figure 34-4). In addition to the fetus, an organ called the *placenta* develops in the uterus. Composed of both maternal and fetal tissues, the placenta is attached to the wall of the uterus and serves as an exchange area between mother and fetus. In a process similar to the diffusion between the alveoli and pulmonary capillaries, oxygen and nutrients (and drugs, nicotine, and alcohol) from the mother's blood vessels are carried across the placenta to the blood vessels of the fetus. Carbon dioxide and certain other waste products cross from fetal circulation to maternal circulation. Since the placenta is an organ of pregnancy, it is expelled after the baby is born.

The mother's blood does not flow through the fetus's body. Instead, the fetus has its own circulatory system. Blood from the fetus is sent through blood vessels in the *umbilical cord* to the placenta where, through diffusion, the blood picks up nourishment from the mother, then returns through the umbilical cord to the fetus's body. The umbilical cord, which is about 1 inch wide and 22 inches long at birth, is fully expelled with the birth of the baby and the delivery of the placenta.

While developing in the uterus, the fetus is enclosed and protected within a thin, membranous "bag of waters" known as the *amniotic sac*. This sac contains almost 1 quart of liquid, called amniotic fluid. It allows the fetus to float during development, acts as a cushion between the fetus and minor injury, and helps maintain a constant fetal body temperature. In the vast majority of cases, the amniotic sac breaks during labor and the fluid gushes from the birth canal. This is a normal condition of childbirth that also provides a natural lubrication to ease the infant's progress through the birth canal.

CORE CONCEPT
Physiologic changes in pregnancy

placenta (plah-SEN-tah) the organ of pregnancy where exchange of oxygen, nutrients, and wastes occurs between a mother and fetus.

umbilical (um-BIL-i-kal) *cord* the fetal structure containing the blood vessels that carry blood to and from the placenta.

amniotic (am-ne-OT-ik) *sac* the "bag of waters" that surrounds the developing fetus.

FIGURE 34-4 | Structures of pregnancy.

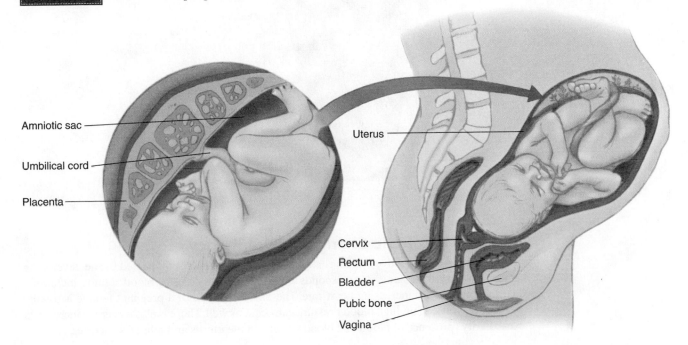

Amniotic sac
Umbilical cord
Placenta
Uterus
Cervix
Rectum
Bladder
Pubic bone
Vagina

Inside/Outside

PHYSIOLOGIC CHANGES OF PREGNANCY

Pregnancy causes numerous physiologic changes (Figure 34-5).

FIGURE 34-5 Physiologic changes in pregnancy.

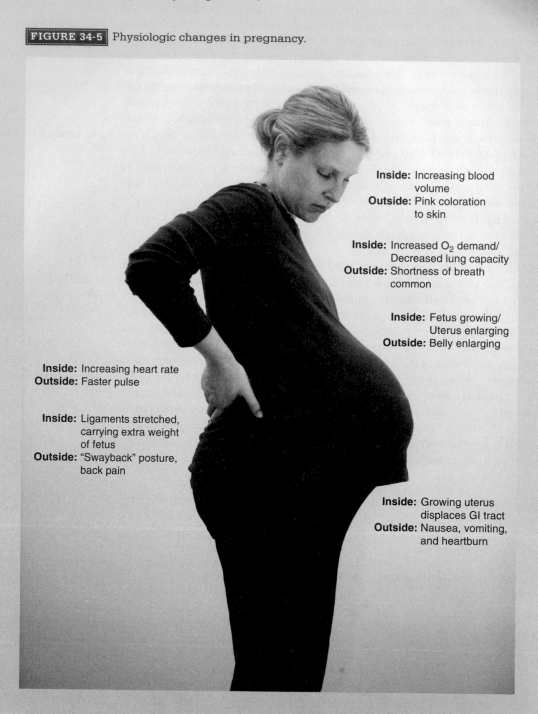

Inside: Increasing blood volume
Outside: Pink coloration to skin

Inside: Increased O$_2$ demand/ Decreased lung capacity
Outside: Shortness of breath common

Inside: Fetus growing/ Uterus enlarging
Outside: Belly enlarging

Inside: Increasing heart rate
Outside: Faster pulse

Inside: Ligaments stretched, carrying extra weight of fetus
Outside: "Swayback" posture, back pain

Inside: Growing uterus displaces GI tract
Outside: Nausea, vomiting, and heartburn

Other Physiologic Changes in Pregnancy

In addition to reproductive system changes, other systems are also impacted by the developing fetus. The cardiovascular system responds to pregnancy by increasing blood volume, increasing cardiac output, and increasing heart rate. The blood pressure of a pregnant female is usually slightly decreased, but high blood pressure can occur as well. There is also a massive increase in vascularity (presence of blood and blood vessels) in the uterus and related structures.

Pregnancy affects the respiratory system by increasing oxygen demand and consumption. In the later stages of pregnancy, the fetus can also put pressure on the woman's diaphragm and decrease the volume of air in her lungs.

In the gastrointestinal system, a growing fetus puts pressure on the stomach and intestines and can slow digestion. Nausea and vomiting are also very common in pregnancy.

Hormones released with pregnancy make the ligaments of a pregnant woman's musculoskeletal system more elastic and therefore more vulnerable to injury. The additional weight can also affect posture and lead to back pain as well as affect balance.

Pregnancy may also impact preexisting medical conditions in the mother. Diseases such as asthma and diabetes both can be made worse with pregnancy.

Supine Hypotensive Syndrome

In the third trimester, near the time of birth, the weight of the uterus, combined with the weight of the infant, placenta, and amniotic fluid, totals approximately 20 to 24 pounds. When the mother is in a supine position, this heavy mass will tend to compress the inferior vena cava, a major blood vessel, reducing return of blood to the heart, thereby reducing cardiac output. The resulting dizziness and drop in blood pressure constitute a set of signs and symptoms known as *supine hypotensive syndrome*. This syndrome is also referred to as vena cava compression syndrome. When it senses the drop in blood pressure, the body begins to compensate by contracting the uterine arteries and redirecting blood to the major organs. This can severely affect the fetus.

Although the drop in blood pressure signals shock, traditional methods of treating shock (hypoperfusion) will not be effective in this instance. To take the weight off the vena cava and counteract or avoid the possible drop in blood pressure, all third-trimester patients should be transported on their left side. A pillow or rolled blanket should be placed behind the back to maintain proper positioning.

supine hypotensive syndrome dizziness and a drop in blood pressure caused when the mother is in a supine position and the weight of the uterus, infant, placenta, and amniotic fluid compress the inferior vena cava, reducing return of blood to the heart and cardiac output.

LABOR AND DELIVERY

The Stages of Labor

Labor is the entire process of delivery. There are three stages of labor (Figure 34-6):

- **First stage.** This stage starts with regular contractions and the thinning and gradual dilation of the cervix and ends when the cervix is fully dilated.
- **Second stage.** This stage is the time from when the baby enters the birth canal until he is born.
- **Third stage.** This stage begins after the baby is born and lasts until the *afterbirth* (placenta, umbilical cord, and some tissues from the amniotic sac and the lining of the uterus) is delivered.

First Stage

The first stage of labor is also called the dilation period. Picture the uterus as a long-neck bottle. In order to expel the contents, the neck of the bottle must be stretched to the size of a wide-mouth jar. Before the cervix can fully dilate, the long neck of the cervix must be shortened and thinned (this process is called effacement) to the wide-mouth-jar shape.

Sometimes, several days or even weeks before the onset of actual labor, the uterine muscles begin mild contractions. These *Braxton-Hicks contractions* are usually irregular and not sustained and they typically do not indicate impending delivery. In contrast, when actual labor begins, the uterus will begin to contract regularly and the cervix will begin to dilate. As this happens, the fetus's head typically moves downward.

Lightening is a term used to describe the fetus's movement from high in the abdomen down toward the birth canal. Some women will describe experiencing this sensation. At times this occurs well before the start of labor, but it can also be an indicator of the beginning of the labor process.

The cycle of contractions starts far apart and becomes shorter as birth approaches. Typically, these contractions range from every 30 minutes at the start down to 3 minutes apart or less near the end.

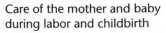

CORE CONCEPT
Care of the mother and baby during labor and childbirth

labor
the three stages of the delivery of a baby that begin with the contractions of the uterus and end with the expulsion of the placenta.

afterbirth
the placenta, membranes of the amniotic sac, part of the umbilical cord, and some tissues from the lining of the uterus that are delivered after the birth of the baby.

Braxton-Hicks (braks-tun-hiks) **contractions** irregular prelabor contractions of the uterus.

lightening
the sensation of the fetus moving from high in the abdomen to low in the birth canal.

FIGURE 34-6 Three stages of labor.

First stage:
beginning of contractions to full cervical dilation

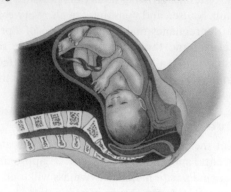

Second stage:
baby enters birth canal and is born

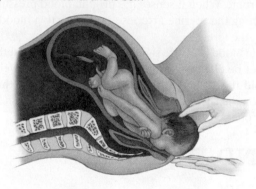

Third stage:
delivery of the placenta

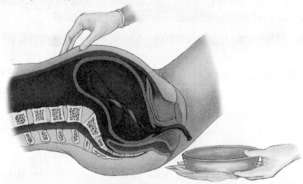

The contractions of the uterus produce normal labor pains. Most women report the start of labor pains as an ache in the lower back. As labor progresses, the pain becomes most noticeable in the lower abdomen, with the intensity of pain increasing. The pains come at regular intervals, lasting from 30 seconds to 1 minute and occur at 2- to 3-minute intervals. When the uterus starts to contract, the pain begins. As the muscles relax, there is relief from the pain. Labor pains may start and stop for a while and then start up again.

As an EMT, you should time the following characteristics of labor pains:

- **Contraction time, or duration.** This is the time from the beginning of a contraction to when the uterus relaxes (from start to end).

- **Contraction interval, or frequency.** This is the time from the start of one contraction to the beginning of the next (from start to start).

When contractions last 30 seconds to 1 minute and are 2 to 3 minutes apart, this indicates delivery of the baby may be imminent.

As contractions continue, the cervix gradually shortens and thins enough (reaching wide-mouth-jar shape) to become flush with the vagina or fully open to the birth canal. The full dilation of the cervix signals the end of the first stage of labor. Women giving birth for the first time will remain in this first stage of labor for an average of 16 hours. However, some women may remain in this stage for no more than 4 hours, especially if this is not their first child.

> **NOTE:** *There is no way to externally assess the dilation of the cervix. As an EMT, you will assess the progression of labor using other findings. EMTs do not do internal cervical examinations.*

As the fetus moves downward and the cervix dilates, the amniotic sac usually breaks. This is commonly referred to as the "water breaking" or the "rupture of membranes." It is often felt by the woman as a gush or trickle of fluid exiting the vagina. Most commonly, it immediately precedes labor. However, it can also happen well before the onset of labor. This is called premature rupture of membranes and can be a serious problem for the fetus.

Normally, the amniotic fluid is clear. Fluid that is greenish or brownish-yellow in color may be an indication of maternal or fetal distress and is called ***meconium staining***.

There may also be a watery, bloody discharge of mucus (not bleeding) associated with the first stage of labor. Part of this initial discharge will be from a mucus plug that helped to keep the cervix closed during pregnancy. This is usually mixed with blood and is called the bloody show. Watery, bloody fluids discharging from the vagina are typical for all three stages of labor.

meconium staining
amniotic fluid that is greenish or brownish-yellow rather than clear as a result of fetal defecation; an indication of possible maternal or fetal distress during labor.

Second Stage

The second stage of labor begins after the full dilation of the cervix. During this time, contractions become increasingly frequent, and labor pains become more severe. In the second stage of labor, the cramping and abdominal pains associated with the first stage of labor are typically still present. As delivery approaches, most women will feel an urge to push or feeling like they need to move their bowels. This occurs as the baby's body moves and places pressure on the rectum. The urge to push is a sign that birth is near, and the EMT will have to decide whether to transport the pregnant patient or keep the mother where she is and prepare to assist with delivery.

Third Stage

The third stage of labor begins immediately after the baby is born. In this stage, the placenta detaches itself from the wall of the uterus and is expelled. Contractions will resume and continue until the placenta is delivered. The contractions and labor pains may be as painful and severe during this stage as they were in the second stage. The third stage usually lasts 10 to 20 minutes and ends as the placenta is delivered.

PATIENT ASSESSMENT

Assessing the Woman in Labor

Although you will assess a woman in labor the same way you would any other patient, there are some specific goals you should keep in mind. You should use your assessment to identify the imminent delivery. Ideally, mothers in labor should be transported to the hospital for delivery; however, it is not always possible to do so. Fortunately, your assessment may reveal some key finding that may indicate that the birth is about to happen.

A simple series of questions, an examination for crowning, and a determination of vital signs will allow you to make the decision for transport. However, do not let the "urgency" of this decision upset the mother. Your patient needs emotional support at this time. Your calm, professional actions will help her feel more at ease and assure her that you will provide the required care for both her and the unborn child.

Assessment of a woman in labor includes all the elements of a traditional patient assessment including checking airway, breathing, and circulation; taking vital signs; and reviewing a SAMPLE history. There are also a few assessment elements that are specific to the pregnancy and labor.

To begin to evaluate the woman in labor:

1. **Ask her name, age, and expected due date.**

2. **Ask if this is her first pregnancy.** The average time of labor for a woman having her first baby is about 16 to 17 hours. The time in labor is typically shorter for subsequent births, unless the mother has given birth to more than four or five babies already. In some women with numerous deliveries, the uterus will continue to act like a well-toned muscle; in others, it will be less effective and delivery will take longer.

3. **Ask her if she has seen a doctor regarding her pregnancy.** This is called prenatal care and is important in identifying such things as multiple gestations (twins, triplets, and so on); known complications or problems with the pregnancy; and possible medical issues with the mother.

4. **Ask her when the labor pains started and how often she is having pains. Ask her if her "bag of waters" has broken and if she has had any bleeding or bloody show.** At this point, with a woman having her first delivery, you may think that you can make a decision about transport. However, you should continue with the evaluation procedure. Also, begin to time the frequency and length of the contractions.

5. **Ask her if she feels the urge to push or if she feels as though she needs to move her bowels.** If she says "Yes," this usually means that the baby has moved into the birth canal and is pressing the vaginal wall against the rectum. However, do not allow the mother to go to the bathroom as she may deliver the infant into the toilet. Birth will probably occur very soon. The mother may tell you that she can feel the baby trying to move out through her vaginal opening. In such cases, birth is likely very near.

6. **Examine the mother for crowning (Figure 34-7).** This is a visual inspection to see if there is bulging at the vaginal opening or if the presenting part of the baby is visible. *Crowning* occurs when the *presenting part* of the baby first bulges from the vaginal opening. The presenting part is defined as the part of the infant that is first to appear at the vaginal opening during labor. Usually, the presenting part of the baby is the head. The normal head-first birth is called a ***cephalic presentation***. If the buttocks or both feet of the baby deliver first, the birth is called a breech presentation or breech birth. If part of the baby's head or presenting part is visible with each contraction, then birth is imminent.

7. **Feel for uterine contractions.** You may have to delay this procedure until the patient tells you she is having labor pains. Tell her what you are going to do, then place the palm of your gloved hand on her abdomen, above the navel. This can be done over the top of

crowning
when part of the baby is visible through the vaginal opening.

cephalic (se-FAL-ik)
presentation when the baby appears head first during birth. This is the normal presentation.

FIGURE 34-7 Crowning of the infant's head.

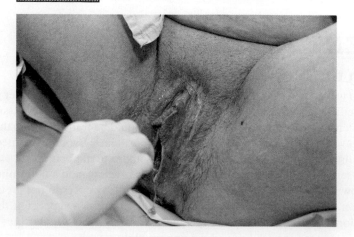

the patient's clothing. You should be able to feel her uterus contract. All contractions should be timed, so keep track of the duration and frequency of the contractions. The uterus and the tissues between this organ and the skin will feel more rigid as the delivery of the baby nears.

8. **Take vital signs.** If you do not have a partner to do it, this is the point to check the patient's vitals.

NOTE: *Do not allow the mother to go to the bathroom, even though she says that she has to move her bowels. Birth is probably only a few minutes away. In addition, do not allow the mother to hold her legs together or use any other method to attempt to delay the delivery.*

Examining for crowning may be embarrassing to the mother, the father, and any required bystanders. For this reason, it is important that you fully explain what you are doing and why. Be certain that you protect the mother from the stares of bystanders. In a polite but firm manner, ask everyone who does not belong at the scene to leave. Carefully help the patient remove enough clothing to allow you an unobstructed view of the vaginal opening.

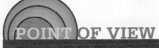POINT OF VIEW

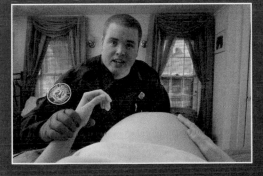

"I had planned to have a very controlled delivery. It was my first baby. And, yes, maybe I was trying to micromanage a natural process . . . when all my plans went to hell. My contractions started, my water broke, and I felt like I was going to have the baby right there.

"My husband and I freaked. All the plans to call people and have a meaningful time together before the hospital went out the window. The only call we made was to 911.

"The EMTs arrived and were great. They calmed us down. Lord knows we needed that. After they asked a few questions and timed the contractions, they thought there would be time to get to the hospital before the baby was born.

"They were right. We did have time. About 8 hours. Did I mention that we totally freaked out? If we ever do this again it will be different. Honest!"

If this is the woman's first delivery, she is not straining, and there is no crowning, there is little reason why she cannot be transported to a medical facility for delivery. (A first delivery typically takes longer than subsequent ones.) However, if this is not her first delivery, and she is pushing, crying out, and complaining about having to go to the bathroom, birth will probably occur too soon for transport. If the mother is having labor pains from contractions that are about 2 minutes apart, birth may be very near. If you determine that delivery is imminent based on the presence of crowning or other signs, local protocol may require you to contact medical direction for the decision to commit to delivery on the site. If delivery does not occur within 10 minutes, contact medical direction again and request permission to initiate transport of the mother.

You may find a patient who is afraid of transport because she believes that her baby's birth will occur along the way. Assure her that you believe there is enough time to get to the hospital before delivery. Let her know that you are trained to assist with the delivery and that the ambulance is well equipped to handle her needs and care for the newborn in case she delivers en route. If crowning occurs during transport, stop the ambulance and prepare for delivery.

If your evaluation of the patient leads you to believe that birth is too near at hand for transport, you and your partner should prepare to assist the mother with delivery. Remember, as part of the preparation, the patient will need emotional support.

- Is delivery of the baby imminent?
- Should I prepare to deliver on scene or move to the ambulance?

    NOTE: *It is best to transport an expecting mother unless, based on your evaluation, you expect delivery within a few minutes.*

Another important assessment goal is predicting the need for neonatal resuscitation. Although the need for resuscitation can never be absolutely predicted, there are some assessment findings that indicate a high probability of that need.

Findings That Might Indicate the Need for Neonatal Resuscitation

- No prior prenatal care. The patient has not seen an obstetrician and therefore has no idea regarding her health or the health of her unborn baby.
- Premature delivery. The earlier the labor, the higher the likelihood of resuscitation.
- Labor induced by trauma or medical conditions affecting the mother.
- Multiple births. Multiple births, like twins and triplets, significantly increase the likelihood of resuscitation.
- History of problems with the pregnancy, especially placenta previa and breech presentations. (We will discuss both these issues later in the chapter.)
- Labor induced by drug use, especially narcotics.
- Meconium staining with the rupture of membranes (water breaking).

The most important outcome of anticipating a neonatal resuscitation is getting help. As you will read later in this chapter, a resuscitation requires a rapid series of actions with full attention focused on the new baby. If that occurs, you will need more help and probably ALS support, if available. Good assessment will enable you to begin assembling these resources prior to delivering the baby.

Decision Point

- Do I need to prepare for multiple births or expect complications?

CRITICAL DECISION MAKING

My Baby Won't Wait!

Childbirth in the field is a rare but very exciting call. For every baby you deliver, you may have dozens of maternity calls in which the mother is transported to the hospital before the baby is delivered. Being able to determine whether the birth is imminent is an important skill for an EMT. For each of the scenarios presented, determine if you should stay and prepare for delivery or transport the patient to the hospital.

1. Your patient states her contractions are severe and about 30 seconds apart. She feels the need to push and suspects she has accidentally moved her bowels. There is significant bulging, and you can see the baby's head crowning. This is her fourth child.

2. Your patient reports contractions are about 5–10 minutes apart but feel strong. This is her first child. You do not observe any crowning or bulging. She is not sure if her water has broken.

3. Your patient reports contractions that are about 2 minutes apart. They have been this way for about 8 hours. Her water broke when the contractions started. She doesn't feel she is progressing through labor and is concerned for her baby.

NORMAL CHILDBIRTH

Role of the EMT

Your primary role in a childbirth will be to determine whether the delivery will occur on-scene and, if so, to assist the mother as she delivers her child.

NOTE: *EMTs do not deliver babies; mothers do!*

Preparing the Mother for Delivery

When your evaluation leads you to believe birth is imminent, you must immediately prepare the mother for delivery. To do so, you should:

1. Control the scene so that the mother will have privacy. (Her birthing coach may remain.) If you are not in a private room and transfer to the ambulance is not practical (crowning is present), ask bystanders to leave.

2. In addition to surgical gloves, you and your partner should put on gowns, caps, face masks, and eye protection since there is a high probability of splashing blood and other body fluids during delivery.

3. Place the mother on a bed, floor, or the ambulance stretcher. Elevate her buttocks with blankets or a pillow. Have the mother lie with knees drawn up and spread apart. You will need about 2 feet of work space below the woman's buttocks to place and initially care for the newborn. Having the patient positioned on the stretcher may speed transport if complications arise.

4. Remove any of the patient's clothing or underclothing that obstructs your view of the vaginal opening. Use sterile sheets or sterile towels to cover the mother, as shown in Figure 34-8. Clean sheets, clean cloths, towels, or materials such as tablecloths can be used if you do not have an obstetrics kit.

5. Position your assistant—your partner, the father, or someone the mother agrees to have assist you—at the mother's head. This person should stay alert to help turn the mother's head in case she vomits. In addition, this person should provide emotional support to the mother, soothing and encouraging her.

6. Position the obstetrics kit near the patient. All items must be within easy reach.

NOTE: *If delivery is to take place in an automobile, position the mother flat on the seat. Arrange her legs so that she has one foot resting on the seat and the other foot resting on the floor.*

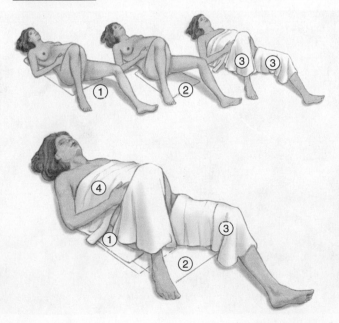

FIGURE 34-8 Preparing the mother for delivery.

Preparing the Obstetrics (OB) Kit

A normal delivery requires some basic equipment that is typically kept in what is called an obstetrics (OB) kit (Figure 34-9). Although supplies will vary, this kit should include:

- Several pairs of sterile surgical gloves to protect you from infection
- Towels or sheets for draping the mother
- 1 dozen 2 × 2 (or 4 × 4) gauze pads (sponges) for wiping and drying the baby
- 1 rubber bulb syringe (3 oz.) to suction the baby's mouth and nostrils if needed
- Cord clamps or hemostats to clamp the umbilical cord (plus extra clamps in case of a multiple birth)
- Umbilical cord tape to tie the cord
- 1 pair of surgical scissors to cut the cord
- 1 baby blanket to wrap the baby and keep him warm
- Several individually wrapped sanitary napkins to absorb blood and other fluids
- Plastic bag

Occasionally, in an off-duty situation, you may need to assist in the delivery of a baby without using a sterile delivery pack. In this case, a few simple supplies can be used to assist the mother:

- Clean sheets and towels to drape around the mother and wrap the newborn
- Heavy flat twine or new shoelaces to tie the cord (Do not use thread, wire, or light string since these may cut through the cord.)
- A towel or plastic bag to wrap the placenta after its delivery
- Clean, unused rubber gloves and eyewear, as the lack of gloves and eyewear will mean possible exposure to infectious diseases

A head covering for the baby may also be helpful as it dramatically reduces heat loss.

A neonatal-sized bag-valve mask (BVM) connected to oxygen should also be prepared prior to the delivery.

Delivering the Baby

Position yourself in such a way that you have a constant view of the vaginal opening. Be prepared for the baby to come at any moment.

FIGURE 34-9 Contents of an OB (obstetrics) kit.

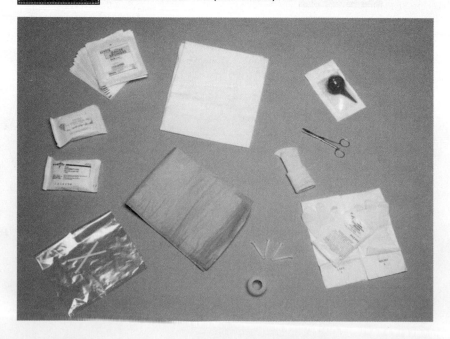

In addition, be prepared for the patient to experience discomfort. Delivering a child is a natural process, but it is accompanied by pain. Your patient may also have intense feelings of nausea. If this is her first child, she may be very frightened. All these factors may cause your patient to be uncooperative at times. You must remember that the patient is in pain and she may feel ill. Therefore, she will need emotional support.

Talk to the mother during the delivery. Encourage her to relax between contractions. Continue to time her contractions from the beginning of one contraction to the beginning of the next. Encourage her not to strain unless she feels she must. Remind her that her feeling of a pending bowel movement is usually just pressure caused by the baby moving into her birth canal. Encourage her to breathe deeply through her mouth. She may feel better if she pants, although she should be discouraged from breathing rapidly and deeply enough to bring on hyperventilation. If her "bag of waters" breaks, remind her that this is normal.

NOTE: *Unless there are signs of complications, consider the delivery to be normal if there is a cephalic presentation. Observe any unusual color in the amniotic fluid.*

NOTE: *Some deliveries are explosive. In this case, do not squeeze the baby, but do provide adequate support. You can prevent an explosive delivery by using one hand to maintain slight pressure on the baby's head, thereby avoiding direct pressure to the infant's soft spots on the skull.*

To assist the mother with a normal delivery Figure 34-10 and Scan 34-1:

1. Continue to keep someone at the mother's head to provide support, monitor vital signs, and be alert for vomiting. If no one is on hand to help, be alert for vomiting and check vital signs between contractions.

2. Position your gloved hands at the mother's vaginal opening when the baby's head starts to appear. Place your hand gently on the baby's head as it bulges out of the vagina to prevent a sudden uncontrolled expulsion of the newborn. Do not touch the area around the vagina except to assist with the delivery. For legal reasons, it is always preferable for both your protection and the patient's to have your partner present at all times when you are touching a woman's vaginal area.

3. Place one hand below the baby's head as it delivers. Spread your fingers evenly, remembering that the baby's skull contains "soft spots," or fontanelles. Support the baby's head, but avoid pressure to these soft areas at the top and sides of the skull. A slight, well-distributed pressure may help prevent an explosive delivery. Keeping one hand on the baby's head and using the other hand to hold a sterile towel to support the tissue between the mother's vagina and anus can help prevent tearing of this tissue during delivery of the head. *Do not pull on the baby!*

4. If the amniotic sac has not broken by the time the baby's head is delivered, use your finger to puncture the membrane. Pull the membranes away from the baby's mouth and

FIGURE 34-10 (A) Delivering the infant's head. (B) Delivering the infant's shoulders.

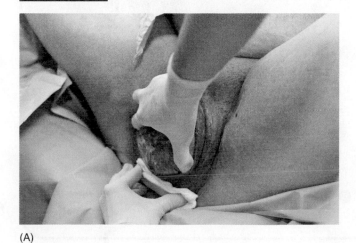

(A)

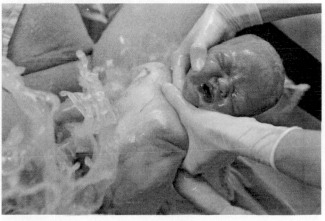

(B)

FIRST TAKE STANDARD PRECAUTIONS.

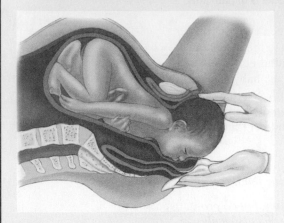

① Support the infant's head. (Assist the mother by supporting the baby throughout the birth process.)

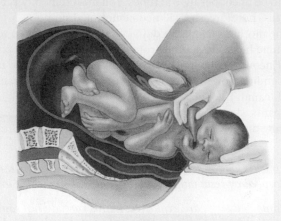

② With the other hand, wipe the mouth and nose with sterile gauze pads. If there are excessive secretions, fluids, or meconium present on the baby's face, use the rubber bulb syringe to suction the baby's mouth, then the nose. Some EMS systems prefer to withhold suctioning at the perineum, waiting until the baby is fully delivered before suctioning. Follow your local protocols.

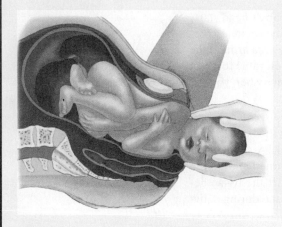

③ Aid in the birth of the upper shoulder.

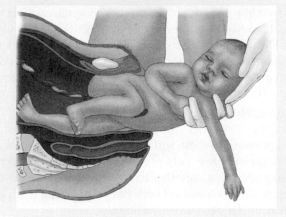

④ Support the trunk.

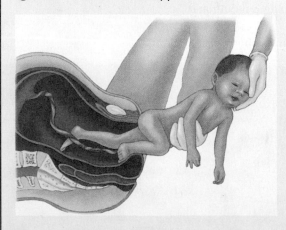

⑤ Support the pelvis and lower extremities.

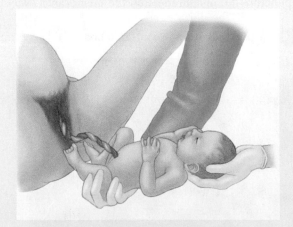

⑥ Keep the infant level with the vagina until the umbilical cord stops pulsating.

nose. The amniotic fluid should be clear. Examine the amniotic fluid for meconium staining, which will appear to be a dark green-black or mustard yellow color. Meconium-stained amniotic fluid is caused by fetal feces (wastes) released during labor, usually because of maternal or fetal distress. If meconium is present, immediately prepare to suction the infant. If the meconium is aspirated (breathed in) by the fetus, the baby can develop pneumonia or other complications.

5. Once the head delivers, check to see if the umbilical cord is wrapped around the baby's neck. Tell the mother not to push while you check. If she can "pant," or take short quick breaths for just a moment, it may help relieve the urge to push while you check. Then gently loosen the cord, if necessary. Even though the umbilical cord is very tough, rough handling may cause it to tear. If the cord is wrapped around the baby's neck, try to place two fingers under the cord at the back of the baby's neck. Bring the cord forward, over the baby's upper shoulder and head.

   If you cannot loosen or slip the cord over the baby's head, the baby cannot be delivered. Therefore, immediately clamp the cord in two places using the clamps provided in the obstetrics kit. Be very careful not to injure the baby. With extreme care, cut the cord between the two clamps. Gently unwrap the ends of the cord from around the baby's neck, and then proceed with the delivery.

6. Help deliver the shoulders. The upper shoulder will deliver next (usually with some delay), followed quickly by the lower shoulder. You must support the baby throughout this entire process. Gently guide the baby's head downward, to assist the mother in delivering the baby's upper shoulder. If the lower shoulder is slow to deliver after the upper shoulder has delivered, assist the mother by gently guiding the baby's head upward (Figure 34-10B).

7. Support the baby throughout the entire birth process. Remember that newborns are very slippery. As the lower extremities are born, grasp them to ensure a good hold on the baby. Never pick up babies by the feet as they are very slippery and you could drop the child. Once the feet are delivered, lay the baby on his side with his head slightly lower than his body. This is done to allow blood, fluids, and mucus to drain from the mouth and nose. Keep the baby at the same level as the mother's vagina until the umbilical cord stops pulsating. (Cutting the cord will be discussed later.) Dry the infant and wrap him in a warm, dry blanket.

8. Assess the airway. Although most active babies will not require suctioning, for some it will be necessary. Suctioning will be important if positive pressure ventilations are necessary or if secretions threaten the airway or obstruct normal breathing. If necessary, use the rubber bulb syringe to suction the baby's mouth, then the nose. Compress the syringe *before* placing it in the baby's mouth. Suction the mouth first, then the nostrils. Carefully insert the tip of the syringe about 1 to 1 1/2 inches into the baby's mouth and release the bulb to allow fluids to be drawn into the syringe. Control the release with your fingers. Withdraw the tip and discharge the syringe's contents onto a towel. Repeat this procedure two or three times in the baby's mouth and once or twice in each nostril. The tip of the syringe should not be inserted more than 1/2 inch into the baby's nostril.

9. Note the exact time of birth. Write the mother's last name and time of delivery on a piece of tape. Fold it so the adhesive does not touch the baby's skin, and place it around the baby's wrist.

THE NEONATE

The term *neonate* is used for a newly born baby and infants less than 1 month old. Remember that a neonate is very different than other infants and must be treated accordingly.

> **NOTE:** A number of terms are often used interchangeably. For clarity and uniformity, it is appropriate to use the following definitions: *fetus*—a baby as it develops in the womb; *neonate*—the baby at the time of birth to 1 month of age; *infant*—a baby in its first year of life.

CORE CONCEPT

Care of the neonate

neonate (NEE-oh-nate)
a newly born infant or an infant less than 1 month old.

Assessing the Neonate

The neonate should be assessed as soon as he is born. If you arrive on scene after the birth, it is still your responsibility to make the assessments based on your first observations. Remember, however, that care for the infant and the mother should not be delayed. The assessment is meant to take place while these other activities are being performed.

Your EMS system may call for a general or a specific evaluation protocol. A general evaluation usually calls for noting the neonate's ease of breathing, heart rate, crying, movement, and skin color. A normal neonate should have a pulse greater than 100/min, be breathing easily, be crying (vigorous crying is a good sign), be moving his extremities (the more active, the better), and show blue coloration at the hands and feet only. Five minutes later, these signs should still be apparent, with breathing becoming more relaxed. The blue coloration may or may not disappear, but it should not spread to other parts of the body.

A specific evaluation protocol that some EMS systems call for is an APGAR score. APGAR scores assign a number value to the neonate's assessment findings. Always remember that the APGAR score does not guide resuscitation efforts, and efforts to determine the APGAR score must never interfere with resuscitation efforts. Table 34-1 shows how an EMT assigns values to different aspects of a neonate's condition. The APGAR score is the total of the five values, and ranges from 0 to 10. It is traditionally determined 1 minute after birth and then again 5 minutes after birth. You should always follow the assessment protocol appropriate to your system.

Caring for the Neonate

Even with a normal delivery, each step in the care of the baby is essential for his survival.

Keeping the Baby Warm

The most important aspect of caring for a neonate is keeping the baby warm. Newly born babies rapidly lose heat. This heat loss not only impacts their comfort, but also can drop their glucose levels and even impact their ability to carry oxygen in their blood. For these reasons, you must consider heat retention a high priority. If the baby is wet, dry her (Figure 34-11). Discard wet blankets and wrap the baby in dry ones. Consider using a commercially available infant swaddler, as these "space blankets" are specially designed to retain warmth. Cover the baby's head.

Cutting the umbilical cord is a relatively low priority. However, if the cord has not yet been cut, raising the baby above the level of the vagina may transfuse blood back into the placenta.

Cutting the Umbilical Cord

In a normal birth, the infant must be breathing on his own before you clamp and cut the cord. Additionally, there is increasing evidence that you should wait at least one minute af-

Table 34-1   The APGAR Score

APGAR SCORE			
	0	**1**	**2**
Appearance	Blue (or pale) all over	Extremities blue, trunk pink	Pink all over
Pulse	0	<100	>100
Grimace (reaction to suctioning or flicking of the feet)	No reaction	Facial grimace	Sneeze, cough, or cry
Activity	No movement	Only slight activity (flexing extremities)	Moving around normally
Respiratory effort	None	Slow or irregular breathing, weak cry	Good breathing, strong cry

FIGURE 34-11 If the baby is wet, dry her. Then wrap her in a warm blanket or swaddler.

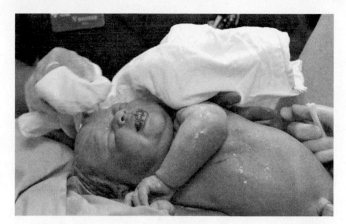

FIGURE 34-11 If the baby is wet, dry her. Then wrap her in a warm blanket or swaddler.

ter birth before clamping and cutting the cord unless there is a need for resuscitation. In most cases cutting the cord should be a relatively low priority and there is no rush to complete this task. Before clamping and cutting the cord, palpate the cord with your fingers to make sure it is no longer pulsating. Pulsation typically stops shortly after delivery.

NOTE: *Do not tie, clamp, or cut the cord of a baby who is not breathing on his own unless you have to do so to remove the cord from around the baby's neck during birth, or unless you have to perform CPR on the infant. Do not cut or clamp a cord that is still pulsating.*

The general procedure for umbilical cord care is as follows:

1. As already noted, keep the infant warm. Turn the heat up in the ambulance or the room you are in. Dry off the baby and wrap him in a baby blanket or infant swaddler, clean towel, or sheet prior to clamping the cord. Do not wash the infant. Sometimes the mother may request you to do so, but it is best to leave the protective coating (called the vernix) on the infant until he reaches the medical facility.

2. Use the sterile clamps or umbilical tape found in the obstetrics kit when cutting the cord. Use extreme care with any tying done to the cord, forming the knot slowly to avoid cutting the cord. Ties should be made using a square knot (right over left, then left over right).

3. Apply one clamp or tie to the cord about 10 inches from the baby. This leaves enough cord for intravenous lines to be used by paramedics or the staff at the hospital if they are needed.

4. Place a second clamp or tie about 7 inches from the baby. The proximal clamp should be about the width of four fingers from the distal clamp.

5. Cut the cord between the clamps or knots using sterile surgical scissors (Figure 34-12). Use caution and protect your eyes when cutting the cord as a spurt of blood is very common. Never untie or unclamp a cord once it is cut. The placental end of the cord should be placed on the drape over the mother's legs to avoid contact with expelled blood, feces, and fluids. Examine the fetal end of the cord for bleeding. Do not attempt to adjust the clamp or retie the knot. If bleeding continues, apply another tie or clamp as close to the original as possible.

6. Be careful when moving the baby so that no trauma is brought to the clamped cord. If the cord does not remain closed off completely, the baby may bleed to death from seemingly little blood loss. In most cases, the cord vessels will collapse and seal themselves.

If you are assisting at a birth when off duty, you will probably be able to find all the items you need to tie and cut the cord. If no clamps or tying devices are on hand, use clean shoelaces or similar soft, clean ties. If you tie the cord, believe it will be some time before you are able to transport and transfer the neonate, and do not have sterile scissors, soak scissors in alcohol for several minutes and use them to cut the cord. If the baby is still attached to the placenta when the organ is delivered, wrap the placenta in a towel and transport the

FIGURE 34-12 Cutting the umbilical cord.

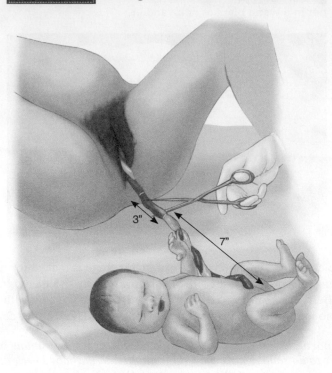

infant and placenta as a unit. The placenta should be placed at the same level as the baby, or slightly higher. Maintain careful monitoring of the baby.

Place the baby on the mother's abdomen (Figure 34-13) and allow the mother to begin breast feeding (if your local protocol allows).

During the birth process, the fetus is passive. However, once the baby is born, he very quickly becomes active. Exposure to the air is usually enough to stimulate the infant to breathe. As you suction, dry, and warm the baby, he is stimulated even more. If the baby is breathing adequately and has a heart rate greater than 100/minute but has central cyanosis (blue coloration of the torso), administer blow-by oxygen (Figure 34-14). If the neonate does not breathe on his own after drying and warming for 30 seconds, begin resuscitation measures.

FIGURE 34-13 Place the baby on the mother's abdomen.

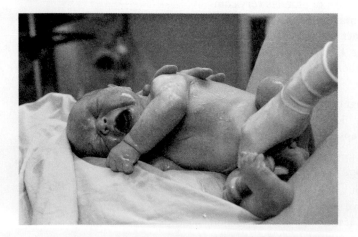

FIGURE 34-14 If the baby is breathing adequately and has a heart rate greater than 100/minute but has a blue coloration to the torso, administer blow-by oxygen.

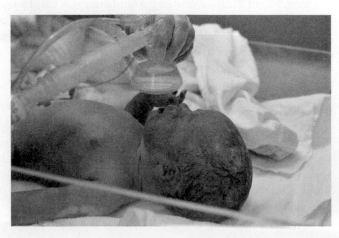

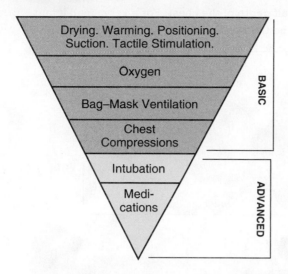

FIGURE 34-15 Inverted pyramid of neonatal resuscitation.

BASIC
- Drying. Warming. Positioning. Suction. Tactile Stimulation.
- Oxygen
- Bag–Mask Ventilation
- Chest Compressions

ADVANCED
- Intubation
- Medications

Neonatal Resuscitation

Neonatal resuscitation follows an inverted pyramid (Figure 34-15). Most neonates with abnormal assessment findings respond to relatively simple maneuvers. Few require CPR or advanced life support measures.

Follow these steps for initial care of the neonate:

1. Provide warmth and assess the baby's airway. If secretions obstruct normal breathing or if positive pressure ventilation is necessary, use a bulb syringe to suction the mouth first and then the nostrils. Squeeze the bulb before inserting the syringe into the baby's mouth. Release the bulb to create suction. It may be necessary to use a sterile gauze pad to clear mucus and blood from around the baby's nose and mouth.

2. Establish that the baby is breathing. Evaluate his respirations, heart rate, and muscle tone. Is the baby crying or breathing? Is the baby active and moving? Usually the baby will be breathing on his own. A neonate should begin breathing within 30 seconds. If he does not, then you must "encourage" the baby to breathe (Figure 34-16). Usually, a gentle but vigorous rubbing of the baby's back will promote spontaneous respiration. If this method fails, snap one of your index fingers against the sole of the baby's foot. Do not hold the baby up by his feet and slap his bottom! You should not become alarmed if the hands and feet of a breathing neonate appear slightly blue. It is not uncommon for this blue color to remain for the first few minutes.

    If assessment of the infant's breathing reveals shallow, slow, gasping, or absent respirations, provide positive pressure ventilation at a rate of 40 to 60 per minute.

NOTE: *Ventilate the neonate only enough to gain chest rise. These ventilations may be only small amounts of air if using mouth to mask, or small squeezes on the bag if using*

FIGURE 34-16 It may be necessary to stimulate the newborn to breathe.

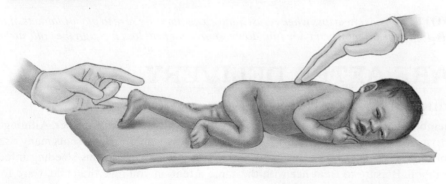

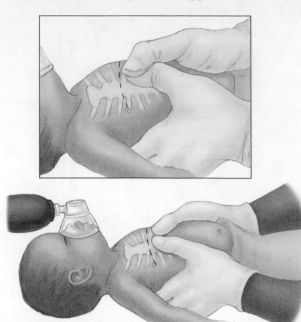

FIGURE 34-17 Deliver chest compressions midsternum with two thumbs, at a depth of one-third to one-half depth of the chest. For a very small infant (inset), the thumbs may be overlapped.

an infant-size bag-valve-mask device. Reassess the infant's respiratory efforts after 30 seconds. If there is no change in the effort of breathing, continue with ventilations and reassessment. It is not necessary to attach supplemental oxygen to the bag mask device during neonatal resuscitation. Use room air to deliver the initial ventilations and consider supplemental oxygen only if oxygen saturations remain low following the resuscitation.

3. Assess the infant's heart rate. If the heart rate is less than 100 beats per minute, then provide artificial ventilations at a rate of 40 to 60 per minute. If the heart rate is less than 60 beats per minute, initiate chest compressions, too, as shown in Figure 34-17. Chest compressions in the neonate should be delivered at a rate of 120 compressions per minute, applied over the lower third of the sternum with two thumbs and using fingers to support the neonate's back. The depth of compression is one-third of the anterior-posterior depth of the chest. Working at a 3:1 ratio of compressions to breaths in the neonate, the EMT should actually be delivering 120 "events" per minute (i.e., 90 compressions and 30 ventilations). Take care to allow full recoil of the chest following compression.

4. If the child has adequate respirations and a pulse rate greater than 100 per minute, reassess the airway. Suction if needed and consider oxygen administration. Supplemental oxygen should be administered if cyanosis persists or if oxygen saturation remains low more than ten minutes after birth. Oxygen is best delivered at 15 liters per minute using a nonrebreather mask or oxygen tubing placed close to, but not directly into, the infant's face.

NOTE: *Consider heat loss when resuscitating a neonate. Be sure to place blankets or towels under the infant when lying him down to prevent heat loss through the cold surface.*

CARE AFTER DELIVERY

Caring for the Mother

CORE CONCEPT

Postdelivery care of the mother

Remember that you have two patients to care for: the infant and the mother. Although it is easy to make the baby your primary focus, remember that childbirth presents many risks for the mother. A woman who has just delivered a baby is at risk for serious bleeding, infection, and emboli. Be sure to treat her with the same attention you give the child. Care for the mother includes helping her deliver the placenta, controlling her vaginal bleeding, and making her as comfortable as possible. Note that in some circumstances, like neonatal resuscitation, you may need additional help to accomplish this goal.

NOTE: *Some EMS systems recommend transport without waiting for delivery of the placenta. There may be a condition in which the placenta does not separate from the uterine wall, and it is important for the mother and baby to get to the hospital. You can always stop the ambulance to deliver the placenta if it crowns en route.*

Delivering the Placenta

The third stage of labor is the delivery of the placenta with its umbilical cord section, membranes of the amniotic sac, and some of the tissues lining the uterus (Figure 34-18). (All of these together are known as the afterbirth.) Placental delivery begins with a brief return of the labor pains that stopped when the baby was born. You will notice a lengthening of the cord, which indicates the placenta has separated from the uterus. In most cases, the placenta will be expelled within a few minutes after the baby is born.

Although the process may take 30 minutes or longer, avoid the urge to put pressure on the abdomen over the uterus to hasten delivery of the placenta. If mother and baby are doing well, and there are no respiratory problems or significant uncontrolled bleeding, transportation to the hospital can be delayed up to 20 minutes while awaiting delivery of the placenta.

Save all afterbirth tissues. The attending physician will want to examine the placenta and other tissues for completeness since any afterbirth tissues remaining in the uterus pose a serious threat of infection and prolonged bleeding to the mother. Try to catch the afterbirth in a container. Place the container in a plastic bag, or wrap it in a towel, paper, or plastic. If no container is available, catch the afterbirth in a towel, paper, or a plastic bag. Label this material "placenta" and include the name of the mother and the time the tissues were expelled.

NOTE: *If the placenta does not deliver within 20 minutes of the baby's birth, transport the mother and baby to a medical facility without delay.*

Controlling Vaginal Bleeding after Birth

Delivery of the baby and placenta is *always* accompanied by some bleeding from the vagina. Although the blood loss is usually no more than 500 cc, it may be profuse, which can lead to shock. Your reassessment of the mother must include evaluation of her bleeding and consideration of shock. To control vaginal bleeding after delivery of the baby and placenta, you should:

1. Place a sanitary napkin over the mother's vaginal opening. Do not place anything in the vagina.
2. Have the mother lower her legs and keep them together. Tell her that she does not have to "squeeze" her legs together. Elevate her feet.

FIGURE 34-18 Guide the placenta out as it begins to appear at the vaginal opening.

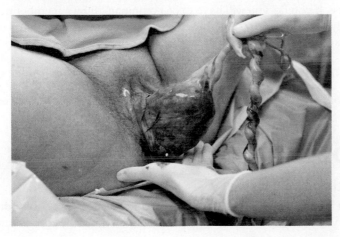

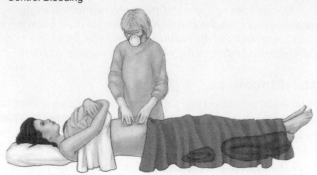

FIGURE 34-19 After delivery of the placenta, massage the uterus to help control vaginal bleeding.

Control Bleeding

3. Massaging the uterus will help it contract (Figure 34-19). This will help control the bleeding. Feel the mother's abdomen until you note a "grapefruit-sized" object. This is her uterus. Rub this area lightly with a circular motion. It should contract and become firm, and the bleeding should diminish. As this action will be very painful for the mother, you must explain that this procedure is necessary to stop serious bleeding.

4. The mother may want to nurse the baby. Although this will aid in the contraction of the uterus, some pediatricians recommend the baby not nurse until a doctor has examined the neonate.

A tearing of tissue can occur in the perineum at the vaginal opening during the birth process. The mother may feel the discomfort from this torn tissue. Let her know that this is normal and that the problem will be quickly cared for at the medical facility. Treat the torn perineum as a wound. Dress by applying a sanitary napkin and applying some pressure.

Providing Comfort to the Mother

Keep in contact with the mother throughout the entire birth process as well as after she has delivered. Your care for the mother does not end when you have completed your duties with the placenta and vaginal bleeding. Frequently take her vital signs. Be aware that she has just undergone a tremendous emotional experience and small acts of kindness will be appreciated and remembered. Childbirth is a rigorous task, and a woman is physically exhausted at the conclusion of delivery. Wiping her face and hands with a damp washcloth and then drying them with a towel will do wonders to refresh her and prepare her for the trip to the hospital. Replace blood-soaked sheets and blankets. Make sure that both she and the baby are warm.

When delivery occurs at home, ask a member of the family or a trusted neighbor to help you clean up. You should clean up whatever disorder EMS care has caused in the house; however, you should not delay transport in order to complete these activities. In some areas, local protocol may have you return to the house after transport in order to complete the clean-up process. If you do, you will have to be accompanied by a member of the family. Be sure to properly dispose of items that have been in contact with blood and other body fluids in a biohazard container.

NOTE: *Keep in mind that birth is an exciting and joyous event. Talking to the mother and paying attention to her new baby are part of total patient care. A good rule to follow is to treat your patient as you would wish a member of your family to be treated.*

CHILDBIRTH COMPLICATIONS

Complications of Delivery

CORE CONCEPT
Complications of delivery

Although most babies are born without difficulty, complications may occur during and after delivery. We have already considered three such complications: the cord around the neck, an

 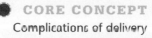

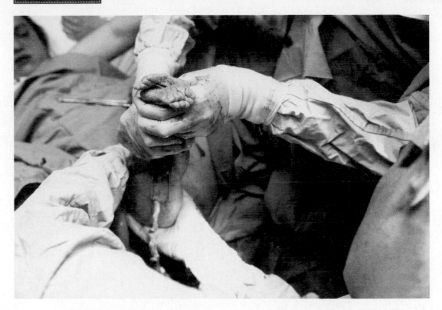

FIGURE 34-20 Breech delivery. *(© Eddie Lawrence/Photo Researchers, Inc.)*

unbroken amniotic sac, and infants who need encouragement to breathe. These problems can be handled by simple procedures. However, there are other complications that can threaten the life of both mother and newborn and for which definitive treatment is beyond the EMT's level of training. For emergencies such as breech presentation, limb presentation, and prolapsed umbilican cord, you will provide high-concentration oxygen and rapid transport to the hospital.

Breech Presentation

Breech presentation, the most common abnormal delivery, involves a buttocks-first or both-legs-first delivery (Figure 34-20). The risk of birth trauma to the baby is high in breech deliveries. In addition, there is an increased risk of prolapsed cord (see the next section). Meconium staining often occurs with breech presentations.

breech presentation
when the baby's buttocks or both legs appear first during birth.

PATIENT ASSESSMENT

Breech Presentation

If you evaluate a woman in labor and find the baby's buttocks or both legs presenting, rather than the head, this is a breech presentation. Breech presentations can spontaneously deliver successfully, but the complication rate is high.

PATIENT CARE

Breech Presentation

Emergency care of a patient with a breech presentation includes the following steps:

1. Initiate rapid transport upon recognition of a breech presentation.
2. Never attempt to deliver the baby by pulling on his legs.
3. Provide high-concentration oxygen.
4. Place the mother in a head-down position with the pelvis elevated.
5. If the body delivers, support it and prevent an explosive delivery of the head. Insert your gloved index and middle fingers into the vagina to form a "V" on either side of the baby's nose to lift it away from the vaginal wall in case the baby begins to spontaneously breathe.
6. Care for the baby, cord, mother, and placenta as in after cephalic delivery.

FIGURE 34-21 Limb presentation.

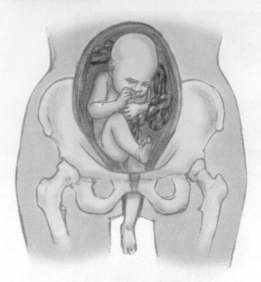 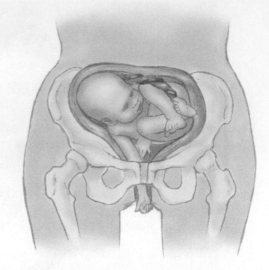

Limb Presentation

limb presentation
when an infant's limb protrudes from the vagina before the appearance of any other body part.

A *limb presentation* occurs when a limb of an infant protrudes from the vagina (Figure 34-21). The presenting limb is commonly a foot when the baby is in the breech position. Limb presentations cannot be delivered in the prehospital setting. In this case, rapid transport is essential to the baby's survival.

PATIENT ASSESSMENT

Limb Presentation

When checking for crowning, you may see an arm, a single leg, an arm and a leg together, or a shoulder and an arm. If one or more limbs present, there is often a prolapsed umbilical cord as well.

PATIENT CARE

Limb Presentation

When you discover a limb presentation, take these emergency care steps:

1. If there is a prolapsed cord, follow the same procedures as you would for any delivery involving a prolapsed cord (discussed next). Remember, you have to keep pushing up on the baby until relieved by a physician. The baby must be kept off of the cord if he is to survive.
2. Transport the mother immediately to a medical facility.
3. Place the mother in a head-down position with the pelvis elevated.
4. Administer high-concentration oxygen with a nonrebreather mask.

NOTE: *For a limb presentation, do not try to pull on the limb or replace the limb into the vagina. Do not place your gloved hand into the vagina unless there is a prolapsed cord.*

Prolapsed Umbilical Cord

prolapsed umbilical cord
when the umbilical cord presents first and is squeezed between the vaginal wall and the baby's head.

Sometimes during delivery, the umbilical cord presents first (this is most common in breech births) and the cord is squeezed between the vaginal wall and the baby's head. This occurrence is known as a *prolapsed umbilical cord*. When this happens, the cord is pinched, and oxygen supply to the baby may be totally interrupted. This is a life-threatening condition to the neonate.

Prolapsed Umbilical Cord

If, upon viewing the vaginal area, you see the umbilical cord presenting, the cord is prolapsed.

Prolapsed Umbilical Cord

Follow these steps when the umbilical cord is prolapsed (Figure 34-22):

1. Position the mother with her head down and pelvis raised with a blanket or pillow, using gravity to lessen pressure on the birth canal.
2. Provide the mother with high-concentration oxygen by way of a nonrebreather mask to increase the concentration carried over to the infant.
3. Check the cord for pulses and wrap the exposed cord, using a sterile towel from the obstetrics kit. The cord must be kept warm.
4. Insert several fingers of your gloved hand into the mother's vagina so that you can gently push up on the baby's head or buttocks to keep pressure off of the cord. You will be pushing up through the cervix. This may be the only chance that the baby has for survival, so continue to push up on the baby until a physician relieves you. You may feel the cord pulsating when pressure is released.
5. Keeping mother, child, and EMT as a unit, transport immediately to a medical facility. Be prepared to stay in this position until you reach the hospital.
6. All patients with prolapsed cords require rapid transport. Have your partner obtain vital signs while en route to the hospital, if possible.

Multiple Birth

When more than one baby is born during a single delivery, it is called a ***multiple birth***. A multiple birth, usually twins, is not considered a complication, provided that the deliveries are normal. However, prematurity and other complications are common with multiple births. Twins are generally delivered in the same manner as a single delivery, with one birth following the other. However, if a multiple birth is encountered, you should have

multiple birth
when more than one baby is born during a single delivery.

FIGURE 34-22 Prolapsed umbilical cord.

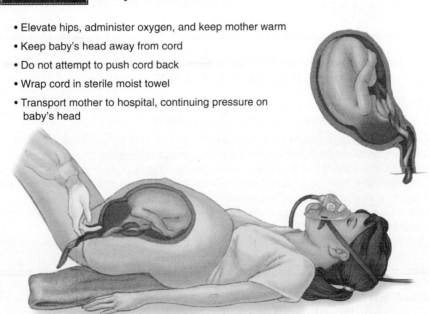

- Elevate hips, administer oxygen, and keep mother warm
- Keep baby's head away from cord
- Do not attempt to push cord back
- Wrap cord in sterile moist towel
- Transport mother to hospital, continuing pressure on baby's head

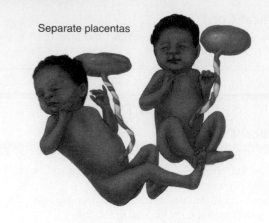

FIGURE 34-23 Multiple births.

Separate placentas

One placenta

enough personnel and equipment available for multiple resuscitations. Call for assistance if needed.

When delivering twins, identify the infants as to order of birth (one and two, or A and B).

PATIENT ASSESSMENT

Multiple Birth

If the mother is under a physician's care, she will probably be aware that she is carrying twins. Without this information, you should consider a multiple birth to be a possibility if the mother's abdomen appears unusually large before delivery, or it remains very large after delivery of one baby. If the birth is multiple, labor contractions will continue and the second baby will be delivered shortly after the first. The second baby may present in a breech position, usually within minutes of the first birth. The placenta(s) are normally delivered (Figure 34-23).

PATIENT CARE

Multiple Birth

When assisting in the delivery of twins, follow these steps:

1. Assure you have appropriate resources on-scene. Assume you will need to conduct multiple neonatal resuscitations simultaneously while still treating the mother.
2. Clamp or tie the cord of the first baby before the second baby is born.
3. The second baby may be born either before or after the placenta is delivered. Assist the mother with the delivery of the second baby.
4. Provide care for the babies, umbilical cords, placenta(s), and the mother as you would in a single-baby delivery.
5. The babies will probably be smaller than in a single birth, so take special care to keep them warm during transport.

---

premature infant
any newborn weighing less than 5 1/2 pounds or born before the 37th week of pregnancy.

Premature Birth

By definition, a ***premature infant*** is one who weighs less than 5 1/2 pounds (2 1/2 kilograms) at birth, or one who is born before the 37th week of pregnancy.

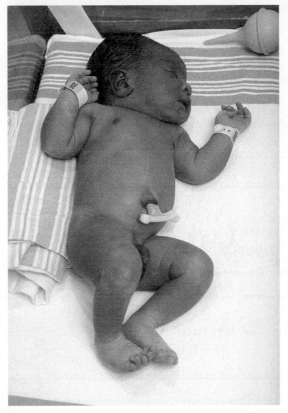

(A)

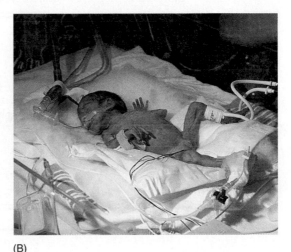

(B)

PATIENT ASSESSMENT

Premature Birth

Since you probably will not be able to weigh the baby, make a determination as to whether the baby is full-term or premature based on the mother's expected due date and the baby's appearance. If the mother is unsure of her due date, you can make a rough estimate by asking her when she had her last menstrual period and adding 40 weeks. Assessment of the baby itself might indicate prematurity. By comparison with a normal full-term baby, the head of a premature infant is much larger in proportion to the small, thin, red body (Figure 34-24).

PATIENT CARE

Premature Birth

Premature babies need special care from the moment of birth. The smaller the baby, the more important is the initial care. You should take the following steps when providing care for the premature infant:

1. Keep the baby warm. Premature infants are at great risk of developing hypothermia. Once breathing, the baby should be dried and wrapped snugly in a warm blanket. Additional protection can be provided by an outer wrap of plastic bubble wrap (keep this away from the infant's face) or a small reflective blanket. Premature babies lack fat deposits that would normally keep them warm. Some EMS systems in cold regions use plastic, bubble wrap, or a bag for the infant, covered by a blanket. This helps maintain warmth and allows for easier visual inspection of the clamped cord to check for bleeding. A stockinet cap should be placed on the baby's head to help reduce heat loss.
2. Keep the airway clear. Continue to suction fluids from the nose and mouth using a rubber bulb syringe. Keep checking to see if additional suctioning is required.

3. Provide ventilations and/or chest compressions as outlined earlier based upon the baby's pulse and respiratory effort. In some cases, resuscitation may not be possible if the baby is extremely premature.
4. Watch the umbilical cord for bleeding. Carefully examine the cut end of the cord. If there is any sign of bleeding, even the slightest, apply another clamp or tie closer to the baby's body.
5. Avoid contamination. The premature infant is susceptible to infection. Keep him away from other people. Do not breathe on his face.
6. Transport the infant in a warm ambulance. The desired temperature is between 90°F and 100°F. Use the ambulance heater to warm the patient compartment prior to transport. In the summer months, the air conditioning should be turned off and all compartment windows should be closed or adjusted to keep the ambulance at the desired temperature.
7. Call ahead to the emergency department and consider transporting to a facility capable of caring for a premature infant.

Meconium

As noted earlier, meconium is a result of the fetus defecating (putting out wastes). It is a sign of fetal or maternal distress.

PATIENT ASSESSMENT

Meconium

Meconium stains amniotic fluid greenish or brownish-yellow in color. Infants born with meconium are at increased risk for respiratory problems, especially if aspiration of the meconium occurs at birth.

PATIENT CARE

Meconium

If the baby requires resuscitation after birth and you see meconium staining in the amniotic fluid or on the baby itself, follow these steps:

1. To reduce the risk of aspiration, do not stimulate the infant before suctioning the oropharynx.
2. Suction the mouth and then the nose.
3. Maintain an open airway.
4. Provide artificial ventilations and/or chest compression as indicated by the infant's effort of breathing and heart rate.
5. Transport as soon as possible.

Emergencies in Pregnancy

CORE CONCEPT
Emergencies in pregnancy

A number of predelivery emergencies can arise in the pregnant patient prior to labor or childbirth. When assessing a pregnant female, consider the changes that have occurred to her body along with the pregnancy. Remember that you are really assessing two people, both the mother and fetus. Always complete a thorough assessment as you would any other patient. You may also consider asking the woman about bleeding or other vaginal discharge as well as syncope as these can indicate serious problems. Ask about the baby's movement. Typically after around 20 weeks a mother will begin to feel movement of the fetus. Although this is not exact, movement or a lack thereof can be a helpful assessment finding.

When treating a pregnant woman (or a potentially pregnant woman), respect her modesty and privacy. Remember that she may not want to share the information you are asking her with the world.

Excessive Prebirth Bleeding

A number of conditions can cause excessive prebirth bleeding late in pregnancy. You should consider any bleeding in late pregnancy a serious emergency. Whether the vaginal bleeding is associated with abdominal pain or not, the risk to both the mother and the unborn child is great.

A pregnant woman does not have to be in labor to have excessive bleeding from the vagina. For example, bleeding in early pregnancy may be due to a miscarriage. If the bleeding occurs late in pregnancy, it may be due to problems involving the placenta.

In one such condition, *placenta previa*, the placenta is formed in an abnormal location (low in the uterus and close to or over the cervical opening) that will not allow for a normal delivery of the fetus. As the cervix dilates, the placenta tears. Another such condition is *abruptio placentae*, in which the placenta separates from the uterine wall. This can be a partial or a complete abruption. Either placenta previa or abruptio placentae may occur in the third trimester. Both are potentially life-threatening conditions for the mother and fetus.

placenta previa (plah-SEN-tah PRE-vi-ah)
a condition in which the placenta is formed in an abnormal location (low in the uterus and close to or over the cervical opening) that will not allow for a normal delivery of the fetus; a cause of excessive prebirth bleeding.

abruptio placentae (ab-RUPT-si-o plah-SENT-ta)
a condition in which the placenta separates from the uterine wall; a cause of prebirth bleeding.

PATIENT ASSESSMENT

Excessive Prebirth Bleeding

The following are common signs and symptoms of excessive prebirth bleeding:

- The main sign is usually profuse bleeding from the vagina.
- The mother may or may not experience associated abdominal pain.
- During your primary assessment, you should look for signs of shock.
- Obtain baseline vital signs. A rapid heartbeat may indicate significant blood loss.

PATIENT CARE

Excessive Prebirth Bleeding

- If signs of shock exist, treat with high-concentration oxygen and rapid transportation.
- Place a sanitary napkin over the vaginal opening. Note the time of napkin placement. *Do not place anything in the vagina.* Replace pads as they become soaked, but save all pads for use in evaluating blood loss.
- Save all tissue that is passed.

Ectopic Pregnancy

In a normal pregnancy, the fertilized egg will begin to divide in the fallopian tube and eventually implant in the wall of the uterus. In an *ectopic pregnancy*, the egg may implant outside the uterus—for example, in the cervix or pelvic cavity. Ectopic pregnancies usually occur in the fallopian tube, which ruptures as the fetus grows. This results in internal bleeding.

ectopic (ek-TOP-ik) *pregnancy*
when implantation of the fertilized egg is not in the body of the uterus, occurring instead in the fallopian tube (oviduct), cervix, or abdominopelvic cavity.

PATIENT ASSESSMENT

Ectopic Pregnancy

The problems related to this condition are seen early in pregnancy. Indeed, some women with an ectopic pregnancy may be unaware that they are even pregnant when the signs and symptoms begin. Women may have signs and symptoms including those indicating shock due to internal bleeding. This condition can be life threatening and, as the saying goes, "Any woman of childbearing age with abdominal pain has an ectopic pregnancy until proven otherwise by the physician in the emergency department."

Be alert to recognize the following signs and symptoms as they develop:

- Acute abdominal pain, often beginning on one side or the other, which can also be referred to the shoulder
- Vaginal bleeding (often accompanies pain)
- Rapid and weak pulse (a later sign)
- Low blood pressure (a very late sign)
- Absent menstrual period, used to indicate a possible pregnancy

PATIENT CARE

Ectopic Pregnancy

Emergency care includes the following steps:

1. Consider the need for immediate transport.
2. Position the patient for shock.
3. Care for shock.
4. Provide high-concentration oxygen by nonrebreather mask.
5. Do not give the patient anything by mouth.

Seizures in Pregnancy

Seizures in pregnancy, sometimes caused by a condition called **eclampsia**, tend to occur late in pregnancy. The seizures are typically a result of a condition called **preeclampsia**. This condition is often related to pregnancy-induced hypertension and may be well known to the patient. Preeclampsia can be recognized by altered mental status; swollen hands, feet, and/or face; and high blood pressure. Seizures in pregnancy pose a serious threat to both the mother and unborn baby.

PATIENT ASSESSMENT

Seizures in Pregnancy

A seizure may be associated with any of the following:

- Existing preeclampsia or pregnancy-induced hypertension
- Elevated blood pressure, which increases the risk of abruptio placentae
- Excessive weight gain
- Extreme swelling of the face, hands, ankles, and feet
- Altered mental status, headache, or other unusual neurologic findings

PATIENT CARE

Seizures in Pregnancy

Emergency care of a pregnant patient with seizures includes the following steps:

1. Ensure and maintain an open airway.
2. Administer high-concentration oxygen by nonrebreather mask.
3. Transport the patient positioned on her left side.
4. Handle the patient gently at all times. Rough handling may induce more seizures.
5. Keep the patient warm, but do not overheat.
6. Have suction ready.
7. Have a delivery kit ready.
8. Contact ALS for immediate assistance.

Miscarriage and Abortion

For a number of reasons, the fetus and placenta may deliver before the 28th week of pregnancy—generally before the baby can live on his own. This occurrence is an **abortion**. When it happens on its own, it is called a **spontaneous abortion**, more commonly known as a **miscarriage**. An **induced abortion** is an abortion that results from deliberate actions taken to stop the pregnancy.

PATIENT ASSESSMENT

Miscarriage and Abortion

Women having a miscarriage that requires them to seek emergency care generally have the following signs and symptoms:

- Cramping abdominal pains not unlike those associated with the first stage of labor

- Bleeding ranging from moderate to severe
- A noticeable discharge of tissue and blood from the vagina

Ask the patient about the starting date of her last menstrual period. If it has been more than 24 weeks, be prepared with an obstetrics kit. Premature infants may survive if they receive rapid neonatal intensive care.

PATIENT CARE

Miscarriage and Abortion

1. Obtain baseline vital signs.
2. If signs of shock are present, provide high-concentration oxygen by a nonrebreather mask. Treatment should be based on signs and symptoms.
3. Help absorb vaginal bleeding by placing a sanitary napkin over the vaginal opening. Do not pack the vagina.
4. Transport as soon as possible.
5. Replace and save all blood-soaked pads.
6. Save all tissues that are expelled. Do not attempt to replace or pull out any tissues that are being expelled through the vagina.
7. Provide emotional support to the mother. Emotional support is very important. When speaking to the patient, her family, or in an area where bystanders may hear you, *always* use the term *miscarriage* instead of *spontaneous abortion*. Most people associate the word *abortion* with an induced abortion, not a miscarriage. It is essential to talk with the patient to gain her confidence and to allow you to provide emotional support.

Trauma in Pregnancy

Obviously the pregnant patient, like any other patient, can sustain injury. However, especially during the last two trimesters, the uterus and fetus are also subject to injuries when the mother is injured. Injuries to the uterus may be blunt or penetrating. In both cases, the greatest danger to the mother and baby is hemorrhage (bleeding) and shock.

The most common cause of blunt trauma is automobile collisions, although falls and assaults also account for many injuries. The uterus is well designed to protect the baby. The fetus is inside a muscular chamber filled with fluid. In this way, the uterus acts as an efficient shock absorber. Thus, most minor trauma to the abdomen, such as a blow or fall, typically does not harm the fetus.

Automobile collisions pose a high risk of injury, as the magnitude of forces in a collision is great. Because of its size and location, the uterus is frequently injured in these collisions. Sudden blunt trauma to the abdomen during the later months of pregnancy may cause uterine rupture or premature separation of the placenta (abruptio placentae). Other blunt trauma injuries, such as a ruptured spleen or liver, may also occur. Rupture of the diaphragm may occur with blunt trauma during later pregnancy. Multisystem trauma with fractures of the pelvis can cause laceration or tearing of the vessels in the pelvis, leading to massive hemorrhage. The common problem with most blunt injuries to the pregnant woman's abdomen or pelvis is massive bleeding and shock.

If a pregnant woman is injured in an incident such as a motor-vehicle collision or a fall, perform a patient assessment and treat her injuries as you would those of any other trauma patient. The best way to keep the fetus alive is to appropriately treat the mother.

PATIENT ASSESSMENT

Trauma in Pregnancy

During a trauma in pregnancy, follow these patient assessment steps:

- During primary assessment and assessment of vital signs, remember the following about the physiology of pregnant women:
  - The pregnant patient has a pulse that is 10 to 15 beats per minute faster than the nonpregnant female. Therefore, vital signs may be interpreted as being suggestive of shock when they are actually normal for the pregnant female.

- A woman in later pregnancy may have a blood volume that is up to 48 percent higher than her nonpregnant state. With hemorrhage, 30 to 35 percent blood loss may occur before otherwise healthy pregnant females exhibit signs or symptoms.
- Although shock is more difficult to assess in the pregnant patient, it is the most likely cause of prehospital death from injury to the uterus.

■ Question the conscious patient to determine if she has received any blows to the abdomen, pelvis, or back.

■ Ask the patient if she has had bleeding or rupture of the bag of waters. When in doubt, examine the vaginal area for bleeding, being certain to provide privacy.

■ Examine the unconscious patient for abdominal injuries, remembering to consider the mechanism of injury.

PATIENT CARE

Trauma in Pregnancy

Remember that maintenance of respiration and circulation and the control of bleeding are vital not only to the mother but also to the fetus. A developing fetus is critically dependent on the uninterrupted oxygenated blood supply that enters the placenta. What is good for the mother is good for the baby. Since the mother-to-be may have undetected internal bleeding or the fetus may be injured, provide the following care to the injured mother:

1. Provide resuscitation, if necessary.
2. Provide high-concentration oxygen by using a nonrebreather mask. (Oxygen requirements of the woman in later pregnancy are 10 to 20 percent greater than normal. If in doubt, give oxygen.)
3. Because of slowed digestion and delayed gastric emptying, there is a greater risk the patient will vomit and aspirate. Be ready with suction.
4. Transport as soon as possible. All pregnant women should be transported in the left lateral recumbent position, supported with pillows or blankets, unless a spinal injury is suspected. If so, first secure the mother to a spine board, then tip the board and patient as a unit to the left, relieving pressure on the abdominal organs and vena cava. Be sure to monitor and record the patient's vital signs.
5. Provide emotional support. A pregnant woman who is a trauma victim will naturally worry about her unborn child. Remind her that the developing baby is well protected in the uterus. Let her know that she is being transported to a medical facility that can take care of her needs and the needs of the unborn child.

Stillbirths

stillborn
born dead.

Some babies die in the uterus several hours, days, or even weeks before birth. Such a baby is called *stillborn*.

It is a tragic time for the parents and other family members when a baby is born dead or dies shortly after birth. Your thoughtfulness may provide the distraught parents with comfort. Never lie to the parents. Many death-and-dying experts believe that parents should be allowed to view the baby if they wish to.

Unless there is obvious death, all resuscitative efforts should be continued until the infant is transferred to the hospital (follow your local protocols). Also, keep accurate records of the time of stillbirth and the care rendered for completion of the fetal death certificate.

PATIENT ASSESSMENT

Stillbirth

When a baby has died some time before birth, death is obvious by the presence of blisters, foul odor, skin or tissue deterioration and discoloration, and a softened head. At other times, a baby may be born in pulmonary or cardiac arrest but in otherwise good condition. These babies have the possibility of being resuscitated.

Stillbirth

Emergency care for a stillborn baby is as follows:

1. Withhold resuscitative efforts from stillborn babies who have obviously been dead for some time before birth.
2. Provide full resuscitation measures for any babies who are born in pulmonary or cardiac arrest.
3. Prepare to provide life support when the baby is alive but respiratory or cardiac arrest appears to be imminent.

Accidental Death of a Pregnant Woman

If a woman in advanced pregnancy dies from trauma and you immediately begin CPR on her, there is a chance of saving the unborn child's life. CPR must be continued until an emergency cesarean section can be performed. Reposition your hands for compressions 1 to 2 inches higher on the sternum to make up for shifting of the heart due to the large fetus. If CPR is delayed 5 to 10 minutes, chances of saving the baby are fair, whereas a 25-minute delay reduces the chances to almost zero. Continue CPR on the mother until you are relieved in the emergency department.

GYNECOLOGICAL EMERGENCIES

Several emergencies may occur that are associated with the reproductive systems of women but not associated with pregnancy, including vaginal bleeding, trauma to the external genitalia, and sexual assault.

CORE CONCEPT
Gynecological emergencies

Vaginal Bleeding

Vaginal bleeding that is not a result of direct trauma or a woman's normal menstrual cycle may indicate a serious gynecological emergency.

Vaginal Bleeding

Since it will be impossible for the EMT to determine a specific cause of the bleeding, it is important that all women who have vaginal bleeding be treated as though they have a potentially life-threatening condition. This is especially true if the bleeding is associated with abdominal pain. The most serious complication of vaginal bleeding is hypovolemic shock due to blood loss. If a woman has been using pads to absorb bleeding, consider asking her how many pads she has used. This count may be helpful in assessing blood loss.

Vaginal Bleeding

1. Take Standard Precautions. Wear gloves, gown, protective eyewear, and mask as indicated.
2. Ensure an adequate airway.
3. Assess for signs of shock.
4. Administer high-concentration oxygen by nonrebreather mask.
5. Transport.

Trauma to the External Genitalia

Trauma to a woman's external genitalia can be difficult to care for because of the patient's modesty and the severe pain often involved with such injuries. You should always consider assault a possibility in this type of trauma as it is the leading cause of external genitalia trauma.

PATIENT ASSESSMENT

Trauma to the External Genitalia

Injuries in this area tend to bleed profusely because of the rich blood supply provided to the area. Injuries to the female external genitalia are frequently the result of straddle-type injuries:

- In sizing up the scene, observe for mechanisms of injury.
- During primary assessment, look for signs of severe blood loss and shock.
- Consider the potential for additional internal injuries.

PATIENT CARE

Trauma to the External Genitalia

1. Maintain a professional attitude.
2. Control bleeding with direct pressure over a bulky dressing or sanitary pad. (If the patient is alert, she will probably prefer to do this herself.) Do not remove the patient's undergarments unless necessary. Do not pack the vagina.
3. If signs of shock are present, treat with high-concentration oxygen.
4. Respect the patient's privacy. Remove unneeded bystanders and expose the patient's body only to the extent necessary to provide appropriate care.
5. Consider the possibility of assault. Contact law enforcement, and consider providing social service referrals.

Sexual Assault

Situations in which a sexual assault has occurred are always a challenge to the EMT. Care of the patient must include both medical and psychological considerations. In addition, law enforcement agencies are also frequently involved.

There is no question that the sexual assault patient is under tremendous stress. Because of this, you must be prepared to deal with a wide range of emotions that the patient may exhibit. The best approach is to be nonjudgmental and to maintain a professional but compassionate attitude. Unless it delays care, it is generally preferable that an EMT of the same sex as the patient establish rapport and be the primary provider of emergency care.

PATIENT ASSESSMENT

Sexual Assault

- Since you may be entering a potential crime scene, ensure that the scene is safe prior to entering. It may be necessary to "stage" your unit near the scene until it is rendered safe by police.

- Be professional and compassionate. Be nonjudgmental in your questioning and do not make promises you cannot keep. For example, avoiding saying things like, "It will be OK," or "He'll definitely go to jail."

- Be conscious of personal space. Explain your examinations and treatments beforehand. Be sensitive to the patient's fears and embarrassment.

- During assessment, identify and treat both the medical and the psychological needs of the patient.

Sexual Assault

1. Treat immediate life threats.
2. Be careful not to disturb potential criminal evidence unless it is absolutely necessary for patient care.
3. Examine the genitals only if severe bleeding is present.
4. Discourage the patient from bathing, voiding, or cleansing any wounds, as this may result in loss of important evidence.
5. Fulfill any reporting requirements that are locally mandated.
6. Learn what social service resources are available in your area. Consider providing referrals.

CHAPTER REVIEW

Key Facts and Concepts

- Although birth is a natural process that usually takes place without complications, the involvement of EMS usually indicates something unusual has happened.

- The EMT's role at a birth is generally to provide reassurance and to assist the mother in the delivery of her baby.

- During the normal delivery, the EMT will evaluate the mother to determine if there should be immediate transport to a medical facility or if birth is imminent and will take place at the scene.

- If birth is to take place at the scene, the EMT must prepare for the worst. Have equipment ready and appropriate resources on hand. Always be prepared for the neonatal resuscitation.

- Complications of delivery represent a true emergency. An EMT must be prepared to initiate rapid transport in the case of breech presentation, prolapsed umbilical cord, limb presentation, premature birth, or meconium staining of the amniotic fluid.

- There may also be predelivery emergencies, or emergencies associated with pregnancy (such as excessive bleeding, ectopic pregnancy, seizures, abortion, or trauma to the pregnant mother) that the EMT must be prepared to treat.

- Stillbirth, death of the mother, and sexual assault are difficult emergencies the EMT is occasionally called upon to manage. Emotional care for these issues may be as important as medical care.

Key Decisions

- Is there time to transport this woman in labor to the hospital or should I prepare for delivery on-scene?

- Should I anticipate a neonatal resuscitation after delivery? Do I have the necessary resources on-scene?

- During neonatal assessment, are there necessary interventions I must perform?

- In a gynecological emergency involving vaginal bleeding, how serious is the vaginal bleeding?

Chapter Glossary

abortion spontaneous (miscarriage) or induced termination of pregnancy.

abruptio placentae (ab-RUPT-si-o plah-SENT-ta) a condition in which the placenta separates from the uterine wall; a cause of prebirth bleeding.

afterbirth the placenta, membranes of the amniotic sac, part of the umbilical cord, and some tissues from the lining of the uterus that are delivered after the birth of the baby.

amniotic (am-ne-OT-ik) *sac* the "bag of waters" that surrounds the developing fetus.

Braxton-Hicks (braks-tun-hiks) *contractions* irregular prelabor contractions of the uterus.

breech presentation when the baby's buttocks or both legs appear first during birth.

cephalic (se-FAL-ik) *presentation* when the baby appears head first during birth. This is the normal presentation.

cervix (SUR-viks) the neck of the uterus at the entrance to the birth canal.

crowning when part of the baby is visible through the vaginal opening.

eclampsia (e-KLAMP-se-ah) a severe complication of pregnancy that produces seizures and coma.

ectopic (ek-TOP-ik) *pregnancy* when implantation of the fertilized egg is not in the body of the uterus, occurring instead in the fallopian tube (oviduct), cervix, or abdominopelvic cavity.

embryo (EM-bree-o) the baby from fertilization to 8 weeks of development.

fallopian (fu-LO-pe-an) *tube* the narrow tube that connects the ovary to the uterus. Also called the *oviduct*.

fetus (FE-tus) the baby from 8 weeks of development to birth.

induced abortion expulsion of a fetus as a result of deliberate actions taken to stop the pregnancy.

labia (LAY-be-uh) soft tissues that protect the entrance to the vagina.

labor the three stages of the delivery of a baby that begin with the contractions of the uterus and end with the expulsion of the placenta.

lightening the sensation of the fetus moving from high in the abdomen to low in the birth canal.

limb presentation when an infant's limb protrudes from the vagina before the appearance of any other body part.

meconium staining amniotic fluid that is greenish or brownish-yellow rather than clear as a result of fetal defecation; an indication of possible maternal or fetal distress during labor.

miscarriage *see* spontaneous abortion.

mons pubis soft tissue that covers the pubic symphysis; area where hair grows as a woman reaches puberty.

multiple birth when more than one baby is born during a single delivery.

neonate (NEE-oh-nate) a newly born infant or an infant less than 1 month old.

ovary (o-vu-RE) the female reproductive organ that produces ova.

oviduct *see* fallopian tube.

ovulation (ov-U-LA-shun) the phase of the female reproductive cycle in which an ovum is released from the ovary.

perineum (per-i-NE-um) the surface area between the vagina and anus.

placenta (plah-SEN-tah) the organ of pregnancy where exchange of oxygen, nutrients, and wastes occurs between a mother and fetus.

placenta previa (plah-SEN-tah PRE-vi-ah) a condition in which the placenta is formed in an abnormal location (low in the uterus and close to or over the cervical opening) that will not allow for a normal delivery of the fetus; a cause of excessive prebirth bleeding.

preeclampsia (pre-e-KLAMP-se-ah) a complication of pregnancy in which the woman retains large amounts of fluid and has hypertension. She may also experience seizures and/or coma during birth, which is very dangerous to the infant.

premature infant any newborn weighing less than 5 1/2 pounds or born before the 37th week of pregnancy.

prolapsed umbilical cord when the umbilical cord presents first and is squeezed between the vaginal wall and the baby's head.

spontaneous abortion when the fetus and placenta deliver before the 28th week of pregnancy; commonly called a *miscarriage*.

stillborn born dead.

supine hypotensive syndrome dizziness and a drop in blood pressure caused when the mother is in a supine position and the weight of the uterus, infant, placenta, and amniotic fluid compress the inferior vena cava, reducing return of blood to the heart and cardiac output.

umbilical (um-BIL-i-kal) *cord* the fetal structure containing the blood vessels that carry blood to and from the placenta.

uterus (U-ter-us) the muscular abdominal organ where the fetus develops; the womb.

vagina (vah-JI-nah) the birth canal.

Preparation for Your Examination and Practice

Short Answer

1. Name and describe the anatomical structures of a woman's body that are associated with pregnancy.

2. Describe the three stages of labor.

3. Explain how to evaluate and to prepare the mother for delivery.

4. Name, in the order of the inverted pyramid, the steps that may be taken to resuscitate a newly born infant.

5. Name and describe several possible complications of delivery.

6. Name and describe several possible predelivery emergencies.

Thinking and Linking

Think back to Chapter 2, "The Well-Being of the EMT," and link information from that chapter with information from this chapter as you consider the following situation:

- While assisting with an emergency out-of-hospital childbirth, you are sprayed with amniotic fluid. Afterwards, you find out that the mother is HIV positive. Who should you go to with this information? What should you do?

Critical Thinking Exercises

Your calm, professional demeanor is very important when you are called to care for a woman in labor. The purpose of this exercise will be to make a key decision for a particular patient: to prepare for delivery at the scene or to transport.

- You are called to respond to a pregnant woman who is in labor. During your evaluation, you find that this is the woman's first pregnancy, the baby's head is not yet crowning, and contractions are 10 minutes apart. You ask the mother if she feels like she needs to move her bowels, and she says she does not. Do you prepare for delivery at the scene? Or do you transport the mother to the hospital? Explain your reasoning.

Pathophysiology to Practice

The following questions are designed to assist you in gathering relevant clinical information and making accurate decisions in the field.

1. How would you expect the vital signs to change in a late-term pregnant female as a result of the pregnancy?
2. How would the changes in pregnancy alter your ability to recognize shock?
3. How should you assess the severity of a vaginal bleed? Why should you assume the worst?
4. What are your priorities in assessing and treating a neonate?

Street Scenes -

Your sleep is interrupted by the tones of the radio and the dispatcher saying, "Bravo 3, stand-by for a call." You swing your feet onto the floor and grab the radio. "Go ahead, dispatch," you reply.

"Bravo 3, respond to 77 Cherry Tree Lane for a pregnant patient in labor. The other dispatcher is still on the phone with the husband. Additional information to follow."

You and your partner head to the ambulance and start toward the scene. About 3 minutes from the patient's house, the dispatcher tells you that the baby appears to be crowning and the husband is still on the phone getting instructions. You and your partner decide you need a plan. You agree that both the adult and pediatric equipment need to be brought in, as well as the OB kit. You also agree that you will focus on the baby after delivery and your partner will provide care to the mother.

Street Scene Questions

1. What should be the first priority when entering the scene?
2. Should ALS assistance be requested?
3. What questions should you ask the mother or the father?

As you move toward the house, you ask the dispatcher if ALS has responded. You are told they are already en route. When you walk into the room, you see the mother on the bed and the father with the telephone cradled on his shoulder as he talks to the dispatcher. The father immediately stands aside, and you and your partner see crowning and realize that the delivery will take place any minute. You put on gloves and set up the OB kit while getting assess-

ment information from the mother. It is her second delivery but it is 2 weeks early. Labor started about an hour ago, and the pains have been more frequent lately and very intense. The water broke just before they called 911. While your partner is obtaining a set of vital signs, the baby starts to deliver. The head comes out and you notice that the umbilical cord is around the baby's neck. You are able to slip it over the baby's head, and the baby continues to deliver. The shoulders and the rest of the baby's body quickly follow.

Street Scene Questions

4. What immediate care should be provided to the newborn?
5. What care should your partner be giving to the mother?

You immediately start down the inverted pyramid for neonate resuscitation. You suction the mouth and then the nose. The baby immediately starts to cry. You dry the baby off and wrap the swaddling blanket around her, making sure that the top of the baby's head is covered. The baby is pink and actively moving. You check the pulse, and it is at least 150 beats per minute. Your partner clamps the cord and makes the cut. You call the dispatcher to log in the time of the delivery and announce that it is a girl. At that time, dispatch reports that ALS has been diverted to a cardiac arrest. After 20 minutes, the placenta still has not delivered and you transport the patient to the hospital without any further delay.

When you arrive back at the station, there is still time to get a couple of hours sleep. However, since you are too excited, you turn on the television instead.

35

Pediatric Emergencies

STANDARD
Special Patient Populations (Pediatrics)

COMPETENCY
Applies fundamental knowledge of growth, development, and aging and assessment findings to provide basic emergency care and transportation for a patient with special needs.

CORE CONCEPTS

— Anatomic and physiologic characteristics of children

— Psychological and personality characteristics of children of different ages

— How to interact with pediatric patients and their supporters and caregivers

— How to assess the pediatric patient

— How to identify and treat special concerns with the ABCs, shock, and potential hypothermia

— How to assess and care for various pediatric medical emergencies, especially respiratory disorders

— How to assess and care for various pediatric trauma emergencies

— How to deal with issues of child abuse and neglect and children with special needs

EXPLORE Resource Central

To access Resource Central, follow directions on the Student Access Card provided with this text. If there is no card, go to **www.bradybooks.com** and follow the Resource Central link to Buy Access from there. Under Media Resources, you will find:

▶ **Immobilization Considerations for Pediatric Patients**
Watch a video to learn how to properly immobilize a pediatric patient; how you should measure a cervical collar, and why it is important to use padding.

▶ **Some Differences between Pediatric and Adult Trauma Patients**
View an animation illustrating the differences between the anatomy of a pediatric and adult patient.

▶ **Communicating with Toddlers**
Watch how to interact with young patients, and their parents, in this video. Learn how you should position yourself and what you should and shouldn't say when communicating with a toddler.

OBJECTIVES

After reading this chapter you should be able to:

35.1 Define key terms introduced in this chapter

35.2 Describe the anatomic and physiologic characteristics of infants and children compared to adults and the implications of each for assessment and care of the pediatric patient. (pp. 878–882)

35.3 Discuss the normal vital signs ranges for infants and children. (p. 880)

35.4 Adapt history-taking and assessment techniques to patients in each pediatric age group. (pp. 882–886)

KEY TERMS

The term **pediatric** generally refers to patients who have not yet reached the age of puberty. Although sometimes this is difficult to determine in the field, puberty can typically be identified by breast development in females and hair observed on the face, chest, or underarms of males.

This population features an enormous range of developmental differences. Consider the significant anatomic differences between a 12-month-old child and a 12-year-old child. Although we would never consider the 12-month-old to be a "little adult," the 12-year-old child is probably more anatomically similar to an adult than to a baby. What this means to you as an EMT is that you must adjust your expectation to the developmental baselines of the age group. You must understand how anatomic differences impact your treatments and adjust your assessment to accommodate a patient who may or may not be old enough to answer your questions.

Dealing with pediatric patients requires specific knowledge, creativity, and patience. This chapter is designed to provide you with the tools you need to manage this special population.

DEVELOPMENTAL CHARACTERISTICS OF INFANTS AND CHILDREN

pediatric (pee-dee-AT-rik)
of or pertaining to a patient who has
yet to reach puberty.

Some important differences should be kept in mind when you are caring for a young patient. For example, since young children do not like to be separated from their parents, you will want to let the child sit in the parent's lap, if possible, during assessment and treatment; however, during transport the child must be appropriately restrained (Figure 35-1). Children will exhibit different characteristics as they grow older, and these will require the EMT to adapt treatment strategies, depending on the patient's developmental age. However, the psychological and social characteristics of infants and children cannot be specifically defined by their age. Often children develop at different rates, even among the same age group.

Just as a 6-year-old child is different from a 35-year-old adult, so is a 4-week-old infant different from a 12-year-old child. Children are constantly growing, learning, and, therefore,

FIGURE 35-1 (A) If at all possible, let a young child sit in the parent's lap during assessment and care. (B) During transport, the child must be appropriately restrained.

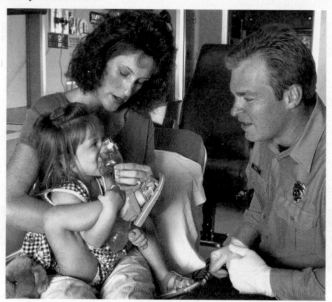
(A)

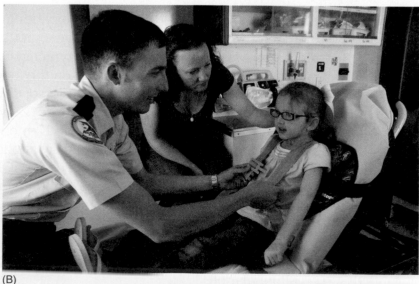
(B)

Table 35-1 Anatomic and Physiologic Characteristics of Infants and Children

ANATOMIC AND PHYSIOLOGIC DIFFERENCES COMPARED TO ADULTS	POTENTIAL IMPACT ON ASSESSMENT AND CARE
Tongue proportionately larger	More likely to partially obstruct the airway
Smaller airway structures	More easily blocked
Abundant secretions	Can block the airway
Deciduous (baby) teeth	Easily dislodged; can block the airway
Flat nose and face	Difficult to obtain good face mask seal
Head heavier relative to body and less-developed neck structures and muscles	Head may be propelled more forcefully than body, creating a higher incidence of head injury
Fontanelle and open sutures (soft spots) palpable on top of young infant's head	Bulging fontanelle can be a sign of intracranial pressure (but may be normal if infant is crying); sunken fontanelle may indicate dehydration
Thinner, softer brain tissue	Susceptible to serious brain trauma
Head larger in proportion to body	Head tips forward when supine, causing flexion of neck, making neutral alignment of cervical spine and airway difficult
Shorter, narrower, more elastic (flexible) trachea	Can close off trachea with hyperextension of neck
Short neck	Difficult to stabilize or immobilize
Abdominal breathers	Reliant on diaphragm to breathe; difficult to evaluate breathing
Faster respiratory rate	Muscles easily fatigue, causing respiratory distress
Newborns/infants typically nose breathers	Nasal obstruction can impair breathing
Larger body surface relative to body mass	Prone to hypothermia
Softer bones	More flexible, less easily fractured; traumatic forces may be transmitted to, and injure, internal organs without fracturing ribs or other bones
More flexible ribs	Traumatic forces may be transmitted to chest cavity without fracturing ribs; lungs easily damaged with trauma
Spleen and liver more exposed	Injury likely with significant force to abdomen

Source: Author: Andrew Stern, NREMT-P, MPA, MA

changing. In an ideal world, we might be able to tell exactly how a 4-year-old will behave. In reality, we have to put children into broad categories according to how children of their age group behave on the average. No system of categorizing children is perfect, but each has advantages for particular uses. This applies to psychological and social characteristics, as well as physical development. Children grow at different rates, and their size may not match their social development. Key anatomic and physiologic characteristics and their potential impact on care are summarized in Table 35-1.

After determining a child's age, if you are able to, attempt to have an age-appropriate conversation with the child. If that doesn't seem to work, then observe the child's interaction with a parent or caregiver for clues that might help you with your assessment and treatment strategies.

For basic life support (rescue breathing and CPR), the American Heart Association defines an infant as ages birth to 1 year, and a child as 1 year to puberty. However, these age ranges do not always apply to the care of children in other medical or trauma cases. In general emergency care, the following age categories are more useful to keep in mind:

- Newborns and infants: birth to 1 year
- Toddlers: 1 to 3 years

Table 35-2   Normal Vital Sign Ranges: Infants and Children

NORMAL PULSE RATE (BEATS PER MINUTE, AT REST)	
Newborn	120 to 160
Infant 0–5 months	90 to 140
Infant 6–12 months	80 to 140
Toddler 1–3 years	80 to 130
Preschooler 3–5 years	80 to 120
School age 6–10 years	70 to 110
Adolescent 11–14 years	60 to 105

NORMAL RESPIRATION RATE (BREATHS PER MINUTE, AT REST)	
Newborn	30 to 50
Infant 0–5 months	25 to 40
Infant 6–12 months	20 to 30
Toddler 1–3 years	20 to 30
Preschooler 3–5 years	20 to 30
School age 6–10 years	15 to 30
Adolescent 11–14 years	12 to 20

BLOOD PRESSURE NORMAL RANGES		
	Systolic:	Diastolic:
	Approx. 80 plus 2 × age	Approx. 2/3 Systolic
Preschooler 3–5 years	Average 99 (78 to 116)	Average 65
School age 6–10 years	Average 105 (80 to 122)	Average 69
Adolescent 11–14 years	Average 114 (88 to 140)	Average 76

NOTE: A high pulse in an infant or child is not as great a concern as a low pulse. A low pulse may indicate imminent cardiac arrest. Blood pressure is usually not taken in a child under 3 years of age. In cases of blood loss or shock, a child's blood pressure will remain within normal limits until near the end, then fall swiftly.

- Preschool: 3 to 6 years
- School age: 6 to 12 years
- Adolescent: 12 to 18 years

Age ranges will vary somewhat in different listings; for example, in vital sign ranges, as shown in Table 35-2. There will be calls when it will not be possible to find out the patient's age and you will have to make a guess, based on the child's physical size and emotional reactions.

Anatomic and Physiologic Differences

CORE CONCEPT

Anatomic and physiologic characteristics of children

Infants and children differ from adults not only in psychology but also in anatomy and physiology. (Review Tables 35-1 and 35-2.) Be sure to review the special characteristics of infants and children in Chapter 5, "Medical Terminology and Anatomy and Physiology." Understanding some of these differences will help you do a better job of assessing and caring for young patients. It is important to keep in mind the key differences in the following major body systems.

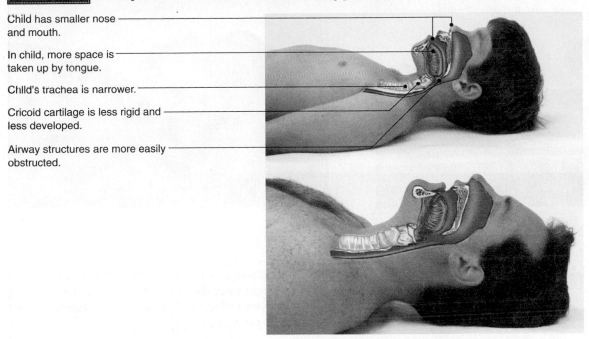

FIGURE 35-2 A comparison of child and adult respiratory passages.

Child has smaller nose and mouth.

In child, more space is taken up by tongue.

Child's trachea is narrower.

Cricoid cartilage is less rigid and less developed.

Airway structures are more easily obstructed.

Head

A child's head is proportionately larger and heavier than an adult's until about the age of 4. Because the head is often the heaviest part of the body, children often fall head first. As a result, you should suspect head injury whenever there is a serious mechanism of injury.

Up to about 1 year to 18 months, infants will have a "soft spot," just anterior to the center of the skull, called the anterior fontanelle. The *fontanelle* is flat and soft while the child is quiet and normally bulges when the infant is crying. A sunken fontanelle may indicate dehydration, whereas a bulging fontanelle may indicate elevated intracranial pressure.

fontanelle (FON-ta-nel)
a soft spot on an infant's anterior scalp formed by the joining of not yet fused bones of the skull.

Airway and Respiratory System

The infant's and child's neck muscles are immature and the airway structures are shorter, narrower, and less rigid than an adult's. There are several other special characteristics about infant's and children's respiratory systems that you should be aware of (Figure 35-2):

- The mouth and nose are smaller and more easily obstructed than in adults.
- The tongue takes up more space proportionately in the mouth than in adults.
- Newborns and infants typically breathe through their noses. Nasal obstruction can impair breathing.
- The trachea (windpipe) is softer and more flexible in infants and children.
- The trachea is narrower and is easily obstructed by swelling or foreign objects.
- The chest wall is softer, and infants and children tend to depend more on their diaphragms for breathing than do adults.

These differences in respiratory anatomy pose several implications for the emergency treatment you provide to an infant or a child:

- Because infants are nose breathers, be sure to suction secretions from the nose as needed to help the patient breathe.
- Hyperextension or flexion of the neck (tipping the head too far back or letting it fall forward) may result in airway obstruction. A folded towel under the shoulders of a supine infant or young child may help to keep the airway in a neutral in-line position (Figure 35-3).

FIGURE 35-3 (A) When an infant or young child is supine, the head will tip forward, obstructing the airway. (B) To keep the airway aligned, place a folded towel under the shoulders.

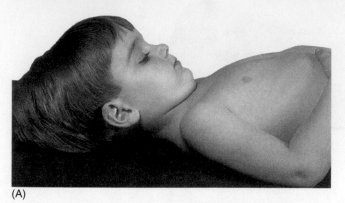

(A)

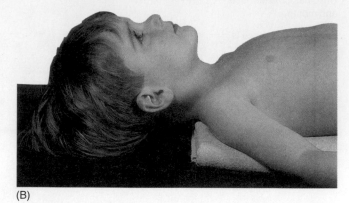

(B)

- "Blind" finger sweeps are not performed when trying to clear an airway obstruction in an infant or child because your finger might force the obstruction back and wedge it in the narrow trachea. An attempt to remove a foreign body airway obstruction should be done only when the obstruction is directly observed.

Chest and Abdomen

The less-developed and more-elastic chest structures of an infant or child make labored or distressed breathing obvious from a distance. The muscles above the sternum and between the ribs, and the ribs themselves, will pull inward when breathing is labored.

Infants and young children are abdominal breathers, using their diaphragms for breathing more than adults. Watch the abdomen as well as the chest to evaluate their breathing.

Abdominal organs are less protected in a pediatric patient. In adults, the rib cage covers more of the abdominal organs. In young pediatric patients, these organs are more exposed and take up proportionately more of the chest and abdomen. Younger patients also have less-developed chest muscles and more flexible bones. Because of this, abdominal organs are more susceptible to injury, and the force of trauma is often transferred throughout the entire abdomen.

Body Surface

A child's body surface area is larger in proportion to the body mass, making the child more prone to heat loss through the skin. This makes infants and children more vulnerable to hypothermia, an abnormally low body temperature. (See Chapter 33, "Environmental Emergencies.") For this reason, temperature should always be a concern when assessing and treating pediatric patients. They must be kept covered and warm. Climate control in the patient compartment of the ambulance is very important.

Because a pediatric patient's head, body, and extremities are proportioned differently from an adult's (the head being larger, for example), the extent of a burn is estimated differently, using a special formula that was described in Chapter 28, "Soft-Tissue Trauma."

Blood Volume

As you would expect, the blood volume of a pediatric patient is less than the blood volume of an adult (Figure 35-4). A newborn does not have enough blood to fill a 12-ounce soda can, and an 8-year-old has only about 2 liters of blood. Blood loss that might be considered moderate in an adult can be a life-threatening situation for a child.

- - - - - - - - - ● CORE CONCEPT
Psychological and personality
characteristics of children of
different ages

Psychological and Personality Characteristics

Each age group has its own general characteristics of psychology and personality that will affect the way you assess and care for the patient. These are outlined in Table 35-3.

FIGURE 35-4 A comparison of infant, child, and adolescent/adult blood volumes.

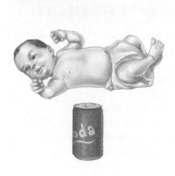
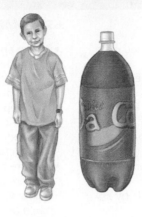
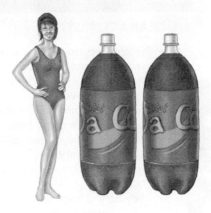

9-pound newborn:
Blood volume equals less than a 12-oz (335 mL) can of a soft drink

60-pound child:
Blood volume equals about a 2-liter bottle of a soft drink

125-pound adult:
Blood volume equals about two 2-liter bottles of a soft drink

Table 35-3 Developmental Characteristics of Infants and Children (continued)		
AGE GROUP	**CHARACTERISTICS**	**ASSESSMENT AND CARE STRATEGIES**
Newborns and infants birth to 1 year 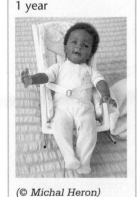 (© Michal Heron)	• Newborns typically have minimal stranger anxiety and do not mind being separated from their parents. Older infants often fear separation. • Infants are used to being undressed but like to feel warm, physically and emotionally. • The younger infant follows movement with his eyes. • The older infant is more active, and is developing a personality. • Infants do not want to be "suffocated" by an oxygen mask.	• Have the parent hold the infant while you examine him. • Be sure to keep him warm—warm your hands and stethoscope before touching the infant. As infants can easily become hypothermic, keep the ambulance compartment warm and the child properly covered during cool or cold weather. • It may be best to observe breathing from a distance, noting the patient's work of breathing, the level of activity, and skin color. • Examine the heart and lungs first and the head last. This is perceived as less threatening to the infant and therefore less likely to start him crying. • A pediatric nonrebreather mask may be held near the face to provide "blow-by" oxygen.
Toddlers 1 to 3 years 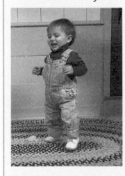 (© Michal Heron)	• Toddlers do not like to be touched or separated from their parents. • Toddlers may believe that their illness is a punishment for being bad. • Unlike infants, they do not like having their clothing removed. • They frighten easily, overreact, and have a fear of needles and pain. • Toddlers may understand more than they communicate. • They begin to assert their independence. • They do not want to be "suffocated" by an oxygen mask. • Toddlers do not like to be restrained.	• When appropriate, have a parent hold the child while you examine him. • Assure the child that he was not bad. • Remove an article of clothing, examine the area, and then replace the clothing. Do your best to respect the child's modesty. • Examine in a trunk-to-head approach to build confidence. (Touching the head first may be frightening.) • Explain what you are going to do in terms the toddler can understand (taking the blood pressure becomes a squeeze or a hug on the arm). • Assert control over the situation, but give the toddler the opportunity to make some decisions: "Which arm would you like me to check your blood pressure on?" • Restrain only when necessary. Restrain well when indicated.

(continued)

AGE GROUP	CHARACTERISTICS	ASSESSMENT AND CARE STRATEGIES
Preschool 3 to 6 years 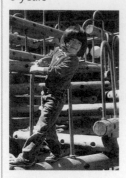 (© Michal Heron)	• Preschoolers do not like to be touched or separated from their parents. • They are modest and do not like their clothing removed. • Preschoolers may believe that their illness is a punishment for being bad. • Preschoolers have a fear of blood, pain, and permanent injury. • They are curious, communicative, and can be cooperative. • They do not want to be "suffocated" by an oxygen mask.	• When appropriate, have a parent hold the child while you examine him. • Respect the child's modesty. Remove an article of clothing, examine the area, and then replace the clothing. • Have a calm, confident, reassuring, respectful manner. Beware of teasing a child. Often children do not understand sarcasm. • Be sure to offer explanations about what you are doing. • Allow simple decision making. Allow the child the responsibility of giving the history. • Explain as you examine. • If desired, hold a pediatric nonrebreather mask near the face to provide "blow-by" oxygen.
School age 6 to 12 years 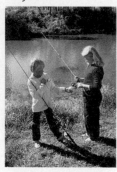 (© Michal Heron)	• This age group cooperates but likes their opinions heard. • They fear blood, pain, disfigurement, and permanent injury. • School-age children are modest and do not like their bodies exposed.	• Allow simple decision making. Allow the child the responsibility of giving the history. • Explain as you examine. • Present a confident, calm, and respectful manner. • Respect the child's modesty.
Adolescent 12 to 18 years 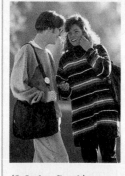 (© Index Stock)	• Adolescents want to be treated as adults. • Adolescents generally feel that they are indestructible but may have fears of permanent injury and disfigurement. • Adolescents vary in their emotional and physical development and may not be comfortable with their changing bodies. • Adolescents are influenced highly by their peers.	• Although they wish to be treated as adults, they may need as much support as children. • Present a confident, calm, and respectful manner. • Be sure to explain what you are doing. • Respect modesty. You may consider assessing adolescents away from their parents. Have the physical exam done by an EMT of the same sex as the patient if possible. • Avoid causing embarrassment in groups. Be sensitive to the adolescent's dignity.

One thing you should note about crying children: To many of your younger patients, you are a scary stranger. To a child who is already injured or ill, a stranger can bring about a strong response in the form of fear and crying. In younger patients, this is an expected response and a lack of it can often indicate an altered mental status. Remember that you can still assess a crying child. Although the noise may make the assessment more difficult, it is still possible. Consider taking steps to gain as much information as you can before approaching the child. When possible, perform a visual assessment from across the room prior to laying hands on the youngster. Consider also your approach. Do you really need six responders in the room with the scared child? Positioning yourself at the child's eye level rather than looming over him may make the young patient less afraid. Speak slowly and quietly to the child to help calm him. Often a certain amount of strategy can improve your interaction.

Never let the potential of upsetting a child prevent you from delivering appropriate treatment. Although many of the things we do will cause the child to cry, for the most part we still need to do those things. Toddlers hate spinal immobilization; however, if it is indicated we need to do it, no matter how much it upsets the child or hurts our ears.

Interacting with the Pediatric Patient

You will not be able to interview infants and most toddlers the same way you would an adult patient. However, parents or care providers can usually provide a history of a small child's illness or injury.

Preschoolers can usually be interviewed if you take your time and keep your language simple. School-age children will be able to describe more clearly how they feel and what happened. They will talk with you honestly, but may feel that the injury or illness is a punishment for something they did. They must be reassured and told it is all right to feel sick or hurt or to cry. Before telling the child something or asking him a question, take a second to think about how the child might interpret what you are about to say. This may help you to minimize the child's confusion or anxiety. Beware of sarcasm and teasing. Often preschoolers do not understand that you are joking. Even older children may feel powerless to answer back or defend themselves.

Include parents, teachers, and/or care providers in your interview. Since they are often the most valuable source of information for your assessment, do not exclude them. Seeing that familiar adults are being included gains the child's confidence if you follow-up by talking directly to the child. If the parents are injured, the child needs to know that someone is caring for him as well.

All patients have some degree of fear at the emergency scene. Infants and children are usually more fearful than adults because they lack experience with illness and injury. In addition to this, children are easily frightened by the unknown. Since so many details of the emergency scene are unknowns, it is easy to see why emergencies can be scary for children. The elements associated with the emergency (pain, noise, bright lights, cold) can set off a panic reaction in infants.

At an emergency, if the child does not understand you, or believes that you do not understand in return, his fear will increase. If the child is to communicate, he must remain calm. Putting the child at ease is a very important part of the care you must provide. Some children, when stressed, will act like a younger child. This is called *regression*.

Any problems faced by the child will be intensified if the parents are not at the scene. Children find security through their parents when facing new problems or emergencies. Asking for mom or dad may be the child's first priority, even above that of having your help.

When dealing with pediatric patients you should:

1. Identify yourself simply by saying, "Hi, I'm Pat. What's your name?"

2. Let the child know that someone has called or will call his parents.

3. Determine if there are life-threatening problems and immediately treat them. If there are no problems of this nature, continue at a relaxed pace. Fearful children cannot take the pressure of a rapidly paced assessment and confusing questions fired at them by a stranger.

4. Let the child have any nearby toy that he may want.

5. Kneel or sit at the child's eye level. Ensure that bright light is not directly behind you and shining into the child's eyes.

6. *Smile*. This is a familiar sign from adults that reassures children.

7. Touch the child or hold his hand or foot. A child who does not wish to be touched will let you know. Do not force the issue; smile and provide comfort through your conversation.

8. Do not use any equipment on the child without first explaining what you will do with it. Many children fear the medical items that are familiar to the EMT, thinking they will cause pain. Always tell the child what you are going to do as you take vital signs and do a physical exam. Do not try to explain the entire procedure at once. Instead, explain each

How to interact with pediatric patients and their supporters and caregivers

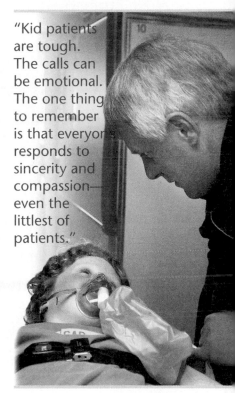

"Kid patients are tough. The calls can be emotional. The one thing to remember is that everyone responds to sincerity and compassion—even the littlest of patients."

step as you do it. Use simple language and remember that children tend to take things literally. If you tell a young child, "I'm going to take your pulse," he may think you are going to take something away from him. Instead say, "I'm going to hold your wrist for a minute." If the child is older, explain why.

9. Let the child see your face, and make eye contact without staring at the child. (Staring makes children uncomfortable.) Speak directly to the child, making a special effort to speak clearly and slowly in words he can understand. Be sure the child can hear you.

10. Stop occasionally to find out if the child understands. Never assume the child understood you, but find out by asking questions if the child is old enough to respond.

11. *Never lie to the child.* Tell him when the examination may hurt. If the child asks if he is sick or hurt, be honest, but be sure to add that you are there to help and will not leave. Let the child know that other people also will be helping.

The Adolescent Patient

In many ways, adolescent patients are almost like adult patients. Certainly they like to be treated as adults and are very sensitive to violations of their dignity or being addressed in a manner they believe is patronizing. However, when they are ill, injured, or frightened, they often regress emotionally and need as much support as younger children (Figure 35-5).

Adolescents should be able to tell you exactly what happened and how they feel. However, in the presence of parents or peers, an adolescent patient may not be completely communicative or cooperative. When injured, scared, or anxious, an adolescent may act immaturely or "act out." He may be embarrassed, intimidated by the attention, trying to hide the fact that he was doing something wrong, or feel pressure to show bravado. Tact may be required to get information from the adolescent patient and assessment may be more productive if this patient can be taken aside or into a private area.

Adolescents are especially sensitive to their peers and what they think. Adolescents may also be intimidated by those in authority, such as parents or teachers. Therefore, it is important to be very discrete when asking sensitive questions about drug or alcohol use and medical issues like a possible pregnancy. Such discussions should take place away from anyone who might overhear the conversation (for example, in the back of the ambulance or, if necessary, by waiting until you arrive at the hospital).

The young adolescent is often embarrassed or worried about the changes occurring to his or her body and uncertain if these changes are "normal." Handling the clothing of a teenager of the opposite sex can be awkward for the EMT as well as for the patient. In most cases, a simple preliminary description of the examination will set the patient at ease. How-

FIGURE 35-5 Treat the adolescent with respect.

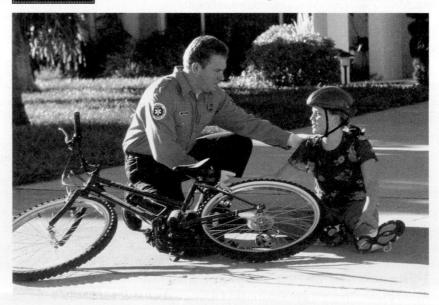

ever, you should make sure that both the adolescent and the parents understand what you are going to do and why it must be done. When possible, have the exam conducted by, or in the presence of, an EMT of the same sex as the patient.

However, do not delay patient evaluation and care because you or the patient may be embarrassed. As a professional, you must put such feelings aside and act in a manner that will allow the patient to relax and understand that there is no need for embarrassment.

SUPPORTING THE PARENTS OR OTHER CARE PROVIDERS

When your patient is young, you will need to make some adjustments in how you proceed with the assessment and care. This is especially true with regard to communicating with parents or other caregivers or providers. Children are very perceptive and will pick up on confidence as well as fear and anxiety in those they trust. What an EMT says, how he says it, and the calming influence he demonstrates can all make a difference in how a parent may respond and ultimately how effectively the EMT can interact with the patient.

Parents may react in one of several ways when their child suffers a sudden life-threatening injury or illness. Their first reaction may be one of denial or shock. Some parents will react by crying, screaming, or becoming angry. Another common reaction is self-blame and guilt. In all of these instances, be calm, reassuring, and supportive. Use simple language to explain what has happened and what is being done to and for their child.

In some cases, an upset parent may interfere with your care of the child. This is a natural reaction to protect the child from further harm. Usually, you can persuade the parent to assist you by asking him to hold the child's hand, give you a medical history, or comfort the child. If the parent is out of control, however, and cannot or will not cooperate, have a friend or relative of the parent remove him from the scene.

At this point, it should be noted that not all children live with two parents in a traditional nuclear family. The child may have a single parent or may be living with a grandparent, another relative, or even someone who is not related to the child. Whoever the child's full-time caretaker or guardian is, that person is likely to have the same emotional responses in an emergency as any parent. The EMT should be sensitive to the fact that the child may or may not call this person "Mommy" or "Daddy" and may be upset if asked about his mother or father. Tact is often required to find out who is responsible for the child and what the child calls that person. Though *parent* or *mom and dad* appear in this chapter, keep in mind that the terms are being used to stand for any person or persons who act as parents, guardians, or principal caretakers to the child.

You need to gain confidence and calm the emotions of all the people around the scene in order to be able to effectively treat the child. If you expect others to be calm, project a calm demeanor. Your interactions with the child will show everyone present your concern, and the manner in which you provide care will show your professionalism.

In general, involving the parent in the child's care helps both the child and the parent. The most effective method of involvement may be to have the parent hold the child in a position of comfort on his lap, if appropriate, during assessment and treatment procedures. Offer as much emotional support as possible to the parent. However, never forget that the child (not the parent) is your patient. Do not allow communication with the parent to distract you from care of the child.

ASSESSING THE PEDIATRIC PATIENT

Patient assessment is an extremely important skill for EMTs to learn, and with pediatric patients it may be even more significant for two reasons: First, the condition of sick and traumatized children can rapidly change. Second, sometimes signs and symptoms in children are subtle and will be missed without close observation.

CORE CONCEPT ●- - - - - - - -
How to assess the pediatric patient

The *pediatric assessment triangle (PAT),* which we will discuss next, helps categorize your assessment from across the room. It addresses three critical assessment elements and helps identify immediate life-threatening problems.

The information you gather using the PAT must be validated by next using the traditional patient assessment sequence you are already familiar with for adults. As already noted, you will need to customize your assessment somewhat to accommodate social and anatomic differences in children. This approach will follow the general format for assessment that was presented in Chapters 11 through 16.

Pediatric Assessment Triangle (PAT)

The pediatric assessment triangle (PAT) (Figure 35-6) is a method of pediatric assessment from two viewpoints. The first is the general impression formed as you approach the child, often referred to as an assessment "from the doorway." The second is the impression based on the remainder of the primary assessment that is done next to the patient. Each of the three sides of the triangle represents a different patient presentation that should be evaluated:

- Appearance
- Work of breathing
- Circulation to skin

The first impressions are those formed as you enter the scene and approach the patient ("from the doorway"). These first few seconds will provide you with a great deal of information that can be important in determining the seriousness of the patient's condition. This view from the door may also reveal information that will not be there if the child begins to cry.

For the first side of the triangle, look at the patient's *appearance.* Consider the child's mental status using the "AV" part of AVPU (alertness, verbal response). Is the child acting appropriately? How is the patient's muscle tone and general interactiveness? Is the child consolable by a parent or caregiver? Is his look or gaze and speech or cry appropriate?

For the second side of the triangle, observe the patient's *breathing (including airway).* Are there any abnormal airway/breathing sounds such as hoarseness, muffled speech, grunting, wheezing, stridor, or crowing? Is there any abnormal body position such as the sniffing position, tripoding, or refusing to lie down? Are there retractions, nasal flaring, "seesaw" breathing, or head bobbing?

For the base of the triangle, look at those signs that might indicate a *circulation* problem, such as pallor, mottling, or cyanosis (a gray-blue coloration).

FIGURE 35-6 The pediatric assessment triangle. *(Used with permission of the American Academy of Pediatrics)*

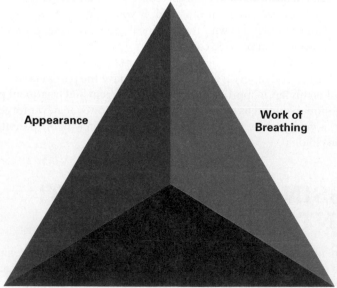

Appearance

Work of Breathing

Circulation to Skin

The remainder of the primary assessment is done up close in a hands-on manner. This confirms what you may already have surmised from your first, from-the-doorway impressions and may identify additional presenting problems requiring immediate interventions. During the hands-on primary assessment, the triangle again looks at appearance, breathing (including airway), and circulation—but with more precision. For *appearance*, you look at mental status using the "PU" part of AVPU (response to pain or unresponsiveness). For *breathing*, you start by ensuring that the airway is open and closely observing the quality of the patient's breathing. For *circulation*, you check for pulse, subtle cyanosis, and capillary refill.

The primary assessment is particularly important in pediatrics as threats to the airway, breathing, and circulation are the most common killers of children. Use primary assessment to identify life threats and treat them as you find them.

Some life threats in children will be subtle. For example, mental status is often difficult to determine in a child that has not started talking yet. Often these subtle indications of instability will be missed in a primary assessment. Therefore, unless you are treating a life threat found in the primary assessment, you should always continue on to a thorough secondary assessment. Identify physical signs that might indicate problems and use a patient history to add information to the situation. Remember that caregivers may often be the most important source of this information.

Keep in mind, assessment is an ongoing process!

The overall sequence of assessment steps is the same for the pediatric patient as for the adult patient. The following sections discuss special concerns for assessment of the pediatric patient.

Scene Size-Up and Safety—Pediatric

When entering an area where there is a pediatric patient, enter slowly and make some important observations. The first is to determine if the scene is safe. Even though it is a rare occurrence, sometimes there may be a risk from violence or abusive behavior, possibly directed toward the child. Look around carefully for any mechanism of injury.

Standard Precautions should be taken as appropriate. Additionally, be aware that ordinary childhood diseases can be devastating when contracted by an adult.

Primary Assessment—Pediatric

Forming a General Impression

A great deal of information can and should be gathered from the doorway, before you approach—and possibly upset—the patient. From across the room, you can gain a general impression of the child. First decide: Is the child well or sick? The child's general appearance and behavior will usually provide the answer.

A child who is alertly watching your approach, squirming and able to talk with you, or vigorously crying obviously has an open airway, is breathing, and has a pulse and blood pressure. If the child is silent, appears to be sleeping deeply, or is unresponsive, the child's airway, breathing, and circulation must be immediately assessed.

As you approach and form your general impression, use the PAT to make the following observations:

- **Mental status.** The well child is alert. Alternatively, the sick child may be drowsy, inattentive, or sleeping.

- **Interaction with the environment or others.** The healthy child exhibits normal behavior for his age. He moves around, plays, is attentive, establishes eye contact, and interacts with his parents. The sick child may be silent, listless, or unconscious.

- **Emotional state.** The well child's emotional state is appropriate to the situation. Crying may be his normal response to pain or fear. A withdrawn child or one who is emotionally flat is probably a sick child.

- **Response to you.** A well child may be interested in you or afraid of you. A sick child will give little attention to a stranger.

- **Tone and body position.** A sick child may be limp, with poor muscle tone. Pediatric patients with respiratory distress often assume characteristic positions that seem to help them breathe (e.g., leaning forward with hands on knees, referred to as tripoding).

retractions

pulling in of the skin and soft tissue between the ribs when breathing. This is typically a sign of respiratory distress in children.

- **Effort of breathing.** The well child's breathing should be unlabored. The sick child will be making a visible effort to breathe, including use of flared nostrils and **retractions** or pulling in of the tissues between the ribs.
- **Quality of cry or speech.** In general, a strong cry or normal speech indicates a well child with good air exchange. The child who can speak only in short sentences or grunts has significant respiratory distress.
- **Skin color.** A sick child may be pale, cyanotic, or flushed.

Assessing Mental Status

Use the AVPU method of assessing mental status, taking the child's age and developmental characteristics into account. You may need to shout to elicit a response to verbal stimulus. If necessary, tap or pinch the patient to test for response to painful stimulus. Never shake an infant or child.

Assessing the Airway

Consider not only whether the airway is open but whether it is endangered. A depressed mental status, secretions, blood, vomitus, foreign bodies, face or neck trauma, and lower respiratory infections may all compromise the airway. Be careful not to hyperextend the child's neck.

Assessing Breathing

First, assess whether or not the patient is breathing. If the patient is not breathing or is breathing inadequately, provide artificial ventilations with supplemental oxygen. If the patient is experiencing respiratory distress, provide high-concentration oxygen by pediatric nonrebreather mask. (See Chapter 19, "Respiratory Emergencies.")

To assess breathing, observe the following:

- **Chest expansion.** There should be equal movement on both sides of the chest.
- **Effort of breathing.** Watch for nasal flaring when the patient inhales, and retractions or "pulling in" of the sternum and ribs with inhalation.
- **Sounds of breathing.** Listen for stridor, crowing, or other noisy respirations. Breath sounds should be present and equal on both sides of the chest. Note the presence of grunting at the end of expiration, which is a worrisome sign.
- **Breathing rate.** Normal respiratory rates for infants and children are as follows: 12 to 20 per minute in an adolescent, 15 to 30 per minute in a child, 25 to 50 per minute in an infant. Breathing that is either faster or slower than normal is inadequate and requires artificial ventilation as well as oxygen.
- **Color.** Cyanosis (blue or gray color) indicates that the patient is not getting enough oxygen.

Assessing Circulation

As with an adult, check for normal warm, pink, and dry skin and a normal pulse as indications of adequate circulation and perfusion. For assessment, check the radial pulse in a child and the brachial pulse in an infant. For basic life support, check the carotid pulse in a child and the brachial or femoral pulse in an infant (Figure 35-7). In infants and children 5 years old or younger, also check capillary refill. When you press on the nail bed or press the top of a hand or foot, the area will turn white (Figure 35-8). If the patient's circulation is adequate, the normal pink color will return in less than 2 seconds, or in less time than it takes to say "capillary refill." Check for and control any blood loss.

Identifying Priority Patients

A patient who is a high priority for immediate transport is one who:

- Gives a poor general impression
- Is unresponsive or listless

FIGURE 35-7 For basic life support, check the (A) brachial pulse or (B) femoral pulse in an infant.

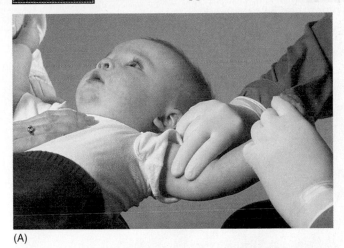

(A)

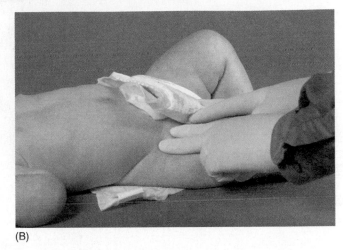

(B)

FIGURE 35-8 (A) Capillary refill—press. (B) Capillary refill—release.

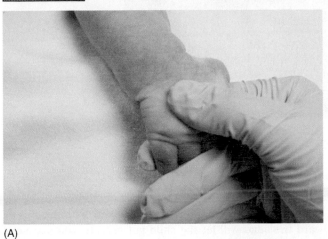

(A)

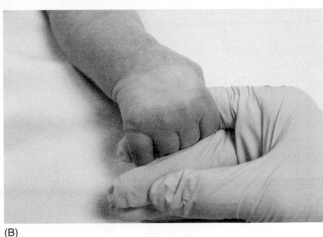

(B)

- Does not recognize the parent or primary caregiver
- Is not comforted when held by a parent but becomes calm and quiet when set down
- Has a compromised airway
- Is in respiratory arrest or has inadequate breathing or respiratory distress
- Has a possibility of shock
- Has uncontrolled bleeding

Secondary Assessment—Pediatric

At times, the child may be the only source of a history. He may be at school or another place where medical records are not kept or where adults who know his medical history are not present. In this case, get as much history as you can from the child by asking simple questions that cannot be answered with a "Yes" or "No." A child who cannot tell you where it hurts can usually point to the area.

Perform a physical exam for a medical patient and a rapid trauma assessment for a trauma patient, as you would for an adult. Explain to the awake child what you are doing, and do the exam in trunk-to-head order to avoid frightening the child.

Take and record vital signs, assessing blood pressure only in children older than age 3, using an appropriately sized cuff (Figure 35-9). Review Table 35-2 for normal ranges of pediatric vital signs. It may be helpful to carry a pocket guide or reference card with pediatric vital signs when responding to pediatric calls.

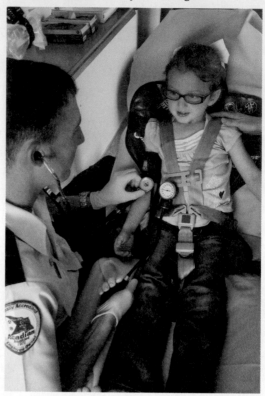

FIGURE 35-9 Take blood pressure in patients older than 3 years of age.

Physical Exam—Pediatric

The EMT normally performs the physical examination or body assessment in head-to-toe order; however, on alert infants and small children this is reversed. Starting with the toes or trunk and working your way toward the head will let the child get used to you and your touch before you attempt to touch him around the head and face. Playing with the infants' feet often puts them at ease.

Unless there are possible injuries that indicate the child should not be moved, a young child should be held on the parent's lap during the physical exam. Many EMS teams carry clean stuffed animals (like teddy bears) that can be given to a child during the physical exam. The toys can provide comfort to the child and allow you to explain the examination by using the toy as a model. Point to an area on the toy to show the child where you must touch and where you will bandage when you need to provide emergency care. This type of one-to-one communication also helps build parent and bystander confidence, letting them know that a professional, compassionate EMT is caring for the child. (If you use a toy, allow the child to keep it.)

Most very young children will suffer no embarrassment when you remove or reposition clothing during the exam. Nonetheless, protect the child from the stares of onlookers. Many children around the age of 5 to 8 go through a stage of intense modesty. You may have to keep explaining why you must remove certain articles of clothing. Many parents, teachers, and day care personnel teach children that strangers should not remove their clothing or touch them. The children that you examine may not understand your intentions and may resist. Some children may become upset because they feel you are taking something away from them. Take your time and do not rush children into accepting all that is happening. Remember that children rapidly lose body heat, so if you expose them, quickly cover them with a blanket.

The assessment of an infant or child is done to look for the same signs of injury and illness as in the case of the adult patient. However, you should take special care with components of the exam as discussed in the following sections (Figure 35-10 and Scan 35-1).

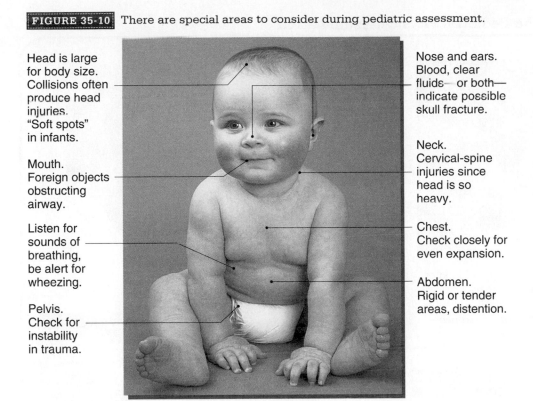

FIGURE 35-10 There are special areas to consider during pediatric assessment.

Head is large for body size. Collisions often produce head injuries. "Soft spots" in infants.

Mouth. Foreign objects obstructing airway.

Listen for sounds of breathing, be alert for wheezing.

Pelvis. Check for instability in trauma.

Nose and ears. Blood, clear fluids— or both— indicate possible skull fracture.

Neck. Cervical-spine injuries since head is so heavy.

Chest. Check closely for even expansion.

Abdomen. Rigid or tender areas, distention.

Head

Do not apply pressure to an infant's "soft spots" (fontanelles). The skin over the anterior fontanelle is normally level with the top of the skull, or slightly sunken. It may bulge naturally when the infant cries or be abnormally sunken if the infant is dehydrated. Meningitis and head trauma cause the fontanelle to bulge due to increased intracranial pressure. Collisions involving infants and children can often produce head injuries.

Nose and Ears

Look for blood and clear fluids coming from the nose and ears. Suspect skull fractures if either fluid is present. Children are nose breathers, so mucus or blood clot obstructions will make it hard for them to breathe.

Neck

Children are vulnerable to spinal cord injuries because of their proportionately larger and heavier heads. The neck offers less support because muscles and bone structures are less developed. In medical emergencies, the neck may be sore, stiff, or swollen.

Airway

Keep the infant's head in the neutral position and the child's head in the neutral-plus or sniffing position (chin thrust forward to maintain an open airway). If there is no suspicion of spinal injury, place a flat, folded towel under the patient's shoulders to get the appropriate airway alignment. Children's airways are more pliable and smaller than an adult's. Hyperextension or hyperflexion may close off the airway. For medical respiratory problems, the child will probably want to sit up.

Chest

Listen closely for even air entry and the sounds of breathing on both sides of the chest. Be alert for wheezes and other noises. Check for symmetry, bruising, paradoxical movement, and retraction of the sternum or the muscles between the ribs. Remember that a child's soft ribs may not break, but there may be underlying injuries to the organs within the chest.

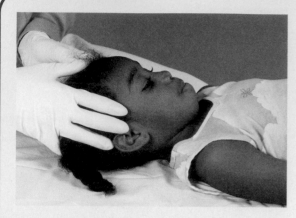

1 Examine the head. Look for bruising or blood or clear fluid draining from the nose or ears. Palpate gently for soft or spongy areas, skull irregularities, or crepitus (feeling of grinding bone fragments). Check the fontanelle in infants.

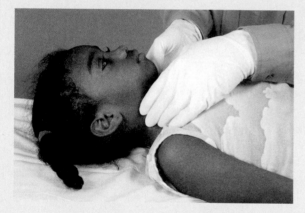

3 Examine the neck. Check for the position of the trachea, swollen neck veins, stiffness, tenderness, or crepitus.

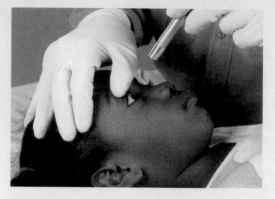

2 Check the eyes. The pupils should be equal in size and reactive to light.

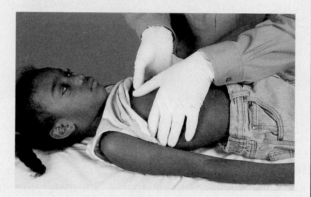

4 Examine the chest. Check for bruising, equal chest rise and fall, and crepitus. Watch for signs of breathing difficulty.

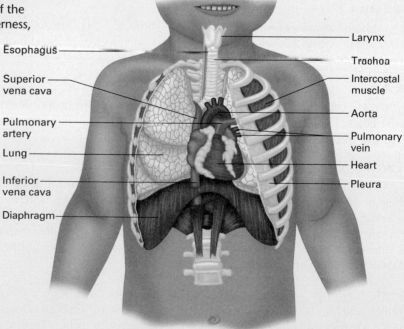

Esophagus

Superior vena cava

Pulmonary artery

Lung

Inferior vena cava

Diaphragm

Larynx

Trachea

Intercostal muscle

Aorta

Pulmonary vein

Heart

Pleura

While examining the chest, be aware of the contents of the thorax.

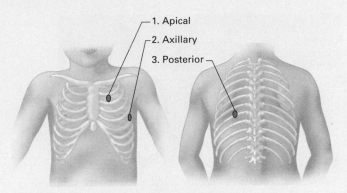

1. Apical
2. Axillary
3. Posterior

Auscultation sites.

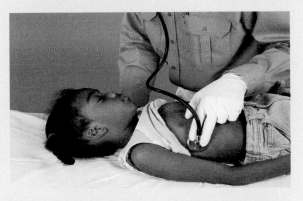

5 Auscultate for breath sounds over all lung fields.

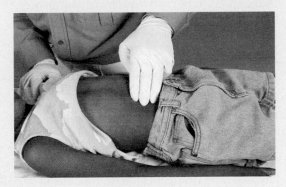

6 Examine the abdomen. Check for bruising, tenderness, or guarding. Look for swelling that may indicate swallowed air.

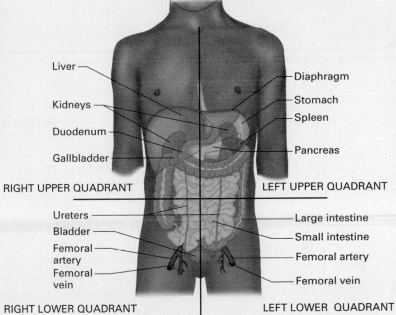

Liver

Kidneys

Duodenum

Gallbladder

Diaphragm

Stomach

Spleen

Pancreas

RIGHT UPPER QUADRANT

LEFT UPPER QUADRANT

Ureters

Bladder

Femoral artery

Femoral vein

Large intestine

Small intestine

Femoral artery

Femoral vein

RIGHT LOWER QUADRANT

LEFT LOWER QUADRANT

Divide the abdomen into quadrants and examine each one, while remembering which organs are located in each quadrant.

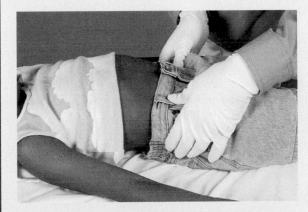

7 Examine the pelvis for tenderness, swelling, bruising, or crepitus. If the patient complains of pain, injury, or other problems in the genital area, assess for bruising, swelling, or tenderness in that area.

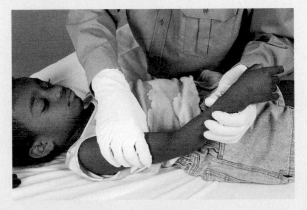

8 Examine the extremities. Evaluate pulses, sensation, and warmth. Look for unequal movement.

(continued)

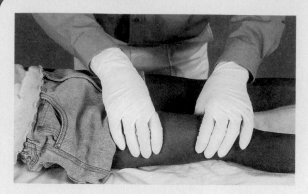

9 If you have immobilized an extremity, check the patient's capillary refill and peripheral pulses and compare them with the other arm or leg.

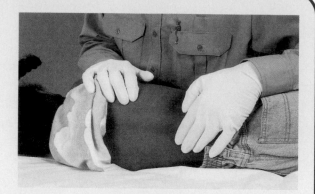

10 Examine the back. Assess for tenderness, bruising, and crepitus. If the child requires immobilization, the back can be checked while the child is being log rolled onto the spine board.

Abdomen

Note any rigid or tender areas and distention. Because a child's abdominal organs (especially the spleen and liver) are large in relation to the size of the abdominal cavity, and because there is little protection offered by the still-undeveloped abdominal muscles, these organs are more susceptible to trauma than an adult's. Because most children 8 years of age or younger are abdominal breathers, any injury that impedes the movement of the diaphragm can compromise a young child's breathing.

Pelvis

In trauma, check for stability of the pelvic girdle.

Extremities

Perform an assessment with capillary refill and distal pulse, including a neurological component for motor function with a sensation check. With an infant or young child, you do not have to press on a nail bed. You can quickly check capillary refill by squeezing a hand or foot, forearm, or lower leg. Check for painful, swollen, and deformed injury sites. (The bones of an infant or child are more pliable so they bend, splinter, and buckle before they fracture.)

Reassessment—Pediatric

Pediatric patients are dynamic—that is, constantly changing. Continual assessment is essential to good patient care. A rule of thumb for infants and children is: Don't take your eyes off them for a minute!

As time permits, you should do the following steps. In some cases in which the patient is seriously ill or traumatized, maintaining the airway and supporting ventilations will keep the EMT from performing a complete physical exam and history:

1. Reassess mental status.
2. Maintain an open airway.
3. Monitor breathing.
4. Reassess the pulse.
5. Monitor skin color, temperature, and moisture.
6. Reassess vital signs:
   - Every 5 minutes in unstable patients
   - Every 15 minutes in stable patients
7. Ensure that all appropriate care and treatment are being given.

COMPARING ASSESSMENTS

The following scenario may help you see the special considerations involved in assessing pediatric patients.

Dispatch

Two ambulance crews, including you and three other EMTs, have been dispatched to care for three victims of carbon monoxide inhalation: Andrea (16 years old), Megan (10 years old), and Eddie (11 months old). You find the patients inside a neighbor's home, Megan supine on the floor, Eddie crying in Andrea's arms.

Assessment of 10-Year-Old Girl (Megan)

Primary Assessment

Your partner's general impression is of a moaning 10-year-old girl. Megan's mental status is awake and crying. Her airway is open and her breathing is adequate in both rate and depth. Your partner's assessment of circulation reveals a strong, rapid radial pulse. Her skin is flushed and dry. There is no apparent external bleeding. Megan's priority is high because of the nature of the illness: carbon monoxide poisoning. Your partner calms the child as she begins administering oxygen by pediatric nonrebreather mask at 15 liters per minute and continues with her assessment.

Secondary Assessment—Medical

At first, like many sick children, Megan is withdrawn and not interested in communicating with your partner, who is a stranger to her. However, by treating Megan in a calm and friendly manner, your partner is able to gain her attention and confidence. The history your partner can gather is scant, however. The firefighter says Megan was found lying on the living room floor, very drowsy, and was quickly carried out of the house. Megan confides that the whole family started feeling sick at the same time and that right now her head hurts. A rapid physical exam reveals no injuries or other abnormalities. Baseline vital signs are pulse 140, regular and strong; blood pressure 100/70; and respirations of 28 and regular.

Assessment of 11-Month-Old Infant (Eddie)

Primary Assessment

The general impression formed by the EMT from the other ambulance is of an infant who appears to be in no acute distress. Eddie's mental status is awake and calm. He is moving energetically in Andrea's arms and looking around curiously at all the activity in the room. His airway is open and his breathing is adequate in both rate and depth. The assessment of circulation reveals a strong, rapid brachial pulse. His skin is warm, pink, and dry. There is no apparent external bleeding. Although Eddie does not appear to be in distress, his priority is high because of the nature of the illness: carbon monoxide poisoning. The EMT starts to administer high-concentration oxygen. Eddie fights the mask, but he tolerates "blow-by" administration with his big sister holding the mask near his face.

Secondary Assessment—Medical

Eddie's history—provided by Andrea—includes the fact that his sister had placed him upstairs in a crib when the family started feeling ill, so he was relatively far from the malfunctioning furnace. The EMT who is assessing Eddie gets him giggling happily by playing with his toes, then conducts a rapid physical assessment in a toe-to-head sequence. The assessment reveals no injuries or other abnormalities. Baseline vital signs are pulse 128, regular and strong; respirations of 30 and regular.

Assessment of 16-Year-Old Girl (Andrea)

Primary Assessment

The general impression is of a teenage girl who appears to be in no acute distress. Andrea's mental status is awake and oriented, although she is quite anxious about her sister and brother. Her airway, breathing, and circulation are all normal. Although she appears to be well, her priority is high because she has been exposed to carbon monoxide. The EMT gives her high-concentration oxygen, but first thinks to enlist Andrea's help in showing the mask to Eddie, smiling, and saying, "Look what I get to put on!" so Eddie won't be frightened by the mask on his sister's face.

En Route

Secondary Assessment—Medical

Andrea's history includes the fact that she had been upstairs with her baby brother and, like him, farther from the furnace than her little sister. The female EMT has gained Andrea's confidence by treating her with professionalism and respect. Andrea admits that she is afraid she has done herself some permanent injury by breathing carbon monoxide and also feels guilty that she didn't do more to help her siblings. The EMT is able to comfort and reassure her. She explains to Andrea the elements of the rapid physical assessment before she conducts it. She is careful to protect Andrea's privacy during the exam, which reveals no injuries or other abnormalities. Baseline vital signs are pulse 70, regular and strong; blood pressure 94/60; respirations of 18 and regular.

Backup drivers have been sent to the scene so members of each ambulance crew can attend to their patients en route. You continue administering oxygen to Andrea. She remains alert and is complaining of a slight headache and some nausea by the time you arrive at the emergency department. Her vital signs remain in the normal range as you turn her care over to the emergency department staff. Megan's head still hurts, but she is far less drowsy and is looking and feeling better. In the other ambulance, Eddie, being comforted by one EMT as the other continues to administer oxygen, seems quite well by the time they arrive at the emergency department.

At the hospital, blood tests on the patients confirm that they all were exposed to carbon monoxide. Megan had a moderate exposure, and Andrea and Eddie had only a minor exposure. All three are expected to make a good recovery.

SPECIAL CONCERNS IN PEDIATRIC CARE

- - - - - - - - - - ● **CORE CONCEPT**
How to identify and treat special concerns with the ABCs, shock, and potential hypothermia

Like adults, infants and children may be subject to either medical problems or trauma. Concerns that frequently apply to both medical emergencies and trauma are airway maintenance, providing supplemental oxygen, supporting ventilations, caring for shock, and protecting the infant or child from hypothermia (Figure 35-11).

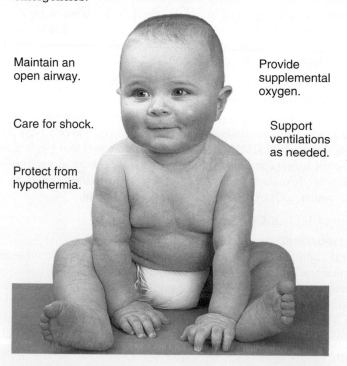

FIGURE 35-11 Special considerations apply to the treatment of many pediatric medical and trauma emergencies.

Maintain an open airway.

Care for shock.

Protect from hypothermia.

Provide supplemental oxygen.

Support ventilations as needed.

Maintaining an Open Airway

Just as with an adult, it is important to position the child's head and neck to align and open the airway. It is important not to hyperextend or to permit flexion of a child's neck. The child's head should be positioned in a more neutral position than an adult's because of the danger of closing the airway when the neck is flexed or hyperextended. Placing a folded towel under the shoulders of a young infant or child will help to keep the airway aligned. To achieve the proper position, perform a head-tilt, chin-lift maneuver if there is no trauma, or a jaw-thrust maneuver with spinal immobilization if trauma is suspected.

Be prepared to suction the airway as needed. Use suction catheters that are sized for infant and child patients. Do not touch the back of the patient's throat, as this may activate the gag reflex, causing vomiting. It is also possible to stimulate the vagus nerve in the back of the throat, which can slow the heart rate. Do not suction for more than a few seconds at a time, as cutting off the body's oxygen supply is especially dangerous to infants and children, causing cardiac arrest more quickly than in adults. You may give a few extra breaths after suctioning.

As with adults, the tongues of infants and children are likely to slide back into the pharynx and obstruct the airway. In fact, airway blockage by the tongue is even more likely with infants and children because their tongues are proportionately larger compared to the size of their mouth and pharynx.

If the patient is unconscious and does not have a gag reflex, you may insert an oropharyngeal airway to prevent the tongue from blocking the airway. To insert an oropharyngeal airway, insert a tongue depressor to the base of the tongue. Push down against the tongue while lifting the jaw upward. Then insert the oropharyngeal airway. An important difference to note is that when an oropharyngeal airway is inserted in an adult, it is inserted with the tip pointing toward the roof of the mouth, then rotated 180 degrees into position. For an infant or child, the oropharyngeal airway is inserted with the tip of the airway pointing downward, toward the tongue and throat, in the same position it will be in after insertion (Scan 35-2).

If the patient is conscious but cannot maintain an open airway, a nasopharyngeal airway can be inserted (Scan 35-3). Note, however, that a nasopharyngeal airway should not be used if the child has facial trauma or head injuries, because the airway could penetrate a breach in the cranium.

Clearing an Airway Obstruction

Infants and children are naturally curious. They explore their environment and often put things in their mouths. Because of this, they can easily choke on a foreign object as well as on a piece of food.

An airway obstruction can be partial or complete. With many partial obstructions, the child is still able to breathe and get enough oxygen. With other partial obstructions or with complete obstruction of the airway, the supply of air is cut off. The assessment and care summaries that follow detail how to determine if an obstruction is partial or complete and how to manage an obstruction.

Inside/Outside

AIRWAY POSITION

Children less than 4 years old often have a proportionately larger head with a larger occiput (the round posterior aspect of the skull). They also have a narrower, more flexible trachea. Laying a small child with altered mental status flat could result in flexion of the airway. Looking from the outside, this position would cause the head and neck to be flexed down toward the chest. On the inside, the airway could be obstructed. Overflexion of the airway causes the pliable trachea to bend unnaturally and kink off the flow of air. Additionally, this position may also cause the proportionately larger tongue to obstruct air movement at its base. Simply padding behind the shoulders can compensate for the large head and move the airway back into an open position. (Review Figure 35-3.)

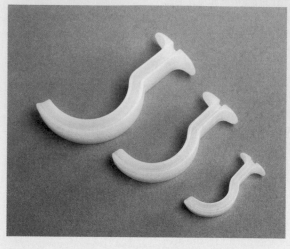

① Oropharyngeal airways come in a variety of sizes.

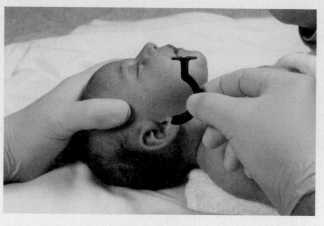

② Size the airway by measuring from the corner of the mouth to the tip of the earlobe

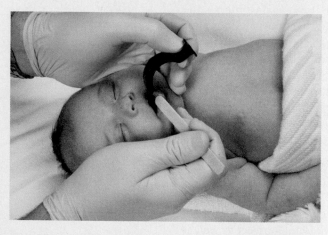

③ Use a tongue depressor to hold the tongue in position. Insert the airway with the tip pointing downward, toward the tongue and throat—the same position it will be in after insertion.

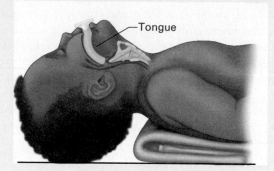

—Tongue

④ The oropharyngeal airway in position.

PATIENT ASSESSMENT

Partial Airway Obstruction

The following are common signs of a partial airway obstruction in a pediatric patient:

- Noisy breathing (stridor, crowing)
- Retractions of the muscles around the ribs and sternum when inhaling
- Normal skin color
- Peripheral perfusion is satisfactory (capillary refill under 2 seconds in a child 5 years old or less)
- Still alert, not unconscious

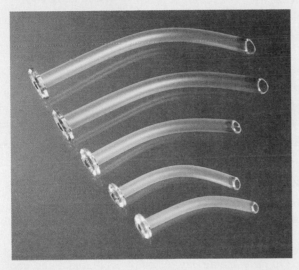

❶ Nasopharyngeal airways come in a variety of sizes.

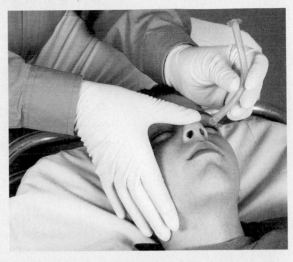

❷ The airway should be about the thickness of the patient's little finger and should measure from the nostril to the tragus (cartilage at the front) of the ear.

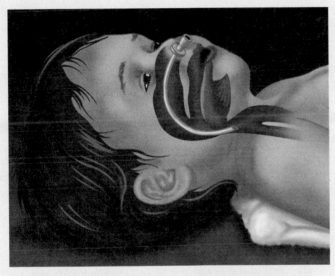

❸ The nasopharyngeal airway in position.

PATIENT CARE

Partial Airway Obstruction

Emergency care of a pediatric patient with a mild airway obstruction is as follows:

1. Allow the child to assume a position of comfort, sitting up, not lying down. Assist an infant or younger child into a sitting position. Allow the child to sit on the parent's lap.
2. Offer high-concentration oxygen by pediatric nonrebreather mask or blow by technique (described later in this chapter).
3. Transport.
4. Do not agitate the child. Limit your examination to avoid upsetting the child. Do not assess blood pressure.

Severe Airway Obstruction

The obstruction may be complete, or a partial obstruction may be severe enough to prevent adequate intake of oxygen. Signs of a severe obstruction are:

- Cyanosis
- Child's cough becomes ineffective; child cannot cry or speak
- Increased respiratory difficulty accompanied by stridor or respiratory arrest
- Altered mental status or loss of consciousness

PATIENT CARE

Severe Airway Obstruction

Follow these steps for emergency care of a severe airway obstruction:

1. Perform airway clearance techniques. For infants less than 1 year old, alternate 5 back blows and 5 chest thrusts (Figure 35-12). If the patient becomes unconscious begin CPR. After 30 compressions, visualize the airway. If an object is visible remove it. *Do not* use blind finger sweeps to clear the airway. Attempt to ventilate and continue chest compressions if necessary. For children older than 1 year, provide subdiaphragmatic abdominal thrusts (the Heimlich maneuver) until they lose conscioussness. If they lose consciousness begin CPR and airway visualization as just explained. (Airway clearance sequences are summarized in Table 35-4.)
2. Attempt artificial ventilations with a pocket mask or bag-valve-mask unit in the appropriate pediatric size and supplemental oxygen (Table 35-5).

Infant and Child BCLS Review

For a review of infant and child basic cardiac life support, including CPR (ventilations and chest compressions) and airway clearance techniques, see Appendix A, "Basic Cardiac Life Support Review."

Providing Supplemental Oxygen and Ventilations

As in adults, high-concentration oxygen should be administered to children in respiratory distress, those with inadequate respirations, or those in possible shock. Hypoxia (oxygen starvation) is the underlying reason for many of the most serious medical problems with

FIGURE 35-12 For a severe airway obstruction in an infant, alternate (A) back blows with (B) chest thrusts.

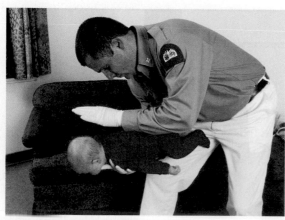

(A)

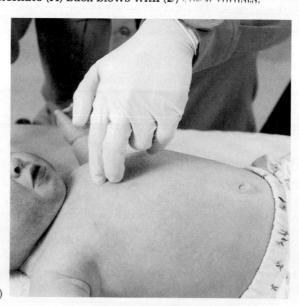

(B)

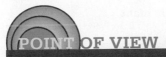
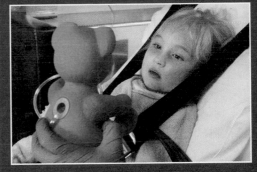

"We don't get a lot of pediatric calls. That's a good thing. When we do get them, it is a bit unnerving. I don't have kids myself so sometimes I think it's harder for me. The EMTs I volunteer with that have kids seem to be more natural.

"Well, wouldn't you know I get a peds call while I am crew chief of the all-bachelor-no-kids crew. The little girl had trouble breathing and had a real barky cough. Her parents were worried. I was, too. But, you know, I did it. I got down on her level and talked with her. She was sitting with her mother and seemed alert. By the time we were headed to the ambulance I think she even liked me.

"What really clinched it was the oxygen bear. There wasn't any way I could have got a mask on her face without freaking her out. She liked the bear, and it gave her some blow-by oxygen.

"Maybe I do have some potential getting along with kids."

Table 35-4   Pediatric Airway Clearance Sequences

	CHILD: 1 YEAR TO PUBERTY	INFANT: BIRTH TO 1 YEAR
Conscious	Ask, "Are you choking?" Perform subdiaphragmatic abdominal thrusts.	Observe signs of choking (small objects or food, wheezing, agitation, blue color, not breathing). Series of five back blows, five chest thrusts.
Loses Consciousness during Procedure	Assist the patient to the floor. Begin 30 chest compressions. Open the airway. Remove any visible objects (*no* blind sweeps). Attempt to ventilate. If unsuccessful, reposition the head and attempt to ventilate again. If unsuccessful, continue CPR. If alone, call for help after 2 minutes.	Begin 30 chest compressions. Open the airway. Remove any visible objects (*no* blind sweeps). Attempt to ventilate. If unsuccessful, reposition the head and attempt to ventilate again. If unsuccessful, continue CPR. If alone, call for help after 2 minutes.
Unconscious When Found	Establish unresponsiveness. Open the airway. Attempt to ventilate. If unsuccessful, reposition the head and attempt to ventilate again. If unsuccessful, perform CPR, attempting compressions to ventilations at a 30:2 ratio. Remove any visible objects from the airway (*no* blind sweeps). Continue CPR until ventilations are successful.	Establish unresponsiveness. Open the airway. Attempt to ventilate. If unsuccessful, reposition the head and attempt to ventilate again. If unsuccessful, perform CPR, attempting compressions to ventilations at a 30:2 ratio. Remove any visible objects from the airway (*no* blind sweeps). Continue CPR until ventilations are successful.

Table 35-5   Artificial Ventilation

	PUBERTY AND OLDER	OVER AGE 1 TO PUBERTY	BIRTH TO 1 YEAR
Ventilation Duration	1 second	1 second	1 second
Ventilation Rate	10 to 12 breaths/minute	12 to 20 breaths/minute	12 to 20 breaths/minute

children. Inadequate oxygen will have immediate effects on the heart rate and the brain, as shown by a slowed heart rate and an altered mental status.

However, infants and young children are often afraid of an oxygen mask. For these patients who will not tolerate a mask, try a "blow-by" technique. In this technique you will hold, or have a parent hold, the oxygen tubing or the pediatric nonrebreather mask 2 inches from the patient's face so the oxygen will pass over the face and be inhaled. Some departments use blow-by oxygen devices that resemble stuffed animals. These commercially made products may be less threatening to a child than traditional oxygen devices. Follow the manufacturer's recommendations regarding liter flow per minute when using these devices. Some children respond well when oxygen tubing is pushed through the bottom of a paper cup, especially if the cup is colorful or has a picture drawn inside it (Figure 35-13). Hand the cup to the child or ask a parent to hold it. Infants and young children instinctively explore

FIGURE 35-13 You can deliver oxygen to an infant using the blow-by method.

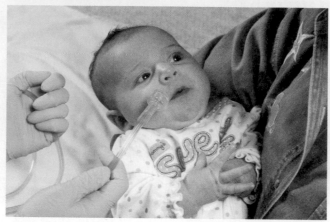

new things by bringing them up to their mouths. As the patient handles and explores the cup, he will breathe in the oxygen. *Do not use a Styrofoam cup.* Styrofoam may flake and the child can inhale the particles.

Remember that a nonrebreather mask will always provide more efficient oxygen delivery, and many children tolerate it well. Use blow-by only if more efficient administration methods fail.

Positive pressure ventilations should be provided at the rate of 12 to 20 per minute (one every 3 to 5 seconds) for an infant or child up to puberty, and at 10 to 12 per minute (one every 5 to 6 seconds) if the child has reached puberty. (Note that the rate is higher when performing a neonatal resuscitation. In that case use a rate of 40–60 breaths per minute) Use a pocket face mask (Figure 35-14) or a bag-valve-mask unit (Figure 35-15) in the correct infant or child size. Follow these guidelines when ventilating the infant or child patient:

- Avoid breathing too hard through the pocket face mask or using excessive bag pressure and volume. Use only enough force to make the chest rise.

FIGURE 35-14 Ventilation of a child using a pocket face mask.

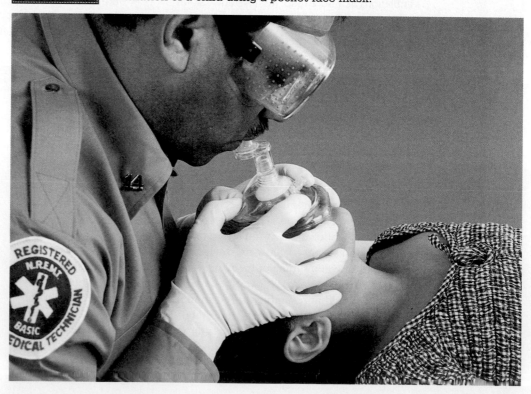

FIGURE 35-15 Ventilation of a child using a bag-valve-mask device. If using one hand to squeeze the bag, achieve a good mask seal with the other hand by placing your fingers in an E-C configuration. The thumb and index finger form a C around the mask chimney whereas the other three fingers form an E along the child's jaw.

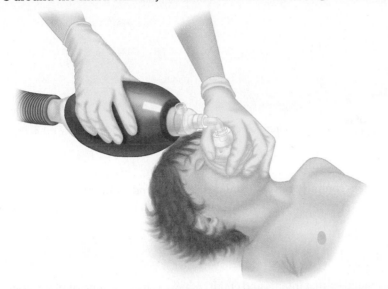
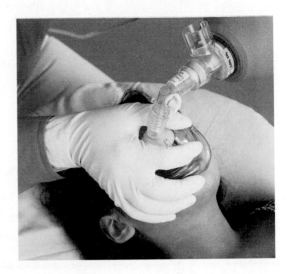

FIGURE 35-16 Correct placement of a properly sized mask is necessary to ensure a good mask seal. (A) This shows correct placement of the mask. (B) This shows the mask placed on a child.

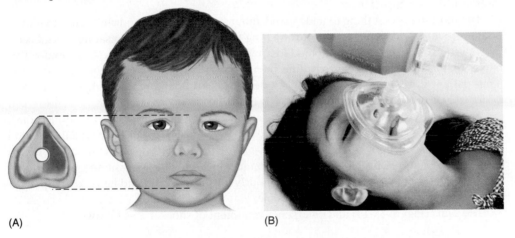

(A)   (B)

- Use properly sized face masks to ensure a good mask seal (Figure 35-16).
- Flow-restricted, oxygen-powered ventilation devices are contraindicated in infants and children.
- If ventilation is not successful in raising the patient's chest, perform procedures for clearing an obstructed airway. Then try to ventilate again. (Review Tables 35-4 and 35-5.)

Caring for Shock

Shock is another term for hypoperfusion, which is the inadequate circulation of blood and oxygen throughout the body. One common cause of shock in adults—a failure of heart function or of the cardiovascular system—is rare in infants and children. The following are some common causes of shock in infants and children:

- Diarrhea and/or vomiting with resulting dehydration
- Infection
- Trauma (especially abdominal injuries)
- Blood loss

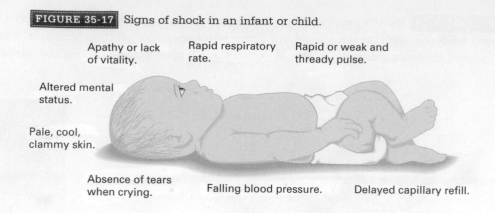

FIGURE 35-17 Signs of shock in an infant or child.

Apathy or lack of vitality.

Rapid respiratory rate.

Rapid or weak and thready pulse.

Altered mental status.

Pale, cool, clammy skin.

Absence of tears when crying.

Falling blood pressure.

Delayed capillary refill.

The following are some less common causes of shock in infants and children:

- Allergic reactions
- Poisoning
- Cardiac events (rare)

It is important to remember that infants and children have a small volume of blood compared to adults (approximately 8 percent of the total body weight). Bleeding that would not be dangerous in an adult may be serious in an infant or child. Shock can develop in the small child who has a laceration to the scalp (with its many blood vessels) or in the 3-year-old who loses as little as a cup of blood.

The most important thing to understand about shock in infants and children is that their bodies are able to compensate for it for a long time. When the compensating mechanisms fail, at approximately 30 percent blood loss, hypovolemic shock develops very rapidly. This means that a child may appear to be fine, then "go sour" in a hurry. This is in contrast to the adult patient in whom hypovolemic shock develops earlier and more gradually, making it easier to assess and treat than in a child.

The definitive care for shock takes place at the hospital (usually in the operating room). Since infants and children are prone to go into hypotensive shock—shock in which the blood pressure has dropped severely—so suddenly, *it is important not to wait for signs of hypotensive shock to develop*. Instead, in any situation in which shock is a possibility, provide oxygen (which boosts the supply of oxygen to poorly perfused tissues and helps keep up heart function) and transport as quickly as possible.

The signs (Figure 35-17) and emergency treatment of shock are as follows.

PATIENT ASSESSMENT

Shock

The following are common signs of shock in pediatric patients:

- Rapid heart rate
- Mental status changes
- Rapid respiratory rate
- Pale, cool, and clammy skin
- Weak or absent peripheral pulses
- Delayed capillary refill, more than 2 seconds (in a child 5 years or younger)
- Decreased urine output (Ask parents about diaper wetting; look at diaper.)
- Absence of tears, even when crying

Decision Point

• Is my pediatric patient developing shock but compensating?

Inside/Outside

Compensatory changes will begin immediately inside the body of a child who is losing blood. For example, the heart will beat faster to improve blood circulation. Increasing heart rate is a key component in pediatric compensation for shock. In addition, the child's blood vessels will constrict to move blood toward the body's core to support the function of essential organs. To compensate for hypoxia, the respiratory rate will increase. If hypoxia persists, brain function may be disrupted.

Outside the child's body, there will be evidence of these compensatory changes. Increased heart rate will be seen as an increased pulse rate (if it can be found peripherally). Vessel constriction will be seen in the form of pale skin and delayed capillary refill. Disrupted brain function will show as altered mental status.

PATIENT CARE

Shock

Follow these steps for emergency care:

1. Ensure an open airway.
2. Manage severe external hemorrhage, if present.
3. Provide high-concentration oxygen. Be prepared to artificially ventilate.
4. Lay the patient flat.
5. Keep the patient warm.
6. Transport immediately. Perform any additional assessment and treatments en route.

Protecting against Hypothermia

Hypothermia, or cooling of the body below its normal temperature, is a life-threatening condition in extreme cases. People lose heat more readily if their clothes are wet, if they are exposed to wind, or if they are submerged in cold water. The body attempts to compensate for a decrease in body temperature, but as these compensatory functions begin to fail, the core body temperature drops. Because children have a large surface area in proportion to their body mass, exposure to cool weather and water can result in hypothermia more easily than with adults. Therefore, hypothermia is always a concern with a pediatric patient.

Other causes of hypothermia, in children as well as in adults, include ingestion of alcohol or drugs that dilate peripheral vessels and cause loss of body heat, metabolic problems such as hypoglycemia, brain disorders that interfere with temperature regulation, severe infection or sepsis, and shock.

Hypothermia may be a concern in both medical and trauma emergencies. For example, a sick child in a cool room or in sheets or nightclothes that have become wet from perspiration or loss of bladder control may be hypothermic. When trauma occurs outdoors, caregivers attending to injuries may forget to protect the patient from a cool or damp environment, and may exacerbate the situation by exposing the patient's body during the physical exam.

Field care for children is the same as for adults. It is important to keep the patient warm, so cover the patient to avoid further loss of body heat. Pay special attention to covering the head, as the head is a major area of heat loss. Also, be aware of the temperature in the patient compartment of the ambulance. Consult medical direction for advice on active rewarming of the body by application of hot water bottles or other heat sources if the patient is awake and responding appropriately. Avoid rough handling and inserting anything in the patient's mouth as these actions may cause ventricular fibrillation or cardiac arrest in the severely hypothermic child. Suction very gently if suctioning is necessary, and be alert to the possibility of cardiac arrest.

PEDIATRIC MEDICAL EMERGENCIES

● CORE CONCEPT

How to assess and care for various pediatric medical emergencies, especially respiratory disorders

Respiratory Disorders

Respiratory disorders are a great concern in infants and children. For example, it is important to remember that, although cardiac arrest in the adult is likely to be caused by a heart problem, the likeliest cause of cardiac arrest in a child, other than trauma, is respiratory failure. For the pediatric patient, it is important to distinguish whether the probable cause of the breathing difficulty is an upper airway problem or a lower airway problem. The care that you would give for an upper airway obstruction is not indicated for a lower airway disorder. Also, because respiratory problems can have such serious consequences in infants and children, it is critical to be alert for early signs of respiratory failure.

Difficulty Breathing

There are a number of respiratory diseases or disorders an infant or child may have that will cause difficulty breathing, ranging from serious ones like epiglottitis to less serious ones like a cold. It is not easy to determine which respiratory problem the child may have. Many signs and symptoms are similar, and age ranges for occurrence overlap.

As an EMT, you do not need to decide what respiratory disorder a child is suffering from. Instead, use the following guidelines for recognizing and managing respiratory distress. It is especially important to recognize the signs of early respiratory distress and treat it before it advances to a life-threatening stage or to respiratory arrest.

Differentiating Upper Airway Problems from Lower Airway Disorders The upper airway starts at the mouth and nose and ends at the opening of the trachea. Upper airway disorders affect structures such as the mouth, the throat (the pharynx and hypopharynx), and the area around the opening of the trachea (the larynx). Common upper airway disorders include foreign body obstructions, trauma, and swelling from burns and infections. In addition to difficulty breathing, upper airway disorders can commonly be identified by the presence of stridor or difficulty speaking.

The lower airway begins at the opening of the trachea and ends at the alveoli. Lower airway disorders affect the large and small bronchiole tubes and the alveoli themselves. Common lower airway disorders include asthma, pneumonia, and other respiratory infections. Lower airway disorders commonly cause difficulty breathing, but the distinguishing sign is

Inside/Outside

RESPIRATORY DISTRESS VS. RESPIRATORY FAILURE

Inside the child with an airway or breathing problem, the body will take steps to compensate for the problem. The pulmonary system will increase respiratory rate and volume. The autonomic nervous system will engage the fight-or-flight response, increase heart rate, and constrict blood vessels. These mechanisms are often successful in temporarily maintaining the body's oxygenation and ventilation despite the challenge to its respiratory system. When these compensatory mechanisms are working, we typically refer to the patient's condition as *respiratory distress*. By that we mean the patient has a respiratory challenge, but the increased respirations and heart rate are temporarily serving to keep the brain oxygenated and ventilated.

On the outside, this patient will present with difficulty breathing. You will observe the compensation by recognizing an increased respiratory rate and an increased pulse. You may note pale skin and/or delayed capillary refill. Most important, respiratory distress can be recognized by the signs of

adequate oxygenation and ventilation. Mental status is a key finding. A normal mental status indicates the brain is receiving oxygen and eliminating carbon dioxide. When this stops or is interfered with, mental status typically changes.

Unfortunately, the body can only compensate for a breathing problem for a limited period of time. If not corrected, the compensatory mechanisms just described will eventually fail, and the respiratory distress will become *respiratory failure*. Inside the body, respiratory failure occurs when the challenge overwhelms the body's ability to compensate. Continued hypoxia tires the muscles of respiration and they begin to fail. As a result, increased carbon dioxide and low oxygen levels begin to interfere with brain function.

Outside, respiratory failure can be identified by all the signs of respiratory distress *plus* cyanosis of the skin, slowing or irregular respirations, and altered mental status.

wheezing lung sounds. It is important to remember, however, that not all lower airway problems will be accompanied by wheezing.

Although you may not be able to identify the root cause of the problem, distinguishing an upper airway problem from a lower airway problem will help you properly target your immediate treatments.

In general, with suspected airway diseases you should transport as quickly as possible if you see or hear wheezing, breathing effort on exhalation, or rapid breathing.

NOTE: *With some diseases, it is dangerous to perform finger sweeps or to place a tongue depressor or any other instrument in the patient's mouth or pharynx, because this may set off spasms along the airway. Do not attempt to clear the airway of a foreign obstruction unless it is clear that this is the problem—that is, the child has been observed ingesting a foreign object or the signs of such ingestion are clear.*

PATIENT ASSESSMENT

Difficulty Breathing

Recognizing respiratory distress or failure is an important goal in the assessment of a pediatric patient with difficulty breathing. Gather information quickly from the parents and do a rapid assessment of the child. Unless there are clear indications of foreign body airway obstruction, do not put a tongue depressor in the child's mouth to examine the airway. This may cause spasms that can totally obstruct the airway.

Recognize the following signs of early respiratory distress (Figure 35-18):

■ Nasal flaring
■ Retraction of the muscles above, below, and between the sternum and ribs

FIGURE 35-18 Signs of respiratory distress.

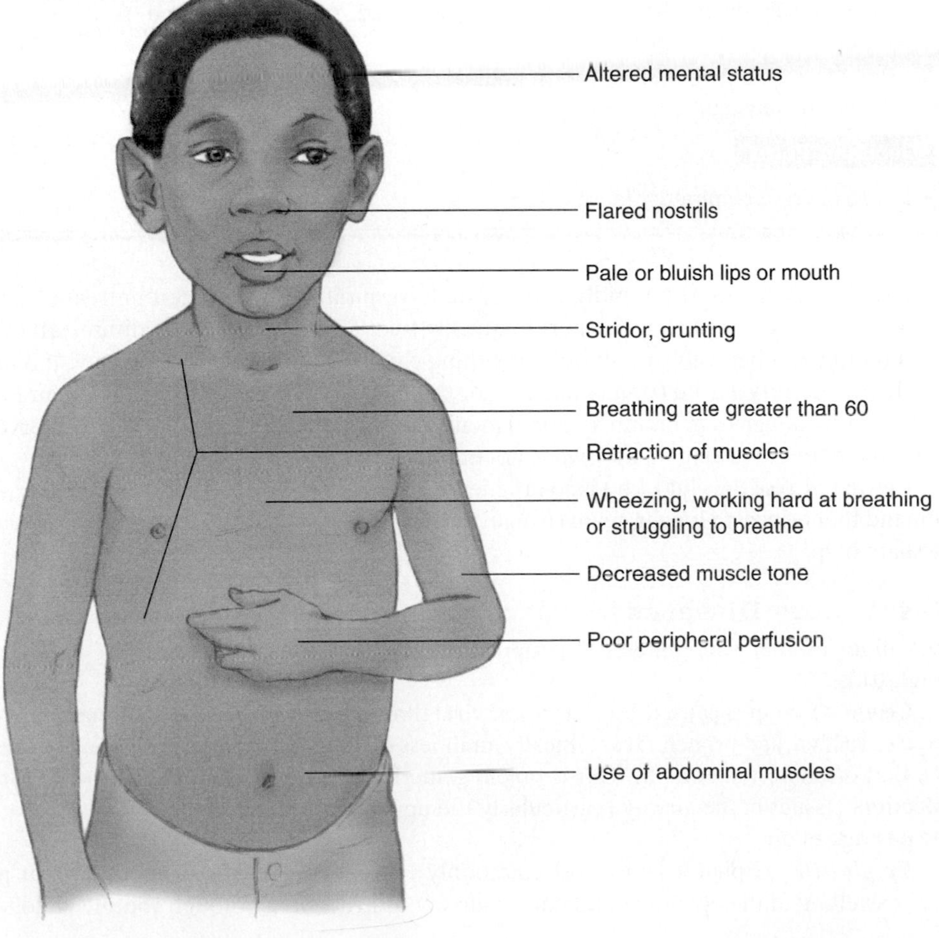

- Altered mental status
- Flared nostrils
- Pale or bluish lips or mouth
- Stridor, grunting
- Breathing rate greater than 60
- Retraction of muscles
- Wheezing, working hard at breathing or struggling to breathe
- Decreased muscle tone
- Poor peripheral perfusion
- Use of abdominal muscles

- Use of abdominal muscles
- Stridor (high-pitched, harsh sound)
- Audible wheezing
- Grunting
- Breathing rate greater than 60

In addition to these signs of early respiratory distress, watch for these additional signs of respiratory failure:

- Altered mental status
- Slowing or irregular respiratory rate
- Cyanosis (especially after the addition of supplemental oxygen)
- Decreased muscle tone
- Poor peripheral perfusion (capillary refill greater than 2 seconds)
- Decreased heart rate (a late sign)

Decision Points

- Is my pediatric patient in early respiratory distress?
- Is my pediataric patient in respiratory failure?

PATIENT CARE

Difficulty Breathing

Provide oxygen to all children with respiratory emergencies.
For children in early respiratory distress:

- Provide oxygen by pediatric nonrebreather mask or blow-by technique if the patient will not tolerate a mask.

For children in respiratory failure (those with respiratory distress and altered mental status, cyanosis even when oxygen is administered, poor muscle tone, or inadequate breathing) or respiratory arrest:

- Provide assisted ventilations with pediatric pocket mask or bag-valve mask and supplemental oxygen.

Decision Point

- Is this child in respiratory failure?

Respiratory failure will rapidly deteriorate to respiratory arrest if left untreated. As an EMT, you must always be on the alert to quickly treat a patient in this condition. Often the decision to use a bag-valve mask on a breathing child is a difficult one. However, it is critical. If you identify a child (or any patient, for that matter) who is not oxygenating and ventilating well enough to maintain a normal mental status, you need to immediately intervene. What the patient is doing on his own is not enough!

Beware also of the child who is so fatigued from the effort to meet increased respiratory demand that he can no longer go on (irregular, slowing respirations). He, too, needs your immediate help.

Respiratory Diseases

Two illnesses that sometimes cause upper airway problems in children are croup and epiglottitis.

Croup Croup is caused by a group of viral illnesses that result in inflammation of the larynx, trachea, and bronchi. It is typically an illness of children 6 months to about 4 years of age that often occurs at night. This problem sometimes follows a cold or other respiratory infection. Tissues in the airway (particularly the upper airway) become swollen and restrict the passage of air.

Epiglottitis Epiglottitis is most commonly caused by a bacterial infection that produces swelling of the epiglottis and partial airway obstruction. Although routine childhood vaccinations have made this disease in children rare, it should be suspected when treating any child with stridor (a high-pitched sound caused by air moving through narrowed passageways), especially in children who are unvaccinated.

NOTE: *All cases of epiglottitis must be considered life threatening, no matter how early the detection.*

PATIENT ASSESSMENT

Croup

During the day, the child with croup will usually have these signs:

- Mild fever
- Some hoarseness
  At night, the child's condition will worsen and he will develop:
- A loud "seal bark" cough
- Difficulty breathing
- Signs of respiratory distress including nasal flaring, retraction of the muscles between the ribs, the child tugging at his throat
- Restlessness
- Paleness with cyanosis

PATIENT CARE

Croup

Emergency care of a pediatric patient with croup is as follows:

1. Place the patient in a position of comfort (usually sitting up).
2. Administer high-concentration oxygen. When possible, this should be from a humidified source. (*Do not delay oxygen administration in order to humidify.*)
3. Move slowly to the ambulance. The cool night air may provide relief as the cool air reduces the edema in the airway tissues.
4. Do not delay transport unless ordered to do so by medical direction.

PATIENT ASSESSMENT

Epiglottitis

The following are common signs of epiglottitis:

- A sudden onset of high fever
- Painful swallowing (the child often will drool to avoid swallowing)
- Patient will assume a "tripod" position, sitting upright and leaning forward with the chin thrust outward (sniffing position) and the mouth wide open in an effort to maintain a wide airway opening.
- Patient will sit very still, but the muscles will work hard to breathe, and the child can tire quickly from the effort.
- Child appears more generally ill than with croup.

PATIENT CARE

Epiglottitis

Emergency care for the pediatric patient with epiglottitis is as follows:

1. Contact ALS (Remember that the hospital may be the closest source of ALS care.)
2. Immediately transport the child, with the child sitting on the parent's lap.
3. Provide high-concentration oxygen from a humidified source. Do not increase the child's anxiety. If he or she resists the mask, let the parent hold it in front of the child's face. (*Do not delay oxygen administration in order to humidify.*)

4. Constantly monitor the child for respiratory distress or arrest and be ready to resuscitate.
5. *Do not place anything into the child's mouth*, including a thermometer, tongue blade, or oral airway. To do so may set off spasms along the upper airway that will totally obstruct the airway.

The child will not want to lie down, and you should not force him to do so. The child must be handled gently, since rough handling and stress could lead to a total airway obstruction from spasms of the larynx and swelling tissues.

All respiratory disorders in children must be taken seriously. Respiratory disease is the primary cause of cardiac arrest not due to trauma. If you treat the respiratory system, the heart will also respond. The EMT's primary concern when caring for infants and children with respiratory problems, whether medical or trauma related, is to establish and maintain an open airway. About one-third of all pediatric trauma deaths are related to airway or respiratory compromise.

Other Pediatric Disorders

Fever

Above-normal body temperature is one of the most important signs of an existing or impending acute illness. Fever usually accompanies infections (ear infections are common) as well as such childhood diseases as chicken pox, mononucleosis, pneumonia, epiglottitis, and meningitis. The fever also may be due to heat exposure, any infection, or some other noninfectious disease.

PATIENT ASSESSMENT

Fever

Never regard a fever as unimportant. Fever can be the most important sign of a variety of serious conditions.

Use relative skin temperature as a sign if you do not have a reliable means to obtain an accurate temperature. Applying the ungloved back of your hand to the patient's forehead or to the abdomen beneath the clothing is another way to determine relative skin temperature. A high relative skin temperature is always enough reason to transport and seek medical opinion. Other signs are:

■ Fever with a rash is a sign of a potentially serious condition.

■ A seizure or seizures may accompany a high fever.

PATIENT CARE

Fever

Children can tolerate a high temperature, and only a small percent will have a seizure due to fever (febrile seizure). It is the rapid rise in temperature rather than the temperature itself that causes seizures. Cooling the child without bringing on hypothermia is an important care objective. If you find an infant or child has a high fever, take the following steps:

1. Remove the child's clothing, but do not allow him to be exposed to conditions that may bring on hypothermia. If the child objects to having clothing removed, let the child keep on light clothing or underwear.
2. If the condition is a result of heat exposure, and if local protocols permit, cover the child with a towel soaked in tepid water. This will quickly cool the child.
3. Monitor for shivering and avoid hypothermia. This may develop quickly in children. If shivering develops, stop the cooling activities and cover the child with a light blanket.
4. If local protocols permit, give the child fluids by mouth or allow him to suck on chipped ice. This may not prevent dehydration but will increase his comfort.
5. Be aware that a mild fever can quickly turn into a high fever that may indicate a serious, if not life-threatening, problem. If the infant or child feels very warm-to-hot to the touch, then prepare the patient for transport. Transport all children who have

suffered a seizure as quickly as possible, protecting the patient from temperature extremes.

There are also some "do nots" in treating an infant or child with fever:

- Do not submerge the child in cold water, or cover with a towel soaked in ice water (which can rapidly cause hypothermia).
- *Do not use rubbing alcohol to cool the patient.* (It can be absorbed in toxic amounts and is a fire hazard.)

Meningitis

Meningitis is a potentially life-threatening infection of the lining of the brain and spinal cord (the meninges). It is caused by either a bacterial or a viral infection and commonly occurs between the ages of 1 month and 5 years. However, it is not uncommon to see meningitis in adolescents.

PATIENT ASSESSMENT

Meningitis

The following are signs and symptoms of meningitis:

- High fever
- Stiff neck
- Lethargy
- Irritability
- Headache
- Sensitivity to light
- In infants, bulging fontanelles unless the child is dehydrated
- Painful movement during which the child does not want to be touched or held
- Seizures
- A rash if the infection is bacterial

PATIENT CARE

Meningitis

It is most important to carefully take appropriate Standard Precautions. Wear appropriate respiratory protection, since meningitis is an airborne disease. When meningitis is suspected, provide the following care:

1. Monitor the patient's airway, breathing, circulation, and vital signs.
2. Provide high-concentration oxygen by nonrebreather mask.
3. Ventilate with a pediatric pocket mask or bag-valve mask with supplemental oxygen, if necessary.
4. Provide CPR, if necessary.
5. Be alert for seizures.
6. Transport immediately. This is a *true emergency*. Do not delay.

NOTE: *Some forms of meningitis may be highly infectious, requiring that EMS personnel be evaluated and provided antibiotic treatment by a physician.*

Diarrhea and Vomiting

Diarrhea and vomiting are common in childhood illness. Either one can cause dehydration that worsens whatever other condition the child may have and may lead to life-threatening shock. Infants are more susceptible to the effects of dehydration because, compared to adults, a greater percentage of their body is water and their fluid maintenance needs are greater.

PATIENT ASSESSMENT

Diarrhea and Vomiting

For any pediatric patient with diarrhea or vomiting:

1. Monitor the airway.
2. Monitor respiration.
3. Be alert for signs of shock.

PATIENT CARE

Diarrhea and Vomiting

Emergency care for diarrhea and vomiting includes the following:

1. Maintain an open airway and be prepared to provide oral suctioning.
2. Provide oxygen if respirations are compromised.
3. If signs of shock are present, contact medical direction immediately and transport.
4. If your protocols or medical direction permits, offer the child sips of clear liquids or chipped ice if only diarrhea is present. Many physicians recommend nothing by mouth if there is nausea or vomiting.
5. Some systems recommend that you save a sample of vomitus and rectal discharge (e.g., a soiled diaper). Follow your local protocols.

Seizures

Fever is the most common cause of seizures in infants and children. Epilepsy, infections, poisoning, hypoglycemia, trauma including head injury, or decreased levels of oxygen can also bring on seizures. Some seizures in children are idiopathic; that is, they have no known cause. They may be brief or prolonged. They are rarely life-threatening conditions in the children who frequently have them. However, *the EMT should consider seizures, including those caused by fever, to be life threatening.* Usually, you will arrive after the convulsion has passed.

PATIENT ASSESSMENT

Seizures

Interview the patient as well as family members and bystanders who saw the convulsion. Ask:

- Has the child had prior seizures?
- If yes, is this the child's normal seizure pattern? (How long did the seizure last? What part of the body was seizing?)
- Has the child had a fever?
- Has the child taken any anti-seizure medication? Other medication?

Assess the child for signs and symptoms of illness or injury, taking care to note any injuries sustained during the convulsion. All infants and children who have undergone a seizure require medical evaluation. The seizure itself may not be serious but it may be a sign of an underlying condition. Be aware that seizures may also be caused by a head injury.

PATIENT CARE

Seizures

If the patient has a seizure in your presence, possibly during transport, provide the following care:

1. Maintain an open airway. Do not insert an oropharyngeal airway or bite stick.
2. Position the patient on his side if there is no possibility of spinal injury.
3. Be alert for vomiting. Suction as needed.
4. Provide oxygen. If the patient is in respiratory arrest, provide artificial ventilations with supplemental oxygen.

5. Transport.

6. Monitor for inadequate breathing and/or altered mental status, which may occur following a seizure.

More information on the treatment of seizures can be found in Chapter 21, "Diabetic Emergencies and Altered Mental Status."

Altered Mental Status

Altered mental status may be caused by a variety of conditions, including hypoglycemia, poisoning, infection, head injury, decreased oxygen levels, shock, or the aftermath of a seizure.

PATIENT ASSESSMENT

Altered Mental Status

Assessment of the patient with altered mental status focuses on life-threatening problems discovered during the primary assessment:

- Be alert for a mechanism of injury that may have caused the altered mental status, such as head injury.
- Be alert for signs of shock.
- Look for evidence of poisoning from ingested, inhaled, or absorbed substances.
- Attempt to quickly obtain a history of any seizure disorder or diabetes.

PATIENT CARE

Altered Mental Status

Emergency care of a pediatric patient with altered mental status includes the following steps:

1. Ensure an open airway. Be prepared to suction.
2. Protect the spine while managing the airway if a head injury or other trauma is present.
3. Administer high-concentration oxygen by pediatric nonrebreather mask or blow-by technique. Be prepared to perform artificial ventilations by pediatric pocket mask or bag-valve mask with supplemental oxygen.
4. Treat for shock.
5. Transport.

Poisoning

Children are often the victims of accidental poisoning, often resulting from the ingestion of household products or medications. Certain poisons can quickly depress the respiratory system, cause respiratory arrest, and cause life-threatening conditions of the circulatory and nervous systems. The airway and gastrointestinal tract can also be burned by corrosive substances upon ingestion and with subsequent vomiting.

Review Chapter 23, "Poisoning and Overdose Emergencies," for information on ingested, inhaled, absorbed, and injected poisons. This information applies to children as well as to adults.

PATIENT ASSESSMENT

Poisoning

Some types of poisonings are not often associated with adult patients but are common to children. These special cases are:

- **Aspirin poisoning.** Look for hyperventilation, vomiting, and sweating. The skin may feel hot. Severe cases cause seizures, coma, or shock.
- **Acetaminophen poisoning.** Many medications have this compound, including Tylenol, Comtrex, Bancap, Excedrin PM, and Datril. Initially, the child may have no

abnormal signs or symptoms. The child may be restless (early) or drowsy. Nausea, vomiting, and heavy perspiration may occur. Loss of consciousness is possible.

- **Lead poisoning.** This usually comes from ingesting chips of lead-based paint. It is often a chronic condition (building up over a long time). Look for nausea with abdominal pain and vomiting. Muscle cramps, headache, muscle weakness, and irritability are often present.

- **Iron poisoning.** Iron compounds such as ferrous sulfate are found in some vitamin tablets and liquids. As little as 1 gram of ferrous sulfate can be lethal to a child. Within 30 minutes to several hours, the child will show nausea and bloody vomiting, often accompanied by diarrhea. Typically the child will develop shock, but this may be delayed for up to 24 hours as the child appears to be getting better.

- **Petroleum product poisoning.** The patient will usually be vomiting with coughing or choking. In most cases, you will smell the distinctive odor of a petroleum distillate (e.g., gasoline, kerosene, heating fuel).

PATIENT CARE

Poisoning

Emergency care for a responsive poisoning patient includes the following steps:

1. Contact medical direction or the poison control center.
2. Consider the need to administer activated charcoal (where protocol allows).
3. Provide oxygen.
4. Transport.
5. Continue to monitor the patient. The patient may become unresponsive.

Emergency care for an unresponsive poisoning patient includes the following steps:

1. Ensure an open airway.
2. Provide oxygen.
3. Be prepared to provide artificial ventilation.
4. Transport.
5. Contact medical direction or the poison control center.
6. Rule out trauma as a cause of altered mental status.

Drowning

As explained in Chapter 33, "Environmental Emergencies," drowning is the process of experiencing respiratory impairment from submersion/immersion in liquid, which may result in death, morbidity (illness or other adverse effects), or no morbidity. Water temperature may affect outcomes from drowning. Patients who have been submerged in *cold* water have been revived 30 minutes or more after submersion.

PATIENT ASSESSMENT

Drowning

If the patient is unresponsive and you suspect he may be in cardiac arrest:

1. Establish unresponsiveness, breathlessness, and pulselessness.
2. If the patient is unresponsive, breathless, and pulseless, perform five cycles of compressions and ventilations (30:2 ratio) at a rate of 100 compressions per minute before activating the emergency response system if this has not already been done.
3. If trauma may have been a cause or result of the submersion incident (such as injury from a dive), maintain spinal stabilization and follow trauma assessment procedures. Remember, however, that resuscitation is your first priority.
4. Consider possible ingestion of alcohol as a cause of the drowning, especially in adolescents.
5. Consider the possibility of "secondary drowning syndrome"—deterioration after normal breathing resumes, minutes to hours after the event.

Drowning

For the drowning patient, provide the following care:

1. Provide artificial ventilation or CPR as necessary. This is your first treatment priority.
2. Protect the airway. Suction, if necessary.
3. Consider spinal immobilization.
4. Protect against possible hypothermia, especially if the patient has been in cool or cold water. As soon as practical, remove wet clothing, dry the skin, and cover with a blanket.
5. Treat any trauma.
6. Transport all drowning patients to the hospital, even if they seem to have recovered.

Sudden Infant Death Syndrome

In the United States, sudden infant death syndrome (SIDS)—the sudden, unexplained death during sleep of an apparently healthy baby in its first year of life—occurs in 2,000 to 2,500 babies each year. These babies were usually receiving proper care and frequently have passed physical examinations within days of their sudden death.

Many possible causes for this syndrome have been investigated but are not well understood. The problem is not caused by external methods of suffocation or by vomiting or choking. The problem may possibly be related to nerve cell development in the brain or the tissue chemistry of the respiratory system or the heart. Some relationships have been drawn to family history of SIDS and respiratory problems, but there is still no accepted reason why these babies die.

When asleep, the typical SIDS patient will show periods of cardiac slowdown and temporary cessation of breathing known as sleep apnea. Eventually, the infant will stop breathing and will not start again on its own. Unless reached in time, the episode can be fatal. The baby's condition is most commonly discovered in the early morning when the parents go to wake the baby.

It is not up to you, as an EMT, to diagnose SIDS. All you or the parents will know is that the baby is in respiratory or cardiac arrest. You will treat the baby as you would any patient in this condition:

1. Unless there is rigor mortis (stiffening of the body after death), provide resuscitation.

2. Be certain that the parents receive emotional support and that they understand that everything possible is being done for the child at the scene and during transport.

Parents who lose a child to SIDS often suffer intense feelings of guilt from the moment they find the child. Whether or not the parents express such guilt, remind them that SIDS occurs to apparently healthy babies who are receiving the best of parental care. Do not speak with a suspicious tone or ask inappropriate questions. Do not be embarrassed to express your sorrow for their loss.

PEDIATRIC TRAUMA EMERGENCIES

Trauma is the number one cause of death in infants and children. Blunt trauma far exceeds penetrating trauma in this age group. Much of this trauma occurs because children are curious and learning about their environment. Exploring often leads to injury from accidental falls (or things falling on them), burns, entrapment, crushing, and other mechanisms of injury.

When providing emergency care for the injured child, always tell him what you are going to do before you do it.

Injury Patterns

Injury management is basically the same for children as for adults (Figure 35-19). However, their anatomic and physiologic differences cause children to have different patterns of injury (Table 35-6).

CORE CONCEPT ●- - - - - - -
How to assess and care for various pediatric trauma emergencies

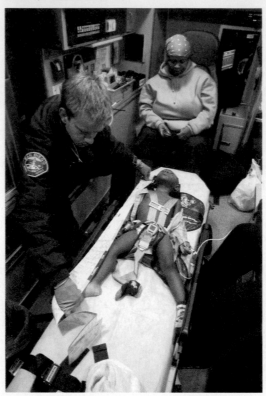

FIGURE 35-19 Infant receiving emergency care. *(© Daniel Limmer)*

During motor-vehicle collisions:

- Unrestrained child passengers (those without seat belts or restraint in a child safety seat) tend to have head and neck injuries.

- Restrained passengers may have abdominal and lower spine injuries.

Children who are struck by autos while bicycle riding often have head, spinal, and abdominal injuries.

The child who has been struck by a vehicle may present with the following triad of injuries:

- Head injury
- Abdominal injury with possible internal bleeding
- Lower extremity injury (possibly a fractured femur)

Other common injuries include diving injuries with associated head and neck injury; sports injuries, which also often involve the head and neck; and injuries from child abuse.

You will need to have a good understanding of pediatric anatomic and physiologic characteristics as they relate to trauma in order to deliver expert emergency care. These include features of the head, chest, abdomen, and extremities, as described in the following paragraphs.

Head

Recall that the head is proportionately larger and heavier in the small child. This leads to head injury when the head is propelled forward in a collision. This is often combined with internal injuries. Suspect internal injuries whenever a child with a head injury presents with shock, since head injury itself is seldom a cause of shock. Respiratory arrest is a common secondary effect of head injury, so be alert to this possibility. Although the most frequent sign of head injury is an altered mental status, nausea and vomiting also often occur.

Chest

The less-developed respiratory muscles of the chest and the more elastic ribs make the pediatric chest more easily deformed. The immature respiratory muscles make breathing

Table 35-6 High-Risk Mechanisms of Injury and Pediatric Injury Patterns

Transport to a trauma center with pediatric care capabilities if any of the following are identified:

HIGH-RISK MECHANISM	TYPE OF INJURY TO PEDIATRIC PATIENT
FALLS **Over age 15:** 20 feet (one story = 10 feet) **Under age 15:** fall > 10 feet or two to three times child's height **Note:** Seriousness depends on (1) height of fall, (2) surface on which child fell, and (3) child's age. (Infants may have serious head injury from falls of 3–4 feet from a changing table.)	Head and upper neck injury and fractures to upper and lower extremities from moderate falls, 5–15 feet Head, neck, spine injury, abdominal and chest injury, and fractures of upper and lower extremities from high falls over 15 feet
AUTO CRASH **Improperly restrained/unrestrained passenger**	Serious head and neck injury, facial abrasions, and lacerations. Soft-tissue injury of the neck from shoulder belt used without lap belt or shoulder belt used on a too-small child. Internal abdominal injury from lap belt used without shoulder belt or lap belt improperly positioned over abdomen. Fracture of lower vertebrae and spinal cord damage from violent flexion at waist when lap belt is used without shoulder belt.
Child struck by deployed air bag	Severe head and neck injury. Burns to the eye and face caused by the caustic powder released when air bag deploys.
Pedestrian or bicyclist struck with significant (> 20 mph) impact **Child thrown onto hood/windshield or minimal distance on impact**	Severe head injury, especially if thrown any distance, by force of high speed at impact. Multiple head, chest, abdominal, and leg injuries. Fracture of long bones, especially the femur. Internal injury and bleeding of the liver and/or spleen. (Kidney, liver—blows to right upper quadrant; spleen—blows to flank and torso.)
Child run over by car	Internal chest injury, often without obvious external damage. Internal abdominal injury, often without obvious external damage. Fractures of upper and lower extremities and the pelvis.

slightly less efficient than in adults. The more elastic ribs rarely fracture; however, there is more likely to be injury to the structures beneath the ribs. You must suspect internal chest injuries when the mechanism of injury is significant, despite the absence of external signs of chest injury.

Abdomen

Infants and young children are abdominal breathers; that is, they rely on their diaphragms for breathing more than adults do. Thus, they may not have significant movement of their chest while breathing. Therefore, watch the abdomen to evaluate breathing. In addition, abdominal muscles are immature and therefore provide less protection to internal organs than do adult abdominal muscles.

The abdomen can be a site of "hidden" injuries. You must suspect an internal abdominal injury when the patient deteriorates even without evidence of external injury. In addition, air in the stomach can distend the abdomen and interfere with artificial ventilation. This may also lead to vomiting. Be prepared to suction the patient.

Extremities

Despite the more flexible bones in the pediatric patient, their extremity injuries are managed the same way as extremity injuries in adults.

Burns

Burns are a common pediatric injury. Review the pediatric differences in the "rule of nines" in Chapter 28, "Soft-Tissue Trauma," as it applies to estimating the extent of burns in children and infants. Follow these guidelines when managing patients with burns:

- Identify candidates for transportation to burn centers. Local protocols should guide your determination.
- Cover the burn with sterile dressings. Nonadherent dressings are the best, but sterile sheets may be used.

Moist dressings should be used with caution in the pediatric patient. Remember that the child's body surface area is larger proportionately to their body mass, making them more prone to heat loss. Burned patients who become hypothermic have a higher death rate. You must keep the infant or child covered to prevent a drop in body temperature.

PATIENT CARE

Trauma

Emergency care steps for the pediatric trauma patient should include the following:

1. Ensure an open airway. Use the jaw-thrust maneuver.
2. Suction as necessary, using a rigid suction catheter.
3. Provide high-concentration oxygen.
4. Ventilate with a pediatric pocket mask or bag-valve mask as needed.
5. Provide spinal immobilization (Scan 35-4).
6. Transport immediately.
7. Continue to reassess en route.
8. Assess and treat other injuries en route if time permits.

SCAN 35-4   Immobilizing a Child Using a KED

Although many pediatric immobilization devices are available, an adult Kendrick Extrication Device (KED) can also be used successfully to immobilize a child if adjusted to suit the child's size and anatomy. *Manually stabilize the child's neck and spine throughout, and apply a cervical spine immobilization collar before securing the child to the KED.*

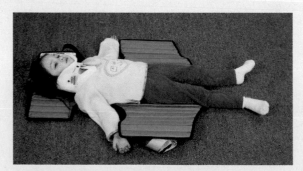

❶ Open the KED and place padding on it to properly position and align the child's head and body. Log roll the child onto the KED.

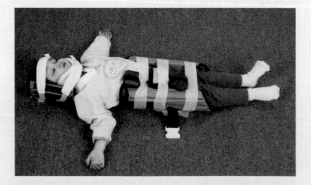

❷ Fold the side pieces inward to provide side padding and support and to allow visualization of the chest and abdomen. Since the torso straps will be rolled to the inside, secure the torso with tape. Fold the head flaps securely against the child's head and tape across the head and chin.

The Little Ones Make Us Nervous

Pediatric patients cause stress because the stakes are high and we (fortunately) don't get a lot of pediatric calls. The decision making in this section will involve your "from-the-doorway" pediatric assessment. With the information provided, determine if the patient is in a serious or a less-serious condition.

1. You are met at the door by an upset mother who is holding a limp 13-month-old child in her arms.

2. A 3-year-old child is reported as having a croupy cough and difficulty breathing. She is screaming and clinging to her mother as you approach.

3. A child has fallen from a high sliding board. You arrive to find the child holding his left forearm against his body while quietly clinging to his mother.

CHILD ABUSE AND NEGLECT

Although the number of known child abuse cases is large, the real number may be even larger than the statistics indicate. Experts believe that for every abused child seen by the emergency department or family physician, there are many more unreported cases who never receive care.

Child abusers are mothers, fathers, sisters, brothers, grandparents, stepparents, baby-sitters and other caregivers, white-collar workers, blue-collar workers, and those who are unemployed, rich, or poor. There is no distinction as to race, creed, ethnicity, or economic background.

Child abuse can take several different forms, often occurring in combination:

- Psychological (emotional) abuse
- Neglect
- Physical abuse
- Sexual abuse

What constitutes neglect is a serious legal question. If a child goes without proper food, shelter, clothing, supervision, treatment of injuries and illnesses, a safe environment, and love, the effects surely will be seen but will seldom directly trigger an emergency call. Physical and sexual abuse are the problems likely to be seen by EMTs. If signs of neglect are observed in the course of a call, they should also be reported to the proper authorities.

Physical and Sexual Abuse

Abusers inflict almost every imaginable kind of injury and maltreatment. Physically abused children—often called "battered" children—are beaten with fists, hair brushes, electric cords, pool cues, pots and pans, and almost any other object that can be used as a weapon. They are intentionally burned by hot water, steam, open flames, cigarettes, and other thermal sources. Battered children may be severely shaken, thrown into their cribs or down steps, pushed out of windows and over railings, and even pushed from moving cars.

Sexual abuse ranges from adults exposing themselves to children to sexual intercourse or sexual torture. Often, cases in which sexual abuse results in serious physical injury are reported to the authorities. However, some cases, especially those in which emotional injury or minor physical injury were done, are not reported, and therefore they are difficult to estimate.

CORE CONCEPT
How to deal with issues of child abuse and neglect and children with special needs

---

PATIENT ASSESSMENT

Physical Abuse

In child physical abuse cases, you will find (Figure 35-20):

- Slap marks, bruises, abrasions, lacerations, and incisions of all sizes and with shapes matching the item used. You may see wide welts from belts, a looped shape from

FIGURE 35-20 Child abuse injuries. (© Robert A. Felter, MD)

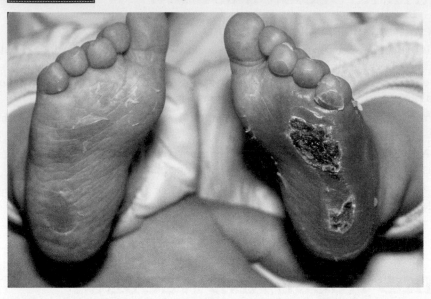

cords, or the shape of a hand from slapping. You may find swollen limbs, split lips, black eyes, and loose or broken teeth. Often the injuries are to the back, legs, and arms.

■ Broken bones are common and all types of fractures are possible. Many battered children have multiple fractures, often in various stages of healing, or have fracture-associated complications.

■ Head injuries are common, with concussions and skull fractures being reported. Closed head injuries occur to many infants and small children who have been severely shaken.

■ Abdominal injuries include ruptured spleens, livers and lungs lacerated by broken ribs, internal bleeding from blunt trauma and punching, and lacerated and avulsed genitalia.

■ Bite marks showing the teeth size and pattern of the adult mouth may be present.

■ Burn marks that are small and round from cigarettes; "glove" or "stocking" burn marks from dipping in hot water; burns on buttocks and legs (creases behind the knees and at the thighs are protected when flexed); and demarcation burns in the shape of an iron, stove burner, or other hot utensil are frequently found.

■ Indications of shaking an infant include a bulging fontanelle due to increased intracranial pressure from the bleeding of torn blood vessels in the brain, unconsciousness, and typical signs and symptoms of head and brain injury. Injuries to the central nervous system from "the shaken baby syndrome" are among the most lethal child abuse injuries.

Sometimes you will treat an injured child and never consider that he has been abused, especially if the child relates well with the parents and there appears to be a strong bond between them. However, there can be certain indications that abuse may be occurring in or outside the home, with the family feeling they must not admit to the problem. Be on the alert for:

■ Repeated responses to provide care for the same child or children in a family. Remember that in areas with many hospitals, you may see the child more frequently than any one hospital.

■ Indications of past injuries. This is one reason why you must do a physical examination and why you must remove articles of clothing. Pay special attention to the child's back and buttocks.

■ Poorly healing wounds or improperly healed fractures. It is extremely rare for a child to receive a fracture, be given proper orthopedic care, and then show angulations and large "bumps" and "knots" of bone at the "healed" injury site.

■ Indications of past burns or fresh bilateral burns. Children seldom put both hands on a hot object or touch the same hot object again (true, some do—this is only an indication, not proof). Some types of burns are almost always linked to child abuse, such as cigarette burns to the body and burns to the buttocks and lower extremities that result from the child being dipped in hot water.

- Many different types of injuries to both sides, or to the front and back, of the body. This gains even more importance if the adults on the scene keep insisting that the child "falls a lot."
- Fear on the part of the child to tell you how the injury occurred. The child may seem to expect no comfort from the parents and may have little or no apparent reaction to pain.
- The parent or caregiver at the scene who does not wish to leave you alone with the child, tells conflicting or changing stories, overwhelms you with explanations of the cause of the injury, or faults the child. These should arouse your suspicions and cause you to more carefully assess the situation.

Pay attention to the adults as you treat the child:

- Do they seem inappropriately unconcerned about the child?
- Do they have trouble controlling their anger?
- Do you feel that at any moment there may be an emotional explosion?
- Do any of the adults appear to be in a deep state of depression?
- Are there indications of alcohol or drug abuse?
- Do any of the adults speak of suicide or seeking mercy for their unhappy children?

Although parents or caregivers may call for help for the child, they may be reluctant to provide a history of the injury and refuse transport. Take note of any parent who refuses to have his child sent to the nearest hospital or to a hospital where the child has been seen before. This may indicate fear of the staff remembering or seeing a record of past injuries. (You cannot transport without parental consent; however, you may be able to convince the parents the child needs to be seen by a doctor because of certain signs and symptoms that are "difficult to determine" in the field.) Be the child's advocate, but do not accuse the parent.

PATIENT ASSESSMENT

Sexual Abuse

Rearrange or remove clothing only as necessary to determine and treat injuries. This will help preserve evidence where possible. Examine the genitalia only if there is obvious injury or the child tells you of a recent injury. The child may be hysterical, frightened, or withdrawn and unable to give you a history of the incident. Be calm and as reassuring as possible. The following are common signs of sexual abuse:

- Obvious signs of sexual assault, including burns or wounds to the genitalia.
- Any unexplained genital injury such as bruising, lacerations, or bloody discharge from genital orifices (openings).
- Seminal fluid on the body or clothes or other discharges associated with sexually transmitted diseases.
- In rare cases, the child may tell you that he was sexually assaulted.

Remain professional and control your emotions. Protect the child from embarrassment. Say nothing that may make the child believe that he is to blame for the sexual assault. (Many believe that they are.)

PATIENT CARE

Physical or Sexual Abuse

Emergency care for physical or sexual abuse includes the following steps:

1. Dress and provide other appropriate care for injuries as necessary.
2. Preserve evidence of sexual abuse if it is suspected:
   Discourage the child from going to the bathroom (for both defecation and urination).
   Give nothing to the patient by mouth.
   Do not have the child wash or change clothes.
3. Transport the child.

NOTE: You must plainly and clearly report to the medical staff any finding or suspicion regarding possible physical or sexual abuse.

Role of the EMT in Cases of Suspected Abuse or Neglect

Remember that you are charged with providing emergency care for an injured child. You are not a police officer, court investigator, social worker, or judge. Gather information from the parents or caregiver away from the child without expression of disbelief or judgment. Talk with the child separately about how an injury occurred. As you assess the patient and provide appropriate care, control your emotions and hold back accusations. Do not indicate to the parents or other adults at the scene that you suspect child abuse or neglect. Do not ask the child if he has been abused. Doing so when others are around could produce stress too great for the injured child to handle.

If you are suspicious about the mechanism of injury, transport the child even though the severity of injury may not warrant such action.

In some states, EMTs are mandated reporters; that is, they are required by law to report suspicions of child abuse or neglect. Commonly, reporting means contacting your state's child abuse reporting hotline. Often just notifying hospital personnel about your suspicions is not enough. Be familiar with your state laws. Even if reporting possible child abuse or neglect is not a legal requirement in your state, it is a professional obligation. As an EMT, you may be the only advocate an abused child has. Be conscientious.

Past responses can be checked and future responses noted in case a pattern develops to indicate possible abuse. However, even when talking to your partner, the hospital staff, the police, and your superiors, use the terms *suspected* and *possible*. Always be objective and report only the facts. Avoid generalizations and assumptions. Do not call someone a child abuser. Keep in mind that the courts can deal harshly with those who provide patient care and then violate the confidentiality of the patient, the family, and the home. Rumors about abuse may, in the long run, cause mental or physical harm to your child patient.

It may be difficult, but remember that the parent or caregiver needs help as well. Your actions, response, and concern directed toward suspected abusers can help them recognize their problem and may encourage them to seek therapy and rehabilitation. Also bear in mind that your suspicions may be unfounded. Not every injury to a child is the result of child abuse. Suspicions should be aroused not by individual injuries but by patterns of injuries and behavior.

INFANTS AND CHILDREN WITH SPECIAL CHALLENGES

Over the years, medical expertise has improved significantly, allowing many children who would formerly have died to live. The following are some common groups of children with special challenges:

- Premature infants with lung disease
- Infants and children with heart disease
- Infants and children with neurological disease
- Children with chronic disease or altered function from birth

Often these children are able to live at home with their parents. This means that you may receive calls to care for children who have complicated medical problems and are dependent on various technologies (Figure 35-21). In fact, children with special challenges living at home constitute a significant percentage of the relatively small number of pediatric emergency calls.

The children's parents will be familiar with the various devices used and can serve as a valuable resource. Common devices include tracheostomy tubes, home artificial ventilators, central intravenous lines, gastrostomy tubes and gastric feeding tubes, and shunts.

Emergency care of children with special challenges has often been complicated by the lack of information that EMTs and emergency department staff are able to quickly obtain about the children's medication, condition, history, precautions needed, and special management plans.

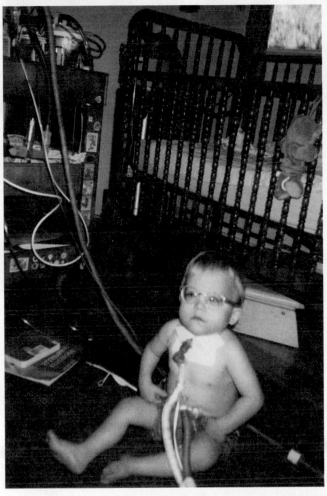

FIGURE 35-21 Children who have complicated medical problems are often dependent on various technologies. *(© Family Voices)*

NOTE: *In 1999, the American College of Emergency Physicians (ACEP) and the American Academy of Pediatrics (AAP) developed the Emergency Information Form for Children with Special Needs that should be kept up-to-date and on hand by the patient's caregivers. If a copy of this form is available at the patient's home, it should be brought along if the child is transported to the hospital.*

More about patients with special challenges and the advanced medical devices they may rely on will be discussed in Chapter 37, "Emergencies for Patients with Special Challenges."

Tracheostomy Tubes

Tracheostomy tubes are tubes that have been placed into the child's trachea to create an open airway (Figure 35-22). They are often used when a child has been on a ventilator for a prolonged time. Although there are various types of tubes, the potential complications are identical. You may be called to help when there is:

- Obstruction
- Bleeding from the tube or around the tube
- Air leaking around the tube
- Infection
- Dislodged tube

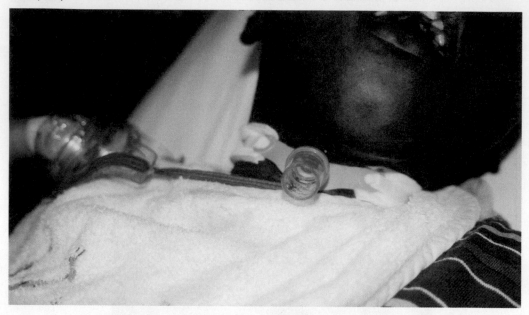

FIGURE 35-22 Various emergencies may arise when a child has a tracheostomy. *(© Fran Nadel, MD)*

Your emergency care will consist of:

- Maintaining an open airway
- Suctioning the tube as needed
- Allowing the patient to remain in a position of comfort, perhaps on the parent's lap
- Transporting the patient to the hospital

Home Artificial Ventilators

Artificial ventilators in the home are becoming more common. Although the parents will be trained in the ventilator's use, they will call EMS when there is trouble. Regardless of the problem, your emergency care will include:

- Maintaining an open airway
- Artificially ventilating with a pocket mask or bag-valve mask with oxygen
- Transporting the patient

Central Intravenous Lines

Central lines are intravenous lines that are placed close to the heart. Unlike most peripheral IV lines, central lines may be left in place for long-term use. Possible complications of the use of central lines are:

- Infection
- Bleeding
- Clotting-off of the line
- Cracked line

Your emergency care will include:

- Applying pressure if there is bleeding
- Transporting the patient

Gastrostomy Tubes and Gastric Feeding

Gastrostomy tubes, tubes placed through the abdominal wall directly into the stomach, are used when a patient is not able to be orally fed. The most dangerous potential problem associated with their use involves respiratory distress. The emergency care will include the following steps:

- Being alert for altered mental status in diabetic patients. They may become hypoglycemic quickly when unable to eat.
- Ensuring an open airway.
- Suctioning the airway as needed.
- Providing oxygen, if needed.
- Transporting the patient in either a sitting position or lying on the right side with the head elevated to reduce the risk of aspiration.

Shunts

A shunt is a drainage device that runs from the brain to the abdomen to relieve excess cerebrospinal fluid. There will be a reservoir on the side of the skull. If the shunt malfunctions, pressure inside the skull will rise, causing an altered mental status. An altered mental status may also be caused by an infection. These patients are prone to respiratory arrest. Your emergency care will include the following steps:

- Maintaining an open airway
- Ventilating with a pocket mask or bag-valve mask and high-concentration oxygen, if needed
- Transporting the patient

THE EMT AND PEDIATRIC EMERGENCIES

Many types of pediatric illnesses and injuries have been discussed in this chapter. The focus has been on the patient. Now we will look at the psychological responses of the EMT.

It is well known that pediatric calls can be among the most stressful for the EMT, even when they are uneventful. EMTs who have children often identify their patients with their own children. Other EMTs have no experience with children and feel anxiety about communicating with them and treating them—even about estimating their ages. However, the skills of communicating with and treating children can be learned and applied. Often, the EMT who starts out "knowing nothing about children" turns out to have a real knack for dealing with them.

Child care mostly consists of applying what you have learned about the care of adult patients and combining it with knowledge of the key differences in developmental characteristics, anatomy, and physiology of children.

Often the most serious stresses an EMT faces result from pediatric calls that involve a very sick, injured, or abused child, or a child who has died or who dies during or after emergency care. Fortunately, such calls are rare and can be prepared for with advance training.

When you have had an experience like this, talk with other EMTs. If your squad or service has a counselor, see this person for advice. You may think that you can handle the stress or sorrow by yourself, but experienced EMTs know better. Unless you resolve the impact of stressful events, the problems created may compound and could lead to "burnout."

CHAPTER REVIEW

Key Facts and Concepts

- The assessment and treatment of children is often different than that of adults.
- Children often differ from adults both anatomically and psychosocially.
- Assessment and treatment procedures must take into account these specific differences.
- As an EMT, you must learn these differences to enable you to better serve this special population.

Key Decisions

- Is this a normal mental status for this child?
- Are the vital signs normal for this age group?
- Can I involve mom/dad in the assessment and treatment of this child?
- Does the pediatric assessment triangle indicate a critical patient?
  - How can I confirm this using the primary assessment?
- Why is this child's heart beating so fast?
  - Is he in shock?

Chapter Glossary

fontanelle (FON-ta-nel) a soft spot on an infant's anterior scalp formed by the joining of not yet fused bones of the skull.

pediatric (pee-dee-AT-rik) of or pertaining to a patient who has yet to reach puberty.

retractions pulling in of the skin and soft tissue between the ribs when breathing. This is typically a sign of respiratory distress in children.

Preparation for Your Examination and Practice

Short Answer

1. Name one psychological/social characteristic that you would be likely to find in a patient of each of the following ages and explain how you would tailor your actions as an EMT to accommodate this characteristic: 2-year-old, 6-year-old, and 15-year old.

2. Describe ways of calming and interacting effectively with the infant or child patient and with the parent or caregiver.

3. Explain some of the elements of a general impression of the infant or child patient that you can obtain "from the doorway"—before you approach the patient.

4. Explain how to differentiate between an upper airway obstruction and a lower airway disease or disorder. Explain how and why the two should be treated differently.

5. Explain the main steps of emergency treatment for any infant or child trauma patient.

6. Explain how suspicion of child abuse should or should not affect the care you provide for an infant or child. Explain the reporting requirements regarding child abuse and neglect in your state or locality.

Thinking and Linking

Think back to Chapter 11, "The Primary Assessment," and link information from that chapter with information from this chapter as you consider the following situation:

- You are called to respond to a "sick baby." When you arrive, you are led to a baby in its crib. The baby's eyes are closed. How do you conduct your primary assessment?

Critical Thinking Exercises

With a pediatric trauma patient, you will need to call on everything you know about injury patterns and the physical and psychosocial development characteristics of different age levels. The purpose of this exercise will be to consider these elements in relation to a pediataric trauma patient.

- You are called to the scene of a collision between a vehicle and a 5-year-old on a bicycle. The child is lying near the curb. Based on what you know about the developmental characteristics of children as well as common injury patterns in children, explain some of the special elements you should take into consideration as you proceed to assess and care for this patient.

Pathophysiology to Practice

The following questions are designed to assist you in gathering relevant clinical information and making accurate decisions in the field.

- Describe key differences in the anatomy and physiology of infants and children with regard to the following:
  1. Head
  2. Airway and respiratory system
  3. Chest
  4. Abdomen
  5. Body surface
  6. Blood volume

- For the previous elements, discuss how you might have to adjust your assessment and/or treatment to account for the difference:
  7. Head
  8. Airway and respiratory system
  9. Chest
  10. Abdomen
  11. Body surface
  12. Blood volume

Street Scenes

The dispatcher sends you to 143 Pine Lane for "a child not breathing. More information to follow." As you head in that direction, you receive additional details. A normally active 2-year-old girl named Shawna had been playing without incident most of the afternoon. After dinner, her face seemed flushed, her forehead was warm, and she was not her usual self. When Shawna's mother got her ready for bed, she noticed Shawna arch her back and start to shake. Shawna did not appear to be breathing. That's when the mother called 911.

Street Scene Questions

1. What is your assessment plan for this patient?
2. What equipment should be brought into the house?
3. Should ALS be dispatched to the scene prior to your arrival?

Your response time is less than 5 minutes. Your partner radios the dispatcher and asks for an ALS response before you arrive at the scene. Dispatch has informed you that the mother is very upset and he has no additional information. About a minute before arriving, you discuss with your partner the equipment that needs to go into the house, and you both agree to take in the pediatric bag that contains the airway equipment, including the bag-valve mask, an oxygen tank, and a suction unit. You volunteer to get the equipment, while your partner goes to the patient. Your partner enters the house just before you and he sees the mother holding a limp child. He takes the child and places her on the couch.

Your partner immediately evaluates the child's airway and breathing. He then performs a head-tilt, chin-lift maneuver, which brings the tongue forward. He sees mucus around the mouth, so he clears the airway by suctioning. Shawna becomes more responsive and cries. Her respirations are deep and adequate. (They would have to be for her to cry that loudly.) You and your partner realize that it is a good sound.

Street Scene Questions

4. What care should be provided next?
5. What additional assessment needs to be done?
6. What information needs to be relayed to the ALS unit?

You administer blow-by oxygen to the patient, while your partner gets a full set of vital signs. You reassure the mother that Shawna is breathing and tell her that she can help by answering some questions. You proceed to ask all the SAMPLE questions. Shawna's mother describes what led up to this event. You radio the ALS unit with this information and are informed of a 2-minute ETA, so you start to package the patient for transport to the hospital. As you are doing this, Shawna opens her eyes. She continues to cry and you ask her mother to hold her hand and talk to her. Although Shawna is not fully alert, she is breathing well and her skin color is improving.

As you arrive at the ambulance, the ALS unit pulls up and a paramedic gets into your patient compartment. She does an assessment and is confident that a BLS transport is all that is required. She calls medical direction and provides a patient history with vital signs. Medical direction concurs that a BLS transport is appropriate. As she returns to her vehicle, the paramedic compliments you and your partner on a job well done.

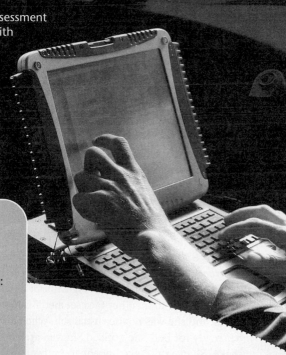

36 Geriatric Emergencies

○ **STANDARD**
Special Patient Populations (Geriatrics)

○ **COMPETENCY**
Applies fundamental knowledge of growth, development, and aging and assessment findings to provide basic emergency care and transportation for a patient with special needs.

○ **CORE CONCEPTS**
— Age-related changes in the elderly

— Communicating with older patients

— Assessing and caring for older patients

— Illness and injury in older patients

EXPLORE Resource**Central**

To access Resource Central, follow directions on the Student Access Card provided with this text. If there is no card, go to **www.bradybooks.com** and follow the Resource Central link to Buy Access from there. Under Media Resources, you will find:

▶ **Information about Alzheimer Disease**
Watch a video to learn about this disease; discover associated risk factors, how the disease progresses, and available treatments.

▶ **Information about Geriatric Trauma**
Read about responding to calls involving geriatric patients, what tools are used in the prehospital environment, and why over-triage may be beneficial.

▶ **Information about Geriatric Cognition**
Be prepared for anything you may encounter when dealing with this population. Watch this video to learn about some usual cognitive changes that occur with age as well as the complications that may result from an undiagnosed mental disorder.

OBJECTIVES

After reading this chapter you should be able to:

36.1 Describe common changes in body systems that occur in older age. (pp. 931–934)

36.2 Discuss adaptations that may be required in communicating with and assessing older patients. (pp. 935–939)

36.3 Discuss the need for awareness of and the special considerations regarding medical conditions and injuries to which older patients are prone, including effects of medications, shortness of breath, chest pain, altered mental status, gastrointestinal complaints, dizziness/ weakness/malaise, depression/suicide, rash, pain, flulike symptoms, and falls, and the possible significance of general or nonspecific complaints in older adults. (pp. 940–944)

36.4 Recommend changes to improve safety in the home of an elderly person. (pp. 944–945)

36.5 Discuss possible indications of elder abuse. (pp. 944–945)

36.6 Discuss psychosocial concerns of older patients, including the fear of loss of independence (pp. 945–946)

of this age-related change may not have an appropriate index of suspicion for shock in an elderly patient when the heart rate is not as rapid as they expect with shock. Table 36-1 describes some of these age-related changes, how they may be apparent in the assessment, and how they may relate to your patient care decisions.

Table 36-1   Effects of Aging and Implications for Assessment and Decision Making

BODY SYSTEM	AGE-RELATED CHANGES	RESULT	ASSESSMENT AND DECISION MAKING
Cardiovascular System	Degeneration of the valves and muscle	Reduced stroke volume and cardiac output may lead to orthostatic hypotension, decreased brain perfusion, and reduced tolerance for activity	Patients may complain of dizziness, fainting, or weakness, especially on changing from a sitting to a standing position. Medicines for high blood pressure and dysrhythmias can contribute to these effects. Prevalence of congestive heart failure increases; assess lung sounds and check for edema.
	Degeneration of conduction system	Dysrhythmias, decrease in maximum heart rate	The heart rhythm may be irregular, or may be abnormally fast or slow. The heart rate may not increase as much in response to blood loss, especially if the patient is taking certain medicines for heart problems or high blood pressure.
	Thickening and narrowing of coronary and systemic arteries	Decreased delivery of oxygenated blood to the tissues; increased risk of heart attack, stroke, aortic aneurysm, and peripheral artery disease	Determine whether any complaints or changes in mental status or neurological problems are new. Remember, a heart attack in the elderly may not present with chest pain.
Respiratory System	Decreased elasticity of lungs; decreased lung volume; decreased activity of cilia	Decreased ability to increase oxygen intake when needed; increased risk of pneumonia	Check patient's oxygenation status, and administer oxygen as needed.
	Diminished cough and gag reflexes	Increased risk of aspiration	Pay particular attention to the patient's ability to swallow secretions; suction as necessary. Patient may not cough, even with pneumonia or other respiratory infections.
Digestive System	Decreased movement of intestinal tract, decreased secretion of stomach acid, decreased sensation of taste, difficulty chewing and swallowing, decreased food absorption	Constipation, bowel obstruction, weight loss, malnutrition	Maintain a high index of suspicion for bowel obstruction, even with vague or minimal complaints of abdominal pain, fullness, constipation, or bloating.
	Changes in gastrointestinal lining, increased risk of cancers, relaxation of sphincters	Increased risk of gastrointestinal bleeding, gastroesophageal reflux (heartburn), and fecal incontinence	When relevant, ask about blood in stools, black tarry stools, or vomiting blood or coffee grounds-appearing material. Be alert to patient hygiene needs.

(continued)

BODY SYSTEM	AGE-RELATED CHANGES	RESULT	ASSESSMENT AND DECISION MAKING
Liver and Kidneys	Decreased breakdown and clearance of medications; decreased production of clotting factors and other blood proteins	Increased risk of drug toxicity and drug interactions; increased edema; decreased blood clotting	Always be suspicious of drug toxicity or interactions as a cause of altered mental status and other complaints. Patients can be more prone to uncontrolled bleeding.
Endocrine System	Diminished thyroid function	Decreased energy metabolism, problems with temperature regulation	Patients are more prone to both heat- and cold-related emergencies, even in relatively mild temperatures, indoors and outdoors.
	Pancreas, changes in insulin production or function	More prone to type 2 diabetes and hyperglycemia	Consider diabetic emergencies as a cause of altered mental status.
Musculoskeletal System	Decreased muscle mass and strength; arthritis	Weakness, more prone to falls, unable to get up from falls, decreased mobility; patients may be less able to care for self	Assess for injuries from falls and immobility. Immobility can lead to decubitus ulcers (bed sores) and increased risk for pulmonary embolism.
	Decreased bone mass and strength; especially a problem in females	Fractures may occur with minimal force, and sometimes with little pain	Handle patients gently; assess for fractures.
Nervous System	Decreased pain sensation	Patients may sustain injury, such as hot water burns, without realizing it; patients may experience diffuse or vague pain, even with serious illness	Take all complaints of pain seriously. Realize that conditions such as myocardial infarction may not have typical pain patterns in elderly patients, or may not result in a complaint of pain at all.
	Decreased reaction and cognitive processing times	Less able to avoid injury	Assess for injuries, allow time for patient to follow instructions.
	Increased risk of dementia	Patients may be prone to injury, wandering away, being taken advantage of, or abused; patients may neglect themselves	Carefully assess the patient's degree of orientation and be aware of signs of neglect and abuse.
	Increased risk of depression and sleep disorders	May attempt suicide, or neglect self; elderly with sleep disorders are more likely to be physically abused	Don't rule out medication overdoses or other types of self-harm in the elderly.
Integumentary System	The skin becomes thin, dry, and fragile; nails become weak and brittle, and hair becomes dry and more sparse	Skin easily bruised and torn	Assess for signs of injury, even with minor trauma, and handle elderly patients carefully.

Sometimes it is difficult for patients to differentiate between expected age-related changes and the onset of disease. A patient may attribute aches and pains or shortness of breath to "old age" when, in fact, these symptoms may indicate an acute problem that should be treated. As EMTs, we must avoid the pitfall of attributing signs and symptoms of disease to the aging process. There are ways you can reduce your chances of misattributing signs and symptoms when determining a patient's normal or baseline condition. One way to do this is to ask the patient how things are different now than they were a week ago. For example, "Mr. Shah, is there anything different about the way you feel today from the way you felt last week?" This information can be very helpful in distinguishing a chronic condition from a new problem.

- How may this patient's age-related changes affect my assessment and care?

Communicating with Older Patients

By no means do all older patients have impairments that interfere with communication. However, changes in hearing, vision, and working memory, as well as changes in dentition (the number and arrangement of teeth), the residual effects of a stroke, or dementia, sometimes interfere with an older person's ability to understand you or to make himself understood. Difficulty communicating is a frustrating situation for anyone, regardless of age. Table 36-2 lists some common causes of communication difficulty and suggests some ways to improve communication.

A few of the elderly have a significant deterioration of memory and overall intellectual ability from dementia, a loss of brain function. The most common cause of dementia in the elderly is Alzheimer's disease, a chronic organic disorder. However, do not assume that confusion in your elderly patient is "normal" or the result of long-term mental deterioration. Unless someone who knows the patient can confirm that this is a chronic condition, suspect that an altered mental status may be the result of the present illness or injury.

Always attempt to communicate directly with an older patient first, rather than assuming she will give an unreliable history and asking others about her (Figure 36-2). You should only rely on others for information if you are unable to get a satisfactory history from the older patient or if you need to confirm information the patient has provided.

When you are speaking to any patient, it is important that the patient see and hear you. This is especially true in the elderly patient who has a hearing impairment or poor peripheral vision. Keep in mind that speaking loudly, slowly, or very clearly to a patient does not mean speaking down to a patient. Treat the patient with respect and dignity. Begin by calling the patient by a title and her last name; for example, Mrs. Sanchez. Ask the patient how she would like to be addressed before assuming that you may use her first name. Never simply call the patient "Honey" or any similarly disrespectful term. Whenever possible, speak to the patient at the same eye level. This may involve crouching, or even kneeling down.

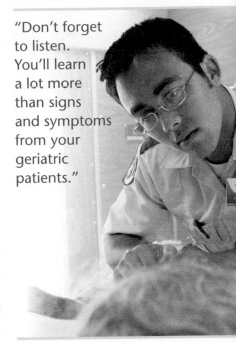

CORE CONCEPT
Communicating with older patients

"Don't forget to listen. You'll learn a lot more than signs and symptoms from your geriatric patients."

History and Assessment of Older Adult Patients

The steps of assessment for older adult patients are the same as those for other patients. During these steps, however, you should be aware of and look for some findings that are of special concern in older patients.

CORE CONCEPT
Assessing and caring for older patients

Table 36-2 Effects of Aging and Implications for Communication			
PROBLEM	**CAUSES**	**POSSIBLE CONSEQUENCES**	**EMT COMMUNICATION STRATEGIES**
Decreased vision, including poor night vision, peripheral vision, and farsightedness; possible blindness	Cataracts, glaucoma, retinal degeneration	Increased risk for falls and other injuries, difficulty reading medication directions, difficulty reading and signing consent forms	Position yourself in front of the patient. Adjust lighting to reduce glare, help patient find glasses, and assist with walking, if needed.
Decreased hearing, especially for higher pitched sounds	Shrinkage of structures in the ear (may also lead to dizziness or difficulty with balance)	Difficulty hearing others	If television or radio is too loud, ask to turn it down. Speak clearly, and assist with hearing aids, if necessary.
Unclear speech	Stroke, poor-fitting dentures	Patient may become frustrated if he cannot make himself understood	Ask patient to put in his dentures, if necessary. Stroke patients with garbled or slurred speech may be able to write; offer a pen and paper.

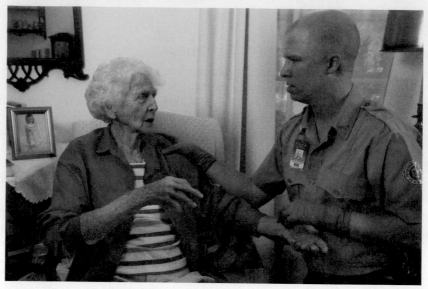

Scene Size-Up and Safety

When you approach an elderly person's residence, look both outside and inside for clues to the patient's physical and mental abilities. Is the outside of the house conscientiously cared for, or is the paint on the house peeling and the garden untended? When you enter the home, besides looking for potential dangers to you and your crew, look at the general condition of the residence. Is half-eaten food sitting in the living room? Is something unrecognizable drying up in a pan on the stove? Is the house dirty? Are items left out in the open where someone can trip on them?

A very important question to ask is, "What is the temperature?" Like infants, older people cannot regulate their body temperatures very well. They need an environment that frequently feels uncomfortably warm to younger people. Even at such temperatures, some older people still wear several layers of clothing to retain sufficient heat. This can become a problem when a heat wave occurs and the older person fails to feel the temperature rising. A life-threatening rise in body temperature can result. (See Chapter 33, "Environmental Emergencies.")

Primary Assessment

Forming a General Impression   Now that you have looked at the patient's surroundings, look at the patient. What is the level of his distress? Is he leaning forward with hands on knees gasping for breath? Is he lying on a hospital bed apparently unresponsive and breathing through an open mouth? Is he sitting in a chair in no acute distress?

Assessing Mental Status   This can be very challenging, because some older people have an abnormal mental status as part of their baseline condition. If family members or caregivers are available, it is important to find out from them what the normal status is for this patient. A recent or sudden onset of confusion or other deterioration in mental status should make you consider a serious underlying medical condition rather than Alzheimer's disease or other forms of dementia.

Assessing the Airway   Evaluating the airway of an older patient is very similar to evaluating the airway of other patients with two major exceptions. You may find it difficult to extend the head and flex the neck of an older patient because of arthritic changes in the bones of the neck. The best thing to do in this case is try not to force the head back but instead to thrust the jaw forward to pull the tongue out of the airway.

The other difficulty you may come across is dentures. If a patient's dentures are secure, there is usually no reason to remove them. If, however, they are loose or ill-fitting, it is best to remove them from the mouth of an unresponsive patient to prevent them from becoming an airway obstruction.

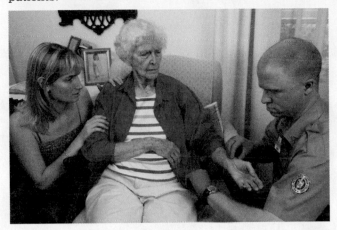

FIGURE 36-3 Finding a radial pulse in an older patient is usually no different from finding a pulse in other patients.

Assessing Breathing Older patients are at higher risk of foreign body airway obstruction. Two major risk factors are large, poorly chewed pieces of food and dentures. If you are unable to ventilate an older patient, reposition the head and try to ventilate again. If this does not work, initiate the sequence of steps to relieve a foreign body airway obstruction.

Assessing Circulation Finding a radial pulse in an older patient is usually no different from finding a pulse in other patients (Figure 36-3). What you may notice in these patients, though, is that the pulse is often irregularly irregular (i.e., completely without any kind of repeated cycle or regularity). This is the result of a very common dysrhythmia (abnormal heart rhythm) in older people. The irregularity is not a reason for concern in itself.

Identifying Priority Patients Older patients are less likely to complain of severe symptoms in certain conditions, so it can be difficult to determine a patient's priority. For example, most people having a heart attack experience significant chest pain. However, an older person is more likely to have just the sudden onset of weakness with no chest pain. Keep a high index of suspicion for serious conditions in elderly patients, even if symptoms are seemingly mild or vague.

Secondary Assessment

History Obtaining a history of the present illness can be challenging when evaluating an elderly patient. He may answer questions very slowly or even inappropriately. It may be difficult to understand his speech, or he may have difficulty understanding your questions. Regardless of the particular circumstances, you must gather as much information as you can from the patient and from other sources. Of particular note when assessing the patient's level of orientation: consider the patient oriented to time if he is able to tell you what year it is. Knowing what day or month it is can be a function of participating in the workforce, reading newspapers, or watching the news on television. A person who does not do these things may not have a good sense of day or month. However, if he knows the year, he can still be considered oriented to time.

When interviewing the patient, be sure to introduce yourself, speak slowly and clearly, and position yourself where the patient can easily see you. If he is answering your questions slowly and your primary assessment did not reveal any immediate threats to life, give him additional time. Be sure to ask just one question at a time. Similarly, if the patient's speech is slurred but still understandable, do not rush him. Doing so could easily fluster him, delaying responses even more, and destroy any rapport you have established. If the patient's speech is difficult to understand because his dentures are not in place, ask him to put them in, if appropriate.

Sometimes a patient will answer questions very slowly because he is clinically depressed, or so sad or blue that his eating and sleeping habits are altered, he feels fatigued, his memory or concentration is impaired, his self-confidence is low, and he may even have thoughts of suicide. Depression is a common problem among the elderly, but the patient may not be

FIGURE 36-4 Older patients often take multiple medications.

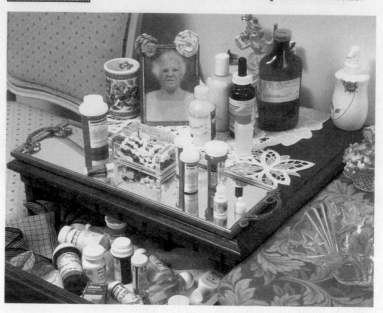

diagnosed or receiving treatment for it. However, do not automatically assume that a depressed patient has no other problems. Depression can both mimic and mask other serious medical problems. In fact, having serious health problems is itself a risk factor for depression.

Another possibility you may find when interviewing a patient is that the family tells you he was wrong in some of his responses. This is sometimes a result of a neurological condition, but it can also be caused by medications the patient is taking, especially if there are many of them (Figure 36-4) or the dose for some is too high.

A variation of this is the patient who gives you a story of having gone out to the movies last night but who, according to family members, has not left the house in years. This is called *confabulation*. The patient is replacing lost circumstances with imaginary ones. These made-up experiences are usually quite believable and the patient is typically very pleasant to talk to. Nonetheless, the experiences are not real and may very well change if you ask the same question a few minutes later. Confabulation can be caused by a number of neurological conditions.

This underscores the importance of gathering information from family members and others who are familiar with the patient's condition. If the patient lives with a spouse or other family members, they can frequently be an excellent source of information about his medications, past medical history, and even the history of the present illness. Similarly, visiting nurses can often provide or confirm a great deal of this information.

Physical Exam   When performing a physical exam on an older person, keep the patient's dignity in mind. Explain what you are going to do before you do it and replace any clothing you remove as soon as possible. Many older people have a high threshold for pain, so an extremity that is obviously fractured may cause very little discomfort to some patients. Others have a very low threshold for pain and will find elements of the physical exam extremely uncomfortable. You will need to be sensitive to these possibilities when doing the exam.

Baseline Vital Signs   Vital signs of the elderly are similar to those of other adults with only a few exceptions. As people age, the systolic blood pressure has a tendency to increase. Many older patients you meet will be on medication for hypertension, usually defined as a diastolic pressure over about 90 mmHg. These medications can have significant side effects, including weakness and dizziness, especially on standing up quickly from a sitting or supine position.

The skin loses much of its elasticity with aging, leading to dry skin that is thin and fragile. Applying pressure that is too heavy, even with just your fingertips, can be enough to cause the skin to tear in some patients. Be careful when pulling or lifting a patient to be as gentle as possible.

The pupils are not round and reactive to light in some older patients. Eye surgery or pre-existing conditions may have given the pupil an abnormal shape or the inability to react normally to light. Certain eye drops can also prevent normal reactions to light. When you find this condition, inquire as to whether it is normal before assuming the patient has a serious condition based on this sign.

Steps of the Physical Exam

The physical exam for older patients is the same as for other adults. However, you may come across some unusual findings because of the patient's age or condition.

Head and Neck   When evaluating the head, be especially attentive. Injuries to the head and face are very common in older patients who have sustained a fall or been involved in a motor-vehicle collision. In fact, falls and motor-vehicle collisions account for the overwhelming majority of injuries in patients over 65 years of age.

The patient's neck may be stiff and the head may be far forward of its normal position because of changes in the spine. This can be a challenge to deal with when you suspect a neck injury and must immobilize the patient. Use folded towels or other materials to keep the head in its normal position, prevent hyperextension, and make the patient more comfortable.

Chest and Abdomen   Although the chest and abdomen are not commonly injured, keep in mind the decreased sensitivity to pain that many older people have. Serious abdominal problems that would cause a younger person agony may produce only slight discomfort for older patients. The elderly may have diminished breath sounds because of decreased lung capacity and decreased movement of the chest wall. Also listen to the lungs for wheezes or crackles, which can be signs of respiratory or cardiac problems. Sometimes, elderly patients can have crackles in the bases of the lungs that disappear after the patient has taken a few deep breaths.

Pelvis and Extremities   The hip or proximal femur is commonly fractured in a fall, especially in women. This is partly because more women than men survive to be old, but even more so because women are more prone to lose calcium from their bones. This leads to so much weakening of the bone that a fracture is sometimes the cause of a fall rather than a result. Other areas on the extremities are also injured sometimes because of this weakening of the bone, most notably the wrists and proximal humerus. Be sure to check the patient's extremities, especially the lower extremities, for edema (swelling). Significant edema can be a sign of underlying heart, vascular, or liver disease.

Spine   The back may occasionally be injured in a fall, but it is very commonly injured in motor-vehicle collisions. Again, because of abnormal curvature that sometimes accompanies aging, immobilizing these patients can be challenging. Do your best to keep the vertebrae in alignment and to reduce the patient's discomfort (Figure 36-5).

Reassessment

Children who deteriorate are likely to exhibit sudden changes in condition. Although that can also happen in elderly patients, it is more common for them to show a slow, steady decline in condition. This can be deceiving because the patient does not suddenly tell you or show sudden signs that his condition is going downhill. Instead, you may be lulled into a false sense of security because there is little or no appreciable change from one minute to the next. Guard against this by reassessing the patient at regular intervals and comparing your findings to those you previously recorded. Look for trends that indicate trouble.

Keep in mind the elements of the reassessment:

1. Reassess mental status
2. Maintain an open airway
3. Monitor breathing
4. Reassess pulse
5. Monitor skin color, temperature, and moisture
6. Reassess vital signs
   - Every 5 minutes in unstable patients
   - Every 15 minutes in stable patients
7. Ensure that all appropriate care and treatments are being given

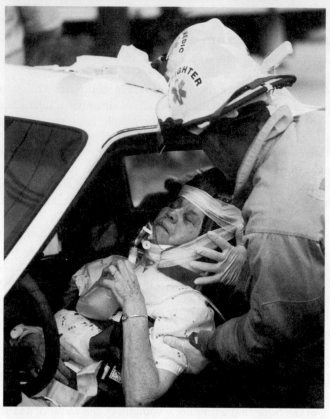

FIGURE 36-5 Extrication of an elderly patient from a motor-vehicle collision. (© *Eddie Sperling Photography*)

Illness and Injury in Older Patients

Older patients are more prone to some problems because of age-related changes in their body systems. For the same reason, these problems may present differently than in younger patients or may present with vague signs and symptoms.

Medication Side Effects and Interactions

The elderly use far more medications than other age groups. This is true not only because of the numerous diseases and conditions they have but also because modern medicine is producing more medications to treat these conditions. A significant number of the elderly take more than just one medication; some take as many as six, eight, ten, or even more. Keeping track of which pill to take and when to take it can be challenging even for the best-organized person. A handy way to help prevent problems like this is the use of a pill organizer with the pills for each day (or for each time of day) in a separate compartment (Figure 36-6). Another potential problem is that pills that have very different effects may have very similar appearances. If someone with vision problems and limited manual dexterity drops several pills, it becomes very easy to mix them up.

Many medications are expensive. Unfortunately, some elderly people must make the choice between food and medication because they cannot afford both. Obviously, this can lead to noncompliance with medication schedules. This can be even worse when a missed pill was one the doctor had prescribed to correct some of the undesirable effects of another drug that the patient is still taking.

Even when a medication is taken as directed, it can have a number of adverse effects. For example, many elderly patients take a medication from a class known as nonsteroidal anti-inflammatory drugs (NSAIDs). These medications, such as ibuprofen and naproxen (both available without a prescription), relieve the pain and inflammation associated with conditions such as arthritis. Unfortunately, these and other NSAIDs are also irritating to the gastrointestinal tract and often cause internal bleeding. More than 16,000 people die

FIGURE 36-6 **FIGURE 36-6** Many elderly persons use a pill organizer to help them remember when to take medications.

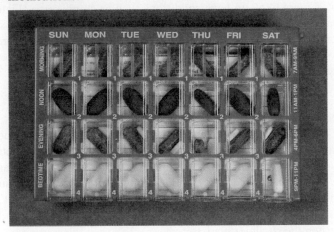

every year in the United States because of gastrointestinal bleeding when these medications are taken for arthritis.

Drug-patient interactions can occur because of the older patient's inability to clear medications from the body as quickly as before. Most drugs are broken down by the liver and kidneys, then excreted. However, liver and kidney function decrease with age. A dose that would be fine for a 30-year-old may be incapacitating to a 75-year-old.

Drug-drug interactions are very common in this age group, especially as the number of medications goes up. When two drugs interact, there are two possibilities: one may block or reduce the effect of the other, or one may increase the effect of the other. This outcome can be so severe that it becomes life threatening. The likelihood of a drug-drug interaction increases when a patient goes to different doctors for different problems and fills prescriptions at different pharmacies. Patients sometimes forget to tell the doctor or pharmacist about the other medications they are taking.

Drug-drug interactions are not limited to just prescription drugs. Prescription medications can have serious interactions with over-the-counter drugs, nutrient or herbal preparations, and even food (for example, grapefruit juice can increase the effects of certain cardiac medications).

Decision Point

- Does this patient take any medications that could alter his presentation or explain his condition?

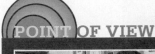

POINT OF VIEW

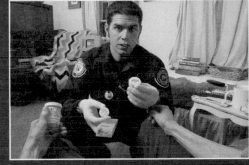

"I wasn't feeling well. It happens at my age—93. I didn't think much of it, but my daughter called the ambulance. She read that it could be a stroke or my heart or something.

"The men and women from the ambulance are always nice to me. A lot of them know my name. Some of them even know my medical problems by heart. This time the man was new. I have so many medications and medical problems it seems like it takes 20 minutes to get them all straight.

"But he listened and wrote things down. Then he listened some more and wrote more down. He was very nice. He actually looked at my medications and reminded me about a condition I forgot I had. Pretty sharp fellow, that youngster.

"It's nothing personal, but I hope I don't see the people from the ambulance again for awhile."

Shortness of Breath

The elderly can experience shortness of breath as a result of the same diseases that cause this symptom in younger patients, such as asthma or pulmonary embolism. The older population, however, is more likely to have conditions such as emphysema (Figure 36-7), heart failure (pulmonary edema), or a combination of these diseases that cause shortness of breath. Shortness of breath is also often the chief complaint of elderly patients having myocardial infarctions (heart attacks). As a patient gets older, the patient experiencing a cardiac problem is more likely to complain of shortness of breath *without* chest pain. The EMT must maintain a high index of suspicion for cardiac problems in these patients.

Chest Pain

A complaint of chest pain can arise from many conditions. Some that are more common in the elderly than other age groups are angina, myocardial infarction, pneumonia, and aortic aneurysm. An aneurysm is an abnormal widening of a blood vessel, usually an artery. As the vessel walls are stretched, they become thinner and weaker, so the vessel can rupture, leading to catastrophic bleeding. The pain from a thoracic aortic aneurysm as it dissects (separates the layers of the artery) is classically described as "tearing" in nature and often radiates to the back between the shoulder blades.

Altered Mental Status

The list of conditions that can cause alteration of mental status is nearly endless. Some of the more common ones in the elderly include adverse effects from medications (many drugs have sedating effects that are more pronounced in the elderly), hypoglycemia (perhaps from taking too much diabetic medication), stroke (from chronic or untreated hypertension), generalized infection in the bloodstream (the immune system may not fend off microbes as well as it used to), and hypothermia (the elderly patient may lose heat at a temperature that is comfortable for others). As already emphasized, do not assume that an altered mental sta-

FIGURE 36-7 Elderly patients with emphysema or other forms of lung disease may depend on a home oxygen unit and nasal cannula. (© *Michal Heron*)

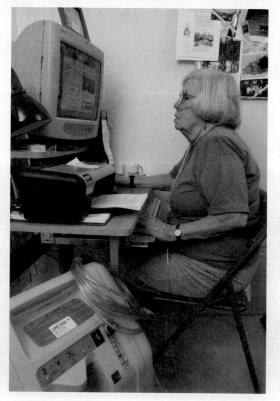

tus is normal for an elderly patient until you check with someone who knows the patient and can describe the patient's baseline status.

Pneumonia, an inflammation in the tissue of the lung, is the fourth leading cause of death in the elderly. Patients in this age group sometimes cannot cough effectively and have immune systems that are not able to combat disease-causing organisms very well, leading to infection in the lung tissue. The patient with pneumonia classically presents with fever and a cough that brings up sputum. In the elderly, however, these signs may be very subtle or entirely absent. An altered mental status, resulting from hypoxia, may be the only outward sign of a problem such as pneumonia. Despite aggressive treatment with antibiotics in the hospital, some of these patients will not survive.

Abdominal Pain and Gastrointestinal Bleeding

Conditions that would cause abdominal pain in a younger patient often do not cause pain in the older patient. Therefore, when an older person complains of abdominal pain, it is often a sign of a serious condition and will be taken very seriously in the emergency department. One of the most serious causes of abdominal pain in this population is an abdominal aortic aneurysm, which you may hear experienced providers refer to as a "triple A." If it is stable in size or growing very slowly, the patient may not even know about it. Like the aneurysm in the thoracic aorta, though, as it grows it sometimes causes pain with a tearing nature. The pain is often excruciating in intensity and will be accompanied by severe shock if the artery has ruptured. If it is leaking slowly, the problem can sometimes be surgically repaired if the patient is able to withstand the stress of surgery.

Another common cause of abdominal pain in the elderly is bowel obstruction or blockage, which can cause severe pain and may require surgery for repair. Also common in this age group is diverticulosis, a condition in which a diverticulum, or outpouching of the intestine, provides a sac where food can lodge and cause inflammation and infection (diverticulitis).

Ask the patient with abdominal pain if he has had black, tarry stools, caused by the remains of red blood cells that have gone through the digestive tract, which is one indicator of internal bleeding. Cancers of the gastrointestinal tract, ulcers, and adverse effects of medications can also cause either upper or lower gastrointestinal bleeding. In addition to asking about blood in the stools, ask the patient about vomiting blood or material that looks like coffee grounds. In some patients, the loss of blood occurs over a prolonged period of time. In this case, the patient's vital signs may be normal, but the patient may be suffering from anemia, which is a decreased number of red blood cells. In this case, the patient's chief complaint may be shortness of breath, weakness, dizziness, or fainting.

Dizziness, Weakness, and Malaise

Dizziness, weakness, and malaise are vague symptoms that are easy for the EMT to take lightly. Don't! These complaints can be associated with a number of serious conditions, including some life-threatening ones. Dizziness, especially upon standing, may be the only indication that a patient is experiencing significant internal bleeding. Weakness can be the result of cardiac dysrhythmias. When an 80-year-old's heart is beating 180 times a minute, there isn't time for the heart to fill between contractions. More commonly in the elderly, the heart experiences bradycardia, a pulse rate less than 60 per minute. Fortunately, either condition can be treated with medications, a pacemaker, or both.

Many other extremely serious conditions may present in an elderly patient with no more than the complaint that "I'm not feeling myself today." Be diligent in your assessment of this seemingly minor problem.

Depression and Suicide

Depression is very common in the elderly, sometimes because of medical conditions that limit activity, medications that sap the patient's energy, loss of friends or a spouse (especially widowers), or just a biochemical imbalance in the brain. For this reason, many elderly patients are on antidepressants. When evaluating a patient's illness or injury, observe the patient's mood, speech, and activity. Referral to an appropriate source of assistance may be lifesaving.

The segment of the population most likely to be successful in a suicide attempt is elderly males. It is not possible to predict accurately who will attempt or complete suicide, so mention any suspicions of this nature to the emergency department staff when you turn over the patient.

FIGURE 36-8 (A) A shingles rash often appears as a narrow beltlike band around the torso. (B) A shingles rash can appear anywhere on the body, including the face. *(Photos A and B: © Edward T. Dickinson, MD)*

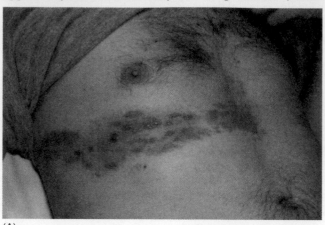

(A)

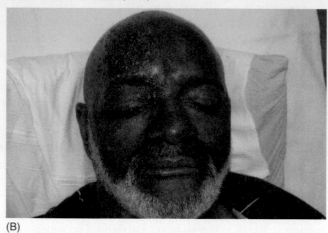

(B)

Rash, Pain, and Flulike Symptoms

A condition much more common in the older population is herpes zoster or shingles. This condition is the result of varicella, the same virus that causes chicken pox. In shingles, the virus reawakens after years of inactivity. The patient experiences pain, often quite severe, on one side of the body over a dermatome, the area associated with one of the nerves coming from the spinal cord. Within a few days, a small rash with blisters over red skin appears in that area. A shingles rash often appears as a beltlike band on the torso extending from the middle back around to the chest on one side (following the path of the affected spinal nerve). However, the rash can appear anywhere on the body, including the face (Figure 36-8). After a few days, the blisters dry out and scab over. Further healing takes a few more weeks. Like the rash already described, the pain of shingles commonly occurs somewhere on one side of the torso, but it also can occur higher up. Symptoms of a shingles outbreak may also, in some patients, include headache, sensitivity to light, and flulike symptoms including stomach pain, diarrhea, chills, and fever. Unfortunately for many older patients, healing of the shingles rash is not the end of the problem. In almost half of the patients over 60 years of age, the area remains quite painful, requiring strong pain medication for relief.

> **NOTE:** *Until the lesions scab over, an EMT who has not had varicella infection can contract it from the fluid. Standard Precautions and attention to hygiene should keep the uninfected EMT healthy.*

Falls

The significance of a fall for an older person should not be underestimated. Of older patients seen in an emergency department for a fall, one-quarter will die within a year. Death may not be a direct result of the fall, but instead may result from complications of the fall. For example, while recuperating from bruised ribs sustained in a fall, a 74-year-old woman may not breathe as deeply as normal because of the pain associated with inhalation. As a result of not being able to cough, as well as other changes in the aging lungs, if this patient comes down with pneumonia she is more likely to die from it.

Often, a fall is just an indication of a more serious problem. A number of older people fall because of abnormal heart rhythms. Others fall because of a stroke or internal bleeding from an ulcer. Whenever possible and when time allows, assess the patient not only for injuries from the fall, but also for a cause of the fall.

EMTs can help prevent falls. When you enter an older person's home, look for potential hazards. Table 36-3 lists a number of hazards and what you or the patient's family or friends can do to correct them.

Elder Abuse and Neglect

Elder abuse and neglect have occurred for many years but have only recently received the attention they deserve. There are essentially three ways in which elders can be abused or neglected: physically, psychologically, and financially. Physical abuse includes pushing, shoving,

Table 36-3 Making a Home Safer for the Elderly

HAZARD	CONSEQUENCE	INTERVENTION
Torn or slippery rugs	Slipping, tripping, falling	Remove, repair, or replace
Chairs without armrests	Patient cannot get leverage to get out of chair	Replace chairs, or install armrests
Chair with low back	Does not support neck; allows patient to fall backward when attempting to get up	Replace with a high-back chair
Chair with wheels or castors	Chair may roll away as patient tries to sit, causing her to fall	Use the brake for wheelchairs; replace chairs with castors
Temperature too low or too high	Patient may develop hypothermia or hyperthermia	Set a temperature of 72°F; ensure adequate ventilation and cooling in summer
Hot water temperature is too high	Burns from washing dishes or bathing	Adjust hot water heater temperature to 120°F or lower
Bathtub or slippery shower	Unable to get out of tub; slipping and falling in the shower	A walk-in tub or shower that allows comfortable sitting, has a nonslip surface, and uses handrails is safest
Stairs without handrails	Risk of falling	Install handrails

hitting, or shaking of an older person. It occasionally includes sexual abuse. Physical neglect includes improper feeding, poor hygiene, or inadequate medical care. Psychological abuse and neglect include threats, insults, or ignoring an older person ("the silent treatment"). Financial abuse and neglect include exploitation or misuse of an older person's belongings or money.

Detecting elder abuse and neglect can be difficult. Don't automatically assume that an injury is the result of a simple fall, even though falls are common among the elderly. Evaluate any injury in this age group with an eye toward recognizing signs of abuse or neglect. Many states have laws that require the reporting of such suspicions. Be aware of the laws in your state and local protocols and take whatever actions you are permitted to take to help the victim of abuse.

Loss of Independence

It is hard for younger adults to understand how disruptive a serious injury or illness can be to an older person. Years of independence can vanish in an instant, leaving the patient in the

CRITICAL DECISION MAKING

Changes with Age

Geriatric patients differ from those in other age groups. This exercise asks you to apply your understanding of these differences to your assessment and decision making.

1. You are treating a geriatric patient who, you suspect, has fractured her hip. The patient is pale and is rapidly breathing. You suspect shock, but her pulse is 84. She is a diabetic, has a cardiac history and hypertension, and takes several medications. If she is in shock, why isn't her pulse rate more rapid?

2. Your geriatric patient hasn't felt well for the past several days. She complains of a cough and flulike symptoms. She has become increasingly weak. Her family suspects the flu, but she doesn't have a fever. Why?

3. You are called to an assisted living facility for a man who is "just not right." He was fine last night. The man complains of suddenly feeling very weak and is having a little difficulty breathing. The nurse wants him sent to the hospital in case he is having a heart attack. Why would she think this?

care of strangers. Even worse, the patient goes to a hospital where many friends and perhaps a spouse have gone, never to return. The EMT can help by treating the patient with dignity. Do not minimize the patient's fears and concerns. Instead, acknowledge them and try to put them in perspective.

Ask the patient if he would like you to lock up before you leave the house. Inquire about the care of any pets and whether there is a trusted neighbor who can take care of them for awhile. If you can honestly say it, reassure the patient that most patients you have seen with this particular problem do well and return home in good condition. A friendly hand on the forearm, if you feel the patient will accept it, can be very reassuring.

Talking with the patient during transport about what he has done over the course of a lifetime can be not only therapeutic for the patient, but enlightening for you as well (Figure 36-9). Above all, treat the patient in a respectful, empathetic manner.

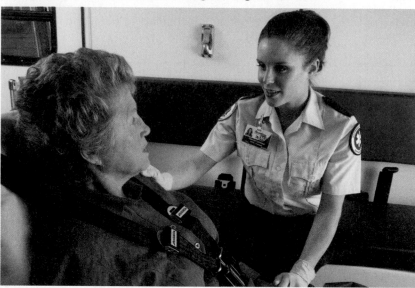

FIGURE 36-9 Talking with the patient during transport can be therapeutic for the patient and enlightening for the EMT.

CHAPTER REVIEW

Key Facts and Concepts

- Although we can make some generalizations about age-related changes, older people are individuals who can differ significantly in their health care needs.

- The prevalence of many diseases increases with age, increasing the proportion of individuals in the older population who require health care.

- Age-related decline in body system function alters the body's response to illness and injury, requiring modified interpretation of assessment findings and complaints.

- Multiple medical problems and multiple medications to treat them can lead to unpredictable problems and drug interactions.

- Changes in the nervous system, along with isolation, financial problems, loss of loved ones, and chronic health problems, all increase the risk for depression in the elderly. Depression can interfere with a person's self-care and ability to communicate.

Key Decisions

- Can this patient give me a reliable medical history?
- How is the patient's condition different from usual?
- Could the patient's vague or nonspecific complaints be symptoms of a serious problem?
- Do I need to adjust my communication strategies to interact effectively with this patient?
- Are there indications that the patient is abused, neglected, or unable to properly care for himself?

Preparation for Your Examination and Practice

Short Answer

1. How would you adjust your history-taking approach for an elderly patient who has vision and hearing impairments?

2. What question should you ask to determine if an elderly patient's condition is normal or a change from baseline?

3. Name some of the most common medical conditions that cause EMS to be called for elderly patients.

4. List some causes of altered mental status in elderly patients.

Thinking and Linking

Elderly patients can pose a number of challenges in assessment and management. This exercise combines material you have learned in this chapter with material from previous chapters. Decide how you would handle each of the following situations.

1. An 85-year-old man has been getting dizzy when he gets up from his chair. His wife wants him to be transported to the hospital, but he does not want to go. What issues must be considered in this situation?

2. A 92-year-old woman has severe curvature of her thoracic spine (kyphosis). When you place her supine on a long backboard, her head remains about 4 inches off the backboard. How can you make the patient comfortable and immobilize her spine?

3. A 78-year-old patient with dementia is agitated during transport. She is screaming, trying to hit you, and spitting at you. What issues must be considered in this situation?

Critical Thinking Exercises

Calls to elderly patients can present complex challenges. Describe how you would handle each of the following situations and explain your reasoning.

1. You respond to an elderly woman who has fallen and injured her hip. When you arrive, you find a 90-year-old woman lying on the kitchen floor, alert and oriented, complaining of hip pain. She is somewhat hard of hearing. Her 91-year-old husband is very upset over what happened and blaming himself for her fall.

2. You respond to the home of an 82-year-old man who lives by himself. His neighbor called EMS, concerned for his welfare because he has not been seen outside the home recently. The patient is confused, wearing clothing soiled with urine and feces, and the home is a mess. The patient appears to have lost weight and has several open sores on his arms and legs. The neighbor tells you that the man's nephew is supposed to check on the patient and provide assistance, but he has not been to the home in a few days.

Pathophysiology to Practice

The following questions are designed to assist you in gathering relevant clinical information and making accurate decisions in the field.

1. In what ways is the elderly patient less able to compensate for blood loss? How would this be reflected in your assessment findings?

2. An elderly patient who is nearly blind and too weak to get out of her chair without assistance tells you she met a handsome young man that looks just like your partner while she was out dancing last night. Can this patient give you any accurate information about her medical history? Explain your answer.

3. An 85-year-old patient who is normally alert and oriented awoke this morning very confused. His skin is very hot and moist, his respiratory rate is 28 per minute, and his heart rate is 118 and irregular. His blood pressure is 102/70, his pulse oximetry reading is 89 percent on room air, and you don't believe you can hear breath sounds in his right lower lung. What is a possible explanation for the patient's condition? How would this lead to a sudden onset of confusion?

4. For each of the following patients, decide which of the three listed conditions is most likely. Although minimal information is presented for each patient, your knowledge of the conditions will guide you to the correct choice and help hone your decision making and intuition in the field.
   - Gastrointestinal bleeding
   - Heart attack
   - Congestive heart failure

   a. A 75-year-old patient complains of weakness and tiredness and states she's been getting worse for 3 days. She sleeps in a recliner at night.

   b. A 72-year-old patient complains of tiredness and shortness of breath which has been getting worse for a week. He takes ibuprofen for his arthritis.

c. A 65-year-old diabetic complains of nausea, vomiting, weakness, and "just not feeling well" which came on early this morning.

d. An 80-year-old patient becomes confused on and off during the day. Some days are worse than others. He has a history of high blood pressure and prostate cancer.

e. A 77-year-old tells you she takes aspirin every day since she had a heart attack 2 years ago. Her chief complaint today is that she is weak and "vomiting up some kind of dark stuff."

Street Scenes

"Unit 10, respond to the senior citizen housing center on Martin Luther King, Jr., Avenue for a patient having difficulty breathing." When you arrive, you stop for a moment at the doorway and notice that the apartment is messy. The patient is a 67-year-old male sitting upright in a chair with rapid respirations and wheezing. You ask why he has called EMS, and he responds in short sentences, telling you that he is having trouble catching his breath and may be having an asthma attack. Your partner tells the patient she wants to give him oxygen. While a nonrebreather mask is set up, you perform a primary assessment.

Street Scene Questions

1. What is your initial priority for providing care to this patient?
2. After the primary assessment is completed, what assessment information should be obtained next?
3. Why is the condition of the apartment significant?

The patient's airway is open and his respirations are 24 per minute with wheezing upon exhalation. Your partner continues to obtain additional vitals, and you get a past medical history. When you ask the patient if he is taking any medications, he asks if you could speak up because he doesn't hear well. You reposition yourself in front of the patient and speak clearly, without shouting, at a greater volume. He responds by pointing to a shoe box full of pill bottles and two inhalers. You ask if he has been taking his medications and, appearing confused, he says he doesn't remember which ones he took today. When asked if someone knows about his medication schedule, he states that he lives alone. Your partner reports the following vital signs: respirations are 28, pulse is 110, blood pressure is 160/100, skin is moist, and pupils are equal and reactive. You and your partner tell the patient that you want to take him to the hospital. He agrees, so you package and move him to the ambulance, bringing his box of medications along.

Street Scene Questions

4. Based on the assessment, would you expect this patient's condition to worsen? How should you be prepared if it does?
5. What additional assessment should be done en route to the hospital? How often should the vital signs be taken?
6. What information about the patient's living situation should you provide to the hospital staff?

You briefly discuss the patient situation with your partner and you decide that a transport with red lights and siren seems appropriate as the patient's breathing rate is increasing and you may need to assist ventilations with a bag-valve mask. You also decide, based on the patient's confused state and inability to breathe deeply, not to assist him with one of his inhalers. As you proceed to the hospital, with your partner driving, you reassess his vital signs and find the patient's respiratory rate has returned to 24 and the patient is starting to talk in longer sentences. You ask some additional medical history questions about previous asthma attacks and the patient seems more lucid. You are communicating well with the patient, and he is hearing you. In fact, he provides the name of his daughter and gives you a telephone number. The patient seems less anxious and, about 5 minutes before arrival at the hospital, he has a respiratory rate of 20 with wheezing still present. You contact the hospital by radio, provide patient information, and give an ETA.

While completing your prehospital care report, you remember the condition of the patient's apartment and that this patient lives alone. Before leaving, you share this information with the charge nurse and suggest that if this patient is sent home, he may need living assistance as well as help with his care, such as medications. The nurse thanks you and tells you that she will ask a case manager to follow up.

Emergencies for Patients with Special Challenges

STANDARD
Special Patient Populations (Patients with Special Challenges)

COMPETENCY
Applies fundamental knowledge of growth, development, and aging and assessment findings to provide basic emergency care and transportation for a patient with special needs.

CORE CONCEPTS
— The variety of challenges that may be faced by patients with special needs

— Types of disabilities and challenges patients may have

— Special aspects of prehospital care for a patient with special challenges

— Congenital and acquired diseases and conditions

— Types of advanced medical devices patients may rely on

— How to recognize and deal with cases of abuse and neglect

EXPLORE Resource Central

To access Resource Central, follow directions on the Student Access Card provided with this text. If there is no card, go to **www.bradybooks.com** and follow the Resource Central link to Buy Access from there. Under Media Resources, you will find:

▶ **Parkinson's Disease**
Watch a video to learn about this disease; discover the cause, signs and symptoms, and current treatments available.

▶ **Fact Sheet about the Homeless**
Get statistics about the homeless population; circumstances that lead to homelessness, a homeless individual's ability to obtain medical care and the prevalence of medical conditions in the homeless.

▶ **Information about Minority Health**
Read what defines a minority, why it is necessary to reduce and eliminate disparities in health care, and discuss ways to modify your usual assessment when dealing with an individual who speaks little or no English.

OBJECTIVES

After reading this chapter you should be able to:

37.1 Define key terms introduced in this chapter.

37.2 Describe special challenges patients may have, including various disabilities, terminal illness, obesity, homelessness/poverty, and autism. (pp. 950–956)

37.3 Describe general consideraitons in responding to patients with special challenges. (pp. 956–959)

37.4 Recognize physical impairments and common medical devices used in the home care of patients

with special challenges, including respiratory devices, cardiac devices, gastrourinary devices, and central IV catheters, and discuss EMT assessment and transport considerations for each. (pp. 959–968)

37.5 Explain why patients with special challenges are often especially vulnerable to abuse and neglect and what the EMT's obligations are in such situations. (p. 969)

autism spectrum disorders
   (ASD), *p. 954*
automatic implanted
   cardiac defibrillator
   (AICD), *p. 962*
bariatrics, *p. 953*

central IV catheter, *p. 967*
continuous positive airway
   pressure (CPAP), *p. 959*
dialysis, *p. 966*
disability, *p. 950*
feeding tube, *p. 964*

left ventricular assist device
   (LVAD), *p. 963*
obesity, *p. 953*
ostomy bag, *p. 966*
pacemaker, *p. 962*
stoma, *p. 960*

tracheostomy, *p. 960*
urinary catheter, *p. 965*
ventilator, *p. 961*

The principles of emergency medical care you have learned so far apply to a wide variety of patients. For some patients with special challenges, you will need to adapt these principles to meet their particular health care needs. Patients with special challenges include patients with sensory impairments, patients with developmental disorders, the terminally ill, patients who are very obese, those who are homeless or living in poverty, and patients who are dependent on advanced medical devices. The health problems associated with these special challenges increase the likelihood that these persons will need EMS at one time or another. In addition, like other vulnerable people, such as the elderly and children, some patients with special needs are at higher risk for abuse and neglect. This chapter focuses on meeting the unique emergency care needs of patients with special challenges.

PATIENTS WITH SPECIAL CHALLENGES

CORE CONCEPT
The variety of challenges that may be faced by patients with special needs

When we speak of patients with special challenges, sometimes referred to as special needs patients or patients with special needs, we are really referring to patients with many different types of challenges that require special considerations. As health care professionals, one of the few generalizations we can make about caring for such a diverse group is that empathy and respect for the patient, the patient's dignity, and the patient's rights are key factors in treatment.

Disability

CORE CONCEPT
Types of disabilities and challenges patients may have

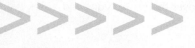

disability
a physical, emotional, behavioral, or cognitive condition that interferes with a person's ability to carry out everyday tasks, such as working or caring for oneself.

Unfortunately, many special needs groups are discriminated against or viewed negatively by others. Because of the stigma that may be associated with certain conditions, and because we are often unsure about what descriptive terms are acceptable, we often feel uncomfortable with these patients or struggle to find the correct terminology to refer to their situation without causing offense.

The term ***disability*** is used to refer to a condition that interferes significantly with a person's ability to engage in activities of daily living, such as working and caring for oneself. Disabilities include vision impairment and loss (Figure 37-1), hearing impairment and loss, loss of mobility, and emotional and cognitive impairments. It is preferable to speak of a person having a disability, rather than using the term *handicapped*.

The Centers for Disease Control uses the term *developmental disability* to mean a chronic (persistent or lasting) mental and/or physical impairment beginning at any age up to 22 years and causing significant impairment in the person's major life activities. Develop-

FIGURE 37-1 (A) A blind patient may wish to touch the EMT's face. (B) If the blind patient has a guide dog, the EMT must never get between the dog and the patient. *(Photos A and B: © Michal Heron)*

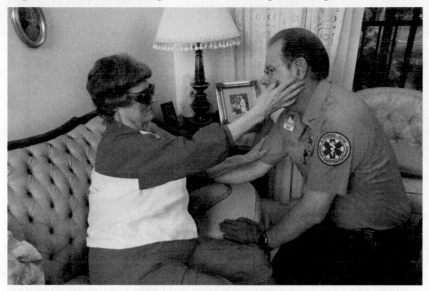

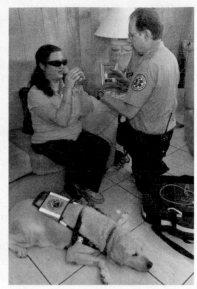

(A)   (B)

mental disabilities include cerebral palsy and Down syndrome (Figure 37-2), among others. Other disabilities are not developmental in nature but may occur from traumatic injury or medical conditions. Multiple sclerosis, Parkinson's disease, stroke, traumatic brain injury, spinal cord injury, and other conditions can result in cognitive, emotional, and/or physical disability. Table 37-1 describes some impairments associated with particular conditions.

Many patients with disabilities can live independently, often with some type of assistive equipment or accommodations. For example, wheelchair ramps, lowered countertops, handrails, and modified bathrooms can allow someone who relies on a wheelchair to live alone. Service animals can also be of great assistance to people with many different disabilities, increasing their independence. Some patients with more severe disabilities live at home but require special assistance, such as ventilators, feeding tubes, and home health care services. You may also encounter patients with special challenges in a variety of group home and institutional settings.

FIGURE 37-2 You may be called to care for a patient with a developmental disability, such as Down syndrome. *(© Daniel Limmer)*

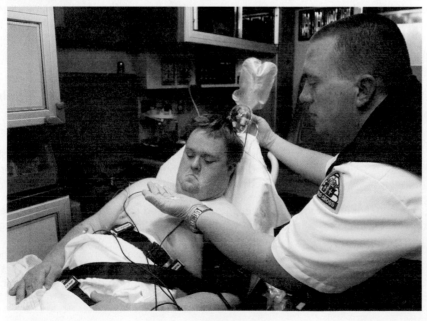

Table 37-1 Selected Conditions for Patients with Special Challenges

CONDITION	DESCRIPTION	IMPLICATIONS
Autism	A developmental disorder in which the patient has impaired social functioning and communication. The patient may have repetitive or restricted behaviors.	There is a wide spectrum of autism disorders. Patients with Asperger's syndrome may have social challenges and unusual behaviors, but normal language and intellect. Patients with classic autism usually have language delays, communication problems, and, often, intellectual disability.
Cerebral palsy	A permanent impairment in motor control, present at birth. Cerebral palsy is not progressive. Movements are characterized by lack of coordination, exaggerated reflexes, and tightness of muscles.	Although some patients with cerebral palsy may also have cognitive impairment, do not assume this is the case.
Cognitive disabilities	These may result from mental retardation due to a variety of genetic and congenital problems; for example, Down syndrome and fetal alcohol syndrome. It may also result from stroke, dementia, or past traumatic brain injury.	Patients have varying levels of impairment in intellectual functioning, including learning, judgment, problem solving, social skills, and communication with others. Some patients may live independently, whereas others have only limited ability to interact with others.
Hearing impairment	This condition may be congenital, due to trauma, or due to age. Hearing loss may be partial or complete.	Patients may have hearing aids, use TTY devices, or use sign language. Some patients can lip-read, so it is important to face the patient and talk to him directly, even if he has complete hearing loss.
Kidney failure	This condition may be a consequence of diabetes, high blood pressure, or other medical problems. Patients can have varying levels of kidney function, and receive dialysis at different frequencies.	Patients are prone to a number of metabolic disturbances, especially if a dialysis appointment is missed. Dialysis access devices (shunts or fistulas) can malfunction and bleed. Don't take a blood pressure in an extremity with dialysis access. Patients with continuous ambulatory peritoneal dialysis will usually know the best way to manage their device.
Neuromuscular disorders	Examples include muscular dystrophy, multiple sclerosis, and Lou Gehrig's disease.	Patients have varying levels of muscular weakness, which can be intermittent or progressive, resulting in paralysis. Complications can include respiratory paralysis, in which the patient depends on a ventilator.
Stroke	Levels of disability vary from mild to incapacitating. Specific problems relate to the area of the brain affected, and may involve emotional, behavioral, communication, intellectual, or physical limitations.	Don't make assumptions about a patient's ability to hear and understand, even though communication skills may be impaired.
Spinal cord injury	With complete spinal cord injury, patients experience lack of sensation and function below the level of injury.	Patients with high spinal cord injuries may be ventilator dependent. This, combined with an inability to cough, increases the chances of pneumonia. Patients with urinary catheters are also prone to infection. Immobility may result in ischemia of compressed tissues, leading to breakdown of the skin and tissue beneath it (decubitus ulcer, pressure sore, or bedsore).
Vision impairment	This condition may be congenital or acquired, and may be either complete or partial.	Often, visually impaired patients cope well and are able to find their way through familiar surroundings. Ask the patient about the best way to help him navigate. If the patient uses a cane or service animal, be sure to transport them with the patient. Always explain what you are going to do before you do it.

Terminal Illness

Terminally ill patients, such as patients with end-stage cancer, heart failure, or kidney failure, or those with progressive fatal diseases such as Huntington's disease or Lou Gehrig's disease, may prefer to stay at home under the care of family, possibly with assistance from hospice or home health care providers. Alternatively, they may spend the final weeks or days of their lives in a specially designated hospice facility. Terminally ill patients may be depending on technology to sustain life or relieve pain. Often, terminally ill patients have advance directives that specify what type of emergency care they are willing to accept (see Chapter 4, "Medical, Legal, and Ethical Issues").

Terminally ill patients and their families also have special emotional needs. (See "Understanding Reactions to Death and Dying" in Chapter 2, "The Well-Being of the EMT.") Unfortunately, the cost of end-of-life care can also create financial problems, compounding the patient's and family's concerns.

Obesity

Bariatrics is the branch of medicine that deals with the causes, prevention, and treatment of obesity. *Obesity* is defined as a *body mass index (BMI)* of 30 or more. Body mass index is calculated by dividing your weight in pounds by the square of your height in inches, and multiplying by 703. For example, for a woman who weighs 135 pounds and is 5 feet, 5 inches tall (65 inches):

$$BMI = 135/(65 \times 65) \times 703 = 22.46$$

A BMI of up to 24.9 is considered healthy for people over 20 years of age. A BMI of 25 to 29 is considered as overweight, while a BMI of 30 or greater is considered obese. Keep in mind that BMI does not measure body fat directly, and that an extremely muscular person could end up with a BMI of 30 or more without being obese. For most people, though, BMI is a good indicator of healthy weight.

Obesity is a significant and growing health concern in America for both adults and children. Obesity increases the risk of some cancers, type 2 diabetes, hypertension, heart attack, stroke, liver and gallbladder disease, arthritis, sleep apnea, and respiratory problems. Because of the prevalence of obesity and because of the serious health issues related to obesity, you will frequently encounter obese patients.

As an EMT, you will need to take special measures to care for the obese patient, as well as special care in lifting to avoid injury to yourself, your coworkers, and the patient. Very obese patients may have difficulty breathing when they are supine, because of the extra weight that must be moved by the diaphragm during inspiration. If possible, allow the patient to assume a comfortable position for breathing. Monitor the patient's oxygen saturation, and provide oxygen and ventilatory assistance as needed. Make sure you have enough assistance when lifting and moving obese patients, and use special equipment if the patient's weight exceeds the maximum load capacity of your stretcher (see Chapter 3, "Lifting and Moving Patients").

Homelessness and Poverty

Homelessness is a state of not having a regular place to live, often because of an inability to afford or otherwise maintain regular, safe, and adequate housing. The homeless may live in vehicles, parks, on the street, in makeshift dwellings, or in abandoned buildings. In many communities, homeless shelters are available but may not have the capacity to provide for the number of homeless seeking shelter. In addition, many homeless individuals choose not to use shelters even when space is available. The homeless include men, women, children, and families. Disproportionate numbers of veterans and minorities make up the homeless population.

Several serious health problems are related to homelessness: mental health problems, malnutrition, substance abuse problems, HIV/AIDS, tuberculosis, bronchitis and pneumonia, environmental emergencies, wounds, and skin infections. The lack of access to health care also means that conditions that begin as minor problems can go untreated until they become emergencies. Underlying chronic health problems and malnutrition can impair the body's ability to respond to injuries and acute illnesses, making these issues of more serious concern than they might be otherwise. Homeless women may be victims of domestic or sexual abuse. A high number of the estimated 1.35 million homeless children suffer from emotional problems.

bariatrics
the branch of medicine that deals with the causes of obesity, as well as its prevention and treatment.

obesity
a condition of having too much body fat, defined as a body mass index of 30 or greater.

Poverty, which may be a cause of homelessness, means that a person's or family's income is not adequate to allow them a standard of living considered acceptable in society. For 2009, the U.S. Department of Health and Human Services determined the poverty guideline for a single person as an income of $10,830 or less, and $22,050 for a family of four. However, there are also large numbers of individuals and families whose incomes are above this, yet not enough to provide all their necessities, including health care, health insurance, prescription medications, and adequate nutrition. Therefore, the poor are prone to many of the same health issues as the homeless.

Autism

Autism spectrum disorders (ASD) are developmental disorders that affect, among other things, the ability to communicate, report medical conditions, self-regulate behaviors, and interact with others to get needs met. This can create serious problems for emergency responders. Traditional assessment techniques and treatment protocols may need to be modified for the ASD patient. With autism spectrum disorders affecting approximately 1 in 91 children and 1.5 million Americans, you are likely to encounter a patient with an ASD.

A mnemonic to use when dealing with patients who have autism is ABCS: awareness, basic, calm, and safety.

Awareness

It is very important for EMTs to understand that people with an ASD will not behave or react in the same manner as most patients. Since they may not be able to adapt to the situation, EMTs will need to change their approach and strategies to meet the needs of the person with autism.

Persons with autism are susceptible to the same medical emergencies as the general population; often have coexisting medical conditions, such as seizure disorders; and are prone to sustaining certain types of injuries, all of which increase the likelihood of an EMS response. However, persons with autism have rigid routines and a strong preference for things to be predictable and as expected. Disruption is not well tolerated.

Communication with the patient with an ASD can be challenging. Persons with autism often have literal perception and difficulty distinguishing patterns of speech such as humor, slang, sarcasm, or idioms from unambiguous statements. Body language, such as gesturing or facial expression, may also not be recognized. Approximately 25 to 30 percent of persons with ASD will stop speaking, usually between 15 and 24 months of age. About a quarter of those will remain nonverbal at age 9. In a stressful situation, even those with good verbal ability may be unable to speak. Consider using a picture card system, which can help the patient express his needs and may assist you in explaining procedures and interventions to the patient.

Escalation and meltdown, which can occur in a person with an ASD, can be described as an *involuntary* increase in tantrum-*like* behaviors that include screaming, swearing, stomping, throwing objects, hitting and/or kicking (people or objects), pushing, and biting. There are several causes of this behavior, with the most common involving sensory, emotional, or cognitive overstimulation, social skills deficits, excessive demands being placed on the individual, interruption of established routines, and being put in a situation that was unexpected or is unpredictable. If a person with an ASD is behaving aggressively or is escalated, it is rarely from what most of us would refer to as malicious or defiant behavior. It is much more likely that the individual is reacting to extreme stress and is out of control. These persons often know that they are out of control but do not have the ability to regain control effectively and may need your help to return to a calm sense of being. Simply put, they want circumstances to change, but do not know how to implement that change.

Basic

One of the most important aspects of interacting with persons with autism is to keep things basic. There are a few ways that this concept applies:

- **Keep your instructions basic.** Simple, clear, precise directions are easiest to follow for persons with autism. For example, say "Sit down here" (pointing at a chair), *not* "Why don't you have a seat?" Don't be sarcastic, use figures of speech, or tell jokes.

- **Ask basic questions.** Many people with autism will do better answering short, closed-ended questions than open-ended questions. Allow extra time to answer even simple questions. If the person still does not answer, he may be nonverbal, may not understand the question, or may not know the answer. People who have an ASD have difficulty asking for clarification when they do not understand questions or instructions.

- **Basic means less "stuff"!** Our radios, pagers, cell phones, and even things like flashlights and stethoscope covers may overstimulate the senses of a person with autism. They frequently have hyperacute responses to stimulations of one or more of the five senses that a majority of people tolerate well or don't even notice. For example, they may be able to see strobelike flickering in fluorescent lights. A gentle touch on the shoulder, intended to be reassuring, may feel like a powerful blow. They may also have difficulty separating loud foreground noise from faint background noise. Your radio, even if turned way down, may be perceived as being as loud as your speech. Sensory stimulus overload can easily be an antecedent to escalation and meltdown. Therefore, it is important to keep as much "stuff" as possible turned off and out of sight. If you are aware that your potential patient is autistic, it also is advisable to discontinue use of lights and siren as you approach the scene.

- **Keep your treatment basic.** Since persons with autism do not adapt well to sudden changes, it is best to minimize as many unplanned experiences as possible. In an emergency, the routines of these patients are interrupted, they are being bombarded with questions, things are being demanded of them from every direction, and an injury or illness may be causing significant pain or discomfort. Their already-heightened levels of anxiety, stress, and frustration are being pushed to the limit. The last thing that they need is to be "attacked" by EMTs wanting to poke them here and put stickers there.

  Although you should not withhold absolutely necessary treatment, it is usually best to defer treatment interventions that are done routinely as precautions or to help the emergency department staff. In other words, ask yourself, "*Must this be done to get the patient to the hospital safely?*" before initiating specific treatments.

  It is critically important to remember, however, that the patient with autism may not offer typical complaints, may have very high pain thresholds (thereby tolerating injuries that most patients would describe as excruciating), and may choose to engage in a pleasurable activity (such as playing with a toy or listening to music) over dealing with an obvious injury or medical condition, despite the amount of discomfort it may be causing. In some cases, these traits may cause serious conditions to be missed. Therefore, careful assessment is always needed and you should never withhold treatment that the patient needs.

Calm

When dealing with a person with autism, particularly if the patient is escalating or having a meltdown, it is imperative that you remain calm. Posturing aggressively, commanding loudly, becoming aggravated—even telling the patient to "calm down"—will be either ineffective or counterproductive. Just because the individual has temporarily lost control of his behavior is no reason for you to do so. Remember: Calm creates calm.

Although a "show of force" may be an effective deterrent against aggressive behavior for many people, this strategy will likely be lost on the patient with autism. If anything, extra people add to confusion, increase frustration, and heighten anxiety, causing negative behaviors to escalate. A better approach is to allow one person to make direct contact with the patient with autism, preferably accompanied by a parent, family member, or caregiver. Keep your tone of voice clear and controlled. Offer empathy and compassion, and reassure the patient that you are there to help him. Allow the patient to express his concerns and frustrations.

Being calm means taking extra time—sometimes a lot of extra time. Don't force your agenda. Unless the patient has an immediately life- or limb-threatening condition, it's the patient's emergency and the patient's timeline. Forcing the patient to move on before he is ready likely will result in escalation and meltdown. If he is already escalated, it may increase the intensity and duration of the event and may break all trust that has already been established. Escalation could exacerbate medical emergencies such as asthma or heart problems. Since physical activity accompanies escalation, his injuries could easily be aggravated.

Safety

Having a sense of safety and security is important to patients with autism. Often the environment where you find the patient offers a feeling of familiarity and security, even if it does not seem apparent to you. On the other hand, your ambulance is a strange and unfamiliar place, representing unpredictability to the patient with autism. Therefore, it is usually best to begin patient interaction where the patient is found. Remove things from around the person that may be aggravating to him (for example, turn off fluorescent lights), and disperse unnecessary personnel and bystanders.

Consider doing the physical exam in toe-to-head instead of head-to-toe order. Move slowly and do one thing at a time, such as assessing a leg or taking a blood pressure. Tell the patient *what* you are going to assess next and *how* you will assess it. Allow time for the patient to ask questions (e.g., some patients might want to know *why*) and make sure he is ready for you to do the next part of the assessment before you do it. If the patient begins to show signs of agitation or discomfort, and if his condition permits, consider taking a break before continuing the assessment. You may need to "segment" your exam and pause several times before completing it.

The concept of preparing the patient at each step along the way is essential to establish a sense of safety. The patient needs to know what to expect next. *What* can he expect to see? *When* will it occur? *How long* will it last? Use solid, descriptive terms to explain how an intervention will feel, as persons with autism often perceive pain quite differently than other people do. For example, when describing how it feels to have a blood pressure taken, don't say "It won't hurt." Instead, say "This cuff is going to tightly squeeze your arm."

Allowing the patient to tell you when he is ready for you to perform procedures or treatments provides the patient with a much-needed sense of control. Let the patient tell you when he is ready to move to the ambulance. He may want to look around the ambulance, look in cabinets and drawers, and even handle equipment before he is comfortable settling down. He may want to sit in a specific seat, such as the captain's chair, or sit in various seats before deciding where he would prefer to sit. Involving the patient in his care and accommodating these needs, when possible, will likely build trust and increase compliance and cooperation.

Even if the person with autism is escalated or having a meltdown, restraining the individual is frightening and terrifying. It should be avoided, used only as a last resort, and performed only when the person is in imminent danger of causing harm to himself or others.

GENERAL CONSIDERATIONS IN RESPONDING TO PATIENTS WITH SPECIAL CHALLENGES

● CORE CONCEPT
Special aspects of prehospital care for a patient with special challenges

In many respects, responding to and caring for a person with special challenges is like any other call for service in that it may be for an emergency such as a fall, general illness, chest pain, seizures, or shortness of breath. What is different for you, the EMT, is that the patient's preexisting condition can complicate and quickly overwhelm your ability to assess and treat the patient. To ensure proper care for such a patient, you must be able to recognize, understand, and evaluate the patient's specific special health care needs in addition to the presenting problem or chief complaint that led to the 911 call. In addition to increasing your knowledge about patients with special challenges in general, you can also take steps to be prepared for specific patients or types of patients in your response area.

Advanced Medical Devices in the Home

In recent years, medical advances and insurance coverage changes have allowed more and more people to have medical devices and care at home that were formerly seen only in the hospital. Patients who previously may have been unable to survive at home are now afforded the opportunity and relative comfort of living and working in a normal, nonhospital environment. As a result, prehospital providers are faced with an increasing number of calls to patients with devices and conditions that EMTs previously did not encounter (Figure 37-3). These calls may be for a problem with the device the patient relies on or it may be for a medical or traumatic problem unrelated to the device.

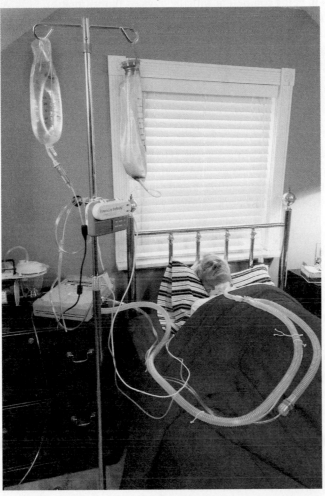

FIGURE 37-3 EMTs are increasingly called to assist patients who rely on advanced medical devices at home. This patient has a feeding line and a home ventilator connected to a tracheostomy. (© Ray Kemp/911 Imaging)

Variety of Health Care Settings

Patients with special care needs can be encountered in a variety of locations. With the proliferation of varied levels of health care settings, an EMT may respond to calls at private residences, nursing homes, specialty rehabilitation centers, and specialized care facilities. As an EMT, you should take the time to become familiar with any special health care settings in your community so you can be better prepared for calls of this nature.

In addition to identifying the locations of such facilities, EMTs should meet and develop plans with facility representatives in order to minimize confusion that could occur during an emergency call. Facility representatives may be able to arrange for you to see various medical devices in operation prior to any problems or medical distress.

Some communities have programs in place through their dispatch system to help identify people who may require additional help with medical devices in case of a disaster or evacuation from a building.

Knowledgeable Caregivers

One of the advantages EMTs have when encountering patients with special challenges is that these patients will often have on site, or will be accompanied by, a person who has been trained in the use of the patient's devices and conditions. This person may be medically trained, such as a Registered Nurse, a Certified Nursing Assistant, or a home health aide; however, more often it will be a family member or friend.

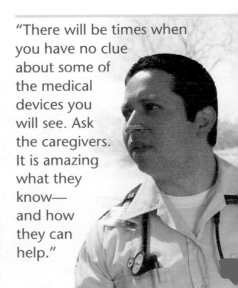

"There will be times when you have no clue about some of the medical devices you will see. Ask the caregivers. It is amazing what they know— and how they can help."

Although family members may not have had formal medical training or certification, they are generally very familiar and comfortable with using the devices the patient relies on. Many learned about the equipment and techniques for using it from medical professionals before their family member (the patient) was discharged from a hospital. Because they have a vested interest in being competent with the devices, family members are very thorough and deliberate with their understanding and application of the devices and their features. Therefore, it is advisable to seek their input on any problem that may be occurring with devices the patient has and to ask if they have been in a similar situation before. Some general questions should include:

Has this problem ever occurred before? If so, what fixed it?

Have you (or other family members/caregivers) been taught how to fix this problem?

Have you tried to fix the problem? If so, what happened?

Additionally, asking questions such as "How do you normally move him?" or "Has she ever been transported by ambulance, and what worked well for the transfer?" will allow family members to be part of the solution. Family members do not necessarily expect the arriving members of EMS to know or be familiar with the patient's medical device, and they can help guide the EMTs in the device's use and function. It is a good idea to assign a member of the EMS team to work with the family member regarding the medical device while others on the team concentrate on assessment, treatment, and moving the patient to the ambulance.

Despite the family's willingness to help you, they will still be apprehensive about the problem that occasioned the EMS call and eager to ensure that the device is not damaged or allowed to malfunction. Therefore, proceed with deliberate steps and explain all of your actions to the family.

A Knowledgeable Patient

The patient may also be a great help to the EMT regarding his condition, need for the device, functioning of the device, and how the device operates. The patient has likely been using and/or watching the use of this device for some time and has most likely been trained by medical providers to correctly use the device. Ask the patient about the device and any problems he may be having with it (Figure 37-4).

This approach will depend greatly on the patient's mental status and baseline level of functioning. If the patient has an altered mental status or if medical conditions dictate otherwise, the family will be the primary source of knowledge. Regardless of the patient's mental status or condition, always explain what you are doing. One of the last senses a patient

FIGURE 37-4 The patient is often an expert on the device or devices she depends on. Enlist the patient's advice as you discuss her condition, special devices, and the assessments and care you plan to perform.

(© Ray Kemp/911 Imaging)

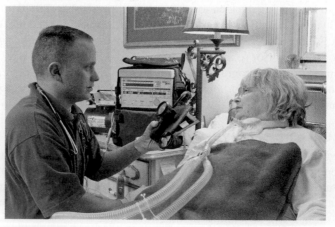

may lose is hearing, so talking and explaining your actions to the patient may help alleviate any stress the patient may be feeling yet unable to show.

Following Protocols

One note of caution is that, as an EMT, your actions fall under specific regional and state scopes of practice. Thus, you should confer with medical direction if the treatment or skill required is not something you are trained in or allowed to do under these protocols. Specific considerations should be given, such as:

Is the problem with the device life threatening?

Do I have the knowledge to fix this problem?

Do I have the supplies needed to fix this problem?

Is this within my protocols or within medical control authorization?

DISEASES AND CONDITIONS

A disease or condition may be congenital or acquired. A *congenital disease* or condition is one that is present at birth. Some congenital diseases may be genetic, others may not. One example of a congenital disease is congenital heart disease (the most common birth defect), where the heart or large blood vessels of the heart are malformed. Other examples include cleft palates and congenital deafness.

An *acquired disease* or condition is one that occurs after birth and may be the result of exposure to a virus or bacteria or the result of another medical condition or trauma. Examples of acquired diseases include COPD, AIDS, and traumatic spinal cord injury.

Some diseases or conditions may be either congenital or acquired, depending on how they occurred. An example of this would be deafness. A patient may be congenitally deaf from a birth defect or may become deaf from a disease or from a loud explosion.

It is important to understand that a patient with a chronic disease, whether it is congenital or acquired, may develop a sudden, acute worsening of the disease that prompts a call to 911. In addition, the patient with a chronic disease may develop an acute illness, and this acute illness may be potentially more devastating than the same disease would be for a patient who did not have a coexisting chronic disease.

CORE CONCEPT
Congenital and acquired diseases and conditions

ADVANCED MEDICAL DEVICES

As an EMT, you may encounter patients of any age or physical condition who have advanced medical devices. Take into consideration what the device is doing for the patient and how important the device is to the patient's survival. Some devices are intended to allow the patient to improve the quality of life or to have the fullest life possible, whereas others actually sustain life. Many patients who rely on such devices for life support have limited life expectancies. Even with proper use of the devices, their diseases or conditions may be terminal.

As already noted, you should include family caregivers, as appropriate, in care decisions and patient transportation.

CORE CONCEPT
Types of advanced medical devices patients may rely on

Respiratory Devices

Continuous Positive Airway Pressure Devices

Continuous positive airway pressure (CPAP) is a form of noninvasive positive-pressure ventilation (NPPV) provided by a device that blows oxygen or air under constant low pressure, through a tube and mask, to prevent airway passages from collapsing at the end of a breath. It is often prescribed to patients who suffer sleep apnea (periods when breathing stops during sleep) to help keep airway passages open as the patient sleeps (Figure 37-5). CPAP can help such patients prevent exacerbation of other medical conditions and conquer the chronic fatigue and irritability that are likely to result from interrupted sleep caused by the apneic

continuous positive airway pressure (CPAP)

a device worn by a patient that blows oxygen or air under constant low pressure through a tube and mask to keep airway passages from collapsing at the end of a breath.

FIGURE 37-5 A continuous positive airway pressure (CPAP) device provides constant pressure to keep airway passages open. It may be prescribed to (A) adults or (B) children.

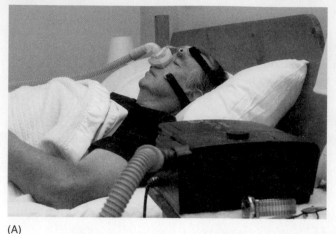

(A)

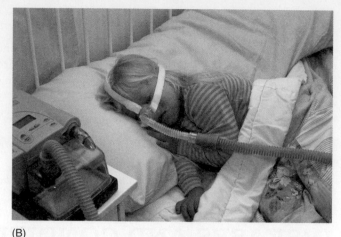

(B)

periods, and may be especially helpful in moderating behavioral problems that can occur in children with sleep apnea. A related device is the biphasic continuous positive airway pressure (BiPAP) device, which provides assistance with both inhalation and exhalation.

Review Chapter 9, "Respiration and Artificial Ventilation," and Chapter 19, "Respiratory Emergencies," for a more complete discussion of CPAP and BiPAP.

EMT Assessment and Transport A patient who uses a CPAP device at night is unlikely to have a medical emergency directly related to the device and will not need the device during transport. However, the patient may wish to bring the device along to the hospital. Hospital personnel should also be alerted that the patient uses a CPAP device during sleep.

Tracheostomy Tubes

tracheostomy
a surgical opening in the neck into the trachea.

stoma
a surgically created opening into the body, as with a tracheostomy, colostomy, or ileostomy.

A ***tracheostomy*** is a surgical opening through the neck into the trachea (Figure 37-6). When the opening created is permanent, it is called a ***stoma***. A tracheostomy is usually created near the second to fourth tracheal ring. A tracheostomy tube (a short breathing tube and flange) is inserted into the airway to allow the patient to breathe through the stoma instead of through the nose and mouth. It is often called a "trach" (prounounced trayk) tube.

Tracheostomy tubes used by older children and adults are usually double-cannula tubes. A double-cannula tube has an inner cannula (a tube within a tube) that can be locked into place and removed periodically for cleaning. Tracheostomy tubes for young children are usually single-cannula tubes that don't have the removable inner cannula. A bag-valve mask can be connected to either type of trach tube—to the inner cannula of a double-cannula tube or directly to a single-cannula tube.

FIGURE 37-6 Various emergencies may arise in a patient with a tracheostomy tube.

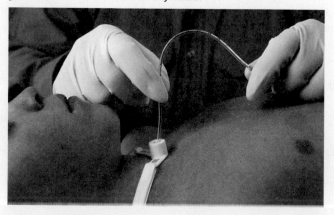

Trach tubes usually come with an obturator, which is a long "plug" that is placed inside the tube to help guide it during insertion and that also prevents material from getting into and clogging the tube during insertion. The obturator is removed after the trach tube is in place.

A tracheostomy procedure may be performed for long-term reasons in patients with neuromuscular disorders, spinal cord injuries, tumors, congenital deformities, coma, and a variety of other conditions that affect the patient's ability to breathe. A patient with a tracheostomy tube may or may not be on a home ventilator. Tracheostomy patients who are on ventilators may be on them all the time or only when sleeping.

Tracheostomy patients range from newborns to the very elderly. A patient with a tracheostomy may or may not be able to speak, depending on his condition. Some are able to speak by covering the tracheostomy tube briefly and making use of a speaker valve attached to the tube or an electronic box applied to the larynx. Do not assume that a patient with a tracheostomy either can or cannot speak.

A frequent problem with tracheostomy tubes is a buildup of mucus that forms in the tube. Because the tube bypasses the upper airway's function of warming, filtering, and humidifying inspired air, suctioning of the tube is needed regularly, often every few hours. This is especially common during times of distress, the first few weeks after tube insertion, or if the patient has an infection. Other problems with the tube can range from dislodgement to infection around the stoma to general respiratory distress.

A patient with a tracheostomy requires extensive care, and their caregivers are given substantial training. Caregivers should be very familiar with the procedures used to suction the tube. They should also know how to change and replace the tracheostomy tube, since it needs to be regularly cleaned. These procedures are outside the scope of practice for most EMTs, so check with your local protocols before attempting them.

EMT Assessment and Transport Carefully assess the tracheostomy tube for any blockage, and clear it (under protocol, or by having caregivers perform this). To clear a blockage, carefully insert a whistle-tip catheter (a soft, flexible catheter used to suction tracheostomy or endotracheal tubes) into the stoma. Determine the correct depth of insertion by measuring the suction tubing against the length of the obturator, which is the same length as the trach tube itself. You will usually be able to find the obturator among the patient's tracheostomy supplies. If you can't locate the obturator for measurement, stop inserting the suction catheter when you feel resistance. Suction as the catheter is being withdrawn, using a twisting motion as it is slowly removed. The patient may "buck" during this procedure.

If the patient requires further suctioning (indicated by visible or audible mucus), insert the suction tip into a container of sterile water to remove any mucus left in the catheter, then repeat. If the patient is on a ventilator, he may need to be ventilated by a bag-valve mask between suctionings. During transport, the patient should be positioned with his head slightly elevated to allow for mucus drainage.

Home Ventilators

A ***ventilator*** is a device that breathes for a patient. A home ventilator weighs anywhere from several pounds to over 20 pounds and can range from the size of a desktop computer to the size of this textbook. It is programmed to take over the functions of inhalation, exhalation, timing, and rate of breathing.

ventilator
a device that breathes for a patient.

The ventilator is attached to a ribbed tube called a ventilator circuit, which may come in various lengths, that enters the trachea. The tube from the ventilator may be attached to a plastic or metal port (called a cannula) that enters through a stoma in the neck. It may also be attached to an endotracheal tube through the mouth.

Although the patient is dependent on the ventilator for breathing, he may still lead an active life. One of the best examples of this was Christopher Reeve, the actor who once played Superman, who was paralyzed from the neck down in a 1995 riding accident. With the assistance of a ventilator, he was able to lead an active professional and family life until his death in 2004.

The patient on a home ventilator may call EMS for a variety of problems with his device. As with a tracheostomy tube, mucus plugs and secretions develop that require suctioning, and the patient may develop infections or respiratory distress. Additionally, the home ventilator depends on AC power, so power failures may be cause for concern. Ventilators do have backup batteries that generally last an hour or more.

Home ventilators are tailored with settings that are the most comfortable for the patient. In the case of a mechanical failure, or during transport of the patient, a bag-valve-mask (BVM) device can take over the function of the ventilator. During this procedure, you should adjust the rate, volume, and pressure of the BVM to the patient's comfort level. This can often be accomplished with guidance from the patient or his caregivers. If the patient or caregivers are unable to provide guidance, you should observe for adequate chest rise and improving skin color.

EMT Assessment and Transport   While caring for a patient with a home ventilator, ensure that the ventilator tube does not have any mucus buildup, and suction as needed. During transport, it may be easier to use a BVM while moving the patient to the ambulance, depending on the location and situation (e.g., stairs or a heavy patient). If you use a BVM at any point, ensure that it is the appropriate size for the patient and that it is connected to oxygen. If the patient has a tracheostomy tube and the BVM does not fit the tube attachment, use the face mask from the BVM to cover the stoma and secure the mask to provide a good seal against the neck, then ventilate as normal.

If the ventilator is left attached to the patient, firmly affix it to the stretcher. Secure the ventilator to prevent movement in the ambulance during transport. Consider transport time versus battery life, and plug the ventilator into the ambulance's inverter if available. If a BVM will be used during transport, obtain extra help so you can continue to provide assessment and care.

Cardiac Devices

Implanted Pacemakers and Cardiac Defibrillators

A patient may have an implanted pacemaker or automatic implanted cardiac defibrillator. These devices are both designed to respond to potentially lethal electrical rhythm changes in the heart.

In the case of a *pacemaker*, a small device is implanted under the skin and wires are implanted into the heart. The pacemaker is designed to prevent the heart rate from becoming too slow. Early pacemakers were set at a fixed rate, but modern pacemakers are "rate-responsive"; that is, they detect what the patient is doing and modify the heart rate accordingly. For example, if the patient is moving around and performing an action, a sensor will detect this and increase the rate to allow for the activity. Additionally, if the breathing rate increases, the pacemaker will increase the heart rate as well. The pacemaker delivers a series of low-energy pulses at set intervals to stimulate the heart to beat at a faster rate. These pulses are not felt by the patient and cannot be detected on the skin or felt by providers. The pacemaker does not squeeze the heart or fix damaged muscle; rather, it helps regulate the timing of each beat.

Like a pacemaker, an *automatic implanted cardiac defibrillator (AICD)* is placed under the skin with wires inserted into the heart. The AICD varies in size from slightly larger

pacemaker
a device implanted under the skin with wires implanted into the heart to modify the heart rate as needed to maintain an adequate heart rate.

automatic implanted cardiac defibrillator (AICD)
a device implanted under the skin of the chest to detect any life-threatening dysrhythmia and deliver a shock to defibrillate the heart.

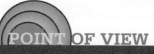

POINT OF VIEW

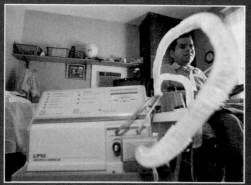

(© AP Photo/Journal Times, Jim Slosiarek/AP Images)

"I went to school with a guy who got into a motorcycle crash. He was hurt pretty bad. He had an injury to his spine that put him in a wheelchair and on a ventilator. I think about him from time to time. When I became an EMT and started transporting patients, it really got me thinking. What if he ever needed an ambulance?

"The logistics of either taking the ventilator, or ventilating him with a BVM, is probably more scary to him than it is to me. But it is pretty intimidating to me, too, let me tell you. I'd do it. But I'd be nervous.

"Do you think it's normal to feel that way?"

than a 9-volt battery to the size of a wallet. It is usually implanted in the upper left chest area, although occasionally it may be implanted in the area of the left upper quadrant of the abdomen. It is generally palpable through the skin.

The implanted defibrillator is designed to detect life-threatening cardiac rhythms (ventricular fibrillation and ventricular tachycardia). Newer models may have a pacemaker feature built in as well. The AICD delivers a single shock when a life-threatening rhythm is detected. This shock is often very painful to the patient, and is generally rated as 6 on a 1-to-10 pain scale. If the single shock does not correct the rhythm, or if the rhythm returns, other shocks will be delivered, one at a time, until the dysrhythmia is resolved or the machine is turned off. The AICD can be turned off only by a special magnet and generally only in a hospital setting.

> **NOTE:** *The occurrence of an AICD shock is often very upsetting to the patient. Be prepared to provide emotional support.*

Although muscle twitches may be seen on the patient, providers and caregivers will not be shocked or harmed if the AICD shocks while they are touching the patient. The AICD is not dangerous if it shocks when the patient is wet. Patients are generally instructed to call their doctor if they feel fine after a shock. However, if they have any symptoms such as dizziness, chest pain, shortness of breath, not feeling well, or if they are shocked more than twice in any 24-hour period, they should go to the hospital or call EMS.

The functioning of pacemakers and AICDs can be affected by certain electromagnetic and radio frequency signals, so people with these devices should not stand still in the doorway of a business with an electronic anti-theft device nor stand still in a walk-through metal detector (although walking through either of these without stopping is not harmful). Stereo speakers and cellular telephones should not be held against a pacemaker or AICD device. Additionally, electric motors (as in power tools) and gas-powered tools (such as chainsaws and snow blowers) must be kept at least 6 inches away from the AICD or pacemaker when they are running.

Most patients who have one or both of these devices have had a significant cardiac medical history. They may be on multiple medications and may carry wallet cards or wear bracelets stating that they have one of these devices in use.

EMT Assessment and Transport   Depending on the nature of the call and chief complaint, the EMT may wish to have ALS transport for a patient with a pacemaker or AICD device. A patient who merely has a pacemaker as part of his medical history may not need ALS, but if the pacemaker is malfunctioning or if an AICD has discharged, this patient is a high-risk cardiac patient and should be treated as such with high-concentration oxygen and frequent reassessment. If the patient goes into cardiac arrest, CPR and an AED should be used as indicated.

Left Ventricular Assist Devices

A recent advance in cardiac care is the ***left ventricular assist device (LVAD)***. The left ventricle is the cardiac chamber that pumps blood through the aorta to the body. When there is severe left ventricular heart failure, a heart transplant may be required. While the patient is waiting for a suitable donor, the LVAD serves as a "bridge to transplant." The LVAD moves blood from the left ventricle through an inserted tube to a pump implanted in the abdomen where the blood is pressurized and sent to the aorta for transport to the body. A tube extends from the LVAD through the abdominal wall to an external pump battery and control panel.

Problems that may be associated with LVADs are infection, air leakage, and battery failure. All require rapid transport to a hospital.

EMT Assessment and Transport   The patient with an LVAD will have an external battery pack that may be the size of a small backpack or briefcase (Figure 37-7). This should be carefully secured and prevented from tugging on the attached tubing. Failures of the battery system should first be addressed by attempting to plug the unit into an AC source in the home, inverter in an ambulance, or other power source. This will begin recharging the battery, and allow functioning of the pump. If the pump itself fails, a hand or foot pump is included with the system as a backup. The pump looks similar to the bulb on a blood pressure cuff and must be squeezed for each beat of the heart. Heart transplant centers will generally provide training to local EMS personnel if someone in the community has an LVAD. The training is specific to the model used by local patients.

left ventricular assist device (LVAD)

a battery-powered mechanical pump implanted in the body to assist a failing left ventricle in pumping blood to the body.

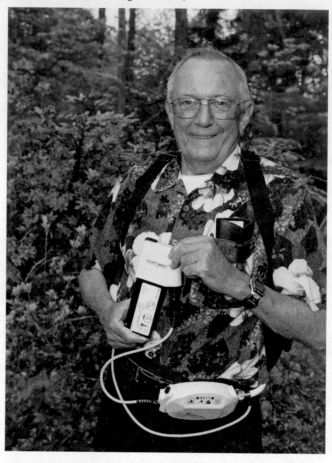

FIGURE 37-7 This patient holds one of the two batteries that powers his implanted left ventricular assist device. The LVAD's controller is attached to his belt. *(© AP Photo/George Widman)*

Gastrourinary Devices

Feeding Tubes

A *feeding tube* is used in a patient who is unable to feed himself or can't swallow. It may be used short term (during recovery from surgery) or long term (for chronic conditions). A feeding tube is most commonly seen in one of two forms: a nasogastric tube or a gastric tube.

A *nasogastric tube (NG-tube)* is a long tube inserted through the nose into the stomach that can be used to deliver nutrients. Additionally, the device can be used in emergency departments and by some ALS providers to suction out the stomach's contents; for example, in the case of certain overdoses. The NG-tube is generally taped to the patient's nose or cheek to prevent the tube from dislodging. A *gastrostomy tube (G-tube)* is a feeding tube surgically implanted through the abdominal wall and into the stomach (Figure 37-8). It is used to provide longer term nutrient delivery than would be provided by an NG-tube. The G-tube is held in place by a balloon inside the stomach. It can also be used by hospital personnel to drain stomach contents. Some feeding tubes are placed through the abdominal wall, directly into the small intestine. For example, a *J-tube* is placed into the jejunum section of the small intestine.

Common problems with both NG-tubes and G-tubes include dislodgement, infection at the site of insertion, or a clog that prevents nutrients from being provided to the patient. All of these conditions warrant transport and evaluation in a hospital setting.

EMT Assessment and Transport Ensure that the feeding tube is secured with tape to the patient's body before transport (Figure 37-9). If protocols allow, and nutrients are being administered during transport, keep the nutrient source higher than the level of the NG-tube or G-tube and hang it like an IV bag. Although the tube is not pressurized when nutrients are not being administered, the protective end cap should be placed on the tube to prevent leakage.

FIGURE 37-8 In her home kitchen, this mother is administering a liquid cornstarch solution to her child through an implanted gastric feeding tube. The child has a rare disease that requires him to ingest cornstarch every 4 hours to avoid seizures and hospitalization. (© AP Photo/The Charlotte Observer, David T. Foster III)

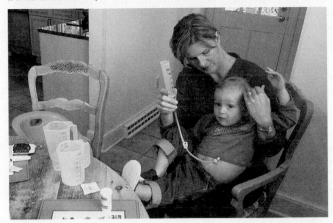

FIGURE 37-9 A gastric tube (G-tube) implanted in a baby's abdomen. Use tape to secure such a feeding tube to the patient's body before transport.

(© Ray Kemp/911 Imaging)

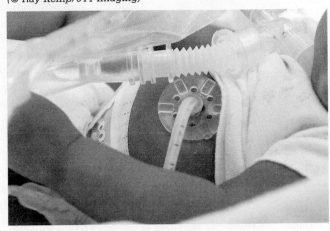

Urinary Catheters

A *urinary catheter* is used for a patient who has lost the ability to urinate or the ability to control when he urinates. Most commonly seen as indwelling Foley catheters, other types include the externally applied condom catheter. Most catheters are inserted into the bladder through the urethra and use a balloon to hold the tubing in place. The external tubing is connected to a collection bag (Figure 37-10), which may be a bag strapped to a leg or a larger

urinary catheter
a tube inserted into the bladder through the urethra to drain urine from the bladder.

FIGURE 37-10 This patient has a urinary catheter that is connected to a collection bag.

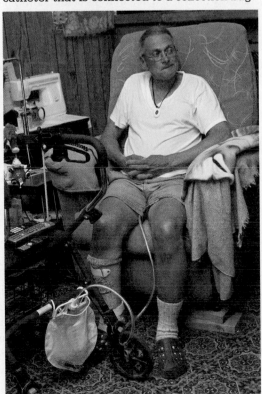

drainage bag, called a down drain, that may hang on the side of a patient's bed. Patients with leg bags are generally those who are more active than patients with down drains, as the leg bag may be hidden under clothing when the patient is in public. Common problems EMTs see with urinary catheters include infection, blockages causing lack of urinary output, discoloration of urine, and dislodgement of the catheter.

EMT Assessment and Transport   During transport, keep the catheter bag lower than the level of the patient (but not on a floor), and use care not to damage the bag with a stretcher or lifting device. Document and report any discoloration of the urine or any odors from the urine itself. Drainage bags should be emptied when they are one-third to one-half full. EMTs may want caregivers to empty the bag before transport to prevent overfilling, which will cause backflow into the bladder. Some patients are required to keep track of their total urine output every day, so document the amount emptied.

Ostomy Bags

ostomy bag
an external pouch that collects fecal matter diverted from the colon or ileum through a surgical opening (colostomy or ileostomy) in the abdominal wall.

As an EMT, you may also encounter a patient who has an ***ostomy bag***, also called an ostomy pouch. An ostomy bag is connected to the site of a colostomy or an ileostomy. A colostomy or ileostomy is the result of a surgery that brings a section of the intestine through the abdominal wall in order to divert the flow of stool away from the normal path to the rectum. An ostomy may be necessary because of a medical condition such as Crohn's disease or ulcerative colitis or cancer, especially colon cancer. An ostomy bag is usually attached to the patient's leg and often will not be visible under clothing. Common problems include infection at the stoma site, blockage, or, in some cases, dislodgement.

EMT Assessment and Transport   Use care when moving a patient if an ostomy bag is present to prevent breakage or dislodgement through rough handling.

Dialysis

dialysis
the process of filtering the blood to remove toxic or unwanted wastes and fluids.

A patient who requires ***dialysis*** has renal failure. The kidneys are unable to remove the buildup of toxins that occurs with the metabolism of daily life. Dialysis removes these toxins and filters the blood, taking over some of the roles the kidneys play in detoxifying the blood. Dialysis serves two important roles: waste removal and fluid removal. There are two forms of dialysis: hemodialysis and peritoneal dialysis.

Hemodialysis is performed by attaching the patient to an external machine called a dialyzer. The procedure is usually performed at a dialysis center, although home units do exist. Hemodialysis requires the use of large needles and tubing to remove and return the blood. The needles are inserted into a site where an artery has been surgically connected to a vein: an arteriovenous (A-V) fistula. Common complications encountered with patients on hemodialysis include bleeding from the A-V fistula site after dialysis and infection at the site of external dialysis catheters.

Peritoneal dialysis requires a permanent catheter that is implanted through the patient's abdominal wall and into the peritoneal cavity. Several liters of a specially formulated dialysis solution are run into the abdominal cavity to be absorbed into the intestines. Peritoneal dialysis can be performed at home. Common complications encountered with patients on peritoneal dialysis include dislodging of the catheter and infection in the peritoneal cavity (peritonitis), which results in the normally clear dialysis fluid turning cloudy.

Review Chapter 26, "Hematologic and Renal Emergencies," for a more complete discussion of dialysis.

EMT Assessment and Transport   Do not take a blood pressure on any arm with an A-V shunt, fistula, or graft, as this can cause damage that requires surgical repair.

If a shunt, graft, or fistula ruptures, significant blood loss (up to 500 mL/minute or more) will occur very quickly. In the case of a bleeding shunt, stop the bleeding by direct pressure. In the case of a fistula or graft bleed, which may be indicated by significant swelling under the skin at the site, apply direct pressure. *Do not* release the pressure until advised by a physician to do so, because the pressure is unlikely to allow clotting that would stop the bleeding. In all cases of bleeding from a shunt, fistula, or graft, the patient should be treated for shock, transported, and carefully monitored.

Central IV Catheters

Sometimes a patient you encounter will have a *central IV catheter*. A patient who receives frequent IV therapy, such as with chemotherapy or total parenteral nutrition, may have one of a variety of such catheters. Inserted in a hospital with surgery or under radiography, central IV catheters prevent patients from having to endure multiple needlesticks in their arms. A common problem with central IV catheters is infection at the site. Central IV catheters are usually inserted via a surgical venous puncture to introduce medications or fluids into the central circulation.

One form of central IV catheter is the *peripherally inserted central catheter (PICC) line*, which has an external tube slightly larger than IV tubing. The catheter is inserted into a peripheral vein, then threaded into the central circulation. A PICC line is often found inserted into the patient's arm.

Another form of central IV catheter is a *central venous line*, which may be inserted through a subclavian, jugular, or femoral vein. Central venous lines carry a variety of brand names, such as a Groshong®, a Hickman®, or a Broviac® catheter. These catheters may have one, two, or three external IV tubes that are attached to the patient's chest.

Finally, a central IV catheter may be in the form of an *implanted port* that can be felt under the skin. This port has no external tubing, and a special needle called a Huber is required to access this port. Brand names for these catheters include Port-a-Cath® and Mediport®.

EMT Assessment and Transport In most cases, neither the EMT nor a family caregiver will use a central IV catheter to administer medications to the patient or for any other purpose. Use of a central IV catheter is usually restricted to hospital personnel. However, awareness of the presence of a central IV device is important for the EMT, who must exercise caution to avoid any tugging or contamination of the catheter site.

central IV catheter
a catheter surgically inserted for long-term delivery of medications or fluids into the central circulation.

Physical Impairments

Patients who call EMS may have a variety of impairments that affect their hearing, sight, or speech. When one of these senses has been adversely affected or removed, you should take extra care and time to help the patient adjust. It is important to remember, however, that these impairments do *not* necessarily affect the patient's ability to think. Each limitation requires different approaches and considerations when you are assessing and treating the patient.

Although hearing loss is more common in the elderly than in younger persons, it is not restricted to the older patient. Approach each patient individually and ascertain his abilities. Not all patients with hearing loss can read lips, and in most cases yelling or slowing down your speech will only make matters worse. One of the easiest ways to communicate with a patient with hearing loss is to write your questions and explain your actions on a piece of paper. Many dispatch centers and communities also have TDD/TTY phones, and may be able to relay information through these devices.

NOTE: *TDD/TTY stands for Telecommunication Device for the Deaf/TeleTYpewriter. The system consists of a keyboard, display screen, and modem connected to an analog telephone line. The user can type in a message and receive a response that is displayed on the screen.*

Impairments to sight can be partial or complete. Determine if the patient has poor vision or no vision. Blind patients may not use lights in their home or may not notice lights that have burned out. It is good practice for the EMT to always carry a small flashlight, even during the day. The patient may know the layout of his home very well, so if anything is moved for transport of the patient, be sure to return it to its original position. If the patient has a guide dog, federal law allows for the patient to bring the dog along in an ambulance, unless the dog is a direct threat to others (for example, if it is barking or growling).

A patient who is unable to speak (aphasic) may need to write answers to your questions, use a TDD/TTY phone, or have a computer that speaks the words he types.

Many elderly persons contend with difficulty walking or standing, but problems with gait and balance can occur at any age. Carefully assist people who have such disabilities, and make sure to bring along any helping devices they want to have with them, such as a cane, a walker, or braces. Patients in wheelchairs may be difficult to assess completely as they may be unable to stand or turn for complete physical assessment. If a patient in a wheelchair is moved to a stretcher, ensure that the patient's wheelchair either safely accompanies them or is secured from theft or loss.

EMT Assessment and Transport Approach and treat each patient with one or more physical impairments by providing whatever extra assistance he requires. Carefully assess to determine if an impairment is the patient's baseline or if it is a new problem (for example, a person suffering a stroke and has lost the ability to speak). Determine the patient's comfort level and any abilities or tools he uses to compensate. During care, carefully explain all of your actions and treatments. Bring any devices the patient uses, such as a walker, a hearing aid, glasses, speech computer, or other items to help communicate with hospital staff, and make his environment more comfortable. If the patient has a wheelchair, consider the use of a wheelchair van if one is available.

ABUSE AND NEGLECT

CORE CONCEPT

How to recognize and deal with cases of abuse and neglect

Keep in mind that patients with special challenges can be more vulnerable to physical or sexual abuse, exploitation, and neglect because of their dependence on others. This vulnerable population can include children and adults, especially the elderly. Be alert to this possibility during your scene size-up, history taking, and assessment. Stories that are inconsistent with injuries, multiple injuries in various stages of healing, repeated injuries, and caregivers' indifference to the patient should bring to mind the possibility of abuse or neglect. As with any suspected case of abuse or neglect, do not make accusations. Do your best to get the patient out of the environment and report your suspicions according to the requirements of your jurisdiction (see Chapter 4, "Medical, Legal, and Ethical Issues").

CRITICAL DECISION MAKING

EMTs Need to Know

Patients with special needs pose challenges for EMTs at all levels. For each of the following situations, explain how you would handle it and where you might turn for help or advice.

1. You are treating an unresponsive diabetic patient when you notice he has an insulin pump. You believe you should turn it off but are not sure how.

2. You are treating a patient who had just performed peritoneal dialysis at home. She complains of excruciating pain with even the least little movement.

3. You are called for a possible respiratory infection in a child. You arrive to find the patient has a trach and a ventilator. You are not sure how to transport the ventilator.

Key Facts and Concepts

- Patients with special challenges include those who are homeless or living in poverty, are very obese, have sensory impairments, are terminally ill, have developmental disorders, and/or are technology-dependent.

- A disability is a condition that interferes with a person's ability to engage in everyday activities, such as working or caring for oneself.

- Although patients with special challenges may require EMS for problems related to their disability or chronic condition, do not assume that this is the case for a particular patient.

- It is critical for EMTs to treat patients with special challenges with empathy and respect.

- The homeless, poor, and very obese are at increased risk of health problems.

- When dealing with a patient who has autism, use the ABCS: *awareness* (that ASD patients behave and react differently from most patients), *basic* (keep instructions, questions, treatments, and the environment simple), *calm* (be calm and patient; don't lose your temper, yell, or try to force the patient), and *safety* (as much as possible, interact with the patient in his familiar surroundings where he feels safe).

- Patients with special challenges, their families, and caregivers are often very knowledgeable about the patient's needs and the function of their special equipment. As much as possible, rely on their expertise and involve them in the patient's care.

Key Decisions

- What is the patient's problem today? Is it a complication of the disability or chronic condition, or is this a new problem?

- Must the patient's special equipment remain with her during transport, or can it stay behind? In either case, what steps are necessary to prepare the patient for transportation?

- How knowledgeable is the patient or his family or caregiver about the situation? What information and assistance can they provide to make the situation easier?

- If the patient has a disability that impairs communication, what is the best way to communicate with her?

Chapter Glossary

autism spectrum disorders (ASD) developmental disorders that affect, among other things, the ability to communicate, report medical conditions, self-regulate behaviors, and interact with others.

automatic implanted cardiac defibrillator (AICD) a device implanted under the skin of the chest to detect any life-threatening dysrhythmia and deliver a shock to defibrillate the heart.

bariatrics the branch of medicine that deals with the causes of obesity, as well as its prevention and treatment.

central IV catheter a catheter surgically inserted for long-term delivery of medications or fluids into the central circulation.

continuous positive airway pressure (CPAP) a device worn by a patient that blows oxygen or air under constant low pressure through a tube and mask to keep airway passages from collapsing at the end of a breath.

dialysis the process of filtering the blood to remove toxic or unwanted wastes and fluids.

disability a physical, emotional, behavioral, or cognitive condition that interferes with a person's ability to carry out everyday tasks, such as working or caring for oneself.

feeding tube a tube used to provide delivery of nutrients to the stomach. A nasogastric feeding tube is inserted through the nose and into the stomach; a gastric feeding tube is surgically implanted through the abdominal wall and into the stomach.

left ventricular assist device (LVAD) a battery-powered mechanical pump implanted in the body to assist a failing left ventricle in pumping blood to the body.

obesity a condition of having too much body fat, defined as a body mass index of 30 or greater.

ostomy bag an external pouch that collects fecal matter diverted from the colon or ileum through a surgical opening (colostomy or ileostomy) in the abdominal wall.

pacemaker a device implanted under the skin with wires implanted into the heart to modify the heart rate as needed to maintain an adequate heart rate.

stoma a surgically created opening into the body, as with a tracheostomy, colostomy, or ileostomy.

tracheostomy a surgical opening in the neck into the trachea.

urinary catheter a tube inserted into the bladder through the urethra to drain urine from the bladder.

ventilator a device that breathes for a patient.

Preparation for Your Examination and Practice

Short Answer

1. List several advanced medical devices you might find when responding to patients with special challenges at home.

2. What health problems are associated with obesity?

3. If a tracheostomy tube is blocked and your protocols allow, describe a method of clearing the blockage.

4. If a ventilator that a patient relies on to breathe malfunctions, what life support care should you perform?

5. What are some specific health problems associated with homelessness?

6. List and briefly describe the "ABCS" for dealing with a patient who has autism.

7. If a patient cannot hear or cannot speak, describe several methods that might facilitate communication with him.

Thinking and Linking

Patients with special needs can pose a number of challenges in assessment and management. This exercise combines material you have learned in this chapter with material from previous chapters. Decide how you would handle each of the following situations.

1. Your patient is a 2-year-old girl having a seizure on only one side of her body. Her father tells you she was born without a corpus callosum, the fibers that connect the left and right sides of the brain. Describe how you will assess and manage the patient. What are some questions you should ask the parents to ensure the patient gets the best care?

2. Your patient is a 30-year-old woman whom you estimate to weigh approximately 600 pounds. She is in her second-floor apartment, which she has not left for over a year. There is no elevator. What resources do you need to get the patient out of her apartment and to the hospital? What are your considerations in moving and transporting the patient?

3. Your patient is a 45-year-old man who receives continuous ambulatory peritoneal dialysis. When you arrive, the patient is allowing fluid to be drained from his abdomen into a collection bag. How should you determine the best way to manage the patient's dialysis process during transport?

4. Your patient is a 12-year-old boy with a severe developmental disability. His teacher says his nose began bleeding and she has not been able to stop it. The patient is frightened of you. He is kicking and screaming and refuses to let you near him. How would you handle this situation?

Critical Thinking Exercises

A call to a patient with special needs may require some creative problem solving. Describe how you would handle each of the following situations—and explain your reasoning.

1. You are called to respond to a patient who has an arteriovenous (A-V) fistula that is used during his triweekly visits to the dialysis center. The patient presents as pale, sweaty, anxious, and almost incoherent. Could the cause of his condition be related to the A-V fistula? How might you determine if this is the case? What actions should you take?

2. You are called to a nursing home to transport a 79-year-old patient who had a severe stroke 6 months ago. She has a feeding tube in place, a colostomy bag, and a urinary catheter. Today she is presenting with a fever, a heart rate of 120, respirations of 24, and a blood pressure of 100/60. What are your primary concerns with this patient? What are your considerations for dealing with her feeding tube, colostomy bag, and urinary catheter?

3. Think back to your training in Basic Life Support. What BLS training might you draw upon to help you deal with a patient with special needs whose life-sustaining equipment has malfunctioned?

4. Your patient is a paraplegic, paralyzed from the waist down after a vehicle collision. She called EMS today because she thinks she has pneumonia. She lives alone and has a service dog that assists her. She insists that she must take the dog with her. How should you handle this situation?

5. Your patient is a 10-year-old girl with autism who does not speak. She has fallen from a chair she was standing on and seems to have injured her ankle. When she sees you coming in, she becomes visibly terrified. How can you best assess and treat this child?

Pathophysiology to Practice

The following questions are designed to assist you in gathering relevant clinical information and making accurate decisions in the field.

1. What risk factors do the homeless and poor have for developing serious health problems? Why might patients in this group be less able to compensate for illness and injury?

2. What is the difference between congenital and acquired diseases? What are examples of each?

3. Why might a patient who is paralyzed be more prone to bedsores, pneumonia, and other infections?

You answer a call for a young girl who has an issue with her tracheostomy tube. Dispatch tells you 18-month-old Amber's parents left her in the care of her Aunt Dorothy for a day. Dorothy is familiar with Amber's tracheostomy but has not had any experience with anything going wrong. Unfortunately, something went wrong. Late in the afternoon, Amber experienced a fever and began to look a little gray. That's when Dorothy called EMS.

Your initial impression as you enter Amber's room is that she is alert but in some respiratory distress with cyanosis around the lips. When you examine her tracheostomy, you see that there is a small amount of mucus coming from her trach tube. Her radial pulse is rapid and weak.

Street Scene Questions

1. What is this patient's priority?
2. What additional information do you need to treat the patient?

Next to Amber you see several small soft suction catheters. You remove one from the package, attach it to your suction device, measure the length to insert by comparing it to the obturator on the table next to the patient, and suction some mucus out of her trach tube. Amber's color begins to improve. Your partner tells you the patient's pulse is 128 and her respiratory rate is 44.

Street Scene Questions

3. How should you reassess the patient?
4. What equipment should you take to the hospital with Amber?

You listen to Amber's breathing through her trach tube and no longer hear the gurgling sounds that were initially audible. She is moving air well. Although her color is better than when you found her, she appears pale and still in some respiratory distress, although less than before you suctioned her. Amber's pulse oximeter reading has increased from 85 percent to 91 percent. You gather Amber's "ready-to-go" bag with her medical records and Emergency Information Form as you prepare her for transport. You administer high-concentration oxygen and suction her trach tube a few more times on the trip to the emergency department.

Later, Amber's parents call your station to thank you for what you did. Amber had a respiratory infection that is responding well to treatment. Dorothy was very impressed with your calm professionalism, and the entire family is very grateful.

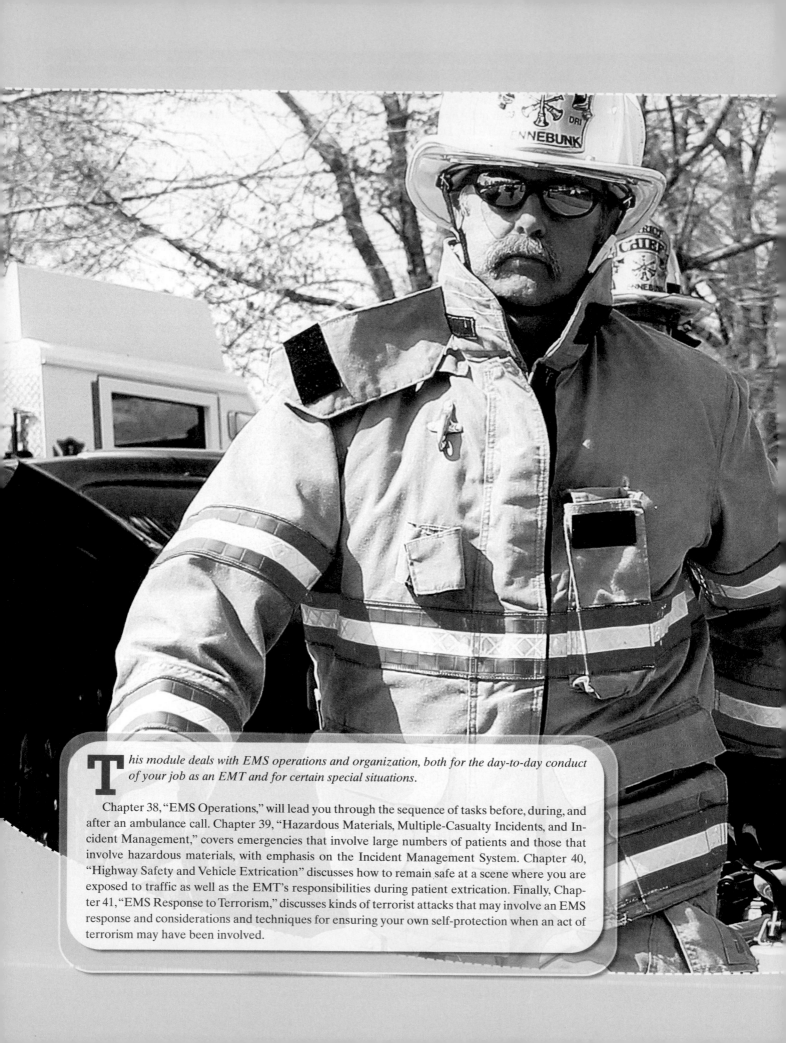

This module deals with EMS operations and organization, both for the day-to-day conduct of your job as an EMT and for certain special situations.

Chapter 38, "EMS Operations," will lead you through the sequence of tasks before, during, and after an ambulance call. Chapter 39, "Hazardous Materials, Multiple-Casualty Incidents, and Incident Management," covers emergencies that involve large numbers of patients and those that involve hazardous materials, with emphasis on the Incident Management System. Chapter 40, "Highway Safety and Vehicle Extrication" discusses how to remain safe at a scene where you are exposed to traffic as well as the EMT's responsibilities during patient extrication. Finally, Chapter 41, "EMS Response to Terrorism," discusses kinds of terrorist attacks that may involve an EMS response and considerations and techniques for ensuring your own self-protection when an act of terrorism may have been involved.

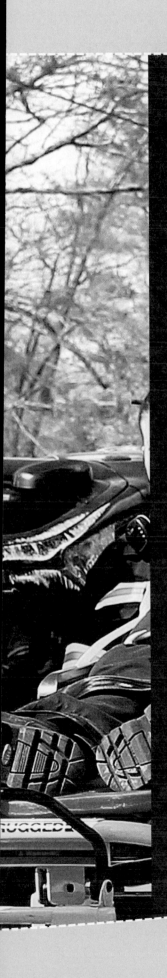

Operations

38

EMS Operations

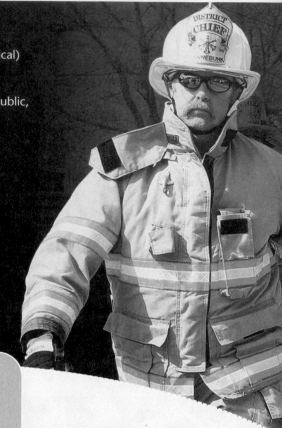

○ **STANDARD**
EMS Operations (Principles of Safely Operating a Ground Ambulance; Air Medical)

○ **COMPETENCY**
Applies knowledge of operational roles and responsibilities to ensure patient, public, and personnel safety.

○ **CORE CONCEPTS**
— Phases of an ambulance call

— Preparation for a call

— Operating an ambulance

— Transferring and transporting the patient

— Transferring the patient to the emergency department staff

— Terminating the call, replacing and exchanging equipment, cleaning and disinfecting the unit and equipment

— When and how to use air rescue

EXPLORE Resource**Central**

To access Resource Central, follow directions on the Student Access Card provided with this text. If there is no card, go to **www.bradybooks.com** and follow the Resource Central link to Buy Access from there. Under Media Resources, you will find:

▸ **Sanitization, Disinfection, and Sterilization**
Watch a video on how to properly disinfect, sanitize, and sterilize equipment.

▸ **Safe Driving Tips**
Read about ways to avoid accidents and learn what is meant by *defensive driving*.

▸ **Some Information about Air Medical Services**
Learn what situations may require requesting air medical services, how you should prepare for these providers, and read about some additional challenges faced by air medical service providers.

OBJECTIVES

After reading this chapter you should be able to:

38.1 Recognize the four types of ambulances currently specified by the U.S. Department of Transportation. (pp. 975, 976)

38.2 Describe the types of equipment required to be carried by EMS response units. (pp. 975, 976–980)

38.3 Describe the components of the vehicle and equipment checks done at the start of every shift. (pp. 975, 980–982)

38.4 Describe the roles and responsibilities of the Emergency Medical Dispatcher. (pp. 982–983)

38.5 Discuss the principles of safe ambulance operation while responding to the scene. (pp. 983–988)

38.6 Explain laws that typically apply to ambulance operations. (pp. 984–985)

38.7 Discuss how to maintain safety at highway incidents. (pp. 988–989)

38.8 Describe the steps necessary for transferring the patient to the ambulance. (pp. 989–991)

38.9 Describe the EMT's responsibilities while transporting a patient to the hospital. (pp. 991–993)

Your responsibilities may differ somewhat depending on the type of EMS agency you join. However, most nonmedical operational responsibilities include the following five phases:

- Preparing for the ambulance call
- Receiving and responding to a call
- Transferring the patient to the ambulance
- Transporting the patient to the hospital
- Terminating the call

PREPARING FOR THE AMBULANCE CALL

The modern ambulance has come a long way from its primitive beginnings. Far more than just a means of transport, today's ambulance is a well-equipped and efficiently organized mobile prehospital emergency department and communications unit.

The U.S. Department of Transportation has issued specifications for Type I, Type II, and Type III ambulances. Because of the extra equipment now placed on ambulances for specialty rescue, advanced life support, and hazardous materials operations, their gross vehicle weight has been easily exceeded in some communities. This has necessitated introduction of a medium-duty truck chassis built for rugged durability and large storage and work areas (Figure 38-1). As needs evolve, ambulance standards will also continue to evolve.

Ambulance Supplies and Equipment

If an ambulance does not have the proper equipment for patient care and transportation, it is just a ride to the hospital. Table 38-1 lists the 2009 recommendations of the American College of Surgeons, the American College of Emergency Physicians, the National Association of EMS Physicians, and the American Academy of Pediatrics. EMS services are regulated in most states, and each state has a list of equipment required to be carried by EMS response units. Please refer to your state or regional office for your specific regulations and an equipment list.

Compare the items listed in Table 38-1—and lists of equipment required by your state or region—with the inventory of your ambulance. Learn where each item is stored, what every item is for, and when it should be used. If the item is a mechanical device, also learn how it works and how it should be maintained.

Ensuring Ambulance Readiness for Service

As a professional rescuer, you are expected by the public and your organization to be ready when an emergency occurs. Therefore, you must be sure that you, your vehicle, and your equipment are ready to respond. Most services require that an inspection of the vehicle and equipment be conducted at the start of every shift to ensure "ready-ness."

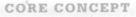
CORE CONCEPT ●
Phases of an ambulance call

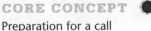
CORE CONCEPT ●
Preparation for a call

FIGURE 38-1 Four types of ambulances: (A) Type I, (B) Type II, (C) Type III, and (D) medium duty.

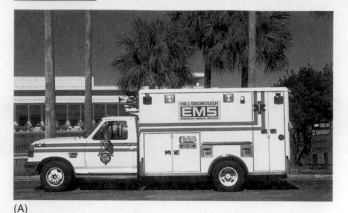
(A)

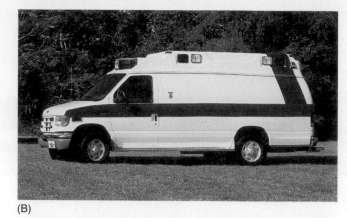
(B)

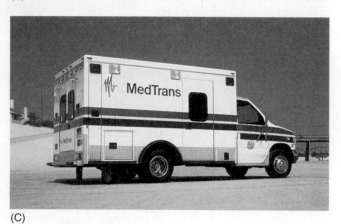
(C)

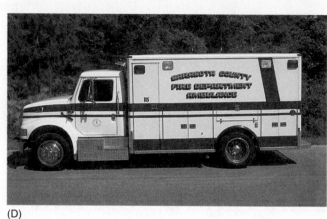
(D)

Table 38-1 Required Equipment for Basic Life Support Ambulances

2009 REQUIRED EQUIPMENT FOR BASIC LIFE SUPPORT AMBULANCES

A. Ventilation and Airway Equipment	1. Portable and fixed suction apparatus with a regulator (per federal specifications; see Federal Specification KKK-A-1822F reference) • Wide-bore tubing, rigid pharyngeal curved suction tip; tonsillar and flexible suction catheters, 6F–16F are commercially available (have one between 6F and 10F and one between 12F and 16F) 2. Portable oxygen apparatus, capable of metered flow with adequate tubing 3. Portable and fixed oxygen supply equipment • Variable flow regulator 4. Oxygen administration equipment • Adequate length tubing; transparent mask (adult and child sizes), both nonrebreathing and valveless; nasal cannulas (adult, child) 5. Bag-valve mask (manual resuscitator) • Hand-operated, self-reexpanding bag; adult (>1,000 mL) and child (450–750 mL) sizes, with oxygen reservoir/accumulator; valve (clear, disposable, operable in cold weather); and mask (adult, child, infant, and neonate sizes) 6. Airways • Nasopharyngeal (16F–34F; adult and child sizes) • Oropharyngeal (sizes 0–5; adult, child, and infant sizes) 7. Pulse oximeter with pediatric and adult probes 8. Saline drops and bulb suction for infants

B. Monitoring and Defibrillation	All ambulances should be equipped with an automated external defibrillator (AED) unless staffed by advanced life support personnel who are carrying a monitor/defibrillator. The AED should have pediatric capabilities, including child-sized pads and cables.

C. Immobilization Devices	1. Cervical collars
	   • Rigid for children ages 2 years or older; child and adult sizes (small, medium, large, and other available sizes)
	2. Head immobilization device (not sandbags)
	   • Firm padding or commercial device
	3. Lower extremity (femur) traction devices
	   • Lower extremity, limb-support slings, padded ankle hitch, padded pelvic support, traction strap (adult and child sizes)
	4. Upper and lower extremity immobilization devices
	   • Joint-above and joint-below fracture (sizes appropriate for adults and children), rigid-support constructed with appropriate material (cardboard, metal, pneumatic, vacuum, wood, or plastic)
	5. Impervious backboards (long, short; radiolucent preferred) and extrication device
	   • Short (extrication, head-to-pelvis length) and long (transport, head-to-feet length) with at least three appropriate restraint straps (chin strap alone should not be used for head immobilization) and with padding for children and handholds for moving patients

D. Bandages	1. Commercially packaged or sterile burn sheets
	2. Triangular bandages
	   • Minimum two safety pins each
	3. Dressings
	   • Sterile multitrauma dressings (various large and small sizes)
	   • ABDs, 10″ × 12″ or larger
	   • 4″ × 4″ gauze sponges or suitable size
	4. Gauze rolls
	   • Various sizes
	5. Occlusive dressing or equivalent
	   • Sterile, 3″ × 8″ or larger
	6. Adhesive tape
	   • Various sizes (including 1″ and 2″) hypoallergenic
	   • Various sizes (including 1″ and 2″) adhesive
	7. Arterial tourniquet (commercial preferred)

E. Communication	Two-way communication device between EMS provider, dispatcher, and medical direction
F. Obstetrical Kit (commercially packaged is available)	1. Kit (separate sterile kit) • Towels, 4″ × 4″ dressing, umbilical tape, sterile scissors or other cutting utensil, bulb suction, clamps for cord, sterile gloves, blanket 2. Thermal absorbent blanket and head cover, aluminum foil roll, or appropriate heat-reflective material (enough to cover newborn)
G. Miscellaneous	1. Sphygmomanometer (pediatric and adult regular and large size cuffs) 2. Adult stethoscope 3. Length/weight-based tape or appropriate reference material for pediatric equipment sizing and drug dosing based on estimated or known weight 4. Thermometer with low temperature capability 5. Heavy bandage or paramedic scissors for cutting clothing, belts, and boots 6. Cold packs 7. Sterile saline solution for irrigation (1-liter bottles or bags) 8. Flashlights (2) with extra batteries and bulbs 9. Blankets

(continued)

G. Miscellaneous (continued)	10. Sheets (minimum 4), linen or paper, and pillows
	11. Towels
	12. Triage tags
	13. Disposable emesis bags or basins
	14. Disposable bedpan
	15. Disposable urinal
	16. Wheeled cot (conforming to national standard at the time of manufacture)
	17. Folding stretcher
	18. Stair chair or carry chair
	19. Patient care charts/forms
	20. Lubricating jelly (water soluble)
H. Infection Control (latex-free equipment should be available)	1. Eye protection (full peripheral glasses or goggles, face shield)
	2. Face protection (for example, surgical masks per applicable local or state guidance)
	3. Gloves, nonsterile (must meet NFPA 1999 requirements found at http://www.nfpa.org/)
	4. Coveralls or gowns
	5. Shoe covers
	6. Waterless hand cleanser, commercial antimicrobial (towelette, spray, liquid)
	7. Disinfectant solution for cleaning equipment
	8. Standard sharps containers, fixed and portable
	9. Disposable trash bags for disposing of biohazardous waste
	10. Respiratory protection (for example, N-95 or N-100 mask—per applicable local or state guidance
I. Injury Prevention Equipment	1. All individuals in an ambulance need to be restrained (there is currently no national standard for transport of uninjured children)
	2. Protective helmet
	3. Fire extinguisher
	4. Hazardous material reference guide
	5. Traffic signaling devices (reflective material triangles or other reflective, nonigniting devices)
	6. Reflective safety wear for each crew member (must meet or exceed ANSI/ISEA performance Class II or III if working within the right of way of any federal-aid highway. Visit http://www.reflectivevest.com/federalhighwayruling.html for more information.)

OPTIONAL BASIC EQUIPMENT

This section is intended to assist EMS providers in choosing equipment that can be used to ensure delivery of quality prehospital care. Use should be based on local resources. The equipment in this section is not mandated or required.

A. Optional Equipment	1. Glucose meter (per state protocol)
	2. Elastic bandages
	• Nonsterile (various sizes)
	3. Cellular phone
	4. Infant oxygen mask
	5. Infant self-inflating resuscitation bag
	6. Airways
	• Nasopharyngeal (12Fr, 14Fr)
	• Oropharyngeal (size 00)
	7. Alternative airway devices (for example, a rescue airway device such as the ETDLA [esophageal-tracheal double lumen airway], laryngeal tube, or laryngeal mask airway) as approved by local medical direction.

A. Optional Equipment (continued)	8. Alternative airway devices for children (few alternative airway devices that are FDA approved have been studied in children. Those that have been studied, such as the LMA, have not been adequately evaluated in the prehospital setting).
	9. Neonatal blood pressure cuff
	10. Infant blood pressure cuff
	11. Pediatric stethoscope
	12. Infant cervical immobilization device
	13. Pediatric backboard and extremity splints
	14. Topical hemostatic agent
	15. Appropriate CBRNE PPE (chemical, biological, radiological, nuclear, explosive personal protective equipment), including respiratory and body protection
	16. Applicable chemical antidote auto-injectors (at a minimum for crew members' protection; additional for patient treatment based on local or regional protocol; appropriate for adults and children)
B. Optional Basic Life Support Medications	1. Albuterol
	2. EpiPens
	3. Oral glucose
	4. Nitroglycerin (sublingual tablet or paste)
C. Interfacility Transport	Additional equipment may be needed by ALS and BLS prehospital care providers who transport patients between facilities. Transfers may be done to a lower or higher level of care, depending on the specific need. Specialty transport teams, including pediatric and neonatal teams, may include other personnel such as respiratory therapists, nurses, and physicians. Training and equipment needs may be different depending on the skills needed during transport of these patients. There are excellent resources available that provide detailed lists of equipment needed for interfacility transfer such as the American Academy of Pediatrics Guidelines for Air and Ground Transport of Neonatal and Pediatric Patients.

APPENDIX: EXTRICATION EQUIPMENT

Adequate extrication equipment must be readily available to the emergency medical service responders, but is more often found on heavy rescue vehicles than on the primary responding ambulance. In general, the devices or tools used for extrication fall into several broad categories: disassembly, spreading, cutting, pulling, protective, and patient-related. The following is necessary equipment that should be available either on the primary response vehicle or on a heavy rescue vehicle.

A. Disassembly Tools	1. Wrenches (adjustable)
	2. Screwdrivers (flat and Phillips head)
	3. Pliers
	4. Bolt cutter
	5. Tin snips
	6. Hammer
	7. Spring-loaded center punch
	8. Axes (pry, fire)
	9. Bars (wrecking, crow)
	10. Ram (4 ton)
B. Spreading Tools	1. Hydraulic jack/spreader/cutter combination cutting tools
	2. Saws (hacksaw, fire, windshield, pruning, reciprocating)
	3. Air-cutting gun kit
C. Pulling Tools/Devices	1. Ropes/chains
	2. Come-along
	3. Hydraulic truck jack
	4. Air bags

(continued)

Table 38-1	Required Equipment for Basic Life Support Ambulances (continued)
D. Protective Devices	1. Reflectors/flares
	2. Hard hats
	3. Safety goggles
	4. Fireproof blanket
	5. Leather gloves
	6. Jackets/coats/boots
E. Miscellaneous	1. Shovel
	2. Lubricating oil
	3. Wood/wedges
	4. Generator
	5. Floodlights

NOTE: *Local extrication needs may necessitate additional equipment for water, aerial, or mountain rescue.*

Source: American College of Surgeons, Committee on Trauma; American College of Emergency Physicians; National Association of EMS Physicians; American Academy of Pediatrics

Do a brief shift report with the off-going crew, if possible. Learn whether they experienced any problems with either the ambulance or its equipment during their shift. Make a thorough bumper-to-bumper inspection of the ambulance (Scan 38-1), using the checklist provided by your service. There are usually two components to the inspection: a vehicle component and an equipment component. In most cases, the EMT assigned to be the driver completes the vehicle component check and the EMT crew leader completes the medical equipment check.

Ambulance Inspection, Engine Off

The following inspection steps can be taken while the ambulance is in quarters:

1. Inspect the body of the vehicle. Report any damage that may be evident.
2. Inspect the wheels and tires. Check for damage or worn wheel rims and tire sidewalls. Check the tread depth. Use a pressure gauge to ensure that all tires are properly inflated. Do not forget to inspect the inside rear tires.
3. Inspect the windows and mirrors. Look for broken glass and loose or missing parts. See that mirrors are clean and properly adjusted for maximum visibility.
4. Check the operation of every door and all latches and locks.
5. Check the level of the fluids: oil, coolant, and brake and transmission fluids.
6. Check the battery. Inspect the battery cable connections for tightness and signs of corrosion.
7. Inspect the interior surfaces and upholstery for damage and cleanliness.
8. Check the windows for operation. See that the interior surface of each window is clean.
9. Test the horn, siren, and emergency lights
10. Adjust the driver's seat and ensure the seat belts are operational.
11. Check the fuel level. Refuel after each call whenever practical.

NOTE: *Allow the engine to cool before removing any pressure caps.*

Ambulance Inspection, Engine On

The next steps require you to start the engine. Pull the ambulance from quarters if engine exhaust fumes will be a problem. Set the parking brake, put the transmission in "park," and have your partner chock the wheels before undertaking the following steps:

1. Check the dash-mounted indicators to see if any light remains on to indicate a possible problem with oil pressure, engine temperature, or the vehicle's electrical system.
2. Check dash-mounted gauges for proper operation.

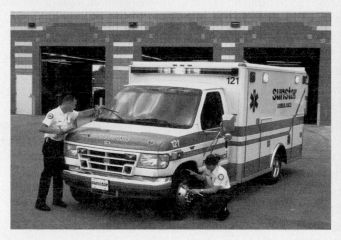

1 Check the ambulance body, wheels, tires, and windshield wipers.

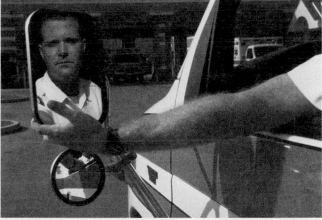

2 Check the windows, doors, and mirrors.

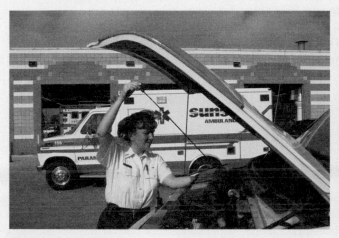

3 Check under the hood.

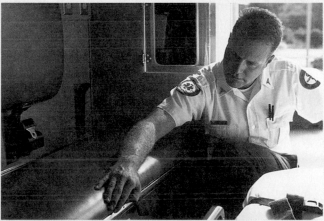

4 Check the interior surfaces and upholstery.

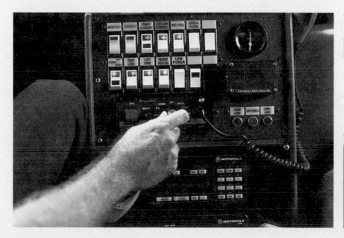

5 Check the dash instruments and communications equipment.

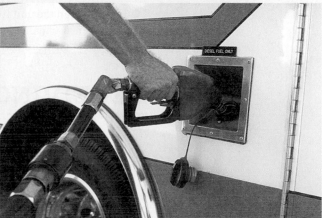

6 Check the fuel level and fill up.

3. Depress the brake pedal. Note whether pedal travel seems correct or excessive. Check air pressure as needed.

4. Test the parking brake. Move the transmission level to a drive position. Replace the level to the "park" position as soon as you are sure that the parking brake is holding.

5. Turn the steering wheel from side to side.

6. Check the operation of the windshield wipers and washers. The glass should be wiped clean each time the blade moves.

7. Turn on the vehicle's warning lights. Have your partner walk around the ambulance and check each flashing and revolving light for operation. Turn off the warning lights.

8. Turn on the other vehicle lights. Have your partner walk around the ambulance again, this time checking the headlights (high and low beams), turn signals, four-way flashers, brake lights, side and rear scene illumination lights, and box marker lights.

9. Check the operation of the heating and air-conditioning equipment in both the driver's compartment and the patient compartment. This is also a good time to check the on-board suction if the engine is running.

10. Check transmission fluid.

11. Operate the communications equipment. Test portable as well as fixed radios and any radio-telephone communications.

Return the ambulance to quarters. While you are backing up, have your partner note whether the backup alarm is operating (if the vehicle is so equipped).

Inspection of Patient Compartment Supplies and Equipment

Shut off the engine and complete your inspection by checking the patient compartment and all exterior cabinets:

1. Using your checklist, conduct a detailed inspection and inventory of the equipment and supplies.

2. Check treatment supplies and equipment and rescue equipment. Items should not only be identified, they should also be checked for completeness, condition, and operation. Check the pressure of oxygen cylinders. Inflate air splints and examine them for leaks. Test oxygen and ventilation equipment for proper operation. Examine rescue tools for rust and dirt. Operate battery-powered devices to ensure that the batteries have a proper charge. Some equipment, such as the AED, may require additional testing. See that an item-by-item inspection of everything carried on the ambulance is done, with findings recorded on the inspection report.

3. When you are finished, complete the inspection report. Correct any deficiencies. Replace missing items. Make your supervisor aware of any deficiencies that cannot be immediately corrected.

4. Finally, clean the unit for infection control and appearance. Maintaining the ambulance's appearance enhances your organization's image in the public's eye. People who take pride in their work show it by taking pride in the appearance of their ambulance.

RECEIVING AND RESPONDING TO A CALL

In many areas of the country, a person needs only to dial 911 to access ambulance, fire, or police services 24 hours a day. A trained Emergency Medical Dispatcher (EMD) records information from callers, decides which service is needed, and alerts that service to respond. (Always say "nine-one-one" when talking to community or school groups. Children cannot find "eleven" on the phone dial or key pad.)

Role of the Emergency Medical Dispatcher

Many cities and communication centers train and certify Emergency Medical Dispatchers (EMDs) based on the medical priority card system. This system originated in 1979 through the leadership of Jeffrey Clawson, MD. An EMD is trained to perform the following tasks:

- Ask questions of the caller and assign a priority to the call
- Provide prearrival medical instructions to callers and information to crews
- Dispatch and coordinate EMS resources
- Coordinate with other public safety agencies

When answering a call for help, the EMD must obtain as much information as possible about the situation that may help the responding crew. The questions the EMD should ask are:

1. **What is the exact location of the patient?** The EMD must ask for the house or building number and the apartment number, if any. It is important to ask for the street name with the direction designator (e.g., North, East), the nearest cross street, the name of the development or subdivision, and the exact location of the emergency.

2. **What is your call-back number?** (Enhanced 911 will show the number.) "Stay on the line. Do not hang up until I (the EMD) tell you to." In life-threatening situations, the EMD will offer instructions to the caller, after the units have been dispatched, that the caller or others on the scene should follow until the units arrive. It is also important for the caller to stay on the line in case a question arises about the location that was given.

3. **What's the problem?** This will provide the chief complaint. It will help the EMD decide which line of questioning to follow and the priority of the response to send.

4. **How old is the patient?** Most ambulances are set up to respond to the scene with a pediatric kit if the patient is a child rather than an adult. If prearrival CPR instructions are given, it will be necessary to distinguish between an infant, a child, and an adult.

5. **What's the patient's sex?** Ask this if it is not obvious from the information given.

6. **Is the patient conscious?** An unconscious patient is a higher response priority.

7. **Is the patient breathing?** If the patient is conscious and breathing, the EMD will often ask many additional questions relative to the chief complaint to determine the appropriate level of response; for example, Emergency Medical Responders, EMTs, or ambulances may respond "cold" (at normal speed—sometimes called Priority 3) or "hot" (an emergency, lights-and-siren mode—sometimes called Priority 1). If the patient is not breathing, or the caller is not sure, the EMD will dispatch the maximum response and begin the appropriate prearrival instructions for a nonbreathing patient, which may also involve telephone CPR if the patient does not have a pulse.

If the call is for a traffic collision, a series of key questions must be asked to help determine the priority and amount of response. With thorough questioning of the caller, it may be possible for the EMD to appropriately dispatch one unit "hot" and backup units "cold," which in turn will help prevent emergency vehicle collisions.

This is how an EMD might dispatch an ambulance to the location of a sick person:

MEDCOM to Ambulance 641 and Medic 640, respond Priority 1 to a 60-year-old unconscious female with breathing difficulty. The location is the Boston Market on Route 9 with Kunker Road on the cross. Time now is 1745 hours.

The EMD may repeat the message to minimize any question as to its content and ensure the ambulance has received the call.

Operating the Ambulance

Even if you will only occasionally be driving an ambulance, you may be mandated to attend emergency vehicle operator training, which has both classroom and in-vehicle road sessions.

CORE CONCEPT ●
Operating an ambulance

Being a Safe Ambulance Operator

To be a safe ambulance operator, you must:

- Be physically fit. You should not have any impairment that prevents you from operating the ambulance or any medical condition that might disable you while driving.
- Be mentally fit, with your emotions under control. The judgment of someone operating an ambulance should not be compromised by the excitement of lights and sirens.
- Be able to perform under stress.

- Have a positive attitude about your ability as a driver but not be an overly confident risk taker.
- Be tolerant of other drivers. Always keep in mind that people react differently when they see an emergency vehicle. Accept and tolerate the bad habits of other drivers without flying into a rage.

Some additional safety tips include:

- Never drive while under the influence of alcohol, illicit or "recreational" drugs such as marijuana or cocaine, medicines such as antihistamines, "pep pills," or tranquilizers.
- Never drive with a restricted license.
- Always wear your glasses or contact lenses if required for driving.
- Evaluate your ability to drive based on personal stress, illness, fatigue, or sleepiness.

Understanding the Law

Every state has statutes that regulate the operation of emergency vehicles. Emergency vehicle operators are generally granted certain exemptions with regard to speed, parking, passage through traffic signals, and direction of travel. However, the laws also state that if an emergency vehicle operator does not drive with due regard for the safety of others, he must be prepared to pay the consequences, such as tickets, lawsuits, or even time in jail.

The following list contains some points typically included in laws regulating ambulance operation:

- An ambulance operator must have a valid driver's license and may be required to complete a training program.
- Privileges granted under the law to the operators of ambulances apply when the vehicle is responding to an emergency or is involved in the emergency transport of a sick or injured person. When the ambulance is not on an emergency call, the laws that apply to the operation of nonemergency vehicles also apply to the ambulance.
- Even though certain privileges are granted during an emergency, the exemptions granted do not provide immunity to the operator in cases of reckless driving or disregard for the safety of others.
- Privileges granted during emergency situations apply only if the operator uses warning devices in the manner prescribed by law.

Most statutes allow emergency vehicle operators to:

- Park the vehicle anywhere if it does not damage personal property or endanger lives.
- Proceed past red stop signals, flashing red stop signals, and stop signs. Some states require that emergency vehicle operators come to a full stop, then proceed with caution. Other states require only that an operator slow down and proceed with caution.
- Exceed the posted speed limit as long as life and property are not endangered.
- Pass other vehicles in no-passing zones after properly signaling, ensuring that the way is clear, and taking precautions to avoid endangering life and property. This does not include passing a school bus with its red lights blinking. Wait for the bus driver to clear the children and then turn off the red lights of the bus.
- With proper caution and signals, disregard regulations that govern direction of travel and turning in specific directions.

If you ever become involved in an ambulance collision, the laws will be interpreted by the court based upon two key issues: (1) Did you use due regard for the safety of others? and (2) Was it a true emergency? The requirement of due regard actually sets a higher standard for drivers of emergency vehicles than for other drivers. This is why an investigation by the district attorney or grand jury, as well as your ambulance service, is not uncommon following a collision.

Most states reserve the emergency mode of operation for a true emergency, defined as one in which the best information available to you is that loss of life or limb is possible. When dispatched to a call, there is often not much information to go on, so a "collision" will get an emergency response. However, once you arrive and find that your patient is stable with no life-threatening injuries or conditions, it is no longer a true emergency. A lights-and-siren, high-speed response to the hospital in such a situation would be improper.

The exemptions described here are just examples of those often granted to ambulance operators. Do not assume that they are granted in your state. Obtain a copy of your state's rules and regulations and carefully study them.

Using the Warning Devices

Safe emergency vehicle operation can be achieved only when proper use of warning devices is coupled with sound emergency and defensive driving practices. Studies show that other drivers do not see or hear an ambulance until it is within 50 to 100 feet, so never let the lights and siren give you a false sense of security.

The Siren Although the siren is the most commonly used audible warning device, it is also the most misused. Consider the effects that sirens have on other motorists, patients in ambulances, and ambulance operators themselves:

- The continuous sound of a siren may cause a sick or injured person to suffer increased fear and anxiety, and his condition may worsen as stress builds up.

- Ambulance operators themselves are affected by the continuous sound of a siren. Tests have shown that inexperienced ambulance operators tend to increase their driving speeds from 10 to 15 miles per hour while continually sounding the siren. In some cases, operators using a siren were unable to negotiate curves that they could pass through easily when not sounding the siren. Sirens also affect hearing, especially if used for long periods with the siren speaker over the cab. The best placement for the speaker is in the vehicle grill.

Many states have laws that regulate the use of audible warning signals. In areas where there are no statutes, ambulance organizations usually create their own policies. If your organization does not, you may find the following suggestions helpful:

- Use the siren sparingly, and only when you must. Some states require use of the siren at all times when the ambulance is responding in the emergency mode. Others require it only when the operator is exercising any of the exemptions discussed earlier.

- Never assume that all motorists will hear your signal. Buildings, trees, and dense shrubbery may block siren sounds. Soundproofing keeps outside noises from entering vehicles, and radios or CD players also decrease the likelihood that an outside sound will be heard.

- Always assume that some motorists will hear your siren but ignore it.

- Be prepared for the erratic maneuvers of other drivers. Some drivers panic when they hear a siren.

- Do not pull up close to a vehicle and then sound your siren. This may cause the driver to jam on his brakes and you may be unable to stop in time. Use the horn when you are close to a vehicle ahead.

- Never use the siren indiscriminately, and never use it to scare someone.

The Horn The horn is standard equipment on all ambulances. Experienced operators find that the judicious use of the horn often clears traffic as quickly as the siren. The guidelines for using a siren apply to the horn as well.

Visual Warning Devices Whenever the ambulance is on the road, night or day, the headlights should be on. This increases the vehicle's visibility to other drivers. In some states, headlights are now required of all vehicles in low visibility conditions or whenever the windshield wipers are in use. Alternating flashing headlights should be used only if they are attached to secondary head lamps. In most states, it is illegal to drive at night with one headlight out.

The large lights on the outermost corners of the box should blink in tandem, or unison, rather than wigwagging or alternating. This helps the vehicle that is approaching from a distance identify the full size of your vehicle. There are several types of lights on ambulances, including rotating lights, flashing lights, strobe lights, and the newer LED (light-emitting diode) lights. When planning the lighting package of an ambulance, check the research before making your decision. In general, it is wisest for the package to combine different types of lights in strategic places rather than just one type of lighting system.

Four-way flashers and directional signals should not be used as emergency lights. This is very confusing to the public, as well as being illegal in some states. Drivers expect a vehicle with four-way flashers on to be traveling at a very slow speed. Additionally, the flashers disrupt the function of the directional signals.

When the ambulance is in the emergency response mode, either en route to the scene or to the hospital with a high-priority patient, all the emergency lights should be used. The vehicle should be easily seen from 360 degrees.

In some communities, ambulances still follow an old tradition of using their emergency lights when returning to the station. However, this practice is very confusing to the public. Do not be surprised if other drivers do not pull over when you are on an emergency run if they constantly see your ambulance with emergency lights on. *Save the use of lights and siren for life- or limb-threatening emergencies.*

Speed and Safety

You are often told to drive in a slow and careful manner. At this point, you may be thinking something like, "How will I ever get a seriously ill or injured person to a hospital if I poke along?" We are not suggesting that you "poke along." However, we do suggest you drive with these facts in mind:

- Excessive speed increases the probability of a collision.
- Speed increases stopping distance, reducing the chance of avoiding a hazardous situation.

Remember that the laws in most states excuse you from obeying certain traffic laws only in a true emergency and only with due regard for the safety of others. Except in these circumstances, obey speed limits, stoplights and signs, yield signs, and other laws and posted limits. Approach intersections with caution, avoid sudden turns, and always properly signal lane changes and turns. Be sure that the ambulance driver and all passengers wear seat belts whenever the ambulance is in motion.

Escorted or Multiple-Vehicle Responses

When the police provide an escort for an ambulance, there are additional hazards. Too often, the inexperienced ambulance operator follows the escort vehicle too closely and is unable to stop when the lead vehicle(s) make an emergency stop. Also, the inexperienced operator may assume that other drivers know his vehicle is following the escort. In fact, other drivers will often pull out in front of the ambulance just after the escort vehicle passes.

Because of the dangers involved with escorts, most EMS systems recommend no escorts unless the operator is not familiar with the location of the patient (or hospital) and must be given assistance from the police.

In multiple-vehicle responses, the dangers can be the same as those generated by escorted responses, especially when the responding vehicles travel in the same direction, close together. A great danger also exists when two vehicles approach the same intersection at the same time. Not only may they fail to yield for each other; other drivers may yield for the first vehicle but not the second. Obviously, great care must be used at intersections during multiple-vehicle responses.

Factors That Affect Response

Most ambulance collisions take place in seemingly safe conditions. In New York State, 18 years of ambulance-collision statistics show that the typical collision happens on a dry road (60 percent) with clear weather (55 percent) during daylight hours (67 percent) in an intersection (72 percent). During this period, there were 5,782 ambulance collisions, which involved 7,267 injuries and 48 fatalities! Additionally, an ambulance response can be affected by several factors:

- **Day of the week.** Weekdays usually have the heaviest traffic because people are commuting to and from work. In resort areas, weekend traffic may be heavier.
- **Time of day.** In major employment centers, traffic over major roads tends to be heavy in all directions during commuter hours.
- **Weather.** Adverse weather conditions reduce driving speeds and thus increase response times. A heavy snowfall can temporarily prevent any response at all. Be careful to lengthen your following distance whenever there is decreased road grip due to inclement weather

- **Road maintenance and construction.** Traffic can be seriously impeded by road construction and maintenance activities. Be aware of area road construction and plan responses as needed.

- **Railroads.** There are still more than a quarter-million grade crossings in the United States with traffic often blocked by long, slow freight trains. Some communities may use a secondary response system on the other side of train tracks that splits the town in half.

- **Bridges and tunnels.** Traffic over bridges and through tunnels slows during rush hours. Collisions—including ambulance collisions—tend to occur when drivers forget that bridges freeze before roadways.

- **Schools and school buses.** The reduced speed limits in force during school hours slow the flow of vehicles. An emergency vehicle should never pass a stopped school bus with its red lights flashing. Wait for the school bus driver to signal you to proceed by turning off the lights. In addition, emergency vehicles attract children, who often venture out into the street to see them. The operator of every emergency vehicle should slow down when approaching a school or playground. Obey the directions given by school crossing guards.

POINT OF VIEW

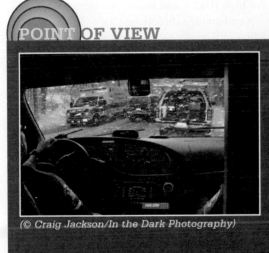

(© Craig Jackson/In the Dark Photography)

"I never realized when I started doing EMS that I'd have to drive in the same stuff that is causing all the crashes.

"We were called for a three-car collision on Highway 17, a road on the outskirts of the city. With the snow that was building up it took us a good 15 white-knuckled minutes to get out there. We drove carefully, and most of the time at less than half the speed we would have used to get there on a clear day. People were sliding all over the road. We just had to tell ourselves we wouldn't do any good if we didn't get there.

"When we did get to the scene we had to be very careful parking so someone didn't hit us. A trooper and a fire engine were parked between our back door and the traffic. We were only at the scene for about 5 minutes when a car spun out of control and almost hit the trooper's car. Crazy.

"You don't have snow days in EMS like you had in school. That's for sure! C'mon spring."

Getting There: Navigating to the Scene

Many EMS services have global positioning satellite (GPS) navigation installed in their emergency vehicles. This is an excellent tool for navigation to emergency scenes and hospitals. However, there is still no substitute for an intimate knowledge of the response area. Often a GPS suggests a route that may not be possible because of recent road construction or other changes in the area. GPS devices can also be a significant distraction! Be careful about attempting to operate the GPS while driving. Driving while distracted increases the chance of a crash.

Obtain detailed maps of your service area. Hang one map in quarters and place another in the ambulance. Even if you have GPS navigation, check the maps before you leave for a call. If you get lost while responding to a call, turn off your emergency lights and siren and pull over. Recheck the map and recheck the GPS. Call the EMD on the radio and obtain additional instructions.

Response Safety Summary

The following list summarizes important points about how to make a safe response.

- Minimize lights-and-siren "hot" responses. Remember: Driving with lights and siren involves high risk.

- Wear your seat belts.

- Know where you are going before you respond. Use the GPS and check the maps. Be familiar with your response area.

- Come to a complete stop at intersections.

- Don't be a distracted driver. Have the crew leader operate the radio, siren, GPS, computer, and other devices.
- Don't eat or drink when responding under emergency conditions. Pay complete attention to the task at hand.
- Don't listen to music, text, talk on cell phones, or indulge in any other distracting activities. Pay 100 percent attention to safe driving.

Safety at Highway Incidents

Operation at highway incidents exposes EMTs to significant danger. EMTs, firefighters, and police officers are injured and killed every year while operating at the scenes of highway incidents. The following are some tips for improving the safety of highway operations.

Keep Unnecessary Units and People Off the Highway   If you are not the primary or first-arriving unit, stay off the highway. Park or stage your unit near the on ramp until the first unit has sized up the incident and determined the resources needed. You don't want to expose people to any more risk than necessary when working on the highway. *The more vehicles and people gathered, the greater the risk.*

Avoid Crossovers Unless a Turn Can Be Completed without Obstructing Traffic Crossovers on limited access highways involve high risk. Avoid using this maneuver if possible. It may be safer to go to the next off ramp and change directions.

If Yours Is the First Unit On-Scene   The first unit on-scene blocks the incident by parking the apparatus "upstream" from the incident. The apparatus is placed to block the crash from traffic by using the vehicle as a barrier. The best vehicle for this is a fire truck because of its size and weight. Ideally, ambulances should be parked "downstream" in a safe loading area (see Figure 38-2).

The EMT should conduct a scene size-up and then transmit an arrival report. At that point, he should cancel or request additional resources, as needed. To avoid overcrowding the site, cancel anything that is not absolutely needed. (*Remember: The more vehicles and people gathered, the greater the risk.*)

Wear Your PPE   If there is no extrication in progress, wear an ANSI Class 2 safety vest and a helmet. If extrication is indicated, then you should wear turnouts. The basic idea is this: *EMS workers should match the level of protection being worn by other responders, such as fire department personnel.*

Place Cones/Flares and Reduce Emergency Lighting   Place cones/flares upstream to warn and direct traffic around the incident. Remember that response lights can blind approaching drivers and increase scene risks. Consider reducing emergency lighting to prevent blinding motorists.

Unit Placement Is Important!   Consider crash scene preservation when placing apparatus. Avoid driving over debris and skid marks, because the police consider these to be crime scene evidence. If extrication is necessary, leave room for placing rescue vehicles that will be needed to do the extrication. Create a "safe area" downstream; place ambulances downstream past the incident. This is also a good area for the placement of Command/staff vehicles. Prevent anyone from blocking the egress of ambulances, and try to keep all ambulances heading in the same direction.

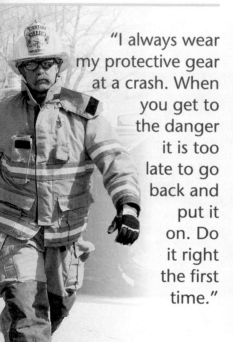

"I always wear my protective gear at a crash. When you get to the danger it is too late to go back and put it on. Do it right the first time."

FIGURE 38-2 Park the ambulance properly at the scene of a collision.

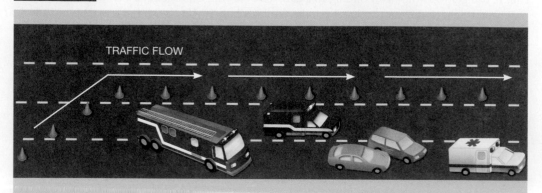

TRAFFIC FLOW

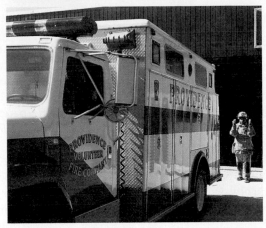

FIGURE 38-3 Use a spotter to help guide the ambulance when backing up.

Try to keep the ambulance on the same side of the road as the incident. It is very dangerous to carry stretchers across lanes of moving traffic. Do not have emergency personnel crossing in traffic (review Figure 38-2).

Backing Up As an operator of an emergency vehicle, you should avoid backing up, if possible, especially during emergencies. There are large blind spots in your mirrors and a danger of striking a pedestrian, an object, or another vehicle. If you must back up, position someone at the rear of the ambulance as a spotter to guide the backing process (see Figure 38-3).

CRITICAL DECISION MAKING

Arriving Safely

Although most of this text has discussed treating the patient at the scene, your response and vehicle placement is an important part of your responsibilities at a call. Proper vehicle placement ensures your safety and that of the vehicle, and its contents are available to you in a convenient location. For each of the following situations, explain where you would park the ambulance if you were first arriving.

1. You are called to a railroad car derailment.

2. You are called to a collision on the interstate. An engine company and trooper are parked at the scene, blocking oncoming traffic.

3. You are called to a scene involving domestic violence. Police are not yet on the scene.

TRANSFERRING THE PATIENT TO THE AMBULANCE

On most ambulance runs, you will be able to reach a sick or injured person without difficulty, assess his condition, carry out emergency care procedures where he lies, and then transfer him to the ambulance. At times, however, dangers at the scene or the priority of the patient will dictate moving the patient before assessment and emergency treatments can be completed. When a spinal injury is suspected, you must manually stabilize the patient's head, apply a cervical collar, and immobilize the patient on a spine board.

Transfer to the ambulance is accomplished in four steps, regardless of the complexity of the operation:

1. Select the proper patient-carrying device.

2. Package the patient for transfer.

CORE CONCEPT ●

Transferring and transporting the patient

3. Move the patient to the ambulance.

4. Load the patient into the ambulance.

The wheeled ambulance stretcher is the most commonly used device for transferring the patient to the ambulance.

The term *packaging* refers to the sequence of operations required to ready the patient to be moved and to combine the patient and the patient-carrying device into a unit ready for transfer. A sick or injured patient must be packaged so that his condition is not aggravated. You must complete all necessary care for wounds and other injuries, stabilize impaled objects, and check all dressings and splints before the patient is placed on the patient-carrying device. The properly packaged patient is covered and secured to the patient-carrying device.

When packaging the severely ill or injured patient, packaging is a balance between expedience and function. The patient should be firmly secured to transport devices and backboards so he will not fall or worsen his current condition in any way. Yet the EMT recognizes that packaging must be done quickly and efficiently in order to promptly and safely get the patient to the hospital.

Covering a patient helps to maintain body temperature, prevents exposure to the elements, and helps ensure privacy (Figure 38-4). A single blanket, or perhaps just a sheet, may be all that is required in warm weather. A sheet and blankets should be used in cold weather. When practical, cuff the blankets under the patient's chin, with the top sheet outside. Do not leave sheets and blankets hanging loose. Tuck them under the mattress at the foot and sides of the stretcher. In wet weather, place a plastic cover over the blankets during transfer. Remove it once you are in the ambulance to prevent overheating. In cold or wet weather, cover the patient's head, leaving the face exposed.

A patient-carrying device should have a minimum of three straps for securely holding the patient. The first should be at the chest level, the second at hip or waist level, and the third on the lower extremities. Sometimes there is a fourth strap if two are crossed at the chest.

Newer stretchers have straps that act as a harness and restrain the upper body (Figure 38-5). By combining over-the-shoulder straps with encircling straps, the patient is more securely held on the stretcher in the event of a collision.

All patients, including those receiving CPR, must be secured to the patient-carrying device before transfer to the ambulance. If your patient is not on a carrying device such as a spine board but instead is just on the ambulance stretcher, some states, as a matter of policy, require shoulder harnesses that secure the patient to the stretcher to prevent him from sliding forward in case of a short stop.

Although much has been said about protecting the patient from a possible ambulance collision, perhaps not enough has been said about protecting the EMT in the patient compartment, who is actually at greater risk. The patient is secured to the stretcher and obtains some safety benefit from that. Most of the time, however, the EMT is unsecured and vulnerable in the event of a collision. When traveling in an ambulance you should remain seated,

FIGURE 38-4 This patient is packaged for cold, wet conditions.

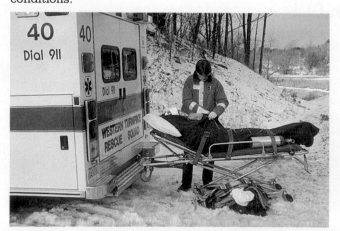

FIGURE 38 5 Stretcher straps that act as a harness restrain the patient's upper body.

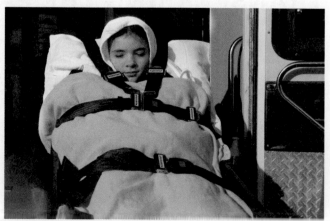

wearing a seat belt or harness when possible. Although it isn't always possible to remain seated, avoid unnecessary movement during emergency response and transport.

Unsecured equipment turns into projectiles upon collision, threatening both the patient and EMT. Always ensure that all equipment in the patient compartment (e.g., oxygen cylinders, kits) has been secured.

TRANSPORTING THE PATIENT TO THE HOSPITAL

Transport involves more than just driving to the hospital. A series of tasks must be undertaken from the time a patient is loaded into the ambulance until he is handed over to hospital personnel.

Preparing the Patient for Transport

The following activities may be required to prepare the patient for transport once he is in the ambulance:

- **Continue your assessment.** Make sure that a conscious patient is breathing without difficulty once you have positioned him on the stretcher. If the patient is unconscious with an airway in place, make sure he has an adequate air exchange once you have moved him into position for transport.

- **Secure the stretcher in place in the ambulance.** Always ensure that the patient is safe during the trip to the hospital. Before closing the door, and certainly before signaling the ambulance operator to move, make sure that the cot is securely in place. Patient compartments are equipped with a locking device that prevents the wheeled stretcher from moving about while the ambulance is in motion. Failure to fully engage the locking device at both ends of the stretcher can have disastrous consequences once the ambulance is in motion.

- **Position and secure the patient.** During transfer to the ambulance, the patient must be firmly secured to a stretcher. This does not mean that he must be transported in that position. Positioning in the ambulance should be dictated by the nature of his illness or injury.
    - If he was not transferred to the ambulance in that position, shift an unconscious patient who has no potential spine injury, or one with an altered mental status, into the recovery position (on his side). This will promote maintenance of an open airway and the drainage of fluids.
    - Remember that the head and foot ends of the ambulance stretcher can be raised. A patient with breathing difficulty and no possibility of spinal injury may be more comfortable being transported in a sitting position. A patient in shock can be transported with the legs raised 8 to 12 inches.
    - A patient with a potential spinal injury must remain immobilized on the long spine board, with the patient and board together being secured to the stretcher. If resuscitation is required, he must remain supine with constant monitoring of the airway and suctioning equipment ready. If resuscitation is not required, the unresponsive patient and spine board can be rotated as a unit and the board propped on the stretcher so that the patient is on his side for drainage of fluids and vomitus from the mouth.

- **Adjust the security straps.** Security straps applied when a patient is being prepared for transfer to the ambulance may tighten unnecessarily by the time he is loaded into the patient compartment. Adjust the straps so they still hold the patient safely in place but are not so tight that they interfere with circulation or respiration or cause pain.

- **Prepare for respiratory or cardiac complications.** If the patient is likely to develop cardiac arrest, position a short spine board or CPR board underneath the mattress prior to starting on the trip. Then, if he does go into arrest, time will not be wasted locating and positioning the board. Riding on a hard board may not be comfortable, but temporary discomfort is better than permanent injury or even death from delayed resuscitation.

- **Loosen constricting clothing.** Clothing may interfere with circulation and breathing. Loosen ties and belts and open any clothing around the neck. Straighten clothing that is bunched under safety straps. Remember that clothing bunched at the crotch may be painful. Before you do anything to rearrange the patient's clothing, however, explain what you are going to do and why.

- **Load a relative or friend who must accompany the patient.** Consider the following guidelines if your service does not prohibit the transportation of a relative or friend with a patient: First, encourage the person to seek alternative transportation, if available. If there is just no other way the relative or friend can get to the hospital, allow him to ride in the operator's compartment—not in the patient's compartment where he may interfere with patient care. Make certain the person buckles his seat belt. If an uninjured child must come along, bring the family's child car seat and use it.

- **Load personal effects.** If a purse, briefcase, overnight bag, or other personal item is to accompany the patient, make sure it is properly secured in the ambulance. If you load personal effects at the scene of a collision, be sure to tell a police officer what you are taking. Follow policies and fill out forms, if any, required by your local system for safeguarding personal effects.

- **Talk to your patient.** Apprehension often mounts in a sick or injured person after he is loaded in an ambulance. Not only is he held down by straps in a strange, confined space, but he may also be suddenly separated from family members and friends. Maintaining a conversation with the patient helps allay his fears and concerns and simply helps pass the time.

- **Avoid letting patients sit on the bench or airway seat.** Unless it's a multiple-casualty incident or there is some other extenuating circumstance, patients belong on the stretcher. Simply put, it's the safest place for them to be. If the patient suddenly becomes uncooperative and wants to jump out of a moving vehicle or assault the EMT, the stretcher and its restraints will slow him down. This restraint might even avert a tragedy.

When you are satisfied that the patient is ready, signal the operator to begin the trip to the hospital. If this is a high-priority patient, most of the preparation steps—loosening clothing, checking bandages and splints, reassuring the patient, even vital signs—can be done en route rather than delaying transport.

Caring for the Patient en Route

Having at least one EMT in the patient compartment is minimum staffing for an ambulance, although having two is preferred. Seldom will you be able to merely ride along with your patient. You may have to undertake a number of activities en route:

- **Notify the hospital.** Most EMS services radio the hospital with a patient report.

- **Continue to provide emergency care as required.** If life-support efforts were initiated prior to loading the patient into the ambulance, they must be continued during transportation to the hospital. Maintain an open airway, resuscitate, administer to the patient's needs, provide emotional support, and do whatever else is required, including updating your findings from the primary patient assessment.

- **Use safe practices during transport.** In most cases, the patient packaging and preparation will be completed prior to loading. En route to the hospital, vitals may need to be repeated, the patient has to be tended to, and the hospital must be called on the radio. Remain seat-belted as much as possible. If a crash occurs, being belted improves your chances of survival and helps reduce injuries. Stow any unnecessary equipment, because equipment can become projectiles in a crash. Probably the most important safety consideration is this: *Is it really necessary to transport this patient with lights and siren on?* When you are running "hot," the chances of a crash significantly increase. In most EMS systems, true emergencies needing a "hot" ride to the hospital constitute less than 5 percent of all transports. Don't use lights and siren for the drive to the hospital unless it is a life-threatening situation!

- **Compile additional patient information.** If the patient is conscious and emergency care efforts will not be compromised, record the patient information. Compiling information during the trip to the hospital serves two purposes. First, it allows you to complete your report. Second, supplying information temporarily takes your patient's mind off his problems. Remember, however, that this is not an interrogation session. Ask your questions in an informal manner.

- **Continue assessment and monitor vital signs.** Keep in mind that vital sign changes indicate a change in a patient's condition. For example, an unexplained increase in pulse rate may signify deepening shock. Record vital signs and be prepared to report changes to an emergency department staff member as soon as you reach the medical facility. Reassess vital signs every 5 minutes for an unstable patient, and every 15 minutes for a stable patient.

- **Notify the receiving facility.** Transmit patient assessment and management information and provide your estimated time of arrival.

PEDIATRIC NOTE

Remember that a toy such as a teddy bear can do much to calm a frightened child. Many ambulance units carry a sanitized, soft or padded, brightly colored toy just for these occasions. It is difficult at best to get information from a young child whose parents may have been injured and transported in another ambulance. Small children do not, as a rule, carry identification. Don't forget, you are a complete stranger in a hostile environment.

The collision scene, confusion, noise, injuries, possible pain, disappearance of a parent, EMTs caring for injuries, and gathering information—all create a terrifying experience for a child. The presence of a female EMT or police officer may be helpful; sometimes young children feel more comfortable talking to a woman. A smile and a calm, reassuring tone of voice are things that cannot be learned from a textbook, yet they may be the most critical care needed by the frightened child.

TRANSFERRING THE PATIENT TO THE EMERGENCY DEPARTMENT STAFF

You should take the following steps to ensure that the patient transfer to the care of emergency department personnel is accomplished smoothly and without incident. Brief as it may be, the transfer is a crucial step during which your primary concern must be the continuation of patient-care activities. The steps of the transfer are illustrated in Scan 38-2.

CORE CONCEPT
Transferring the patient to the emergency department staff

- **In a routine admissions situation or when an illness or injury is not life threatening, check first to see what is to be done with the patient.** If emergency department activity is particularly hectic, it might be better to leave your patient in the relative security and comfort of the ambulance while your operator determines where he is to be taken. Otherwise, the patient may be subjected to distressing sights and sounds and perhaps be in the way. (If you do this, make sure an EMT remains with the patient at all times.) *Under no circumstances should you simply wheel a nonemergency patient into a hospital, place him in a bed, and leave him!* This is an important point. Unless you transfer care of your patient directly to a member of the hospital staff, you may be open to a charge of abandonment.

  Staff members may be treating other seriously ill and injured persons, so suppress any urge to demand attention for your patient. Simply continue emergency care measures until someone can assume responsibility for the patient. When properly directed, transfer the patient to a hospital stretcher.

- **Assist emergency department staff as required and provide a verbal report.** Stress any changes in the patient's condition that you have observed.

- **As soon as you are free from patient-care activities, prepare the prehospital care report.** Remember, the job is not over until the paperwork is complete. Find a quiet spot and complete your prehospital care report (PCR).

- **Transfer the patient's personal effects.** If a patient's valuables or other personal effects were entrusted to your care, transfer them to a responsible emergency department

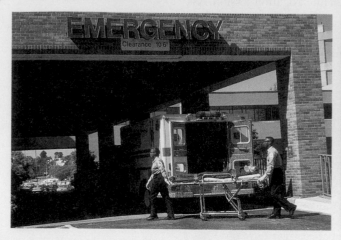

1 Transfer the patient as soon as possible. Stay with the patient until transfer is complete.

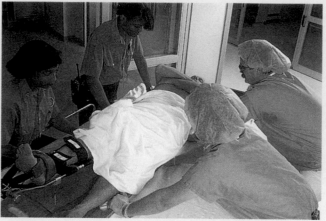

2 Assist the emergency department staff as required.

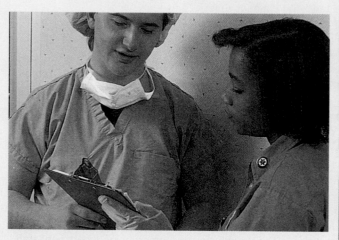

3 Transfer patient information as a verbal report and in a written prehospital care report.

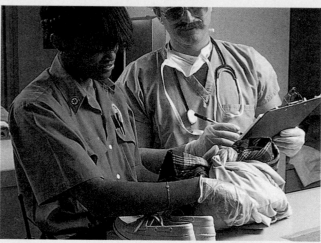

4 Transfer the patient's personal effects.

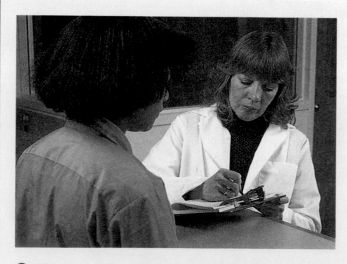

5 Obtain your release from the hospital.

staff member. Some services have policies that involve obtaining a written receipt from emergency department personnel as protection from a charge of theft.

- **Obtain your release from the hospital.** This task is not as formal as it sounds. Simply ask the emergency department nurse or physician if your services are still needed. In rural areas where not all hospital services are available, it may be necessary to transfer a seriously ill or injured person to another medical facility. If you leave and have to be recalled, the patient will lose valuable time.

TERMINATING THE CALL

An ambulance run is not really over until the personnel and equipment that comprise the prehospital emergency care delivery system are ready for the next response. The functions of EMTs in this final phase of activity include more than just changing the stretcher linen and cleaning the ambulance. A number of tasks must be accomplished at the hospital, during the return to quarters, and after arrival at the station.

CORE CONCEPT ●--------

Terminating the call, replacing and exchanging equipment, cleaning and disinfecting the unit and equipment

At the Hospital

While still at the hospital, the ambulance crew should begin making the ambulance ready to respond to another call. Time, equipment, and space limitations sometimes preclude vigorous cleaning of the ambulance while it is parked at the hospital. However, you should make every effort to quickly prepare the vehicle for the next patient (Scan 38-3):

1. **Quickly clean the patient compartment while taking appropriate Standard Precautions.** Follow biohazard disposal procedures according to your agency's OSHA exposure control plan. Examples of biohazards are contaminated dressings and used suction catheters.
   - Clean up blood, vomitus, and other body fluids that may have soiled the floor. Wipe down any equipment that has been splashed. Place disposable towels used to clean up blood or body fluids directly in a red bag.
   - Remove and dispose of trash such as bandage wrappings, open but unused dressings, and similar items.
   - Sweep away caked dirt that may have been tracked into the patient compartment. When the weather is inclement, sponge up water and mud from the floor.
   - Bag dirty linens or blankets to be appropriately laundered.
   - Use a deodorizer to neutralize odors of vomit, urine, and feces. Various sprays and concentrates are available for this purpose.

2. **Prepare respiratory equipment for service.**
   - Clean and then properly disinfect nondisposable, used bag-valve-mask units and other reusable parts of respiratory-assist and inhalation-therapy devices to keep them from becoming reservoirs of infectious agents that can easily contaminate the next patient. Disinfect the suction unit.
   - Place used disposable items in a plastic bag and seal it. Replace the items with similar ones carried in the ambulance as spares.

3. **Replace expendable items.**
   - If you have a supply replacement agreement with the hospital, replace expendable items from hospital storerooms on a one-for-one basis—such as sterile dressings, bandaging materials, towels, disposable oxygen masks, disposable gloves, sterile water, and oral airways.
   - Do not abuse this exchange program. Keep in mind that the constant abuse of a supply-replacement program usually leads to its discontinuation. At the very least, abuse places a strain on ambulance-hospital relations.

4. **Exchange equipment according to your local policy:**
   - Exchange items such as splints and spine boards. Several benefits are associated with an equipment exchange program: There is no need to subject patients to injury-aggravating movements just to recover equipment, crews are not delayed at the hospital, and ambulances can return to quarters fully equipped for the next response.

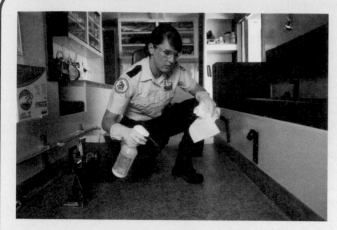

1 Clean the ambulance interior.

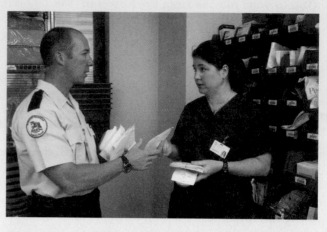

2 Replace disposable equipment per local protocols.

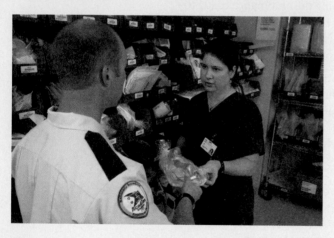

3 Replace airway equipment per local protocols.

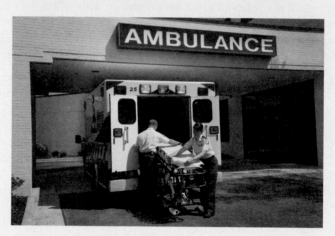

4 Make up the ambulance stretcher.

- When equipment is available for exchange, quickly inspect it for completeness and operability. Parts are sometimes lost or broken when an immobilizing device is removed from a patient.
- If you do find that a piece of equipment is broken or incomplete, notify someone in authority so the device can be repaired or replaced.

5. Make up the ambulance cot. The following procedure is one of many that can be used to make up a wheeled ambulance stretcher:

- Raise the stretcher to the high-level position, if possible; this makes the procedure easier. The stretcher should be flat with the side rails lowered and straps unfastened.
- Remove unsoiled blankets and pillows, and place them on a clean surface.
- Remove all soiled linen, and place it in the designated receptacle.
- Clean the mattress surface with an appropriate EPA-approved, low-level disinfectant unless there is visible blood, which should be cleaned up using a 1:100 bleach/water solution.
- Turn the mattress over; rotation adds to the life of the mattress.
- Center the bottom sheet on the mattress and fully open it. If a full-sized bed sheet is used, first fold it lengthwise.
- Tuck the sheet under each end of the mattress; form square corners and then tuck under each side.

- Place a disposable pad, if one is used, on the center of the mattress.
- Fully open the blanket. If a second blanket is used, open it fully and match it to the first blanket. This task should be done with an EMT at each end of the stretcher.
- Open a top sheet in the same way, placing it on top of the blanket. Fold the blanket(s) and top sheet together lengthwise to match the width of the stretcher; fold one side first, then the other.
- Tuck the foot of the folded blanket(s) and sheet under the foot of the mattress.
- Tuck the head of the folded blanket(s) and sheet under the head of the mattress.
- Place the slip-covered pillow lengthwise at the head of the mattress and secure it with a strap.
- Buckle the safety straps and tuck in excess straps.
- Raise the side rails and foot rest.

NOTE: *A neatly prepared stretcher inspires the patient's confidence. Do not use stained linen, even though it might be clean. Always make the presentation of your stretcher a matter of personal and professional pride.*

The stretcher is now ready for the next patient. It must be reemphasized that this is one of many techniques for preparing a wheeled ambulance stretcher for service. Whatever the method, it should meet the following objectives:

- Prepare for the next call as soon and as quickly as possible.
- Store all linens, blankets, and pouches neatly on the stretcher.
- Fold or tuck all linens and blankets so that they will be contained within the stretcher frame.
- Replace the cot in the ambulance.
- Replace any nondisposable patient-care items.
- Check for equipment left in the hospital.

En Route to Quarters

When heading back to quarters, your emphasis should be on a safe return. An ambulance operator may practice every suggestion for safe vehicle operation while en route to the hospital and then totally disregard those suggestions during the return to quarters. Defensive driving must be a full-time effort. Do not forget that the driver and all passengers must wear seat belts.

1. **Radio the EMD.** Let him know that you are returning to quarters and that you are available (or not available) for service. Valuable time is lost if an EMD has to locate and alert a backup ambulance when he does not know that a ready-for-service unit is on the road. Be sure that you notify the EMD if you stop and leave the ambulance unattended for any reason during the return to quarters.

2. **Air the ambulance, if necessary.** If the patient just delivered to the hospital has an airborne communicable disease, or if it was not possible to neutralize disagreeable odors while at the hospital, make the return trip with the windows of the patient compartment partially open, weather permitting. If the unit has sealed windows, use the air-conditioning or ventilating system (do not set on "recirculate") to air the patient compartment out.

3. **Refuel the ambulance.** Local policy usually dictates the frequency with which an ambulance is refueled. Some services require the operator to refuel after each call regardless of the distance traveled. In other services, the policy is to refuel when the gauge reaches a certain level. At any rate, the fuel should be at such a level that the ambulance can respond to an emergency and then to the hospital without fear of running out.

In Quarters

When you return to quarters, a number of activities need to be completed before the ambulance can be placed in service and before it is ready for another call (Scan 38-4).

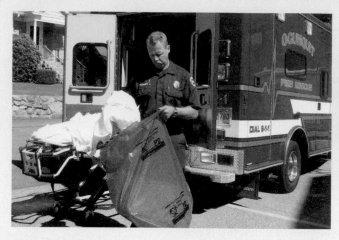

1 Place contaminated linens in a biohazard container, and noncontaminated linens in a regular hamper.

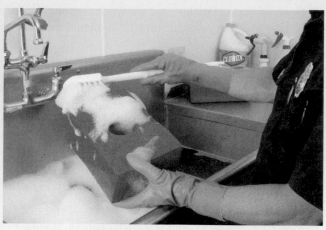

2 Remove and clean patient-care equipment as required.

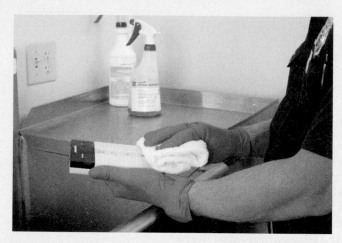

3 Clean and sanitize respiratory equipment as required.

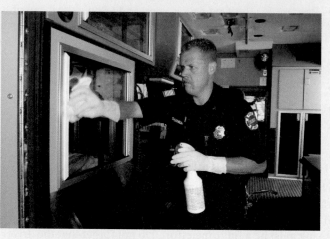

4 Clean and sanitize the ambulance interior as required. Use germicide on devices or surfaces that were in contact with blood or other body fluids.

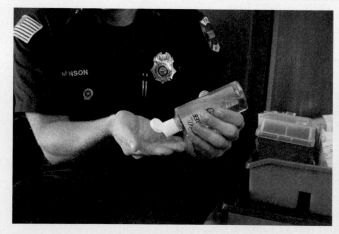

5 Wash your hands thoroughly, and change soiled clothing. Do this first if exposed to a communicable disease.

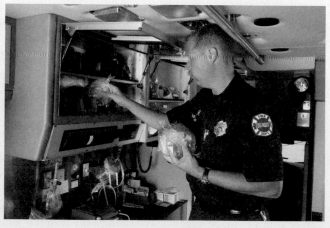

6 Replace expendable items as required.

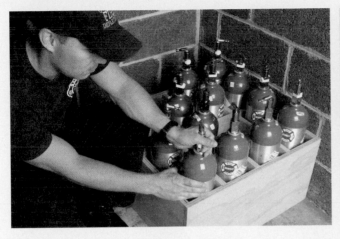

7 Replace oxygen cylinders as necessary.

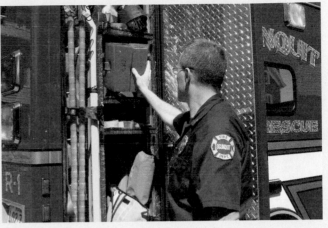

8 Replace patient-care equipment as needed.

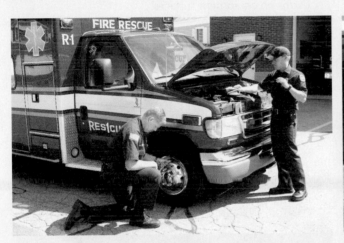

9 Maintain the ambulance as required. Report problems that will take the vehicle out of service.

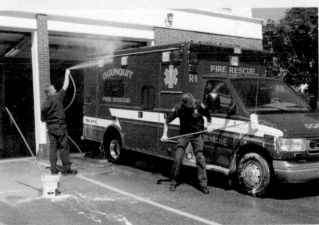

10 Clean the ambulance exterior as needed.

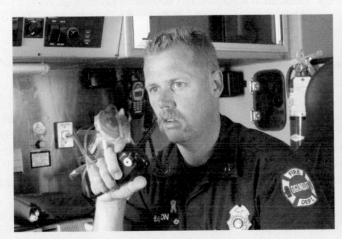

11 Report the unit ready for service.

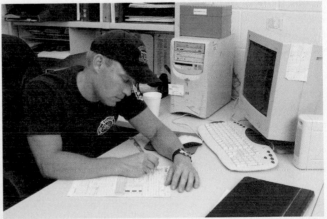

12 Complete any unfinished report forms as soon as possible.

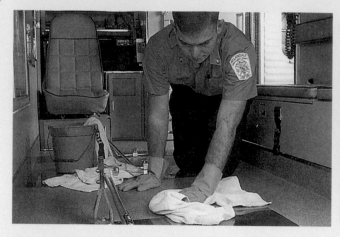

1 A low-level disinfectant approved by the U.S. Environmental Protection Agency (for example, a commercial product such as Lysol) will clean and kill germs on ambulance floors and walls.

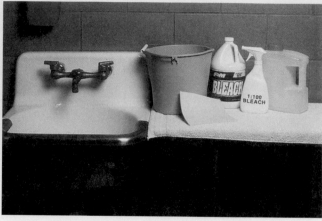

2 An intermediate-level disinfectant, such as a mixture of 1:100 bleach-to-water, can be used to clean and kill germs on equipment surfaces.

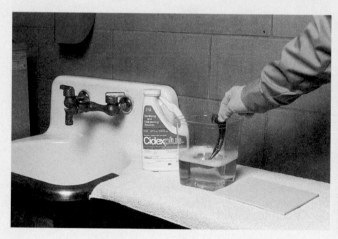

3 A high-level disinfectant, such as Cidex Plus, will destroy all forms of microbial life except high numbers of bacterial spores.

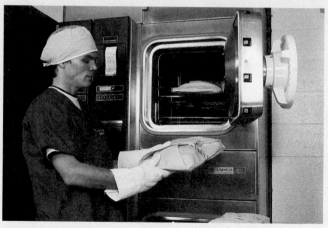

4 Sterilization is required to destroy all possible sources of infection on equipment that will be used in an invasive way.

With the emphasis today on protection from infectious diseases, you need to take every precaution to protect yourself. It is essential that you follow your agency's OSHA exposure control plan. Always wear gloves when handling contaminated linen, cleaning the equipment, handling the respiratory equipment, and cleaning the ambulance interior (there may be many hidden nooks and crannies where the patient's blood or body fluids could be gathered).

Once in quarters, you are ready to complete the cleaning and disinfecting chores. Consult Scan 38-5 for the levels of reprocessing to be used for equipment.

1. **Place badly contaminated linens in a biohazard container, and noncontaminated linens in a regular hamper.**

2. **As necessary, clean any equipment that touched the patient.** Brush stretcher covers and other rubber, vinyl, and canvas materials clean, then wash them with soap and water.

3. **Clean and disinfect used nondisposable respiratory-assist and inhalation therapy equipment.**
   - Disassemble the equipment so that all surfaces are exposed.
   - Fill a large plastic container with the cleaning solution outlined in your service's infection control plan.
   - Clean the inner and outer surfaces with a suitable brush. Inner surfaces can be cleaned with a small bottle brush, whereas outer surfaces can be cleaned with a hand or nail brush. Make sure all encrusted matter is removed.
   - Rinse the items with tap water.
   - Soak the items in an EPA-approved germicidal solution. An inhalation therapist at a local hospital can suggest a germicide suitable for respiratory equipment. Follow directions for dilution, safe handling, and soaking time. Gloves are recommended when using some germicides.
   - After the prescribed soaking period, hang the equipment in a well-ventilated clean area and allow it to dry for 12 to 24 hours.

4. **Clean and sanitize the patient compartment.** Use an EPA-approved germicide to clean any fixed equipment or surfaces contacted by the patient's body fluids.

5. **Prepare yourself for service.**
   - Wash thoroughly, paying attention to the areas under your fingernails. Remember that contaminants can collect there and become a source of infection not only to you but also to the persons whom you touch.
   - Change soiled clothes. Clean contaminated clothing as soon as possible, especially if you were exposed to someone with a communicable disease. It is a good policy to bring a spare uniform to work, and each EMS agency should have a washer and dryer. It is against OSHA regulations for blood- or body fluid-soiled clothes to be taken home to be washed.

6. **Replace expendable items.** Exchange them with items from the unit's storeroom.

7. **Replace or refill oxygen cylinders.** Do this in accordance with your service's procedures.

8. **Replace patient-care equipment.**

9. **Carry out post-operation vehicle maintenance procedures as required.** If you find something wrong with the vehicle, correct the problem or make someone in authority aware of it.

10. **Clean the vehicle.** A clean exterior lends a professional appearance to an ambulance. Check for broken lights, glass and body damage, door operation, and other parts that may need repair or replacement.

11. **Complete your paperwork.** Complete any unfinished report forms as soon as possible, and report the unit ready for service.

AIR RESCUE

In some circumstances, it is best for a patient to be transported by an air rescue helicopter (Figure 38-6) or fixed-wing aircraft. The following are some considerations for use of this kind of transport. Since geographic and other circumstances, as well as the availability of such transport, will vary in different localities, follow your local protocols.

CORE CONCEPT
When and how to use air rescue

When to Call for Air Rescue

Air rescue may be required for any of the following reasons:

- **Operational reasons.** Operational reasons for air rescue include: (1) to speed transport to a distant trauma center or other special facility, (2) when extrication of a high-priority patient is prolonged and air rescue can speed transport, or (3) when a patient must be rescued from a remote location that can only be reached by helicopter. Follow your local protocols.

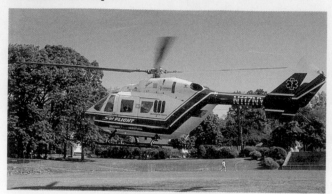

FIGURE 38-7 Helicopter landing zone.

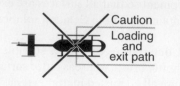

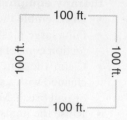

- **Medical reasons.** Medical reasons for air rescue primarily affect patients who are high priority for rapid transport; for example, a patient in shock, a patient with a Glasgow Coma Scale total of less than 10, a patient who has a head injury with altered mental status, a patient with chest trauma and respiratory distress, a patient with penetrating injuries to the body cavity, a patient with an amputation proximal to the hand or foot, a patient with extensive burns, or a patient with a serious mechanism of injury.

Patients with certain medical conditions may also be flown by helicopter. Cardiac patients requiring catheterization or surgery, stroke patients, and those patients requiring hyperbaric oxygen treatment (e.g., after carbon monoxide poisoning) are examples of medical patients who may also be flown by air. In many cases, you will transport these patients to your local hospital for stabilization and the helicopter will transfer the patient from one hospital to another. Cardiac-arrest patients are usually not transported by air rescue unless they are hypothermic. Follow your local protocols.

How to Call for Air Rescue

In some areas, rescue may be called for by any law enforcement, fire, or EMS command officer at the scene of an incident. In addition, as an EMT, you may radio dispatch for advice if you think such a service is needed. When calling an air rescue service, give your name and call-back number, your agency name, the nature of the situation, the exact location including crossroads and major landmarks, and the exact location of a safe landing zone. Follow your local protocols.

How to Set Up a Landing Zone

A helicopter requires a landing zone, or LZ, approximately 100-by-100 feet (approximately 30 large steps on each side) on ground that has a slope of less than 8 degrees. The landing zone and approach/departure path should be clear of wires, towers, vehicles, people, and loose objects (Figure 38-7). The landing zone should be marked with one flare in an upwind position. During night operations, *never* shine a light into the pilot's eyes during landing or takeoff or while the aircraft is running on the ground. Keep emergency red lights on.

Describe the landing zone to the air rescue service:

- **Terrain.** "The landing zone is located on top of a hill." "The landing zone is located in a valley."

- **Major landmarks.** "There is a river (major highway, factory, water tower) to the north (or other direction) of the landing zone."

- **Estimated distance to nearest town.** "The landing zone is approximately 12 miles west of Centerville."

- **Other pertinent information.** "There are wires on the east side of the landing zone." "There is a deep ditch to the west." "Winds are out of the north-northeast at about 10 mph."

How to Approach a Helicopter

Do not approach a helicopter unless escorted by the flight personnel. Allow the helicopter crew to direct the loading on-board of the patient. Stay clear of the tail rotor at all times. Keep all traffic and vehicles 100 feet or more distant from the helicopter. Do not smoke within 200 feet of the aircraft. Be aware of the danger areas around helicopters, as shown in Scan 38-6. *Never* walk around the tail rotor area.

SCAN 38-6 Danger Areas around Helicopters

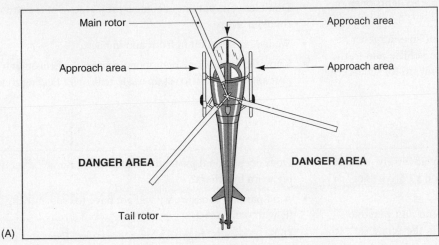

(A)

A. The area around the tail rotor is extremely dangerous. A spinning rotor cannot be seen.

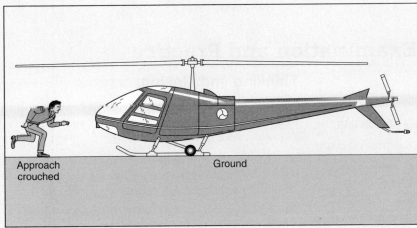

(B)

B. A sudden gust of wind can cause the main rotor of a helicopter to dip to a point as close as 4 feet from the ground. Always approach a helicopter in a crouch when the rotor is moving.

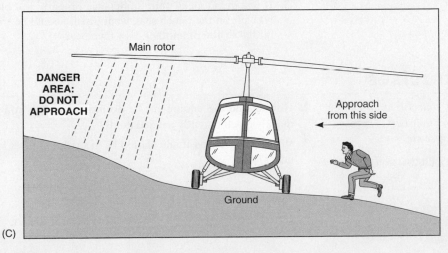

(C)

C. Approach the aircraft from the downhill side when a helicopter is parked on a hillside.

Key Facts and Concepts

- Inspect the vehicle to assure that it is complete and that critical items can be easily located.

- A "hot" response means using lights and siren. Hot responses involve high risk. A "cold" response means no lights or siren. Cold responses decrease risk.

- The laws in most states allow the driver of an emergency vehicle running "hot" to break some of the vehicle and traffic laws. However, it must be done with due regard for the safety of others.

- Pay attention! Do not text, make cell phone calls, drink beverages, or be in any way distracted while driving.

- Secure all gear. It can become a projectile in a crash!

- Don't let your patient become a projectile. Use the stretcher shoulder straps.

- Wear your seat belt in front and in back.

- Know the medical and operational reasons for helicopter transport and know how to set up a safe helicopter landing zone.

Key Decisions

- Does this patient have a true emergency adversely affected by time? How will this affect my decision to drive "hot" or "cold" to the hospital?

- How can I park to best protect the scene and personnel? Can I create a safe zone from traffic? Is the scene safe to enter?

- Does my personal protective equipment "match" what is being worn by others?

- Am I parking to assure we will not have to cross moving traffic with patients?

- Helicopters are "high risk" transportation. Does this patient really need one?

Preparation for Your Examination and Practice

Short Answer

1. List the five phases of an ambulance call.

2. List activities you perform at the beginning of each shift.

3. List three ways to prevent collisions when driving an emergency vehicle.

4. What types of stretcher straps are essential to restrain a patient and prevent him from becoming a projectile in a collision?

5. Describe the steps that should be followed when air rescue is required.

Thinking and Linking

Think back to Chapter 1, "Introduction to Emergency Medical Services and the Health Care System," where you read about the roles and responsibilities of the EMT.

1. How do your daily roles and responsibilities as an EMT as described in Chapter 1 relate to the various phases of an ambulance call as described in this chapter?

Think back to Chapter 2, "The Well-Being of the EMT."

2. If you didn't clean your ambulance properly and blood was left on the bench seat, what disease could be transmitted to you or another crew member?

Critical Thinking Exercises

Organizing your equipment is a key part of your job as an EMT. The purpose of this exercise will be to consider how best to manage the equipment you will need at the emergency scene.

1. What equipment should you include in a kit that you carry to the scene?

2. How should the equipment be positioned so that you can quickly reach urgently needed items?

3. What special items, if any, should be in the kit to meet local needs?

You receive a Priority 1 call. "Ambulance 19, respond to 1901 Greentop Road for a report of a cardiac arrest." You acknowledge, get into the ambulance, and buckle up. Your partner does the same and turns on the red lights and siren. The dispatcher tells you that there is no additional information from the caller, and you will be the first unit to arrive. You know it will be a long response because the call is at the far end of your district, and you feel pressured to hurry. As you approach an intersection, your partner changes the siren from wail to yelp and goes through without slowing down. "That light was red," you tell him. He doesn't respond and keeps driving at the same speed. When he starts to weave through traffic, you suggest an alternative route to avoid the approaching rush-hour congestion.

Street Scene Questions

1. When operating an ambulance using the red lights and siren, what precautions do you need to take?
2. How can speed affect the safety of ambulance operation?
3. What driving techniques might be used to make driving to this scene safer?

All of a sudden, a car comes out of a driveway and into your path. Your partner hits the brakes, performs an evasive move, and just misses the other vehicle. You notice that a box of tissues and a stethoscope landed on the floor in the patient compartment. "What would have happened if I had been back there with a patient?" you ask. Your partner finally realizes he is driving too fast and slows down. At the next intersection, he slows down even more and makes sure that traffic has come to a stop before going through. During the rest of the response, you focus on preparing for your arrival on the scene.

You have decided to load all your equipment on the stretcher and wheel it to the front door as soon as the ambulance is parked. As you pull up to the scene, your partner finds a good spot to park where the ambulance will not create a hazard. He leaves the warning lights on for visibility.

Street Scene Questions

4. What should you do first for patient care?
5. What information should you provide to the dispatcher?

Your patient is in his bedroom, sitting on his bed, and greets you as you approach. You immediately ask him why EMS was called. "My wife called because I passed out. It's happened before, but my doctor isn't sure what causes it." Your partner radios dispatch that the patient is alert and that another unit is not needed. You assess the patient, obtain a patient history, and get a set of vital signs. The patient is alert and oriented, his pulse is 82 with a blood pressure of 130/82, respirations are 20, and skin is unremarkable. The patient says that he takes a medication because his cholesterol is "way up there." The patient's wife reports that he was sitting in a chair and slumped over. She did not see any seizure activity. He did not respond to verbal stimulus, so she moved him to the floor. He regained consciousness within 2 minutes.

The patient consents to transport to the hospital for further evaluation. You move him by stair chair from the bedroom to the stretcher. You place the patient on the stretcher and fasten all the safety straps. You place the stretcher into the ambulance compartment and, after it is in the bracket, you recheck to make sure it is properly secured. Your partner puts the stair chair away in its compartment and asks what the priority is to the hospital. "Priority 2," you answer. "Based on the assessment, there is no need to use the red light and siren."

39

Hazardous Materials, Multiple-Casualty Incidents, and Incident Management

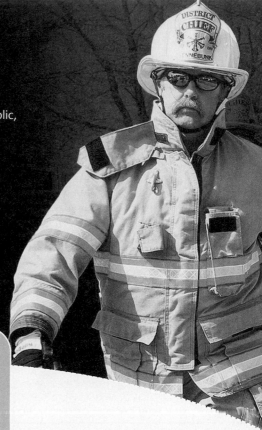

STANDARD
EMS Operations (Incident Management; Multiple-Casualty Incidents; Hazardous Materials)

COMPETENCY
Applies knowledge of operational roles and responsibilities to ensure patient, public, and personnel safety.

CORE CONCEPTS
— How to identify and take appropriate action in a hazardous materials incident
— How to identify a multiple-casualty incident
— The Incident Command System
— Triage
— Transportation and staging logistics
— Psychological aspects of multiple-casualty incidents

EXPLORE Resource**C**entral

To access Resource Central, follow directions on the Student Access Card provided with this text. If there is no card, go to **www.bradybooks.com** and follow the Resource Central link to Buy Access from there. Under Media Resources, you will find:

▶ **Mass Casualty Information from the CDC**
Learn to identify situations that may result in mass casualties, what happens to patients involved in blast injuries, and what you can do to manage the stress from a mass casualty incident.

▶ **Information about Resources for Emergency Workers**
Discover resources that may benefit an EMT when you encounter different types of stressful situations and learn what you can do to maintain your own health.

▶ **Information about Children during Disasters**
View a video on dealing with children in disaster situations; identify different types of disasters and why children are more vulnerable.

OBJECTIVES

After reading this chapter you should be able to:

39.1 Define key terms introduced in this chapter.

39.2 Anticipate situations in which hazardous materials may be involved. (pp. 1007–1008)

39.3 Describe the roles in hazardous materials response of providers trained at each of the four levels of hazardous materials training specified by OSHA. (pp. 1008–1009)

KEY TERMS

ou have already learned how to deal with many situations in which an individual patient needs emergency care. However, you also need to know what to do if you are called to the scene of an explosion, an airline crash, a multiple vehicle pile-up, an earthquake, or some other situation in which there may be many known or potential patients. Although you are not trained to deal with all the complexities of such emergencies, you must be able to recognize them and call for the appropriate assistance. This chapter offers the essentials that every EMT should know about special operations involving multiple patients and/or hazardous materials.

HAZARDOUS MATERIALS

Hazardous materials (hazmats) are everywhere, and EMS frequently responds to incidents involving them. Because many incidents begin as routine EMS calls, it will be up to you to recognize a hazmat early, be familiar with your local plan for management of a hazardous materials incident, and understand your role in such an incident.

According to the U.S. Department of Transportation (DOT), a ***hazardous material*** is "any substance or material in a form which poses an unreasonable risk to health, safety, and property when transported in commerce." One of the undesirable aspects of our modern

hazardous material
any substance or material in a form which poses an unreasonable risk to health, safety, and property when transported in commerce.

Table 39-1 Examples of Hazardous Materials

MATERIAL	POSSIBLE HAZARD
Benzene (benzol)	Toxic vapors; can be absorbed through the skin; destroys bone marrow
Benzoyl peroxide	Fire and explosion
Carbon tetrachloride	Damages internal organs
Cyclohexane	Explosive; eye and throat irritant
Diethyl ether	Flammable and can be explosive; irritant to eyes and respiratory tract; can cause drowsiness or unconsciousness
Ethyl acetate	Irritates eyes and respiratory tract
Ethylene chloride	Damages eyes
Ethylene dichloride	Strong irritant
Heptane	Respiratory irritant
Hydrochloric acid	Respiratory irritant; exposure to high concentration of vapors can produce pulmonary edema; can damage skin and eyes
Hydrogen cyanide	Highly flammable; toxic through inhalation or absorption
Methyl isobutyl ketone	Irritates eyes and mucous membranes
Nitric acid	Produces a toxic gas (nitrogen dioxide); skin irritant; can cause self-ignition of cellulose products (e.g., sawdust)
Organochloride (Chlordane, DDT, Dieldrin, Lindane, Methoxyclor)	Irritates eyes and skin; fumes and smoke toxic
Perchloroethylene	Toxic if inhaled or swallowed
Silicon tetrachloride	Water-reactive to form toxic hydrogen chloride fumes
Tetrahydrofuran (THF)	Damages eyes and mucous membranes
Toluol (toluene)	Toxic vapors; can cause organ damage
Vinyl chloride	Flammable and explosive; listed as a carcinogen

CORE CONCEPT

How to identify and take appropriate action in a hazardous materials incident

world is the growing number of such materials (Table 39-1). Hazardous materials are used for the manufacture of products and also can be the waste products of manufacturing. Even though safety procedures have been established and are followed for the most part, accidents involving hazardous materials do occur. Hazardous materials incidents are especially likely to take place at factories; along railroads; and on local, state, and federal highways.

As an EMT, you will be highly skilled in emergency care. However, without specialized training, you are still a layperson when it comes to hazardous materials. Special training is required to understand hazmats, to work at the scene of incidents involving these materials, and to render the scene safe. You cannot judge the state of a container or the probability of explosion without the benefit of such training. Do not assume that you can use safety equipment unless you are trained in the care, field testing, and use of the equipment. With hazmat incidents, you may be able to do nothing more than stay a safe distance away from the scene until expert help arrives.

Training Required by Law

Two federal agencies—the Occupational Safety and Health Administration (OSHA) and the Environmental Protection Agency (EPA)—have developed regulations to deal with the increasing frequency of hazmat emergencies. These regulations are meant to enhance the knowledge, skills, and safety of emergency response personnel, as well as to bring about a more effective response to hazmat emergencies. The regulations are described in the OSHA publication "29 CFR 1910.120—Hazardous Waste Operations and Emergency Response Standard."

According to the regulations, employers are responsible for determining, providing, and documenting the appropriate level of training for each employee. Training is required for "all employees who participate, or who are expected to participate, in emergency response to hazardous substance accidents."

The regulations identify four levels of training:

- **First Responder Awareness.** Rescuers at this level are likely to witness or discover a hazardous substance release. They are trained only to recognize the problem and initiate a response from the proper organizations. There are no minimum training hours required.

- **First Responder Operations.** This level of training is for those who initially respond to releases or potential releases of hazardous materials in order to protect people, property, and the environment. They stay at a safe distance, keep the incident from spreading, and protect others from any exposures. A minimum of 8 hours of training is required.

- **Hazardous Materials Technician.** This level is for rescuers who actually plug, patch, or stop the release of a hazardous material. A minimum of 24 hours of training is required.

- **Hazardous Materials Specialist.** This level of rescuer is expected to have advanced knowledge and skills and to command and support activities at the incident site. A minimum of 24 hours of additional training is required.

Most of the training levels outlined by OSHA have a fire-service focus. EMS responders should be trained to the awareness level and perhaps the operations level but in different skills. Responding to this difference, the National Fire Protection Association has published Standard #473, which deals with competencies for EMS personnel at hazardous materials incidents.

Regardless of agency affiliation, as an EMT you play an important role. You are usually among the first on the scene for all types of hazmat calls. Your initial decisions and actions lay crucial groundwork for the remainder of the incident.

Responsibilities of the EMT

Your responsibilities as an EMT at a hazardous materials incident include recognizing that a hazardous materials incident exists, controlling the scene, and identifying the substance.

Recognize a Hazmat Incident

Whether hazmat incidents are very obvious or very subtle, you must quickly recognize one for what it is. It helps to be aware of the locations where hazmats are likely. They include highway incidents involving common carriers, trucking terminals, chemical plants or places where chemicals are used, delivery trucks, agriculture and garden centers, railway incidents, and laboratories.

Every community has chemical hazards. Identification starts with awareness and knowledge of what exists in the community. Spend some time with local police and fire agencies, and learn about or develop preincident plans for common hazardous materials.

When you arrive at a potential incident as an EMT, you must restrain your natural impulse to take action. Never assume the scene is safe. After the initial patients, EMTs are the most likely to become injured or killed because they tend to quickly react. Therefore, assess the situation first. Take a Command position and stay a safe distance from the site before you take action. Once a hazmat is recognized, only those personnel trained to the technician level and equipped with the proper personal protective equipment should enter the immediate site. All patients leaving the site of the incident should be considered contaminated until proven otherwise.

Control the Scene

Your primary concerns at the scene of a hazardous materials incident are your safety and the safety of your crew, the patient, and the public. If you arrive first at the scene of a hazardous materials incident, establish a "danger zone" and a "safe zone." Keep all people out of the danger zone, and try to convince them to leave the immediate area. Stay in the safe zone until expert help arrives and makes other areas safe to enter.

The safe zone should be on the same level as, and upwind from, the hazardous materials incident site. Avoid being downhill in case there are flowing liquids or gases that are burning or otherwise unsafe. Avoid low-lying areas in case fumes are escaping and hanging close to the ground. Avoid placing yourself higher than the accident scene so that you will not be in the path of escaping gases or heated air. Also be aware that a sewer system can rapidly spread hazardous materials over a large area.

Call for the help that you will need. The support services required at the scene of a hazardous materials incident may include fire services, special rescue personnel, local or state hazardous materials experts, and law enforcement personnel for crowd control. If the incident has taken place at an industrial site or along a railway, the company experts in hazardous materials need to be notified. Much of this can be done by a single call to your dispatcher.

Implement your agency's Incident Management System. Establish and remain in Command until you are relieved by someone higher in the chain of command.

The situation must be prevented from becoming worse. Establish a perimeter, evacuate people if necessary, and direct bystanders to a safe area. It cannot be overemphasized that EMTs should not risk personal safety by initiating rescue attempts.

While help is on the way, establish control zones. Isolate the *hot zone* (the area of contamination or the area of danger). Establish a decontamination corridor (area where patients will be decontaminated) in the *warm zone*, an area immediately adjacent to the hot zone. Equipment and other emergency rescuers should be staged in the next adjacent area— the *cold zone*. Station yourself in the cold zone.

Identify the Substance

As a responding EMT, you may be the first to recognize that a hazardous materials situation exists. For example, you may answer a call to a business where four employees are ill after being in the warehouse. When there are multiple medical patients, "think hazmat."

You must make an attempt to identify the hazardous material and assess the severity of the situation. Until that is done, it will be difficult to determine the risk to the public, rescuers, patients, and the environment. You must try to find out what the substance is and what its properties and dangers might be; whether or not there is imminent danger of the contamination spreading; what you can hear, see, and smell; how many patients are involved; and if there is any danger of secondary contamination from the patients. (Secondary contamination occurs when a contaminated person makes contact with someone who previously was "clean.")

Because it is not safe to approach the scene, you must obtain information indirectly or from a distance. Ways of obtaining information safely may include the following:

- **Use binoculars to look for identifying signs, labels, or placards from a safe distance** (Figure 39-1). In many cases, there will be a colored placard (Figure 39-2) on the storage container, vehicle, tank, or railroad car.

NOTE: *Do not approach the scene to obtain this information.*

hot zone
area immediately surrounding a hazmat incident; extends far enough to prevent adverse effects outside the zone.

warm zone
area where personnel and equipment decontamination and hot zone support take place; it includes control points for the access corridor and thus assists in reducing the spread of contamination.

cold zone
area where the Incident Command post and support functions are located.

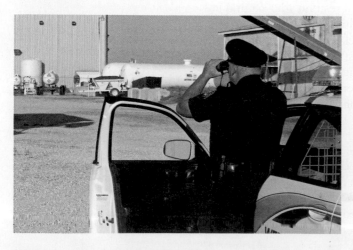

FIGURE 39-1 Binoculars will allow a visual inspection of the hot zone from a safe distance.

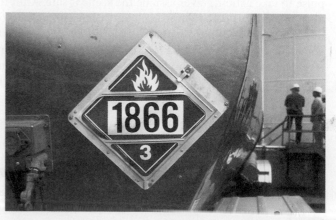

FIGURE 39-2 Vehicles carrying hazardous materials are required to display placards that communicate the nature of their cargo.

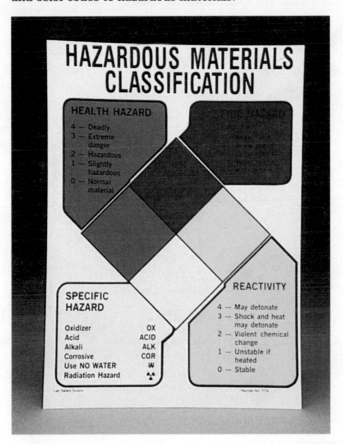

- **Search for placards.** A commonly used placarding system is the National Fire Protection Association (NFPA) 704 System. It uses numerical and color coding to show the type and degree of health hazard, fire hazard, reactivity, and specific hazard contained within a fixed facility (Figure 39-3).

  NOTE: *Studies by the Office of Technology Assessment have shown that some states report 25 to 50 percent of identification placards are incorrect. These same studies indicate that many shipping documents also are inaccurate or incomplete.*

- **Look for labels.** The U.S. Department of Transportation requires that packages, storage containers, and vehicles containing hazardous materials bear labels or placards with markings that identify the nature of the contents (Figure 39-4). Diamond-shaped placards used in the transportation of dangerous goods not only show the hazard class, such as "explosives," "flammable gas," "poison," or other, they also bear a division number which provides more specific information on the material, as shown in Table 39-2. In addition, a four-digit identification number may appear on the placard itself or on a panel near the placard. Older placards are usually orange and have an identification number preceded by the letters UN or UA. Your dispatcher may have access to the name of the material through this identification number.

- **Check invoices, bills of lading (trucks), and shipping manifests (trains).** If you can safely obtain them, these documents will identify the exact substance being transported, the exact quantity, its place of origin, and its destination.

- **Review material safety data sheets (MSDS).** MSDS must be provided on hazardous materials by all manufacturers. These sheets must be maintained at the work site by the employer and available to all employees on the grounds that employees working with hazardous materials have a right to know about them. If you can safely obtain these sheets,

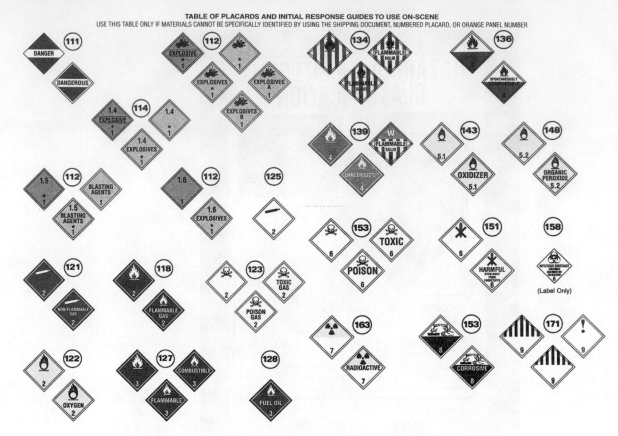

TABLE OF PLACARDS AND INITIAL RESPONSE GUIDES TO USE ON-SCENE
USE THIS TABLE ONLY IF MATERIALS CANNOT BE SPECIFICALLY IDENTIFIED BY USING THE SHIPPING DOCUMENT, NUMBERED PLACARD, OR ORANGE PANEL NUMBER

they generally name the substance, its physical properties, fire and explosion hazard information, health hazard information, and emergency first aid treatment.

- **Interview workers or others leaving the hot zone.** These people may be good sources of information about the substance involved. Vehicle drivers, plant and railroad personnel, and perhaps even bystanders may be able to tell you the name of the hazardous material. Workers at a manufacturing site often understand very well what chemicals are used, the processes, and their reactions. However, note that workers may identify a substance by its trade name and not realize that it is a mixture of many chemicals.

EMTs are only expected to understand some of the common substance-identifying systems available and to make a preliminary identification based on this information. On the basis of this preliminary information, you can obtain advice about what initial actions should be taken at the scene from your dispatcher, a hazardous materials expert, or one of the following sources:

FIGURE 39-5 Have the latest edition of the *Emergency Response Guidebook* in your vehicle at all times.

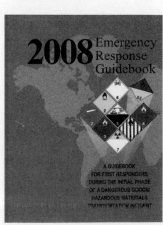

- **Emergency Response Guidebook** (ERG2008) (Figure 39-5). This essential booklet, published by the U.S. Department of Transportation, Transport Canada, and the Secretariat of Communications and Transportation of Mexico, provides the names of chemicals and concise but thorough descriptions of the actions that should be taken in case of a hazmat emergency. Be sure to have the latest edition in your vehicle at all times.

- **Chemical Transportation Emergency Center (CHEMTREC).** This group has been established in Washington, DC, as a service of the Chemical Manufacturers Association. They can provide your dispatcher or you with information about the hazardous material through a 24-hour toll-free telephone number for the United States and Canada, which is 800-424-9300. For calls originating elsewhere and for collect calls, the number is 703-527-3887. When you call, keep the line open so that changes at the scene can be reported to CHEMTREC and the center can confirm that they have contacted the shipper or manufacturer. CHEMTREC will be able to direct you as to your initial course of action

Table 39-2 Hazard Classification System

CLASS 1—EXPLOSIVES

Division 1.1	Explosives with a mass explosion hazard
Division 1.2	Explosives with a projection hazard
Division 1.3	Explosives with predominantly a fire hazard
Division 1.4	Explosives with no significant blast hazard
Division 1.5	Very insensitive explosives; blasting agents
Division 1.6	Extremely insensitive detonating articles

CLASS 2—GASES

Division 2.1	Flammable gases
Division 2.2	Nonflammable, nontoxic, compressed gases
Division 2.3	Gases toxic by inhalation
Division 2.4	Corrosive gases

CLASS 3—FLAMMABLE LIQUIDS AND COMBUSTIBLE LIQUIDS

CLASS 4—FLAMMABLE SOLIDS; SPONTANEOUSLY COMBUSTIBLE MATERIALS; AND DANGEROUS-WHEN-WET MATERIALS

Division 4.1	Flammable solids
Division 4.2	Spontaneously combustible materials
Division 4.3	Dangerous-when-wet materials

CLASS 5—OXIDIZERS AND ORGANIC PEROXIDES

Division 5.1	Oxidizers
Division 5.2	Organic peroxides

CLASS 6—TOXIC MATERIALS AND INFECTIOUS SUBSTANCES

Division 6.1	Toxic materials
Division 6.2	Infectious substances

CLASS 7—RADIOACTIVE MATERIALS

CLASS 8—CORROSIVE MATERIALS

CLASS 9—MISCELLANEOUS DANGEROUS GOODS

Division 9.1	Miscellaneous dangerous goods
Division 9.2	Environmentally hazardous substances
Division 9.3	Dangerous wastes

- **CHEM-TEL, Inc.** This emergency response communication service can be reached 24 hours a day at 800-255-3924 in the United States and Canada. For calls originating elsewhere or collect calls, use 813-979-0626.

- **A current list of state and federal radiation authorities.** These organizations provide information and technical assistance on handling incidents involving radioactive materials. The list is maintained by both CHEMTREC and CHEM-TEL, Inc.

- **Regional poison control centers.** This source is often overlooked during a hazardous materials situation. Using their reference and medical resources, they can provide essential guidance in the decontamination and treatment of patients affected by hazardous materials.

When you call one of the previously named sources for advice, do the following:

1. Give your name, call-back number, e-mail address, and FAX number.
2. Explain the nature and location of the problem.
3. Report the identification number(s) of the material(s) involved, if there is a safe way for you to obtain this information.
4. Give the name of the carrier, shipper, manufacturer, consignee, and point of origin.
5. Describe the container type and size.
6. Report if the container is on rail car, truck, open storage, or housed storage.
7. Estimate the quantity of material transported and released.
8. Report local conditions (e.g., the weather, terrain, and proximity to schools or hospitals).
9. Report injuries and exposures.
10. Report local emergency services that have been notified.
11. Keep lines of communication open at all times.

NOTE: *Do not take hasty action because you think you have identified the nature of the substance. Seek and follow expert advice. Do only what you have been trained to do.*

If there is no identification number and no one knows what is being carried, you may have no other choice but to wait for experts to arrive at the scene. When a hazmat team arrives, they will identify and deal with unknown substances, using the necessary computer and textbook resources.

Establish a Treatment Area

All EMS personnel and equipment must be staged in the cold zone. EMS personnel have two responsibilities at a hazmat incident: to monitor and rehabilitate the hazmat team members and to take care of the injured.

Rehabilitation Operations

In order to safely enter the hot zone, the hazmat team members must wear chemical-protective clothing and breathing apparatus that both slows heat loss and prevents heat stress. Team members must be carefully monitored prior to, during, and after emergency operations. This is done to make sure that their condition does not deteriorate to a point where safety or the integrity of the operation is jeopardized. To address this need, you should establish an area of operations called rehabilitation (rehab). Although the rehab area supervisor may not be an EMS provider, all rehab operations must include EMTs or advanced-level EMTs.

The characteristics of the rehab area must include the following:

- Located in the cold zone
- Protected from weather (shielded from rain or snow, a warm area in a cold environment, a cool area in a warm environment)
- Large enough to accommodate multiple rescue crews
- Easily accessible to EMS units
- Free from exhaust fumes
- Allows for rapid reentry into the emergency operation

While suiting up in chemical-protective equipment, hazmat team members should have their baseline vital signs taken. When the hazmat team members show signs of fatigue or when they have had 45 minutes of work time, they are sent to rehab. As soon as possible after exit from the hot zone, reassess their vital signs. If a member's heart rate exceeds 110 beats per minute, take an oral temperature. If a member's temperature exceeds 100.6°F, the rescuer must stay in rehab until his pulse slows and temperature returns to normal. Always follow your local protocols and consult medical direction. All preentry and exit vitals should be tracked on a flow sheet.

In addition to medical monitoring, rehab should be set up for prehydration and hydration, rest, and in some cases nourishment of hazmat team members. Proper hydration is an important element in preventing heat stress and promoting optimal physical performance. Heat injury is usually caused by imbalances of water and electrolytes during periods of high heat stress and physical exertion. During physical exertion, members should consume at least 1 quart of water per hour. For short-duration emergency operations, electrolyte sport drinks usually are not necessary. However, if they are used they should be diluted to half strength. Coffee and caffeinated beverages should be avoided because they promote dehydration.

When incidents will be of extended duration, some type of nourishment may be provided in rehab. Foods low in salt and saturated fats are ideal. Bananas, apples, oranges, and other fruits are excellent for fast nourishment. In cold environments, soups and stews are more easily eaten and digested than sandwiches.

Care of Injured and Contaminated Patients

Hazardous materials or terrorist incidents (see Chapter 41, "EMS Response to Terrorism") involve civilians and/or EMRs. Prompt, safe, and effective decontamination procedures are essential to protect against, or reduce the effects of, exposure to both patients and EMRs. Decontamination is performed to protect citizens, personnel, equipment, and the environment from the harmful effects of the contaminants.

The National Fire Protection Association (NFPA) defines **decontamination** as a chemical and/or physical process that reduces or prevents the spread of contamination from persons or equipment. According to the Occupational Safety and Health Administration (OSHA), decontamination is the removal of hazardous substances from employees and their equipment to the extent necessary to preclude foreseeable health effects.

EMTs must work with Incident Command and hazmat team members to determine the most appropriate course of action. The decision to stay at the scene and decontaminate or to begin evacuation must be made after careful consultation with CHEMTREC, the poison control center, and other reference sources.

In the decontamination (decon) corridor in the warm zone, the hazmat team will decontaminate hazmat team members and any patients rescued. EMS is responsible for setting up the medical treatment area in the cold zone to receive decontaminated patients. Unless EMS personnel are trained to the hazmat technician level, they must remain in the cold zone.

The field decon process is designed to remove contaminants and deliver a relatively "clean" patient to EMS personnel for care and transportation (Figure 39-6). However, there is a chance of secondary contamination from patients to EMS personnel. It is important that EMS personnel work closely with the decon officer and consult with medical direction on both treatment and appropriate protection during transportation.

The following points are important when treating and transporting hazmat patients:

- Field-decontaminated patients are not completely "clean." Chemicals that pose a risk of secondary contamination to rescuers sometimes settle in hard-to-clean areas of the body. These areas are typically the scalp/hair, groin, buttocks, between fingers and toes, and the armpits.

- Personal protective equipment or clothing (PPE/PPC) is needed to prevent secondary contamination of rescuers. EMS personnel need to wear PPE such as Tyvek coveralls and booties to prevent contamination and exposure. They may also need to wear a double layer of gloves. Often nitrile or neoprene is best, because these are more resistant to chemicals than standard latex or vinyl gloves. Consult with the decon officer to determine if your PPE is suitable or if they have more appropriate PPE.

- Protect vehicles from contamination. In the decon process, patients are washed and are usually dripping wet. Since they cannot be completely decontaminated in the field, some of their water runoff could contaminate an emergency vehicle. To prevent this, the water runoff must be contained by either placing the patient in a disposable decontamination pool or covering the inside of an ambulance with plastic.

- Consider used equipment as disposable. When an item such as a spine board, splint, blood-pressure cuff, or stethoscope is used, it may not be able to be decontaminated and may require disposal.

decontamination
a chemical and/or physical process that reduces or prevents the spread of contamination from persons or equipment; the removal of hazardous substances from employees and their equipment to the extent necessary to preclude foreseeable health effects.

FIGURE 39-6 An example of a field decontamination process.

9-Station Decontamination Procedure

STEPS

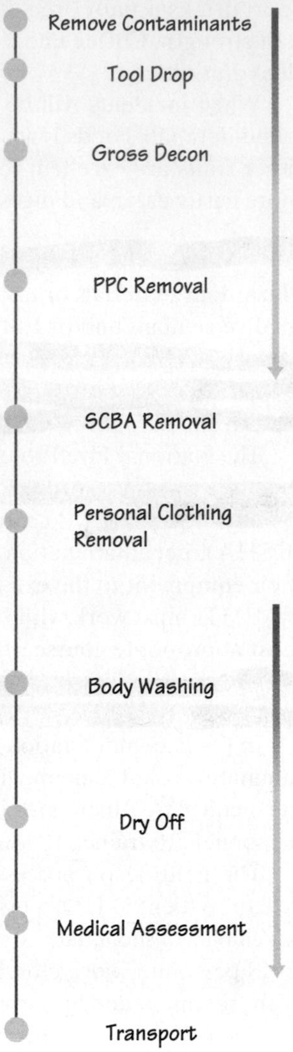

Station 1. Rescuers enter decon areas and mechanically remove contaminants from victims. Tools are dropped in tool drop area. Rescuers are in SCBA and protective clothing. **Proceed to Station 2.**

Station 2. *Gross Decontamination*: Victims and rescue personnel are showered and/or scrubbed by decon personnel. Dilution is conducted inside diked area. Victims may be transported directly to Station 6. **Proceed to Station 6.**

Station 3. *Protective Clothing Removal*: Rescuers remove protective clothing, clothing is isolated and labeled for later disposal. Clothing is placed on contaminated side. **Proceed to Station 4.**

Station 4. *SCBA Removal*: Rescue personnel remove and isolate their SCBA. If re-entry is necessary, personnel don new SCBA from non-contaminated side. **Proceed to Station 5.**

Station 5. *Personal Clothing Removal*: All clothing and personal items are removed. Victims who have not been undressed are undressed here. All clothing and personal items are isolated in plastic bags and labeled for later disposal. **Proceed to Station 6.**

Station 6. *Body Washing*: Full body washing is performed using soft scrub brushes or sponges and soap or mild detergent. Cleaning tools are bagged for later disposal. **Proceed to Station 7.**

Station 7. *Dry Off*: Towels and sheets are used to dry off. Rescuers and victims are dressed in clean clothes. Towels/ sheets are bagged for later disposal. **Proceed to Station 8.**

Station 8. *Medical Assessment*: Rapid patient assessment is conducted by rescuers. Necessary stabilization procedures are accomplished. **Proceed to Station 9.**

Station 9. *Transport*: Transfer of patient to hospital for medical attention or to recovery areas for rest and observation.

Station flow (right column):
- Remove Contaminants
- Tool Drop
- Gross Decon
- PPC Removal
- SCBA Removal
- Personal Clothing Removal
- Body Washing
- Dry Off
- Medical Assessment
- Transport

- Structural firefighting clothing is not designed or recommended for use when working in hazardous materials environments. If personnel in firefighting gear encounter a hazardous chemical environment, they should take precautions to minimize the chance of contamination. A team in bunker gear can stand back and apply a fog stream to contaminated persons.

When treating a contaminated patient is unavoidable, it is crucial to identify the hazardous material. Follow the treatment instructions given in the *Emergency Response Guidebook* or by the poison control center.

Four types of patients are likely to be encountered by EMTs:

- Uninjured and not contaminated
- Injured and not contaminated
- Uninjured and contaminated
- Injured and contaminated

If you are confronted with contaminated patients prior to the arrival of the hazmat team, do the following.

1. Take precautions appropriate to the substance as listed in the *Emergency Response Guidebook*. This usually means isolation from the substance. Be sure to use personal protective equipment similar to what you would use for splash protection from blood-borne pathogens.

2. Follow the first aid measures listed in the *Emergency Response Guidebook*.

3. Manage the patient's critical needs. Do not forget to manage the ABCs.

4. If treatment calls for irrigation with water, remember that water only dilutes most substances. It does not neutralize them. Cut the patient's clothing off and irrigate the patient's body with large amounts of water. Try to contain the runoff. If possible, use tepid or warm water to prevent hypothermia. Try to avoid flushing contaminants directly into open wounds. Pay particular attention to cleaning areas such as dense body hair, ear canals, navel, fingernails, crotch, armpits, and so on. Use disposable equipment whenever possible. Discard it later.

5. After treating the patient, decontaminate yourself. Your clothing may need disposal.

Remember that the severity of any poisoning depends on the substance, route of entry, dosage, and duration of contact. Immediate emergency care measures as listed in the *Emergency Response Guidebook* may decrease the severity of the poisoning and save lives. Whenever possible, the entire decontamination process should be carried out by qualified personnel from the hazmat team before the EMT touches the patient.

Contaminated personnel (injured or not) pose a secondary contamination risk and should be decontaminated prior to leaving the scene. If scene decontamination is not performed, patients must be decontaminated at an appropriate hospital decon site before they enter the emergency department.

Phases of Decontamination

The two major phases of decontamination are gross decontamination and secondary decontamination. (There is usually a third or tertiary decontamination phase, but it generally occurs at a medical facility and may involve such processes as sterilization or debridement.)

Gross decontamination is the removal or chemical alteration of the majority of the contaminant. It must be assumed that some residual contaminant will always remain on the host after gross decontamination. This residual contamination can cause cross-contamination. *Secondary decontamination* is the alteration or removal of most of the residual product contamination. It provides a more thorough decontamination than the gross effort. However, some contaminant may still remain attached to the host.

Mechanisms for Decontamination

There are seven common mechanisms for performing decontamination. They are:

- **Emulsification.** This is the production of a suspension of ordinarily immiscible (unmixable)/insoluble materials using an emulsifying agent such as a surfactant, soap, or detergent.

- **Chemical reaction.** This is a process that neutralizes, degrades, or otherwise chemically alters the contaminant. Normally, a chemical reaction does not ensure that all hazards have been eliminated, and reaction procedures can be both difficult and dangerous to perform. Chemical reaction is therefore not recommended for use on living tissue.

- **Disinfection.** This is a process that removes the biological (etiological) contamination hazards as the disinfectant destroys microorganisms and their toxins.

- **Dilution.** This is a process that simply reduces the concentration of the contaminant. It is most commonly used for substances that are miscible (mixable)/soluble. Huge quantities of solvent may be required to dilute even small volumes of some solute contaminants.

- **Absorption and adsorption.** This is the penetration of a liquid or gas into another substance. An example is water soaking into a sponge.

- **Removal.** This is the physical process of removing contaminants by pressure or vacuum. Most efforts involve the use of water, though solids can be removed with brushes and wipes; even air can be used.

- **Disposal.** This is the aseptic removal of a contaminated object from a host, after which the object is disposed of. (*Aseptic* means using sterile instruments and/or otherwise preventing the spread of the contaminant.)

Decontamination Procedures

The objectives of the responders assigned to decontamination are to:

- Determine the appropriate level of protective equipment based on materials and associated hazards
- Properly wear and operate in PPE
- Establish operating time log
- Set up and operate the decontamination line
- Prioritize the decontamination of patients according to a triage system
- Perform triage in PPE
- Be able to communicate while in PPE

A basic list of equipment required for decontamination is:

- Buckets
- Brushes
- Decontamination solution
- Decontamination tubs
- Dedicated water supply
- Tarps or plastic sheeting
- Containment vessel for water runoff
- Pump to transfer wastewater from decontamination tubs to a containment vessel
- A-frame ladder (to reach the top of the responder's suit)
- Appropriate-level PPE for responders performing decontamination

Decontamination for Patients Wearing PPE   Take the following steps to decontaminate a patient who is wearing PPE:

1. Rinse, starting at the head and working down.
2. Scrub the suit with a brush, starting at the head and working down. Pay special attention to heavily contaminated areas (e.g., hands, feet, front of suit).
3. Rinse again, starting at the head and working down.
4. Assist the responder in removing PPE.
5. Contain the runoff of hazardous wastewater.

Decontamination for Patients Not Wearing PPE   The decontamination of patients not wearing PPE proceeds in a different manner. As always, the first and foremost consideration is responder safety. If responders are incapacitated, they are unable to help others.

You should use a public address system to direct ambulatory patients to a decontamination line. This provides a rapid form of triage. Patients should be instructed to begin decontamination by removing their clothing. Have people remove shoes, socks, jewelry, watches, and other items that trap materials against the skin. They should also remove contact lenses as soon as possible. Double-bag their clothing for disposal or decontamination later. Valuables and identification should be bagged and may (based on hazards) be carried by the patients.

Next, the patients should receive a 2- to 5-minute water rinse. Solid or particulate contaminants should be lightly brushed off (dry decontamination) as completely as possible prior to washing (wet decontamination). Viscous liquid contaminants (including vesicants, which are blistering agents) should be blotted off prior to washing. If the material is water reactive, it must be brushed off prior to the application of water. Rinsing is done as needed to flush remaining chemicals that may react with the moisture of the skin and eyes. You should also use an appropriate decontamination solution.

Washing and rinsing should start at the head to reduce contamination on or near the nose, mouth, ears, and eyes. If the patient has removed his contact lenses, the eyes should be irrigated. Open wounds should be irrigated starting from the area nearest the body core and working outward. You may use plastic wrap to isolate the wound once it has been cleaned. Use a low-water-pressure system to avoid aggravating soft-tissue injuries and to avoid over-spray and splashing. A low-pressure system will also help prevent the creation of an aerosol out of dry product.

During decontamination, patients should be given some type of cover for modesty and protection from the elements.

Although not strictly a form of self-protection, "decon" is vital to prevent, reduce, and remove contamination for both responders and patients.

MULTIPLE-CASUALTY INCIDENTS

A *multiple-casualty incident (MCI)*—or, in some areas, a multiple-casualty situation (MCS)—is an event that places a great demand on EMS equipment and personnel resources. The number of patients required before an MCI can be declared varies in practice. Some jurisdictions will declare an MCI for as few as three patients on the grounds that practice with smaller-scale incidents will help EMTs prepare for larger ones. Other jurisdictions reserve the MCI designation for five, seven, or more patients (Figure 39-7). The most common MCI is an automobile collision with three or more patients. You will likely respond to

CORE CONCEPT ●
How to identify a multiple-casualty incident

multiple-casualty incident (MCI)
any medical or trauma incident involving multiple patients.

FIGURE 39-7 Multiple-casualty incidents may range from small to large. (A) A car crash with as few as three to five patients will be declared a multiple-casualty incident by many EMS jurisdictions. (B) In this bus crash, all passengers were triaged and 44 patients were transported to area hospitals. *(Photos A and B: ©Mark C. Ide)*

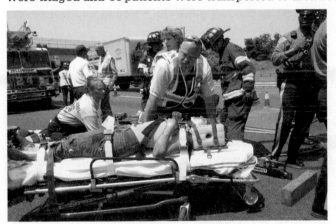

(A)

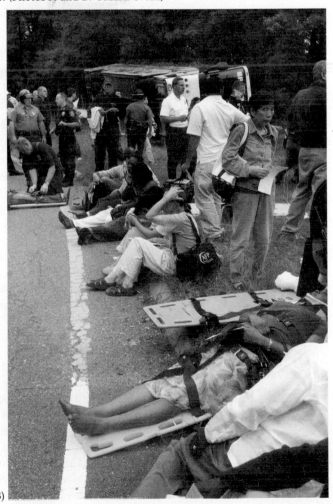

(B)

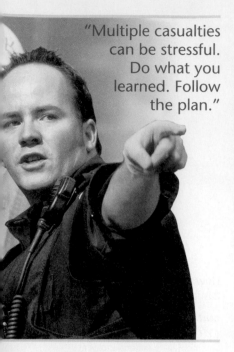

"Multiple casualties can be stressful. Do what you learned. Follow the plan."

many incidents with 3 to 15 potential patients. Incidents with large-scale casualties are rare and apt to be "once in a career" events.

The important ingredient in defining an MCI is that, for whatever reason, the EMS system's ability to respond to the situation is challenged or hampered by the situation itself. For any MCI plan to be effective, it must be flexible and expandable enough to be used from small three-patient incidents to large-scale incidents of 15 or more patients. In other words, the plan for "the big one" should be a logical extension of the same plan used to manage smaller incidents.

Multiple-Casualty-Incident Operations

Though the principles of managing small- and large-scale MCIs are generally the same, large-scale MCIs unfold over a longer period of time and require greater support from outside agencies. Well-trained and practiced EMTs can usually cope with a small-scale MCI pretty well. However, experience has shown that even the best-trained EMTs have a difficult time managing an incident of greater magnitude.

One way to minimize the operating difficulties of a large-scale MCI is for every EMT to be familiar with the local *disaster plan.* A disaster plan is a predefined set of instructions that tells a community's various emergency responders what to do in specific emergencies. Although no disaster plan can address every problem that could arise, there are several features common to every good disaster plan. The disaster plan should be:

disaster plan
a predefined set of instructions for a community's emergency responders.

- **Written to address the events that are conceivable for a particular location** (e.g., Kansas needs to plan for tornadoes, not hurricanes).

- **Well publicized.** Each emergency responder should be familiar with the plan and how it is to be put into operation.

- **Realistic.** The plan must be based on the actual availability of resources.

- **Rehearsed.** Experience has proven that the only way to get a plan to work correctly is to exercise it and, in so doing, work out the unforeseen "bugs."

It is beyond the scope of this text to teach you how to write a disaster plan or even to impart enough knowledge for you to be in charge of a disaster operation. However, it is important to introduce basic information about your potential roles in such an incident.

Incident Command System

● CORE CONCEPT
The Incident Command System

National Incident Management System (NIMS)
the management system used by federal, state, and local governments to manage emergencies in the United States.

Incident Command System (ICS)
a subset of the National Incident Management System (NIMS) designed specifically for management of multiple-casualty incidents.

Command
the first on the scene to establish order and initiate the Incident Command System.

By federal declaration, the *National Incident Management System (NIMS)* is the management system used by federal, state, and local governments to manage emergencies in the United States (Figure 39-8). A subset of the NIMS system is also known as the *Incident Command System (ICS).* Although not specifically a plan designed for MCI management, it provides a clear management framework for all types of large-scale incidents. In addition, it is mandated by law for the management of some types of incidents, such as those involving hazardous materials.

ICS originated in California, where it was designed as a management plan to handle large-scale firefighting operations involving multiple agencies and jurisdictions. A flexible tool for managing people and resources, the system components include Command, Operations, Logistics, Planning, and Finance. The most commonly used components are Command and Operations.

Command

Command, which must be established at all incidents, is the person who assumes responsibility for incident management. This individual stays in Command unless that function is transferred to another person or until the incident is brought to a conclusion.

IMS systems recognize that the manageable span of control is six people. As the MCI escalates and becomes more complex, the number of people and span of control become too large for one person to effectively manage. At this point, Command designates people to handle the specific functions needed to manage the operation. The basic elements of the Incident Management System—with sections such as Operations being subordinate to Command—are:

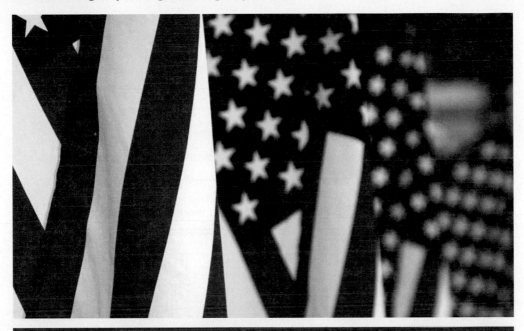

NATIONAL INCIDENT MANAGEMENT SYSTEM

December 2008

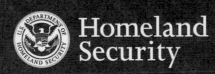 Homeland
Security

- Operations
- Planning
- Logistics
- Finance

Command assumes all incident management functions except those that Command may delegate to someone else. Unless an incident is very complex, the most common function designated is Operations.

Two methods of Command defined under NIMS are single incident command and unified command. In *single incident command*, a single agency controls all resources and operations. In many communities, for example, EMS is managed by fire services. Accordingly, single incident command is often used at fire and rescue incidents with the Incident

single incident command
command organization in which a single agency controls all resources and operations

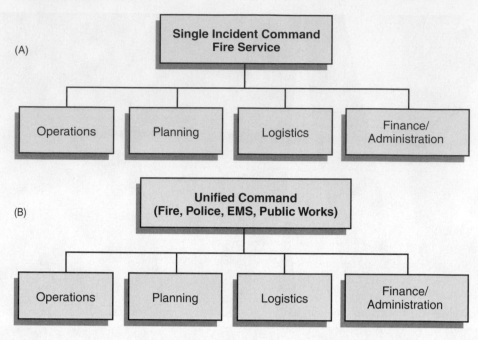

FIGURE 39-9 (A) A single incident command organization. (B) A unified command organization.

(A)

**Single Incident Command
Fire Service**

Operations

Planning

Logistics

Finance/
Administration

(B)

**Unified Command
(Fire, Police, EMS, Public Works)**

Operations

Planning

Logistics

Finance/
Administration

unified command
command organization in which several agencies work independently but cooperatively.

Incident Command
the person or persons who assume overall direction of a large-scale incident.

Commander provided by the fire service (Figure 39-9A). However, if police agencies have major involvement, if there is a separate EMS provider, or if other agencies are involved, **unified command** is more appropriate (Figure 39-9B). In unified command, several agencies work independently but cooperatively rather than one agency exercising control over the others. In most communities, unified command is the best way to manage resources. It recognizes that large-scale incidents tend to be complex and that the right agency must take the lead at the right time, with Command officers from all agencies cooperating.

Command Functions

Initially, **Incident Command** is assumed by the most senior member of the first service on the scene. Very often, this will be an EMS unit. Depending on jurisdiction, laws, or protocols, Incident Command may be later transferred to another individual or may be continued by whoever established it.

Two modes or phases of action must then be undertaken: scene size-up/triage and organization/delegation. First, Command and the crew do an initial scene size-up, start the triage process, and call for backup. While waiting for help, initial triage is completed and Command gets ready for arriving resources.

When reinforcements arrive, there are two options for the person who initially assumed Command: Continue to be in Command or transfer Command to someone of higher rank. In a unified system, Incident Command would be assumed cooperatively by the Command of each service. Command is positioned at a location close enough to allow observation of the scene but secure enough to permit management of incoming resources and communication with others. In a unified command system, EMS, Police, and Fire Command establish one field command post together and stay there. Some plans call for the field command vehicle or command post to be designated by placing two traffic cones on top of the vehicle being used. In a single incident command mode, one person acts as Command, and EMS would typically be a group under the Operations section.

Scene Size-Up

Size-up the scene by making a sweep to determine what needs must be met:

1. Arrive at the scene and establish Incident Command. Put on the proper identification.

2. Do a quick walk through the scene (or, if it is a hazmat scene, observe from a safe distance) and assess the number of patients, hazards, and degree of entrapment. Identify the

number of patients, including the "walking wounded," apparent priority of care, need for extrication, number of ambulances needed, other factors affecting the scene and corresponding resources needed to address them, and areas where resources can be staged.

3. Get as calm and composed as possible to radio in an initial scene report and call for additional resources.

CRITICAL DECISION MAKING

We Have *How Many* Patients???

One of the key elements of this chapter is handling the multiple-casualty incident. The concepts that were described in Chapter 10, "Scene Size-Up," return here with increased importance. For each of the following scenarios, determine what resources you would call for in your initial report to the dispatcher.

1. You are called to a shopping mall for "sick people." You arrive to find dozens of people standing outside the mall, coughing and rubbing their eyes. Looking around the parking lot, you see hundreds of cars.

2. You arrive at a motor-vehicle crash in which two cars collided at an intersection with considerable force. One patient has been ejected. Three others don't appear to be moving.

3. You are treating a woman in her home for flulike symptoms. You notice that her husband and one child are also sick. You check on another child sleeping in the same residence and find that he won't wake up.

Communications

Once scene size-up has been done, you should make an initial scene report to the communications center. Keep the report short and to the point, but give enough information for the communications center and other responders to understand the severity of the situation and react accordingly. Give yourself a unique Command name to distinguish yourself and your incident location from other personnel and incidents that may be using the same radio system. Example:

> MEDCOM, this is Medic 640. We are on the scene of a two-car MVA with severe entrapment of four Priority 1 patients. Dispatch a rescue company and four paramedic ambulances. I will now be called Franklin Avenue Command. Police are needed at the scene to assist with traffic and crowd control as soon as possible.

If the disaster plan is to be put into operation, it is critical that other responding units be informed of this fact. Your communications may also include telling other units what equipment to bring, what they should plan on doing once they arrive, how best to access the scene, and where to park.

As help begins to arrive, control of on-scene communication is important. Once units arrive, as much face-to-face communication as possible should be used, especially between Command and Command's direct subordinates. This will help to reduce radio channel crowding. If you feel you are getting too tied up in radio communications, designate a radio aide.

Basically, the flow of communications at the scene should correspond to the organizational chart being used. Accordingly, the only unit talking to the communications center and requesting resources is Command. The only ones who talk to Command are those directly subordinate to Command. All others talk only to the officer or supervisor they are assigned to.

Organization

Getting organized early and aggressively is very important. You must have a plan to deploy resources when they arrive. In addition, you must decide what subordinate officers will be needed and where resources will be placed. A common mistake is to underestimate the resources that will be needed. Somehow new patients not found during scene size-up have a way of appearing. Think big. Order big. Put resources in the staging area if they are not needed

FIGURE 39-10 An example of an incident tactical worksheet.

INCIDENT TACTICAL WORKSHEET

Location _____
Med. Command _____

___ Establish underlined command with fire & police   ___ Put bib on   ___ Advise inbound units where to stage
___ Place 2 cones on command vehicle   ___ Designate triage officer   ___ Advise crews to stay with units until given instructions
                                                                          ___ Advise units to switch to EMS Admin., 265 or 715

LEVEL 1 *(3-10 Patients)*	LEVEL 2 *(11-25 Patients)*	LEVEL 3 *(over 25 Patients)*	FIRE	RESCUE
___ Declare MCI	___ Declare MCI	___ Declare MCI	___ Assess # of Units Needed	___ Establish Perimeter
___ EMS All Call	___ EMS All Call	___ EMS All Call	___ EMS All Call Req. 619	___ Request Speciality Units
___ Request # of Units Needed	___ Request # of Units Needed	___ Request # of Units Needed	___ Designate Triage	___ Triage Officer Handles Inner
___ Cover Town/Sr. Medic Act 615	___ Cover Town/Sr. Medic Act 615	___ Cover Town/Sr. Medic Act 615	___ Set up Rehab at Air Bank	___ Circle
___ Roll Call Hospitals	___ Roll Call Hospitals	___ Roll Call Hospitals	___ Use 619 as ALS Unit	
___ Transport Officer?	___ Get Mutual Aid Units	___ Get Mutual Aid Units		
	___ Designate Treatment Officer	___ Designate Treatment Officer	**HAZ-MAT**	
	___ Designate Transport Officer	___ Designate Transport Officer	___ Req. # of Units Needed	
	___ Designate Staging Officer	___ Designate Staging Officer	___ EMS All Call	
	___ REMO MD to Scene	___ REMO MD to Scene	___ Est. Command in Cold Zone	
	___ Consider Rehab & CISD	___ Request Bus to Scene	___ Designate Triage	
(2-5 Amb. Needed)	*(5-13 Amb. Needed)*	*(over 13 Amb. Needed)*	___ Identify Agent	
			___ Research Decontamination	
			___ Research Med.	

HOSPITAL ROLL CALL	AMCH	St. PETERS	MEMORIAL	VA	ELLIS	St. CLARE'S	LEONARD	St. MARY'S	SAMARITAN
CAN TAKE									
# PATIENTS SENT									

UNITS RESPONDING

620	621	622
630	631	632
640	641	642
650	651	652
610	611	605
TSU-1	TSU-2	
619	___	
Guild.	___	
CPHM	___	
Albany	___	
Mohawk	___	
Empire	___	

UNITS IN STAGING

620	621	622
630	631	632
640	641	642
650	651	652
610	611	605
TSU-1	TSU-2	
619	___	
Guild.	___	
CPHM	___	
Albany	___	
Mohawk	___	
Empire	___	

 # OF PATIENTS BY PRIORITY

1 *(Red)*	2 *(Yellow)*	3 *(Green)*	0 *(Black)*	TOTALS

right away. In urban/suburban incidents, backup can be fast and overwhelming. If you do not think about supply and staging areas early, you take the chance of being overrun.

It is important to prevent "freelancing." Freelancing is uncoordinated or undirected activity at the scene. Given the opportunity, most rescuers will arrive on the scene and begin setting their own priorities. Command can prevent this problem. When Command is established early, people and crews are assigned to tasks as they arrive.

Often it is helpful to have some personal tools to help get organized. For example, many organizations have distilled the major points of their plans into a "tactical worksheet" they can use in the field. With enough use, the plan can become committed to memory (Figure 39-10).

Scene Management

The senior person on the first-arriving EMS unit will likely assume Incident Command (known simply as Command). He will establish a command post to oversee the incident's medical aspects and the safety of all personnel, designate area supervisors, and work closely with the fire and police commanders. On larger incidents, Command may have an aide to assist with communications as well as a public information officer and a safety officer.

It is important to keep uninjured people from becoming injured. This will probably require restricting access to the scene to only those personnel performing triage (explained later), extrication from wreckage, and patient care. As resources arrive at the scene, police officers or safety officers may take over this function.

EMS Branch Functions

Under NIMS, in a very large and complex multiple-casualty incident, EMS will function as a branch under the Operations section. For smaller MCIs, the EMS person who has assumed Incident Command may be able to handle all aspects of management without delegating tasks to others. However, as an incident increases in size and complexity, additional staff and area supervisors will be needed (Figures 39-11 through 39-13). EMS operations generally include the following:

- Mobile command center
- Extrication (in cases of entrapment)
- Staging area
- Triage area
- Treatment area
- Transportation area
- Rehabilitation area

Individuals and agencies on the scene will be assigned particular roles in one or more areas. Most systems use brightly colored reflective vests that can be worn over protective clothing to make each incident sector officer easy to identify. Any EMT arriving at the scene at this time would be expected to report to an area supervisor for assignment of specific duties. Once assigned a specific task, the EMT should complete the task and report back to the area supervisor.

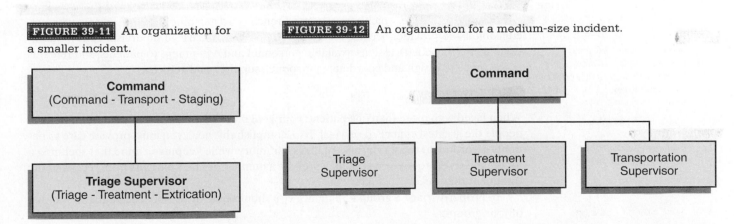

FIGURE 39-11 An organization for a smaller incident.

Command
(Command - Transport - Staging)

Triage Supervisor
(Triage - Treatment - Extrication)

FIGURE 39-12 An organization for a medium-size incident.

Command

Triage Supervisor

Treatment Supervisor

Transportation Supervisor

FIGURE 39-13 An organization for a major incident.

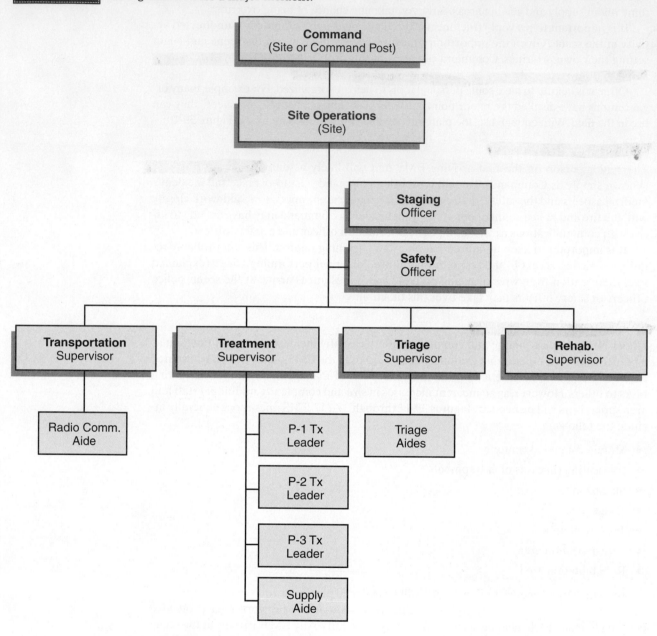

Triage

Once organization has been established, the next task is to quickly assess all the patients and assign each a priority for receiving emergency care or transportation to definitive care. This process is called *triage*, which comes from a French word meaning "to sort." The most knowledgeable EMS provider becomes the *triage supervisor*. The triage supervisor calls for additional help (if needed), assigns available personnel and equipment to patients, and remains at the scene to assign and coordinate personnel, supplies, and vehicles.

Primary Triage

When faced with more than one patient, your goal must be to afford the greatest number of people the greatest chance of survival. To accomplish this goal, you must provide care to patients according to the seriousness of illness or injury while keeping in mind that spending a lot of time trying to save one life may prevent a number of other patients from receiving the treatment they need.

To properly triage a group of patients, you should quickly classify each patient into one of four groups.

triage
the process of quickly assessing patients at a multiple-casualty incident and assigning each a priority for receiving treatment; from a French word meaning "to sort."

triage supervisor
the person responsible for overseeing triage at a multiple-casualty incident.

- **Priority 1: Treatable Life-Threatening Illness or Injuries.** Patients with airway and breathing difficulties, uncontrolled or severe bleeding, decreased mental status, severe medical problems, shock (hypoperfusion), and/or severe burns.

- **Priority 2: Serious but Not Life-Threatening Illness or Injuries.** Patients who have burns without airway problems, major or multiple bone or joint injuries, and/or back injuries with or without spinal cord damage.

- **Priority 3: "Walking Wounded."** Patients with minor musculoskeletal injuries or minor soft-tissue injuries.

- **Priority 4 (sometimes called Priority 0): Dead or Fatally Injured.** Examples include patients with exposed brain matter, cardiac arrest (no pulse for over 20 minutes except with cold-water drowning or severe hypothermia), decapitation, severed trunk, and incineration.

Patients in arrest are considered Priority 4 (or 0) when resources are limited. The time that must be devoted to rescue breathing or CPR for one person is not justified when there are many patients needing attention. Once ample resources are available, patients in arrest become Priority 1.

How triage is performed depends on the number of injuries, the immediate hazards to personnel and patients, and the location of backup resources. Local operating procedures will give you more guidance on the exact method of triage for a given situation. Basic principles of triage are presented here.

The first triage cut can be done rapidly by using a bullhorn, PA system, or loud voice to direct all patients capable of walking (Priority 3) to move to a particular area. This has a two-fold purpose. It quickly identifies the individuals who have an airway and circulation, and it physically separates them from patients who will generally need more care.

You must rapidly assess each remaining patient, stopping only to secure an airway or stop profuse bleeding. It is important that you not develop "tunnel vision"—spending time rendering additional care to any one patient and thus failing to identify and correct life-threatening conditions of the remaining patients. If Priority 3 patients are nearby and well enough to help, they may be employed to assist you by maintaining an airway or direct pressure on bleeding wounds of other patients. Priority 3 patients who have been reluctant to leave ill or injured friends or relatives may be permitted to stay near them where they can be of possible help later.

Once all patients have been assessed and treated for airway and breathing problems and severe bleeding, more thorough treatment can be initiated. You will need to render care to the patients who are most seriously injured or ill but who stand the best chance of survival with proper treatment. This requires treating all the Priority 1 patients first, Priority 2 patients next, and Priority 3 patients last. Priority 4 patients do not receive treatment unless no other patients are believed to be at risk of dying or suffering long-term disability if their conditions go unattended.

Usually patients will be immobilized on backboards, if necessary, and carried by "runners" to the appropriate secondary sector (as described later). Extensive treatment does not occur at the incident site since it is in a hazard zone and could impede rescue and initial treatment of other patients.

START Triage: A National Standard for Rapid Primary Triage

The most commonly used method of prioritizing patients in the United States is the START method of triage (Figure 39-14). It was developed by the Newport Beach, California, Fire Department and the Hoag Hospital in Newport Beach, California. *START* stands for *Simple Triage and Rapid Treatment.* The foundation of the system is the speed, simplicity, and consistency of its application. It relies on some simple commands and the following physiologic parameters that can be remembered by the mnemonic *RPM:*

Respiration

Pulse

Mental Status

START triage is intended to be completed in about 30 seconds per patient.

FIGURE 39-14 START triage.

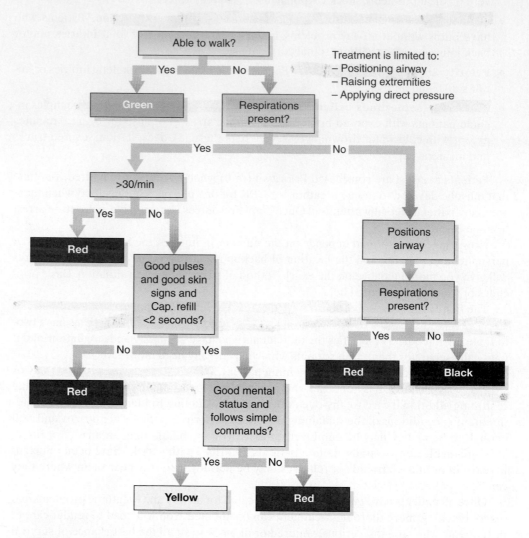

START Triage

Treatment is limited to:
– Positioning airway
– Raising extremities
– Applying direct pressure

Begin by asking all patients who can walk to get up and go to a collection point such as an ambulance or a building. Since those who can do this are . . .

• Conscious
• Able to follow commands
• Able to walk

. . . they obviously are perfusing their brain, are breathing, have a pulse, and have a nervous system that is currently working. All of these patients are considered to be Priority 3 (*green tag*) patients for right now. (They are often called the "walking wounded.") This also leaves people at the site who are unable to hear, walk, or follow commands and are the Priority 0, 1, or 2 patients. Among these patients, you must now focus your attention on those who are likely to be of higher priority.

Start making your triage sweep methodically by avoiding patients who are obviously conscious. The only three treatments provided during START triage are to:

• Open an airway and insert an oropharyngeal airway
• Apply pressure to bleeding
• Elevate an extremity

Assess Respiration (Breathing Status) First If the patient is *not breathing* and your attempts to open the airway do *not* start breathing, tag the patient as a Priority 0 (*black tag*) patient. If the patient *starts breathing* after the airway is opened, then tag as a Priority 1 (*red tag*). Is the patient breathing more than 30 times per minute? If so, tag the patient as a Priority 1 (*red tag*) patient. Is the patient breathing less than 30 times per minute? If so, go to the next step.

Assess Radial Pulse Second If the patient is *unresponsive, not breathing*, and has *no pulse*, tag the patient as a Priority 0 (*black tag*) patient. If the patient is *breathing* but has *no pulse*, tag as a Priority 1 (*red tag*) patient. If the patient is *breathing* and *has a pulse, good skin signs*, and *capillary refill less than 2 seconds*, go to the next step.

Assess Level of Consciousness (Mental Status) Third If *alert*, tag as a Priority 2 (*yellow tag*) patient. If there is any *altered mental status*, tag as a Priority 1 (*red tag*) patient.

Now Re-Triage the Priority 3 "Walking Wounded" Patients Just because they could initially walk does not mean some of the Priority 3 patients do not have serious medical conditions! Many could have an altered mental status, be bleeding, and have significant signs of shock, which could cause them to be recategorized as a higher priority patient. Move methodically using the same START assessment of (1) respiration, (2) pulse, and (3) mental status.

A START Summary A quick summary of START is as follows:

1. Order the walking wounded to some type of temporary collection point. They are considered Priority 3 (*green*) for now.

2. Assess all others for RPM (respiration, pulse, and mental status) and tag as follows:
   Priority 1 (red) are patients who have:
   - Altered mental status, or . . .
   - Absent radial pulse, or . . .
   - Respirations of greater than 30/minute
   Priority 2 (yellow) are patients who:
   - Are alert, and . . .
   - Have radial pulses present, and . . .
   - Have respirations less than 30/minute
   Priority 0 (black) are patients who:
   - Are not breathing (after an attempt to open the airway), or . . .
   - Have no pulse and are not breathing

3. Re-triage all walking wounded.

Patient Identification

By now, it should be clear that a system will be required to group and identify patients by treatment priority. A widely used system is to color-code patients according to their priority. The START system, discussed previously, is one example of a color-coding system. Other systems' color codes may be slightly different. For example, Priority 1 might be red; Priority 2, yellow; Priority 3, green; and Priority 4 (if a separate category) might be black or gray.

Since different localities have different systems, it is important that you know and understand the system used in your area. It is equally important that different services in the same region use the same coding system. This is because many MCIs are multiple-agency events. If each agency were to use a different system, there would be no way to correctly coordinate the order in which patients are to receive care.

As you move among patients to conduct initial triage, you should affix a *triage tag* to each patient, indicating the priority group to which that patient has been assigned. Triage tags are color-coded and may have space in which limited medical information can be recorded (Figures 39-15, 39-16, and 39-17).

triage tag
color-coded tag indicating the priority group to which a patient has been assigned.

There are some local variations of the triage tag. Some use adhesive-backed colored shipping labels. Others use colored surveyor's tape or duct tape to classify patients. Surveyor's tape can be quickly tied on as an arm band. Duct tape will stick to just about anything in any kind of weather. For this reason, it is particularly useful in an MCI setting. It is also useful to have a laundry marker or wax pencil handy for wet conditions when a standard pen or pencil will not write well.

Whatever system you use, it is vital that the color coding be easily located and identified. When properly performed, this coding allows a later EMT to quickly identify which treatment group patients belong to and to institute treatment in that manner.

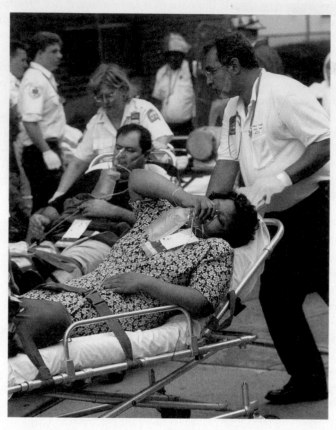

FIGURE 39-15 The triage tag indicates the priority group to which that patient has been assigned.

(© Black Star)

Secondary Triage and Treatment

As more personnel arrive at the incident scene, they should be directed to assist with the completion of initial triage. If triage has been completed, these EMTs can initiate treatment.

Secondary triage is generally performed at a patient collection point or ***triage area*** from which patients are assigned to a treatment group.

Patients are physically separated into treatment groups based on their priority level as designated by a triage tag. Some systems call for vehicles to carry red, yellow, and green tarps, which are used to designate these areas. An area to which triaged patients are removed is referred to as a ***treatment area***. Each treatment area should have its own ***treatment supervisor***, an EMT responsible for overseeing the triage and treatment within that area. The treatment supervisor should re-triage the patients in that area to determine the order in which they will receive treatment. Secondary triage is important to ensure that patients are treated and transported according to their priority.

During secondary triage, it may be necessary to recategorize a patient whose condition has deteriorated or improved, or who was incorrectly triaged, to a higher or lower priority group than was medically warranted. This will necessitate moving the patient to the proper treatment area as resources permit. Some systems use a different disaster tag during secondary triage on which more detailed information about the patient can be recorded (Figure 39-17).

The treatment area EMTs will need supplies and equipment from the ambulances such as bandages, blood pressure cuffs, and oxygen.

Transportation and Staging Logistics

Once patients have been properly assessed and triaged, and once treatment for the patients has been initiated according to their priority, consideration must be given to the order in which the patients will be transported to a hospital. Again, this is done according to triage priority.

triage area
the area where secondary triage takes place at a multiple-casualty incident.

treatment area
the area in which patients are treated at a multiple-casualty incident.

treatment supervisor
person responsible for overseeing treatment of patients who have been triaged at a multiple-casualty incident.

● CORE CONCEPT
Transportation and staging logistics

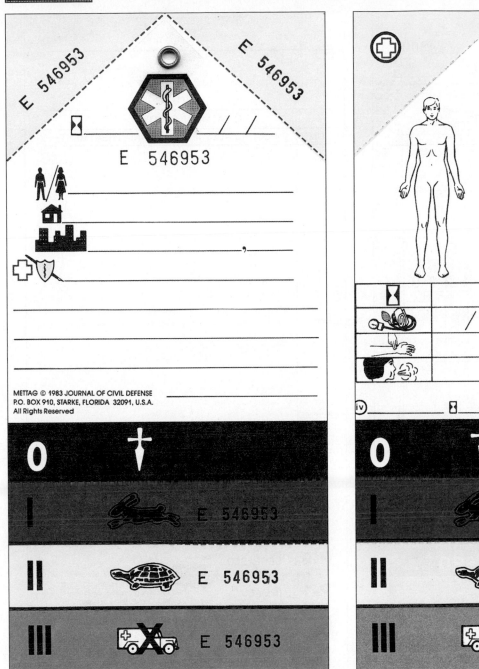

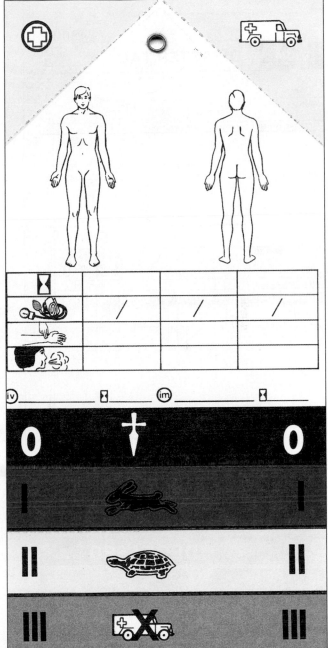

It is advisable to have a **staging area** from which ambulances can be called to transport patients. The staging area will be the responsibility of the **staging supervisor**, who must keep track of the ambulance vehicles and personnel. In large-scale incidents, the staging supervisor may need to arrange for certain human needs, such as rest rooms, meals, and rotation of crews.

No ambulance should proceed to a treatment area unless requested by the **transportation supervisor** and directed by the staging supervisor. The staging supervisor is responsible for communicating with each treatment area regarding the number and priority of the patients in that area. This information can then be used by the transportation supervisor to arrange for transport of patients from the scene to the hospital in the most efficient way.

It is vital that no ambulance transport any patient without the approval of the transportation supervisor, since the transportation supervisor is responsible for maintaining a list of patients and the hospitals to which they are transported. This information is relayed from the

staging area
the area where ambulances are parked and other resources are held until needed.

staging supervisor
person responsible for overseeing ambulances and ambulance personnel at a multiple-casualty incident.

transportation supervisor
person responsible for communicating with sector officers and hospitals to manage transportation of patients to hospitals from a multiple-casualty incident.

FIGURE 39-17 EMS disaster tag (front and back).

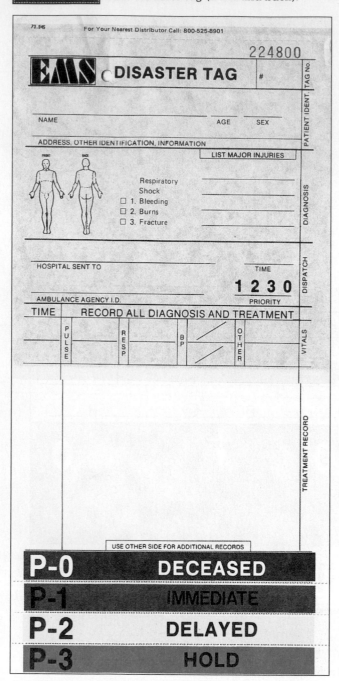

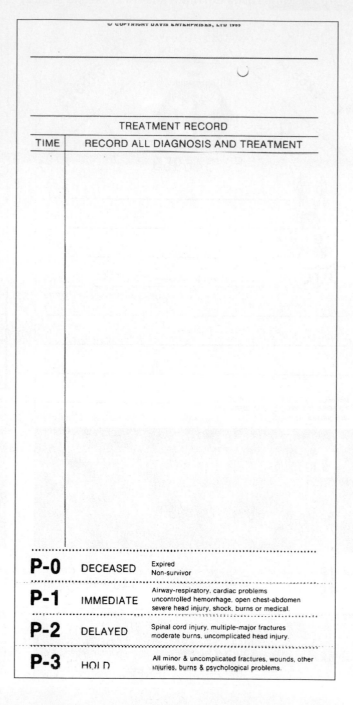

transportation supervisor to each receiving hospital. (In a large-scale incident, the transportation officer may actually have an aide who does nothing but speak to hospitals.) In this way, the hospitals know what to expect and receive only the patients they are capable of handling. It is critical that the EMTs on the ambulance comply with the instructions of the transportation supervisor. Failure to do so may result in patients being transported to the wrong facilities.

Once an ambulance has completed its run to a hospital, it will probably be directed to return to the staging area, perhaps bringing needed supplies, to await its next instructions from the staging supervisor.

Communicating with Hospitals

It is important that receiving hospitals be alerted to the nature of the MCI or disaster as soon as the magnitude of the incident is known. This allows the hospitals to call in additional personnel or to clear beds as necessary to accept the anticipated number of patients.

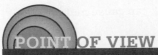

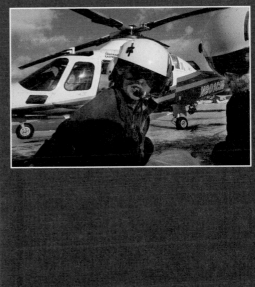

"You know how you figure if you ever get into a car crash it'll be a fender bender? Not me. I had to do it big. Real big.

"I was on the freeway, coming over the crest of a hill. Fortunately, I was going slow enough so I was able to stop just before a big wreck on the other side. There must've been 10 or 12 cars all over the road. Sounds like I did good, right? Nope. The tractor-trailer behind me couldn't stop fast enough. He hit me so hard he pushed me into the car in front of me and then into three others. Squished my little car like an accordion.

"While that was really the pits, I never realized that there would be injured people all over the place. I mean, this road was littered with crashed cars and injured people. When the rescue people finally got to my car, they tied a red ribbon around my wrist and put a red sticker on my windshield. I was starting to feel bad. I asked an EMT what the red meant. He smiled at me very nicely and said, 'You'll be heading out first.'

"OK, great, I thought. Things were getting a little fuzzy. Then I saw spacemen heading my way. They had helmets on. They took me to a helicopter. I couldn't believe it. I thought maybe I was hallucinating, but sure enough, they loaded me in and flew me to the gosh-darned hospital.

"Too bad I couldn't have flown that helicopter to work and missed that whole crash thing. I'd probably still have my spleen!"

Because radio communication channels will be heavily used, the transportation officer, not individual EMTs, should communicate with the hospitals. This will keep unnecessary radio usage to a minimum. It will also ensure that the proper information is recorded at both ends of the ambulance ride. In large-scale MCIs, it is not necessary to give a patient report for each patient since the treating and transporting EMTs will most likely be different and there will generally be too many patients to allow EMTs to give a good patient radio report under the circumstances. In these instances, the hospital may be told only basic information; for example, that they are receiving a Priority 1 patient with respiratory problems.

Psychological Aspects of MCIs

During MCIs, EMTs often encounter another, frequently overlooked condition: psychologically stressed patients. Although they may outwardly exhibit few signs of injury or emotional stress, people involved in MCIs have been subjected to devastating circumstances with which they are normally unprepared to cope. Proper early management of the psychologically stressed patient can support later treatment and help ensure a faster recovery.

Adequately managing a patient during an MCI may require you to administer "psychological first aid." This may take the form of talking with a terrified parent, child, or witness. You should not attempt to engage in psychoanalysis and should not say things that are untrue in an attempt to calm a patient. However, a caring, honest demeanor can reassure a patient, as will listening to the patient and acknowledging his fears and problems. Often this is all the patient will need.

Patients are not the only ones subject to emotional stress during a multiple-casualty incident; emergency responders are as well. It is very important that you understand that large-scale or horrific MCIs (Figures 39-18 and 39-19) may affect rescuers as much as, if not more than, non-rescuers.

EMTs who become emotionally incapacitated should be treated as patients and removed to an area where they can rest without viewing the scene. These patients must be monitored by an EMS provider until a clinically competent provider can take over. These EMTs should not be allowed to return to duty without first being evaluated by someone professionally trained to do so.

CORE CONCEPT
Psychological aspects of multiple-casualty incidents

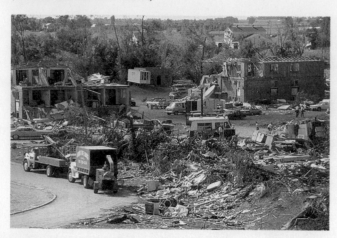

FIGURE 39-18 A tornado can cause great devastation.
(© Steve Leonard/Black Star)

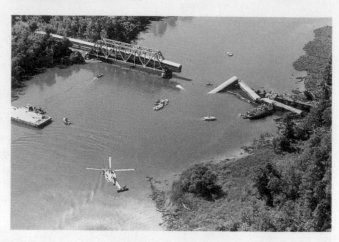

FIGURE 39-19 A train wreck can cause multiple casualties. (© Black Star)

CHAPTER REVIEW

Key Facts and Concepts

- Be suspicious. Many hazmat incidents start out as routine EMS calls.

- The biggest problem in most hazmat incidents is identifying the offending substance. Look for the shipping placard and the MSDS sheets. Use the *Emergency Response Guide* to help determine your initial actions.

- Remember hot zone-warm zone-cold zone. Once you realize it's a hazmat incident, get to the cold zone and call for help.

- Keep responders in rehab until they are rested, hydrated, and vitals return to normal.

- Patients who have been "decontaminated" almost always still have some contamination.

- Patients being transported must be cared for by EMS responders with "Operations" level training and equipment.

- Use your MCI plan and procedure at small incidents, as this will make managing larger ones easier.

- NIMS and Incident Management are the national standard for incident management.

- Learn and practice START triage essentials.

- Be alert for signs of stress after incidents and seek help as necessary.

Key Decisions

- What is the hazardous substance? What risk does it pose to me, the other rescuers, and the public?

- Does anyone need immediate evacuation?

- If a patient has some contamination, can we safely start decontamination?

- Is this incident at a level where I should institute the Incident Management System?

- Should I start using triage tags?

- What additional resources should I call for?

Chapter Glossary

cold zone area where the Incident Command post and support functions are located.

Command the first on the scene to establish order and initiate the Incident Command System.

decontamination a chemical and/or physical process that reduces or prevents the spread of contamination from persons or equipment; the removal of hazardous substances from employees and their equipment to the extent necessary to preclude foreseeable health effects.

disaster plan a predefined set of instructions for a community's emergency responders.

hazardous material any substance or material in a form which poses an unreasonable risk to health, safety, and property when transported in commerce.

hot zone area immediately surrounding a hazmat incident; extends far enough to prevent adverse effects outside the zone.

Incident Command the person or persons who assume overall direction of an incident.

Incident Command System (ICS) a subset of the National Incident Management System (NIMS) designed specifically for management of multiple-casualty incidents.

multiple-casualty incident (MCI) any medical or trauma incident involving multiple patients.

National Incident Management System (NIMS) the management system used by federal, state, and local governments to manage emergencies in the United States.

single incident command command organization in which a single agency controls all resources and operations.

staging area the area where ambulances are parked and other resources are held until needed.

staging supervisor person responsible for overseeing ambulances and ambulance personnel at a multiple-casualty incident.

transportation supervisor person responsible for communicating with sector officers and hospitals to manage transportation of patients to hospitals from a multiple-casualty incident.

treatment area the area in which patients are treated at a multiple-casualty incident.

treatment supervisor person responsible for overseeing treatment of patients who have been triaged at a multiple-casualty incident.

triage the process of quickly assessing patients at a multiple-casualty incident and assigning each a priority for receiving treatment; from a French word meaning "to sort."

triage area the area where secondary triage takes place at a multiple-casualty incident.

triage supervisor the person responsible for overseeing triage at a multiple-casualty incident.

triage tag color-coded tag indicating the priority group to which a patient has been assigned.

unified command command organization in which several agencies work independently but cooperatively.

warm zone area where personnel and equipment decontamination and hot zone support take place; it includes control points for the access corridor and thus assists in reducing the spread of contamination.

Preparation for Your Examination and Practice

Short Answer

1. List the information contained in an initial report of a hazardous materials incident.

2. Explain how to identify a hazardous material and how to obtain information about that material.

3. Describe the general assessment and emergency care of a patient with a hazardous materials injury.

4. Describe the major components and benefits of an Incident Management System.

5. Define the basic role of the EMT at a multiple-casualty incident.

6. Explain why patients are assigned priorities during triage.

7. Identify four priority categories of triage.

Thinking and Linking

Think back to Chapter 2, "The Well-Being of the EMT," and link information from that chapter with information from this chapter as you consider the following situations:

1. At an MCI, one EMT, who was among the first to arrive and has been working at peak level ever since, looks really tired. As Incident Commander, you ask if she wants a break. She says she is fine and doesn't need a break. What should you do?

2. Several weeks after working an MCI, you start having trouble sleeping, are having trouble concentrating, and find you are snapping at your family and coworkers. You realize the symptoms may be related to that MCI but figure you'll get over it. Right? Wrong? What should you do?

Critical Thinking Exercises

When you are first on-scene at a possible multiple-casualty incident with possible hazardous materials involvement, what should you do? The purpose of this exercise will be to think through your actions at such an incident.

- Your call is to a motor-vehicle collision with an unknown number of injuries. As your unit approaches the scene, you see that three cars and downed wires are involved. You get a whiff of gasoline as you pass by. The drivers are visible in each vehicle—one appears to be conscious and the other two are bent forward or slumped back. There are passengers visible in two vehicles, one or more of whom may need extrication. How should you proceed?

It's raining hard and there's a loud noise on the station PA system with the dispatcher saying: "Ambulances Alpha 2, Alpha 5, Bravo 1, and Charlie 10, respond to a three-car motor-vehicle crash at the intersection of Avenues A and B. Unknown how many occupants. Timeout of 1933 hours." You turn to your partner and say, "This call is only about 10 blocks away. We should be the first on-scene." As you head toward the scene, you are notified by dispatch that the police are on-scene and report a total of nine occupants. Additional ambulances are being dispatched.

You and your partner agree that you will establish Incident Command and he will do triage. "Dispatch, Bravo 1 is on-scene and establishing Incident Command." The first thing you do is put on the Command bib for identification. Your partner puts on the triage bib and takes triage tags to check on the occupants. You briefly tell the police officer you are Incident Command and he informs you that his captain is responding and has three units handling traffic control. He has also requested heavy rescue from the fire department in case extrication is needed.

With flashlight in hand and while trying to keep the rain out of your eyes, you perform a scene size-up. You realize that you need a place to stage the other ambulances for easy access and so they don't get blocked in. You see a location and quickly share your idea with the police officer. He agrees. He will tell his units to make sure that area is accessible for the ambulances. You call dispatch on the radio using the identifier "Incident Command" and ask that they instruct all responding ambulances to stage in the parking lot of the insurance company.

Street Scene Questions

1. As Incident Command, what are some of the things you need to do?
2. What information do you expect first from the triage officer?
3. How will you decide what patients go to what hospitals?

Your partner advises you that three patients are Priority 1, five are Priority 2, and one is Priority 3. You radio dispatch with this information. You are told that a canvass of local hospitals has already been done and the trauma center can handle all Priority 1 patients. The other patients can be divided between the other three area hospitals. You ask that they call the trauma center back and confirm that they will be getting three patients and the other hospitals will be getting two each.

You then ask dispatch to tell you how many ambulances have been dispatched. You are informed there are a total of five. Remembering that one of the ambulances is yours, you request two more ambulances. Two ambulances are on-scene and parked in the staging area. You tell them to each take a Priority 1 patient. The next ambulance is assigned to the last Priority 1 patient. You ask the triage officer if some of the Priority 2 or 3 patients can be doubled up, which seems appropriate for four of the patients.

Street Scene Questions

4. Is there a need for a safety officer on this scene?
5. How should patient information be transmitted to the hospitals?
6. What information should you be sharing with Police Command and Fire Command?

The fire captain tells you that his crew has disconnected the batteries of all the vehicles and will stand by to assist with extrication. Access has been gained to all patients using hand tools. You ask if his safety officer can continue in that role until all the patients are off the scene.

The first ambulance is loaded and en route to the trauma center. The second will shortly be en route. You advise these crews to notify the hospital directly but tell them to keep the transmission short.

The last Priority 1 patient is out of the car, and you tell the triage supervisor that the other hospitals get two patients each. He should coordinate this with crews and tell them to call the patient information directly into the hospital.

Within 30 minutes of the call notification, every patient is en route to a hospital. You let Police and Fire Command know. Your partner looks at you and says, "Not bad for someone who looks like a drowned rat."

Highway Safety and Vehicle Extrication

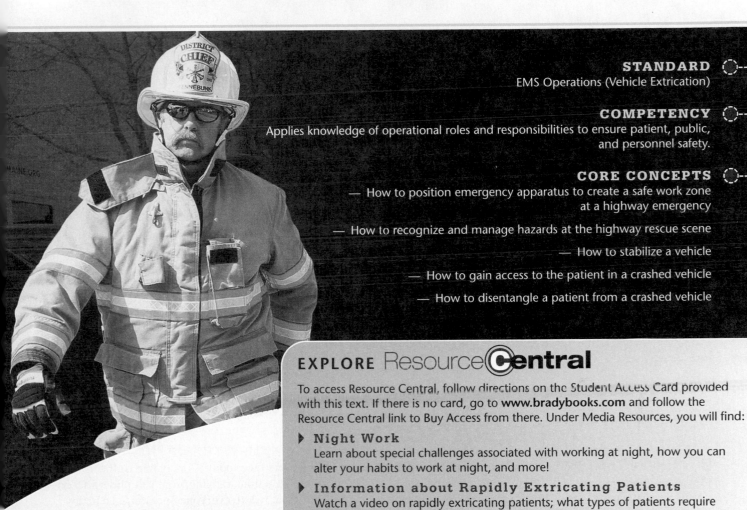

STANDARD ⭘------
EMS Operations (Vehicle Extrication)

COMPETENCY ⭘------
Applies knowledge of operational roles and responsibilities to ensure patient, public, and personnel safety.

CORE CONCEPTS ⭘------
— How to position emergency apparatus to create a safe work zone at a highway emergency

— How to recognize and manage hazards at the highway rescue scene

— How to stabilize a vehicle

— How to gain access to the patient in a crashed vehicle

— How to disentangle a patient from a crashed vehicle

EXPLORE ResourceCentral

To access Resource Central, follow directions on the Student Access Card provided with this text. If there is no card, go to **www.bradybooks.com** and follow the Resource Central link to Buy Access from there. Under Media Resources, you will find:

▶ **Night Work**
Learn about special challenges associated with working at night, how you can alter your habits to work at night, and more!

▶ **Information about Rapidly Extricating Patients**
Watch a video on rapidly extricating patients; what types of patients require rapid extrication and what types of tools and equipment is needed.

▶ **Information about Traffic Safety**
Read about the importance of traffic safety during an emergency and what you can do to protect yourself and others on the scene.

OBJECTIVES

After reading this chapter you should be able to:

40.1 Describe the risks to EMS providers during highway emergency operations.

40.2 Given a variety of highway response scenarios, describe how to create as safe a work area as possible. (p. 1038)

40.3 Discuss particular considerations in ensuring safety during night operations. (pp. 1040–1041)

40.4 List the 10 phases of vehicle extrication and rescue operations. (pp. 1041, 1043)

(continued)

40.5 In a rescue situation, recognize and manage hazards by wearing appropriate protective gear, safeguarding your patient, managing traffic, safely dealing with deployed air bags and energy-absorbing bumpers, managing spectators, and exercising safe practices around electrical hazards. (pp. 1044–1050)

40.6 Describe actions taken at a rescue scene by those trained to do so regarding control of vehicle fires, stabilizing a vehicle, and gaining access to patients. (pp. 1050–1060)

A t least 10 types of specialty rescue teams may be available in various communities, depending on each community's hazards. Each specialty requires a significant amount of additional training over and above your EMT course. These specialties include vehicle rescue, water rescue, ice rescue, high-angle rescue, hazardous materials response, trench rescue, dive rescue, back-country or wilderness rescue, farm rescue, and confined space rescue. Training that is available in each of these specialties often depends on the types of emergency responses that might be required in your community.

The focus of this chapter is the EMT's role at a vehicle collision where extrication of the patient is required, since this is the most common type of rescue across the United States (Figure 40-1).

HIGHWAY EMERGENCY OPERATIONS

CORE CONCEPT

How to position emergency apparatus to create a safe work zone at a highway emergency

One of the greatest hazards emergency responders face today is oncoming traffic at highway incidents. Drivers are in quiet cars with distractions ranging from cell phones to onboard video players. Distracted drivers pose a great risk to everyone operating at a highway incident. It requires a team effort of police, fire, and EMS to ensure a work area that is as safe as possible from as many hazards as possible. EMTs are not typically in charge of highway incidents but play a key role, because they are called to treat the injured who are likely to be entrapped in wreckage.

The care of the injured and safety of the responders are both high priorities at a highway incident. To achieve these goals, it is important that:

- EMS response should be limited to only the manpower and vehicles needed to accomplish the mission and should not expose more people than necessary to the risks of highway operations.

- The first-arriving unit should institute "blocking" to protect the work area. Because of its size and weight, fire apparatus is preferred for this purpose.

- If it is necessary to block lanes of traffic, they should be cleared as quickly as possible so the flow of traffic can return to normal.

Initial Response

On limited-access highways, only the primary or first-due units should proceed directly to the scene. Units sent for backup should stage off the highway until they are requested to the scene.

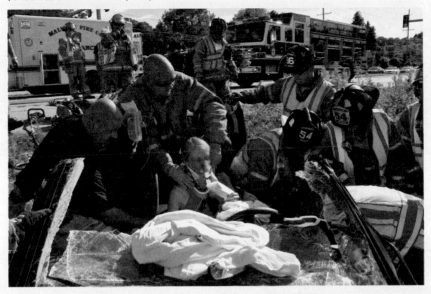

FIGURE 40-1 A vehicle collision where extrication of the patient is required is the most common type of rescue across the United States. *(© Edward T. Dickinson, MD)*

The first-arriving units should:

- Establish Command and confirm the exact location of the incident with the dispatch center.
- Use apparatus to institute "upstream blocking" of the scene to protect the work area. Although fire apparatus is ideal, as already noted, any first-arriving unit can institute blocking. If fire apparatus responds subsequently, they can be placed behind the lighter units.
- Rescue trucks (police or EMS) arriving to perform extrication should be positioned downstream of the initial blocking vehicle.

Congestion at incidents is a big problem. To minimize scene congestion, units should park in the same direction and remain in single file, if possible. Again, larger units should provide upstream blocking whereas Command and EMS units are downstream in the "safe zone." Responding units need to exercise extreme caution in performing turnarounds on limited-access highways. These should be done only when a turn can be completed without obstructing the flow of traffic in either travel direction or when all traffic movement has stopped.

EMS personnel should avoid parking their units and conducting ambulance loading on the side that is across traffic flow from the side where the crashed vehicle or vehicles are located. Unless a roadway is completely shut down, EMS crews should avoid crossing over lanes of traffic on foot, especially when they are trying to move patients. Doing so is extremely dangerous. Whenever possible, park downstream from the crash in a safe zone created by blocking from upstream apparatus.

Positioning Blocking Apparatus

The apparatus that is used to block should be positioned to create one-and-a-half to two lanes of blockage (Figure 40-2). This will usually create a large enough work zone. The driver of the apparatus must also consider preservation of the crash scene and must avoid running over road debris or crash evidence.

Ideal blocking placement has the fire apparatus positioned at an angle, with its working side toward the work zone to protect the crew. The front wheels are rotated away from the incident. In the event that a motorist strikes the engine, the engine will be a barrier. If the engine is pushed by the striking vehicle on impact, the unit will move away from the work zone. Some incidents may require more than one piece of blocking apparatus.

It is important to leave space in the area immediately next to the crash to position vehicle extrication units (Figure 40-3). Ambulances, command vehicles, and other units should

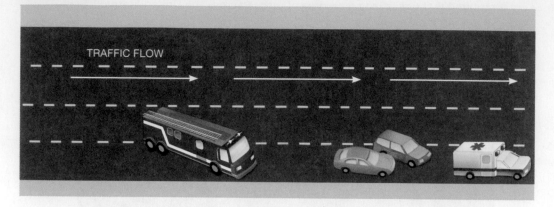

FIGURE 40-2 Blocking with no extrication.

TRAFFIC FLOW

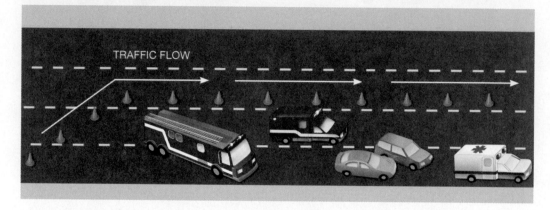

FIGURE 40-3 Blocking with placement of a rescue truck.

TRAFFIC FLOW

be positioned downstream from the crash. Positioning units in this manner allows for safer patient loading and rapid departure from the scene.

Exiting the Vehicle Safely

Responders who are exiting apparatus are at high risk of being struck by a passing vehicle. They should always exit into the safe zone, if possible, after checking to be sure that traffic has stopped. Be sure everyone in the responding vehicle is communicating, looking out for traffic, and being aware of when it is safe to exit the unit.

Be Seen and Warn Oncoming Traffic

Before exiting the vehicle, all responders should be in full protective clothing or, at a minimum, ANSI Class 2 traffic safety vests and helmets (Figure 40-4).

To help slow oncoming traffic, flares, traffic cones, or other devices should be placed to channel traffic away from the incident and establish a safe work zone. Cones and/or flares should be placed on an angle across the road and around the site (Scan 40-1). Some apparatus have amber flashing directional arrows to direct traffic that should be activated to assist in alerting oncoming traffic.

If it is necessary to channel traffic around a curve, hill, or ramp, the first cone or flare must be placed before the hill or curve. The intent is to warn oncoming traffic of a hazard ahead. The rest of the cones, as already noted, should be placed diagonally across the lanes and around the work zone.

Night Operations

At night, headlights or flashing lights can temporarily blind drivers that are approaching an emergency scene, preventing them from seeing emergency workers. In this circumstance, re-

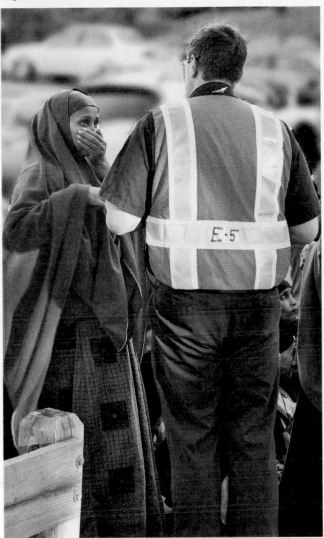

FIGURE 40-4 An EMT wears a highly visible vest at a high-traffic scene.

flective safety vests become ineffective. Therefore, drivers of emergency apparatus parked at highway incidents should turn off vehicle headlights. In addition, they should shut off any white response lighting that could blind oncoming drivers.

The best combination of lights to provide maximum visibility is:

- Red/amber warning lights—on
- Headlights—off
- Fog lights—off
- Traffic directional boards operating

VEHICLE EXTRICATION

Extrication is the process by which entrapped patients are rescued from vehicles, buildings, tunnels, or other places. There are 10 phases of the extrication or rescue process that you, as an EMT, should understand:

1. Preparing for rescue
2. Sizing up the situation
3. Recognizing and managing hazards

Posted speed (mph)	Stopped distance for that speed		Posted speed (in feet)		Distance of the farthest warning device
20 mph	50 feet	+	20 feet	=	70 feet
30 mph	75 feet	+	30 feet	=	105 feet
40 mph	125 feet	+	40 feet	=	165 feet
50 mph	175 feet	+	50 feet	=	225 feet
60 mph	275 feet	+	60 feet	=	335 feet
70 mph	375 feet	+	70 feet	=	445 feet

Cones or flares are positioned according to a formula that includes the stopping distance for the posted speed plus a margin of safety.

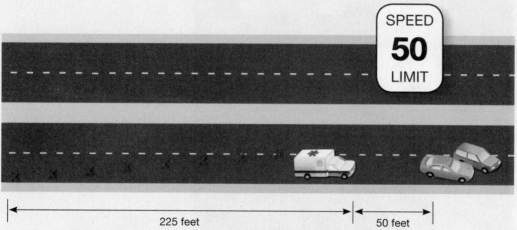

Cones or flares positioned on a straight road. Approaching vehicles are moved into the correct lane before they reach the edge of the danger zone.

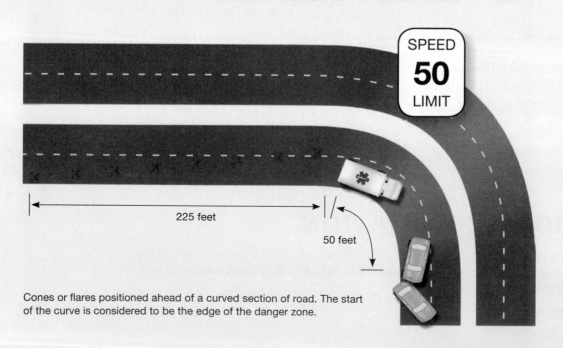

Cones or flares positioned ahead of a curved section of road. The start of the curve is considered to be the edge of the danger zone.

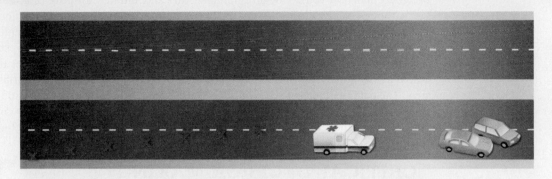

Cones or flares positioned on a hill. The flares slow approaching vehicles and make them turn into the correct lane before they reach the top of the hill.

4. Stabilizing the vehicle prior to entering

5. Gaining access to the patient

6. Providing primary patient assessment and a rapid trauma assessment

7. Disentangling the patient

8. Immobilizing and extricating the patient from the vehicle

9. Providing assessment, care, and transport to the most appropriate hospital

10. Terminating the rescue

As an EMT, you are responsible for the medical component of the rescue process; others are responsible for the mechanical or physical components. As you carry out your responsibilities, attention to safety must be your highest priority to help minimize the potential for injury to yourself and the other rescuers as well as any additional injury to your patient. Although you may never personally perform disentanglement, it is important for you to understand the rescue process so you can keep your patient informed and anticipate any dangerous steps in the extrication action plan.

Preparing for Rescue

Modern rescue is a sophisticated process. It requires preparation that is a combination of training, practice, and the right protective gear and tools. As previously noted, training and practice for specific types of rescue, including vehicle rescue, will be above and beyond your basic EMT course. The availability of such training will depend to a great extent on the kinds of rescues most likely to be required in your area. The kinds of protective gear and tools that should be available for vehicle rescue will be discussed throughout this chapter.

Sizing Up the Situation

As you arrive on the scene of a vehicle crash, it is important to conduct a good "size-up" to evaluate hazards and assess the need for additional resources. Quickly determine how many patients are involved, their priority, and the mechanisms of injury. Will additional ambulances be needed? If so, call them right away. You can always cancel them if they are not actually needed. What is the extent of the patient's entrapment? Conduct an initial triage sweep and, using START triage, as was explained in Chapter 39, "Hazardous Materials, Multiple-Casualty Incidents, and Incident Management," sort and tag the patients as soon as possible.

During scene size-up, you must be able to assess the extrication needs well enough to communicate with the extrication team and anticipate what they will be doing. Effective rescue requires a balance of medical and mechanical skills, with the right amount of each applied at the right time.

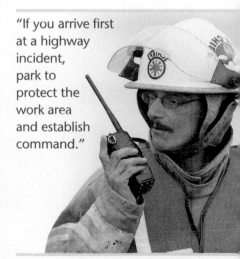

"If you arrive first at a highway incident, park to protect the work area and establish command."

During all of this, you will keep in mind that the most seriously injured patients must reach the hospital or trauma center for lifesaving surgery as quickly as possible. As the EMT, you must plan how you can begin emergency care and initiate transport as rapidly as possible.

Although a low-priority trauma patient has time for elective packaging and more time-consuming elective extrication procedures, a critical patient does not. For example, a stable patient complaining of neck pain has the time for careful short spine board or vest immobilization, whereas a high-priority trauma patient cannot afford the 15 to 20 minutes this may take. Rapid extrication to a long spine board, taking 2 minutes, may be more appropriate for this patient. The patient's medical needs must always drive the process of extrication and patient care. The principles of spinal immobilization remain the same whether the patient is low or high priority, although the requirements for speed of removal will dictate the specific technique you use.

CRITICAL DECISION MAKING

When Minutes Count, Decisions Matter

Patient priority is an important consideration in rescue operations. More time is available to gain access to a stable patient than to an unstable one who needs quick transport. Scene decisions are based both on the type of entrapment and on the patient's condition. Your responsibility as an EMT is to represent the patient's needs in the rescue effort. For each patient described here, determine whether the extrication must be done quickly because the patient is unstable or if more time is available.

1. Your patient was involved in a head-on crash. The patient is unresponsive with a rapid pulse.

2. Your patient was driving a car that was rear-ended. She is alert and oriented. Her pulse is 80, respirations are 16. The car's frame has shifted so none of the doors will open.

3. Your patient was a front-seat passenger who was thrown into the back seat. You can only reach the patient's upper body, but you find a rapid pulse and clammy skin. The patient is alert and talking with you.

Recognizing and Managing Hazards

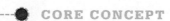

CORE CONCEPT

How to recognize and manage hazards at the highway rescue scene

As explained in the following sections, some collision-related hazards must be managed, if not eliminated, even before any attempt is made to reach injured persons in damaged vehicles.

Protective Gear for EMS Responders

At a crash, any personnel who are working in the "inner circle"—that is, the area immediately around and including the vehicle—should wear full protective gear to avoid being injured. Figure 40-5 shows an EMT dressed for a rescue operation with minimal hazards.

Protective gear is important. Get your own if your service does not provide it (most states require it on ambulances), and use it! Consider reviewing the following National Fire Protection Association standards when purchasing protective gear and uniforms: NFPA 1951 (USAR Protective Equipment), NFPA 1973 (Gloves for Structural Firefighting), and NFPA 1975 (Station/Work Uniforms).

EMS personnel have a wide selection of personal protective equipment (PPE) available to them. Until recently, most PPE was designed for structural firefighting and not for rescue/EMS operations. Today, rescuers have a wide variety of compact lightweight helmets with integral eye protection. There are now PPE garments designed for urban search and rescue (USAR) operations that are ideal for EMS. They are lightweight, breathable, and provide protection from flame, fluids, and common chemicals. This is in stark contrast to firefighter PPE, which is designed with greater insulation to provide protection from heat/flame. As a result, firefighter PPE is much heavier and more bulky.

Working in Traffic As discussed at the beginning of this chapter, being struck by a vehicle while working in traffic is a major hazard facing the EMT. As of 2009, federal highway standards require that all emergency responders wear ANSI safety vests when working in

FIGURE 40-5 An EMT dressed for rescue operations.
(© Jon Politis)

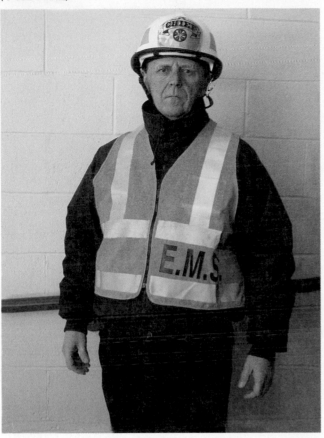

highway operations. To enhance safety, they should also wear helmets. Safety vests greatly enhance both day and night visibility, giving rescuers added protection because motorists can see them. The best way to understand this is to study Figures 40-6A and 40-6B, which show clothing with reflective elements in daytime and nighttime settings.

During Extrication Operations When extrication is in progress at a motor-vehicle collision, the rescuer has an increased exposure to flame, glass, fluids, and sharp objects. The best practice is to wear EMS or firefighter turnout clothing, including a helmet and eye protection (Figure 40-7).

FIGURE 40-6 EMTs working in traffic should be dressed for both daytime and nighttime visibility. Photo (A) shows EMTs dressed for daytime visibility. Photo (B) shows how the same clothing would appear in approaching headlights at night. *(Photos A and B: © Jon Politis)*

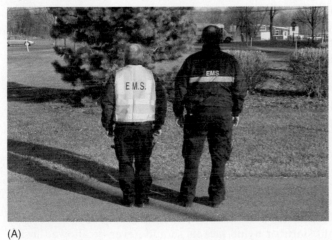

(A)

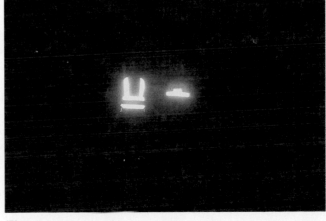

(B)

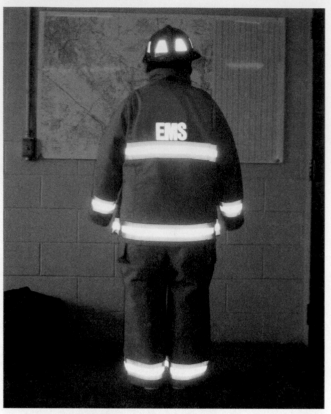

FIGURE 40-7 Full turnout gear should be worn at an extrication. *(© Jon Politis)*

Matching the Level Others Are Wearing One of the easiest ways to determine the correct PPE is to look at what other workers are doing in the industry and "match" their level of PPE. A typical construction site is a "hard hat" job. In other words, workers there are required to wear a hard hat and safety glasses. Therefore, the rescuer should wear that level of PPE, too. The highway level of PPE is a hard hat and safety vest, and at extrications one should wear full turnouts.

Helmets Wearing effective head protection is essential. One good piece of headgear that offers adequate protection is a rescue helmet that meets NFPA 1951 Standards for USAR PPE. Many EMTs prefer a model that does not have a rear brim, which can be awkward in tight spaces. Helmets with rear brims designed for fire suppression are also effective, and many EMTs prefer to use that type of PPE instead. All helmets should be brightly colored with reflective stripes and lettering to make the wearer visible both day and night, and should display the Star of Life on each side to identify the wearer as an EMS provider. The helmet should also indicate the level of training to make scene management easier when many EMS and rescue units are on hand.

Eye Protection Eye protection is vital. Hinged plastic helmet shields do not provide adequate protection; flying particles can strike the eyes from underneath or from the side. Protection is best provided by safety goggles with a soft vinyl frame that conforms to the face and provides indirect venting to keep them fog-free, or safety glasses with large lenses and side shields.

Hand Protection Because EMTs stick their hands into all sorts of unfriendly places, every EMT should have optimal hand protection. Good protection is afforded by wearing disposable vinyl or other synthetic gloves underneath either firefighter's gloves or leather gloves.

Firefighter's gloves will protect your hands from a variety of sharp, hot, cold, and dangerous surfaces. They are bulky, but can be worn in most rescue situations. If greater dexterity is needed, you can wear intermediate-weight leather gloves. Fabric garden or work gloves are too thin to offer adequate protection.

Body Protection An EMT will often protect his head, eyes, and hands but leave the body virtually unprotected. Light shirts or nylon jackets should never be allowed inside the inner circle because they do little to protect the EMT from jagged metal, broken glass, or flash fires.

Good upper body protection is offered by wearing either a short or mid-length turnout coat that meets Occupational Safety and Health Administration (OSHA) requirements. A heavy-duty EMS or rescue jacket can be used to protect you from bad weather and minor injury. As with helmets, bright colors and reflective material will help make your jacket more visible.

Good lower body protection can be provided by wearing either turnout pants with cuffs wide enough to pull over work shoes or fire-resistant trousers or jumpsuits. Serious consideration should be given to wearing high-top, steel toe work shoes with extended tops to protect the ankles.

Safeguarding Your Patient

When your patients have been injured in a collision, it is your responsibility to see to it that further injuries are not inflicted during the rescue operation. You can minimize the chance of such additional injuries by shielding the patient and exercising care. The following items can be used to protect the patient from heat, cold, flying particles, and other hazards:

- *An aluminized rescue blanket* offers protection from bad weather and, to a degree, from flying particles. A paper blanket does not afford this protection; it merely hides the patient's view of the debris that is about to strike him.

- *A lightweight vinyl-coated paper tarpaulin* can protect the patient from bad weather.

- *A wool blanket* should be used to protect the patient from cold. Cover the wool blanket with an aluminized blanket or a salvage cover whenever glass must be broken near a patient, since glass particles are just about impossible to remove from wool blankets.

- *Short and long spine boards* can shield a patient from contact with tools and debris.

- *Hard hats, safety goggles, industrial hearing protectors, disposable dust masks, and thermal masks* (in cold weather—and unless the patient has airway or breathing problems or is on oxygen) will protect a patient's head, eyes, ears, and respiratory passages.

Managing Traffic

Collisions almost always produce traffic problems. Often the wreckage blocks lanes of traffic. Even if it does not, backups are caused when curious drivers slow down to "rubberneck," or stare at the scene. Rescuers, firefighters, and police usually handle traffic control. However, what if the ambulance EMTs are responding alone or ahead of other emergency service units?

Obviously, personal safety, rescue, and emergency care have priority. However, an ambulance crew should still initiate basic traffic control, channeling vehicles past the scene. Remember to be extremely watchful and careful when you work to control traffic to be sure that you are not struck by an approaching or passing vehicle.

Your ambulance and its warning lights will serve as the first form of traffic control. However, you should position other warning devices as soon as possible. Bad weather, darkness, vegetation, and curved or hilly roadways may keep approaching motorists from seeing your ambulance soon enough to safely stop.

Using Flares for Traffic Control   Although some argue that flares are unsafe, when used properly they are still a good device for warning motorists of dangerous conditions. Moreover, several dozen flares can be carried behind the front seat of an ambulance, whereas battery-powered flashing lights—an alternative to flares—take up valuable compartment space.

Review Scan 40-1, which shows the proper positioning of cones or flares at collision scenes, including a straight road, a curved road, and a hill. Keep in mind that the stopping distance for large trucks is much greater than for cars. When the road carries truck traffic, extend the flare strings beyond the distances shown.

Remember the following points when you place flares:

- Look for and avoid spilled fuel, dry vegetation, and other combustibles before you ignite and position flares, especially at a road edge.

- Do not throw flares out of moving vehicles.

- Position a few flares at the edge of the danger zone as soon as the ambulance is parked. They will supplement the ambulance warning lights.

- Take a handful of flares and walk (carefully) toward oncoming traffic.
- Position the flares every 10 feet, if possible, to channel vehicles into an unblocked lane. (Do not turn your back to traffic while placing flares.)
- If the collision has occurred on a two-lane road, position flares in both directions.
- Never use a flare as a traffic wand; flares can spew molten phosphorous, which can cause third-degree burns to the skin.

Supplemental Restraint Systems: Air Bags

Auto air bag systems have revolutionized automobile safety. Manufacturers emphasize that air bags are not designed to replace seat belts but rather to be used in conjunction with seat belts; consequently, air bags are often referred to as *supplemental restraint systems* (SRS). Air bags are designed to inflate on impact, dissipate kinetic energy, and minimize trauma to the body. During rescue, it is important to see if an air bag has deployed.

Witnesses may have noticed "smoke" inside the vehicle during air bag deployment. This is not actually smoke but rather dust from the cornstarch or talcum used to lubricate the bag as well as from the seal and particles within the bag. The powder may contain sodium hydroxide, which can irritate the skin. For this reason, it will be important to wear protective gloves and eyewear when you gain access to the passenger compartment. It also will be important to protect the patients from getting additional dust in their eyes or wounds. Experts recommend that the EMT lift a deployed air bag and examine the steering wheel and dash, which may reveal if the patients struck any of these areas with enough energy to damage them.

One hazard to watch for is an air bag that remains undeployed after a crash. If an air bag deploys during the extrication process, it can seriously injure rescuers. To disable the air bags, the battery must be disconnected. Disconnecting the power will cause the system to power off in 2 to 3 minutes, depending on the type of system. Keep in mind that turning off the ignition alone may not disable the system, because most systems operate independently of the ignition.

Energy-Absorbing Bumpers

Most cars are equipped with 5-mile-per-hour bumpers designed to absorb low-speed front and rear-end collision forces. If the bumpers were involved in the collision, you may notice that the bumper's shock absorber system is compressed, or "loaded." Never stand in front of a loaded bumper. If it springs out and strikes your knees, it could cause serious injury. Some rescuers chain the shock absorber to prevent an uncontrolled release.

Spectators

Spectators do more than just create problems for passing motorists. If allowed to wander freely, they will close in on the wreckage just to get a better view. In fact, they may get so close that they interfere with rescue and emergency care efforts. Rescue squads, police, and fire units have personnel and equipment for crowd control; ambulances usually do not. However, an EMT can usually initiate some crowd-control measures. If local policies permit it, ask for assistance from one or more responsible-looking bystanders. Ask the persons you recruit to keep the spectators away from the danger zone. Give them a roll of barricade tape if you have one. Be sure not to put the recruited personnel in unsafe positions such as near spilled fuel or an unstable vehicle.

Electrical Hazards

Electricity poses many dangers at vehicle-collision scenes. When there is an electrical hazard, establish a danger zone and a safe zone. The danger zone should only be entered by individuals responsible for controlling the hazard, such as power company personnel or specialty rescue. The safe zone should be sufficiently far away to ensure that an arcing or moving wire could not possibly injure any of the rescue personnel or bystanders.

Keep in mind the safety points in the following list. Many have to do with taking precautions around conductors. A conductor is a wire or any other object or material that will carry electricity.

- High voltages are not as uncommon on roadside utility poles as people often think. In some areas, wood poles support conductors of as much as 500,000 volts.

- Assume that the entire area is extremely dangerous. Conductors may have touched and energized any part of the system, including electrical, telephone, cable TV, and other wires supported by the utility pole, guy wires, ground wires, the pole itself, the ground surrounding the pole, and nearby guard rails and fences. Assume that severed or displaced conductors may be touching and energizing every wire and conductor at the highest voltage present. Dead wires may be reenergized at any moment. Energized conductors may arc to the ground.
- Ordinary protective clothing does not protect against electrocution.

Remembering these points and the following procedures may keep you alive at the scene of a collision where unconfined electricity is a hazard.

Broken Utility Pole with Wires Down A broken utility pole with wires down is very dangerous. You probably cannot work safely in the area until a power company representative assures you that the power is off and the scene is safe. If you discover that a utility pole is broken and wires are down:

- Park the ambulance outside the danger zone.
- Before you leave the ambulance, be sure that no portion of the vehicle, including the radio antenna, is contacting any sagging conductors.
- Order spectators and nonessential emergency service personnel from the danger zone. Use perimeter tape to set up a large safety zone.
- Discourage occupants of the collision vehicle from leaving the wreckage.
- Prohibit traffic flow through the danger zone.
- Determine the number of the nearest pole you can safely approach, and ask your dispatcher to advise the power company of the pole number and its location.
- Do not attempt to move downed wires. Metal implements will, of course, conduct electricity, but even implements that may not appear to be conductive, such as tools with wood handles or natural fiber ropes, may have a high moisture content that will conduct electricity and may electrocute a well-intentioned rescuer.
- Stand in a safe place until the power company cuts the wires or disconnects the power.

Be especially careful when approaching a collision located in a dark area such as a rural roadside at night. As you walk from the ambulance, sweep the area ahead of you, to each side and overhead, with the beam of a powerful hand light. An energized conductor may be dangling just at head level. If you discover that a wire is down, leave the area immediately and notify the power company.

Sometimes, especially in wet weather, a phenomenon known as ground gradient may provide your first clue that a wire is down. Voltage is greatest at the point where a conductor touches the ground, then diminishes with distance from the point of contact. That distance may be several inches or many feet. Being able to recognize and respond properly to energized ground can save your life.

Stop your approach immediately if you feel a tingling sensation in your legs and lower torso. This sensation means that you are on energized ground. Current is entering one foot, passing through your lower body, and exiting through your other foot. If you continue on, you risk being electrocuted!

Turn 180 degrees and take one of two escape measures. Hop to a safe place on one foot. Alternatively, shuffle away from the danger area with both feet together, allowing no break in contact between your two feet or between your feet and the ground. Either technique helps prevent your body from completing a circuit with energized ground, which can cause electrocution. (A circuit is a circular path for electrical flow, such as up one leg, down the other, and through the ground. Hopping on one leg or keeping your feet together creates a straight path rather than a circular circuit, which may prevent electrocution.)

Broken Utility Pole with Wires Intact Even if wires are intact, a broken utility pole is still dangerous. Wires that are still holding up the pole can break at any time, dropping the pole and wires onto the scene. If you arrive to find such a situation:

- Park the ambulance outside the danger zone.
- Notify your dispatcher of the situation.

- Stay outside the danger zone until power company representatives can deenergize the conductors and stabilize the pole.
- Keep spectators and other emergency service personnel out of the danger zone.

Damaged Pad-Mounted Transformer When electrical cables run underground, the transformer may be mounted on a pad above ground (Figure 40-8). When an aboveground pad-mounted electrical transformer is struck and damaged, it poses a serious threat. In such a situation:

- Request an immediate power company response.
- Do not touch either the transformer case or a vehicle touching it, and warn other emergency service personnel not to touch it, either.
- Stand in a safe place until the power company deenergizes the transformer.
- Keep spectators out of the danger zone.

Vehicle Fires

When you find a vehicle on fire, always request the response of firefighting apparatus. Do not assume that someone else has called the fire department. In fact, fire apparatus should always stand by during vehicle extrication.

Extinguishing a vehicle fire is the responsibility of persons who are trained and equipped for the job: firefighters. Nonetheless, there are some measures that trained EMTs can take when they arrive before fire units (Scan 40-2).

For small fires, a 15- or 20-pound class A:B:C dry chemical fire extinguisher can extinguish virtually anything that may be burning in a vehicle, including upholstery, fuel, and electrical components. Only burning magnesium and other flammable metals cannot be extinguished by an A:B:C extinguisher. Before you try to put out a fire, always put on a full set of protective gear.

Fire in the Engine Compartment If the hood is fully open, stand close to an A-post (front roof-supporting post) of the vehicle and, if possible, with your back to the wind to guard against the agent blowing back into your face or entering the passenger compartment. (Dry chemical extinguishing agents irritate respiratory passages and may contaminate open wounds.) Then sweep the extinguisher across the base of the fire with short bursts. Use no more than necessary to extinguish the fire. You will need what is left if there is a subsequent flare-up.

If the hood is open to the safety latch, do not raise the hood farther—leave it where it is. This will help to restrict air flow and deprive the fire of oxygen. Direct the agent through any opening to the engine compartment: between hood and fender, around the grill, under a wheel well, or through a broken head lamp assembly. Again, use no more agent than is needed.

If the hood is closed tight, let the fire burn under the closed hood, leaving its extinguishment to the fire department, and continue to get the patients out of the vehicle. The firewall should protect the passenger area long enough to get the patients out of the vehicle, using emergency moves.

FIGURE 40-8 A pad-mounted transformer, if damaged, poses a serious threat.

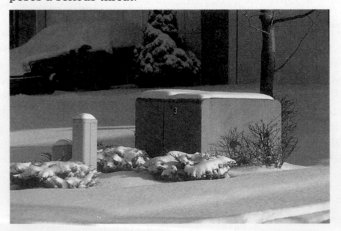

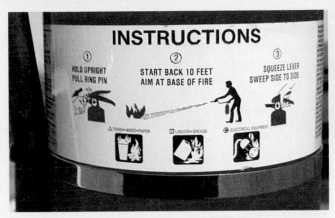

Markings that identify an extinguisher that can be used for Class A, B, and C fires.

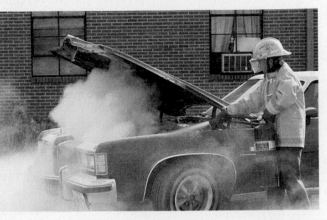

Extinguishing a fire in the engine compartment when the hood is fully open.

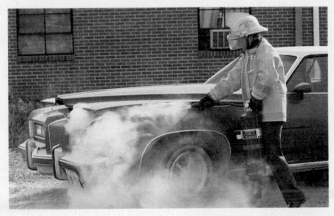

Extinguishing a fire in the engine compartment when the hood is partially open.

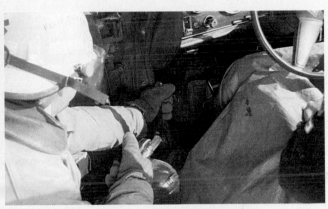

Extinguishing a fire under the dash. Care must be taken not to fill the vehicle's interior with a cloud of agent.

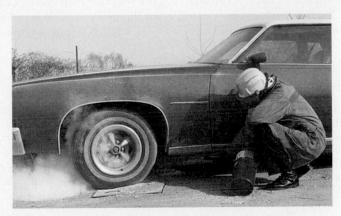

Extinguishing fuel burning under a vehicle. Flames are swept away from the vehicle.

Fire in the Passenger Compartment or Trunk   If the fire is under the dash or in upholstery or other combustibles, carefully apply the agent directly to the burning material. Apply sparingly to avoid creating a cloud of powder that may be harmful to occupants. If there is fire in the trunk, as with fire under a closed hood, leave extinguishment to the fire department and continue working to get patients out of the vehicle.

Fire under the Vehicle   Using a portable unit to extinguish burning fuel under a vehicle may be an exercise in futility when the spill is large. However, when people are trapped in the vehicle, you may feel the urge to try. Attempt to sweep the flames from under the passenger compartment as you apply the agent. If you do extinguish the fire, be sure that sources of ignition are then kept away. The vehicle's own catalytic converter (usually found in the area under the front passenger's feet) can be an ignition source since its temperature can reach over 1,200 degrees.

Truck Fires   An A:B:C extinguisher can also be used to combat truck fires. Be aware, however, that burning truck tires are especially dangerous. Flames can quickly spread to the vehicle's body and its cargo, or the tires can blow apart when heated by fire. *Never* stand directly in front of a truck wheel when there is a fire; instead, approach from a 45-degree angle.

NOTE: *At times you will find that fuel is leaking from a damaged vehicle but is not on fire. If you discover that a fuel tank is leaking, call for fire department response. The decision to continue the rescue effort should be governed by your perception of the danger. You should not be expected to continue rescue operations if gasoline is pooled under the vehicle or flowing toward a source of ignition. Warn spectators away from flowing fuel. Do not use flares near spilled fuel or in the path of flowing fuel. Watch where you park your vehicle, as your ambulance's catalytic converter can easily ignite spilled fuel or other combustibles.*

Disabling a Vehicle's Electrical System

Many rescue units routinely disable the electrical system of every collision vehicle by cutting a battery cable. Unless gasoline is pooled under a vehicle or undeployed air bags need to be disabled, cutting the battery out of the electrical system may not only be a waste of time, it may actually hinder the rescue operation. Remember that many cars have electrically powered door locks, window operators, and seat adjustment mechanisms. Being able to lower a window rather than breaking it eliminates the likelihood of spraying occupants with glass. Being able to operate door locks may eliminate the need to force doors open. And being able to operate a powered seat will create space in front of an injured driver.

If there is a reason to disrupt the electrical system, disconnect the negative cable from the battery. In this way, you will not be likely to produce a spark that can drop onto spilled fuel or ignite battery gases. Such a spark can be created when the positive cable is pulled away from the battery terminal, or when a tool touches a metal component while in contact with the positive terminal or cable.

Stabilizing a Vehicle

CORE CONCEPT
How to stabilize a vehicle

Unstable collision vehicles pose a hazard to rescuers and patients alike. Scan 40-3 shows methods for stabilizing a vehicle involved in a collision.

NOTE: *Rescuers often fail to stabilize a collision vehicle because it appears to be stable. Rather than taking the chance of incorrectly "reading" a collision vehicle's stability— and having the vehicle move during rescue with disastrous results—you should consider any collision vehicle from which patients need to be extricated to be unstable and act accordingly.*

If your ambulance is equipped with stabilization equipment, you should attend a formal vehicle rescue course that includes basic stabilization procedures taught by a qualified instructor. If the ambulance is not equipped for stabilization procedures, or if you are not trained, stand by until a rescue unit has stabilized the vehicle, even if roof posts are intact and the vehicle appears to be stable.

The information on vehicle stabilization that follows is intended only to help you, as an EMT, understand the process that trained personnel will be following. It is not a substitute for formal training in stabilization procedures.

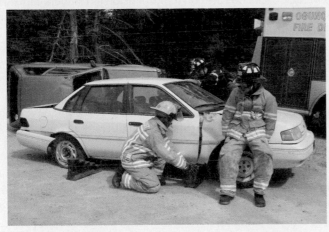

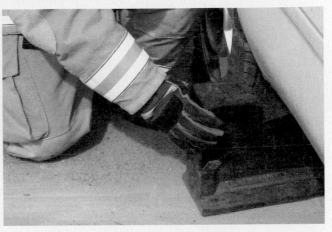

Stabilizing a car on its wheels with cribbing while patient contact is initiated.

A vehicle on its side stabilized with cribbing.

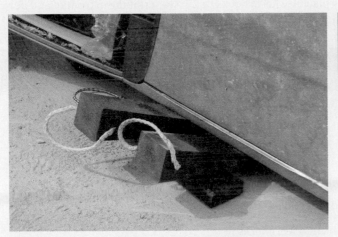

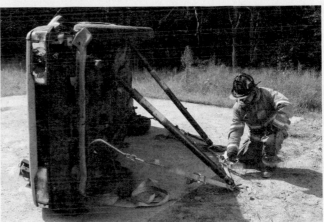

Placing a step chock. Keep the hands clear of the vehicle while placing the chock.

A vehicle on its side stabilized with struts.

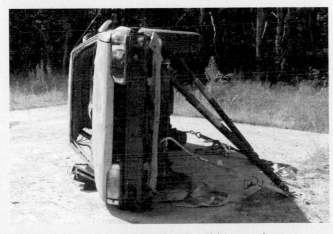

A vehicle on its side stabilized with cribbing and struts.

Vehicle on Its Wheels

A collision vehicle that is upright on four inflated tires looks stable. However, it is easily rocked up and down, side to side, and back and forth on its suspension as rescuers climb into and over it. These motions can seriously aggravate occupants' injuries. First, if rescuers have access to the inside of the vehicle, they should make sure the engine is turned off, the vehicle is in park, the keys are removed from the ignition, and the parking brake is set. The best method of stabilizing a vehicle on its wheels is using three step chocks, one on each side and a third under the front or back of the vehicle.

Then—in situations where significant "tool work" must be done to extricate, such as door or roof removal—all the tires should be deflated. This can be accomplished by simply pulling the valve stems from their casing with pliers. (Slashing the tires is an inappropriate technique for deflating tires.) A police officer should be told the tires have been deflated so investigators will not think that the tires are flat as a result of the collision.

> **NOTE:** *Tires do not need to be deflated in all crashes—only in situations where significant "tool work," such as door or roof removal, must be done to extricate a patient or patients.*

A listing of the equipment that can be carried to stabilize a vehicle and gain access appears in Table 40-1. If the ambulance is not equipped with step chocks, a degree of stabilization can be accomplished by placing wheel chocks or 2" × 4" cribbing in front of and behind two tires on the same side.

Table 40-1 Supplies and Equipment for Vehicle Stabilization and Gaining Access

QUANTITY	ITEM
10	2" × 4" × 8" cribbing
10	4" × 4" × 18" cribbing
4	Step chocks
6	Wood wedges
2	Vehicle wheel chocks
100 feet	Nylon 1/2" utility rope
2 sets	Struts
1	"Door-and-window kit" with hand tools such as. . . 1 pair, battery pliers 1 12" adjustable wrench 1 3- or 4-pound drilling hammer 1 spring-loaded center punch 2 hacksaws with spare blades 1 10" locking-type pliers 1 10" water-pump pliers Several 12" to 15" flat prybars 1 8" flat blade screwdriver 1 12" flat blade screwdriver 1 spray container of power steering fluid as a lubricant
1	Flathead ax
1	Glas-Master windshield saw
1	Combination forcible entry tool such as a Halligan or Biel tool
500 feet	Perimeter tape

If a car has rolled over several times and comes to rest on its wheels, the roof may be crushed, which may preclude access through windows. In this case, the roof may need to be raised before doors can be opened or the roof can be removed.

> **NOTE:** *When placing cribbing, never kneel on both knees. Always squat, so you can quickly move away from the vehicle if you have to. Once the vehicle is stabilized, if a door must be opened, tie it in the fully open position before you try to crawl inside.*

Vehicle on Its Side

When a vehicle is on its side, spectators will often attempt to push it back onto its wheels. They fail to realize that this movement may injure, or more severely injure, the vehicle's occupants. Instead, the vehicle should be stabilized on its side. If the vehicle is on its side, do not attempt to gain access before it is stabilized using ropes, stabilization struts, and/or cribbing. Although a car on its side may appear stable, simply climbing onto one side in an attempt to open a door may cause the vehicle to drop onto its roof or wheels. Moreover, you can be trapped under the vehicle when it topples.

A person who will act as a safety guide can be placed at each end of the vehicle to "feel" the vehicle's movement and quickly warn the rescuers who are placing cribbing, struts, or ropes to get back if the vehicle begins to fall over. Some services will deploy two ropes looped around the same wheel in both directions so that personnel can temporarily hold the vehicle stable while placing struts and/or cribbing. There are many ways to stabilize a vehicle on its side, from using manpower alone to using hydraulic rams and pneumatic jacks. The objective is to increase the number of contacts with the ground to make the vehicle on its side more stable.

Vehicle on Its Roof

If the vehicle is resting on its roof, roof posts are intact, and the vehicle appears stable, it may be tempting to try to reach the vehicle's occupants by gaining access through window or door openings—immediately, and without stabilizing the vehicle. However, if the posts collapse, as is often the case when the windshield integrity has been broken, the vehicle may come crashing down and injure the EMT who is attempting to climb into the vehicle or who has an arm in a window opening. You must wait to gain access until the rescue crew has stabilized the vehicle. This is usually accomplished by building a box crib with 4 × 4s under the vehicle.

A vehicle on its roof is likely to be in one of four positions:

- Horizontal, with the roof crushed flat against the vehicle's body and both the trunk lid and hood contacting the ground
- Horizontal, resting entirely on the roof, with space between the hood and the ground and space between the trunk lid and the ground
- Front end down, with the front edge of the hood contacting the ground and the rear of the car supported by the C-posts (rear posts)
- Front end up, with the trunk lid contacting the ground and much of the weight of the vehicle supported by the A-posts (front posts)

If the vehicle is tilted with the engine, which is the heaviest part of the vehicle, on the ground and the trunk in the air, it can often be stabilized by using two step chocks upside down under the trunk.

When the roof is crushed flat against the body, as when all the roof posts have collapsed, the car is essentially a steel box resting on the ground with the occupants completely trapped inside. Unless the vehicle is on a hill or perched precariously on debris or another vehicle, this is the one time when stabilization is unnecessary. The structure is rigid. In such a situation, it may be impossible to gain access through a window, door, or the roof. However, it may be possible to cut through the floor pan and have an EMT either crawl inside, if the opening is big enough or the EMT small enough, or to reach through the opening to touch and offer emotional support to the occupants until rescue personnel can lift or open the vehicle.

If the vehicle is unstable and cannot be safely approached by an EMT, get as close as you safely can so you can talk or signal to the occupants to reassure them that help is on its way and begin getting an idea of their condition.

Remember that when the vehicle is found in any of the previously described positions, it should be considered unstable and must be stabilized by trained personnel prior to entry by an EMT.

Gaining Access

CORE CONCEPT

How to gain access to the patient in a crashed vehicle

Why does a car door not fly open in a crash? The answer is the Nader pin (named for Ralph Nader, the consumer advocate who lobbied for the device), a case-hardened pin in an automobile door. In a collision, the cams in the door locks grasp the pin to keep the door from flying open, preventing occupants from being thrown from the vehicle. All cars sold in the United States since 1966 have the Nader pin.

The Nader pin is a safety device, since being thrown from a vehicle is far more dangerous than being kept inside during a crash. However, the device does make gaining access to vehicle occupants more difficult. Prior to the Nader pin, rescue personnel could open a door with a crowbar. Subsequently, rescuers had to start using a hydraulic spreader to peel the cams off the pins. Ironically, safety features designed to keep occupants inside wrecked vehicles were keeping rescuers out! Each new safety improvement to vehicles created a new challenge to rescue personnel.

Vehicle rescue training became a complicated business, and rescuers were asked to learn dozens of techniques, some of which could be used only on certain models of cars. The need for effective but simplified procedures became evident. The next few pages will describe a procedure that has been developed to meet this need.

Simple Access

First, remember that, as an EMT, your responsibility is not to rescue the vehicle but to rescue the patient. You will usually assume that an occupant or occupants of the vehicle have sustained life-threatening injuries, and that at least one EMT needs to gain quick access to the patient, even while rescuers are working to gain a more wide-open access, create exitways, and disentangle occupants.

After the vehicle is stable enough for you to approach it safely, check to see if a door can be opened or if an occupant of the vehicle can roll down a window or unlock a door. (Try Before You Pry!) Such ordinary ways of getting into the vehicle are known as simple access.

Complex Access

If simple access fails, you may need to use tools or special equipment to break a window and gain access even while the rescue crew is dismantling the vehicle for extrication of the occupants (Figure 40-9). When tools or equipment are used for this purpose, the process is known as complex access.

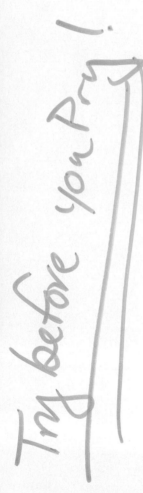

FIGURE 40-9 Complex access involves the use of tools and equipment to reach and extricate the patient. (© Edward T. Dickinson, MD)

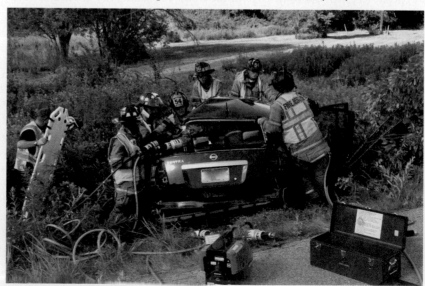

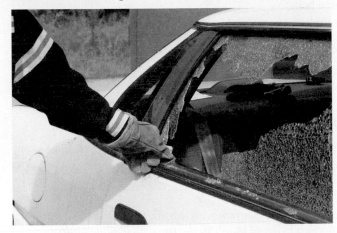

FIGURE 40-11 A Glas-Master saw can aid in windshield removal.

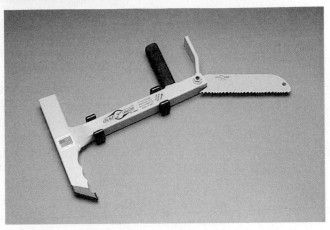

All automotive glass is one of two types: laminated or tempered. Windshields and some side and rear van and truck windows are laminated safety glass—two sheets of plate glass bonded to a sheet of tough plastic like a glass-and-plastic sandwich. Most passenger car side and rear windows are tempered glass. They are very resilient, but when they do break, rather than shattering into sharp fragments, they break into small, rounded pieces.

You will usually try to gain access through a side or rear window as far as possible from the passengers. Use a spring-loaded center punch against a lower corner to break the glass (Figure 40-10). Punch out finger holds in the top of the window and use your gloved fingers to pull fragments away from the window.

A flathead ax is usually required to break through a windshield. This can also be done very quickly using a Glas-Master saw (Figure 40-11). Although a windshield is usually not broken to gain access, the rescue squad may need to remove it if they plan to displace the dash or steering column or remove the roof. Before breaking the windshield, cover the passengers with aluminized rescue blankets or tarps, if possible. Avoid the use of hospital-style blankets that will allow the tiny slivers of glass to pass through and come in contact with the patient.

Once you gain an entry point, at least one EMT, who is properly dressed, should crawl inside the vehicle and immediately begin the primary assessment and rapid trauma assessment, as well as manual cervical stabilization. Do not forget to explain what is going on and provide emotional support to the patient by talking and reassuring him that everything that can be done for him is being done. Access holes are usually small, so do not be tempted to pull a patient out of an access hole prior to spinal immobilization.

Disentanglement: A Three-Part Action Plan

In most instances, EMTs will not be directly involved in disentanglement other than to act as the patient's advocate and be the EMT inside the vehicle. However, it is helpful to understand the plan for complex access that may be used by rescue personnel to free the trapped patient.

The following is a description of a three-part procedure that can be accomplished by fire, rescue, and EMS personnel with the appropriate equipment. The procedure is not vehicle-specific; that is, it can be used on virtually any car or truck. Furthermore, the procedure does not include a lot of techniques that require special equipment. Personnel can be trained in a short course. Most important to EMS personnel, there is no need to fill several compartments of the ambulance with rescue equipment.

Steps One and Two: Gain Access by Disposing of Doors and the Roof For more than 25 years, emergency service personnel have been trained to carry out a progression of procedures to reach the occupants of a wrecked vehicle: first try the doors; if that fails, unlock and unlatch the doors by nondestructive or destructive means; when all else fails, gain access through window openings. However, this multipart procedure is time-consuming and requires a number of tools.

CORE CONCEPT

How to disentangle a patient from a crashed vehicle

A quicker and far more efficient procedure is first to dispose of the doors and then to dispose of the roof as soon as hazards have been controlled and the vehicle is stable. Disposing of the doors and roof has three benefits:

- It makes the interior of the vehicle accessible. EMS personnel can stand beside or climb into the vehicle and pursue emergency care efforts while rescuers carry out disentanglement procedures.

- It creates a large exitway through which an occupant can be quickly removed when he has a life-threatening injury or when fire or another hazard is threatening the operation.

- It provides fresh air and helps cool off the patient when heat is a problem.

Scan 40-4 illustrates procedures for removing the doors and roof using hydraulic tools. If you don't have a hydraulic rescue tool, you can accomplish these procedures with ordinary hacksaws and a spray container of lubricant.

NOTE: *After roof posts are cut and/or doors removed, ensure that all sharp edges are covered with appropriate protection to avoid injury to the rescuers and the patient.*

Step Three: Disentangle Occupants by Displacing the Front End Most vehicle rescue training courses include procedures for displacing or removing seats, dash assemblies, steering wheels, steering columns, and pedals. A quicker and more efficient way to disentangle an injured driver and/or passenger from these mechanisms of entrapment is to displace the entire front end of the vehicle. Although the task sounds difficult, it is not. Scan 40-5 illustrates a procedure for displacing the front end of a passenger car with a hydraulic rescue tool. A dash displacement can also be accomplished with heavy-duty jacks and hacksaws.

If the steering wheel hub is large and rectangular, the car probably has an air bag or bags (the passenger-side bag being in the glove compartment area). If the bags have not deployed, they are not likely to deploy now unless extrication involves displacing the dash or steering wheel. If such displacement is to be done, air bag manufacturers recommend following these guidelines:

- Disconnect the battery cables, starting with the negative terminal.
- Avoid placing your body or objects against an air bag module or in its path of deployment. (Even after disconnecting the battery cables, a slight electrical charge capable of deploying an air bag remains.)
- Do not displace or cut the steering column until the system has been fully deactivated.
- Do not cut or drill into an air bag module.
- Do not apply heat in the area of the steering wheel hub.

You may wonder, must the three-part procedure just described be used for all extrication operations? Must the three procedures always be accomplished in the same order? Must these procedures always be used? Not at all. In some cases, it may be necessary only to force a door open to reach a single patient and create an exitway for his removal. In other cases, it may be prudent to open doors before disposing of the roof or to dispose of the roof before displacing the doors. In still other situations, there may be no need to displace the front end of a collision vehicle.

The extent to which you, as an EMT, will participate in vehicle rescue procedures depends on the role your EMS unit plays in vehicle rescue and whether or not your ambulance arrives ahead of fire and rescue units. The main purpose for the EMT to know extrication procedures is to incorporate them into the patient care plan.

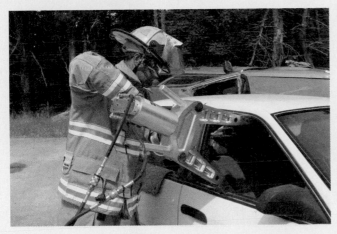

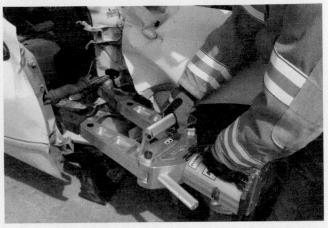

Displace the door to expose hinges and move the door away from the patient compartment.

Remove the door.

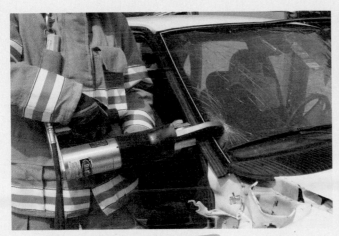

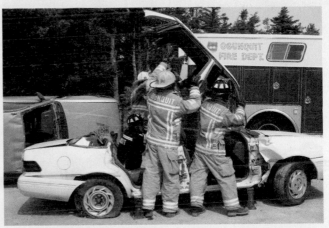

Cut the A-post to begin roof removal.

With B- and C-posts cut, roll the roof away while a rescuer enters the rear seat to stabilize the patient's head and neck.

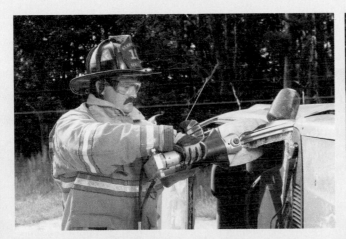

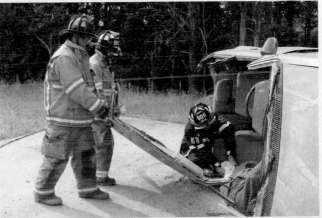

For a vehicle on its side, cut the posts.

Then remove the roof to expose and extricate the patient.

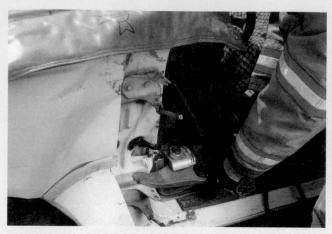

Make cuts for the spreader tool.

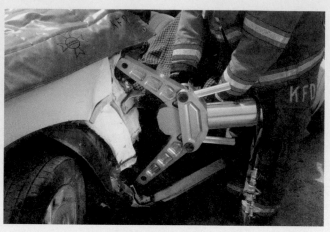

Use the spreader to roll back the dash.

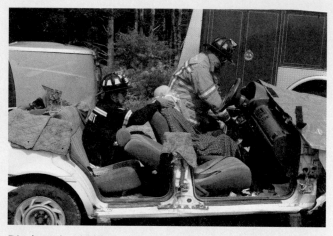

Displace the dashboard to gain access to the patient.

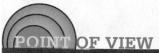

POINT OF VIEW

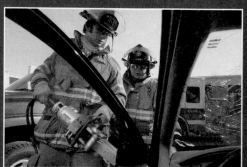

"I was driving along, minding my own business, when a truck pulled out from a side street in front of me. It was a horrible crash. I can still hear the loud crunch and breaking glass. I should say I can still feel it. It was awful. My air bags went off. I was sitting in a cloud of dust.

"I tried to get out and I couldn't. The door wouldn't open. Then I noticed that my ankle was killing me. My foot was wedged under the gas pedal.

"I was upset. OK, I was freaking out. In fact, I was pretty irrational when the ambulance got there. They tried to calm me down and told me the fire department was on the way to get me out. I was getting calmer until I saw and heard those giant whatchamacallits they were going to use to cut—yes, cut—me out. Then they put a blanket over me so I'd be safe. I was never claustrophobic—until then. I don't mean to be a whiner, but that really shook me!

"They got me out of the car on a board and into the ambulance, but by the time I got to the hospital I was shaking and spent. What an ordeal. I don't want to imply for a minute that the EMTs and firefighters were any less than professional. They were great. But let me tell you, that was a day I don't ever want to live through again.

"Oh, no. I never thought about my car. I'll bet it's in pieces. Oh, no...."

Key Facts and Concepts

- Remember, highway operations are *high risk*. Take these precautions:
  - Wear high-visibility garments.
  - Position the ambulance for blocking until fire apparatus arrives. Then position ambulances "downstream" in the safe zone.
  - Reduce lighting that may blind passing drivers.
  - Avoid crossing traffic lanes with patients.
- Scene size-up is key. How many patients are there? What is the triage status? Are additional resources needed?
- Protect yourself. Look out for:
  - Traffic
  - Undeployed air bags (Disconnect the battery to deactivate the air bag system.)

- Loaded bumpers
- Sharp metal

  Match the level of PPE being worn by other public safety responders.

- Ensure scene safety:
  - If wires are down, keep spectators back! If wires are over an occupied car, don't allow the occupants to exit until the power company deactivates the wires.
  - Make sure the vehicle is stable! Be sure it won't roll away or tip over.
- First try simple means to gain access.
- Protect your patient during the extrication process.

Key Decisions

- What is the best access to the scene for my unit? Is my unit needed on the limited-access highway?
- What level of PPE and what high-visibility garments do I need at this scene?
- If I am first in, where should I park the apparatus?

- How many patients are there? What are the triage priorities?
- Can patients be accessed and extricated by simple means?
- Does the battery need to be disconnected?
- Does the vehicle need to be stabilized?

Preparation for Your Examination and Practice

Short Answer

1. If your EMS unit is first to arrive on the scene, what initial actions should you take?
2. What gear should be worn at the scene of a highway incident to improve your visibility to others?
3. What gear should be worn during a vehicle extrication?
4. What must be done to deactivate automobile air bags?
5. You have arrived at a crash and all the doors look jammed. What steps should you take to gain access? In what order?

Thinking and Linking

Think back to Chapter 39, "Hazardous Materials, Multiple-Casualty Incidents, and Incident Management," and link information from that chapter with information from this chapter as you consider the following situations:

1. One of the vehicles involved in a highway crash is a tanker that is now leaking some unidentified substance. What steps are required at this scene that would not be necessary at a "simple" two-car crash?
2. The highway crash you are dispatched to is a seven-car pile-up. Your unit is first on-scene. What steps are required that would differ from those for crashes involving one car striking a tree?

Critical Thinking Exercises

Rescue scenes require decision making of a type that more "normal" calls may not require. The purpose of this exercise will be to consider how you might make decisions specific to a rescue scene.

1. With knowledge of your own community, which of the 10 types of rescue specialty teams are needed and who provides the service?

2. After considering the safety of yourself and others, what should be your primary goal at the scene of a vehicle collision?

You're on the scene of a one-car crash into a telephone pole. You position the ambulance about 50 feet behind the crash site with warning lights on, and both you and your partner put on full turnout gear including helmet, gloves, eye protection, and a reflective vest.

To control traffic, your partner places flares over a 200-foot section leading to the scene. You look around to make sure that there are no wires in the area and none on the vehicle. The scene appears to be safe. You go to the patient, notice the passenger side is intruded 2 feet, and see only one passenger, the driver. Two wheels of the vehicle are up on the sidewalk and the car appears to be unstable. You identify yourself to the occupant but don't get a response. Next, you try to open the door, but it is jammed. You decide the car must have spun around as you observe more damage on the driver's side of the vehicle. You advise dispatch that heavy rescue is needed.

Street Scene Questions

1. What are the scene safety issues that you need to address?
2. What techniques should you consider for extrication?

Heavy rescue has an ETA of 10 minutes. The patient isn't responding, so you and your partner agree that entry is needed now. First, you put blocks at the wheels to make sure the car doesn't shift. Next, you pick a spot on the window that seems to place the patient at lowest risk, use a punch, and start removing glass. Once inside, you observe that your patient is a male about 30 years old with snoring respirations. You perform a primary assessment and find he is only responsive to painful stimuli. The snoring respirations stop when you move his jaw forward and manually stabilize his head and neck, but his breathing remains irregular. You administer oxygen, and you suspect that you may need to start assisting respirations. At that moment, heavy rescue arrives and you report the scene status and patient condition.

Street Scene Questions

3. Should rapid extrication be considered for this patient?
4. Describe assessment for this patient.

The lieutenant of heavy rescue tells you he will handle the battery disconnect and have his crew check to see if more cribbing is needed for vehicle stability. You maintain an airway and manual stabilization of the patient from inside the vehicle while your partner applies a cervical collar and leaves to prepare the backboard. Rescue is able to pop a door open and allow full access to the patient. You are just about to say that the patient is clear when you see his foot is caught under a pedal. You tell the lieutenant from heavy rescue about the patient's trapped foot, and his crew sets up a small hydraulic jack. You make sure the patient is protected.

Once the foot is free, you and your partner decide that a rapid extrication is the best approach and move the patient to the board. When the patient is outside the vehicle, your partner is able to perform a rapid trauma assessment while you maintain manual stabilization. He checks the chest and it seems okay (the patient was wearing a seat belt).

The patient's respiration rate is about 28 and slightly irregular; ventilatory assistance is not needed yet. His pulse is 90 and regular. The patient is secured to the board and taken to the ambulance for further assessment and transport to the hospital. Considering the damage to the vehicle, you're surprised that the only injuries you find are a bump on the left side of the patient's head and a swollen left ankle. By the time you get to the hospital, the patient is responding to verbal stimuli.

Later that day you are curious about this patient and call the hospital. The charge nurse tells you the patient suffered only a concussion and a bruised ankle and he will stay overnight for observation.

EMS Response to Terrorism

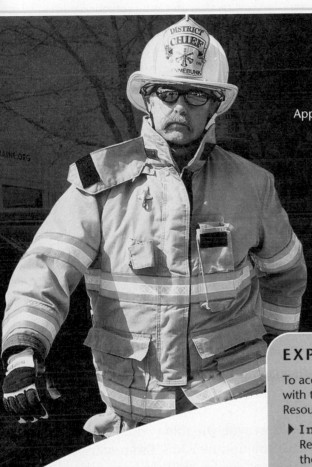

41

STANDARDS ◯------

EMS Operations (Terrorism and Disaster)

COMPETENCY ◯------

Applies knowledge of operational roles and responsibilities to ensure patient, public, and personnel safety.

CORE CONCEPTS ◯------

— Types of terrorism and terrorist events

— How to identify the type of threat posed by a terrorist event

— Use of time/distance/shielding for protection at a terrorist event

How to respond to and deal with harms from a terrorist event

— Applying strategy and tactics at a terrorist event

— Self-protection at a terrorist event

EXPLORE Resource Central

To access Resource Central, follow directions on the Student Access Card provided with this text. If there is no card, go to **www.bradybooks.com** and follow the Resource Central link to Buy Access from there. Under Media Resources, you will find:

▶ **Information Pertaining to Terrorist Threats**
Read about terrorist threats in our nation and what is being done to combat these threats.

▶ **Information about Blast Injuries**
Learn how to identify a patient with a blast lung injury and what the protocol is for treating this patient in the prehospital environment.

▶ **Adoption of Standards for Hazardous Materials/WMD**
Find out what standards have been established for EMTs dealing with hazardous materials and weapons of mass destruction and how you can benefit from these guidelines.

OBJECTIVES

After reading this chapter you should be able to:

41.1 Define key terms introduced in this chapter.

41.2 List the "CBRNE" agents, also called weapons of mass destruction, that are often involved in terrorist incidents. (p. 1066)

41.3 Describe the risks to first responders in terrorism incidents. (pp. 1066–1067)

41.4 Discuss clues, such as occupancy or location, type of event, timing of events, and on-scene warning signs that help with identificaiton of suspicious events. (pp. 1067–1069)

41.5 Given a scenario involving a terrorism incident, predict the types of harm that may occur. (pp. 1069–1070)

(continued)

41.6 Discuss the principles of time, distance, and shielding that may minimize exposure to harm from terrorism incidents. (p. 1070)

41.7 Discuss types of harm and self-protection measures for each of the following:
  a. Chemical incident (pp. 1070–1071)
  b. Biological incident (pp. 1071–1074)
  c. Radiological/nuclear incident (p. 1074)
  d. Explosive incident (p. 1075)

41.8 Discuss how chemical and biological agents can be disseminated and weaponized. (pp. 1075–1077)

41.9 Describe the characteristics associated with the following:
  a. Chemical agents (pp. 1077–1078)
  b. Biological agents (pp. 1079–1087)
  c. Radiological/nuclear devices (pp. 1087–1088)
  d. Incendiary devices (p. 1088)

41.10 Describe blast injury patterns and treatment for blast injuries. (pp. 1088–1089)

41.11 Discuss strategy, tactics, and self-protection with regard to a terrorist incident. (pp. 1089–1095)

KEY TERMS

Terrorism is nothing new on the planet. Its history dates back hundreds of years to the Dark Ages. Just since the early 1900s, there have been thousands of bombings and incendiary devices used for terrorist purposes. Of course, EMS has had a prominent part in responding to violent acts since its inception in the early 1970s.

Since the terrorist attacks of September 11, 2001, however, the role of emergency responders has been redefined. Emergency services provided by EMS, fire rescue, and law enforcement are now defined by the U.S. government as one of five parts of the National Critical Infrastructure—the infrastructure considered to be critical to the continued operation of our nation.

EMS is a key part of the public safety net, the support network that ensures the safety and health of our citizens (Figure 41-1). Thus, the evolution of EMS involves not only improvements in emergency medical care but a constant refinement of the response mission as well.

>>>>>> DEFINING TERRORISM

CORE CONCEPT
Types of terrorism and terrorist events

The U.S. Department of Justice, Federal Bureau of Investigation (FBI), defines *terrorism* as "the unlawful use of force or violence against persons or property to intimidate or coerce a government, the civilian population or any segment thereof, in furtherance of political or social objectives."

The Federal Bureau of Investigation further defines two types of terrorism that occur in the United States: domestic terrorism and international terrorism.

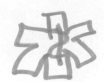

FIGURE 41-1 After the September 11, 2001 terrorist attacks, the U.S. Department of Homeland Security inaugurated color codes to indicate current threat levels. (The yellow "elevated" level, shown here outside the Portland, Maine, Police and Fire building, was the middle of five levels.) In 2011, the color code system was abandoned and replaced with a more specific public alert system.

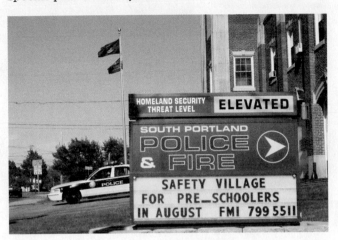

Domestic Terrorism

Domestic terrorism involves groups or individuals whose terrorist activities are directed at the government or population, without foreign direction. Domestic terrorism is changing, moving away from structured organizations to a fragmented, leaderless phenomenon in which individuals or small groups act independently in planning and executing their attacks.

Although we usually associate terrorism with those of foreign birth, a disturbing trend has been the radicalization of some American citizens by certain elements of Islam and other religions and political groups. Some American would-be terrorists are indoctrinated overseas in terrorist training camps; for example, the "shoe bomber," who attempted to blow up an American Airlines flight in 2001, as well as the man who attempted to detonate a car bomb in Times Square in 2010. Others, such as the shooter on the Fort Hood army base in Texas who killed 13 people and wounded 30 others in 2009 (Figure 41-2), have seemingly become radicalized via the Internet. Radicalization is also a growing phenomenon among prison populations in the United States. Since the 9/11 attacks, there have been over 46 publicly reported cases of radicalization, involving over 125 American citizens.

Domestic terrorist groups or individuals can be fueled by a range of motivations. A wide variety of domestic terrorist groups and individuals have been identified, including environmental terrorists, survivalists, militias, racial-hate groups, and groups with extreme political, religious, or other philosophies or beliefs.

International Terrorism

International terrorism involves groups or individuals whose terrorist activities are foreign-based and/or directed by countries or groups outside the targeted country or whose activities cross national boundaries. One trend in international terrorism is the shift from well-organized, state-sponsored localized groups to loosely organized, international networks of terrorists. The Al Qaeda network is an example.

These loosely networked individuals and groups have increasingly turned to a variety of sources of funding, including private sponsorship, drug trafficking, crime, and illegal trade. Concurrently, there is a growing trend away from terrorism that is politically motivated to terrorism that is religiously or ideologically motivated.

terrorism
the unlawful use of force or violence against persons or property to intimidate or coerce a government, the civilian population, or any segment thereof, in furtherance of political or social objectives (U.S. Department of Justice, FBI, definition).

domestic terrorism
terrorism directed against the government or population without foreign direction.

international terrorism
terrorism that is foreign-based or directed.

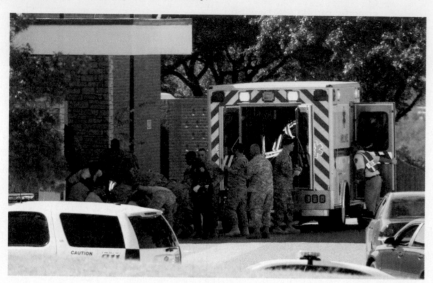

FIGURE 41-2 In this image released by the U.S. Army, wounded are prepared for transport in waiting ambulances outside Fort Hood's Soldier Readiness Processing Center, Thursday, November 5, 2009, in Fort Hood, Texas. Army psychiatrist Major Nidal Malik Hasan was accused of firing more than 100 rounds at the base, killing 13 and wounding others, in the soldier processing center at Fort Hood.
(© AP Photo/U.S. Army, Jeramie Sivley)

Types of Terrorism Incidents

In addition to armed attacks, incidents of terrorism may involve what are often called the CBRNE agents:

Chemical

Biological

Radiological

Nuclear

Explosive

The CBRNE agents are considered to be technological hazardous agents—a broad field, of which hazmats (the types of hazardous materials that were discussed in Chapter 39, "Hazardous Materials, Multiple-Casualty Incidents, and Incident Management") are a subcategory. The CBRNE agents, often called ***weapons of mass destruction (WMD)***, are intended to cause widespread harm and/or fear among a population.

Terrorism incidents can also encompass criminal activities. In such acts as arson, environmental crime, and industrial sabotage, criminal and technological incidents overlap. Of course, terrorism can also be committed by conventional or unanticipated means, such as flying an airplane into a building.

Although the Department of Justice, as noted earlier, uses a narrow definition of terrorism, EMS has responsibilities for violent incidents that go well beyond that limited scope. This chapter will principally cover terrorism involving CBRNE agents.

TERRORISM AND EMS

Emergency Medical Responders as Targets

Emergency Medical Responders are often the principal targets of a terrorist attack, as will be discussed in more detail later. Responders must stay alert and never assume the incident scene is safe until this is verified by appropriate agencies or authorities. Responders must

---

weapons of mass destruction (WMD)

weapons, devices, or agents intended to cause widespread harm and/or fear among a population.

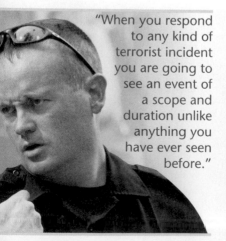

"When you respond to any kind of terrorist incident you are going to see an event of a scope and duration unlike anything you have ever seen before."

weigh the threat or risk of their actions against the benefit of their actions. This is true at all emergency scenes, of course, but even more true at the scene of a terrorist attack.

NOTE: *Always remember: The EMS provider's safety is the most important consideration when responding to a potential terrorist incident. The responder who gets hurt cannot help others.*

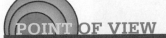
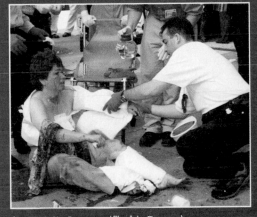

"When you take your EMT class you learn about a lot of things. You even learn about what to do at multiple-casualty incidents.

"I had some minor MCIs in my early days. Car crashes with five patients, a fire with a lot of smoke inhalation. But nothing could prepare me—no class and no experience—for the real "big one." A terrorist incident.

"I'm not going to tell stories. All I can say is that sometimes things are of a magnitude that you can't even conceive until you are there. You are a small cog in a big wheel. You feel like you are both so small in a big incident, and yet so important for being there. The injuries and specific things you see actually become secondary to the hugeness of it all.

"It was tough. It was enormous. It was mass humanity and mass confusion at the same time. It'll happen again somewhere. It may happen to you. It will be tough, but you'll be glad you were there to do your job. Someone has to."

(© Ciniglio Lorenzo/Corbis Sygma)

Identify the Threat Posed by the Event

EMS response to a terrorist event is complicated. You may be dealing with a hazardous materials or mass-casualty incident, using recognized protocols such as the hazmat procedures and Incident Management System discussed in Chapter 39, "Hazardous Materials, Multiple-Casualty Incidents, and Incident Management." A terrorist incident, however, may involve two additional factors that all responders will have to take into account: deliberate targeting of responders and crime scene considerations.

Terrorists have a history of utilizing *secondary devices* and/or booby traps to target emergency responders. In January 1997, a bomb went off outside an Atlanta family planning clinic. One hour after the initial detonation, a second bomb went off close to the point where the Incident Command post had been established, which resulted in several injuries to responders and could have caused deaths.

If the incident is a potential act of terrorism, it is also a crime scene. Although there will be similarities between terrorist events and nonterrorist mass-casualty incidents (such as major transportation collisions and hazmat incidents), crime scene considerations, such as the need to preserve evidence and the need to guard against further criminal activity, will complicate responder operations.

Regardless of the mechanism or motive behind an incident, responders should remain focused on reducing the impact of the event as efficiently and safely as possible. Whether dealing with a terrorist or a nonterrorist event, all responders should follow their agency's established operating guidelines. All responders on the scene should operate under an Incident Command System and utilize some type of staff-personnel accountability system that is compatible with those used by all participating agencies.

Although recognizing suspicious incidents may be difficult, being alert to clues, surroundings, and events will greatly assist in identification. Clues such as the OTTO signs, discussed in the following list, will help with this process:

Occupancy or location

Type of event

Timing of the event

On-scene warning signs

CORE CONCEPT
How to identify the type of threat posed by a terrorist event

secondary devices
destructive devices, such as bombs, placed to be activated after an initial attack and timed to injure emergency responders and others who rush in to help care for those targeted by an initial attack.

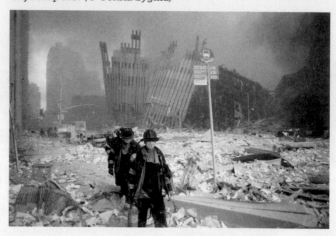

FIGURE 41-3 The Twin Towers of the World Trade Center in New York City were destroyed, and thousands were killed, on September 11, 2001, when terrorists flew hijacked jetliners into those famous skyscrapers. *(© Corbis/Sygma)*

Occupancy or Location

The following clues regarding the event's occupancy or location may indicate a terrorist incident:

- **Symbolic and historical targets.** These include targets that represent some organization or event that is particularly offensive in the minds of an extremist individual or group. Examples might include Bureau of Alcohol, Tobacco, and Firearms (BATF) offices for those who oppose all forms of gun control; Internal Revenue Service (IRS) offices for tax resisters; or a national monument such as the Statue of Liberty for anti-Americans. The World Trade Center (Figure 41-3), with its great height and location at the financial hub of New York City, became such a target twice, in 1993 and on September 11, 2001.

- **Public buildings or assembly areas.** These areas provide the opportunity for attention-getting mass casualties. Some of these public buildings are also symbolic targets, so the terrorist can cause massive casualties and link the owner/operator of the building or assembly area with danger in the minds of the public. These targets include shopping malls, convention centers, entertainment venues, and tourist destinations.

- **Controversial businesses.** These businesses usually have a history of attracting the enmity of extremist groups. Family planning clinics, nuclear facilities, and furriers all fall into this category.

- **Infrastructure systems.** These operations are necessary for the continued functioning of our society. Major cities are full of targets such as bridges, power plants, phone companies, water treatment plants, mass transit, and hospitals. Attacks on any of these have the potential to disrupt entire regions and cost hundreds of millions of dollars to correct.

Type of Event

Certain types of events should raise your awareness of possible terrorist involvement. In general, they can be categorized as follows:

- **Explosions and/or incendiaries.** These are among the favorite weapons of terrorists. Any bombing or suspicious fire may raise suspicions of terrorist involvement, especially when combined with the previously listed location or occupancy factors.

- **Incidents involving firearms.** These should always be treated as suspicious. If they occur in conjunction with other indicating factors, terrorism is a definite possibility.

- **Nontrauma mass-casualty incidents.** These incidents have occurred as the arsenal of terrorism increases in sophistication. When large numbers of victims are generated without obvious (physical) injury, but with symptoms of illness, you may suspect terrorist involvement.

Timing of the Event

For many years to come, April 19 will be a day around which government facilities operate at a heightened state of security awareness. It is the anniversary of both the fire at the Branch Davidian compound in Waco, Texas, and the bombing of the Alfred P. Murrah building in Oklahoma City, and so has become a rallying point for anti-government extremists. National holidays are also possible target dates.

Aside from significant anniversaries and holidays, events that occur on specific days of the week and times of day are worth treating with suspicion. A fire in a subway tunnel at the height of rush hour, aimed at harming a large number of people and alarming the public, may indicate terrorism.

On-Scene Warning Signs

When you arrive on the scene, you should always watch for signs that you are dealing with a suspicious incident. Unexplained patterns of illness or deaths can be attributed to chemical, radiological, or biological agents. Some of these substances have recognizable odors and/or tastes. Unexplained signs and symptoms of skin, eye, or airway irritation may be linked to chemical contamination, as may unexplained vapor clouds, mists, and plumes.

Always remain on the lookout for chemical containers, spray devices, or lab equipment in unusual locations. Watch for items or containers that appear out of place at unusual incidents, which might contain a secondary device. Large fires, spot fires, and fires of unusual behavior may also arouse suspicion, as can anything that appears abnormal for a given incident scene.

Recognize the Harms Posed by the Threat

To implement self-protection measures, you must first understand the types of harm to which you can be exposed. These types of harm—Thermal, Radiological, Asphyxiation, Chemical, Etiological, Mechanical, and Psychological—can be categorized utilizing the acronym TRACEM-P.

The TRACEM-P Harms

- **Thermal harm.** This refers to harm caused by either extreme heat, such as that generated by burning liquids or metals, or extreme cold from cryogenic materials such as liquid oxygen. Radiant heat can melt protective clothing and other equipment if an individual is too near the heat source.

- **Radiological harm.** This refers to danger from alpha particles, beta particles, or gamma rays, which are generally produced by sources such as nuclear fuels, byproducts of nuclear power production, or nuclear bombs. Figure 41-4 shows the relative penetrating power of the three types of radiation.

- **Asphyxiation.** This is caused by a lack of oxygen in the atmosphere. One common cause of this is heavier-than-air gases such as argon, carbon dioxide, or chemical vapors in a confined space. Extremely dusty situations such as the site of the World Trade Center towers' collapse create additional problems. An oxygen level of 19.5 percent is required for normal breathing.

FIGURE 41-4 The relative penetrating power of alpha, beta, and gamma radiation.

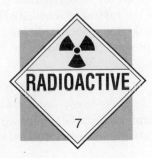

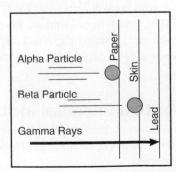

- **Chemical harm.** This harm is posed by toxic or corrosive materials. These can include acids such as sulfuric acid, caustics such as lye, and chemical toxins ranging from cyanides to nerve agents.

- **Etiological harm—etiology.** Etiology concerns the causes of disease—whether it comes from disease-causing organisms such as bacteria and viruses or toxins derived from living organisms.

- **Mechanical harm.** This is any sort of physical trauma such as gunshot wounds, slip-trip-and-fall injuries, and injury from bomb fragments or shrapnel.

- **Psychological harm.** This can, of course, result from any violent or traumatic event. Terrorist events are designed to create fear, invoke panic, reduce faith in government, and (as the name indicates) cause terror. In fact, psychological harm is generally the purpose of a terrorist attack. Responders and patients will be subject to posttraumatic stress and survival guilt. These effects may occur during or right after the event or may manifest themselves at a much later time.

Professional counseling is available to responders in many local communities.

TIME/DISTANCE/SHIELDING

CORE CONCEPT

Use of time/distance/shielding for protection at a terrorist event

Protection of the EMR is based on avoiding or minimizing exposure through the principles of time, distance, and shielding.

- **Time.** Minimize your time at a dangerous scene, such as a crime scene or a hazmat scene. Spend the shortest amount of time possible in the dangerous area or exposed to a hazardous material, a biological agent, or radiation. An example of utilizing time constraints would be executing rapid entries to perform reconnaissance or rescue. The less time you spend in the affected area, the less likely you are to become injured. Minimizing the time you spend in the affected area will also reduce your chances of contaminating a crime scene.

- **Distance.** Maximize your distance from the hazard area or the projected hazard area. One example of utilizing distance would be avoiding contact by following the recommended guidelines regarding hazardous materials in the current edition of the *Emergency Response Guidebook*. You can determine the safe distances from vehicles suspected of containing explosives from the recommendations in *Vehicle Bomb Explosion Hazard and Evacuation Distance Tables* obtainable from the Bureau of Alcohol, Tobacco, and Firearms.

- **Shielding.** Use appropriate shielding to address specific hazards. Shielding can consist of vehicles, buildings, fire-protection clothing, hazmat suits, positive-pressure self-contained breathing apparatus, and personal protective equipment (PPE). Also consider the vaccinations recommended by your service to provide immunization against specific diseases.

Responders should use all three forms of protection whenever possible. Just because you feel properly shielded does not mean that you can spend excessive time in close proximity to a contaminated site.

RESPONSES TO TERRORISM

CORE CONCEPT

How to respond to and deal with harms from a terrorist event

The following sections will cover the TRACEM-P harms for the CBRNE terrorism categories. The TRACEM-P harms that are not listed are not relevant to the CBRNE category (chemical, biological, radiological/nuclear, explosive) that is being discussed. In each CBRNE category, each harm listed is identified as primary or secondary for that specific type of agent.

Responses to a Chemical Incident

Chemical incidents can include many classes of hazardous materials. Materials can be inhaled, ingested, absorbed, or injected. These materials can include industrial chemical or warfare-type agents.

NOTE: *It is important to attain a weather report from the dispatch center when responding to suspected chemical incidents to ensure you approach upwind from any potential airborne chemicals.*

Types of Harm from Chemical Incidents

The following types of harm can result from chemical incidents:

- **Thermal harm.** This is a secondary harm since many chemical reactions create heat. The chemicals involved may also be flammable.
- **Asphyxiation.** This is a secondary harm and is possible because some chemical reactions may deplete oxygen or create gases that displace oxygen.
- **Chemical harms.** These are the primary harm and include a wide variety of effects such as corrosivity and reactivity. They may also have a variety of systemic effects that may attack the central nervous system, cardiovascular system, respiratory system, and other body systems.
- **Mechanical harm.** This is a secondary harm that must be taken into account because corrosive chemicals like strong acids can weaken structural elements.
- **Psychological harm.** This is a secondary harm because many individuals will react emotionally to a possible chemical exposure.

Self-Protection Measures at a Chemical Incident

Because of the wide variety of hazards posed by chemical agents, responders should take care to use the principles of time, distance, and shielding to minimize exposure risks under all circumstances. Specialized teams are available in most areas to deal with chemical incidents. It is important to use self-protection measures including respiratory protection and protective clothing. In the Tokyo subway attack involving the chemical nerve agent sarin (discussed later in the chapter), there was secondary contamination of a rescuer who performed CPR on a patient and later died from the exposure.

Responses to a Biological Incident

Biological incidents (Figure 41-5) will present as either a focused emergency or a public health emergency. A focused emergency is a situation in which a potential or actual point of origin or source of a disease is located (such as a single case or a small and localized number of cases of a disease) and attempts are made to prevent or minimize damage and spread. A public health emergency manifests itself as a sudden demand upon the public health infrastructure with no apparent explanation for the occurrence. Causative agents may be

FIGURE 41-5 In Baltimore, a specialized team trains to handle a bioterrorism incident. *(© AP Images/ Alex Dorgan-Ross)*

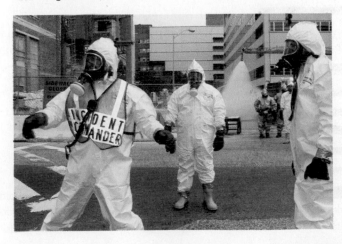

bacteria, viruses, or toxins. These agents may cause harm by being inhaled or ingested into the body.

- **Bacteria.** These single-celled organisms can grow in a variety of environments. Dangers to humans come from two directions: disease-causing bacteria growing in the human body, and bacteria that grow outside of the body but produce toxins that may pose a danger. (*Rickettsia* are sometimes classified as a genus of bacteria, and sometimes as organisms that share characteristics of both bacteria and viruses. Like bacteria, they can be destroyed by antibiotics. Like viruses, they can only live and multiply inside cells. They cause diseases such as Q fever and typhus. In the remainder of this chapter, rickettsia will be grouped with bacteria.) Anthrax, a bacterium, has been the weapon of choice in several American bioterrorist events.

- **Viruses.** These are the smallest known entities capable of reproduction. They only grow inside of living cells and cause those cells to produce additional viruses.

- **Toxins.** These are poisons produced by living organisms. The organisms may be bacteria, fungi, flowering plants, insects, fish, reptiles, or mammals. Often, toxins are distilled from plant material. For example, the extremely potent toxin ricin is distilled from the castor bean plant. A tiny drop of ricin can be deadly. The FBI has disrupted terrorist attempts to use ricin, such as a 2009 event in Las Vegas, Nevada, in which a police officer was sickened by secondary contamination from ricin at a crime scene.

Critical Information about Biological Incidents

What Is an Exposure? *Exposure* equals the *dose* or the *concentration* of the agent multiplied by *time* (the duration of the exposure).

- **Chemical doses.** These are generally measured in milligrams per kilograms of body weight. *Biological doses* are measured in fractions of micrograms per kilograms of body weight.

- **Concentration.** The concentration of an agent is measured in parts per million.

NOTE: *If you reduce the dose, concentration, or time near the agent, you will reduce the exposure.*

Remember that infectious dose data are standardized. They are typically based on a 70-kg or 150-pound male in good health. Individuals who fall below these parameters may become infected at lower doses. Examples include the elderly, who are often in poor health, and young children, whose body weight is less than 150 pounds.

Four Major Routes of Entry *Routes of entry* are critical concepts that must be understood prior to studying individual WMD agents. Exposures occur through "routes" or pathways into the body. Biological agents can enter the body through four routes:

- Absorption (skin contact)
- Ingestion (mouth)
- Injection (needles or projectiles)
- Inhalation (breathing)

Biological agents seldom enter the body through *the skin*. The exception is T2 mycotoxins, which can be absorbed through the skin. Items that affect skin absorption are:

- Injury to the skin
- Skin temperature/blood flow
- Higher concentration = greater exposure
- Area with more hair = more exposure
- Length of exposure
- Type of agent

Ingestion is a common route to infection. Ingestion includes swallowing biological agents in food or drink or accidentally swallowing the agent by itself. One highly likely way to become infected is to eat or drink before completing decontamination procedures.

exposure
the dose or concentration of an agent multiplied by the time, or duration.

routes of entry
pathways into the body, generally by absorption, ingestion, injection, or inhalation.

Injection or puncturing can be accidental or purposeful. Vectors (such as mosquitoes or fleas) can carry biological agents from one host to another. Personnel can become infected with biological agents by accidentally injecting themselves through improper handling of a needle or puncturing themselves with a jagged piece of debris. Common infection routes for biological infection are:

- Vector (a disease-carrying organism)
- Jagged glass or metal
- Syringes
- High-pressure devices

Inhalation has the potential to cause more biological agent infection than any other route of exposure, provided the particle is small enough to reach the lower respiratory tract. The degree of infection is based on:

- Rate of breathing
- Depth of breathing

Decontamination after inhalation is only psychologically beneficial.

What Is Contamination? *Contamination* is caused by contact with or presence of a *contaminant*, which is material that is present where it does not belong and that is somehow harmful to persons, animals, or the environment. As contaminants, biological agents may be in the solid, liquid, or aerosol form. Dealing with each of these requires a different set of skills and operations.

Things that can be contaminated include:

- Hard and soft surfaces
- Skin and hair
- Clothing

contamination
contact with or presence of a material (contaminant) that is present where it does not belong and that is somehow harmful to persons, animals, or the environment.

Exposure versus Contamination Exposure occurs when a substance is taken into the body through one of the routes of exposure. Contamination occurs when a substance clings to surface areas of the body or clothing.

Clothing and other materials can become *permeated* with a contaminant. (*Permeation* is the movement of a substance through a surface or, on a molecular level, through intact materials. In general, it means penetration, or spreading.) However, biological agents can usually be washed out of clothing. In most cases, clothing and personal protective equipment (PPE) can be reused after decontamination. The removal of clothing removes most of the contamination. It is important to ensure that a patient's dignity is protected during the decontamination operation. Many services carry extra Tyvek suits or a box of oversized trash bags to cover patients whose clothing has been removed.

permeation
the movement of a substance through a surface or, on a molecular level, through intact materials; penetration, or spreading.

Types of Harm from Biological Incidents

The following types of harm can result from biological incidents:

- **Chemical harm.** This could be a secondary hazard; for example, at the scene of a clandestine laboratory.
- **Etiological harm.** This is the primary type of harm. These materials are classified as Class 6 Hazardous Materials (Poison) by the U.S. Department of Transportation.
- **Mechanical harm.** This is a possible secondary hazard where explosives have been used to disperse the agent.
- **Psychological harm.** This is a secondary harm. Just the thought of possible exposure to, or contamination by, a biological agent can cause stress, even if the person has not actually come in contact with the agent.

Self-Protection Measures at a Biological Incident

Take care to limit exposure and contamination if a biological incident is suspected. Personal protective equipment provides a shield to isolate a person from the hazards that can be encountered at an incident. Such equipment includes both personal protective clothing and respiratory protection. Adequate personal protection equipment should protect the respiratory system, skin, face, hands, feet, head, and body.

Limiting exposure and contamination can be accomplished by responders prioritizing protective measures at any incident. It is important to get as much information as possible to be prepared for what you are going into. The order of protection priorities should be:

- Self-protection (*Respiratory protection is the priority*. Always protect yourself first. You don't need to become one more patient at the scene.)
- Using the buddy system
- Availability of Rapid Intervention Teams
- Civilian protection (Moving civilians to an area of refuge may be their best protection.)

Responses to a Radiological/Nuclear Incident

As rogue nations continue to acquire and sell nuclear technology, the possibility of a nuclear detonation cannot be dismissed. Small nuclear devices known as "suitcase bombs" were developed during the Cold War and remain in stockpiles with the potential to fall into the wrong hands. A more practical possibility is the use of a radiological dispersion device that would involve the use of a conventional explosive containing radiological material, such as medical waste or low level radioactive sources. Such a device is commonly called a "dirty bomb." Spreading of radioactive materials might also be accomplished by sabotaging or attacking a nuclear power facility.

Identifying a nuclear incident may be difficult, because radiation cannot be detected by the senses. Furthermore, symptoms of radiological exposure are generally delayed for hours or days. Exposure to radiation can, however, be treated if it is diagnosed early.

Types of Harm from Radiological/Nuclear Incidents

The following types of harm can result from radiological/nuclear incidents:

- **Thermal harm.** This is the primary harm from a nuclear explosion.
- **Radiological harm.** This is the primary danger from radiological materials. Because of the nature of the materials, this will represent an ongoing hazard, the scope of which will only be determined when the amount and identity of the substance involved is ascertained. Radiological exposure is generally more dangerous to children, pregnant women, and the elderly. The first signs and symptoms are often nausea, vomiting, and diarrhea.
- **Chemical harm.** This secondary harm is a concern because many radiological substances are also chemical hazards. This is an area often overlooked by responders who are concentrating on radiation effects.
- **Mechanical harm.** This is a primary harm from a nuclear explosion.
- **Psychological harm.** This is a secondary harm. As in all terrorist incidents, a sudden traumatic occurrence can cause immediate or delayed emotional or psychological reactions.

Self-Protection Measures at a Radiological/Nuclear Incident

Time, distance, and shielding are the mainstays of self-protection at a radiological incident. The use of radiological detection equipment is the best method of determining whether your self-protection measures are appropriate and effective.

As noted in the following section, *all* explosive incidents should be treated as potential disseminations of radiological (or biological or chemical) materials. This will ensure you take the appropriate protective measures, even before the nature of the explosion can be ascertained. Additionally, review the information on decontamination procedures in Chapter 39, "Hazardous Materials, Multiple-Casualty Incidents, and Incident Management."

NOTE: *Keep in mind that a bombing may have been a suicide bombing, and one of the bomb victims may be the bomber. For this reason, search all patients at the scene for weapons prior to transport.*

Responses to an Explosive Incident

Explosive incidents can involve a wide variety of devices, from small pipe bombs to large vehicle bombs. The incident may involve an attack against a fixed target or against a group of people such as emergency responders. The incident may be an isolated event or may involve secondary devices, booby traps, or suicide bombers.

The materials involved will always include some form of explosives. However, as noted earlier, the detonation may also be designed to disperse biological, chemical, or radiological materials. The type of explosive may be improvised or commercially manufactured. The bomb itself may be equipped with switches or controls that can be activated by light, pressure, movement, or radio transmission. For this reason, untrained personnel should never attempt to neutralize an unexploded device.

Explosives are categorized as high-order explosives (HE) or low-order explosives (LE). HE explosives produce a defining supersonic overpressurization shock wave. Examples of HE include TNT, C-4, Semtex, nitroglycerin, dynamite, and ammonium nitrate fuel oil (ANFO). LE explosives create a subsonic explosion and lack the overpressurization wave produced by HE. Examples of LE include pipe bombs, gunpowder, and most pure petroleum-based bombs such as Molotov cocktails or aircraft used as guided missiles. HE and LE cause different injury patterns. Bombs and explosives have been, and probably will continue to be, the weapons used most frequently by terrorists.

Types of Harm from Explosive Incidents

The following types of harm can result from explosive incidents:

- **Thermal harm.** This is a primary hazard to those exposed to the heat generated by the detonation. It is usually not an ongoing risk unless unexploded materials are present.
- **Asphyxiation.** This is a potential secondary harm because of the possibility of extremely dusty conditions that can aerosolize a variety of toxins, such as asbestos.
- **Chemical hazards.** These hazards are created as a result of the explosive reaction either from chemicals already present at the detonation site or if chemicals have been included in the device for dispersal.
- **Mechanical harm.** This is another primary harm typically seen at bombing incidents. It can result from blast overpressure, shock waves, and fragmentation. (Review the information on types of blast injuries in Chapter 28, "Soft-Tissue Trauma.")
- **Psychological harm.** This often results, as happens in any violent incident. A stunned response could last seconds or minutes, causing individuals to "freeze" and be temporarily unable to think or act. Delayed reaction shows up later in the form of posttraumatic stress.

Self-Protection Measures at an Explosive Incident

With explosive incidents, the responder needs both preblast and postblast protection. Preblast is defined as that portion of operations that occurs after a written or verbal warning is received but before an explosion takes place. Postblast refers to operations occurring after at least one detonation has occurred.

DISSEMINATION AND WEAPONIZATION

It is important to be familiar with the potential methods for *dissemination* of CBRNE materials, particularly chemical, biological, and radiological/nuclear agents (Figure 41-6). Responders also must not forget that many industrial materials can be used just as effectively as military agents.

dissemination
spreading.

The Respiratory Route

The most effective and most common means of dissemination is to enable the material to enter through the respiratory tract. As you have learned in the respiratory care sections of this text, the respiratory tract has a vast and delicate surface area that is exposed to the

FIGURE 41-6 CBRNE agents can be weaponized and disseminated in an enormous variety of ways. In 1995, as an example, members of Aum Shinrikyo, a Japanese religious cult, released sarin, a deadly nerve agent, into the Tokyo subway system, killing 12 people and sending thousands to the hospital. Their purpose, according to experts, was to hasten the end of the world. They transported liquid sarin in tightly sealed packages made to look like lunch boxes or bottled drinks, then punctured the packages with umbrellas and left them in subway cars and stations where the volatile substance escaped and permeated the atmosphere as a gas. Its quick dispersal in the atmosphere meant fewer deaths than the perpetrators probably intended. The photo shows a clean-up crew at work in the subway. *(© Neville Elder/Corbis Sygma)*

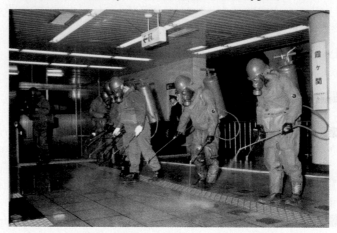

outside environment through respiration. The deeper into the passageways of the lungs that a terrorist can "place" a harmful material, and the longer the material remains there, the more effective it will be.

The passageways of the respiratory system become smaller and smaller as they progress deeper into the lungs. Particulates, gases, and vapors will be trapped and held at various levels based upon factors such as the size of the particles, the depth and rate of respiration, and whether or not the material is water or lipid (nonwater) soluble.

Other routes of exposure, as discussed in the following text, can be harmful or lethal. However, remember that the most effective means of achieving mass casualties is to have the materials enter the body through respiration.

Other Routes

Other means of dissemination depend upon the agent used. For example, the effectiveness of the ingestion, or alimentary, route of exposure depends on whether the agent can survive the stomach's acidic environment. Many bacteria cannot live in low pH conditions, although others can. An example would be anthrax, a bacterium that can survive for long periods of time and in harsh environments as dormant spores. (Anthrax can infect a person through contact with the skin, ingestion, or inhalation—inhalation being the most lethal route.)

Some have raised concerns over a terrorist's ability to contaminate a domestic water supply as an ingestion route of exposure. Processes such as dilution, filtration, and chlorination greatly reduce this potential threat. Additionally, the fact that only 1 percent of a domestic water supply is consumed through ingestion further reduces the potential effectiveness of this means of dissemination.

The dermal, or percutaneous, route of exposure (through the skin) is very effective with the blister agents, or vesicants, but less effective with many of the biological agents. Nerve agents such as sarin, soman, or taban with an organophosphate base easily penetrate the skin and cause systemic efforts. Only a few biological materials are dermally active, because healthy, intact skin provides an excellent barrier. The use of vectors such as fleas to disseminate biological agents (e.g., bubonic plague) presents significant logistical difficulties to the terrorist and is therefore not likely to be a readily selected means of dissemination.

Some bacterial, and many viral, agents can be disseminated effectively by human-to-human contact. With such agents, especially when there is a delayed incubation period, it is possible to infect a large population prior to detection. These factors are of particular concern with smallpox, pneumonic plague, and viral hemorrhagic fevers, to name a few.

Weaponization

In summary, *weaponization* of *most* of the agents we will discuss is most effective when targeted through the inhalation route. If the terrorist can get the materials into a respirable form—that is to say, in particles no more than approximately 3 to 5 microns in diameter—he can achieve the greatest number of casualties. Such airborne dissemination can be created by applying various forms of energy to the material. Energy such as heat would cause a liquid to evaporate faster, resulting in a higher airborne concentration. Explosives or sprayers could also be used to aerosolize and disseminate the materials.

weaponization
packaging or producing a material, such as a chemical, biological, or radiological agent, so that it can be used as a weapon; for example, by dissemination in a bomb detonation or as an aerosol sprayed over an area or introduced into a ventilation system.

CHARACTERISTICS OF CBRNE AGENTS

Characteristics of the various CBRNE agents (chemical, biological, radiological/nuclear, and explosive) are discussed in the following sections.

Chemical Agents

Chemical Agent Considerations

Physical Considerations Known agents cover the whole range of physical properties. Under various ambient conditions, their physical state may be gaseous, liquid, or solid. Their vapor pressures vary from high to negligible. Their vapor densities vary from slightly lighter than air to considerably heavier. The range of odors varies from none to highly pungent or characteristic. They may be soluble or insoluble in water. These varied physical properties affect the agent's behavior in the field with respect to such considerations as vapor hazard, persistency, and possible means of decontamination.

Volatility Considerations Agents that have a low boiling point and high vapor pressure tend to be nonpersistent; that is, they will evaporate more readily. Evaporation presents good news and bad news. The bad news is that the more volatile (easily evaporable) a material, the greater the airborne concentration that will be released. The good news is that the more volatile a material, the less time it will remain on a surface area. Agents that have a high boiling point (therefore, a lower vapor pressure) tend to be more persistent.

Chemical Considerations The only general characteristic of the known chemical agents is that they are sufficiently stable to survive dissemination and transport to the site of their action. However, their inherent reactivity and stability can widely vary. Some chemically reactive agents naturally lose their potency at a rapid rate, whereas other, less-reactive agents require, for example, bleach solutions to inactivate them. Solid adsorbents (e.g., Fuller's earth) are also very effective decontaminants.

Toxicological Considerations Keep in mind that not all individuals of a species react in the same way to a given amount of agent. Some are more or less sensitive as a result of various factors, including genetic background, race, and age. The route of entry can also influence the effect. Toxicological studies estimate the potential biological effects of chemical agents by different routes of entry. The physical properties of the materials may alter the toxicological effects and the response of the affected system.

Some nerve agents act on the parasympathetic nervous system. For example, the enzyme acetylcholinesterase is inhibited by the nerve agent and fails to break down the neurotransmitter acetylcholine. This causes an overstimulation of the parasympathetic nervous system and a specific set of signs and symptoms.

SLUDGEM is a mnemonic used to remember the signs and symptoms of nerve agent poisoning. The letters stand for:

Salivation—due to stimulation of the salivary glands

Lacrimation—due to stimulation of the lacrimal glands

Urination—due to relaxation of the internal sphincter muscle of the urethra

Defecation—due to relaxation of the anal sphincter

GI upset—changes to smooth muscle tone in the GI tract

Emesis—vomiting because of GI system effects

Miosis—abnormal contraction of the pupils

Classifications of Chemical Agents

Chemical weapons can be classified broadly in the following manner:

- **Choking agents.** These predominately respiratory irritants can be found not only as weaponized materials but also as commonly encountered industrial chemicals. Many of these common industrial chemicals are classified as simple asphyxiants such as chlorine.

- **Vesicating agents (blister agents).** These agents cause chemical changes in the cells of exposed tissues almost immediately on contact. However, in many cases, the effects are not felt or realized until hours after the exposure.

- **Cyanides.** Formerly referred to as "blood agents," these actually have no impact on the blood. They work by preventing the use of oxygen within the body's cells and therefore are cellular asphyxiants.

- **Nerve agents.** These agents inhibit an enzyme that is critical to proper nerve transmission, allowing the parasympathetic nervous system to run out of control. Many agencies carry nerve agent antidote kits for their emergency response personnel (Figure 41-7). Many of these nerve agents are stronger versions of common pesticides from the organophosphate family and are easily absorbed through the skin. Most have a smell of petroleum and have a milky off-white color. They produce the signs and symptoms that make up the mnemonic SLUDGEM (see Inside/Outside feature).

- **Riot control agents.** These agents include irritating materials and lacrimators (tear-flow increasers). The effects of these materials seldom last more than several minutes after exposure has ended, although pepper spray can trigger asthmatic reactions. Riot control agents such as mace, pepper spray, and CS gas have the ability to trigger respiratory distress in people with a history of asthma.

FIGURE 41-7 Many emergency response agencies provide nerve agent antidote kits to their personnel.

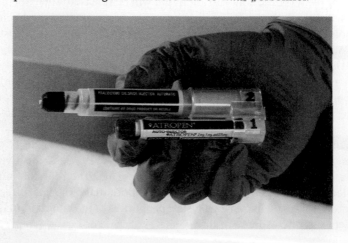

Biological Agents

Biological agents are defined as microorganisms or toxins that can cause disease processes. Most commonly, the biological agents are bacteria, viruses, or toxins, and a wide variety of biological agents are of concern as possible agents of terrorism. Virtually any biological material can be weaponized and disseminated; some are just more effective than others.

It is important to understand the differences between a bacterium, a virus, and a toxin. The differences can influence the ease of manufacture as well as the availability of antidotes and, to some extent, their effectiveness. Some characteristics of the three were noted earlier in the chapter. Additional characteristics are discussed in the following text.

A *bacterium* is a small, free-living microorganism. "Free-living" means that it can live outside of a host cell. Many bacteriological agents respond to antibiotic therapies and, for the most part, are treatable conditions if detected early enough. The EMT should be on alert for fever, nausea, vomiting, and diarrhea of a sudden onset or in a normally healthy person. Multiple patients in the same area in a short period of time is often an indicator of an acute poisoning of a population. Normal flu or seasonal illnesses have a period of spread that is much slower. In addition, an illness usually travels from one person to another. In contrast, multiple people may be exposed to a biological agent all at once and therefore may display the same signs and symptoms in a short period of time.

A *virus* is an organism that requires a host cell inside which to live and reproduce; thus, it is intimately dependent upon the cell that it infects. The diseases that viruses produce generally do not respond to antibiotics, which cannot reach them inside their host cells. However, some may be responsive to the few antiviral compounds that exist.

In contrast to bacteria and viruses, *toxins* are not living organisms. Simply put, a toxin is a poisonous chemical compound that is produced by or derived from a living organism. The producing organism could be a plant, an animal, or a microorganism. Examples include ricin, which is derived from the castor bean; mycotoxins, which are produced by fungi; or the botulinum toxin, which is produced by the bacterium *Clostridium botulinum*.

Although other types of biological agents exist, bacteria, viruses, and toxins are the most common.

Biological Agent Considerations

The biological weapons of greatest concern are listed in Table 41-1. As you review this table, note that the primary concern for all of the biological agents is personal protection if the agent is transmitted from human to human. The role of EMS in patient care and treatment will be primarily supportive in nature as most bacteria agents and many of the viral agents have treatment regimens.

Regardless of whether the agent is a bacterium, a virus, or a toxin, there are certain features that influence their potential for use as weapons. They are:

- Infectivity
- Virulence
- Toxicity
- Incubation period
- Transmissibility
- Lethality
- Stability

Unique to many of these biological agents, and distinct from their chemical counterparts, is the ability to multiply over time and actually increase their effect. Therefore, biological material that can readily replicate itself has a greater potential to be transmitted from person to person. The potential epidemiological impacts of such a biological weapon are obvious.

These factors are discussed in more detail in the following list.

- **Infectivity.** The infectivity of an agent reflects the relative ease with which the microorganisms involved establish themselves in a host species. Pathogens with high infectivity cause disease with relatively few organisms, whereas those with low infectivity require a larger number. High infectivity does not necessarily mean that the symptoms

Table 41-1 Biological Agent Quick Reference Guide

DISEASE (CLASS)	ROUTE OF INFECTION	INCUBATION PERIOD/ ONSET TIME	HUMAN-TO-HUMAN TRANSMISSION
BACTERIA			
Anthrax (Bacterium)	S, D, R	1 to 6 days	No, except for cutaneous infection
Cholera (Bacterium)	D, DC	1 to 5 days	Rare
Plague, Bubonic (Bacterium)	V, R	2 to 10 days	High
Plague, Pneumonic (Bacterium)	V, R	2 to 3 days	High
Q Fever (Bacterium)	V, R	2 to 10 days	Rare
Tularemia (Bacterium)	V, R, D	2 to 10 days	No

V = vector, R = respiratory, D = digestive, DC = direct human-to-human contact, S = skin

and signs appear more quickly nor that the illness will be more severe. Instead, it simply means that it takes only a small number of organisms to produce symptoms, regardless of timing or severity.

- **Virulence.** An agent's virulence reflects the relative severity of the disease produced by a microorganism. Different strains of the same microorganism may cause diseases of different severity.
- **Toxicity.** An agent's toxicity reflects the relative severity of the illness or incapacitation produced by a toxin.
- **Incubation period.** A sufficient number of microorganisms or a sufficient quantity of toxin must penetrate the body to produce infection (the infective dose) or intoxication (the intoxicating dose). Infectious agents then must multiply (replicate) to produce disease. The time between exposure and the appearance of symptoms is known as the incubation period. This is governed by many variables, including the initial dose, virulence, route of entry, rate of replication, and host immunological factors.

SIGNS AND SYMPTOMS	DECONTAMINATION OR INFECTION CONTROL PROCEDURES	PREHOSPITAL CARE
BACTERIA		
Fever, malaise, and mild chest discomfort, followed by severe respiratory distress with difficulty breathing, sweating, stridor (harsh breathing sounds), and cyanosis (bluish skin color); shock and death within 24 to 36 hours of severe symptoms.	Universal body decontamination with low-pressure, soap and water wash, then 0.5 percent hypochlorite solution, then second soap and water wash.	Supportive according to local protocol.
Range of no symptoms to severe symptoms with sudden onset, vomiting, abdominal distension, and pain with little or no fever followed rapidly by diarrhea. Fluid loss can exceed 5 to 10 liters per day.	Enteric precautions, soap and water washes, and a hypochlorite solution for equipment. Personal contact rarely causes infection.	Supportive care directed at rapid fluid replacement.
High fever, chills, malaise, tender lymph nodes (buboes), which may progress to infection throughout the bloodstream, with spread to the central nervous system, lungs, and elsewhere.	Isolation precautions, secretion, and lesion (open sore or skin infection) precautions. Use of soap and water for personnel decon; use heat, UV rays, or disinfectants for equipment.	Supportive care and respiratory and circulatory support.
High fever, chills, headache, coughing up blood, and blood poisoning, with rapid progression to breathing difficulty, stridor (harsh breathing sounds), and cyanosis (bluish skin color); death is due to respiratory failure or circulatory collapse.	Strict isolation precautions. Use of soap and water for personnel decon, heat, UV rays, and disinfectants for equipment.	Supportive care and respiratory and circulatory support.
Fever, cough, and sharp chest pain.	Use of soap and water or a weak 0.5 percent hypochlorite solution.	Supportive care.
Local ulcer and regionally enlarged lymph nodes that may develop into abscesses, fever, chills, headache, and malaise. Signs include fever, headache, malaise, discomfort behind the breastbone, weight loss, nonproductive cough.	Secretion and lesion precautions, strict isolation not required, use of heat or disinfectants renders the organism harmless.	Supportive care.

(continued)

- **Transmissibility.** Some biological agents can be transmitted directly from person to person. Indirect transmission (for example, via vectors, such as insects) may be a significant means of spread as well. In the context of biological warfare casualty management, the relative ease with which an agent is passed from person to person (its transmissibility) constitutes the principal concern.

- **Lethality.** Lethality reflects the relative ease with which an agent causes death in a susceptible population. We can quantify a material's relative lethality by determining its "lethal dose" or "lethal concentration" (LD or LC).

- **Stability.** The viability of a biological agent is affected by various environmental factors, including temperature, relative humidity, atmospheric pollution, ultraviolet light, and sunlight. A quantitative measure of stability is an agent's decay rate (e.g., "aerosol decay rate").

Additional factors that may influence the suitability of a microorganism or toxin as a biological weapon include ease of production, stability when stored or transported, and ease of dissemination.

Table 41-1   Biological Agent Quick Reference Guide (continued)

DISEASE (CLASS)	ROUTE OF INFECTION	INCUBATION PERIOD/ ONSET TIME	HUMAN-TO-HUMAN TRANSMISSION
TOXINS			
Botulinum (Toxin)	D, R	24 hours to several days	No
Ricin (Toxin)	D, R	24 to 72 hours	No
Staphylococcal Enterotoxin B (SEB) (Toxin)	D, R	4 to 6 hours	No
Trichothecene Mycotoxins (T2) (Toxin)	R, S, DC, D	Minutes to hours	Yes
VIRUSES			
Smallpox (Virus)	R, S, DC	10 to 12 days	High
Venezuelan Equine Encephalitis (VEE) (Virus)	R, V	2 to 6 days	Low
Viral Hemorrhagic Fevers (VHFs) (Virus)	DC, V, R	3 to 21 days	Moderate

V = vector, R = respiratory, D = digestive, DC = direct human-to-human contact, S = skin

Bacteria

As noted earlier, bacteria are single-celled organisms that can grow in a variety of environments. Like the cells of the human body, they have an internal cytoplasm surrounded by a rigid cell wall. Unlike human body cells, they lack an organized nucleus and other intracellular structures. They can reproduce independently, but they require a host to provide food and other support. To obtain this, they bind to the outsides of host cells in the body.

For purposes of weaponization, bacteria are relatively easy to grow, reproduce, and spread.

Anthrax   Anthrax is a naturally occurring *zoonotic* disease (a disease that can move through the animal-human barrier) found commonly in livestock. As carriers of anthrax, cattle, sheep, and horses can infect humans naturally, particularly those who handle the hair, wool, hides, or excrement of infected animals.

The most common human form of anthrax seen in natural cases is the cutaneous form of anthrax, which is also known as *woolsorter's disease.* This condition is found in those per-

zoonotic

able to move through the animal-human barrier; transmissible from animals to humans.

SIGNS AND SYMPTOMS	DECONTAMINATION OR INFECTION CONTROL PROCEDURES	PREHOSPITAL CARE
TOXINS		
Drooping eyelids, weakness, dizziness, dry mouth and throat, blurred vision and double vision, impaired speech, hoarseness, difficulty swallowing, followed by symmetrical descending paralysis and respiratory failure.	0.5 percent hypochlorite solution and/or soap and water.	Aggressive respiratory support, and supportive care for other symptoms.
Weakness, fever, cough, and fluid in the lungs 18 to 24 hours postexposure, followed by severe respiratory distress and death from lack of blood oxygen in 36 to 72 hours.	0.5 percent hypochlorite solution and/or soap and water.	Supportive care with aggressive airway management. Volume replacement of gastrointestinal fluid loss.
Sudden onset, with fever, chills, headache, muscle pain, and nonproductive cough. Some may develop respiratory distress and pain behind the breastbone. If ingested, nausea, vomiting, and diarrhea may occur.	0.5 percent hypochlorite solution and/or soap and water.	Supportive care directed at respiratory support.
Skin pain, itching, redness, blisters, tissue death; nose and throat pain, nasal discharge, sneezing, cough, breathing difficulty, wheezing, chest pain; and coughing up blood; lack of muscle coordination, shock, and death.	Soap and water, after clothing has been removed. Eye exposure—copious saline irrigation.	Supportive care directed at respiratory and circulatory support.
VIRUSES		
Malaise, fever, chills, vomiting, headache, backache; 2 to 3 days later, sores which develop into pus-filled blisters, more abundant on face and extremities.	Strict quarantine with respiratory isolation for a minimum of 16 to 17 days following exposure for all contacts. Patients are infectious until all scabs heal.	Supportive care.
Sudden onset, with malaise, spiking fever, chills, severe headache, intolerance of light, and muscle pains. Nausea, vomiting, cough, sore throat, and diarrhea may follow.	Standard Precautions; infectious through mosquito bites.	Pain relievers for headache and muscle pain, anticonvulsants and respiratory support.
Fever, easy bleeding, purplish beneath-the-skin hemorrhage spots, low blood pressure, shock, swelling, malaise, muscle pain, headache, vomiting, and diarrhea.	Decontamination with hypochlorite or phenolic disinfectants. Use Standard Precautions.	Supportive care directed at respiratory and circulatory support.

sons who have had open sores or lacerations contaminated with anthrax spores during the handling of hides or shearing of wool.

Anthrax also can be transmitted by contaminated meat. However, this is extremely rare because cooking the meat will destroy the anthrax. If transmitted in this way, the gastrointestinal form of anthrax is seen.

As noted earlier, anthrax can survive the acids of the stomach when so many other biological agents will not readily survive the ingestion route of exposure. Anthrax is a *sporulating bacterium.* Simply put, sporulating (spore-producing) bacteria create a hard seedlike shell over themselves that makes them very resistant to breakdown by UV light and other insults. Therefore, areas contaminated by anthrax can remain contaminated for long periods of time. This is why special sporicidal soaps are best used as decontamination materials.

The form of anthrax that is of greatest concern is the inhalational form. If anthrax can be aerosolized in small enough particles (3 to 5 microns in diameter) so that they can be inhaled and retained in the deeper portions of the respiratory tract, then this form of anthrax can be transmitted by the respiratory route. This form of anthrax is very lethal.

With all forms of anthrax, antibiotic therapy works well to counteract the effects, provided that antibiotics are given early enough in the disease process. The problem with inhalational anthrax, however, is that it commonly presents with nonspecific respiratory symptoms and may not be recognized as anthrax. Therefore, the start of antibiotics may be delayed and, if they are not started before the "anthrax eclipse," such therapy may have little benefit. The eclipse is a brief, 12- to 41-hour period during the disease process in which recovery seems to be occurring and the patient feels much better. However, shortly after the eclipse, the symptoms return and death follows in 2 to 3 days.

Cholera Outbreaks of cholera typically are seen in developing nations, particularly those without effective sanitary systems. This gastroenteritic agent is more incapacitating than it is lethal if proper care is rendered.

Essentially, cholera is a diarrheal disease caused by the bacterium *Vibrio cholera*. This bacterium readily multiplies within the small intestines and releases an enterotoxin that causes the intestines to release large volumes of fluids, causing severe diarrhea and a characteristic "rice water" stool. Death generally occurs from the secondary effects of severe dehydration and electrolyte imbalances.

Proper supportive care aimed at correcting these dehydration-related problems and the use of antibiotics is generally very effective. From a personal protection standpoint, responders should avoid direct contact with bodily fluid and excrement. Otherwise, human-to-human transmission is low.

Plague We know it best as the "Black Death" of the Middle Ages, which was a naturally occurring form of the plague. The plague bacterium (*Yersinia pestis*) is a zoonotic bacterium carried by rats and ground squirrels. It is transmitted to humans by fleas.

In this naturally occurring infection of the human, the plague begins as the bubonic form (*bubo-* referring to a swollen or enlarged lymph node), primarily in the legs. With lack of treatment, it progresses to the systemic form, which develops into the highly contagious pneumonic plague. Pneumonic plague is the primary syndrome seen if plague is aerosolized and inhaled, whereas bubonic plague is seen first in natural occurrences or if weaponized via vectors such as fleas.

The incubation period for plague is 2 to 10 days, depending upon the form. The pneumonic form has an incubation period of as little as 2 to 3 days. As with many aerosolized biological weapons, the initial symptoms are fever, weakness, and nonspecific respiratory symptoms. As the pneumonia rapidly progresses, bloody sputum, severe dyspnea (breathing difficulty), and cyanosis (bluish skin color) are found. Definitive diagnosis can only be made by laboratory tests and is impossible to determine in the field.

Since the pneumonic form is highly transmissible from human to human by aerosolized droplets generated by coughing, respiratory precautions are indicated. Field care consists of self-protection and supportive treatment of the patient. Again, antibiotics are required and are most effective if started within 24 hours of the onset of the pneumonic form.

Q Fever Q fever is a zoonotic rickettsial disease caused by *Coxiella burnetii*. The natural disease results from exposure to domestic livestock. Q fever in spore form can withstand harsh environments and remain viable for months. As a biological weapons agent, Q fever is similar to anthrax.

The incubation period for Q fever is about 10 to 20 days with uneventful recovery as a rule. It has multiple symptoms including fever, chills, and headache. Q fever pneumonia is a frequent complication. Other symptoms can include sweating, malaise, fatigue, loss of appetite, and weight loss. The fatality rate is low.

Q fever is diagnosed through serology testing. Other laboratory findings may not be helpful due to the difficulty in isolating rickettsia. Treatment consists of antibiotics and support therapy.

Tularemia Tularemia is a zoonotic disease caused by *Francisella tularensis* (gram-negative bacillus). It is also known as rabbit fever or deer fly fever. Natural exposure to tularemia is usually from the bites of infected animals, deer flies, ticks, or mosquitoes. Tularemia has been weaponized in aerosol form.

The symptoms of tularemia include fever, headache, and weight loss. A patient may have respiratory symptoms, substernal discomfort, and a nonproductive cough. Pneumonia may also be present. Natural tularemia has a mortality rate of 5 to 10 percent.

Tularemia is diagnosed by laboratory serology. The treatment of tularemia is antibiotics with appropriate support therapy. Isolation is not required.

Toxins

As discussed earlier, toxins are not living organisms but rather chemical compounds produced by living organisms. Toxins, including botulinum toxin, shiga toxin, shellfish toxin, and ricin, are some of the most deadly compounds known.

Toxins are not volatile; that is, they do not vaporize or aerosolize without the application of energy such as an explosive. In addition, most toxins are not dermally active, so intact skin provides an effective barrier. (An exception is the T2 mycotoxin, which is derived from a fungus.) Since toxins do not replicate themselves, they are not human-to-human transmissible. The best method of weaponization varies with the particular toxin. As examples, botulinum is best disseminated through ingestion, whereas the T2 mycotoxin is most effective when aerosolized.

Botulinum The botulinum toxin is one of the deadliest compounds known. It has an LD (50) (lethal dose for 50 percent of the test population) of 0.001 mcg/kg or 0.1 mcg for a 220-pound human. By weight, botulinum is 15,000 to 100,000 times more toxic than the nerve agents.

Ricin Ricin is a potent protein toxin that is derived from the beans of the castor plant. Ricin has gained a lot of attention in recent years because some groups in the United States have manufactured the material with the specific intent of killing law enforcement officers and public officials. In addition, the recipe for ricin has been published (along with others) on the Internet and in various books. Around the world, assassinations, as well as nonterrorist murder attempts, have occurred using ricin.

The major effect of ricin is to interrupt the body's protein manufacturing process at the cellular level by altering the RNA needed for proper proteins. This results in cellular death and necrosis, or tissue death. It is readily available and easily made. It is very effective by any route of exposure and is most effective through inhalation. The patient will present with symptoms characteristic of the route of exposure. Treatment is supportive, depending upon the route of exposure.

Staphylococcal Enterotoxin B (SEB) SEB is a toxin that most commonly affects the gastrointestinal tract, when ingested, to produce a form of food poisoning. After aerosolization and inhalation, SEB produces a potentially deadly syndrome.

As with most of the biological toxins, the respiratory form normally presents in the early stages with fever, general weakness, and nonspecific respiratory symptoms. Later, fevers ranging from 103°F to 106°F (39°C to 41°C), retrosternal chest pain (pain behind the breastbone), and pulmonary edema (fluid in the lungs) may be seen. Severe cases can be fatal, but more often SEB, especially after ingestion, is incapacitating in nature. Treatment is supportive and no specific antitoxin is available.

Trichothecene Mycotoxins (T2) Trichothecene mycotoxins (T2) are produced from fungal metabolism (usually molds). T2 is soluble in water, heat resistant, and can penetrate intact skin. Natural trichothecene has caused moldy corn toxicosis in animals. There is a suspicion that some groups have weaponized T2.

The symptoms of T2 exposure include weight loss, vomiting, diarrhea, weakness, dizziness, hypotension, and shock. The onset of illness occurs within hours of exposure, and death occurs within 12 hours. There is currently no vaccine for T2 exposure. Skin decontamination is recommended using soap and water or hypochlorite. These solutions remove the toxin, but do not neutralize it.

The treatment for T2 exposure is based on the symptoms. Absorbic acid has been proposed to reduce lethality. Dexamethasone has also been shown to reduce lethality. Superactive activated charcoal will adsorb the remaining toxin and reduce lethality for ingested T2 poisons.

Viruses

Viruses are the simplest microorganisms and are obligatory intracellular parasites; that is, they replicate only inside host cells. In contrast to human body cells—which contain a nucleus, the nucleic acids DNA and RNA, and various structures necessary for life and reproduction—a virus contains only one nucleic acid, either DNA or RNA.

A virus replicates by attaching itself to a host cell and then penetrating the cell with its own genetic code, DNA or RNA. The viral genetic code then instructs the host cell to produce the necessary components to allow the virus to replicate. During this process, the host cell might then release the virus or might be destroyed.

Since the replication of a virus depends on a complicated process using host cells, it is not easy to manufacture viruses in large quantities. A terrorist organization trying to grow them would have to meet significant logistical demands. The organization would need to have well-educated personnel and be very well financed compared to those attempting to make weapons using either bacteria or biological toxins. Therefore, although possible, the weaponization of a virus is less likely than the weaponization of a bacterium or toxin.

Smallpox In 1980, the World Health Organization (WHO) declared the smallpox virus eradicated worldwide through immunization efforts. The last eight cases of smallpox occurred in the United States in 1949. The last documented case of smallpox anywhere in the world occurred in 1978 in Birmingham, England, when the virus accidentally escaped its containment and infected and killed an unimmunized medical photographer.

Today, there are only two known repositories of the virus: the Centers for Disease Control and Prevention (CDC) in Atlanta, Georgia, and the Russian equivalent, Vector, in Novizbresk, Russia. However, clandestine stockpiles may exist in other parts of the world. If they exist, we do not know their extent or location.

Immunization against smallpox in the United States stopped in the 1970s and those immunizations given had an effective duration estimated at only 10 years. Therefore, the majority of U.S. citizens today have no immunity to the virus.

Smallpox is a highly contagious disease with an incubation period that averages 12 days. Early signs and symptoms include acute-onset fever, weakness, headache, backache, and vomiting. This is followed in 2 to 3 days by the development of a rash and chicken pox-like blisters starting in the area of the mouth, throat, and face, which spread to the hands and forearms. Although the blisters also form on the trunk of the body, they are more prominent on the face and extremities than are the blisters found in chicken pox (an important diagnostic distinction). The patient should be considered contagious until all of the scabs separate from the skin. The mortality rate for smallpox in the unvaccinated patient is 30 percent.

Transmission of smallpox occurs by respiratory droplets, therefore requiring respiratory isolation. Furthermore, a strict 17-day quarantine is required for any person in contact with a smallpox patient.

Encephalitis Encephalitis (inflammation of the brain) has numerous forms: eastern, western, St. Louis, and others. The weaponization concern is the Venezuelan Equine Encephalitis, or VEE. This zoonotic disease is, as the name indicates, endemic to the geographical region of Venezuela. An outbreak of this form of encephalitis must be closely scrutinized.

Naturally occurring encephalitis is a disease found in birds and wild animals. It is transmitted to horses and humans by mosquitoes. Thus, any naturally occurring VEE outbreak should be associated with an outbreak in animals. If humans only are infected with VEE without the corresponding effects on indigenous animals, then the potential for an unnatural occurrence should be investigated.

Since encephalitis causes swelling of the brain, the patient will present with neurological symptoms. VEE onset is sudden with fever and the profound central nervous system effects of headache, photophobia (intolerance of light), and altered consciousness.

It is estimated that 90 to 100 percent of persons exposed to VEE are susceptible to its effects. However, because the fatality rate is 1 percent or less, VEE is far more likely to be incapacitating than lethal. Human-to-human transmission is possible, so people should take appropriate body substance precautions, including respiratory protection (HEPA or N-95 respirator) in the case of any patient with a productive cough.

The Viral Hemorrhagic Fevers (VHFs) The names of these diseases are commonly heard and, in the public's perception, are associated with deadly diseases. In fact, VHF is a classification of a group of diseases that includes ebola, dengue fever, Marburg, lassa fever, and many more. What these diseases have in common are their effects. Caused by viruses, they change the clotting characteristics of the blood and the permeability of the capillaries. This results in systemic hemorrhage and liquefaction of solid organs, all in association with a fever (hence, the name *viral hemorrhagic fevers*).

These highly contagious and highly lethal diseases present with a rapid onset of fever, weakness, and easy bruising and bleeding. Many times the effects can be seen first in the sclera of the eyes (the fibrous tissue covering the "whites" of the eyes). In this area, bleeding and leaking of the capillaries may be easily observed. This is then followed by the involvement of all mucous membranes.

The method of transmission to humans varies as much as the number of diseases included in the classification of viral hemorrhagic fevers. Definitely, contact with blood and other secretions is a mode. The respiratory portal of entry is even more likely. Therefore, Standard Precautions and aggressive respiratory precautions must be taken. With few exceptions, there are no vaccines and no cures, and the use of antiviral therapies has met with only limited success. The field treatment of patients will be directed to preventing the spread of the disease and providing supportive care and treatment for hypovolemia (decreased blood pressure caused by capillary permeability and hemorrhage). Depending upon the disease, the mortality rate will range between 5 and 90 percent. An intravenous serum is available to treat many strains of VHF.

Radioactive/Nuclear Devices

Potential Scenarios

When considering the possibility of a terrorist organization using a nuclear weapon, four potential scenarios should be evaluated: (1) the use of a military nuclear weapon; (2) the use of an improvised nuclear weapon; (3) the use of a "dirty bomb," or radiological dispersal device; and (4) the sabotage of a nuclear facility.

Military Nuclear Devices   Although not unheard of, it is highly unlikely that any terrorist organization could both (1) successfully obtain a military nuclear device, and (2) successfully deploy and activate the device without detection by intelligence-gathering agencies. In addition, the potential of a retaliatory response by the United States (or any other nation with nuclear weapons) is a powerful deterrent.

Improvised Nuclear Devices   It's a common belief that the basic information needed to construct a nuclear device is easily obtained. This might very well be the case. However, knowing how to construct the device to the exacting specifications necessary to make it work is another issue. In addition, the physical act of assembling the weapon—that is, placing the radioactive material into the device without the proper shielding—would expose the individual to unsurvivable levels of radiation. Even if all of these obstacles could be overcome, the intelligence community more than likely would detect the acquisition of the prerequisite materials and information before the device could be constructed.

Radiological Dispersal Device (RDD) or "Dirty Bomb"   An RDD is any device that disseminates a radioactive material; for example, a conventional bomb that spreads a radioactive substance upon exploding. This is a more likely scenario than the first two possibilities, which involve using an actual atom-splitting nuclear bomb. However, an RDD poses many of the same logistical problems in getting the radioactive material out of its containment and into the device without killing oneself. And, if we as emergency responders learn to regard all explosive incidents as a potential dissemination means for radioactive materials (as well as for chemical and biological materials), we can use very readily available detection equipment to confirm or rule out the presence of radioactive materials. Medical waste, radiological cameras, and sources from industrial processes such as food sterilization are all common sources for radiological materials that can cause injury.

Sabotage   From the standpoint of nuclear terrorism, the most likely scenario is the sabotage of an existing facility. However, nuclear power plants within the United States are highly hardened facilities. With close regulation, the security at these facilities can be tightened significantly if intelligence-gathering activities indicate credible threats. Furthermore, the checks and balances and redundant safety measures used at such plants make it very difficult for an act of sabotage to occur without being detected in advance. The more likely target is the less hardened, small-scale facilities such as those found in universities.

None of this is to say that there is no potential for an act of nuclear terrorism. However, the possibility of success is limited.

Effects of Radiation

If a terrorist were to use a radiological material, three body systems would be most severely affected: the blood-forming system (specifically the bone marrow), the gastrointestinal system, and the central nervous system. These effects and the *rem* (roentgen equivalent [in] man, a measure of radiation dosage) dose necessary to produce them are summarized in Table 41-2.

rem
roentgen equivalent (in) man; a measure of radiation dosage.

Table 41-2 Systemic Effects of Rem Dosages

STARTING DOSE	SYSTEM AFFECTED	EFFECTS
150 rem*	Blood	• Suppression of the blood-forming characteristics of the bone marrow. • Opportunistic diseases after the white blood cells die and are not replaced (7 days). • Anemia as red blood cells die off (in approximately 30 days). • Clotting difficulties as platelets are not replaced (30–60 days).
500 rem	Gastrointestinal system	• Death of the tissues of the gastrointestinal (GI) tract. • Nausea and vomiting with profound fluid loss. • Hypovolemia (fluid loss) and shock. • Prognosis is poor if symptom onset is within 2 hours of the exposure.
1,000 rem	Central nervous system	• Damage to the vascular bed of the central nervous system (CNS). • Results in cerebral edema (swelling of the brain) and profound CNS effects (headaches, blurred vision, strokelike symptoms, and death). • Prognosis is poor for radiological exposures with CNS effects.

*rem = roentgen equivalent (in) man; a measure of radiation dosage

Incendiary Devices

The use of incendiary devices by terrorists is more plausible than the use of nuclear devices. Obviously, it is not hard either to obtain or to initiate items like Molotov cocktails, propane bombs, or even small, shaped charges on existing storage containers of flammable gases or liquids. In addition, the terrorist may elect to initiate the weapon with complicated chemical, electronic, or mechanical initiation devices. In these cases, the impacts of the initiation items themselves must be considered (chemicals, the use of radios, and remote control devices for toys or models).

Specialized teams are generally available to deal with incendiary devices. These teams are often affiliated with the military or with law enforcement agencies (Figure 41-8). Since even seemingly small devices can cause considerable damage, know how to contact the agency that is responsible for dealing with incendiary devices in your area.

Blast Injury Patterns

Review the information on blast injuries in Chapter 28, "Soft-Tissue Trauma." Primary and secondary blast injuries create specific injury patterns. There are two mechanisms: a high-energy overpressurization, usually a blast wave, and a low-energy blast wind. Parts of the body that are especially vulnerable to blast injuries are the lungs, ears, abdomen, and brain.

FIGURE 41-8 (A) A specialized truck contains equipment for handling explosives, including (B) a robot that can be rolled out to deactivate an explosive device, allowing crew members to remain at a safe distance. *(Photos A and B: © Ray Kemp/911 Imaging)*

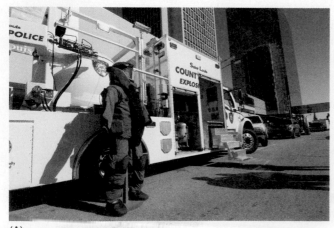

(A)

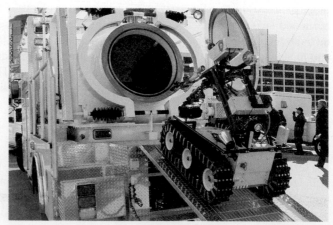

(B)

Lung Injury

"Blast lung" is a direct consequence of the HE overpressurization wave and the most common cause of death. It is the most common fatal primary blast injury among initial survivors. Signs of blast lung are usually present at the time of primary assessment or triage, but they have been reported as late as 48 hours after the explosion. Blast lung is characterized by three signs: apnea, bradycardia, and hypotension (cessation or pauses in breathing, slow heart rate, and low blood pressure). Blast lung should be suspected for anyone with breathing difficulty, cough, coughing up blood, or chest pain following blast exposure.

Ear Injury

Primary blast injuries of the auditory system cause significant injury, but are easily overlooked. Injury is dependent on the ear's orientation to the blast. The rupture of the typanic membrane is the most common injury to the middle ear. Signs of ear injury are usually present at the time of primary assessment and should be suspected for anyone presenting with hearing loss, ringing in the ears, or bleeding from the external canal.

Abdominal Injury

Gas-containing sections of the GI tract are most vulnerable to primary blast effects. This can cause immediate rupture of the large or small intestines, hemorrhage, mesenteric shear injuries, solid organ lacerations, and testicular rupture. Blast abdominal injury should be suspected in anyone exposed to an explosion who has abdominal pain, nausea, vomiting of blood, testicular pain, unexplained hypovolemia, or any findings suggestive of an acute abdomen. Clinical findings may be absent until the onset of complications hours or days later.

Brain Injury

Primary blast waves can cause concussions or mild traumatic brain injury (MTBI) without a direct blow to the head. Consider the patient's proximity to the blast, particularly when given complaints of headache, fatigue, poor concentration, lethargy, depression, anxiety, insomnia, or other constitutional symptoms. The symptoms of concussion and posttraumatic stress disorder can be similar.

Treatment for Blast Injuries

The treatment for patients who incur thermal and blast injuries from these weapons is no different from the treatment for patients of any other thermal or blast injury. Local protocols must be followed. As appropriate, follow your system's hazmat and multiple-casualty incident procedures, as discussed in Chapter 39, "Hazardous Materials, Multiple-Casualty Incidents, and Incident Management."

STRATEGY AND TACTICS

EMS responders should understand how to apply tactical considerations to isolate the incident site, notify the appropriate authorities, identify agent indicators, and protect critical assets. The DOT *Emergency Response Guidebook* provides additional information for the common terrorist weapons:

- Nerve agents (Guide #153)
- Blister agents (Guide #153)
- Blood agents (Guides #117, 119, 125)
- Choking agents (Guides #124, 125)
- Irritant agents (riot control) (Guides #153, 159)

Use of an Incident Command System was discussed in Chapter 39, "Hazardous Materials, Multiple-Casualty Incidents, and Incident Management."

Priorities for responders are:

- Life safety
- Incident stabilization
- Protection of property

CORE CONCEPT

Applying strategy and tactics at a terrorist event

Additional critical asset considerations include:

- Responders
- Responders' equipment
- Organizational function continuity

Strategies are broad general plans designed to achieve desired outcomes. **Tactics** are specific operational actions responders take to accomplish their assigned tasks. This section will discuss tactics for:

- Isolation
- Notification
- Identification
- Protection

Isolation

Initial Considerations

Approaching an act of terrorism (which is also a criminal event) presents unique challenges to the EMS responder. To effectively implement scene control and ensure public safety, emergency responders must quickly and accurately evaluate the incident area and determine the severity of danger. Once the magnitude of the incident is realized, attempts to isolate the danger can begin. Establishing control (work) zones early will enhance public protection and facilitate medical treatment.

Initially, when response resources are limited, isolating the hazard area and controlling a mass exodus of panicked and contaminated people will likely overwhelm the best efforts of first-arriving responders (Figure 41-9). Responders must use any and all available resources effectively and efficiently to prepare the scene for ongoing operations.

Responders must be aware that terrorists may still be lurking nearby, waiting for responders to arrive. In fact, as noted earlier, the responders could be the actual targets. Terrorists may also be among the injured. If this is suspected, initial scene control will likely be delayed and dictated by law enforcement activities.

As in all hazardous situations, self-protection is a top priority. A responder who becomes a patient only adds to the burden on available resources. Responders must anticipate the potential for multiple hazard locations.

Responders may have to define outer and inner operational perimeters. There may be several hazards within the outer perimeter that must be isolated, especially when patients are scattered throughout the boundaries of the incident or when there have been multiple targets that contain dangers.

FIGURE 41-9 Panicked, contaminated people can overwhelm the best efforts of first-arriving responders when response resources are limited. (© AP Images/ Amy Sancetta)

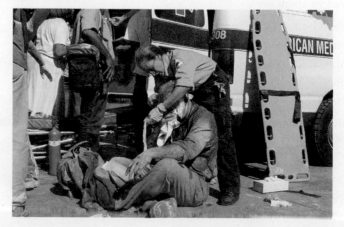

Controlling the scene, isolating hazards, and attempting to conduct controlled evacuations will be resource intensive and require law enforcement personnel. Inordinate security may be needed for the event, so responders should request additional assistance early.

After a bombing, access to the scene may be limited due to rubble or debris. Police activity may also interfere with establishing access and exit avenues for EMS operations. Another problem may involve large numbers of contaminated patients and would-be rescuers moving in and out of the exclusion zone in an uncontrolled manner. In chemical, biological, and radiological/nuclear incidents, secondary contamination is a major risk.

Establishing Perimeter Control

Law enforcement agencies should establish perimeter control at terrorist incidents by following recognized methods or standard operating procedures. Maintaining control of the perimeter may be difficult due to the design of the terrorist or panic among the patients.

Responders need to recognize and evaluate dangers critical to implementing perimeter control. Adequate evaluation of potential harm will guide decisions and considerations for setting stand-off distances or establishing work zones. In order to perform this task efficiently and effectively, responders should first take time to perform an adequate size-up of the situation.

When initially determining your operating perimeter, it is better to overestimate the size of the perimeter than to underestimate. Once you establish a perimeter, it is often easier to reduce than to increase the perimeter after operations are set up. Depending on the size and complexity of the incident, you may need to divide the boundaries or identify them as having outer and inner perimeters.

The *outer perimeter,* the most distant control point or boundary of the incident, is used to restrict all public access to the incident. For example, the outer perimeter established after the bombing of the Alfred P. Murrah Federal Building in Oklahoma City enclosed 20 square blocks. The World Trade Center footprint was over 16 acres with the perimeter encompassing all of lower Manhattan. The *inner perimeter* (or hot zone) isolates known hazards within the outer perimeter. It is often used to control movement of responders. Inner perimeters are established when several suspicious parcels are sighted. The locations of these items are isolated until such time as specialists have rendered the area safe.

Several types of terrorist incidents may require outer and inner perimeter controls. Incidents involving improvised explosive devices should always have responders thinking about secondary devices. Use inner perimeters to control access to any suspicious area. In cases involving chemical or biological dispersion devices, you may need to use inner perimeters to isolate areas highly suspected of contamination as well as of possible secondary devices. In cases of radioactive contamination, inner perimeters may be necessary to isolate possible areas of contamination until specialists with radiation meters have determined the actual level of danger to responders.

Perimeter Control Factors

Perimeter control may be influenced by a variety of factors. These factors should all be considered and weighed in relation to each other when attempting to determine the next course of action.

The amount and type of resources on hand will provide a rough estimate of what is possible to accomplish. The capability of available resources must also be considered. People should not attempt actions beyond their training. The ability of the resources to self-protect is a related factor. No matter how well trained personnel are, if they are unable to properly protect themselves, they cannot function in a hazardous environment. The size and configuration of the incident, as well as the stability of the incident, will also come into play.

These factors are the same whether you are dealing with a noncriminal hazardous materials incident or a terrorist attack.

NOTE: *Never lose sight of the fact that the behavior of a material is not determined by whether the release was accidental or deliberate.*

Notification

In a terrorism event, it is critical that appropriate response and support agencies (at local/state/federal levels) be notified. Notification is usually required by established directives, procedures, or statutes. The appropriate agencies and points of contact should be noted in local EMS or emergency management plans.

It is not the on-scene EMT's responsibility to perform notification functions. Notification is usually done by a dispatch center or emergency operations center. However, an initial radio report by an EMT is often the "trigger event" that starts the notification process. For example, notification that a possible improvised explosive device (IED) is involved generates a notification of federal law enforcement agencies.

Identification

Identify any indicators of a particular agent (Figures 41-10A to D). Note the presence of any chemical containers or lab materials, especially those that seem out of place at the site or for which hazardous materials data sheets or shipping manifests are missing. Observe placards and labels on storage tanks or vehicles from a safe distance with binoculars. Obtain the correct spelling of a chemical or biological agent. Consult your current edition of the *Emergency Response Guidebook*. Contact a poison control center or a CHEMTREC or CHEMTEL hotline, as appropriate, to help identify and deal with the substance. (Review Chapter 39, "Hazardous Materials, Multiple-Casualty Incidents, and Incident Management," with regard to hazardous materials incidents.)

If there is an unusual pattern or incidence of illness, document the numbers of patients involved, their signs and symptoms, and any other relevant information, including pertinent negatives (for example, the absence of an obvious cause for the outbreak). Transmit this information to the appropriate authorities.

FIGURE 41-10 Some emergency and rescue services carry detectors to help identify the presence of various CBRNE agents. Examples include: (A) a chemical agent monitor; (B) a detector kit for gases, vapors, and aerosols; (C) a radiation detector; and (D) a detector kit for multiple agents including nerve agents, blister agents, and blood agents. *(Photos A, B, C, and D: © Pearson Education, courtesy of Ogunquit, Maine, Fire-Rescue)*

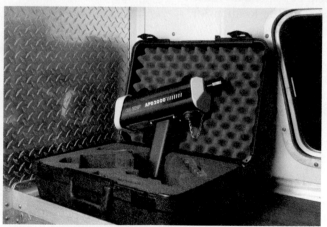

(A)

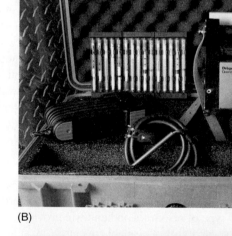

(B)

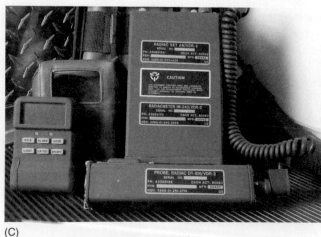

(C)

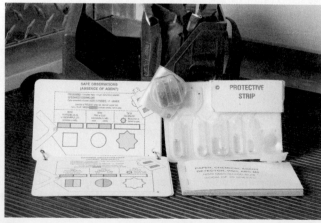

(D)

Protection

Protection of critical assets is an important function in terrorism or other criminal incidents. EMS critical assets include people, vehicles, and equipment/supplies. An applicable military term is *force protection*. Force protection means that EMS forces are protected to ensure mission accomplishment.

Effective protection requires a partnership between EMS responders and security agencies (e.g., law enforcement, private security, and National Guard units). Security agencies provide protection through perimeter protection, entry control, and traffic control.

EMTs are not armed or trained in security protection; they do not directly engage in security operations. As an EMT, your protection responsibilities include the following:

- Make an initial scene size-up to determine security threats.
- Request protection (read security) via radio as soon as practical.
- Establish vehicle staging and triage/treatment areas in protected locations.
- Advise EMS Command about protection/security concerns.
- Immediately report suspicious people or activities.

Decontamination

NFPA 473 lists as a competency for EMS personnel "Gross Decontamination. The initial phase of the decontamination process during which the amount of surface contamination is significantly reduced. This phase can include mechanical removal and initial rinsing."

Review the information on decontamination procedures in Chapter 39, "Hazardous Materials, Multiple-Casualty Incidents, and Incident Management."

SELF-PROTECTION AT A TERRORIST INCIDENT

At this point, it is a good idea to review and reinforce what you have learned about protecting yourself in the event that you are called to respond to a terrorist incident.

CORE CONCEPT
Self-protection at a terrorist event

Protect Yourself First

As always, remember that if you, the EMT, are injured, you cannot help anyone else. For self-protection, you can rely mostly on what you already know about multiple-casualty incidents, the Incident Management System, personal protective equipment (PPE), crime scenes, hazardous materials incidents, and decontamination procedures. Scene size-up and situational awareness are important reassessments in a response to a potential terrorist incident. For example:

- Are patients displaying signs and symptoms of hazardous substance exposure?
- Are there unconscious patients with minimal or no trauma?
- Are there patients exhibiting SLUDGEM? signs/seizures?
- Is there blistering, reddening of skin, discoloration, or skin irritation?
- Are the patients having difficulty breathing?

It is important to look for physical indicators and other outward warning signs. When responding, consider if there is evidence of the following:

- Medical mass casualties or fatalities with minimal or no trauma
- Responder casualties
- Dead animals and vegetation
- Unusual odors, color of smoke, vapor clouds

A few elements may be involved in a terrorist incident that would not necessarily be involved in the usual range of EMS calls. These include the fact that EMRs are often targets of a terrorist attack, that an unusual incidence or pattern of illness may result from a deliberately disseminated biological agent that cannot immediately be identified, and that an explosive device may have been detonated not only for the purpose of causing physical damage but also to spread chemical, biological, or radiological agents.

How to Protect Yourself

Given the wide range of possible agents and devices that can be used in terrorist attacks, how can you best protect yourself? Review the following guidelines, summarized from the text of this chapter.

Recognize a Possible Terrorist Event

Remember the OTTO clues that should arouse suspicion of terrorist involvement:

- Occupancy or location (a place or business that terrorist groups might target)
- Type of event (perhaps one with large crowds)
- Timing (a national holiday or an anniversary date important to terrorist organizations)
- On-scene clues (chemical containers or other out-of-place items, an unexplained pattern of illness)

Don't Rush In!

When terrorist involvement is possible (for example, at a bombing or explosion):

- Wait until the appropriate authority says the scene is safe to enter.
- Follow your Incident Command protocols.
- Wear appropriate personal protective equipment (PPE).
- Beware of possible secondary explosive devices or booby traps.
- Search all patients for explosives or weapons—or wait for police to do so—since a suicide bomber may be one of the patients.

Understand the TRACEM-P Harms

Understand what kind of harm is most likely to result from any given type of terrorist weapon or agent and focus your self-protective measures accordingly. The TRACEM-P harms are:

- Thermal
- Radiological
- Asphyxiation
- Chemical
- Etiological (disease-causing)
- Mechanical
- Psychological

Time, Distance, and Shielding

These three elements—time, distance, and shielding—can be put to use to reduce exposure to every type of terrorist agent. Don't forget to use all three, when possible.

The following paragraphs will summarize the likely TRACEM-P harms, as well as appropriate time/distance/shielding measures, for each type of CBRNE (chemical, biological, radiological/nuclear, explosive) agent.

At a Chemical Incident

Chemical harm is the primary potential harm. Keep exposure *time* to a minimum (for example, rotate teams for short periods; decontaminate yourself as quickly as possible). Remain at a *distance*, outside the contaminated area, unless trained and equipped to enter it. *Shield* yourself by wearing protective clothing and respiratory protection such as self-contained breathing apparatus (SCBA).

At a Biological Incident

Etiological harm is the primary potential harm—that is, the possibility of contracting the disease yourself. Limit exposure and contamination. Keep exposure *time* at a minimum, except as needed to assess and treat patients. Promptly take recommended decontamination measures (review Table 41-1). Stay at a *distance* from contaminated areas as much as possible. *Shield* yourself by keeping recommended vaccinations and inoculations up-to-date and by wearing clothing and equipment that protects your skin, face, hands, feet, head, body, and respiratory system (for example, a HEPA or N-95 mask).

At a Radiological/Nuclear Incident

Radiological harm is the primary potential harm, with potential *thermal harm* and *mechanical harm* as well if an explosive device was involved. Limit your *time* in the contaminated area. Local protocols should define your exact time limits for exposure. Follow your local decontamination procedures promptly after any exposure. Remain at a *distance* from the contaminated area unless you are trained and equipped to enter it. *Shield* yourself behind structures or materials that are impervious to penetration by alpha, beta, and gamma radiation (review Figure 41-4).

At an Explosive Incident

Thermal and *mechanical harms* are the primary potential harms at an explosive incident. *Etiological harm* is possible if the device was used to disperse biological agents; *chemical harm* is possible if used to disperse chemical agents. If an explosion has already occurred, limit the *time* you spend in the hazardous area, since the possibility exists of secondary explosions or attacks on EMRs. For the same reasons, remain at a *distance* from the scene until authorities declare it safe to enter. *Shield* yourself by wearing proper turnout gear, including hard hat, protective gloves, fire-protection clothing—or as necessary for a scene where structural collapse has occurred or may occur. Also wear PPE appropriate for a chemical, biological, or radiological incident if there is any possibility that the explosive device was used to disperse such agents.

CRITICAL DECISION MAKING

It Could Happen to You . . .

Terrorism can come from many sources and on many scales—from local to nationwide. Your safety from a number of hazards is vital. In each situation, explain what hazards you may suspect and how to keep yourself safe. It is the most important decision you can make.

1. You are called to respond with the police and fire department to an office complex where a worker opened an envelope containing white powder.

2. There was an explosion in a downtown office complex. You respond with the police and fire department to treat patients from the blast.

CHAPTER REVIEW

Key Facts and Concepts

- There have been terrorist attacks throughout history. However, since the events of September 11, 2001, the modern world has been a different place because of the threat of terrorism.

- There are many different types of agents and weapons that can be used by terrorists. CBRNE is used to remember the different types. TRACEM-P is used to remember the types of hazards posed by these agents.

- You must be sure to protect yourself from terrorist attacks as well as secondary attacks which are designed to injure or kill rescuers and further the physical and psychological impact of the attack.

Key Decisions

- Is this a terrorist incident or a potential terrorist incident?
- What type of agent is being used?
- Am I in danger from the initial attack or from secondary attacks?
- How can I best protect myself from danger and hazards?
- How do I fit into the incident response plan for this incident?

Chapter Glossary

contamination contact with or presence of a material (contaminant) that is present where it does not belong and that is somehow harmful to persons, animals, or the environment.

dissemination spreading.

domestic terrorism terrorism directed against the government or population without foreign direction. *See also* terrorism; international terrorism.

exposure the dose or concentration of an agent multiplied by the time, or duration.

international terrorism terrorism that is foreign-based or directed. *See also* terrorism; domestic terrorism.

permeation the movement of a substance through a surface or, on a molecular level, through intact materials; penetration, or spreading.

rem roentgen equivalent (in) man; a measure of radiation dosage.

routes of entry pathways into the body, generally by absorption, ingestion, injection, or inhalation.

secondary devices destructive devices, such as bombs, placed to be activated after an initial attack and timed to injure emergency responders and others who rush in to help care for those targeted by an initial attack.

strategies broad general plans designed to achieve desired outcomes.

tactics specific operational actions to accomplish assigned tasks.

terrorism the unlawful use of force or violence against persons or property to intimidate or coerce a government, the civilian population, or any segment thereof, in furtherance of political or social objectives (U.S. Department of Justice, FBI, definition).

weaponization packaging or producing a material, such as a chemical, biological, or radiological agent, so that it can be used as a weapon; for example, by dissemination in a bomb detonation or as an aerosol sprayed over an area or introduced into a ventilation system.

weapons of mass destruction (WMD) weapons, devices, or agents intended to cause widespread harm and/or fear among a population.

zoonotic able to move through the animal-human barrier; transmissible from animals to humans.

Preparation for Your Examination and Practice

Short Answer

1. List and briefly describe the five most common types of terrorism incidents.

2. What is a secondary device? What precautions should be taken by an EMT regarding secondary devices?

3. List several types of events that should trigger an EMT's suspicion of possible terrorism involvement.

4. List the seven types of harm that result from a terrorism incident—and the seven-letter acronym for these types of harm.

5. Briefly discuss the concept of time, distance, and shielding.

6. Discuss several self-protection measures for biological incidents.

7. Discuss the tactics for isolation, notification, identification, and protection.

Thinking and Linking

Think back to Chapter 39, "Hazardous Materials, Multiple-Casualty Incidents, and Incident Management." Link the information on multiple-casualty incidents, hazmats, and decontamination from that chapter with information in this chapter as you consider the following situation:

- Multiple medic units are called to a "possible mass-casualty incident" at the main airport terminal. The first-arriving unit reports that there is a mass exodus of people from the terminal. Many of the patients have some type of fluid on their clothing with an unusual odor. They are clearly contaminated with an unknown substance. What immediate actions should be taken? What protection measures are critical? What decontamination procedures should be implemented?

Critical Thinking Exercises

When responding to a terrorist incident, remember that dangers to the responders may be as great as the dangers for the initial victims of the attack. The purpose of this exercise will be to consider how you might respond to such an incident.

1. You respond to an explosion in a crowded public market. Your supervisor tells you to wait before entering. You see injured people all around and wonder why you aren't allowed in to help. Why would you be held back?

2. You are one of a group of EMTs treating a group of patients that may have been exposed to a nerve agent in a public transportation system. You notice one, then another, of the EMTs you are working with develop an altered mental status. What should you do?

3. You are picking up a friend at the bus station when you notice a man acting suspiciously. The man turns away every time a police officer or employee walks by. He has a large wheeled suitcase which he pushes into a crowd and then runs away. What should you do? What are the possibilities of terrorist weapons that would fit in the suitcase? Does the ethnic background of the man make a difference?

Street Scenes

So far, it's been a slow Wednesday afternoon for your unit, Medic 15. At 14:45, things change. The dispatcher announces, "Medic 15, Engine 11, respond to 5565 Baypoint Boulevard at the Conference Center construction site, worker down from unknown injuries." You and your partner suspect some type of construction injury. One minute later, the dispatcher states, "Medic 15, Engine 11, additional information, two more workers are down; we are now receiving multiple calls."

Your partner reminds you that the Conference Center project was vehemently opposed by the Environmental Life Movement (ELM) because the site was on previously protected wetlands.

On arrival, you are met by the construction manager. He is extremely emotional and says, "There's guys collapsing all over the place. We noticed a funny smell; then it got hard to breathe."

Street Scene Questions

1. What are the indicators that this may be a suspicious incident?
2. What steps should be taken to isolate the area?
3. What steps should be taken to identify a possible mechanism of injury?
4. Identify the critical personal protection issues on this scene.

You follow your service's hazmat and multiple-casualty incident procedures and wait in the cold zone while a rescue team with hazmat suits and self-contained breathing apparatus brings the construction workers out from the toxic environment and the decon team conducts decontamination procedures. With proper personal protection in place, you then perform assessment/triage, treatment, and transport.

Officials suspect that the cause of the incident was a deliberate—rather than an accidental—release of a toxic agent, but the exact substance involved and its source are still under investigation.

Street Scenes

At 03:30, your medic unit responds to a "car fire with possible injuries." The dispatcher reminds you that the location is near the headquarters of Stop American Imperialism, an organization that opposes America's involvement in the Middle East and other parts of the world. A group called Patriots United is suspected of recently vandalizing the storefront from which Stop American Imperialism operates.

You and Engine 15 simultaneously arrive. There is a car on fire in a dead-end alley. You can't see a patient or a bystander, so you stand by while the engine pulls a line into the alley. Suddenly, the engine crew stops and retreats. The lieutenant states, "We see some type of wire stretched across the alley!"

Street Scene Questions

1. What are the indicators that this is a suspicious incident?
2. What protection precautions should be initiated—and by whom?
3. Discuss the proper notification procedures. What support agencies are required on this scene?

The incident turns out to be not a simple car fire or collision but, instead, a bombing. The alley where the car was bombed runs directly behind the Stop American Imperialism storefront, and the bombed-out car is registered to one of that organization's leaders. Neither he nor anyone else was in the car when it was bombed, so officials believe the bombing was intended to lure emergency responders to the scene where they would be killed or injured by the secondary device, a trip-wired booby trap. Investigators are following various clues at the scene, including components of the bomb device, to track down the perpetrators.

EMT PRACTICE EXAMINATION

Whether you are preparing for the National Registry of EMTs (NREMT) examination or your state examination, you are likely anxious about the test that will ultimately hold the key to beginning your experience as an EMT.

You are not alone.

In their 2009 annual report, the National Registry of EMTs noted that 69 percent of the people that took the exam passed on the first try. While this may seem discouraging, this number improves significantly with those who take the exam again.

There are several reasons for this. It is a difficult exam, but those who do not pass probably study a lot more before the next try. They also go back with the experience of having already taken the examination on computer under their belt, which may relieve some of their test-taking anxiety.

People who take the NREMT examination feel that the exam questions are different from some of the questions they see in class. They seem more difficult because the NREMT is written in a "best" answer format. You may go in and think that all of the possible answers look right—or all of them look wrong. Although this is possible, one answer is designed to be the best answer. Look for that best answer, and don't get distracted by this format. This style of question is much different from the "one correct" answer exams you may have had in class.

Also remember that there are a lot of ways to say the same thing. Your instructor may have used one acceptable term, whereas another instructor uses something different—same meaning, different words. Exams are designed to be acceptable for all instructors, all students, and all textbooks. This is why you should read each question carefully and determine exactly what the question is asking before you answer it.

The NREMT examination creates its exam based on the following guidelines:

CONTENT AREA	PERCENT OF EXAM CONTENT
Airway, Respiration, and Ventilation	17–21%
Cardiology and Resuscitation	16–20%
Trauma	19–23%
Medical and OB/Gyn	27–31%
EMS Operations	12–16%

Source: NREMT Newsletter Spring, 2010.

You may think some things are missing, such as patient assessment or pediatrics. This is because they are mixed in with the specific content areas. Patient assessment concepts are often used as part of the question in each section. In all sections (except EMS Operations) you will find that 85 percent of the questions have to do with adults and 15 percent will be pediatric questions.

Finally, your instructor has likely given you advice throughout your class: Read each question carefully. Then read each answer carefully before selecting one. This is the simplest and perhaps the most valuable advice when taking an exam. If you get flustered, stop for a minute. Compose yourself and move on again.

This 100-question examination isn't easy. It isn't designed to be. You need an exam that will help you determine where you stand. We encourage you to take this exam just like you would if it were the real thing. Take it in one sitting and without looking back to your textbook.

We are happy to be able to offer you this practice exam at the end of your class. We wish you the best on your examination—and in your practice as an EMT.

Section: Airway/Respiration/Ventilation

1. Upon insertion of an oropharyngeal airway (OPA), the distal tip of the device should be positioned in what anatomical space?
   a. Oropharynx
   b. Nasopharynx
   c. Hyperpharynx
   d. Laryngopharynx

2. The administration of a beta$_2$ specific drug to a patient with respiratory distress is done to effect a change to what portion of the respiratory tree?
   a. Alveoli
   b. Vocal cords
   c. Bronchioles
   d. Mainstem bronchi

3. Which of the following statements from the patient would BEST indicate severe difficulty in breathing?
   a. "I . . . . can't . . . . b-breathe."
   b. "I feel like I'm breathing through a straw."
   c. "I am struggling to catch my breath . . . . . real bad."
   d. "I can't breathe regular cause my chest is hurting."

4. Which of the following patients is most likely about to lose total airway patency, thereby requiring immediate intervention by the EMT?
   a. A 98-year-old female with brain cancer who is confused
   b. A 52-year-old male who is intoxicated and has recurrent vomiting
   c. A 29-year-old female in active labor who is complaining of severe pain
   d. A 68-year-old male seizing with sonorous sounds heard with each breath

5. Upon assessment of the patient's airway, you note significant gurgling with each breath. What would be the next appropriate airway intervention the EMT should perform to eliminate this finding?
   a. Head tilt–chin lift
   b. Modified jaw thrust
   c. Oropharyngeal suctioning
   d. Insertion of a nasopharyngeal airway

6. You are managing a female patient who has been in an auto accident and is now unresponsive. As you manage her airway, which of the following interventions would you likely NOT employ?
   a. Insertion of an OPA
   b. Upper airway suctioning
   c. A modified jaw-thrust maneuver
   d. Application of a head tilt-chin lift

7. When sizing an OPA for insertion in a 48-year-old male, which sizing technique is most appropriate?
   a. You should measure the OPA from the tip of the nose to the angle of the jaw.
   b. You should measure the OPA from the center of the mouth to the angle of the jaw.
   c. The OPA should fit between the corner of the mouth and the angle of the jaw.
   d. The OPA should be large enough that the lips do not seal shut when properly inserted.

8. During your initial airway management, your patient needs suctioning for prolonged vomiting. How long should you provide this oral suctioning?
   a. For 5 to 10 seconds
   b. No greater than 10 seconds
   c. Less than 25 seconds initially
   d. For as long as needed to remove vomitus

9. The mechanical process of respiration (i.e., ventilation) occurs in two phases. Which phase sees a negative pressure inside the thorax in order to make the ventilation process work?
   a. Inhalation
   b. Exhalation
   c. Pause before inhalation
   d. Pause before exhalation

10. A patient with severe asthma is having trouble breathing and adequately ventilating. What portion of normal tidal volume is this patient most likely experiencing the greatest disturbance in?
    a. Base respiratory rate
    b. Dead space ventilation
    c. Alveolar space ventilation
    d. Overall ventilation per minute

11. A patient with a change in his ventilation status secondary to a severe chest wall injury will likely display what specific early finding indicative of poor alveolar ventilation?
    a. Altered mental status
    b. Absent breath sounds in the bases of the lungs
    c. Poor pulse oximetry and a change in the heart rate
    d. Dropping systolic blood pressure and narrowing pulse pressure

12. A patient is found with a respiratory rate of 8 per minute, absent basal breath sounds, a pulse ox reading of 83 percent, and cyanotic lips and fingernails. This patient is in immediate need of what intervention?
    a. Ventilation
    b. Oxygenation
    c. Airway suctioning
    d. Semi-Fowler's positioning

13. Which of the following findings would still be present in a patient suffering from respiratory distress?
    a. Cyanotic nail beds
    b. Full speech patterns
    c. Altered mental status
    d. Pulse oximeter of 85 percent

14. You are managing a patient who was in a fight and was struck in the head with a large pipe. You find the patient to be unresponsive, apneic, bradycardic, bleeding from the head, and bleeding into the airway from oral trauma. Assuming you had all your EMT equipment available to you, what should be the initial action?
    a. Suction the airway
    b. Immobilize the patient
    c. Provide positive pressure ventilation
    d. Administer high-flow oxygen at 15 lpm

15. Which of the following clinical indications would first appear to indicate that the patient is being adequately ventilated manually with a BVM?
    a. The chest wall moves with each breath.
    b. The ventilations are at a rate of 12/minute.
    c. The patient has breath sounds in all lung fields.
    d. The vital signs and pulse oximeter start to normalize.

16. If the EMT wishes to deliver the highest concentration of oxygen possible to the patient with spontaneous breathing, what oxygenation adjunct should she use?
    a. Venturi mask
    b. Simple face mask
    c. Nonrebreather mask
    d. Partial nonrebreather mask

17. You are preparing to treat a patient with CPAP for respiratory distress. Upon assessment, however, you observe the following findings. Which of these would serve as a contraindication for the use of CPAP?

a. Respiratory rate of 22/minute
b. Pulse oximeter reading of 86 percent
c. Heart rate of 112/minute and irregular
d. Systolic blood pressure of 88 mmHg

18. Which of the following patients has a ventilatory status that would MOST benefit from a prescribed inhaler?
    a. A patient with right lower lobe pneumonia
    b. A patient with dyspnea following a heart attack
    c. Someone with wheezing from an asthma attack
    d. An apneic patient following a traumatic brain injury

19. What childhood respiratory disease is characterized by the production of thick mucus from the airways that may lead to respiratory distress?
    a. Asthma
    b. Emphysema
    c. Cystic fibrosis
    d. Chronic bronchitis

20. A patient complaining of respiratory distress is also found to have chest pressure, crackles to the chest with auscultation, distended neck veins, and edema of the lower extremities. This clinical picture BEST fits what field diagnosis?
    a. Pulmonary edema
    b. Acute asthma attack
    c. Myocardial infarction
    d. Spontaneous pneumothorax

Section: Cardiac and Resuscitation

1. If a patient has suffered a myocardial infarction to the right ventricle, blood flow to what structure may become impaired initially?
   a. Aorta
   b. Lungs
   c. Brain
   d. Pulmonary veins

2. The best known and most common finding associated with a patient suffering an acute coronary syndrome is what?
   a. Nausea
   b. Dyspnea
   c. Sweating
   d. Chest pain

3. A patient experiencing bradycardia would have what finding?
   a. A heart rate of 48/min
   b. A pulse rhythm that is irregular
   c. A respiratory rate that is 6/min
   d. A pulse pressure less than 20 mmHg

4. Of the following segments of the population, which is most likely to experience atypical presentations of a myocardial infarction?
   a. Asian males
   b. Elderly females
   c. Younger African Americans
   d. American Indian descendants

5. EMTs are treating a patient suspected of experiencing a myocardial infarction. Of the following options, which one should the EMT perform first (assuming all could be done immediately)?
   a. Apply oxygen
   b. Administer nitro
   c. Administer baby aspirin
   d. Attach the AED and hit "analyze"

6. The patient's use of which drug class of medications can be problematic if the EMT wishes to help an MI patient administer a sublingual nitro?
   a. Anti-anginals
   b. Erectile dysfunction
   c. Metered-dose inhalers
   d. Cholesterol-lowering drugs

7. Which of the following conditions is LEAST likely to be present in a patient suffering a myocardial infarction?
   a. Headache
   b. Diaphoresis
   c. Tachycardia
   d. Respiratory distress

8. An elderly male patient is experiencing a myocardial infarction. Which one of the following interventions should the EMT NOT perform?
   a. Administer oxygen
   b. Have the patient chew baby aspirin
   c. Allow the patient to take his wife's nitro
   d. Place the patient in a semi-Fowler's position

9. Assuming all of the following patients were experiencing an MI, which patient's medical history would preclude her from receiving aspirin administration?
   a. Stroke
   b. Asthma
   c. Diabetic
   d. Hypertension

10. A patient with coronary artery disease is predisposed to what coronary event?
    a. CVA
    b. Seizures
    c. Tachycardia
    d. Myocardial infarction

11. Expedient transport of a patient experiencing an MI to the hospital is recommended so the hospital can administer what kind of medication in the hopes of stopping the MI progression?
    a. Fibrinolytic
    b. Beta$_2$ specific
    c. Antidysrhythmic
    d. Antihypertensive

12. A patient with cardiac-type complaints asks the EMTs why they are administering a nitro to him. What would be an appropriate response?
    a. "Nitro makes it easier to breathe."
    b. "Nitro makes the blood pressure drop."
    c. "Nitro increases blood flow to your heart muscle."
    d. "Nitro causes the heart to beat harder and raise blood pressure."

13. A patient with a history of congestive heart failure is likely to have what other emergency when she deteriorates?
    a. Pulmonary edema
    b. Hypertensive crisis
    c. Cerebral vascular accident
    d. Severe headache with visual disturbances

14. You are caring for a 59-year-old male thought to be experiencing a heart attack. The patient initially described the pain as substernal and dull in characteristics. The patient now, however, is becoming more and more lethargic and difficult to wake up. You also note the patient's heart rate is becoming irregular. Vitals are blood pressure 112/92, heart rate is 82 and irregular, and respirations are 20. During the ongoing management of this MI, what part of normal MI management should you elect NOT to perform?
    a. Administer oxygen
    b. Ready the AED for application

c. Provide four 81-mg baby aspirin

d. Contact ALS for intercept en route to the hospital

15. What is the most common reason that an AED may shock a patient inappropriately?

a. Human failure in proper use

b. Inappropriate sensing of electrodes on the chest

c. Inability of the machine to charge quick enough to defibrillate V-fib

d. Failure on the AED processor to determine V-fib is either present or absent

16. The most common lethal cardiac rhythm a patient experiencing sudden cardiac arrest displays is what?

a. Asystole

b. Atrial fibrillation

c. Ventricular fibrillation

d. Sinus tach with ventricular ectopy

17. You arrive on-scene and find a patient who is unresponsive with no palpable pulse and no breathing. Bystanders state the patient has been in this condition for about 7 or 8 minutes. Assuming the EMT has all of his equipment immediately available, what should be done first?

a. Administer oxygen

b. Initiate compressions

c. Provide two positive pressure ventilations

d. Call medical direction to pronounce the patient

18. You are using an AED on an adult patient in cardiac arrest. After one particular analysis the AED indicates "no shock advised." What is your next immediate action?

a. Remove the AED pads

b. Assess for a carotid pulse

c. Charge the AED capacitors

d. Start compressions immediately

Section: Trauma

1. You are assessing a patient who fell from a tree. The patient is conscious and complains primarily of pain to his right arm, although he admits to having dyspnea as well. You note he has an open fracture of the right humerus with moderate bleeding controlled with pressure. He also has diminished breath sounds to the right thorax, a pulse of 92 percent on ambient air, and a narrowing pulse pressure. Of the above findings, which is so severe that it would categorize the patient as a "high priority"?

a. Pain to the right leg

b. Open humerus fracture

c. Narrowing pulse pressure

d. Diminished breath sounds

2. A patient has injured the index finger of her left hand while trying to drive a nail with a hammer, accidentally hitting her finger instead. Other than the soft-tissue trauma and skeletal deformity, no other signs of trauma are present. How should the secondary assessment proceed on this patient?

a. Focus only on the injury site

b. Complete a full head-to-toe assessment

c. There is no need to perform a secondary assessment

d. Assess both arms and hands, but not the torso or lower extremities

3. While orienting a new EMT hire to your EMS system, you quiz him over general knowledge and ask him to define what the mnemonic "DCAP-BTLS" stands for. Which of the new EMT's answers below is incorrect?

a. Painful

b. Swelling

c. Contusions

d. Lacerations

4. A teenage patient has sustained soft-tissue trauma while using woodworking tools in shop class. The patient, upon your arrival, has a damp cloth held over his forearm. When he removes this cloth, bright red blood comes spurting out. This would be what kind of bleeding?
    a. Venous
    b. Arterial
    c. Capillary
    d. Arteriovenule

5. A patient with soft-tissue trauma has lost a significant amount of blood. If this patient enters into a hypoperfusion syndrome (shock), what is the likely etiology?
    a. Neurologic
    b. Distributive
    c. Cardiogenic
    d. Hypovolemic

6. You are managing an elderly patient who has sustained a deep laceration to the leg with bleeding. The patient has the following vitals: blood pressure 102/88, heart rate is 98/min, respirations are 22/min, and the skin is cool and clammy. Which of the above findings BEST represents a developing shock state?
    a. Heart rate
    b. Skin findings
    c. Blood pressure
    d. Respiratory rate

7. Of the following types of soft-tissue trauma, which one could present as either an open soft-tissue injury or a closed soft-tissue injury?
    a. Contusion
    b. Crush injury
    c. Arterial laceration
    d. Superficial abrasion

8. You are treating a patient who has sustained a high pressure injection injury to the hand while at his construction job. Prior to transport you have provided oxygen and immobilized the hand. As the EMT, what additional intervention should you provide en route?
    a. Apply heat
    b. Apply cold
    c. Elevate the limb above the heart
    d. Lower the limb below the heart

9. Which of the following interventions should always be provided to any patient suffering from a soft-tissue injury?
    a. Treat for shock
    b. Extremity immobilization
    c. Full spinal immobilization
    d. Transport the patient with lights and sirens

10. A child was running with a broken stick in her hand when she suddenly fell, and the stick she was carrying became impaled through her mouth and into her hard palate. Including proper positioning and stabilization of the object, how should the EMT apply oxygen?
    a. Nasal cannula at 6 lpm
    b. Simple face mask at 10 lpm
    c. Pediatric face mask at 12 lpm
    d. Nonrebreather mask at 15 lpm

11. A 32-year-old male patient has sustained a burn to his entire left arm, the front of his chest and abdomen, and half of his right arm. What is the approximate percentage of his burned skin?
    a. 18 percent
    b. 30 percent
    c. 32 percent
    d. 36 percent

12. During an MCI where your equipment is limited, you are treating a chest trauma patient and you elect to apply an occlusive dressing to an open chest wound. The normal occlu-

sive dressings for this purpose have already been used up. What other type of material could substitute for this purpose?

a. Trauma dressing
b. Sterile burn sheet
c. 4" × 4" gauze pads
d. Material such as plastic wrap

13. What is the most important clinical reason that a flail segment should be properly stabilized as early as possible?

a. To reduce pain
b. To maintain good lung expansion
c. To prevent a hemothorax from forming
d. To prevent a pneumothorax from forming

14. Of the following chest injuries, which one would have the LEAST effect on the quality of breath sounds heard with a stethoscope?

a. Hemothorax
b. Pneumothorax
c. Commotio cordis
d. Traumatic asphyxia

15. Which of the following isolated fractures would be best treated with a traction splint?

a. Tibia
b. Pelvis
c. Femur
d. Humerus

16. You are caring for a patient who fell off the back of a dirt bike. The patient has blood in the airway and an obvious fracture to the thigh. His breathing is labored and his mental status is deteriorating rapidly. What treatment should the EMT render first?

a. Apply oxygen
b. Suction the airway
c. Immobilize the fractured femur
d. Treat the patient's altered mental status

17. In a trauma patient, what is typically the first finding that is consistent with a brain injury?

a. Altered mental status
b. Systolic hypertension
c. Neuromuscular deficit
d. Slowing of the pulse rate

18. Which of the following patients' clinical conditions meets the physiologic criteria for determining if the patient is a high priority?

a. GCS of 15
b. Systolic pressure of 86 mmHg
c. Pupils are 2 to 3 mm in diameter
d. The patient demonstrates weakness to one extremity

19. You are caring for a multisystem trauma victim who is unresponsive. You are currently 10 minutes from an urgent care facility, 35 minutes from a small community hospital, and 1.5 hours from a trauma center. Aeromedical transport could be at your location in 10 minutes, with a 20-minute transport time to the trauma center. What is the best way to provide transport?

a. Transport to the urgent care facility
b. Transport to the trauma center by ground
c. Transport to the small community hospital
d. Call for aeromedical transport to the trauma center

20. If a patient falls through the ice on a lake into the cold water, the patient will lose the majority of her body heat through what mechanism?

a. Elimination
b. Respiration
c. Conduction
d. Evaporation

21. You are caring for a male patient who was found sitting in the stands at a baseball game. The patient is disoriented, skin is warm to the touch, the pulse is strong and bounding, sweating is absent, and the skin is reddened. Along with oxygen and moving the patient out of the sun, what other intervention should you perform as the EMT?
    a. Attach the AED
    b. Provide cool fluids by mouth
    c. Initiate active external cooling
    d. Allow the patient to drink an electrolyte solution

Section: Medical and OB/GYN

1. While assessing a medical patient, what mnemonic will assist the EMT with finding out particularities of the chief complaint?
   a. AVPU
   b. OPQRST
   c. SAMPLE
   d. DCAP-BTLS

2. Which of the following is NOT considered to be one of the components of the secondary exam in a responsive patient with a medical emergency?
   a. Baseline vital signs
   b. Focused physical exam
   c. History of the present illness
   d. Determination of patient priority

3. Upon initial questioning of a patient, the patient is complaining of multiple things: chest pain, dyspnea, and abdominal pain. What should be the next course of action for the EMT?
   a. Ask the patient which thing bothered him first
   b. Ask the patient which thing is bothering him the most
   c. Treat the patient as if he has three chief complaints
   d. Assume that the chest pain is the chief complaint due to its potential severity

4. Which of the following medical patients will the EMT perform a rapid physical exam on?
   a. An 86-year-old unresponsive diabetic patient
   b. A 9-year-old boy with asthma who is scared
   c. A 32-year-old male with respiratory distress
   d. A 60-year-old psych patient threatening to kill himself

5. A patient with an injury or dysfunction to what region of the brain may have problems staying awake or paying attention?
   a. Cerebellum
   b. Hypothalamus
   c. Foramen magnum
   d. Reticular activating system

6. The patient with diabetes has a pathophysiologic problem with what hormone?
   a. Insulin
   b. Glucose
   c. Dopamine
   d. Norepinephrine

7. A diabetic patient takes her insulin medication regularly and watches what she eats. However, one day she is not feeling well and she vomits a few times after breakfast. What medical emergency related to diabetes could this cause?
   a. Hypertension
   b. Hypotension
   c. Hypoglycemia
   d. Hyperglycemia

8. Within the body of the diabetic patient, what organ is most sensitive to lowered levels of glucose?
   a. Liver
   b. Brain

c. Heart

d. Pancreas

9. A diabetic patient may be considered hypoglycemic if he has an altered mental status and a blood sugar level less than what value?

a. 60 mg/dL

b. 80 mg/dL

c. 100 mg/dL

d. 120 mg/dL

10. You are caring for a diabetic patient with low blood sugar. The patient is unresponsive with sonorous airway sounds. He has a rapid pulse and peripheral perfusion is intact. Which of the following interventions is of utmost concern for this patient?

a. Manual airway technique

b. Suctioning out the airway

c. Providing high-flow oxygen

d. Administration of oral glucose

11. A patient with what type of seizure is most likely to present as unresponsive?

a. Partial

b. Generalized

c. Focal motor

d. Jacksonian seizures

12. You are caring for a patient who is experiencing a generalized seizure. During the tonic-clonic phase, which of the following management strategies should you employ?

a. Apply high-flow oxygen via nonrebreather mask and position the patient supine

b. Loosen restrictive clothing and protect the patient from injury

c. Apply oral glucose and place the patient in the recovery position

d. Restrain the patient physically to avoid harm and transport immediately

13. You are assessing a patient who has confusion, difficulty in speaking, and is unable to get out of bed due to left-sided weakness. The symptoms, the family states, occurred very suddenly. The blood pressure is 210/130, the pulse is 98, and respirations are 18. As an EMT, what should be your most likely field impression for the patient's condition?

a. Stroke

b. Seizure

c. Hyperglycemia

d. Hypoperfusion

14. A patient that has recurrent episodes of unilateral weakness, headaches, vision disturbances, or confusion that resolves on its own in a short period of time is likely experiencing what emergency?

a. MI

b. CVA

c. HTN

d. TIA

15. You are working with a new EMT on your squad. After a call for an MI patient who became unresponsive, the EMT asks you how a heart attack could cause such a thing. Which of the following most correctly answers this question?

a. "Increased blood flow due to tachycardia."

b. "A drop in blood flow to the brain from a failing heart."

c. "The heart was extracting too much oxygen from the bloodstream, leaving an insufficient amount for the brain to use."

d. "The patient's lungs were failing due to the drop in left ventricular contraction."

16. You are assessing a known seizure patient that "passed out" according to bystanders. During your assessment, which clinical clue would help you identify that the patient had a syncopal episode rather than a seizure?

a. The patient bit his tongue.

b. The patient was conscious upon your arrival.

c. The patient "woke up" seconds after going supine.

d. The patient took his antiseizure medications today.

17. You have a patient experiencing an anaphylactic reaction. Which chemical mediator function is responsible for the edema to the airway that can rapidly cause the patient's death?

a. Dilation of blood vessels

b. Capillaries start to seep fluid

c. Bronchoconstriction to the lungs

d. Production of thick mucus in the airways

18. You have a male patient who was stung by a bee 5 minutes ago. Of the various signs and symptoms consistent with an allergic reaction, which one would be the most suggestive of a severe allergic reaction (anaphylaxis)?

a. Tachycardia

b. Rapid onset

c. Bilateral wheezing

d. Stridorous breathing

19. The administration of epinephrine to an anaphylactic patient will not have any effect on which of the following clinical conditions?

a. Wheezing

b. Airway edema

c. Itching and hives

d. Low blood pressure

20. You are completing a PCR on an anaphylactic patient you just transported to the hospital. During transport, you had to assist the patient with the administration of her Epi-Pen®. As you complete this task, what adult dose of drug would you document for the epinephrine?

a. 0.15 mg

b. 0.30 mg

c. 0.45 mg

d. 0.60 mg

21. Following the management of a patient with an acute allergic reaction, you have administered epinephrine, given oxygen, and placed him in a position of comfort. Which of the following findings is most consistent with marked patient improvement?

a. The blood pressure increased 10 mmHg.

b. Bilateral wheezing has diminished greatly.

c. The patient is now able to speak in full sentences.

d. The heart rate decreased from 132 to 108/minute.

22. Of the following mechanisms of entry for a poison to enter the body, which is most likely to occur to the pediatric patient?

a. Injection

b. Ingestion

c. Inhalation

d. Absorption

23. You are caring for a male patient who is complaining of severe global abdominal pain. The abdomen is also rigid to the touch. The patient has a history of blunt abdominal trauma from 5 days earlier during a sporting event that he did not seek medical treatment for. What condition is this presentation most consistent with?

a. Peritonitis

b. Pancreatitis

c. Appendicitis

d. Gastroenteritis

24. Which of the following strategies would be MOST beneficial in establishing a rapport with a psychologically disturbed patient who is displaying a behavioral emergency?

a. Avoid eye contact

b. Speak slow and clear

c. Do not listen to her stories

d. Speak to her sternly for clarity

25. During the management of a patient known to have sickle cell anemia, the patient is complaining of shortness of breath. This could be due to what change in her red blood cells?

a. Inability to carry oxygen
b. Inability for the heart to pump the sickle-shaped cells
c. Inability for the lungs to take in oxygen and produce carbon dioxide
d. Inability of the red blood cells to use oxygen for energy production

26. While assisting another ambulance with off-loading a patient at the hospital who is immobilized on a backboard, the EMT states that they can't maintain the blood pressure in this 30-year-old, near-term, pregnant female. As you quickly scan the patient over, what would alert you to a cause for the hypotension?
a. The patient is immobilized supine.
b. The patient is only on low-flow oxygen.
c. The patient has a traction splint applied to the left leg.
d. The patient has backboard straps across the body tightly.

27. You arrive at the scene of a medical patient. You are shown to the patient's bedroom where the patient is found lying on the bed. You immediately see the patient wearing a CPAP mask. Given this, what is one expected medical diagnosis you'll probably see in the patient's history?
a. Sleep apnea
b. Hypertension
c. Severe pneumonia
d. Neuromuscular disorder

28. You are assessing a patient who is on a home ventilator secondary to a traumatic brain injury years earlier. The family is afraid the ventilator is failing. What is the best assessment parameter to let the EMT know that the ventilator is still working properly?
a. The patient has no cyanosis.
b. The heart rate is <100/minute.
c. The patient's pulse ox is >95 percent.
d. The patient still has bilateral breath sounds.

Section: EMS Operations

1. What agency has established national EMS standards as well as an assessment program to achieve these recommended standards?
a. NHTSA
b. NREMT
c. NAEMT
d. NAEMSE

2. Which of the following national certification levels is designed for the first person likely to be on the scene of an accident or illness?
a. Advanced Emergency Medical Technician
b. Emergency Medical Responder
c. Emergency Medical Technician
d. Paramedic

3. You are going to help in the self-administration of an MDI in a patient with COPD that has a prescribed inhaler. If the EMT provides this care without first contacting medical direction, what kind of protocols is he employing?
a. On-line medical direction
b. Off-line medical direction
c. Patient-directed medical care
d. Evidence-based medical direction

4. Organisms that can cause diseases in humans when in contact with the infected patient's blood, such as the HIV virus, are known by what name to the EMT?
a. Cross contamination
b. Airborne pathogens
c. Bloodborne pathogens
d. Parasite-host relationship

5. You are exiting the ambulance for a patient who has called EMS for recurrent vomiting. At a bare minimum, what type of protective equipment should you employ prior to patient contact?
   a. Gown
   b. Gloves
   c. HEPA mask
   d. Eye protection

6. Which of the following lifting techniques is best for maintaining good body mechanics to avoid potential injury?
   a. Keep the weight as close to your body as possible when lifting
   b. Use a backboard for moving patients down stairs whenever possible
   c. When given the choice, pull a wheeled cot rather than push it
   d. Carry, rather than use a wheeled device, for moving patients a distance

7. What type of patient move would the EMT employ if the patient was in a building in danger of collapse that would certainly kill the patient?
   a. Emergency
   b. Non-urgent
   c. Delayed
   d. Urgent

8. An adult patient is suing an EMS provider for not properly immobilizing his leg, leading to a permanent neurologic injury. In a court of law, what legal tenet must the patient's attorney prove in order to show that the EMTs were at fault?
   a. Guilt
   b. Assault
   c. Battery
   d. Negligence

9. During an MCI where there are multiple people injured due to a large industrial building collapse, what type of communication technology may become easily overwhelmed by the sudden usage?
   a. Repeaters
   b. Mobile phone
   c. Mobile radios
   d. Base stations

10. You are at the scene of an MVA where a patient is going to be flown to the hospital due to her injuries. You are serving as the landing zone coordinator for your fire department. As you set up the landing zone, what is the minimum recommended size?
    a. 50' by 50'
    b. 100' by 100'
    c. 150' by 150'
    d. 200' by 200'

11. What would be the recommended training level for EMS responders as it relates to responding to hazardous materials incidents?
    a. First Responder Awareness
    b. First Responder Operations
    c. Hazardous Materials Specialist
    d. Hazardous Materials Technician

12. Although not entirely possible at all MVA incidents, the EMS responders should exit the emergency vehicles to what side?
    a. With oncoming traffic
    b. Against oncoming traffic
    c. Toward the curb side of the road
    d. Toward the centerline of the road

13. You and your partner are attending an in-house continuing education session on terrorism. The presenter has used the term "CBRNE" multiple times, but hasn't explained it completely. Your partner leans over and asks you what the "B" stands for. What would be your response?

a. Burns
b. Bombs
c. Biological
d. Bionuclear

Answers

Section: Airway/Respiration/Ventilation

1. Answer: D

Rationale: The OPA airway works by lifting the base of the tongue off the posterior pharynx. With proper insertion, the tip should rest in the laryngopharynx so it can fully support the tongue. The nasopharynx is where the nasal cavity empties into the pharynx and would be too superior, as would the oropharynx as this is where the oral cavity connects with the pharynx. There is no location referred to as the hyperpharynx.

2. Answer: C

Rationale: A beta$_2$ specific drug will relax smooth muscle, the kind that wraps the bronchioles of the lungs. This relaxation will allow better air flow to the alveoli for gas exchange. The vocal cords are comprised of fibrous tissue that is unresponsive to beta$_2$ stimulation, and the bronchi are supported by cartilage which is also unresponsive to beta$_2$ stimulation. Finally, there are no smooth muscle fibers in the alveoli; hence, this drug will not have an effect at that level.

3. Answer: A

Rationale: A key ability of the EMT is to recognize the difference between adequate and inadequate breathing. A patient that can speak in full sentences (multiple words in one breath) is typically breathing adequately. A patient who cannot speak in full sentences (usually less than two to three words per breath) is not breathing adequately and will need oxygen (and probably PPV support).

4. Answer: D

Rationale: Airway patency is an absolute requirement for patient survival. An indication of partial upper airway occlusion is sonorous breath sounds (snoring). While the unresponsive female and intoxicated male may deteriorate more, as of yet they are not showing indications of partial airway occlusion. The active labor patient also does not show indications of acute airway deterioration.

5. Answer: C

Rationale: The upper airway sound described as "gurgling" is secondary to fluid accumulation in the pharynx that has air passing through it while the patient breathes (think about blowing air through a straw in water). The only intervention listed that will remove the fluid from the airway is suctioning. The other interventions are more appropriate if the tongue is blocking the airway (commonly, this causes snoring sounds with each breath).

6. Answer: D

Rationale: A patient who has potential cervical-spinal trauma, such as this patient who was in an auto accident, should not have cervical manipulation due to the possibility of spinal trauma. The insertion of an OPA, airway suctioning, and a jaw-thrust maneuver are all airway interventions that can be applied without cervical manipulation.

7. Answer: B

Rationale: There are two measuring techniques for the OPA; either is appropriate. The first is to measure the OPA from the center of the mouth to the angle of the jaw. The other is to measure from the corner of the mouth to the earlobe on the same side of the face. While the length is measured, there is no measuring technique for the size as it relates to the mouth opening.

8. Answer: D

Rationale: During airway management, the guideline is to suction for no longer than 10 seconds; however, in a patient who has prolonged vomiting as this patient did, the suctioning should proceed until the vomit has been removed. Failure to do so will allow the patient to aspirate the vomit with detrimental effects. Generally speaking, when doing routine suctioning of small fluid amounts, the patient should be preoxygenated pre- and post-suctioning, with suctioning lasting only about 10 seconds.

9. Answer: A

Rationale: Ventilation occurs due to a changing of pressure within the thorax as compared to atmospheric pressures. During inhalation, the diaphragm drops and the rib cage flares up and out, creating a larger intrathoracic cavity which causes the development of a negative pressure (Boyle's law). The negative pressure then causes air to flow from outside the body (higher pressure) to inside the lungs (lower pressure) in order to equalize. During exhalation there is a positive pressure in the thorax forcing air out. Pauses that occur before a phase of ventilation are non-material to the process or to pressure changes.

10. Answer: C

Rationale: Tidal volume is comprised of the amount of air in one ventilation. For the average person, this volume is roughly 500 mL. Of this 500 mL though, not all of it participates in gas exchange because it fills the dead space regions of the respiratory tree (roughly 150 mL). The balance of the tidal volume is alveolar ventilation. In situations of impaired breathing, the alveolar ventilation normally suffers because the dead space volume does not change (i.e., the body has to fill the dead spaces in order to reach the alveolar space).

11. Answer: B

Rationale: When a patient has poor alveolar ventilation, the first thing that will always be noted is an absence of breath sounds over the lungs' periphery (apical and basal regions). This is from an absence of ventilation making it to the alveoli in order to create a breath sound. Eventually, the absence of diffusion of gases through the alveoli will cause changes in mental status, pulse rate, blood pressure, and pulse oximeter. Basically, once the breath sounds go off-line, then everything else starts to fail from a lack of oxygenation and ventilation.

12. Answer: A

Rationale: The patient in this scenario is in immediate need of ventilation. Although he has a spontaneous respiratory rate of 8/minute, if the depth of breathing is not sufficient enough to create alveolar breath sounds, then the rate really doesn't matter—the patient is still breathing inadequately. There is no indication in the scenario that the patient needs suctioning, and changing the body position may help with breathing, but does not inherently infer that breathing will become adequate.

13. Answer: B

Rationale: A patient with respiratory distress is still able to maintain adequate ventilation with the body's compensatory mechanisms—as such, his speech patterns should remain essentially the same. During respiratory distress, the pulse oximeter and mental status finding also should remain normal, and no cyanosis to the nail beds should be present. Altered mental status, cyanosis, and low pulse oximeter readings are more consistent with respiratory failure and arrest, not simply distress.

14. Answer: A

Rationale: The patient in this scenario needs multiple interventions, almost simultaneously. However, the patient is certainly in dire need of positive pressure ventilation since he is not breathing. However, since there is blood in the airway, this will need to be suctioned out first. After suctioning, positive pressure ventilation can be initiated with high-flow oxygen. Immobilization of the patient should occur following treatment of life threats, but prior to moving the patient.

15. Answer: C

Rationale: When a patient is being adequately ventilated, one of the first things to ensure is that the patient is being ventilated deep enough to create breath sounds bilaterally. Although chest wall motion is an indication, you may still see some chest wall motion even though the patient is not being ventilated deep enough (i.e., just dead space ventilation is being done). The rate of ventilation is not a key finding since ventilating at the right rate but insufficient depth is of no use to the patient. Finally, changes in the vital signs and pulse oximeter will occur only after good ventilations are being performed—their presence is a good finding, but not as reliable or as early as the presence of bilateral breath sounds in all lung fields.

16. Answer: C

Rationale: A nonrebreather face mask has a reservoir bag to collect oxygen used during inhalation as well as butterfly valves that port exhaled gases out of the mask while allowing the inhalation of 100 percent oxygen. This provides the greatest oxygenation to the patient who is spontaneously breathing. The Venturi mask, nasal cannula, and partial nonrebreather mask all allow the patient to entrain room air, which will dilute the oxygen being supplied and lower the overall percentage of oxygen in the inhaled gases.

17. Answer: D

Rationale: CPAP is a treatment intervention in which "back-pressure" is provided to the patient via a mask applied to the face, which helps to stent open the alveoli and small airways to aid in exhalation. The problem, however, is that the back-pressure keeps the alveoli inflated, which in turn makes it more difficult for blood to pass from the right side of the heart to the left. The end result is a potential drop in blood pressure. As such, this intervention should not be used on patients with a systolic blood pressure less than 90 mmHg.

18. Answer: C

Rationale: The medication within a prescribed inhaler is designed to relax the smooth muscle found in the respiratory bronchioles. As such, patients with bronchoconstriction are the main beneficiaries of this drug. Patients with conditions such as asthma and COPD are commonly prescribed this med. The use of the drug with a heart attack or brain injury patient is irrelevant since the cause for dyspnea is not mediated by bronchoconstriction. In addition, pneumonia is an alveolar disease process, which is not aided with an inhaler since there is not smooth muscle tissue in the walls of the alveoli.

19. Answer: C

Rationale: Cystic fibrosis is a genetic childhood disease in which thick sticky mucus accumulates in the digestive tract and the respiratory tract. The respiratory accumulation results in plugging, respiratory distress, recurrent respiratory infections, and in severe cases may cause respiratory failure. Asthma is a disease that causes bronchoconstriction of the airways, and is commonly precipitated by some type of exposure. Emphysema and chronic bronchitis happen most often to adults and elderly people. Where emphysema results in alveolar damage, chronic bronchitis results in mucus production and scarring of the lung tissue.

20. Answer: A

Rationale: Pulmonary edema is a condition commonly caused when the left ventricle begins failing (CHF), causing a backing-up of blood into the lungs. The result is fluid leaking into the alveoli causing dyspnea, crackles, distended neck veins, and other respiratory distress findings. Asthma commonly causes wheezing and has a different history of events. Myocardial infarctions can cause pulmonary edema, but it is not common to every infarction. Finally, a spontaneous pneumothorax causes specific pleuritic pain, diminished or absent unilateral breath sounds, and no presence of crackles.

Section: Cardiac and Resuscitation

1. Answer: B

Rationale: The right ventricle pumps blood to the lungs for reoxygenation. As such, if the right side of the heart is failing from an infarction, then lung perfusion could falter. This commonly causes the patient to experience dyspnea, but the lung sounds are often clear. The brain and aorta are perfused by blood flow coming from the left ventricle, and the pulmonary veins carry oxygenated blood from the lungs to the left atrium.

2. Answer: D

Rationale: Although it may not be present in every single MI, and at times it may present as chest "pressure" rather than chest "pain," chest pain is the most common and most readily recognized finding when a person experiences some type of acute coronary syndrome event. This commonly signals heart muscle that is starving for more oxygen than the diseased arteries can provide. Nausea, dyspnea, and sweating may all be present during an MI (commonly from stimulation of the sympathetic nervous system), but they individually are not more common than chest pain.

3. Answer: A

Rationale: Bradycardia is a term that is used to describe a heart rate that is less than 60 beats per minute. That's not to say the bradycardia is detrimental to the patient's condition, but simply that it is less than 60/minute. An irregular heart rhythm is described exactly like that—irregular. Bradypnea describes a slow respiratory rate, and a narrow pulse pressure is used to describe the finding of a pulse pressure that is too low.

4. Answer: B

Rationale: Females and the elderly are the most common segments of the population to not have typical presentations of an MI. Many times they will not experience outright chest pain; rather, they may complain of fatigue, swollen ankles, and mild dyspnea. The other segments of the population listed do not have a specific predisposition to alterations in MI presentation.

5. Answer: A

Rationale: Although research has never clearly defined the appropriateness of oxygen in "stable" MI patients, its use early on for any patient experiencing an ACS is still advocated. The use of baby aspirin typically occurs after taking the SAMPLE and OPQRST histories, as is the administration of nitro. An AED should only be applied when the patient is unresponsive, apneic, and pulseless (i.e., in cardiac arrest).

6. Answer: B

Rationale: Erectile dysfunction drugs work, in part, by causing vasodilation of certain tissue to facilitate an erection. The problem, however, is that if a patient needs nitro for an MI or angina, and has taken an erectile dysfunction drug within the last 24 to 72 hours, the combination of these two medications can lower the blood pressure critically (and even fatally) low. The other medications listed do not share this precaution with the concurrent use of nitro.

7. Answer: A

Rationale: When a patient experiences a heart attack, there are a multitude of symptoms that are commonly present. For example, the patient typically becomes diaphoretic and tachycardic from the sympathetic discharge that often accompanies an MI. Respiratory distress could be from concurrent failure of the right or left ventricle during the MI. A headache, however, is not a commonly consistent finding in a patient with an MI.

8. Answer: C

Rationale: Although nitroglycerin may be warranted in a patient such as this, the EMT cannot assist in the administration of a medication that is not prescribed for that patient. The EMT can only assist with the administration of medications that are prescribed to the patient for use with its appropriate indication, and it must be given via the correct route, at the correct redosing schedule, and be a current prescription (i.e., not expired). The other interventions are things the EMT can do based off of medications on the ambulance (oxygen and aspirin), as well as positioning for comfort.

9. Answer: B

Rationale: Aspirin administration is contraindicated in the asthma patient because aspirin has been known to induce bronchoconstriction, which is not desirable in an asthmatic patient. However, there is no detrimental relationship associated with aspirin administration in a patient with a stroke, diabetes, or hypertension.

10. Answer: D

Rationale: Coronary artery disease is a disease process in which the interior lumen of the coronary blood vessels becomes clogged and possibly occluded. When this occurs, a myocardial infarction or ischemic episode may occur. While the same disease process can occur in the rest of the arterial system, causing things like seizures or strokes, occlusion of coronary blood vessels will result in damage to the coronary muscle.

11. Answer: A

Rationale: One goal of MI management is to restore blood flow to the injured heart as soon as possible. This is done in the hospital by one of two methods: the use of drugs to dissolve the clot (fibrinolytics) or the insertion of a catheter into the artery to reopen the blocked blood vessel (balloon angioplasty). While the use of antidysrhythmics and antihypertensive agents may be used during an MI, neither treatment reopens an occluded blood vessel. Finally, beta$_2$ specific agents are used to dilate bronchial smooth muscle and have nothing to do with coronary dilatation.

12. Answer: C

Rationale: Nitroglycerin is a coronary and peripheral smooth muscle relaxer of the muscles that surround the blood vessels. This results in coronary vasodilation which increases blood flow to an ischemic heart. Although the relief of chest pain may ease breathing, this is not why nitro is given. Likewise, nitro can cause the blood pressure to drop, but again this is not its desired effect during an MI. Finally, nitro does not cause the heart to beat harder, nor does it cause an elevation in blood pressure.

13. Answer: A

Rationale: Congestive heart failure occurs when the heart weakens to a point where it fails to pump all the blood it receives. When fluid starts to back up, especially behind the left ventricle, the fluid will seep into the alveoli, causing pulmonary edema. A hypertensive crisis and CVA can both occur from the same pathology as CHF, but CHF does not in and of itself cause either. Finally, a severe headache with visual disturbances is more common with certain types of strokes.

14. Answer: C

Rationale: Although it may be evident to the EMT that this patient has physical findings consistent with an MI, warranting the use of aspirin (and nitro), the fact that the patient's mental status is declining serves as a contraindication since the patient may aspirate on the med if the EMT cannot control the patient's airway normally. Otherwise, the use of oxygen, preparing (but not applying) the AED, and contacting ALS for intercept are all appropriate interventions if the patient's status remains unchanged or declines further.

15. Answer: A

Rationale: The technology that has gone into AED research, revision, and production has made this device almost flawless when used properly. In fact, the biggest contributor to inappropriate shocks is when it is used incorrectly by the EMT (i.e., the EMT did not confirm the patient was pulseless prior to application). Otherwise, when used appropriately, the device is almost flawless in its execution.

16. Answer: C

Rationale: There are two ventricular rhythms that the AED may shock when it identifies them: ventricular fibrillation and ventricular tachycardia. Since V-tach may or may not have a pulse, it requires the EMT to assure pulselessness prior to AED application. The AED categorizes all rhythms into two categories: "shockable" (v-tach and v-fib) and "nonshockable" (all other rhythms).

17. Answer: B

Rationale: If the patient is found in cardiac arrest, and there are no signs of obvious death, then compressions should be initiated *first* at a 30:2 ratio with ventilations until an AED is available. Although the patient should be assessed from an "A-B-C" approach, the management flows from a "C-A-B" management sequence. If there are signs of obvious death, then medical direction is called.

18. Answer: B

Rationale: When the AED indicates a "no shock" scenario, then the patient either does, or does not, have a pulse. The EMT will need to assess for either case since this information is needed to determine if the next step is compressions or ongoing airway/ventilatory assessment. Removal of the AED is not advised since the post-arrest patient may again arrest en route to the hospital. Finally, charging the AED is unwarranted because the unit just told you "no shock" was advised.

Section: Trauma

1. Answer: D

   Rationale: The most important concern with this question is determining which finding can actually cause the patient to die if it persists or gets worse. Pain to the arm hurts, but pain is not fatal. An open humerus fracture is graphic, but generally broken bones with controlled bleeding don't kill, either. A narrowing pulse pressure is an indication of body compensation, not a clinical syndrome causing death. Finally, diminished breath sounds mean the patient is not going to oxygenate well—this can potentially cause death and should be treated as a high priority.

2. Answer: A

   Rationale: When a patient has a local injury with no or minimal likelihood of deterioration, the EMT can perform a focused assessment of the injury site during the secondary exam. Part of this assessment may be comparing the two hands and assessing for size and symmetry, but it would not need to include assessing the opposite arm. Likewise, it would not require assessing the body in a head-to-toe format.

3. Answer: A

   Rationale: The mnemonic "DCAP-BTLS" stands for the following: deformities, contusion, abrasions, punctures/penetrations, burns, tenderness, lacerations, swelling. *Painful* is not part of this mnemonic; rather, it is used in the AVPU mnemonic.

4. Answer: B

   Rationale: Arterial bleeding has two major characteristics: it is bright red (oxygenated blood), and it often is very heavy or sometimes spurting. Venous bleeding is typically slower and is a darker red, owing to it being deoxygenated. Capillary bleeding is typically slow and oozing. Arteriovenule bleeding is not a type of bleeding; rather, this is the point in the vascular system where the arterioles and venules interface with the capillary bed.

5. Answer: D

   Rationale: In order to maintain normal perfusion pressures, the body has to have an intact pump (heart), pipes (vascular system), and volume (blood). If the disturbance is a loss of volume, or blood, the type of shock is termed hypovolemic. Cardiogenic shock occurs when the heart fails to pump adequately. Neurologic shock occurs when the pipes, or blood vessels, dilate excessively. Finally, distributive shock is also from widespread vasodilation but it can be from blood infections, anaphylactic reactions, and other processes that result in widespread vasodilation.

6. Answer: C

   Rationale: All the aforementioned findings could be consistent with a shock state as many of them occur while the body starts to compensate for the blood loss. The key is to look at the narrow pulse pressure. This indicates if the systolic pressure is being maintained at a large expense, from peripheral vasoconstriction (pulse pressures less than 20 mmHg typically represent this).

7. Answer: B

   Rationale: A crush injury is one that occurs when a region of the body is injured by a strong blunt-trauma mechanism. When the tissues and underlying structures arc damaged (i.e., crushed), they can bleed internally and cause other tissue or organ dysfunctions. This injury can occur with no break in the overlying skin (closed crush injury), or with a break in the overlying skin (open crush injury). Lacerations and abrasions are both open injuries, whereas a contusion is a closed injury.

8. Answer: C

   Rationale: Elevation of a high pressure injury is considered appropriate treatment prehospitally. The application of heat may vasodilate and cause increased systemic absorption of material, and the application of cold can promote vasoconstriction which further limits blood flow to the injured area, possibly worsening the injury. Placing the injury site below the heart will slow venous drainage, which can contribute to swelling and increased pressures in the limb (it also may change the perfusion status).

9. Answer: A

Rationale: Any patient, whether or not he has a traumatic event or medical emergency, should be treated for shock. Basically, this includes providing oxygen therapy, maintaining body warmth, and placing him in an appropriate position. The use of immobilization is based upon need, not just because there is a soft-tissue injury to the body. Finally, transport of the patient with lights and sirens should be reserved for the unstable or the potentially unstable patient, not all patients.

10. Answer: A

Rationale: If an impaled object enters through the mouth, the EMT will have to stabilize the end of it that is protruding through the mouth. This will undoubtedly make the application of any type of face mask impossible. As such, the use of a nasal cannula could provide oxygenation while not becoming entangled or impaired with the impaled object.

11. Answer: C

Rationale: Using the "rule of nines" for burn estimation, the following would apply: entire left arm = 9 percent, entire front of chest and abdomen = 18 percent, half of right arm 4–5 percent. This then totals approximately 32 percent of the body surface area burned.

12. Answer: D

Rationale: The whole benefit of an occlusive dressing is the inability for air to pass through the material (the dressing needs to be nonporous). This prevents air from getting inside the body through the area of the soft-tissue trauma. If there is no commercial product available, the EMT could use material such as plastic wrap, or the wrapper from a trauma pad or oxygenation device. A trauma dressing, burn sheet, and gauze pad are all porous to air, and will not "seal" the wound they are applied upon.

13. Answer: B

Rationale: In a flail segment, where multiple ribs are fractured in multiple locations, there is a loss of structural integrity that helps support the lungs. As a result, the chest wall is unable to facilitate normal lung expansion and the patient can hypoventilate, which leads to inadequate breathing. The splinting does help to reduce pain, but that is not what will save the patient's life. Finally, the patient may form either a hemothorax or pneumothorax as a result of a flail segment, but again, the most immediate danger is the inadequate lung expansion it causes.

14. Answer: C

Rationale: Commotio cordis is a heart condition in which the patient may go into cardiac arrest after a sharp blow or strike to the chest. The strike causes the heart to go into ventricular fibrillation, after which the patient collapses. This condition, though, does not affect the quality of breath sounds as it does not result in lung collapse. In the other conditions, the lung tissue is collapsed due to air (pneumothorax), blood (hemothorax), or a heavy physical weight (traumatic asphyxia).

15. Answer: C

Rationale: A femoral fracture can be a life-threatening injury due to the concurrent vascular trauma that results in significant blood loss into the muscles surrounding the femur. To help prevent this, a traction splint will draw the broken bone ends apart from each other and help minimize additional vascular trauma. In addition, the stretching will help limit blood loss. Fractures of the tibia and humerus are managed with rigid splints, and the pelvis is commonly immobilized with a pelvic wrap or, at a minimum, by immobilization on the backboard.

16. Answer: B

Rationale: Given the types of injuries this patient has, the first thing the EMT should do is manage the airway with suctioning. The use of oxygen when the airway is occluded is not beneficial; the airway must be cleared first. Treatment of the fracture will occur early on, but will likely not cause immediate death of the patient as the occluded airway could. Finally, an altered mental status is not an "injury" that can be treated; rather, it is the result of other bodily failures that must be managed.

17. Answer: A

Rationale: When a patient suffers a brain injury, a common finding is some type of neural deficit, most often an altered mental status. That does not mean the patient is unresponsive; rather, he may have amnesia, confusion, drowsiness, and so on. Systolic hypertension could indicate a severe brain injury, or a host of other medical conditions. It's not an early sign nor consistent sign either (same goes for the slowing of the pulse rate). Neuromuscular deficit could be from a brain injury, but it could also be from peripheral trauma, so it loses some of its value at predicting brain injury.

18. Answer: B

Rationale: There are three major physiologic criteria for determining a high priority patient: systolic hypotension (<90 mmHg), GCS <14, and a gross disturbance in the respiratory rate (too slow or too fast). A GCS of 15 is normal, pupils of 2 to 3 mm are normal, and weakness to a limb does not automatically mean a stroke or injury as other conditions that are not fatal can cause weakness as well.

19. Answer: D

Rationale: Often the best treatment for a trauma patient can only occur in the surgical suite and, to some extent, within the trauma bay of a large trauma center designed and experienced to handle these types of patients. Given this, the best transport option for this patient would be to the trauma center via aeromedical transport. The urgent care and small community hospital could offer only minimal help, and to drive to the trauma facility is trumped by the speed in which aeromedical could deliver the patient there.

20. Answer: C

Rationale: Conduction occurs when heat is carried away from the body through direct contact with a colder surface, such as water. Respiration is heat loss through breathing, but this will not be the major contributor to heat loss. Evaporation is the loss of heat through sweating and evaporation of the liquid, which obviously cannot happen when someone is submerged in water. Finally, elimination is not a "type" or mechanism for heat loss.

21. Answer: C

Rationale: The patient is presenting in heat stroke; therefore, he needs to be actively cooled to a lower temperature. You should not provide anything by mouth as the patient may aspirate on it, and attaching the AED should only occur on patients who are not breathing, who are pulseless, and who are unresponsive.

Section: Medical and OB/GYN

1. Answer: B

Rationale: The "OPQRST" mnemonic will assist the EMT with exploring the chief complaint. It consists of onset, provocation/palliation, quality, radiation, severity, and time. The AVPU deals with ascertaining the mental status, the SAMPLE deals more globally with the patient's background (i.e., meds, history, allergies), and the DCAP-BTLS is used when assessing for traumatic injuries or conditions.

2. Answer: D

Rationale: The determination of patient priority is actually more of a clinical outcome of completing the assessment of a patient and determining that the patient's status is critical. Most commonly it is determined at the end of the primary survey, although it could be determined at any point in time. The other parameters mentioned—vitals, physical exam, and history—are all normal parts of the secondary assessment. The fourth component of the secondary exam is the history of the present illness.

3. Answer: B

Rationale: Asking the patient for clarity of the chief complaint (i.e., which thing is bothering him the most) will allow the EMT to focus care interventions on the thing that is troubling the patient the greatest. Although what is bothering him first is important, it will not necessarily direct patient care. Treating the patient for three chief complaints may lead to multiple interventions that may contradict each other, and assuming the chief complaint is chest pain will not be true in all instances.

4. Answer: A

Rationale: The rapid physical exam is performed on medical patients when they have an altered mental status and cannot provide reliable answers to the EMT's questions. The focus of the exam is to find life-threatening conditions, or evidence that can help the EMT determine what is wrong with the patient. The other patients listed were conscious, and hence would probably not receive the rapid physical exam; rather, they would receive a focused physical exam.

5. Answer: D

Rationale: The reticular activating system is a region of nerve fibers deep in the brain that controls consciousness by way of staying awake, paying attention, and indicating when sleeping should occur. Thus, an injury or dysfunction here can easily cause the patient to be unresponsive. The hypothalamus is part of the endocrine system and the cerebellum is basically the involuntary control of voluntary muscles. The foramen magnum is actually a part of the skull.

6. Answer: A

Rationale: A diabetic patient's fundamental problem is that insulin is either not being produced, or it is not working as efficiently as it was intended to (type 1 and type 2 diabetes, respectively). Glucose is not a hormone; actually, it is the dietary fuel used to create energy. Dopamine and norepinephrine are both hormones, but they operate within the sympathetic nervous system.

7. Answer: C

Rationale: The diabetic's regulation of sugar can become problematic if she is not stringently watching her diet and medication use. In this situation where the meds are taken to lower the sugar, but the patient vomits the food up, there will be an inadequate amount of sugar in the blood for the insulin and the sugar will drop drastically and dangerously low (hypoglycemia). Hyperglycemia usually happens when the insulin levels are too low, and changes in blood pressure are really not part of the diabetic disease process.

8. Answer: B

Rationale: Almost all tissues of the body can store a certain amount of glucose that can help temporarily buffer a drop in glucose levels. The only organ that cannot do this is the brain. As such, if sugar drops too low, the neurons of the brain start to malfunction, which essentially causes changes in the mental status. Hence, the brain is the most sensitive organ to decreasing glucose levels.

9. Answer: B

Rationale: When a diabetic patient starts to become hypoglycemic, there is usually a change in mental status: he becomes sweaty and his heart rate increases. The blood sugar can complete this clinical picture as a value less than 80 mg/dL is considered to be hypoglycemic in the symptomatic patient. Naturally, levels lower than this further demonstrate hypoglycemia, but 80 mg/dL is when the suspicion becomes confirmed. Levels higher than 80 (up to 120 mg/dL) are consistent with normal glucose levels.

10. Answer: A

Rationale: A hypoglycemic patient is in dire need of glucose to return normal brain activity. However, in this patient, the glucose level has dropped so low that the patient is now unable to maintain his own airway. As such, the airway now becomes the immediate concern and a manual technique is needed to open the airway. The use of oxygen is important, but that will come after the airway is open. The use of oral glucose is not warranted now due to the patient's inability to keep his airway open.

11. Answer: B

Rationale: There are two types of seizures: partial seizures and generalized seizures. Partial seizures (also known as focal-motor seizures) occur when the seizure activity is occurring to one side of the brain and, hence, one side of the body. Generalized seizures affect both sides of the brain, and also cause the patient to be unresponsive. Jacksonian seizures are a type of partial seizures in which muscle tremors are a progressive format (i.e., fingers, hands, arm, etc.).

12. Answer: B

Rationale: A patient experiencing a generalized seizure will need multiple interventions employed quickly. This includes placing the patient on her side for drainage of fluids (if no c-spine injury is noted), loosening of restrictive clothing, removing objects from around the patient that she may fall upon or that might injure her, and protecting the patient from bodily injury without physically restraining her. The best answer described is loosening the clothing and protecting the patient from harm.

13. Answer: A

Rationale: A stroke occurs when a region of the brain is underperfused due to either an occluded blood vessel or a ruptured blood vessel. The brain tissue involved starts to malfunction, which causes changes in mental status and often weakness or paralysis on one-half of the body. Oftentimes, the blood pressure is high in these patients. Hyperglycemia does not have the unilateral findings and is usually a slow onset; in addition, hypoperfusion is unlikely given the blood pressure. Finally, seizures have a rapid onset, but their unilateral findings when present are muscular tremors or convulsions, not weakness.

14. Answer: D

Rationale: A transient ischemic attack (TIA) is a medical emergency in which there is a temporary diminishment or cessation of blood flow to an area of the brain, causing neurological impairment and possible headaches—much like a stroke. The small clot blocking the blood flow breaks up and normal blood flow returns, as does the neurological deficit. Often a TIA is considered an indication of an impending stroke. HTN refers to hypertension which does not cause unilateral signs. The same is true for a heart attack (MI). A CVA is a cerebral vascular accident, which is an older name for a stroke.

15. Answer: B

Rationale: When a person is experiencing an MI, a portion of the heart is dying due to a lack of oxygen. That section will eventually stop contracting normally and will contribute to a drop in cardiac output to the brain and body. If this drop is too great, the patient's mental status can deteriorate due to poor blood flow. Increased blood flow generally is not consistent with brain dysfunction as the brain autoregulates its own blood flow. Also, the heart does not extract so much oxygen that the other organs fail (it takes only what it needs), and the right ventricle (not left) pumps blood to the lungs.

16. Answer: C

Rationale: Both a seizure and syncopal episode can start while the patient is in a standing position. Since syncope commonly occurs from a temporary drop in cerebral blood flow for some reason, as soon as the patient goes supine, blood flow to the brain improves and the patient wakes back up. A seizure patient, however, will continue with the seizure activity when he goes supine, often biting his tongue, which is followed by a post-ictal period. Some patients may still experience a "breakthrough" seizure even though they are taking their meds regularly.

17. Answer: B

Rationale: During an anaphylactic reaction, capillaries start to leak out fluid (termed increased capillary permeability) that causes edema and swelling of surrounding tissues. This is critical in the airway structures where there is not much room for swelling. Bronchoconstriction and mucus production occur to the lungs, but neither causes the airway to occlude shut. Finally, the vascular dilation causes blood pressure to drop, leading to poor peripheral perfusion syndrome.

18. Answer: D

Rationale: All of the above findings can be found in a severe allergic reaction. However, three of them (tachycardia, bilateral wheezing, and rapid onset) can also be seen in a mild or moderate reaction. In contrast, the stridorous breathing, an indicative sign of airway closure, is a critical finding as this infers the airway is nearing complete closure due to edema.

19. Answer: C

Rationale: Epinephrine is used in a severe allergic reaction to counter the easily fatal effects of the chemical mediators released during the syndrome. These include reversing airway edema, as well as bronchiole constriction and vasoconstricting the blood vessels in order to raise the blood pressure. The use of epinephrine will not have a significant effect on the hives and itching that is often present, but that's OK as the hives and itching are not fatal.

20. Answer: B

Rationale: The correct adult dose of epinephrine contained within an epi auto inject pen (Epi-Pen®) is 0.30 mg. The pediatric dose is 0.15 mg. There is no correct dose of either 0.45 or 0.60 mg of drug for an Epi-Pen®.

21. Answer: C

Rationale: Although the airway swelling, bronchiole constriction, or peripheral vasodilation could all be fatal, the fastest among them is the airway swelling and bronchiole constriction. As such, if the patient is now able to talk in full sentences, that means the airway is open and the patient is able to draw in a full breath. As an EMT, you should expect that the blood pressure will improve, the wheezing will improve, and the heart rate will drop. These are not as reliable for immediate patient improvement as simple speech patterns.

22. Answer: B

Rationale: Infants and children have a tendency to place things into their mouths—whether it's a food product or not. As such, this habit makes them more susceptible to poisoning from ingestion (i.e., swallowing). The poison is then absorbed across the GI tract and enters the bloodstream. Inhalation occurs when they inhale the poison, absorption occurs when it crosses the skin to get inside the body, and injection occurs when the poison is injected directly into the tissues or bloodstream.

23. Answer: A

Rationale: Peritonitis is an inflammation of the peritoneal lining of the abdominal cavity. When this occurs, the abdomen becomes rigid and very painful. This condition can occur from irritation to the peritoneum from free blood in the abdomen following abdominal trauma. The other abdominal conditions (appendicitis, gastroenteritis, and pancreatitis) all typically result in localized pain during the syndrome development.

24. Answer: B

Rationale: There are general rules that should always apply when dealing with patients with behavioral emergencies. These include identifying yourself, speaking slowly and clearly, maintaining eye contact, always listening to the patient's words, not being judgmental, using positive body language, acknowledging the patient's feelings, and being alert for sudden changes in the patient's emotional status.

25. Answer: A

Rationale: Very simply, the disease process causes the red blood cells (which are normally doughnut shaped) to assume a sickle shape that has abnormal hemoglobin molecules that do not carry oxygen well, and the shape makes them difficult to pump through blood vessels. As such, they often have episodes of hypoxia and chest pain termed "acute chest syndrome." The heart can still pump the blood and the lungs can still diffuse gas; the problem lies in the inability of the diseased red blood cells to carry (not improperly use) oxygen.

26. Answer: A

Rationale: In a pregnant female near term who is lying supine, the full weight of the gravid uterus will put pressure on the inferior vena cava and can pinch it nearly shut against the posterior pelvis. This reduces preload to the right side of the heart, ultimately leading to systolic hypotension. To prevent this, the EMT should position the supine pregnant female on one side, preferably on the left side or tilted to the left side. The fact the patient is or isn't on oxygen, has a traction splint applied, or is secured by straps is irrelevant to the perfusion pressure.

27. Answer: A

Rationale: Sleep apnea is a condition in which, due to the patient's weight and other pulmonary factors, the patient is unable to keep the small respiratory airways open during sleep. The use of CPAP (continuous positive airway pressure) helps the patient to breathe better while at sleep. Its use is not warranted by hypertension, nor by severe pneumonia. Finally, to use CPAP the patient must have competent breathing muscles; the patient with a neuromuscular disorder does not have this.

28. Answer: D

Rationale: Beyond a normal ventilatory rate, the EMT should gauge the quality of each ventilator breath by its ability to move the chest wall and create alveolar breath sounds. If the vent breath is too minimal to make breath sounds, the vent is simply working ineffectively. The heart rate, pulse ox, and skin color will all change if the vent fails—but not until *after a period* of poor ventilation. The breath sounds, however, change immediately if the vent fails, and can serve as an early warning to the EMT.

Section: EMS Operations

1. Answer: A

   Rationale: The National Highway Traffic Safety Administration (NHTSA) has established EMS system standards. In addition, the NHTSA Technical Assistance Program has been devised to help EMS systems achieve these. The National Registry of EMTs (NREMT) designs a validated EMS certification exam. The National Association of EMTs (NAEMT) is a professional organization that provides current information and CE opportunities to EMS providers. The National Association of EMS Educators (NAEMSE) represents EMS educators working together to increase the quality of EMS education nationally.

2. Answer: B

   Rationale: The Emergency Medical Responder (EMR), formerly known as the *First Responder*, is the training level geared for the people who are likely to arrive first at the scene of an emergency. These people are commonly fire personnel, law enforcement, and industrial health personnel. The EMT is the entry level position with transport capability. The Advanced EMT provides certain advanced skills, and the paramedic is the highest certification level with the most involved training and expectations.

3. Answer: B

   Rationale: There are two types of medical direction the EMT uses: on-line and off-line. On-line occurs when the EMT is required to call the hospital prior to some intervention, whereas off-line occurs when the EMT can do so based on standing orders (typically written), saying that the EMT can exercise his own judgment on the appropriateness of the treatment. Patient-directed and evidence-based treatment are both versions of overall treatment perspectives, but neither are what the EMT must follow while working in EMS.

4. Answer: C

   Rationale: A bloodborne pathogen is one that can cause disease in another human being who comes into contact with blood from the infected person. Airborne pathogens are just that: they can be communicated between people by traveling through the air. Cross contamination actually infers the process by which a person contracts a disease another has, and the parasite-host relationship deals with situations in which one organism is living off another organism (think of a flea and a dog).

5. Answer: B

   Rationale: At a bare minimum, at any and every patient call or patient contact scenario, the EMT should don at least a pair of protective examination gloves. The use of additional PPE equipment (goggles, gowns, face mask, etc.) is dependent upon the exposure to potential splattering of blood or body fluids and the likelihood of inhaling a pathogen the patient releases into the air by way of exhaling, coughing, or spitting.

6. Answer: A

   Rationale: Carrying weights close to the body allows for better lifting mechanics and reduces injuries and accidents. The EMT should always use a stair chair if possible when moving patients down steps. In addition, pushing a wheeled cot is safer to the body than pulling with one arm, which can cause uneven loading on the spine. Finally, always use a wheeled device for moving a patient, especially over distances, rather than carrying her manually.

7. Answer: A

   Rationale: An "emergency" move is one that is employed to get the patient to a safe location for assessment and management. Prior to the move, there is no real assessment done on the patient, nor is there any real treatment. If the patient and the EMT are both in peril, then an emergency move is appropriate. An urgent move is used when initial management steps are completed, but the patient still needs to be moved rapidly for ongoing assessment and care. Finally, a non-urgent move is one undertaken with a slower pace and with more care. A non-urgent move is the type performed most commonly in EMS.

8. **Answer: D**

Rationale: The prosecution must show that negligence led to the defendant's injury. This generally indicates that the EMT had a duty to act, she breached that duty, there were damages (injury) from that breach, and that the breach could be predicted or prevented by the EMT's actions. If found negligent, then the EMT is liable for the injury and often pays a financial penalty to the defendant. Assault and battery deal with unlawful threatening or touching of a patient. Guilt has to do with responsibility for an action, but it is reserved for criminal (not civil) cases.

9. **Answer: B**

Rationale: Although any type of communication technology can be overwhelmed, mobile phone technology use is of particular concern to emergency services. While it may be able to handle the daily volumes of EMS use, if the system is suddenly used by many (i.e., EMS as well as the public), the mobile phone system may start to fail. This happened in some areas after the 9/11 attacks. EMS does not receive special preferential treatment by mobile phone services; as a result, they may suffer from the inability to "get through." Radio technology rarely has this type of failure.

10. **Answer: B**

Rationale: In terms of the pilot's preference, the larger the landing zone, the better. However, unlimited size is not always possible. At a bare minimum, the landing zone should be 100′ by 100′ in size, on level ground, and devoid of any overhead wires or trees. This size will accommodate the vast majority of airframes used in modern day aeromedical transport services.

11. **Answer: A**

Rationale: Although an EMS responder may be educated at the highest level of HAZ-MAT response, every EMS responder should at least become educated at the lowest level, which is First Responder Awareness. Simply put, at this level the responder is trained to recognize and initiate a response from proper organizations. In each of the other levels, portions of the training will include managing the hazardous materials or being responsible for the containment.

12. **Answer: C**

Rationale: The safest location for EMS personnel to exit the emergency units and to operate is between the properly positioned rescue unit and the curb of the road. This will diminish or eliminate any pedestrian or vehicle traffic between the EMS responders and the emergency vehicles you are retrieving equipment from or loading the patient into.

13. **Answer: C**

Rationale: The mnemonic "CBRNE" refers to common mechanisms for terrorist attacks: chemical, biological, radiological, nuclear, and explosive.

BASIC CARDIAC LIFE SUPPORT REVIEW

Some EMT students learned cardiopulmonary resuscitation (CPR) before they began their EMT course. Others learn it in their EMT course. This section reviews the elements of CPR in accordance with the American Heart Association's *2010 Guidelines for Cardiopulmonary Resuscitation and Emergency Cardiovascular Care*.

Before Beginning Resuscitation

When a patient's breathing and heartbeat stop, *clinical death* occurs. This condition may be reversible through CPR and other treatments. However, when the brain cells die, *biological death* occurs. This usually happens within 10 minutes of clinical death, and it is not reversible. In fact, brain cells will begin to die after 4 to 6 minutes without fresh oxygen supplied from air breathed in and carried to the brain by circulating blood. *Cardiopulmonary resuscitation (CPR)* consists of the actions you take to revive a person—or at least temporarily prevent biological death—by keeping the person's heart and lungs working.

Although you may perform CPR alone for a short period, at some point you will work with other EMS and health care providers. An essential element of success in any resuscitation effort is *teamwork*. Rescuers perform many tasks during a resuscitation effort and to be successful, they must work together in a coordinated, organized and efficient manner. Many of these tasks are time-sensitive and quite specific in how they must be performed, so working together is vital. This is especially true since many things happen simultaneously when the resuscitation effort is proceeding well. A team leader must be knowledgeable about resuscitation techniques, skilled in patient assessment, and clear in his or her directions to the team. Communication between members of the team must be accurate and timely to give the patient the best chance of revival.

Another element of successful resuscitation efforts is the ability to tailor the approach to the patient based on the circumstances. A patient who was submerged under water will receive the same general sequence of assessment steps as a patient who suddenly collapsed at home, but the specifics of treatment may be quite different. A good team adapts its approach to the apparent cause of a cardiac arrest. Table B-1 lists the initial steps in basic life support resuscitation, including assessing the patient, activating EMS, positioning the patient, and ensuring an open airway.

Assessing the Patient

Patient assessment is crucial. Initiate resuscitation after determining that the patient needs it. The required assessments are often described as determining unresponsiveness, breathlessness, and pulselessness—or the ABCs (airway, breathing, and circulation). As Table B-1 shows, these categories overlap and treatment may not occur in ABC sequence. For example, a patient in cardiac arrest should receive chest compressions before rescue breaths, i.e., CAB sequence.

Determining Unresponsiveness

When you encounter a patient who has collapsed, your first action is to determine unresponsiveness. Tap or gently shake the patient (being careful not to move a patient with possible spinal injury) and shout, "Are you okay?" The patient who is able to respond does not require resuscitation.

If the patient is unresponsive, immediately activate EMS unless the patient's condition is likely caused by a problem other than heart disease, e.g., submersion, injury, or drug overdose. If the patient is a child or an infant, activate EMS after 2 minutes of resuscitation unless you

Table B-1   Basic Life Support Steps

ASSESSMENT	SPECIAL CONSIDERATIONS
<ul><li>As you approach the patient, observe for signs of life: rise and fall of the chest, moaning, wheezing, coughing, or other sounds or movements.</li><li>When you reach the patient, assess for unresponsiveness by tapping the patient on the shoulder and shouting.</li><li>Palpate the carotid pulse at the same time that you put your head close to the patient's mouth to observe more closely for chest movement and listen for sounds of breathing.</li></ul>	<ul><li>If the patient has signs of life, proceed in **ABC sequence.** Open the **Airway** with the head-tilt, chin-lift, then evaluate **Breathing** and **Circulation.**</li><li>If the patient may have a spine injury, use the jaw thrust.</li><li>In an infant, check the brachial pulse.</li></ul>
MANAGEMENT	**SPECIAL CONSIDERATIONS**
<ul><li>If there are no signs of life and no pulse (or questionable pulse), activate the emergency response system if not already done and, if there is no AED available, proceed in **CAB sequence.** Administer 30 **Chest compressions**.</li><li>Open the **Airway** with the head-tilt, chin-lift and restore **Breathing** by giving two ventilations.</li><li>Repeat the cycle of 30:2 compressions to ventilations.</li></ul>	<ul><li>Tailor your actions to the cause of the patient's condition and the resources available. If there is reason to believe the patient arrested because of a respiratory problem, e.g., drowning or overdose, make ventilations a higher priority. If more than one rescuer is available, work in a coordinated fashion to perform actions simultaneously or as efficiently as possible.</li><li>If a child or infant has a pulse, but it is less than 60, begin ventilations and compressions. Children and infants usually arrest because of respiratory, not cardiac, problems.</li><li>If the patient may have a spine injury, use the jaw thrust.</li><li>If a pulse is present, but breathing is absent or abnormal, ventilate the patient at the rate appropriate for his or her age.</li></ul>

have reason to think the patient's condition is caused by heart disease. Then position the patient and open the airway with the head-tilt, chin-lift or the jaw-thrust maneuver.

Determining Breathlessness

The American Heart Association no longer recommends a separate step of "look, listen, and feel" for breathing. This takes time that delays compressions. Make a quick scan of the patient for signs of life or breathing (e.g., purposeful moving, chest wall movement). If these signs are absent, check the pulse. You will still be able to look for signs of breathing while you are checking the pulse. The patient who is breathing adequately does not require resuscitation. Gasps are not effective breaths.

If the patient is not breathing but definitely has a pulse, provide two ventilations (as explained later).

Determining Pulselessness

At the same time that you evaluate breathing, determine pulselessness by feeling for the carotid artery in an adult or a child, by feeling for the brachial artery in an infant. The adult patient who has a pulse does not require chest compressions. If an infant or child has a pulse slower than 60 beats per minute, begin CPR (ventilations and chest compressions).

If the patient has a pulse but is not breathing, provide rescue breathing (artificial ventilations). Even experienced providers sometimes have difficulty evaluating the presence of a pulse, so, unless you definitely feel a pulse in the adult patient begin chest compressions.

Assessing the ABCs

Assessments of the ABCs are included in the steps just described. Keep the ABCs in mind throughout every patient encounter, whether or not resuscitation is underway. If the answer to any of the ABC questions that follow is no, take the appropriate steps to correct the situation, *keeping in mind that the proper treatment will not necessarily occur in ABC order.*

Is the patient's *airway* open?

Is the patient *breathing*?

Does the patient have *circulation* of blood (a pulse)?

Activating EMS

If you have assistance, the other person should call 911 or otherwise activate the EMS system as soon as a patient collapses or is discovered in collapse. The quicker a defibrillator can reach the patient, the greater the patient's chances of survival.

If you are alone, and the patient is an adult, first determine unresponsiveness and breathing (as described earlier) and then activate EMS before returning to the patient to initiate the next steps. If the patient is a child or an infant, perform 2 minutes of resuscitation before activating EMS.

The reason for the difference in timing of EMS activation is that cardiac arrest in an adult is likely to be the result of a disturbance of the heart's electrical activity that will require defibrillation; so getting defibrillation equipment to the patient takes precedence over starting CPR. When cardiac arrest is probably not the result of a disturbance of the heart's electrical activity, however, (e.g., submersion, injury, or drug overdose), it is more important to perform rescue breathing, so you perform CPR briefly before activating EMS.

Children and infants generally have healthy hearts, and cardiac arrest is likely to have resulted from respiratory arrest. In this situation, rescue breathing is more likely to be helpful in a child than in an adult, and defibrillation will not help. When the child has heart disease, however, cardiac arrest is more like that of an adult, so calling for a defibrillator is more important than performing rescue breathing.

So, in most cases, 2 minutes of resuscitation before activating EMS is recommended for children and infants, but immediate activation of EMS is recommended for adults.

Positioning the Patient

As soon as you have determined unresponsiveness and activated EMS, make sure that the patient is lying supine (on his back). If you find the patient in some other position, help him to the floor or stretcher. If the patient is already lying on the floor, move him onto his back. If you suspect that the patient may have been injured, you or a helper must support the patient's neck and hold the head still and in line with his spine while you are moving, assessing, and caring for him.

Opening the Airway

Most airway problems are caused by the tongue. As the head tips forward, especially when the patient is lying on his back, the tongue may slide into the airway. When the patient is unconscious, the risk of airway problems is worsened because unconsciousness causes the tongue to lose muscle tone and the muscles of the lower jaw (to which the tongue is attached) to relax.

Two procedures can help to correct the position of the tongue and thus open the airway. These procedures are the head-tilt, chin-lift maneuver and the jaw-thrust maneuver.

Head-Tilt, Chin-Lift Maneuver

The head-tilt, chin-lift maneuver (Figure B-1) provides for maximum opening of the airway. It is useful on all patients who need assistance in maintaining an airway or breathing. It is one of the best methods for correcting obstructions caused by the tongue. However, since it involves changing the position of the head, the head-tilt, chin-lift maneuver should be used only on a patient who you can be quite sure has not suffered a spinal injury.

Follow these steps to perform the head-tilt, chin-lift maneuver:

1. Once the patient is supine, place one hand on the forehead and the fingertips of the other hand under the bony area at the center of the patient's lower jaw.

2. Tilt the head by applying gentle pressure to the patient's forehead.

3. Use your fingertips to lift the chin and support the lower jaw. Move the jaw forward to a point where the lower teeth are almost touching the upper teeth. Do not compress the soft tissues under the lower jaw, which can press and close off the airway.

4. Do not allow the patient's mouth to close. To provide an adequate opening at the mouth, you may need to use the thumb of the hand supporting the chin to pull back the patient's lower lip. For your own safety (to prevent being bitten), do not insert your thumb into the patient's mouth.

FIGURE B-1 The head-tilt, chin-lift maneuver, side view. Insert shows EMT's fingertips under bony area at center of patient's lower jaw.

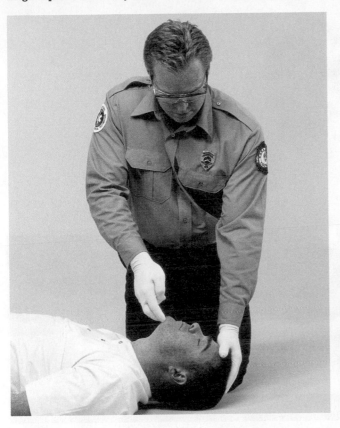
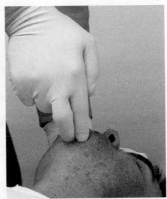

Jaw-Thrust Maneuver

The jaw-thrust maneuver (Figure B-2) is most commonly used to open the airway of an unconscious patient or one with suspected head, neck, or spinal injuries.

Follow these steps to perform the jaw-thrust maneuver.

1. Carefully keep the patient's head, neck, and spine aligned, moving him as a unit, as you place him in the supine position.

2. Kneel at the top of the patient's head. For greater comfort, you might rest your elbows on the same surface the patient is lying on.

3. Reach forward and gently place one hand on each side of the patient's lower jaw, at the angles of the jaw below the ears.

4. You can help to stabilize the patient's head by using your wrists or forearms.

5. Using your index fingers, push the angles of the patient's lower jaw forward.

6. You may need to retract the patient's lower lip with your thumb to keep the mouth open.

7. Do not tilt or rotate the patient's head. *Remember: The purpose of the jaw-thrust maneuver is to open the airway without moving the head or neck.*

NOTE: *The jaw-thrust maneuver is the only widely recommended procedure for use on patients with possible head, neck, or spinal injuries.*

Initial Ventilations and Pulse Check

The reason most apneic (nonbreathing) adults are not breathing is that the heart stopped. You will see very few adults with a pulse but with no breathing. Oxygen is often still in the patient's bloodstream. Since this is so common, you should start CPR with chest compressions, not ventilations, under ordinary circumstances. When the cause of the cardiac arrest is respiratory in nature, it may be reasonable to take a different approach and start with ventilations. In this case, deliver 2 breaths, each delivered over 1 second and of sufficient volume to make the chest rise

FIGURE B-2 The jaw-thrust maneuver, side view. Insert shows EMT's finger position at angle of jaw just below the ears.

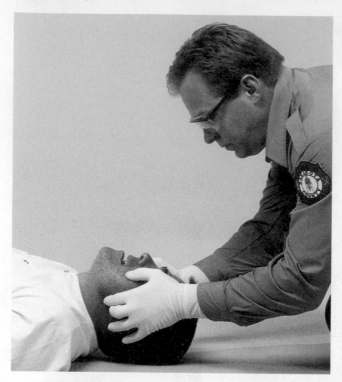
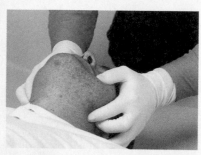

Table B-2	Rescue Breathing		
	ADULT	**CHILD**	**INFANT**
Age	Puberty and older	1 yr–puberty	Birth–1 yr
Ventilation duration	1/sec	1/sec	1/sec
Ventilation rate	10–12 breaths/min	12–20 breaths/min	12–20 breaths/min

(Table B-2). If the first breath is unsuccessful, reposition the patient's head before attempting the second breath. If the second ventilation is unsuccessful, assume that there is a foreign-body airway obstruction and perform airway clearance techniques (as described later).

If the initial ventilations are successful, you have confirmed an open airway and should feel for a pulse. If the patient has no pulse, begin chest compressions with ventilations (as described later under CPR). If the patient has a pulse but breathing is absent or inadequate, perform rescue breathing.

Rescue Breathing

Mouth-to-Mask Ventilation

Mouth-to-mask ventilation is performed using a pocket face mask with a one-way valve. The pocket face mask is made of soft, collapsible material and can be carried in your pocket, jacket, or purse. The steps of mouth-to-mask ventilation are illustrated in Scan B-1 and summarized in Table B-2.

Gastric Distention

Rescue breathing can force some air into the patient's stomach, causing the stomach to become distended. This may indicate that the airway is blocked, that there is improper head position, or that the ventilations being provided are too large or too quick to be

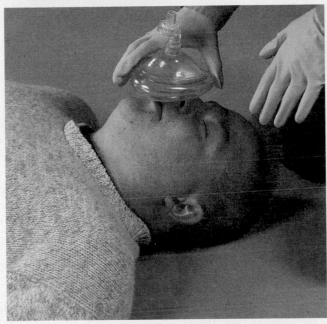

1 Position the patient and prepare to place the mask.

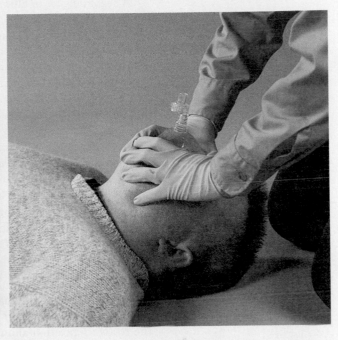

2 Seat the mask firmly on the patient's face.

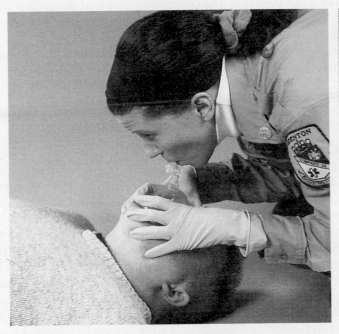

3 Open the patient's airway and watch the chest rise as you ventilate through the one-way valve.

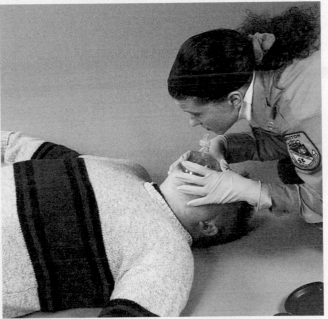

4 Watch the patient's chest fall during exhalation. Ventilate the adult patient 10 to 12 times a minute, a child or infant 12 to 20 times a minute. If the pocket mask has an oxygen inlet, provide supplemental oxygen.

accommodated by the lungs or the trachea. This problem is seen more frequently in infants and children but can occur with any patient.

A slight bulge is of little worry, but major distention can cause two serious problems. First, the air-filled stomach reduces lung volume by forcing the diaphragm upward. Second, regurgitation (the passive expulsion of fluids and partially digested foods from the stomach into the throat) or vomiting (the forceful expulsion of the stomach's contents) is a strong possibility. This could lead to additional airway obstruction or aspiration of vomitus into the patient's lungs. When this happens, lung damage can occur and a lethal form of pneumonia may develop.

The best way to avoid gastric distention, or to avoid making it worse once it develops, is to position the patient's head properly, avoid too forceful and too quickly delivered ventilations, and limit the volume of ventilations delivered. The volume delivered should be limited to the size breath that causes the chest to rise. This is why it is so important to watch the patient's chest rise as each ventilation is delivered and to feel for resistance to your breaths.

When gastric distention is present, be prepared for vomiting. If the patient does vomit, roll the entire patient onto his side. (Turning just the head may allow for aspiration of vomitus as well as aggravation of any possible neck injury.) Manually stabilize the head and neck of the patient as you roll him. Be prepared to clear the patient's mouth and throat of vomitus with gauze and gloved fingers. Apply suction if you are trained and equipped to do so.

Recovery Position

Patients who resume adequate breathing and pulse after rescue breathing or CPR, and who do not require immobilization for possible spinal injury, are placed in the recovery position. The recovery position allows for drainage from the mouth and prevents the tongue from falling backward and causing an airway obstruction.

The patient should be rolled onto his side. This should be done moving the patient as a unit, not twisting the head, shoulders, or torso. The patient may be rolled onto either side; however, it is preferable to have the patient facing you so that monitoring and suctioning may be more easily performed.

If the patient does not have respirations that are sufficient to support life, the recovery position must not be used. The patient should be placed supine and his ventilations assisted.

CPR

Checking for Circulation

Before beginning CPR, you should confirm that the patient is pulseless. In an adult or child (not infant), check the carotid pulse (Figure B-3). While stabilizing the patient's head and maintaining the proper head tilt, use your hand that is closest to the patient's neck to locate his "Adam's apple" (the prominent bulge in the front of the neck). Place the tips of your index and middle fingers directly over the midline of this structure. Slide your fingertips to the side of the patient's neck closest to you. Keep the palm side of your fingertips against the patient's neck. Feel for a groove between the Adam's apple and the muscles located along the side of the neck. Very little pressure needs to be applied to the neck to feel the carotid pulse. Keep in mind that laypeople are taught not to check for a pulse, but to look for signs of circulation: normal breathing, coughing, or movement. In an infant, check for a brachial pulse (Figure B-4). If the adult patient is pulseless, begin CPR. If an infant or child has a pulse slower than 60 beats per minute, begin CPR (ventilations and chest compressions).

To provide chest compressions, place the patient supine on a hard surface and compress the chest by applying downward pressure with your hands. This action causes an increase of pressure inside the chest and possible actual compression of the heart itself, one or both of which force the blood out of the heart and into circulation. When pressure is released, the heart refills with blood. The next compression sends this fresh blood into circulation and the cycle continues.

How to Perform CPR

CPR is a method of artificial breathing and circulation. When natural heart action and breathing have stopped, we must provide an artificial means to oxygenate the blood and keep it in circulation. This is accomplished by providing chest compressions and ventilations.

FIGURE B-3 Check the carotid pulse to confirm circulation.

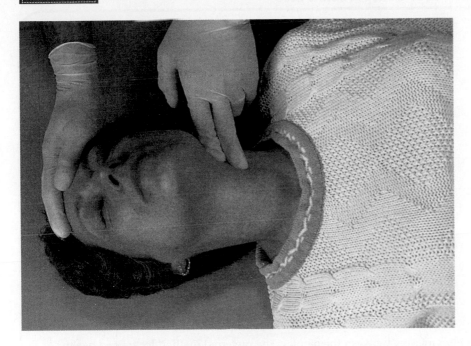

FIGURE B-4 For infants, determine circulation by feeling for a brachial pulse.

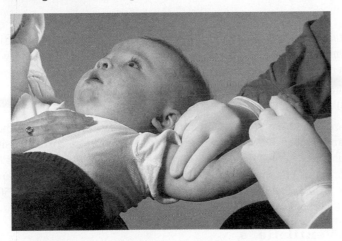

CPR can be done by one or by two rescuers. All of the information under "Providing Chest Compressions," and "Providing Ventilations" applies to both one-rescuer and two-rescuer CPR. Specific information about each type of CPR follows under "One-Rescuer CPR" and "Two-Rescuer CPR." Scans B-2 and B-3 can help you follow and review these procedures as they are described below. These procedures are for an adult patient. Procedures for infants and children will be described later.

NOTE: *Do not initiate CPR on any adult who has a pulse.*

Providing Chest Compressions

After you have placed the patient supine on a hard surface and your hands are properly positioned on the CPR compression site:

1. Place the heel of your hand on the sternum between the nipples. Put your other hand on top of the first with your fingers interlaced. Straighten your arms and lock your elbows. You must not bend the elbows when delivering or releasing compressions.

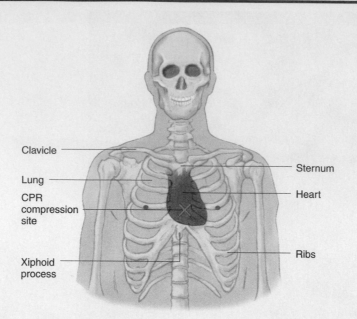

The compression site for CPR is on the sternum midway between the nipples. The preferred method for trained health care providers is outlined in steps 1 to 3 under "Providing Chest Compressions."

2. Make certain that your shoulders are directly over your hands (directly over the patient's sternum). This will allow you to deliver compressions straight down onto the site. Keep both of your knees on the ground or floor.

3. Deliver compressions STRAIGHT DOWN, with enough force to depress the sternum of a typical adult at least 2 inches.

4. Fully release pressure on the patient's sternum, but *do not* bend your elbows and *do not* lift your hands from the sternum, which can cause you to lose correct positioning of your hands. Your movement should be from your hips. Compressions should be delivered in a rhythmic, not a "jabbing," fashion. *The amount of time you spend compressing should be the same as the time for the release.* This is known as the 50:50 rule: 50 percent compression, 50 percent release.

Providing Ventilations

Ventilations are given between sets of compressions. The mouth-to-mask techniques described earlier for rescue breathing are used.

One-Rescuer and Two-Rescuer CPR

Scan B-3 shows the techniques of one-rescuer CPR and two-rescuer CPR for the adult patient and describes compression rates and ratios for CPR on adults, children, and infants.

CPR Techniques for Children and Infants

The techniques of CPR for children and infants are essentially the same as those used for adults. However, some procedures and rates differ when the patient is a child or an infant. (If younger than 1 year of age, the patient is considered an infant. Between 1 year and puberty, the patient is considered a child. Over the age of puberty, adult procedures apply to the patient. Keep in mind that the size of the patient can also be an important factor. A very small 10-year-old who has reached puberty may have to be treated as a child.)

ONE RESCUER	FUNCTIONS	TWO RESCUERS
	• Establish unresponsiveness • Position patient • If there's no response, call 911 • Call for an AED	
	• Check carotid pulse . . . (5–10 seconds) If no pulse . . . • Begin chest compressions	
	DELIVER COMPRESSIONS At least 2 inches At least 100/min.	
	DELIVER VENTILATIONS Compression: Ventilation ratio 30:2	
	• Continue compressions and ventilations • Switch every 5 cycles to prevent fatigue • Limit pulse checks **CONTINUE PERIODIC ASSESSMENT**	

NOTE: Wear gloves and use either a pocket mask with one-way valve or bag-valve mask

---

The techniques of CPR for an infant are shown in Scan B-4. For a child, CPR is conducted as for an adult, the chief difference in procedure being the hand position—using the heel of one or two hands—for chest compressions (Figure B-5). To compare adult, child, and infant CPR, see Table B-3.

When CPR must be performed, adults, children, and infants are placed on their back on a hard surface. For an infant, the hard surface can be the rescuer's hand or forearm. For an infant or a child, use the head-tilt, chin-lift or the jaw-thrust maneuver, but apply only a slight tilt for an infant. Too great a tilt may close off the infant's airway; however, make certain that the opening is adequate (note chest rise during ventilation). Always be sure to support an infant's head. Take these steps to establish a pulse in an infant or a child:

• *For an infant,* you should use the brachial pulse.

• *For a child,* determine circulation in the same manner as for an adult.

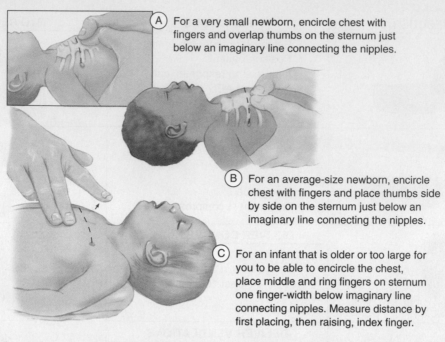

(A) For a very small newborn, encircle chest with fingers and overlap thumbs on the sternum just below an imaginary line connecting the nipples.

(B) For an average-size newborn, encircle chest with fingers and place thumbs side by side on the sternum just below an imaginary line connecting the nipples.

(C) For an infant that is older or too large for you to be able to encircle the chest, place middle and ring fingers on sternum one finger-width below imaginary line connecting nipples. Measure distance by first placing, then raising, index finger.

Position fingers for chest compressions according to the age and size of the infant. The two thumb-encircling hands method is preferred when two rescuers are present.

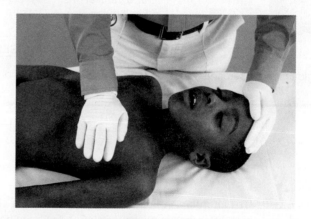

FIGURE B-5 Performing chest compressions on a child.

Special Considerations in CPR

How to Know if CPR Is Effective

To determine if CPR is effective, *if possible have someone else feel for a carotid pulse* during compressions and watch to see the patient's chest rise during ventilations. *Listen for exhalation of air,* either naturally or during compressions, as additional verification that air has entered the lungs.

In addition, any of the following indications of effective CPR may be noticed:

- Pupils constrict.
- Skin color improves.
- Heartbeat returns spontaneously.
- Spontaneous, gasping respirations are made.

	ADULT	CHILD	INFANT
Age	Puberty and older	1 yr–puberty	Birth–1 yr
Compression depth	At least 2 inches	1/3 to 1/2 depth of chest (2 inches)	1/3 to 1/2; depth of chest (1 1/2 inches)
Compression rate	at least 100/min	at least 100/min	at least 100/min (newborn 120/min)
Each ventilation	1 second	1 second	1 second
Pulse check location	carotid artery (throat)	carotid artery (throat)	brachial artery (upper arm)
One-rescuer CPR compressions-to-ventilations ratio	30:2	30:2 15:2 (2 rescuers)	30:2 (alone) 15:2 (2 rescuers) 3:1 (newborn)
When working alone: Call 911 or emergency dispatcher	After establishing unresponsiveness—before beginning resuscitation unless submersion, injury, or overdose	After establishing unresponsiveness and 2 minutes of resuscitation unless heart disease present	After establishing unresponsiveness and 2 minutes of resuscitation unless heart disease present

- Arms and legs move.
- Swallowing is attempted.
- Consciousness returns.

Interrupting CPR

Once you begin CPR, you may interrupt the process for no more than a few seconds to check for pulse and breathing or to reposition yourself and the patient.

In addition to these built-in interruptions, you may interrupt CPR to:

- Move a patient onto a stretcher.
- Move a patient down a flight of stairs or through a narrow doorway or hallway.
- Move a patient on or off the ambulance.
- Suction to clear vomitus or airway obstructions.
- Allow for defibrillation or advanced cardiac life support measures to be initiated.
- Assess the patient for signs of life when taking over CPR from someone else.
- Switch positions to minimize fatigue. (When practical, no one on the team should compress the chest for more than 2 minutes at a time. Compressing the chest is very tiring and rescuers are poor judges of when their compressions are no longer deep enough or fast enough.)

Whenever you must interrupt compressions, it is very important that you do it quickly to minimize the amount of time during which the patient is not circulating blood. When CPR is resumed, begin with chest compressions rather than with ventilations.

When Not to Begin or to Terminate CPR

As discussed earlier in this chapter, CPR should not be initiated when you find that the patient—even though unresponsive and perhaps not breathing—does have a pulse. Usually, of course, you will perform CPR when the patient has no pulse. *However, there are special circumstances in which CPR should not be initiated even though the patient has no pulse:*

- **Obvious mortal wounds.** These include decapitation, incineration, a severed body, and injuries that are so extensive that CPR cannot be effectively performed (e.g., severe crush injuries to the head, neck, and chest).

- **Rigor mortis.** This is the stiffening of the body and its limbs that occurs after death, usually within 4 to 10 hours.
- **Obvious decomposition.**
- **A line of lividity.** Lividity is a red or purple skin discoloration that occurs when gravity causes the blood to sink to the lowest parts of the body and collect there. Lividity usually indicates that the patient has been dead for more than 15 minutes unless the patient has been exposed to cold temperatures. Using lividity as a sign requires special training.
- **Stillbirth.** CPR should not be initiated for a stillborn infant who has died hours prior to birth. This infant may be recognized by blisters on the skin, a very soft head, and a strong disagreeable odor.

In all cases, if you are in doubt, seek a physician's advice. Once you have started CPR, you must continue to provide CPR until:

- Spontaneous circulation occurs ... then provide rescue breathing as needed.
- Spontaneous circulation and breathing occur.
- Another trained rescuer can take over for you.
- You turn care of the patient over to a person with a higher level of training.
- You are too exhausted to continue.
- You receive a "no CPR" order from a physician or other authority per local protocols. There are three criteria that have been extremely accurate in determining when it is reasonable to stop CPR, without missing anyone who has a chance of survival:
  1. The arrest was not witnessed by EMS personnel or first responders.
  2. There has been no return of spontaneous circulation (patient regains a pulse) after three rounds of CPR and rhythm checks with an automated external defibrillator (AED).
  3. The AED did not detect a shockable rhythm and so did not deliver any shocks.

If you turn the patient over to another rescuer, this person must be trained in basic cardiac life support.

The Trained Healthcare Provider versus the Lay Provider CPR

As an EMT you will be regarded as a "trained health care provider" with regard to CPR. The training you receive is more in-depth than a lay rescuer or bystander might receive. The course for people who wish to learn CPR and have no medical background differs from the training an EMT receives in the following ways:

- Lay rescuers are not trained to check for a pulse before beginning compressions in CPR. If the patient is not breathing and does not otherwise respond (breathing, cough, or movement), the lay rescuer is supposed to begin compressions.
- As an EMT you will be taught additional techniques that are not taught to lay rescuers, such as the two-thumbs-encircling-hands technique for two-rescuer compression in infants.
- Lay rescuers may be reluctant to do rescue breathing, especially on a stranger. Also, coordinating and timing both compressions and respirations is likely to be beyond the abilities of a lay provider. For these reasons, the current American Heart Association Guidelines recommend that the lay rescuer perform compressions without respirations.

It is possible for you to come upon a bystander performing CPR and see some of these differences in practice. If you ask the bystander "Does the patient have a pulse?" he might not have checked, nor was he required to do so.

Remember that performing CPR is quite stressful for the lay person or bystander. In many cases, CPR will be performed by one family member on another member of his own family. It is important to be supportive and use a nonjudgmental tone about the efforts undertaken by the lay person or bystander.

Clearing Airway Obstructions

Not every airway problem is caused by the tongue (the situation in which you would use the head-tilt, chin-lift maneuver or the jaw-thrust maneuver, described earlier, to open the airway). The airway can also be blocked by foreign objects or materials. These can include pieces of food, ice, toys, or vomitus. This problem is often seen with children and with patients who have abused alcohol or other drugs. It also happens when an injured person's airway becomes blocked by blood or broken teeth or dentures or when a person chokes on food.

Airway obstructions are either partial or complete. Partial and complete obstructions have different characteristics that may be noted during assessment, and each type has a different procedure of care. It is important to understand the differences between partial and complete obstruction and the correct care for each.

Mild Airway Obstruction

A conscious patient trying to indicate an airway problem will usually point to his mouth or hold his neck. Many do this even when a partial obstruction does not prevent speech. Ask the patient if he is choking, or ask if he can speak or cough. If he can, then the obstruction is mild.

For the conscious patient with an apparent mild airway obstruction, have him cough. A strong and forceful cough indicates he is exchanging enough air. Continue to encourage the patient to cough in the hope that such action will dislodge and expel the foreign object. *Do not* interfere with the patient's efforts to clear the obstruction by means of forceful coughing.

In cases where the patient has an apparent mild airway obstruction but he cannot cough or has a very weak cough, or the patient is blue or gray or shows other signs of poor air exchange, treat the patient as if there is a severe airway obstruction, as described below.

Severe Airway Obstruction

Be alert for signs of a severe airway obstruction in the conscious or unconscious patient:

- *The conscious patient* with a severe airway obstruction will try to speak but will not be able to. He will also not be able to breathe or cough. Sometimes he will display the distress signal for choking by clutching the neck between thumb and fingers.

- *The unconscious patient* with a severe airway obstruction will be in respiratory arrest. When ventilation attempts are unsuccessful, it becomes apparent that there is an obstruction.

Abdominal Thrusts

The use of abdominal thrusts to clear a foreign body from the airway of an adult or child (not infant) patient is performed as follows:

For the conscious adult or child (not infant) who is standing or sitting

1. Make a fist, and place the thumb side of this fist against the midline of the patient's abdomen between waist and rib cage. Avoid touching the chest, especially the area immediately below the sternum.

2. Grasp your properly positioned fist with your other hand and apply pressure inward and up toward the patient's head in a smooth, quick movement. Deliver rapid thrusts until the obstruction is relieved.

For the unconscious adult or child (not infant) or for a conscious patient who cannot sit or stand, or if you are too short to reach around the patient to deliver thrusts

Place the patient in a supine position and begin CPR. Every time you open the airway, look in the mouth for an object. If, and only if, you see an object, remove it by sweeping your fingers in the patient's mouth from one side to the other.

If the obstruction is not relieved after a series of five thrusts, reassess your position and the patient's airway (if the patient is unconscious, also attempt finger sweeps to attempt to remove the obstruction). Attempt to ventilate the patient and, if unsuccessful, repeat the series of thrusts. Repeat the sequence until the obstruction is relieved.

Chest Thrusts

Chest thrusts are used in place of abdominal thrusts when the patient is in the late stages of pregnancy, or when the patient is too obese for abdominal thrusts to be effective. The use of chest thrusts to relieve an airway obstruction is described below.

For the conscious adult who is standing or sitting

1. Position yourself behind the patient and slide your arms under his armpits, so that you encircle his chest.

2. Form a fist with one hand, and place the thumb side of this fist on the midline of the sternum about 2 to 3 finger widths above the xiphoid process. This places your fist on the lower half of the sternum but not in contact with the edge of the rib cage.

3. Grasp the fist with your other hand and deliver chest thrusts directly backward toward the spine until the obstruction is relieved.

For the unconscious adult

1. Place the patient in a supine position.

2. Perform CPR. Every time you open the airway, look in the mouth for an object. If, and only if, you see an object, remove it by sweeping your fingers in the patient's mouth from one side to the other.

Airway Clearance Sequences

Table B-4 lists sequences of procedures to use in the event of a severe airway obstruction or a mild airway obstruction. Note that, as discussed earlier, you should activate the EMS system as soon as unresponsiveness is determined, before carrying out the remainder of the airway clearance procedures.

Airway clearance procedures are considered to have been effective if any of the following happens:

- Patient re-establishes good air exchange or spontaneous breathing.
- Foreign object is expelled from the mouth.
- Foreign object is expelled into the mouth where it can be removed by the rescuer.
- Unconscious patient regains consciousness.
- Patient's skin color improves.

If a person has only a mild airway obstruction and is still able to speak and cough forcefully, do not interfere with his attempts to expel the foreign body. Carefully watch him, however, so that you can immediately provide help if this partial obstruction becomes a complete one.

Table B-4	Airway Clearance Sequences		
	ADULT	**CHILD**	**INFANT**
Age	Puberty and older	1 yr–puberty	Birth–1 yr
Conscious	Ask, "Are you choking?" Abdominal thrusts maneuver until obstruction is relieved or patient loses consciousness	Ask, "Are you choking?" Abdominal thrusts until obstruction is relieved or patient loses consciousness	Observe signs of choking (small objects or food, wheezing, agitation, blue color, not breathing). Series of: 5 back blows and 5 chest thrusts
Unconscious	Establish unresponsiveness.	Establish unresponsiveness.	Establish unresponsiveness.
	If alone, call for help. Then open airway. Attempt to ventilate. If unsuccessful, perform CPR. Remove visible objects (NO blind sweeps).	Open airway. Attempt to ventilate. If unsuccessful, perform CPR. Remove visible objects (NO blind sweeps). After 2 minutes, call for help if alone.	Open airway. Attempt to ventilate. If unsuccessful, perform CPR. Remove visible objects (NO blind sweeps). After 2 minutes, call for help if alone.

Procedures for a Child or Infant

The procedure for clearing a foreign body from the airway of a child is very similar to that used for an adult. The airway clearance procedure for an infant uses a combination of back blows and chest compressions as shown in Scan B-5.

For both a child and an infant, a major difference from adult procedures is:

- If the child or infant becomes unconscious, send someone else to activate the EMS system. If no one else is available, wait until you have either relieved the obstruction or you have attempted the airway obstruction sequence for 2 minutes.

SCAN B-5 | Clearing the Airway—Infant

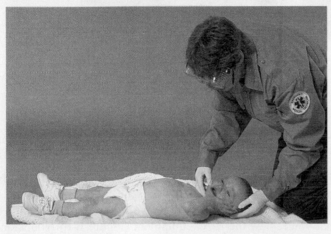

1 Recognize and assess for choking. Look for breathing difficulty, ineffective cough, and lack of strong cry.

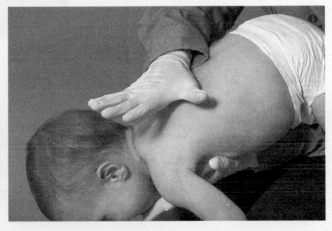

2 Give up to 5 back blows and . . .

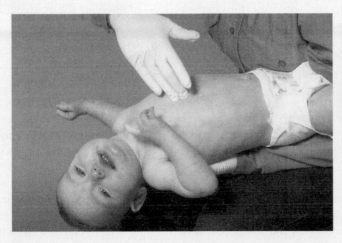

3 . . . 5 chest thrusts.

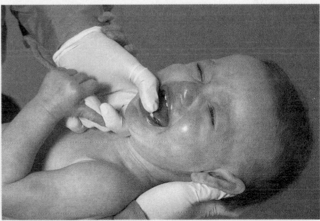

4 If the infant becomes unresponsive, open the airway and look for a foreign body. If you see one, use a finger sweep to remove it. (Never do blind finger sweeps.) Attempt to ventilate. If this fails, reposition the head and try again. If you are not successful, start CPR. If you are working alone, after 2 minutes activate the EMS system and continue airway clearance and ventilation efforts. Transport as quickly as possible.

Note: For realism, the photo sequence above shows airway clearance procedures being performed on a real baby. The baby is awake. In practice, of course, a baby with an airway obstruction is likely to be unresponsive.

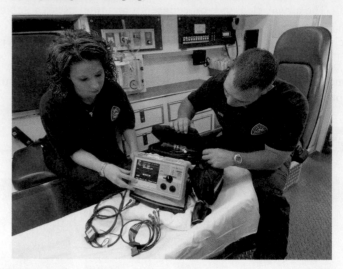

Applying ECG Electrodes

An electrocardiogram (ECG) provides data on the heart's electrical activity. In the field, it is used to alert EMS personnel to life-threatening rhythm disturbances. Interpretation of an ECG has traditionally been a paramedic skill. However, to save time on calls you may be asked to assist. Make sure that you review the ECG equipment (Figure B-6). You should know how to turn on the monitor, how to record an ECG strip, how to change the battery, and how to change the roll of ECG paper. (These are the things that most often need to be done while the paramedic is involved with the patient.)

You also may be asked to carry out four steps in the process of applying the electrodes:

1. Turn on the ECG monitor.
2. Plug in the monitoring cables or "leads."
3. Attach the monitoring cables to the electrodes.
4. Apply the electrodes to the patient's body.

Become familiar with the electrodes used by the paramedics with whom you work. There are two types: monitoring electrodes (with smaller pads) and combination monitoring/defibrillator electrodes (with larger pads). The one most commonly used by paramedics is the monitoring electrode.

If you are asked to apply monitoring electrodes to the patient's body, you will need three or four (depending on the device)—each one giving a different "view" of the heart's electrical activity. First prepare the patient's skin. The best connection is on dry, bare skin, so it may be necessary to shave excessive hair and dry the area. Use a wash cloth to remove oil from the skin and consider using an antiperspirant on patients with very sweaty skin. Become familiar with the monitoring configuration (where to place the electrodes) used by ALS personnel in your system. The most common setup is placing the negative (white) electrode under the center of the right clavicle, the positive (red) electrode on the left lower chest, and the ground (black or green) electrode under the center of the left clavicle or the right lower chest (Figure B-7A).

The abbreviations on the cables that attach to the electrodes have the initials LA, RA, LL, and RL for left arm, right arm, left leg, and right leg. Some ALS providers prefer the electrodes to be placed on the actual extremities (Figure B-7B) rather than on the corresponding portion of the torso as shown in Figure B-7A. Procedures for this vary, so follow the directions from the ALS provider you are assisting or the protocols of your EMS system.

Some ALS systems have moved toward the routine use of a 12-lead ECG in the field. These machines usually provide a computerized interpretation of the patient's cardiogram that can easily be transmitted to the emergency department via cellular phone. A 12-lead

FIGURE B-7A The most common positioning of electrodes for an ECG is shown here. Become familiar with the monitoring configuration used by ALS personnel in your system.

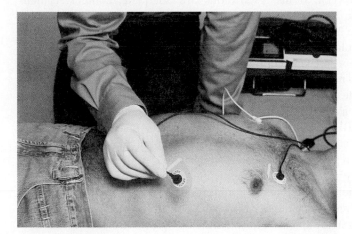

FIGURE B-7B Some ALS providers prefer placing electrodes on the extremities.

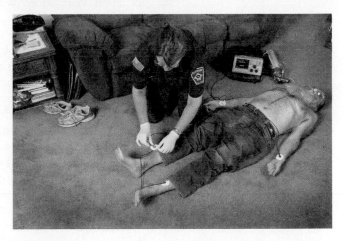

FIGURE B-8 (A) 12-lead ECG lead placement. (B) 12-lead electrodes in place.

Lead V₁ The electrode is at the fourth intercostal space just to the right of the sternum.
Lead V₂ The electrode is at the fourth intercostal space just to the left of the sternum.
Lead V₃ The electrode is at the line midway between leads V₂ and V₄.
Lead V₄ The electrode is at the midclavicular line in the fifth interspace.
Lead V₅ The electrode is at the anterior axillary line at the same level as lead V₄.
Lead V₆ The electrode is at the midaxillary line at the same level as lead V₄.

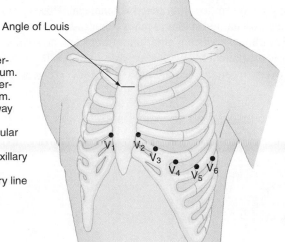

Chest Lead Placement

(A)

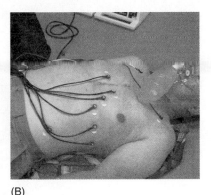

(B)

ECG is used to assist in the diagnosis of an acute myocardial infarction (AMI). In the case of an AMI, "time is muscle." As the clock ticks, more and more heart muscle becomes dysfunctional and finally dies in the absence of oxygenated blood. With field diagnosis of AMI made possible by the 12-lead ECG, the time from AMI to hospital treatment with drugs or procedures to break up the clots causing the AMI can be reduced.

If 12-lead ECG monitors are used in your system, ask the paramedics to review the lead placement with you as this is slightly more complex than the simple three electrodes you may be used to. Figure B-8 demonstrates lead placement for the 12-lead ECG, and shows the 12-lead electrodes in place.

Post Cardiac Arrest Care

In the event that your cardiac arrest patient has a return of spontaneous circulation (ROSC), i.e., a pulse, there are several things you should do. This patient is in a precarious position and will need all of your attention. He is at high risk of arresting again, so leave the AED pads in place and be prepared to defibrillate again.

Unless you were able to defibrillate within a minute or two after the patient went into cardiac arrest, he will probably remain unconscious and will need respiratory support. The patient may breathe less frequently than a normal patient, so judge the adequacy and rate of breathing to determine your next steps. If the patient's breathing is inadequate, ventilate or assist ventilations with oxygen. If his respirations are adequate, administer high-concentration oxygen by mask.

Monitor the patient's pulse frequently, at least every 30 seconds or so if that is practical. Since you will probably be ventilating the patient, it may be difficult to tell if he has gone back into cardiac arrest. If you are not sure whether the patient has a pulse, look for other signs of circulation, like movement. Do not mistake gasping agonal respirations for adequate breathing. If you are not sure, ventilate, compress the chest, and have the AED check the rhythm.

If ALS is available, this is a circumstance where you want to get such assistance. ALS providers, and in some areas BLS providers, too, may have specific instructions regarding the patient's temperature. Therapeutic hypothermia is a treatment that may increase the patient's chance of survival with a good neurological outcome.

ALS can be helpful not only in caring for the patient, but also in determining the transport destination. When there is a choice of hospitals, it is important to go to one that has the specialized facilities and staff necessary to care for a patient who is recovering from cardiac arrest.

The issue of how much oxygen to administer to patients who were in cardiac arrest but now have a spontaneous pulse is a potentially complicated one. Ideally, if the patient is perfusing sufficiently for you to get a pulse oximeter reading, you should reduce the amount of oxygen the patient is getting to attain an oxygen saturation reading of at least 94%, but less than 100%. There is some theoretical reason to believe that too much oxygen may be harmful, so adjusting the oxygen flow rate may be beneficial. This is a significant challenge in a moving ambulance with limited staff and many other tasks to perform for an unstable patient. If you can do this without sacrificing other important steps, do so in accordance with local protocols. Do not allow the patient to become hypoxic, however. If you must make a choice, it is probably better to over-oxygenate the patient than to under-oxygenate the patient.

RESEARCH AND EMS

Ⓐll providers that step foot onto an ambulance would like to believe that what they are doing is really going to make a difference in the lives of their patients. We all hope that the therapies and interventions we deliver will be meaningful. Moreover, as budgets tighten and managers look for ways to control costs, it is as important as ever to ensure that what we do is both meaningful and cost effective.

Yet, in EMS these are not simple issues. We spend nearly $3 billion each year delivering care, but little of what we do has ever been truly evaluated. This presents some significant problems. How do we know we are being helpful? How do we know the tools we use are effective? As EMS matures as a profession, the scientific experimentation to establish facts or measure outcomes, otherwise known as *research,* will offer us an opportunity to answer some of these questions factually and help guide our progress to better benefit our patients.

This change is not simple. EMS is not an easy field to gather research in, and serious challenges exist. As a provider, you should understand the value of research not only to your profession but to your everyday practice. There are simple steps you can take to improve your understanding and to help move EMS toward a more evidence-based approach. In this chapter we will discuss how EMS research can be valuable and how you as a provider can improve the role of research in health care.

EMS Research and You

Knowledge is power. Throughout health care, medicine is moving to a more *evidence-based* approach. That means that outcomes of therapies and interventions are carefully measured to ensure they have the intended results. When changes are made, decisions are based on clear indications and outcomes that point to meaningful improvements in patient care (Figure C-1). As the health care profession matures, more and more progress is based on an evidence-based approach. The interventions we perform and the therapies we deliver must be meaningful and should be measurable. To assess the value of our care we must turn to research. Quality studies and experimentation will separate important, relevant strategies from frivolous, wasteful endeavors. Consider the following situation:

> You work as an EMT for an ambulance service that has 20 ambulances. Staffing is tight and the budget is tighter. Tomorrow a new device used to treat cardiac arrest will be released at a cost of $1,500 each. The company that created the device says it's the most important device the company has ever released and that it will significantly increase cardiac arrest survival rates. As your company's leaders decide whether to buy the device, they must weigh the idea of improving survival rates against the high cost of the device. Of course, everyone would like to see patient care improve, but there is a significant cost in implementing this new device. If they choose to outfit the entire fleet of 20 ambulances, they will spend $30,000. If the devices truly work, it makes a great deal of sense to purchase them, but if they don't work, $30,000 could pay for an additional EMT.

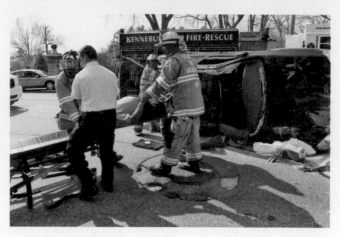

How can your service make the correct decision? The answer comes through quality EMS research. If unbiased scientific experimentation had been done that showed this device really did double survival rates of cardiac arrest patients, then this decision would be easy to make. Similarly, if a quality study demonstrated that the device did not improve cardiac arrest survival, then the service could invest its money in more meaningful areas.

If, as a profession, we were committed to an evidence-based approach, we could avoid spending time and money on ineffective therapies and focus our budgets on the elements of care that mean the most. Although the previous example was hypothetical, EMS agencies are faced with similar dilemmas every day. In addition to spending money, consider the issues EMS leaders and providers are faced with in developing protocols, adopting new medications and devices, allotting staffing resources, and myriad other questions that desperately need thoughtful answers.

In an age of slick marketing and ever-burgeoning technology, quality research and an evidence-based approach will help us answer key questions and expend our resources wisely.

But what about the local level? How does EMS research impact the practice of a single EMT? Consider your state, regional, or even service-level protocols. Decisions regarding scope of practice, equipment, and medications are made every day. Medical Directors, state officials, and local services consult relevant research to aid in choosing the paths and procedures that make the most sense. Consider also the dynamic nature of health care. We know for sure that many of the treatments and therapies you are learning today may prove to be inappropriate on further examination in the future. The history of EMS is littered with ideas, medications, and other therapies that were considered state of the art until they were thoroughly examined and determined to be incorrect. Understanding how to interpret research will help you as a provider stay on the cutting edge of patient care. Decisions are made every day about how we conduct our business. Understanding research can help you contribute to these discussions.

The bottom line is that EMS decision makers are consulting research to make choices about your profession. EMS providers at every level are involved in making these decisions; however, without a basic understanding of research, providers are routinely excluded from the conversation. Understanding research, even at a very simple level, allows you to speak the language of health care and can get you a seat at the table. The best possible care results from an open dialogue between physicians, administrators, and providers and is best achieved by reviewing quality research.

The Basics of EMS Research

Someone once said, "Not everything that is researched is true, and not everything that is true has been researched." This statement certainly applies in the world of EMS. The dynamic nature of our treatment setting makes research difficult at best. We encounter many obstacles to research that simply are not there in other arms of the health care field. The environment we work in is often unstable, our encounters are often brief, and our data collection is frequently disjointed and lacks centralization. Furthermore, we face many ethical dilemmas. Obtaining consent from a critical patient is often challenging at best. We do have many opportunities to create valid and important studies on prehospital care, but to do so we must promote the best practices of research so that our outcomes can truly guide us to high-quality care.

Not all research is created equal. There are good studies and there are bad studies. As we evolve in an evidence-based environment, we should strive to embrace the best practices of conducting and evaluating research. The finer points of medical research are by no means a simple topic, and a thorough examination of how to evaluate research is beyond the scope of this text. However, there are broad concepts that can be helpful to consider.

Remember that the process of research is the same whether you are an EMS researcher or a scientist in a laboratory. We all rely on the *scientific method,* a process of experimentation for answering questions and acquiring new knowledge that was developed by Galileo almost 400 years ago. In this method, general observations are turned into a *hypothesis* (or unproven theory). Predictions are then made, based on the hypothesis, and these predictions are tested to either prove or disprove the theory. For example, you might note that applying a bandage seems to control minor external bleeding. To use the scientific method, you might hypothesize that bandages do indeed control bleeding better than doing nothing at all. You could conduct a randomized control study to test your hypothesis by randomly assigning patients to the "bandage group" or to the "do nothing group." You could then measure the amount of bleeding in each group and compare your results. Although there might be some ethical issues with your study, this experiment would help you prove or disprove the value of bandaging. Furthermore, if your experiment was done properly, your results would hold up if the study was repeated, regardless of who conducted the experiment. That is the value of quality research. Unfortunately, not all research can live up to these quality markers.

In medicine, exacting and comprehensive studies are both difficult and time consuming to conduct. In most cases, we make decisions based on a broad variety of different sources. Unfortunately, much of what we do still relies on the "best guess strategy"; however, as we progress, we rely more and more on research studies. When making decisions based on evidence (especially patient care decisions), it is clearly best to base the decision on many studies, not just a single work. The strength of your conclusion is significantly increased when a variety of studies point to the same conclusion.

The key is to obtain an objective opinion. When more than one study points to the same conclusion, it is more likely to be free from opinion and *bias*. Many individual studies are clouded by bias. Bias occurs when research is influenced by prior inclinations, beliefs, or prejudices. Bias influences a study when the outcomes are manipulated to fit an expected outcome instead of measured objectively against the hypothesis. Although this can occur when researchers have a financial gain in a particular outcome, it more commonly occurs simply from poor methods used to conduct the research. In the true scientific method, outcomes are not bent to conform to previously held notions but rather are examined objectively and evaluated based solely on the facts. Valid research embraces this idea and uses methods designed to limit outside influences.

Some methods of research are considered more valid than others. Research methods are typically judged by how well they avoid potential bias and exclude the possibility of error. Consider the following strategies:

Prospective vs. Retrospective

Retrospective reviews look at events that have occurred in the past. Health care has frequently used retrospective reviews to consider the outcomes of therapies previously performed. In contrast, prospective studies are designed to look forward. Methods are designed to test therapies and outcomes that will occur in the future. Prospective studies are generally easier to control than retrospective studies, as rules and regulations can be put in place in advance to control errors and prevent bias. Retrospective studies cannot be controlled in such a way. Retrospective studies can certainly be considered valid, but a prospective method is generally considered more valid.

Randomization

High-quality studies use randomization. In medicine, this type of study typically compares one therapy against another, and bias is controlled by assigning patients to one therapy or the other randomly, as opposed to having predetermined groups. Randomization also improves objectivity when analyzing outcomes. In high-quality studies, the researcher and the patients may not even know which therapy is being received by whom. This process is called *blinding* and can be either single blinded (the researcher know who gets what therapy but the patients don't) or double blinded (neither the patient nor the researcher knows what therapy is being used on that particular patient). When a study is blinded, it is very difficult to influence outcomes in any way, and the results are far more likely to be objective.

Control Groups

The use of a control group helps to evaluate outcomes fairly. In medicine, a control group is usually a group of patients who are receiving a therapy that is already commonly known or commonly used. The control group outcomes can be compared to the outcomes of the test group that is receiving a new therapy, showing whether or not the new therapy has better outcomes than the old one. In our previous bandaging study, we compared the bandaging group against a "do nothing" group. In that case, the "do nothing" group would be our control group. By including this group, we can not only evaluate the outcome of bandaging, but also compare those outcomes against a different (do nothing) strategy. This comparison of test-group outcomes to control-group outcomes adds weight and value to the analysis.

Study Group Similarity

If a group of patients is being used to test a new treatment, it is important that subjects in that group have a certain degree of similarity. Let's say, for example, that we want to test a new airway device's impact on survival in trauma patients. We have designed and implemented a study to compare the use of the new device against a group of patients that received care without using the device. In our study, let's say that the EMTs were allowed to choose who they wanted to use the new device on. When we look at our results, we find that the group that the device was used on had a much higher mortality rate. At face value, we might assume that this means the device did not work. However, as we analyze the results we find that the group assigned to the new device was much sicker than the group that did not receive the device. In this case, the EMTs thought it would be best to use the new device only in the worst-off patients. Did more people in the test group die because of the device, or did more people die simply because they were hurt worse from the beginning? It is difficult to say, and therein is the difficulty in comparing a therapy used with two vastly different groups. Consider also the challenges in comparing different age groups, different treatment protocols, or different genders.

Types of Medical Research

No study can be completely free from bias; however, as you have seen, certain methods help to minimize the impact of subjectivity. Because of the dynamic and often sensitive nature of medicine, a large variety of research is used to reach conclusions on therapies and treatment. Ideally systematic reviews guide our most important decisions, but more commonly a combination of research studies and research methods guides the decisions that are made. Consider the following types of medical research:

- **Systematic review.** In a systematic review, a series of studies pertaining to a single question are evaluated. Their results are reviewed, summarized, and used to draw evidence-based conclusions. It is important to remember that a systematic review is made up of not one but many different research experiments.

- **Randomized controlled trials (RCTs).** In an RCT, researchers randomly assign eligible subjects into groups to receive or not receive the intervention being tested. A control group is used to compare the tested theory against a known outcome. In 2000, Marianne Gausche-Hill and her colleagues looked at pediatric intubation in Los Angeles County, California. In their study, children needing airway management were randomized, based on the day of the week, to either an intubation group or a bag-mask group. Outcomes of these patients were then studied. Objectivity was improved because subjects were randomized, and the results were more meaningful, because they could compare outcomes of the intubation group against those of the control BVM group.

In medicine, drugs are frequently tested in randomized studies using a placebo for the control group. Patients are often randomized to receive either the real drug that is being tested or a "sugar pill" that has no effect. Frequently, these studies also use a blinding process so that neither the providers carrying out the study nor the patients know who is taking which path. In this type of study, the results for those receiving the new medication can be compared against those in the placebo control group to accurately assess the effect of the new therapy.

- **Cohort/concurrent control/case-control studies.** In these types of studies, two therapies or groups of patients are compared, but subjects are not necessarily randomized. For example, you might compare the outcomes of one service that uses CPAP against the outcomes of another service that does not. A cohort study might follow patients who have a specific disease and compare them to a group of patients that does not have the disease. In both these studies, you are comparing two groups and have a control group, but the results are not randomized. Frequently, case-control studies are retrospective, looking at two groups of events or outcomes that occurred in the past. All of these studies can be valid and yield important information, but they also can be prone to bias in that it is difficult to control all aspects of similarity and methods among the different groups.

- **Case studies/case reports.** Case studies and case reports review the treatment of a single patient or a series of patients. Frequently, they report on unusual circumstances or outcomes. There is no control group, and these reports are always retrospective. They are certainly not as valid as randomized studies, but they often help us formulate larger questions to be investigated.

- **Meta-analysis.** A meta-analysis is not a study itself, but rather is a compilation of different studies looking at a single topic. A meta-analysis will summarize the work of those other studies and frequently will comment on outcomes of those studies. In many cases, these are similar to a systematic review but frequently are much smaller in scale.

It is important to remember that every study should be reviewed independently. The fact that it is a randomized control study does not ensure that its results are valid. That said, methodology does play a role in evaluations of a study's importance. The American Heart Association qualifies the validity of research in a linear fashion using a "Level of Evidence" designation. It assigns varying levels of importance based on how a study was conducted. This progression is useful in evaluating the importance of data and can be used as a framework for considering the utility of a particular study.

- **Level of Evidence 1.** In this sliding scale, the highest level (most valuable) set of data would result from *randomized controlled trials (RCTs)* or meta-analyses of RCTs.

- **Level of Evidence 2.** These studies use concurrent controls without true randomization. Because they are often retrospective and because the methods are more difficult to control without randomization, these types of studies are often less reliable.

- **Level of Evidence 3.** These studies use retrospective controls. There is little control of these experiments, as the testing is based on events that have already occurred. Because of this, it is difficult to ensure similar circumstances among research subjects. Although the data from retrospective studies may be useful, it can be prone to bias.

- **Level of Evidence 4.** These are studies without a control group (e.g., case series). In these studies, only one group is looked at and it is not compared to a second group. Here there is no control group to examine the results against. Important information may be gained, but outcomes are difficult to truly evaluate without comparing to a similar patient who received a different therapy.

- **Level of Evidence 5.** These studies are not directly related to the specific patient/population (e.g., different patient/population, animal models, mechanical models, and so on). These studies are common in EMS and are frequently used to evaluate prehospital treatments. Unfortunately, their data are prone to a wide range of interpretation as we must make assumptions that what works in different populations or under different circumstances would also work in the world of EMS.

How to Evaluate a Research Study

Regardless of the type of study you are reading, you should always review research in a way that helps you identify bias or flaws in the methodology. There is certainly a great deal more to learn about the evaluation of medical research, but there are some important questions to consider when reading a study. Consider the following questions:

1. Was the study randomized and was the randomization blinded?

2. If more than one group was reviewed, were the groups similar at the start of the trial?

3. Were all eligible patients analyzed? If some were excluded, why were they excluded? Bias often occurs by removing data that leads in a different direction from your hypothesis. Often the removal of patients from a study can identify potential problems.

4. Were the outcomes really due to the therapy? Consider the previously discussed example of the new airway device only being used in the sickest patients. Occasionally outcomes can be measured that would have happened randomly. For example, a company could invent a new device that, they say, would make the sun rise tomorrow at 6:00 A.M. Although they could certainly produce a study that demonstrates the predicted outcome, that outcome would have occurred whether the device was used or not. A powerful study is one that can be reproduced with the same results in relatively different circumstances.

5. Is the outcome truly relevant? Many studies show differences among treatments but no real relevance. For example, a study might show that a new medication increases the return of spontaneous circulation in sudden cardiac arrest compared to a placebo control group. Getting a pulse back in more patients is important, but that result is not really relevant if exactly the same number of patients die at the conclusion of care as compared to the control group.

There are many good resources on evaluating evidence-based medicine, and there is a great deal more information available about evaluating research. Learning more about this topic as a provider will help you understand the decisions and discussions that are ongoing both in EMS and in health care in general. Classes, textbooks, and many other tutorials can improve your capability to read and evaluate research. However, there is no better way to learn about research than to become involved in a research study.

Your Role in EMS Research

As previously stated, medicine in general is moving rapidly in a direction guided by evidence-based studies. In EMS, we face a future where insurance reimbursements for specific treatments may be based on validated outcomes. Therefore, your role as an EMS provider in research is especially important. Aside from reading and discussing research, the EMS provider of the future will be on the front line of conducting research. We now know that the only way to truly prove our worth and prove the importance of our prehospital therapies is to evaluate them through clinical trials. As a provider, there are a variety of ways you may be involved in EMS research.

At the most basic level, your good documentation may help improve future studies. As EMS systems begin to collaborate and centralize run-report data, this information may help guide any number of potential studies. EMS leaders will consider skills used, locations, times of day, and many other reported outcomes as they design the EMS practices of the future. The time you take to accurately and thoroughly document your call may be an essential component of evidence-based medicine and may significantly impact the decisions that are made regarding how you do business.

You may also take part in a research study. Your service, local hospital, or region may participate and enroll patients into a specifically designed experiment. In this case, it is important to follow all the instructions you are given. Making exceptions or not following the instructions can insert bias or even eliminate your data from being considered. Participating in a study such as this is an important way to learn more about medical research. Not only might your service benefit from the information learned in the study, but participation often gives you valuable insight into research methods and procedures.

As you progress as a provider, perhaps you will take part in designing a study. As an EMT, you are on the forefront of prehospital medicine and can play an important role in shaping the future of prehospital medicine. Many hospitals and EMS systems conduct research routinely. Your Medical Director or local state official may be able to offer opportunities if you would like to get involved.

Conclusions

EMS research is an important part of the future of our profession. Understanding the basic concepts of research allows you to take a role in shaping that direction. Remember that not all research is created equal. If you take the time to learn more about reading and evaluating research literature, and about actually conducting research, you will enhance your own importance to your chosen field. Remember that every EMS provider must play a role in conducting EMS research. Beyond just participating, becoming involved in research development offers a rewarding pathway for enlightened providers.

Anatomy and Physiology Illustrations 1150

- - - - - - - - - - - - - -

Skeletal System

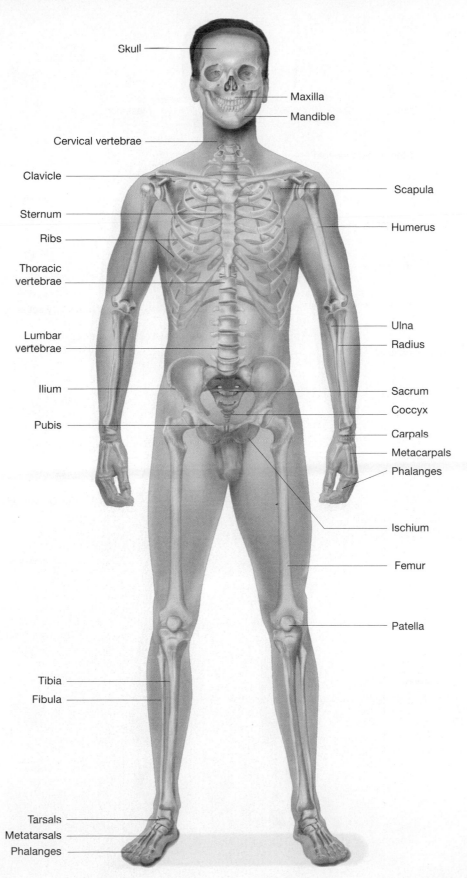

Skull

Maxilla

Mandible

Cervical vertebrae

Clavicle

Scapula

Sternum

Humerus

Ribs

Thoracic vertebrae

Lumbar vertebrae

Ulna

Radius

Ilium

Sacrum

Coccyx

Pubis

Carpals

Metacarpals

Phalanges

Ischium

Femur

Patella

Tibia

Fibula

Tarsals

Metatarsals

Phalanges

Muscular System

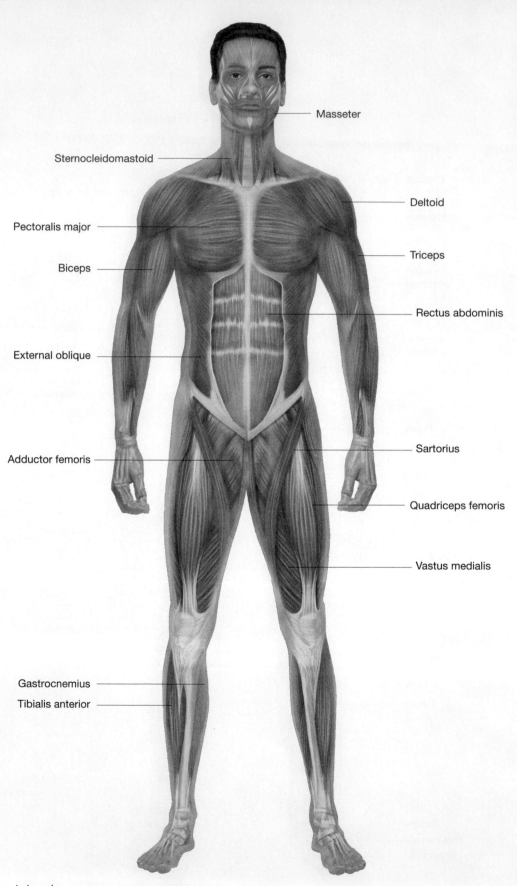

Masseter

Sternocleidomastoid

Deltoid

Pectoralis major

Triceps

Biceps

Rectus abdominis

External oblique

Adductor femoris

Sartorius

Quadriceps femoris

Vastus medialis

Gastrocnemius

Tibialis anterior

Respiratory System

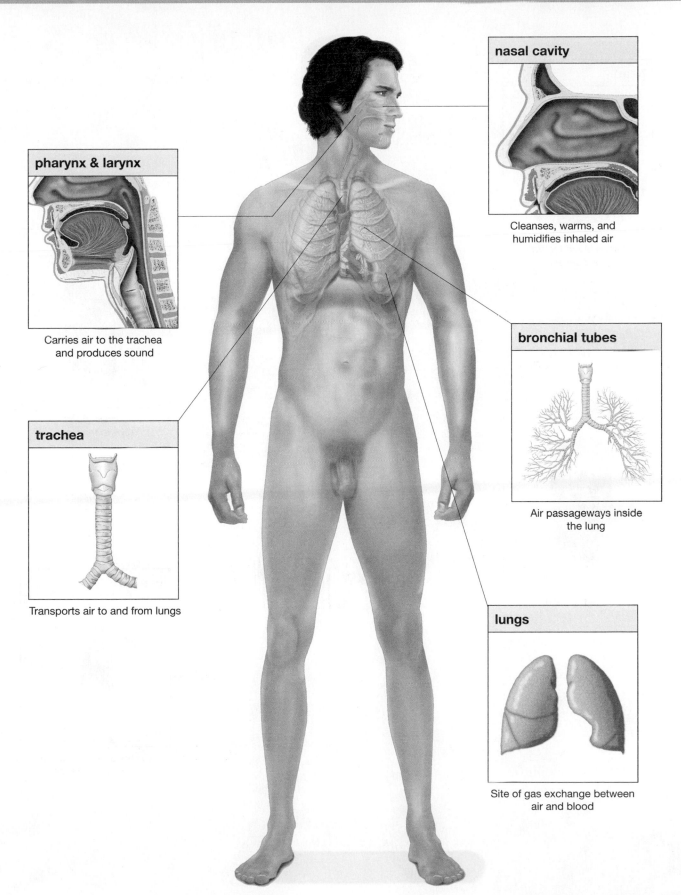

nasal cavity

Cleanses, warms, and humidifies inhaled air

pharynx & larynx

Carries air to the trachea and produces sound

trachea

Transports air to and from lungs

bronchial tubes

Air passageways inside the lung

lungs

Site of gas exchange between air and blood

Cardiovascular System

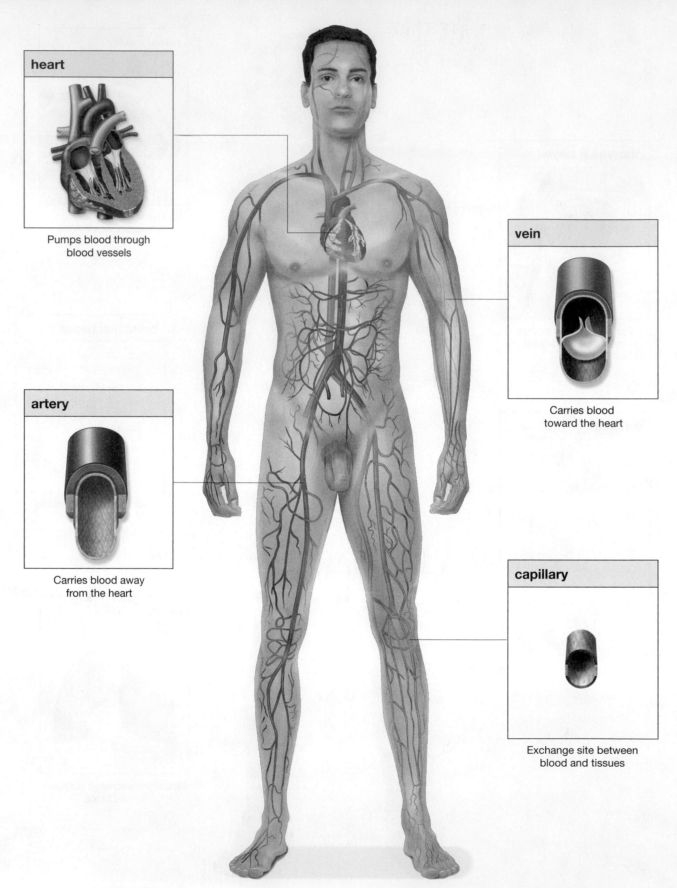

heart
Pumps blood through
blood vessels

vein
Carries blood
toward the heart

artery
Carries blood away
from the heart

capillary
Exchange site between
blood and tissues

Nervous System

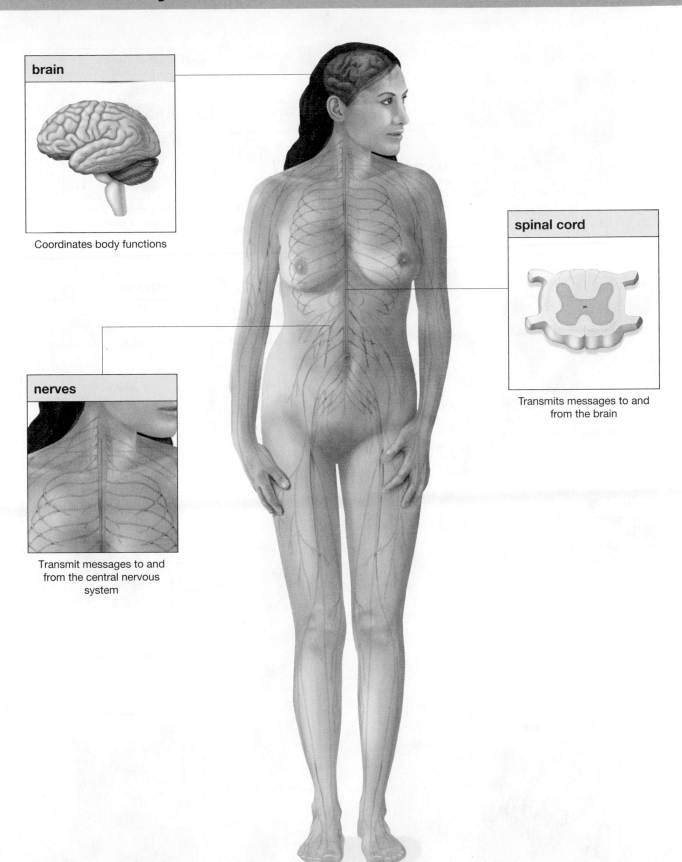

brain

Coordinates body functions

nerves

Transmit messages to and from the central nervous system

spinal cord

Transmits messages to and from the brain

Digestive System

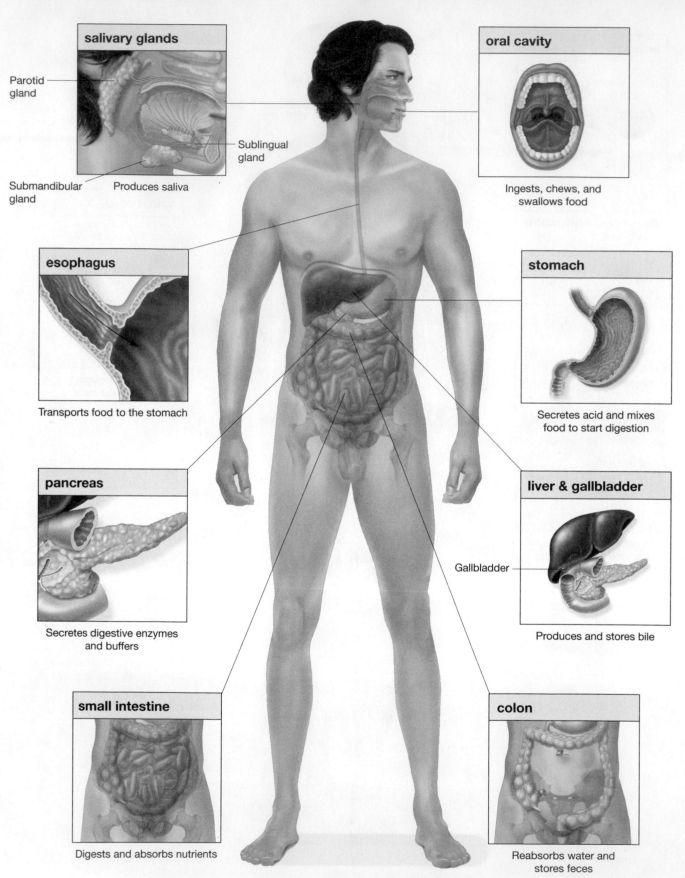

salivary glands

Parotid gland

Submandibular gland

Sublingual gland

Produces saliva

oral cavity

Ingests, chews, and swallows food

esophagus

Transports food to the stomach

stomach

Secretes acid and mixes food to start digestion

pancreas

Secretes digestive enzymes and buffers

liver & gallbladder

Gallbladder

Produces and stores bile

small intestine

Digests and absorbs nutrients

colon

Reabsorbs water and stores feces

Integumentary System

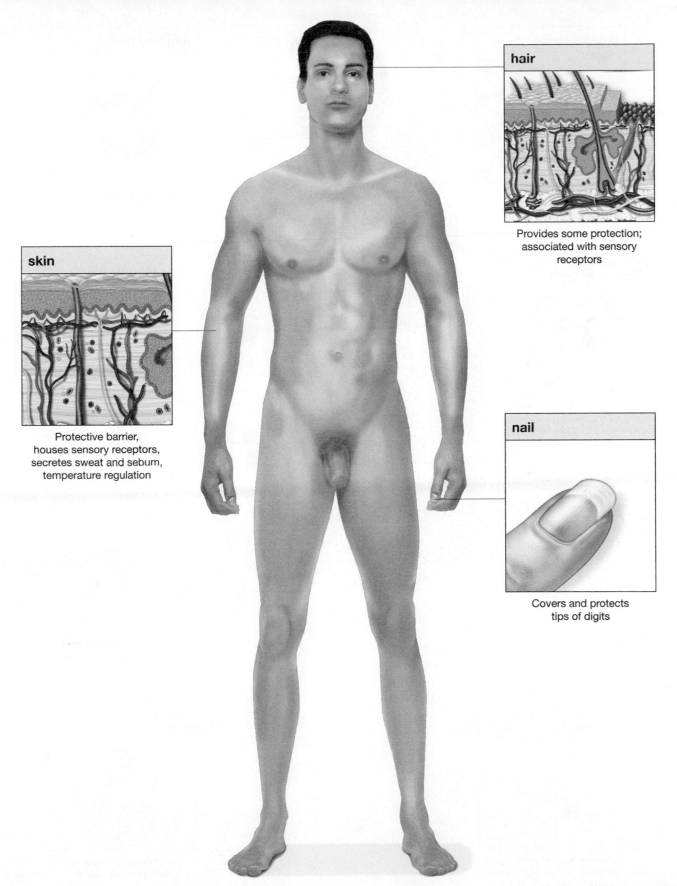

skin

Protective barrier, houses sensory receptors, secretes sweat and sebum, temperature regulation

hair

Provides some protection; associated with sensory receptors

nail

Covers and protects tips of digits

Endocrine System

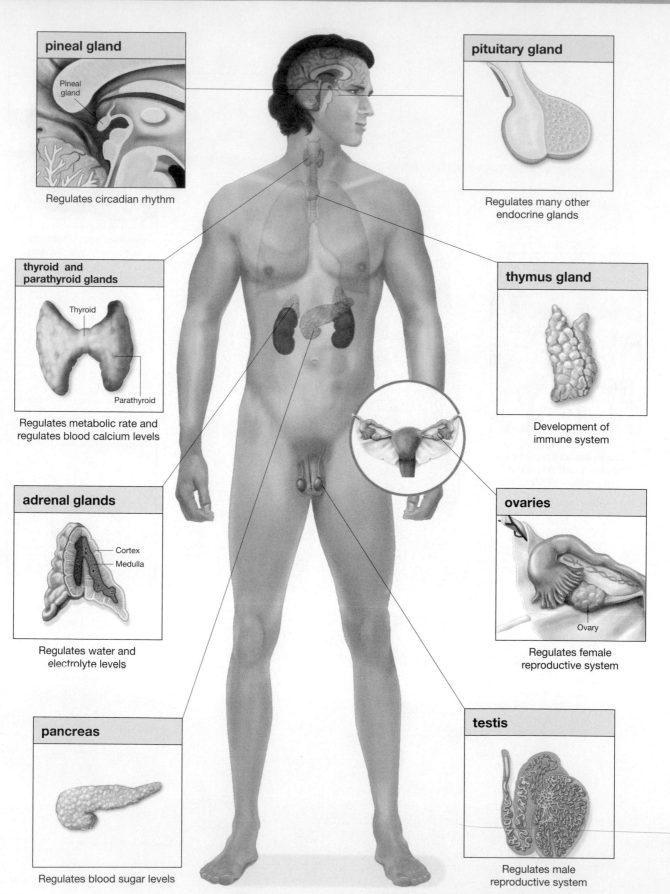

pineal gland

Pineal gland

Regulates circadian rhythm

pituitary gland

Regulates many other endocrine glands

thyroid and parathyroid glands

Thyroid

Parathyroid

Regulates metabolic rate and regulates blood calcium levels

thymus gland

Development of immune system

adrenal glands

Cortex

Medulla

Regulates water and electrolyte levels

ovaries

Ovary

Regulates female reproductive system

pancreas

Regulates blood sugar levels

testis

Regulates male reproductive system

Renal System

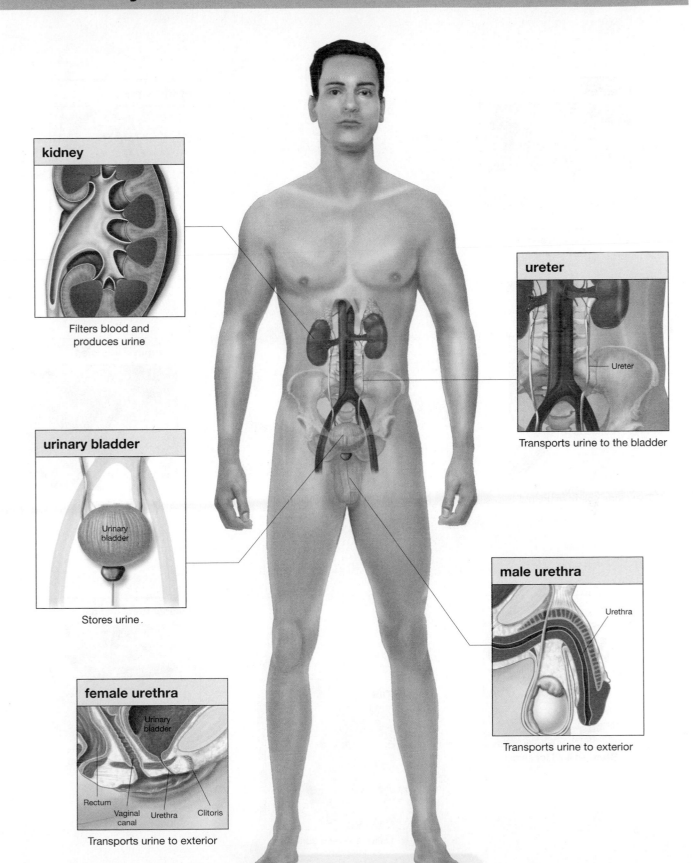

kidney

Filters blood and produces urine

ureter

Ureter

Transports urine to the bladder

urinary bladder

Urinary bladder

Stores urine

male urethra

Urethra

Transports urine to exterior

female urethra

Urinary bladder

Rectum Vaginal canal Urethra Clitoris

Transports urine to exterior

Male Reproductive System

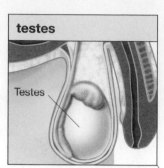

testes

Testes

Produces sperm and secretes testosterone

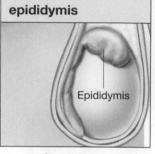

epididymis

Epididymis

Stores sperm

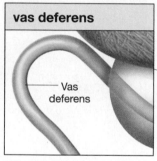

vas deferens

Vas deferens

Transports sperm to urethra

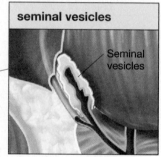

seminal vesicles

Seminal vesicles

Secretes fluid for semen

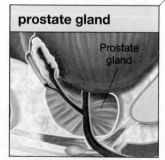

prostate gland

Prostate gland

Secretes fluid for semen

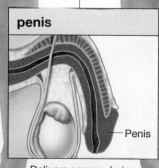

penis

Penis

Delivers semen during intercourse

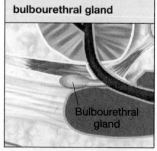

bulbourethral gland

Bulbourethral gland

Secretes fluid for semen

Female Reproductive System

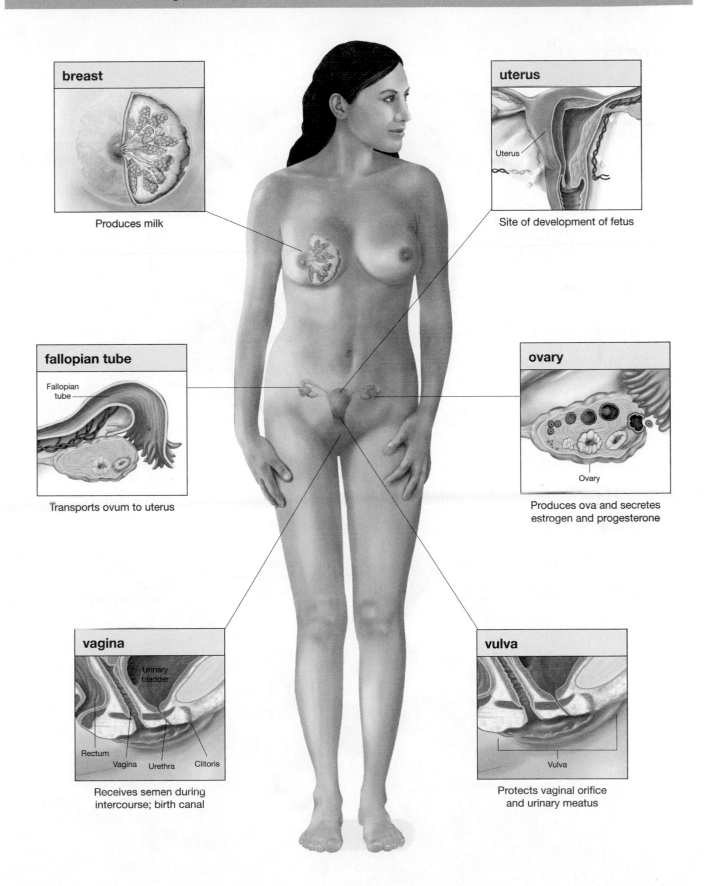

breast

Produces milk

uterus

Uterus

Site of development of fetus

fallopian tube

Fallopian tube

Transports ovum to uterus

ovary

Ovary

Produces ova and secretes estrogen and progesterone

vagina

Urinary bladder

Rectum   Vagina   Urethra   Clitoris

Receives semen during intercourse; birth canal

vulva

Vulva

Protects vaginal orifice and urinary meatus

Special Senses

The Eye

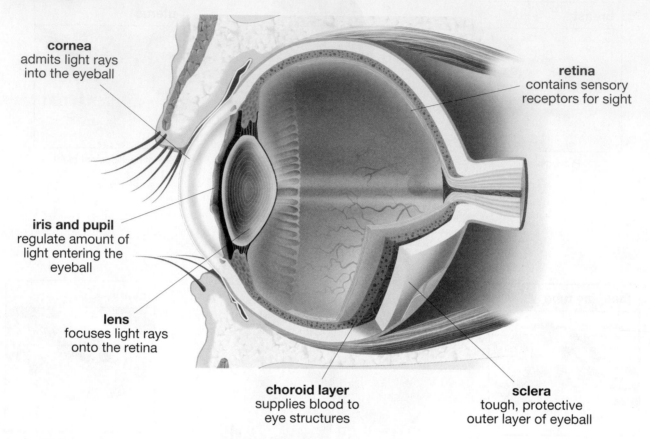

cornea
admits light rays
into the eyeball

retina
contains sensory
receptors for sight

iris and pupil
regulate amount of
light entering the
eyeball

lens
focuses light rays
onto the retina

choroid layer
supplies blood to
eye structures

sclera
tough, protective
outer layer of eyeball

The Ear

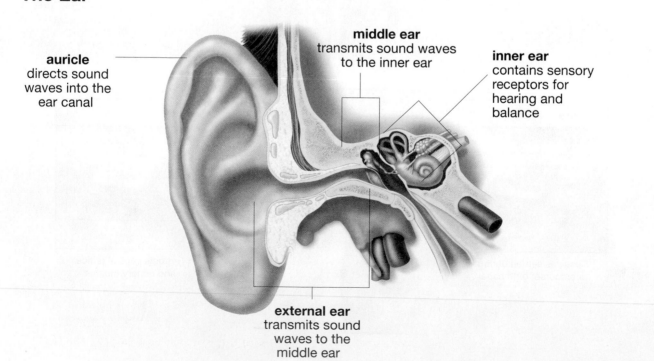

auricle
directs sound
waves into the
ear canal

middle ear
transmits sound waves
to the inner ear

inner ear
contains sensory
receptors for
hearing and
balance

external ear
transmits sound
waves to the
middle ear

MEDICAL TERMINOLOGY

As an EMT, you will probably never have to use more than a few medical terms in the course of your prehospital emergency care activities, and most of them will probably deal with parts of the body. Physicians and nurses prefer EMTs to speak in common layperson language rather than medical terms. However, if you are an avid reader, much of what you read is likely to be freely sprinkled with medical terms; if you cannot translate them, you may not understand what you are reading.

Medical terms are comprised of words, roots, combining forms, prefixes, and suffixes—all little words, if you will, and each with its own definition.

Sometimes medical terms are made up of two whole words. For example, the word *small* is joined with the word *pox* to form the medical term *smallpox*, the name of a disease. However, it is not always so simple!

Roots are the foundations of words and are not used by themselves. For example, *therm* is a root that means heat; to use it alone would make no sense. However, when a vowel is added to the end of the root to make it the *combining form* *therm/o*, it can be joined with other words or roots to form a compound term. *Therm/o* and *meter* (an instrument for measuring) combine to form *thermometer*, an instrument for measuring heat or temperature.

More than one root or combining form can be joined to form medical terms; *electrocardiogram* is a good example. The combining forms *electr/o* (electric) and *cardi/o* (heart) are joined to the suffix *-gram* (a written record) to form the term that means a written record of the heart's electrical activity.

Prefixes are used to modify or qualify the meanings of roots. They usually tell the reader what kind of, where (or in what direction), or how many.

The root *-pnea* relates to breathing, but it says nothing about the quality or kind of breathing. Adding the prefix *dys-* qualifies it as difficult breathing.

Abdominal pain is a rather broad term; it gives the reader no clue as to exactly where the pain is located either inside or outside the abdomen. Adding the prefix *intra-* to *abdominal* pinpoints the location of the pain, for *intra-abdominal pain* means pain within the abdomen. The root *plegia* refers to paralysis of the limbs. The prefix *quadri-* tells the reader how many limbs are paralyzed. *Quadriplegia* means paralysis of all four limbs.

Suffixes are word endings that form nouns, adjectives, or verbs. Medical terms can have more than one suffix, and a suffix can appear in the middle of a compound term affixed to a combining form. A number of suffixes have specialized meanings. The suffix *-itis* means inflammation; thus, *arthritis* means inflammation of a joint. The suffix *-iac* forms a noun indicating a person afflicted with a certain disease, such as *hemophiliac*.

Some suffixes are joined to roots to form terms that indicate a state, quality, condition, procedure, or process. *Pneumonia* and *psoriasis* are examples of medical conditions, whereas *appendectomy* and *arthroscopy* are examples of medical procedures. The suffixes in each case are underlined.

Some suffixes combine with roots to form adjectives, words that modify nouns by indicating quality or quantity or by distinguishing one thing from another. *Gastric*, *cardiac*, *fibrous*, *arthritic*, and *diaphoretic* are all examples of adjectives formed by adding suffixes (underlined) to roots.

Some suffixes, such as *-ole* and *-ule*, are added to roots to express reduction in size. For example, an *arteriole* is smaller than an *artery*, and a *venule* is smaller than a vein.

When added to roots, *-e* and *-ize* form verbs. *Excise* and *catheterize* are examples.

Finally, some of what are commonly accepted as suffixes are actually the combination of a root and a suffix. For example, *-megaly* (enlargement) results from the combination of the root *megal* (large) and the suffix *-y* (which forms the term into a noun). *Cardiomegaly* means enlargement of the heart.

Standard Terms

The following terms are used to denote direction of movement, position, and anatomical posture.

abduction movement away from the body's midline.

adduction movement toward the body's midline.

afferent conducting toward a structure.

anterior the front surface of the body.

anterior to in front of.

caudad toward the tail.

cephalad toward the head.

circumduction circular movement of a part.

craniad toward the cranium.

deep situated remote from the surface.

distal situated away from the point of origin.

dorsal pertaining to the back surface of the body.

dorsiflexion bending backward.

efferent conducting away from a structure.

elevation raising a body part.

extension stretching, or moving, jointed parts into or toward a straight condition.

external situated outside.

flexion bending, or moving, jointed parts closer together.

inferior situated below.

internal situated inside.

laterad toward the side of the body.

lateral situated away from the body's midline.

lateral rotation rotating outward away from the body's midline.

left lateral recumbent lying horizontal on the left side.

mediad toward the midline of the body.

medial situated toward the body's midline.

medial rotation rotating inward toward the body's midline.

palmar concerning the inner surface of the hand.

peripheral away from a central structure.

plantar concerning the sole of the foot.

posterior pertaining to the back surface of the body.

posterior to situated behind.

pronation lying face downward or turning the hand so the palm faces downward or backward.

prone lying horizontal, face down and flat.

protraction pushing forward, such as happens with the mandible.

proximal situated nearest the point of origin.

recumbent lying horizontal, generally speaking.

retraction drawing back, such as happens with the tongue.

right lateral recumbent lying horizontal on the right side.

rotation turning around an axis.

superficial situated near the surface.

superior situated above.

supination lying face upward or turning the hand so the palm faces forward or upward.

supine lying horizontal, flat on the back and face up.

ventral the front surface of the body.

Planes

A plane is an imaginary flat surface that divides the body into sections.

coronal or frontal plane an imaginary plane that passes through the body from side to side and divides it into front and back sections.

midsagittal plane an imaginary plane that passes through the body from front to back and divides it into right and left halves.

sagittal plane an imaginary plane parallel to the median plane. It passes through the body from front to back and divides the body into right and left sections.

transverse plane an imaginary plane that passes through the body and divides it into upper and lower sections.

Word Parts

Prefixes are generally identified by a following dash (*ambi-*). Combining forms have a slash and a vowel following the root (*arthr/o*). Suffixes are generally identified by a preceding dash (*-emia*).

a- (not, without, lacking, deficient) *afebrile*, without fever.

ab- (away from) *abduct*, to draw away from the midline.

abdomin/o (abdomen) *abdominal*, pertaining to the abdomen.

-able, -ible (capable of) *reducible*, capable of being reduced (as a fracture).

ac- (to) *acclimate*, to become accustomed to.

acou (hear) *acoustic*, pertaining to sound or hearing.

acr/o (extremity, top, peak) *acrodermatitis*, inflammation of the skin of the extremities.

acu (needle) *acupuncture*, the Chinese practice of piercing specific peripheral nerves with needles to relieve the discomfort associated with painful disorders.

ad- (to, toward) *adduct*, to draw toward the midline.

aden/o (gland) *adenitis*, inflammation of a gland.

adip/o (fat) *adipose*, fatty; fat (in size).

aer/o (air) *aerobic*, requiring the presence of oxygen to live and grow.

af- (to) *afferent*, conveying toward.

ag- (to) *aggregate*, to crowd or cluster together.

-algesia (painful) *hyperalgesia*, overly sensitive to pain.

-algia (painful condition) *neuralgia*, pain that extends along the course of one or more nerves.

ambi- (both sides) *ambidextrous*, able to perform manual skills with both hands.

ambl/y (dim, dull, lazy) *amblyopia*, lazy eye.

amphi-, ampho- (on both sides, around both) *amphigonadism*, having both testicular and ovarian tissues.

amyl/o (starch) *amyloid*, starchlike.

an- (without) *anemia*, a reduced volume of blood cells.

ana- (upward, again, backward, excess) *anaphylaxis*, an unusual or exaggerated reaction of an organism to a substance to which it becomes sensitized.

andr/o (man, male) *android*, resembling a man.

angi/o (blood vessel, duct) *angioplasty*, surgery of blood vessels.

ankyl/o (stiff) *ankylosis*, stiffness.

ant-, anti- (against, opposed to, preventing, relieving) *antidote*, a substance for counteracting a poison.

ante- (before, forward) *antecubital*, situated in front of the elbow.

antero- (front) *anterolateral*, situated in front and to one side.

ap- (to) *approximate*, to bring together; to place close to.

apo- (separation, derivation from) *apoplexy*, sudden neurologic impairment due to a cardiovascular disorder.

-arium, -orium (place for something) *solarium*, a place for the sun.

arteri/o (artery) *arteriosclerosis*, thickening of the walls of the smaller arteries.

arthrio (joint, articulation) *arthritis*, inflammation of a joint or joints.

articul/o (joint) *articulated*, united by joints.

as- (to) *assimilate*, to take into.

at- (to) *attract*, to draw toward.

audi/o (hearing) *audiometer*, an instrument to test the power of hearing.

aur/o (ear) *auricle*, the flap of the ear.

aut/o (self) *autistic*, self-centered.

bi- (two, twice, double, both) *bilateral*, having two sides; pertaining to two sides.

bi/o (life) *biology*, the study of life.

blephario (eyelid) *blepharitis*, inflammation of the eyelid.

brachi/o (upper arm) *brachialgia*, pain in the upper arm.

brady- (slow) *bradycardia*, an abnormally slow heart rate.

bronch/o (larger air passages of the lungs) *bronchitis*, inflammation of the larger air passages of the lungs.

bucc/o (cheek) *buccal*, pertaining to the cheek.

cac/o (bad) *cacosmis*, a bad odor.

calc/o (bad) *calculus*, an abnormal, hard inorganic mass such as a gallstone.

calcane/o (heel) *calcaneus*, the heel bone.

calor/o (heat) *caloric*, pertaining to heat.

cancr/o (cancer) *cancroid*, resembling cancer.

capit/o (head) *capitate*, head-shaped.

caps/o (container) *capsulation*, enclosed in a capsule or container.

carcin/o (cancer) *carcinogen*, a substance that causes cancer.

cardi/o (heart) *cardiogenic*, originating in the heart.

carp/o (wrist bone) *carpal*, pertaining to the wrist bone.

cat-, cata- (down, lower, under, against, along with) *catabasis*, the stage of decline of a disease.

-cele (tumor, hernia) *hydrocele*, a confined collection of water.

celi/o (abdomen) *celiomyalgia*, a pain in the muscles of the abdomen.

-centesis (perforation or tapping, as with a needle) *abdominocentesis*, surgical puncture of the abdominal cavity.

cephal/o (head) *electroencephalogram*, a recording of the electrical activity of the brain.

cerebr/o (cerebrum) *cerebrospinal*, pertaining to the brain and spinal fluid.

cervic/o (neck, cervix) *cervical*, pertaining to the neck (or cervix).

cheil/o, chil/o (lip) *cheilitis*, inflammation of the lips.

cheirio, chir/o (hand) *cheiralgia*, pain in the hand.

chlor/o (green) *chloroma*, green cancer, a greenish tumor associated with myelogenous leukemia.

chol/e (bile, gall) *choledochitis*, inflammation of the common bile duct.

chondr/o (cartilage) *chondrodynia*, pain in a cartilage.

chrom/o, chromat/o (color) *monochromatic*, being of one color.

chron/o (time) *chronic*, persisting for a long time.

-cid- (cut, kill, fall) *insecticide*, an agent that kills insects.

circum- (around) *circumscribed*, confined to a limited space.

-cis- (cut, kill, fall) *excise*, to cut out.

-clysis (irrigation) *enteroclysis*, irrigation of the small intestine.

co- (with) *cohesion*, the force that causes various particles to unite.

col- (with) *collateral*, secondary or accessory; a small side branch such as a blood vessel or nerve.

col/o (colon, large intestine) *colitis*, inflammation of the colon.

colp/o (vagina) *colporrhagia*, bleeding from the vagina.

com- (with) *comminuted*, broken or crushed into small pieces.

con- (with) *congenital*, existing from the time of birth.

contra- (against, opposite) *contraindicated*, inadvisable.

cor/e, core/o (pupil) *corectopia*, abnormal location of the pupil of the eye.

cost/o (rib) *intercostal*, between the ribs.

crani/o (skull) *cranial*, pertaining to the skull.

cry/o (cold) *cryogenic*, that which produces low temperature.

crypt/o (hide, cover, conceal) *cryptogenic*, of doubtful origin.

cyan/o (blue) *cyanosis*, bluish discoloration of the skin and mucous membranes.

cyst/o (urinary bladder, cyst, sac of fluid) *cystitis*, inflammation of the bladder.

-cyte (cell) *leukocyte*, white cell.

cyt/o (cell) *cytoma*, tumor of the cell.

dacry/o (tear) *dacryorrhea*, excessive flow of tears.

dactyl/o (finger, toe) *dactylomegaly*, abnormally large fingers or toes.

de- (down) *descending*, coming down from.

dent/o (tooth) *dental*, pertaining to the teeth.

derm/o, dermat/o (skin) *dermatitis*, inflammation of the skin.

dextr/o (right) *dextrad*, toward the right side.

di- (twice, double) *diplegia*, paralysis affecting like parts on both sides of the body.

dia- (through, across, apart) *diaphragm*, the partition that separates the abdominal and thoracic cavities.

dipl/o (double, twin, twice) *diplopia*, double vision.

dips/o (thirst) *dipsomania*, alcoholism.

dis- (to free, to undo) *dissect*, to cut apart.

dors/o (back) *dorsal*, pertaining to the back.

-dynia (painful condition) *cephalodynia*, headache.

dys- (bad, difficult, abnormal, incomplete) *dyspnea*, labored breathing.

-ectasia (dilation or enlargement of an organ or part) *gastrectasia*, dilation (stretching) of the stomach.

ecto- (outer, outside of) *ectopic*, located away from the normal position.

-ectomy (the surgical removal of an organ or part) *appendectomy*, surgical removal of the appendix.

electr/o (electric) *electrocardiogram*, the written record of the heart's electrical activity.

-emia (condition of the blood) *anemia*, a deficiency of red blood cells.

en- (in, into, within) *encapsulate*, to enclose within a container.

encephal/o (brain) *encephalitis*, inflammation of the brain.

end-, endo- (within) *endotracheal*, within the trachea.

ent-, ento- (within, inner) *entopic*, occurring in the proper place.

enter/o (small intestine) *enteritis*, inflammation of the intestine.

ep-, epi- (over, on, upon) *epidermis*, the outermost layer of skin.

erythr/o (red) *erythrocyte*, a red blood cell.

esthesia (feeling) *anesthesia*, without feeling.

eu (good, well, normal, healthy) *euphoria*, an abnormal or exaggerated feeling of well-being.

ex- (out of, away from) *excrement*, waste material discharged from the body.

exo- (outside, outward) *exophytic*, to grow outward or on the surface.

extra- (on the outside, beyond, in addition to) *extracorporeal*, outside the body.

faci/o (face, surface) *facial*, pertaining to the face.

febr/i (fever) *febrile*, feverish.

-ferent (bear, carry) *efferent*, carrying away from a center.

fibr/o (fiber, filament) *fibrillation*, muscular contractions due to the activity of muscle fibers.

-form (shape) *deformed*, abnormally shaped.

-fugal (moving away) *centrifugal*, moving away from a center.

galact/o (milk) *galactopyria*, milk fever.

gangli/o (knot) *ganglion*, a knotlike mass.

gastr/o (stomach) *gastritis*, inflammation of the stomach.

gen/o (come into being, originate) *genetic*, inherited.

-genesis (production or origin) *pathogenesis*, the development of a disease.

-genic (giving rise to, originating in) *cardiogenic*, originating in the heart.

gloss/o (tongue) *glossal*, pertaining to the tongue.

glyc/o (sweet) *glycemia*, the presence of sugar in the blood.

gnath/o (jaw) *gnathitis*, inflammation of the jaw.

gnos/o (knowledge) *prognosis*, a prediction of the outcome of a disease.

-gram (drawing, written record) *electrocardiogram*, a recording of the heart's electrical activity.

-graph (an instrument for recording the activity of an organ) *electrocardiograph*, an instrument for measuring the heart's electrical activity.

-graphy (the recording of the activity of an organ) *electrocardiography*, the method of recording the heart's electrical activity.

gynec/o (woman) *gynecologist*, a specialist in diseases of the female genital tract.

hem/a, hem/o, hemat/o (blood) *hematoma*, a localized collection of blood.

hemi- (one-half) *hemiplegia*, paralysis of one side of the body.

hepat/o (liver) *hepatitis*, inflammation of the liver.

heter/o (other) *heterogeneous*, from a different source.

hidr/o, hidrot/o (sweat) *hidrosis*, excessive sweating.

hist/o (tissue) *histodialysis*, the breaking down of tissue.

hom/o, home/o (same, similar, unchanging, constant) *homeostasis*, stability in an organism's normal physiological states.

hyal/o (glass) *hyaline*, glassy, transparent.

hydr/o (water, fluid) *hydrocephalus*, an accumulation of cerebrospinal fluid in the skull with resulting enlargement of the head.

hyper- (beyond normal, excessive) *hypertension*, abnormally high blood pressure.

hypn/o (sleep) *hypnotic*, that which induces sleep.

hypo- (below normal, deficient, under, beneath) *hypotension*, abnormally low blood pressure.

hyster/o (uterus, womb) *hysterectomy*, surgical removal of the uterus.

-iasis (condition) *psoriasis*, a chronic skin condition characterized by lesions.

iatr/o (healer, physician) *pediatrician*, a physician that specializes in children's disorders.

-id (in a state, condition of) *gravid*, pregnant.

idio (peculiar, separate, distinct) *idiopathic*, occurring without a known cause.

il- (negative prefix) *illegible*, cannot be read.

ile/o (ileum) *ileitis*, inflammation of the ileum.

ili/o (ilium) *iliac*, pertaining to the ilium.

im- (negative prefix) *immature*, not mature.

in- (in, into, within) *incise*, to cut into.

infra- (beneath, below) *infracostal*, below a rib, or below the ribs.

inter- (between) *intercostal*, between two ribs.

intra- (within) *intraoral*, within the mouth.

intro- (within, into) *introspection*, the contemplation of one's own thoughts and feelings; self-analysis.

ir/o, irid/o (iris) *iridotomy*, incision of the iris.

ischi/o (ischium) *ischialgia*, pain in the ischium.

-ismus (abnormal condition) *strabismus*, deviation of the eye that a person cannot overcome.

iso- (same, equal, alike) *isometric*, of equal dimensions.

-itis (inflammation) *endocarditis*, inflammation within the heart.

kerat/o (cornea) *keratitis*, inflammation of the cornea.

kinesi/o (movement) *kinesialgia*, pain upon movement.

labi/o (lip) *labiodental*, pertaining to the lip and teeth.

lact/o (milk) *lactation*, the secretion of milk.

lal/o (talk) *lalopathy*, any speech disorder.

lapar/o (flank, abdomen, abdominal wall) *laparotomy*, an incision through the abdominal wall.

laryng/o (larynx) *laryngoscope*, an instrument for examining the larynx.

lept/o (thin) *leptodactylous*, having slender fingers.

leuc/o, leuk/o (white) *leukemia*, a malignant disease characterized by the increased development of white blood cells.

lingu/o (tongue) *sublingual*, under the tongue.

lip/o (fat) *lipoma*, fatty tumor.

lith/o (stone) *lithotriptor*, an instrument for crushing stones in the bladder.

-logist (a person who studies) *pathologist*, a person who studies diseases.

log/o (speak, give an account) *logospasms*, spasmodic speech.

-logy (study of) *pathology*, the study of disease.

lumb/o (loin) *lumbago*, pain in the lumbar region.

lymph/o (lymph) *lymphoduct*, a vessel of the lymph system.

-lysis (destruction) *electrolysis*, destruction (of hair, for example) by passage of an electric current.

macr/o (large, long) *macrocephalous*, having an abnormally large head.

malac/o (a softening) *malacia*, the morbid softening of a body part or tissue.

mamm/o (breast) *mammary*, pertaining to the breast.

-mania (mental aberration) *kleptomania*, the compulsion to steal.

mast/o (breast) *mastectomy*, surgical removal of the breast.

medi/o (middle) *mediastinum*, middle partition of the thoracic cavity.

mega- (large) *megacolon*, an abnormally large colon.

megal/o (large) *megalomaniac*, a person impressed with his own greatness.

-megaly (an enlargement) *cardiomegaly*, enlargement of the heart.

melan/o (dark, black) *melanoma*, a tumor comprised of darkly pigmented cells.

men/o (month) *menopause*, cessation of menstruation.

mes/o (middle) *mesiad*, toward the center.

meta- (change, transformation, exchange) *metabolism*, the sum of the physical and chemical processes by which an organism survives.

metr/o (uterus) *metralgia*, pain in the uterus.

micr/o (small) *microscope*, an instrument for magnifying small objects.

mon/o (single, only, sole) *monoplegia*, paralysis of a single part.

morph/o (form) *morphology*, the study of form and shape.

multi- (many, much) *multipara*, a woman who has given two or more live births.

my/o (muscle) *myasthenia*, muscular weakness.

myc/o, mycet/o (fungus) *mycosis*, any disease caused by a fungus.

myel/o (marrow, also often refers to spinal cord) *myelocele*, protrusion of the spinal cord through a defect in the spinal column.

myx/o (mucous, slimelike) *myxoid*, resembling mucus.

narc/o (stupor, numbness) *narcotic*, an agent that induces sleep.

nas/o (nose) *oronasal*, pertaining to the nose and mouth.

ne/o (new) *neonate*, a newborn infant.

necr/o (corpse) *necrotic*, dead (when referring to tissue).

nephr/o (kidney) *nephralgia*, pain in the kidneys.

neur/o (nerve) *neuritis*, inflammation of nerve pathways.

noct/i (night) *noctambulism*, sleepwalking.

norm/o (rule, order, normal) *normotension*, normal blood pressure.

null/i (none) *nullipara*, a woman who has never given birth to a child.

nyct/o (night) *nycturia*, excessive urination at night.

o/o- (egg) *ooblast*, a primitive cell from which an ovum develops.

ob- (against, in front of, toward) *obturator*, a device that closes an opening.

oc- (against, in front of, toward) *occlude*, to obstruct.

ocul/o (eye) *ocular*, pertaining to the eye.

odont/o (tooth) *odontalgia*, toothache.

-oid (shape, form, resemblance) *ovoid*, egg-shaped.

olig/o (few, deficient, scanty) *oligemia*, lacking in blood volume.

-oma (tumor, swelling) *adenoma*, tumor of a gland.

onych/o (nail) *onychoma*, tumor of a nail or nail bed.

oophor/o (ovary) *oophorectomy*, a surgical removal of one or both ovaries.

-opsy (a viewing) *autopsy*, postmortem examination of a body.

opthalm/o (eye) *opthalmic*, pertaining to the eyes.

opt/o, optic/o (sight, vision) *optometrist*, a specialist in adapting lenses for the correcting of visual defects.

or/o (mouth) *oral*, pertaining to the mouth.

orch/o, orchid/o (testicle) *orchitis*, inflammation of the testicles.

orth/o (straight, upright) *orthopedic*, pertaining to the correction of skeletal defects.

-osis (process, an abnormal condition) *dermatosis*, any skin condition.

oste/o (bone) *osteomyelitis*, inflammation of bone or bone marrow.

ot/o (ear) *otalgia*, earache.

ovari/o (ovary) *ovariocele*, hernia of an ovary.

ov/i, ov/o (egg) *oviduct*, a passage through which an egg passes.

pachy- (thicken) *pachyderma*, abnormal thickening of the skin.

palat/o (palate) *palatitis*, inflammation of the palate.

pan- (all, entire, every) *panacea*, a remedy for all diseases, a "cure-all."

para- (beside, beyond, accessory to, apart from, against) *paranormal*, beyond the natural or normal.

path/o (disease) *pathogen*, any disease-producing agent.

-pathy (disease of a part) *osteopathy*, disease of a bone.

-penia (an abnormal reduction) *leukopenia*, deficiency in white blood cells.

peps/o, pept/o (digestion) *dyspepsia*, poor digestion.

per- (throughout, completely, extremely) *perfusion*, the passage of fluid through the vessels of an organ.

peri- (around, surrounding) *pericardium*, the sac that surrounds the heart and the roots of the great vessels.

-pexy (fixation) *splendopexy*, surgical fixation of the spleen.

phag/o (eat) *phagomania*, an insatiable craving for food.

pharyng/o (throat) *pharyngospasms*, spasms of the muscles of the pharynx.

phas/o (speech) *aphasic*, unable to speak.

phil/o (like, have an affinity for) *necrophilia*, an abnormal interest in death.

phleb/o (vein) *phlebotomy*, surgical incision of a vein.

-phobia (fear, dread) *claustrophobia*, a fear of closed spaces.

phon/o (sound) *phonetic*, pertaining to the voice.

phor/o (bear, carry) *diaphoresis*, profuse sweating.

phot/o (light) *photosensitivity*, abnormal reactivity of the skin to sunlight.

phren/o (diaphragm) *phrenic nerve*, a nerve that carries messages to the diaphragm.

physi/o (nature) *physiology*, the science that studies the function of living things.

pil/o (hair) *pilose*, hairy.

-plasia (development, formation) *dysplasia*, poor or abnormal formation.

-plasty (surgical repair) *arthroplasty*, surgical repair of a joint.

-plegia (paralysis) *paraplegia*, paralysis of the lower body, including the legs.

pleur/o (rib, side, pleura) *pleurisy*, inflammation of the pleura.

-pnea (breath, breathing) *orthopnea*, difficult breathing except in an upright position.

pneum/o, pneumat/o (air, breath) *pneumatic*, pertaining to the air.

pneum/o, pneumon/o (lung) *pneumonia*, inflammation of the lungs with the escape of fluid.

pod/o (foot) *podiatrist*, a specialist in the care of feet.

-poiesis (formation) *hematopoiesis*, formation of blood.

poly- (much, many) *polychromatic*, multicolored.

post- (after, behind) *postmortem*, after death.

pre- (before) *premature*, occurring before the proper time.

pro- (before, in front of) *prolapse*, the falling down, or sinking of a part.

proct/o (anus) *proctitis*, inflammation of the rectum.

pseud/o (false) *pseudoplegia*, hysterical paralysis.

psych/o (mind, soul) *psychopath*, one who displays aggressive antisocial behavior.

-ptosis (abnormal dropping or sagging of a part) *hysteroptosis*, sagging of the uterus.

pulmon/o (lung) *pulmonary*, pertaining to the lungs.

py/o (pus) *pyorrhea*, copious discharge of pus.

pyel/o (renal pelvis) *pyelitis*, inflammation of the renal pelvis.

pyr/o (fire, fever) *pyromaniac*, compulsive fire setter.

quadri- (four) *quadriplegia*, paralysis of all four limbs.

rach/i (spine) *rachialgia*, pain in the spine.

radi/o (ray, radiation) *radiology*, the use of ionizing radiation in diagnosis and treatment.

re- (back, against, contrary) *recurrence*, the return of symptoms after remission.

rect/o (rectum) *rectal*, pertaining to the rectum.

ren/o (the kidneys) *renal*, pertaining to the kidneys.

retro- (located behind, backward) *retroperineal*, behind the perineum.

rhin/o (nose) *rhinitis*, inflammation of the mucous membranes of the nose.

-rrhage (abnormal discharge) *hemorrhage*, abnormal discharge of blood.

-rrhagia (hemorrhage from an organ or body part) *menorrhea*, excessive uterine bleeding.

-rrhea (flowing or discharge) *diarrhea*, abnormal frequency and liquidity of fecal discharges.

sanguin/o (blood) *exsanguinate*, to lose a large volume of blood either internally or externally.

sarc/o (flesh) *sarcoma*, a malignant tumor.

schiz/o (split) *schizophrenia*, any of a group of emotional disorders characterized by bizarre behavior (erroneously called split personality).

scler/o (hardening) *scleroderma*, hardening of connective tissues of the body, including the skin.

-sclerosis (hardened condition) *arteriosclerosis*, hardening of the arteries.

scoli/o (twisted, crooked) *scoliosis*, sideward deviation of the spine.

-scope (an instrument for observing) *endoscope*, an instrument for the examination of a hollow body, such as the bladder.

-sect (cut) *transsect*, to cut across.

semi- (one-half, partly) *semisupine*, partly, but not completely, supine.

sept/o, seps/o (infection) *aseptic*, free from infection.

somat/o (body) *psychosomatic*, both psychological and physiological.

son/o (sound) *sonogram*, a recording produced by the passage of sound waves through the body.

spermat/o (sperm, semen) *spermacide*, an agent that kills sperm.

sphygm/o (pulse) *sphygmomanometer*, a device for measuring blood pressure in the arteries.

splen/o (spleen) *splenectomy*, surgical removal of the spleen.

-stasis (stopping, controlling) *hemostasis*, the control of bleeding.

sten/o (narrow) *stenosis*, a narrowing of a passage or opening.

stere/o (solid, three-dimensional) *stereoscopic*, a three-dimensional appearance.

steth/o (chest) *stethoscope*, an instrument for listening to chest sounds.

sthen/o (strength) *myasthenia*, muscular weakness.

-stomy (surgically creating a new opening) *colostomy*, surgical creation of an opening between the colon and the surface of the body.

sub- (under, near, almost, moderately) *subclavian*, situated under the clavicle.

super- (above, excess) *superficial*, lying on or near the surface.

supra- (above, over) *suprapubic*, situated above the pubic arch.

sym-, syn- (joined together, with) *syndrome*, a set of symptoms that occur together.

tachy- (fast) *tachycardia*, a very fast heart rate.

-therapy (treatment) *hydrotherapy*, treatment with water.

therm/o (heat) *thermogenesis*, the production of heat.

thorac/o (chest cavity) *thoracic*, pertaining to the chest.

thromb/o (clot, lump) *thrombophlebitis*, inflammation of a vein.

-tome (a surgical instrument for cutting) *microtome*, an instrument for cutting thin slices of tissue.

-tomy (a surgical operation on an organ or body part) *thoracotomy*, surgical incision of the chest wall.

top/o (place) *topographic*, pertaining to special regions (of the body).

trache/o (trachea) *tracheostomy*, an opening in the neck that passes to the trachea.

trans- (through, across, beyond) *transfusion*, the introduction of whole blood or blood components directly into the bloodstream.

tri- (three) *trimester*, a period of 3 months.

trich/o (hair) *trichosis*, any disease of the hair.

-tripsy (surgical crushing) *lithotripsy*, surgical crushing of stones.

troph/o (nourish) *hypertrophic*, enlargement of an organ or body part due to the increase in the size of cells.

ultra- (beyond, excess) *ultrasonic*, beyond the audible range.

uni- (one) *unilateral*, affecting one side.

ur/o (urine) *urinalysis*, examination of urine.

ureter/o (ureter) *ureteritis*, inflammation of a ureter.

urethr/o (urethra) *urethritis*, inflammation of the urethra.

vas/o (vessel, duct) *vasodilator*, an agent that causes dilation of blood vessels.

ven/o (vein) *venipuncture*, surgical puncture of a vein.

ventr/o (belly, cavity) *ventral*, relating to the belly or abdomen.

vesic/o (blister, bladder) *vesicle*, a small fluid-filled blister.

viscer/o (internal organ) *visceral*, pertaining to the viscera (abdominal organs).

xanth/o (yellow) *xanthroma*, a yellow nodule in the skin.

xen/o (stranger) *xenophobia*, abnormal fear of strangers.

xer/o (dry) *xerosis*, abnormal dryness (as of the mouth or eyes).

zo/o (animal life) *zoogenous*, acquired from an animal.

The following are text questions and answers/discussion suggestions for Critical Decision Making, a feature within the narrative, and for end-of-chapter Short Answer questions, Critical Thinking Exercises, Pathophysiology to Practice questions, and Street Scene questions.

Chapter 1 Introduction to Emergency Medical Care
Critical Decision Making

1. There are several pieces of information you must gather in order to determine which hospital is most appropriate for your patient. For example, is the patient requesting transport to a particular hospital because his physician practices there? Whenever possible, try to make provisions for patient choice. Or, is the patient's condition too unstable to bypass a closer facility in favor of a hospital a little farther away? In many cases, your local jurisdiction will have specific policies that direct patient transport and hospital destination. These policies often include provisions for transporting patients to specialty centers such as burn and trauma centers. Hospitals are increasingly specializing in managing certain areas of care like cardiac and stroke emergencies, but transport to these facilities should always be considered under the direction of local policy or medical control.

2. Rendering care to your patient, especially something invasive like medication administration, requires the completion of a comprehensive physical assessment and patient history. Understanding the risks and benefits of the treatment you provide and basing your decisions on the facts and evidence revealed during your assessment of the patient will help you develop a treatment plan that meets the needs of the patient without doing harm.

Short Answer

1. The components of the EMS system are 911 and emergency medical dispatchers, Emergency Medical Responders, EMTs (all levels) and ambulances, emergency department, and other hospital units.
2. Special designations of hospitals include trauma centers, burn centers, pediatric care centers, poison control centers, cardiac centers, and stroke centers.
3. The four national levels of EMS training and certification are Emergency Medical Responder (EMR), Emergency Medical Technician (EMT), Advanced Emergency Medical Technician (AEMT), and Paramedic.
4. The roles and responsibilities of the EMT include safety of the crew, patient, and bystanders; patient assessment; patient care; lifting and moving; transport; transfer of care; patient advocacy; and promotion of public health and safety.
5. Some of the desirable personal and physical attributes of the EMT include being in good health and able to lift and carry up to 125 pounds; having good eyesight and hearing; being able to clearly communicate in written and oral form; and being pleasant, sincere, cooperative, resourceful, a self-starter, emotionally stable, able to lead, and neat and clean.
6. Quality improvement is a process of continuous self-review with the purpose of identifying and correcting aspects of the system that require improvement.

7. The difference between on-line and off-line medical direction is that in on-line medical direction, the on-duty physician gives orders directly to the EMT by telephone or radio. In off-line medical direction, the EMT carries out written standing orders from the Medical Director.

Critical Thinking Exercises

1. Some of the desirable personal traits that EMTs should strive to exemplify include a pleasant, sincere, and cooperative attitude around his patients and customers. Being able to step up as a leader and remain emotionally stable during stressful situations is important. Effective listening and communication skills are essential if you want to be successful in the health care industry. Because your patients come from such a diverse population of different cultures and backgrounds—many that may be different from your own—it is critical that you are open-minded and nonjudgmental of your patients and the people you care for. You can strive to incorporate these traits into your everyday care by thinking about them daily and approaching each patient (regardless of the circumstances) with the same approach.

2. You can continually refresh your knowledge and skill performance by taking advantage of conferences, seminars, lectures, classes, videotapes and DVDs, and demonstrations. Review literature and study evidence-based research.

Street Scene Questions

1. It's important to understand that Chuck Hartley has a professional responsibility to set a good example for the new EMT. He should arrive in a well-kept uniform and involve the new EMT in all aspects of the job. For example, a new EMT should help check the ambulance and equipment at the start of the shift. Chuck should also provide an explanation of operating procedures. In other words, a new EMT needs to know what is expected of him.

2. Chuck Hartley exhibits numerous unprofessional behavior characteristics, such as an unkempt uniform, telling the new EMT to sit until he is needed, failure to introduce himself to the patient, using insulting or derogatory terms such as "Hon" in addressing the patient, loudly criticizing the new EMT, and dismissal of patient concerns, such as instructing her to "tell it to the doctor."

3. Some of the characteristics you should expect from someone providing initial field training might include the following:
- Good communication skills
- Neat and well-kept appearance
- Polite and courteous behavior, both with other EMTs and with patients
- Willingness to explain the job
- Understanding the needs of a new EMT (empathy)
- Good patient skills
- Willingness to act as a team player

4. Susan Miller came to work in a well-pressed uniform. She expressed an obvious interest and memory of the new EMT and communicated job expectations in a clear manner. She set an example by providing an orientation to the ambulance, equipment, and agency procedures. She made the new intern a part of the call and provided numerous examples of professional patient care. She monitored actions taken by the new EMT, making every effort not to belittle the person. When the call was completed, Susan took time to critique the run, reinforcing the skills needed to become a good EMT.

5. Susan obviously set a good professional standard and served as a role model for the EMT to follow. The student intern will have a much more positive experience in that type of learning environment.

6. There are many personal traits that you should work to develop as a professional EMT, such as always striving to be pleasant, sincere, cooperative, neat, respectful, and a good listener.

Chapter 2 The Well-Being of the EMT

Critical Decision Making

1. through 5. For discussion: What similar situations would call for these or other Standard Precautions?

Short Answer

1. Some situations that may cause stress for an EMT include multiple-casualty incidents, injuries to infants and children, severe injuries, abuse and neglect, the death of a coworker, or personal situations unrelated to work.

2. The CISD debriefing/defusing model is meant to assist emergency care workers in dealing with the stress experienced in relation to a major incident. It is held within 24 to 72 hours after an incident and is an open discussion of the feelings experienced during and after the call. All information is confidential. Follow-up is provided by a peer member of the team within 24 hours after the CISD.

3. The stages of grief are: denial—the patient denies the fact that he is dying; anger—the patient becomes angry; bargaining—the patient tries to postpone death, even if only briefly; depression—the patient is sad or in despair over things left undone; and acceptance—the patient is ready to die. Understanding what the families and the patients go through can help an EMT deal with the stress they feel as well as his own emotions.

4. Examples of personal protective equipment include: protective gloves—used with controlled bleeding, suctioning, artificial ventilation, CPR; eye protection—used with splashing, spattering, or spraying body fluids; masks—used with infections spread by airborne droplets (measles); and gowns—used with arterial bleeding, childbirth.

Critical Thinking Exercises

Unless you stay safe yourself, you will not be able to help your patient and you may suffer serious injury—or die. Retreat to a safe place and call for a response by law enforcement. Approach the patient only when they inform you that the scene is safe.

Pathophysiology to Practice

1. Common colds, viruses, and influenza are typically spread by tiny droplets when an infected person breathes, coughs, or sneezes on you. These "bugs" can also be transmitted by touching something contaminated and then touching your nose or eyes.

2. The body's response to stress is to activate the sympathetic nervous system. This causes an increased heart rate, increased respiratory rate and dilated bronchial passages, and an increased blood pressure. All of this is part of the body's compensatory mechanism to handle the stress.

3. The difference between good stress and bad stress on the body often comes down to one's own resistance and ability to cope with stress. Stress impacts different people differently; for example, two EMTs on the same call may have opposite responses. More simply, the stress of jogging 2 miles will obviously have a much different impact on the body than the cumulative stress of running back-to-back multiple-casualty incidents.

Street Scene Questions

1. It's essential for you to wear protective gloves on this call because the patient has bad facial injuries that may bring you into contact with blood and other body fluids. Gloves help minimize possible exposure to bloodborne pathogens. Intact skin can offer some protection in case of accidental exposure. In this case, however, you are aware of a partially healed cut on his hand, making the potential risk of exposure even greater if no gloves are worn.

2. Occupational injuries and exposures often don't seem like a big deal—until they happen to you. Don't underestimate the devastating effects of occupational exposure, especially the possibility of transferring a disease to family members and/or fellow EMS workers. In addition, occupational exposure can cause considerable anxiety as an EMT waits to

determine if he has actually contracted the disease, during which time he will often be taking powerful prophylactic medications that have significant side effects.

3. Anytime a potential exposure occurs, it is critical to immediately notify your supervisor. This is not the time to hide the incident or minimize what occurred. Supervisory personnel are typically trained to manage just these situations and determine the extent of the exposure. It is always better to be safe than sorry, which may include an occupational evaluation at the emergency department, physical examination, and baseline blood tests.

4. The anxiety of waiting for test results is often the worst part of an occupational exposure. This anxiety can lead to a strained marital relationship and tension with coworkers developing from an inability to talk about the situation, out of either fear or embarrassment.

5. Hand washing is a first-line defense against infection. Even though you wear gloves, you must still wash your hands after your gloves are removed.

6. At a minimum, all EMTs should have two sets of gloves and eye protection immediately available. Wear the gloves and eye protection on every patient encounter. Gowns and additional protective gear (masks, etc.) may be necessary depending upon your assessment of the situation.

Chapter 3 Lifting and Moving Patients

Critical Decision Making

1. A patient complaining of severe respiratory distress in an upstairs back bedroom should probably be moved by a stair chair unless his difficulty breathing is so severe he can't sit up or he requires ventilation. In those situations, a Reeves-type stretcher is a better option.

2. A patient thrown from an ATV several hundred yards into the woods should be placed on a backboard (long spine board) in full spinal immobilization, and then in a Stokes (wire frame) basket for extrication.

3. A patient with neck and back pain who fell down several stairs onto concrete should be placed on a backboard (long spine board) in full spinal immobilization.

4. An unresponsive medical patient found down in a narrow hallway would likely benefit from rapid extrication using a Reeves-type device, allowing two EMTs to carry the patient out of the hallway to the stretcher.

Short Answer

1. Body mechanics is the proper use of the body to facilitate lifting and moving. Principles of body mechanics include:
   - Position your feet properly, shoulder-width apart.
   - When lifting, use your legs, not your back, to do the lifting.
   - When lifting, never twist or attempt to make any moves other than the lift.
   - When lifting with one hand, do not compensate.
   - Keep the weight as close to your body as possible.
   - When carrying a patient on stairs, use a stair chair instead of a stretcher when possible.

2. A number of situations may require the emergency move of a patient, including when the scene is hazardous, when care of life-threatening conditions requires repositioning, and when other patients must be reached for immediate treatment.

3. Lifts include the extremity lift; the direct ground lift, the draw-sheet method; and the direct carry method. Drags include the shoulder drag, the foot drag, the "fireman's drag," the incline drag, the clothes drag, and the blanket drag.

4. A long-axis drag is a drag from the shoulders of the patient that causes the remainder of the body to assume its natural anatomical position, with the spine and all limbs in normal alignment. This emergency move minimizes or prevents aggravation of a spinal injury.

Critical Thinking Exercises

1. A patient who has fallen 18 feet with suspected spinal injuries should be lifted and moved with a spine board in full spinal immobilization.

2. A patient with chest pain and no spine injury who lives on an upper floor of a building with no elevator should be moved with a stair chair.

3. A patient found in an environment where there is risk of immediate explosion should be moved emergently with a shoulder drag.

Street Scene Questions

1. Remove the patient from the vehicle by applying a cervical collar and a short immobilization device. After conducting the necessary neurological exams, you should rotate the patient onto a long board.

2. When using an extrication device, keep in mind that they can have a negative impact on the patient's airway or breathing and can cause significant patient discomfort. The cervical collar should not be applied too tightly and the short board straps should not restrict the patient's respirations. When rotating the patient onto the long board, the leg straps of the short immobilization device may need to be loosened to reduce patient discomfort.

3. The key to moving any patient, especially in an extrication, is a well-coordinated team effort. The EMT providing head stabilization is responsible for announcing all the moves. For example, he might say, "Slide the patient onto the long board on the count of three." The crew must continually monitor the patient, especially the ABCs and any change in the level of consciousness. A quick neurological exam should be done both before and after the move.

4. In this scenario, the equipment included a cervical collar, short immobilization device (vest-type extrication device), long board, straps, head immobilizer, stretcher, and stretcher-locking device. The equipment was selected based on the mechanism of injury and for maximum patient safety to protect against possible neck or spinal injury.

5. Before moving this patient again, you should continue talking to the patient to make sure her level of responsiveness has not changed and no breathing difficulty has developed. A member of the crew should also perform another quick neurological exam, checking that the patient has pulses, movement, and sensation in all four extremities. Check straps to make sure that the patient is secured to the long board and that everyone knows what he should do to secure a smooth move.

6. When moving the long board to the wheeled stretcher, always make sure the wheeled cot is locked and secured so it does not move and ensure that personnel carrying the backboard all face in the same direction. If somebody needs to back up while placing the board on the stretcher, the person should be guided by placing a hand at his back. There should be sufficient personnel carrying the long board, and each person should keep a firm grip on the board until it is placed completely on the stretcher. The straps of the wheeled cot must be buckled and secured before the patient is moved.

Chapter 4 Medical, Legal, and Ethical Issues
Critical Decision Making

1. Overhearing a colleague admit to a serious clinical error means that you have an ethical responsibility to tell the truth about what you heard. If this event isn't reported, harm could come to the patient. While reporting fellow EMTs is not popular, it might be possible to talk to the provider who made the mistake and encourage him to tell the truth.

2. Providing care while you are intoxicated is a recipe for disaster. Considering how large the drinks were and how long ago you had them would help to determine if you were intoxicated. Some recommend not stopping if you have consumed any alcohol. How would you feel as a patient if you smelled alcohol on the breath of an EMT treating you?

3. A patient is telling you a suspicious story. Unfortunately, you have no way of knowing if the patient is even telling the truth. Most would recommend reporting this to the police. Follow your local guidelines and protocols.

Short Answer

1. The difference between expressed and implied consent is significant because a patient offering expressed consent is an adult that is mentally competent to make decisions, is informed of the risks associated with the care he is about to receive, and is making an expressed decision to receive the care. In implied consent, patients are typically unconscious or incapacitated in some way such that you must assume they would agree to be treated if they were conscious.

2. A finding of negligence requires that all of the following circumstances be proved: the EMT had a duty to the patient (duty to act), the EMT did not provide the standard of care (committed a breach of duty), and by not providing the standard of care, the EMT caused harm to the patient (proximate causation) (the harm can be physical or psychological).

3. Your first priority is always patient care, but it is still possible to preserve evidence and minimize your impact on the scene during the course of your actions. Remember how you found the scene, avoid unnecessarily moving or touching things, remember what you touch, do not cut through holes left in clothing by bullets or knives, and avoid moving or wandering around the scene whenever possible. Work closely with law enforcement.

4. If an EMT has initiated care and then leaves a patient without ensuring that the patient has been turned over to someone with equal or greater training, it constitutes abandonment. The fact that this patient was left in a hospital bed doesn't matter; there must still be a transfer of care.

5. Leaving a copy of the run report on the bulletin board at the station for everyone to review is a violation of the law (HIPAA). Any information you obtain about a patient's history, condition, or treatment is considered confidential and must not be shared with anyone else. Sharing the information with another caregiver involved with the continuing care of the patient (like the nurse receiving the patient at the hospital) is allowed, but tacking a run report up on a bulletin board for all crews (and potentially the cable guy) to see is illegal.

Critical Thinking Exercises

1. This may not fit the strict definition of "duty to act" because you were not officially dispatched to this call, but you still have a moral and ethical obligation to render aid since you are on duty and you are trained providers. In general, if you follow your conscience and provide care, you will incur less liability than if you do not act. Always follow your local protocols and laws.

2. Think back about your care of the patient and your actions on the call. Were the actions of your crew so obviously responsible for the patient's death that a lawsuit is in order? Does *res ipsa loquitur* apply? If not, evaluate your care and actions on the call against the three tests of negligence: (1) Did you have a duty to act? (2) Did you provide the standard of care or commit a breach of duty? (3) If you failed to provide the standard of care, did your actions cause harm to the patient (also known as proximate causation)? In order for negligence to be proven, all three must apply. Remember that proximate causation cannot be applied to patients who are so seriously injured that they cannot be saved.

3. A critical decision like withholding CPR should not be made based on hearsay; it should be made based on an actual legal document. Without the actual DNR present, you should continue CPR and consider making contact with medical direction for further guidance.

Street Scene Questions

1. Radio transmissions can be easily monitored by a curious public, so you should only share information over the radio that is directly related to immediate care. In this particular situation, the presence of AIDS has no direct bearing on the care steps initiated in the field. As a result, the hospital staff does not need to know about the presence of AIDS at the time of the radio report.

2. All patient information should be treated as confidential and should not be released except with written permission or upon request by legal subpoena. It's very simple: It's the law and you must abide by it.

3. The fact that the patient has AIDS is definitely part of her medical history and should be shared, discreetly, with the staff member receiving the patient at the hospital. Keep in mind that if this very private information about the patient becomes public against her wishes, it may impact more than just her treatment. There are many areas where AIDS discrimination still occurs in employment and housing, even though it is illegal.

   Informing all of the hospital staff of the patient's condition is highly inappropriate and is irrelevant because infection control precautions should be the standard in any medical institution and should not rely upon information supplied by an EMT. You assume every patient you encounter has the potential to be an occupational exposure and so you approach every patient encounter the same: with Standard Precautions.

4. Sharing the patient's health history with other EMS providers constitutes a breach of patient confidentiality. Not only is this action inappropriate, but sharing information may carry some legal consequences, especially if it has a negative impact on the patient.

5. The principles of patient confidentiality can be described very simply: If there is not a need to know, then don't share it. In other words, if a colleague is not directly involved in patient care, then that colleague has no need to know anything about the patient or the patient's information. This standard applies to personnel at the hospital, fire department, police department, and, of course, members of the public and media. It is your professional responsibility to protect the patient's information from breach of confidentiality. Failure to do so could mean civil and criminal penalties.

Chapter 5 Medical Terminology and Anatomy and Physiology
Critical Decision Making

1. A patient who has fractured the bones of the arm just above the wrist has likely broken the radius and ulna.

2. The spleen is often injured in blunt trauma and can cause severe internal bleeding. It is located in the left upper quadrant.

3. The large bone in the thigh is the femur. Because this is the largest bone in the body, blood loss can be significant and can exceed 1 liter.

Short Answer

1. The following anatomical terms are defined as:
   • Medial–toward the midline of the body
     Lateral–to the side, away from the midline of the body
   • Anterior–the front of the body or body part
     Posterior–the back of the body or body part
   • Proximal–closer to the torso
     Distal–farther away from the torso

2. The musculoskeletal system functions to give the body shape, to protect vital internal organs, and to provide for body movement.

3. The five divisions of the spine and their locations are:
   • Cervical–neck
   • Thoracic–upper back
   • Lumbar–lower back
   • Sacral–posterior pelvis
   • Coccyx–distal spine, posterior pelvis

4. During inhalation, the muscles of the rib cage and the diaphragm contract. The diaphragm lowers, and the ribs move upward and outward. This expands the size of the chest and thereby creates a negative pressure inside the chest cavity. This negative pressure pulls air into the lungs. During exhalation, the intercostal muscles and the diaphragm relax. The ribs move downward and inward, while the diaphragm rises. This movement causes the chest

to decrease in size and positive pressure to build inside the chest cavity. This positive pressure pushes air out of the lungs.

5. The four places where a peripheral pulse may be palpated are the radial artery, brachial artery, carotid artery, and femoral artery.

6. The central nervous system is composed of the brain and the spinal cord. The brain receives information from the body and, in turn, sends impulses to different areas of the body to respond to internal and external changes. The spinal cord rests within the spinal column and stretches from the brain to the lumbar vertebrae. Nerves branch from each part of the cord and reach throughout the body. The peripheral nervous system consists of two types of nerves: sensory and motor. The sensory nerves pick up information from throughout the body and transmit it to the spinal cord and brain. The motor nerves carry messages from the brain to the body.

7. The functions of the skin include protection, water balance, temperature regulation, excretion, and shock absorption.

Critical Thinking Exercises

The patient has a laceration on his lateral left arm midway between the shoulder and elbow. He has another laceration on the medial aspect of his left arm proximal to the wrist. He has an open, angulated mid-shaft femur fracture of his left leg.

Street Scene Questions

1. Knowledge of the patient's anatomy will guide your assessment and care. The mechanism of injury will point to anatomic locations of potential injury. Understanding underlying structures will help you predict the potential damage and its severity. Understanding airway anatomy will help you better manage the airway. Pediatric anatomy will also have to be considered as there are many anatomical differences in a child compared to an adult.

2. When assessing the child's abdomen, be alert for signs of internal bleeding such as bruising, rigidity, and tenderness.

3. The child's decreased mental status is significant. He also has an airway problem that you are correcting. Furthermore, his abdominal assessment points to additional underlying injuries and the potential for internal bleeding.

4. Altered mental status has many causes. It could be caused by internal bleeding from the abdomen or it could be a traumatic brain injury. Consider also other fractures and wounds associated with high energy trauma.

Chapter 6 Principles of Pathophysiology

Critical Decision Making

This scenario serves as a reminder of how calling on your knowledge of pathophysiology can help you as you consider not only what the patient's physical findings are (including vital signs) but also what may be going on inside the patient's body to cause these findings.

Short Answer

1. Metabolism is the conversion of glucose and other nutrients into energy in the form of adenosine triphosphate. Necessary components include oxygen and glucose.

2. Three types of respiratory dysfunction are disruption of respiratory control, disruption of pressure, and disruption of lung tissue. Disruption of respiratory control occurs when the brain fails to appropriately control breathing. Without regulatory messages being sent, breathing can cease or become ineffective. Disruption of pressure occurs when the integrity of the chest cavity is broken and air passes in and out through the chest wall. This interferes with the pressure changes necessary to move air in and out through the glottic opening. Disruption of lung tissue occurs when lung tissue is displaced or destroyed by disease or mechanical force. Injured or diseased tissue cannot exchange oxygen and carbon dioxide.

3. Dilation and constriction of blood vessels help maintain the necessary pressure in the cardiovascular system to pump blood. These changes give the body the capability to adapt to changes in the volume of circulating blood.

4. Cardiac output is the amount of blood pumped by the heart each minute. Components include stroke volume and heart rate.

5. The body compensates for cardiopulmonary challenges in predictable ways. Commonly, the autonomic nervous system engages the "fight-or-flight" mechanism of its sympathetic arm. This causes blood vessels to constrict and the heart to beat faster and stronger. The sympathetic nervous response also causes pupils to dilate and the skin to sweat. Chemoreceptors in the brain and blood vessels sense increasing carbon dioxide and hypoxia and stimulate the respiratory system to breathe faster and deeper. Signs and symptoms include increased pulse and respirations, delayed capillary refill, and pale skin. Pupils may be dilated and the patient may be sweaty even in cool environments.

Critical Thinking Exercises

1. Normal metabolism requires adequate amounts of oxygen and glucose. When adequate amounts of either are not available, the body changes the process. Anaerobic metabolism occurs in low oxygen states. This inefficient form of metabolism produces less energy and far more waste products.

2. The respiratory system delivers oxygen from room air to the bloodstream. The circulatory system delivers oxygen and glucose to the cells. The blood vessels dilate and constrict to provide sufficient pressure in the cardiovascular system to move blood, and the blood components carry the oxygen and glucose.

Pathophysiology to Practice

1. With a damaged heart, the body's ability to compensate by managing cardiac output is impaired. Cardiac injuries can limit the ability to change heart rate and stroke volume and therefore limit increases in cardiac output.

2. A patient with a loss of tone in his blood vessels would lose the ability to control pressure within the cardiovascular system. This person could not adapt to blood loss by vasoconstriction. Furthermore, excessive dilation of blood vessels can drop blood pressure and cause shock.

3. Red blood cells carry oxygen. A deficit in the number of these cells disrupts the body's ability to move oxygen in the cardiovascular system. Under normal circumstances, this patient will have a difficult time transporting enough oxygen. In times of challenge, this deficit may seriously affect the body's ability to compensate. A loss of red blood cells also limits the body's ability to remove waste products such as carbon dioxide from the tissues. This can be damaging to the tissues.

Street Scene Questions

1. You will want to know how long his problem has been going on. Does he have any history of GI-related problems? Does he have any other medical problems or take any medications?

2. His fast heart rate and pale skin point to compensated shock. With the history he has presented, this person has the potential to be critically ill.

3. This person has no radial pulse because the pressure in the cardiovascular system is very low. His heart rate and respiratory rate have increased to compensate for poor perfusion.

4. The low blood pressure was predictable based on the weak radial pulse.

5. This person's low blood pressure is likely caused by internal bleeding in the GI tract. Clues that indicate this diagnosis include the dark stools and the tender abdomen.

6. ALS should be contacted. Advanced personnel can administer intravenous fluid to help increase cardiovascular pressure and perfusion.

Chapter 7 Life Span Development
Critical Decision Making

1. A 3-year-old boy that is groggy with a pulse of 60/minute is abnormal. He should be alert and active with a pulse of 80-120/minute.

2. A 65-year-old man describing a feeling of "skipping heart beats" and a pulse of 130/minute is abnormal. A normal rate for his age is 70/minute. He may be suffering from any number of fast heart rhythms.

3. A 42-year-old man who fell off a curb and hurt his ankle with a respiratory rate of 16 is normal.

4. A 77-year-old woman complaining of dizziness with a pulse of 56/minute is likely abnormal. A normal heart rate for her age is 70/minute. However, further assessment of her other vital signs (blood pressure, etc.) will give you a clearer impression of her condition.

5. A 3-month-old baby with a respiratory rate of 30 is normal.

Short Answer

1. The following descriptions fit with the following age groups:
- Decreased metabolism: Late adulthood (61 years and older)
- Toilet trained: Toddler (average age 28 months)
- Empty nest syndrome: Middle adulthood (41 to 60 years)
- Noticeable development of external sex organs: Adolescence (13 to 18 years)
- Rooting reflex: Infant (birth to 1 year)
- Self-destructive behaviors common: Adolescence (13 to 18 years)
- Peak physical condition: Early adulthood (19 to 40 years)
- Twilight years: Late adulthood (61 years and older)

2. Your ability to communicate with younger patients will depend on their stage of development. An infant is often perfectly charming, compliant, and willing to cooperate. However, as children develop separation anxiety and fear of strangers, your approach will have to be more delicate. Later, among the adolescent age group, kids strive for independence. Body image and privacy are a big concern. Most adolescents want you to treat them like an adult yet still want to fully indulge in the comforts of childhood.

Critical Thinking Exercises

A 16-year-old girl hesitant to open up or answer your questions in front of her friends is not unusual. Kids go through an often painful process of discovering their own identities during their adolescent years and don't want to risk embarrassing themselves in front of their peers. Body image is a great concern at this point in life and eating disorders can also be an issue. The patient has become sexually mature by this age and may be sexually active. Try to overcome her hesitancy by limiting or removing bystanders. If a female crew member is available to conduct the interview and assessment, the patient may feel more comfortable offering information to her.

Pathophysiology to Practice

1. After suffering a mechanism of injury like the one described, the patient's elevated heart rate is likely due to the excitement of the incident and the stimulation of the patient's sympathetic nervous system, which causes a faster heart rate and higher blood pressure. There is no way to know whether the patient might have suffered internal injuries or bleeding without performing a further assessment.

2. Knowing what medications a patient is taking can help determine a patient's preexisting medical conditions. It's often through your questions about the patient's medications that you get much of your history about illnesses and conditions the patient has had in the past.

Street Scene Questions

1. A child that is 3 or 4 years old is expected to cling fiercely to his mother, especially in a stressful and traumatic incident like this. Kids at this age fear separation from their parents and the incident has most likely magnified his fears all the more.

2. Given the patient's level of anxiety, you should use a very gentle approach and calm voice with the patient. Even with a gentle approach, kids at this age seldom tolerate being strapped down and placed in spinal immobilization. Make sure you have plenty of help and try to limit how many people talk to the child at once. Be sure the patient's mother is allowed to stay with him at all times.

3. The patient's mother is key to your successful management of this patient. By keeping her calm and involved in his care, you will in turn help keep the patient calm and cooperative. Make sure she understands that you are doing everything possible to help her son and make him comfortable. If at all possible, avoid separating the mother and son.

4. All of his vital signs appear to be normal for a patient of this age.

5. Many caregivers carry a quick reference card with them that list normal vital sign ranges for different ages.

6. Keep it very basic and explain what you plan to do prior to doing it. Avoid surprises and never lie to the patient or "sugar-coat" things; if you do, you will lose his trust. Telling a child that something won't hurt only for it to be painful is the surest way to create an uncooperative patient for the rest of your transport. Be truthful without scaring him and provide lots of encouragement for his bravery.

Chapter 8 Airway Management
Critical Decision Making

1. The 16-year-old asthma patient's airway will not likely stay open. Although asthma is primarily a breathing problem, his attack is leading to a decrease in mental status which threatens his airway.

2. The 72-year-old female patient's airway will likely stay open unless her condition significantly worsens. Her problem is likely a breathing issue and not related to her airway. She may be critical as a result of her pneumonia, but at this moment her airway is stable.

3. The 35-year-old male patient's airway is seriously threatened. His position and drooling indicate a difficulty keeping his airway open and are classic signs of edema as a result of an infection in the larynx. This patient has a high probability of losing that airway.

4. The 16-month-old's barking cough indicates an upper airway issue and certainly concerns you. However, in small children the subglottic edema that causes the seal-like bark is often well tolerated and may not truly threaten the airway. On the other hand, there are some children who do not tolerate this well at all. If this is the case, this infection can significantly threaten the airway. Observe these children for signs of adequate oxygenation and assess on a case-by-case basis.

Short Answer

1. The main structures of the airway are the mouth, nose, tongue, nasopharynx, oropharynx, hypopharynx, glottis, trachea, bronchi, bronchioles, and alveoli.

2. Airway care is typically the highest priority because without a patent airway, oxygenation and ventilation cannot occur. Lack of oxygenation will quickly lead to patient death.

3. Signs of an inadequate airway include no air movement, choking, stridor, snoring, and gurgling.

4. The head-tilt, chin-lift maneuver should be used to open the airway on patients who are not at risk of spinal injury. This maneuver moves the head and neck and therefore violates the in-line neutral position. The jaw-thrust maneuver should be used on patients with the potential for spinal injury as it theoretically does not move the neck.

5. Airway adjuncts help maintain an open airway by moving the tongue (and therefore the epiglottis) forward and creating a channel for air to move within. Suctioning removes liquids and loose substances from the airway to prevent them from obstructing air movement and to prevent aspiration.

Critical Thinking Exercises

1. This patient needs immediate airway intervention including suctioning, positioning, and potentially the insertion of an airway adjunct. Further treatment will include positive pressure ventilation and probably advanced life support assistance.

2. Stridor indicates a partially obstructed airway. Your immediate concern is the threat of the airway occluding completely. Rapid transport is necessary.

3. Snoring respirations indicate turbulent air flow through the airway. In an injured or ill patient, it generally indicates a decreased capability to maintain the airway as consciousness decreases. Corrective actions include positioning the head, opening the airway, and potentially inserting an airway adjunct.

Pathophysiology to Practice

1. The signs of a partially obstructed airway include difficulty breathing, difficulty speaking, stridor, snoring, choking, and coughing.

2. An altered mental status can impact the patient's airway because as mental status decreases, control of the muscles that keep the airway open can be impaired. The loss of tone in these muscles can lead to the epiglottis falling back and obstructing the glottic opening. Altered mental status can also cause a loss of the gag reflex. Without this protective reflex, patients are at risk for aspiration.

3. Neck trauma can immediately impact the airway by disrupting pathways and destroying structures, but it might also threaten long-term patency by causing swelling to occur in the airway passages. This swelling can obstruct the movement of air.

Street Scene Questions

1. Once safety has been assured, the first priorities are to establish responsiveness and, if necessary, open the airway and check for breathing.

2. For an unconscious person, you should be prepared to open the airway, support breathing, and potentially begin CPR.

3. Necessary equipment should include personal protective equipment, airway management tools such as suction and airway adjuncts, and breathing support devices such as a bag-valve mask and supplemental oxygen.

4. After determining the scene is safe, you should immediately assess the airway and breathing. After those have been assessed and treated, you should perform a pulse check. Consider also a scene assessment to determine the mechanism of injury.

5. In an unresponsive person, you should first open the airway and then "look, listen, and feel" for air movement. Look at the chest for rise and fall; listen for the sounds of air movement; feel for air moving and for the rise of the chest.

6. The patient should be rapidly turned on his side (if it is safe to do so) to allow gravity to assist with clearing fluid from his airway. You should employ suction to further clear any remaining vomit.

7. Because of the possibility of spinal injuries, the patient's airway should be opened with a jaw-thrust maneuver. Consider using an airway adjunct to help maintain the airway.

Chapter 9 Respiration and Artificial Ventilation

Critical Decision Making

1. A patient found on the floor with no pulse or respirations must be immediately ventilated with a bag-valve mask and high-concentration oxygen.

2. A 14-year-old patient with a fractured femur and strong but mildly rapid pulse and respirations is likely experiencing significant pain. Administer oxygen and help relieve her pain by stabilizing the broken extremity.

3. A 64-year-old alert patient with chest pain and stable vital signs needs oxygen administration and the presence of a calm environment.

4. A 78-year-old COPD patient with rapid, shallow respirations who is no longer oriented should be manually ventilated with high-concentration oxygen to ensure that the patient's tidal volume can be improved with each manual respiration. Because the patient is still somewhat awake, his respirations need to be "tracked" in a manner so as to not agitate the patient and produce gastric insufflation.

Short Answer

1. Signs of respiratory distress include rapid respirations, accessory muscle use, anxiety, pursed lip breathing, and the tripod position. In the case of respiratory distress, the patient should have a relatively normal pulse oximetry and have a relatively normal mental status as increased respiratory efforts are meeting the metabolic needs of the body.

2. Signs of respiratory failure include all the signs of respiratory distress plus signs that the body is no longer compensating for the respiratory challenge. These signs include altered mental status, dropping pulse oximetry, cyanosis, slowing/irregular respirations, and respiratory fatigue.

3. The techniques of artificial ventilation are:
   - Mouth-to-mask–Connect oxygen to the inlet on the mask and run at 15 liters per minute. Position the mask on the patient's face. Hold the mask firmly in place while maintaining head tilt. Take a breath and exhale into the mask port or one-way valve at the top of the mask port with just enough volume to make the chest rise. Remove your mouth from the port and allow for passive exhalation.
   - BVM–Position yourself at the patient's head and establish an open airway. Suction and insert an airway adjunct as necessary. Select the correct size mask for the patient. Position the mask on the patient's face. Form a "C" around the ventilation port with your thumb and index finger. Use the middle, ring, and little fingers under the patient's jaw to hold the jaw to the mask. With your other hand, squeeze the bag once every five seconds, causing the patient's chest to rise. Release pressure on the bag and let the patient passively exhale.
   - FROPVD–Follow the same procedures for mask seal as recommended for the BVM. Trigger the device until the chest rises and repeat every five seconds.

4. A lone rescuer will need to perform all the tasks of BVM ventilation. With two rescuers, however, one person will hold the mask seal on the patient's face while the other squeezes the bag. For a patient with suspected trauma, the provider holding the mask must perform a jaw-thrust maneuver. For a patient with no suspected trauma, the head-tilt, chin-lift maneuver may be used to open the airway.

5. Under normal circumstances, the body flexes the diaphragm and expands the chest cavity to create a negative pressure and pull air in through the glottic opening. Artificial ventilation, such as BVM ventilation, relies upon positive pressure to "push air in."

6. Any condition that causes hypoxia will benefit from supplemental oxygen. These conditions include bronchospasm, acute pulmonary edema, and shock. Hypoxic patients most commonly benefit from high-concentration oxygen delivered through a nonrebreather (NRB) mask, but in some cases these patients may not tolerate high-concentration rates. In cases where patients will not tolerate a NRB mask, lower flow delivery devices such as a nasal cannula may be a better choice. Some EMS systems may also allow providers to use alternative devices such as venturi masks or titrate the level of oxygen administration based on patient condition and oxygen levels (always follow local protocol).

Critical Thinking Exercises

1. After assuring the scene is safe, the EMT should open this patient's airway and, if necessary, support it with an airway adjunct. Her altered mental status, slow respiratory rate, and cyanosis all point to respiratory failure. This patient needs immediate respiratory assistance with a bag-valve mask and supplemental oxygen.

2. At a minimum, this patient needs immediate supplemental oxygen. Further assessment will be necessary to identify respiratory failure, but his inability to speak and position certainly point to at least impending failure. If your assessment identifies further indications of respiratory failure, then immediate artificial ventilation is necessary.

3. Although this patient may just be anxious after the motor-vehicle crash, a thorough assessment must be completed to assure the fast rate is not due to an injury. Rapid respiratory rates can indicate inadequate breathing, but further assessment will be necessary to identify respiratory failure.

Pathophysiology to Practice

1. To identify respiratory failure, both oxygenation and ventilation must be assessed. Mental status, skin color, and pulse oximetry all can be used to assess oxygenation. Listening to lung sounds, observing respiratory effort, and looking for accessory muscle use help assess ventilation. If no deficits in oxygenation or ventilation are noted during these assessments, the patient is breathing adequately. Any deficits with either element point to inadequate breathing and respiratory failure.

2. A breathing patient may need artificial ventilation if his breathing is deemed to be inadequate. Signs include altered mental status, cyanosis, slowing or irregular respirations, and respiratory fatigue.

3. When using a bag-valve mask, watch for chest rise to assure adequate volume.

Street Scene Questions

1. After assuring scene safety and gathering a general impression, you should complete a primary assessment. If problems are found, immediate treatment must be initiated.

2. The essential elements of assessing this patient's breathing include observing his effort and mental status; assessing his skin color; listening to his chest for air movement and unusual lung sounds; and obtaining a pulse oximetry reading.

3. Immediate treatment must include supplemental high-concentration oxygen. It may also be important to assist this patient with his inhaler (if protocol allows). Assessment may also indicate respiratory failure. As such, you should be prepared to provide artificial ventilations.

4. The breathing is not adequate. Fatigue, cyanosis, and difficulty speaking all point to respiratory failure.

5. This patient requires artificial ventilations.

Chapter 10 Scene Size-Up
Critical Decision Making

1. The possibility that the truck is carrying hazardous materials and the stability of the truck are initial concerns. Safety from traffic at the scene is a major concern. After determining if it is safe to approach, you should assess the number of patients (make sure no other vehicles are involved or under the truck) and determine if extrication is needed.

2. Do not walk in or along the highway until you are safe from traffic. Look for leaking gas and other safety hazards. Determine the number of patients and if extrication is needed.

3. There are multiple safety concerns here. The mass exodus from the building could be caused by anything from a person who is shooting to an explosion of some sort. In this case you may be too close to the scene. Plan for an extended multiple-casualty incident.

4. Maintain a safe distance from the residence. Do not enter the house for any reason due to the risk of explosion. Determine if the man believes there is anyone in the residence and report it to incoming fire units. Request the gas company if it hasn't already been done.

5. Watch for unstable construction equipment or buildings. Determine the number of patients and if any special rescue teams will be necessary to access the patient.

Short Answer

1. In the case of leaking gasoline or a vehicle fire, consider the danger zone to be 100 feet in all directions from the wreckage. Park outside the danger zone, upwind, and uphill, if possible. Avoid gutters, ditches, and gullies that can carry fuel to the ambulance. Do not use flares. Use orange traffic cones during daylight and reflective triangles at night. In the case of hazardous materials, check with a hazardous materials reference to determine the danger zone. In all cases, park upwind. Park uphill if liquid is flowing, but on the same level if there are gases that may arise. Park behind a natural or an artificial barrier. In the case of downed power lines, consider the danger zone as the area in which people or vehicles might be contacted by energized wires if the wires pivot around their points of attachment.

2. Indicators of violence or potential violence include fighting or loud voices, weapons visible or in use, signs of alcohol or drug use, unusual silence, and knowledge of prior violence.

3. Protective gloves—controlled bleeding, suctioning, artificial ventilation, CPR. Eye protection—splashing, spattering, or spraying body fluids. Masks—infections spread by airborne droplets. N-95 or HEPA respirator—disease spread by airborne particles.

4. Injuries to bones and joints are common following falls and vehicle collisions. Burns are common injuries from fires and explosions. Penetrating soft-tissue injuries can be associated with gunshot wounds.

5. Sources of information about the nature of the patient's illness could come from the patient, family members, or bystanders at the scene.

6. There are countless scenarios where both medical and trauma calls can tax the available resources and prompt you to summon additional assistance. Whether the situation involves lifting a large patient, assessing or transporting multiple patients, or calling resources with additional training (ALS or law enforcement), it's important to be proactive and call early whenever possible.

Critical Thinking Exercises

First, make certain the police have secured the scene before you enter it. If you fail to do so, you could easily find yourself and your partner hostages or shooting victims. Once the scene is secure, you will proceed with normal scene size-up steps: Take Standard Precautions. Confirm the mechanism of injury (reported to be a gunshot in this case). Establish the number of patients (there might be several shooting victims or persons injured by falls or other actions, or even a person suffering a heart attack from the stress of the event). Decide if more resources are needed to handle the call.

Pathophysiology to Practice

1. A patient with stab wounds to the lower anterior and posterior ribs would have wounds to the internal organs as follows:
   - A penetrating injury to the area of the lower left lateral ribs could potentially puncture any of the organs in the left quadrants including the liver, spleen, intestines, and pancreas.
   - A penetrating injury to the area of the lower right lateral ribs could potentially puncture any of the organs in the right quadrants including the liver, intestines, pancreas, and gallbladder.
   - A penetrating injury to the posterior side of the patient on either side is more likely to penetrate either of the kidneys. Depending on the length of the penetrating object, other organs (listed above) may be impacted as well.

2. If the patient were able to protect himself somewhat by lying in a fetal position, he might be able to shield the liver, spleen, intestines, pancreas, and gallbladder. However, the kidneys are more likely to be exposed to penetrating trauma because of their location on the posterior side.

Street Scene Questions

1. Issues might include a quick check for the number of patients, identification of the mechanism of injury, rapid assessment to determine the severity of injuries, need for additional resources, and so on. The placard on the side of the truck also needs to be identified to determine the contents of the truck and the potential need for a special hazmat team.

2. Although the crew has donned protective gear and made efforts to limit traffic hazards, they must wait until the vehicles are stabilized and the placard is identified before safely approaching the patients.

3. Standard Precautions should include, at a minimum, disposable gloves and eye protection—especially because of the high probability of cuts and open wounds from this type of collision.

4. The second ambulance should be parked in a staging area that is upwind from the scene and at a safe distance. Safeguards should also be taken so that the ambulance is away from moving traffic and has an easy means of egress after the patient is loaded.

5. The patients need to be properly covered and protected during the extrication process. Also, a member of the crew should remain with the patients to calm their fears, answer questions, and monitor their status.

6. You can help ensure the patient safely gets from the scene to the ambulance by considering whether the ambulance should be moved closer to the patient to facilitate loading.

Chapter 11 The Primary Assessment

Critical Decision Making

1. A responsive patient with difficulty breathing who is sitting up is <u>high priority</u>.

2. A man who "passed out" at a wedding and is still unresponsive is <u>high priority</u>.

3. A responsive child who got his foot caught in bike spokes and may have broken his foot is <u>lower priority</u>.

4. A responsive patient who describes severe pain in his abdomen is <u>high priority</u>.

5. A patient who only moans and appears to have ingested alcohol is <u>high priority</u>.

Short Answer

1. When forming a general impression, look at the patient's environment, whether the patient is medical or trauma, whether there are any mechanisms of injury, and the patient's age and sex. Overall, you should form the general impression by looking, listening, and smelling. It is gathered through direct observation and through your feelings and intuition.

2. Assess the patient's mental status using AVPU as follows:
   - <u>A</u>lert—The patient is awake if he can answer your questions. The patient is oriented to person if he can tell you his name. The patient is oriented to place if he can tell where he is. The patient is oriented to time if he can tell you the day, date, and time.
   - <u>V</u>erbal—If the patient appears to have a depressed level of consciousness, determine if the patient responds to verbal stimuli like talking or shouting.
   - <u>P</u>ainful—If the patient does not respond to verbal stimuli, determine if he responds to painful stimuli by rubbing your knuckles across his sternum or by pinching his toe.
   - <u>U</u>nresponsive—The patient will not respond to verbal or painful stimuli.

3. Assess airway breathing and circulation as follows:
   - Airway—If the patient is talking or crying, the airway is open. If the airway is not open, the patient is not alert, or the patient is breathing noisily, open the airway by using the jaw-thrust maneuver for trauma patients and the head-tilt, chin-lift maneuver for medical patients. Suction the airway and insert an airway adjunct. If the airway is blocked, perform the Heimlich maneuver, or back blows and chest thrusts, as appropriate.
   - Breathing—If the patient is not alert, use the technique you learned in CPR class to listen, look, and feel for breath. Perform rescue breathing if necessary. If the patient is breathing, count the breathing rate. If a conscious patient is breathing at a rate of less than 8 breaths per minute or more than 24 breaths per minute, administer oxygen using a nonrebreather mask.
   - Circulation—Take the patient's pulse. Start with the radial pulse in adults and the brachial pulse in infants. If you cannot feel these peripheral pulses, check the carotid pulse. If the pulse is absent, administer CPR and apply an automated external defibrillator. Check for bleeding and control any major bleeding. Check the skin for temperature, moisture, and color. Warm, pink, dry skin indicates good circulation. Pale, cool, and moist skin indicates poor circulation.

4. The CAB approach puts the "C" (circulation/compressions) step of primary assessment before the "A" and "B" (airway and breathing) steps. The CAB approach is performed only on apparently lifeless patients with no breathing or agonal breathing and involves an immediate pulse check and initial compressions when the pulse is absent.

5. ABC is the traditional approach to the patient in the primary assessment. It is performed on most patients you encounter in this sequence: airway, breathing, circulation.

6. The statement that the order of interventions depends on the patient's condition and number and priority of conditions means that "ABC" is a mnemonic to remind you of

the three main things you must assess and treat, as necessary, during the primary assessment. However, "ABC" does *not* indicate the *order* in which you must do these steps. For example, a patient with vomit in the airway would be suctioned first. A patient with arterial bleeding would get bleeding control first. You will consider the ABCs on every call, but the order may differ depending on the patient's needs.

7. The statement "Multiple EMTs can accomplish multiple priorities simultaneously" means that when there are two or more EMTs or other trained personnel on-scene, many tasks can be carried out at the same time. This is often the case. For example, one EMT could stabilize the patient's c-spine while another suctions the patient. In another call, one EMT could control bleeding while the other EMT opens the airway.

8. Making a priority decision means determining whether a patient has a life-threatening condition that requires immediate transport to the hospital.

9. A trauma patient needs manual stabilization of the head and spine during the primary assessment. To further protect the spine, a jaw-thrust maneuver should be used to open the airway rather than the head-tilt, chin-lift maneuver. An unresponsive patient needs high-concentration oxygen by nonrebreather mask or bag-valve mask and transport as a high-priority patient. In fact, any level of responsiveness below that of "alert" may indicate the possibility of a life-threatening problem.

Critical Thinking Exercises

Questions 1 to 3 ask you to state whether the patient's priority is stable, potentially unstable, or unstable. Question 4 asks you to decide, for each patient, which portion of the primary assessment should be performed first (CAB approach or ABC approach).

1. One might be inclined to minimize this patient's condition because of where he was found–outside a bar–and simply assume he's intoxicated. But that is very risky. At this point, you only know that he has been unconscious and better control of his airway has improved his condition. His condition remains unstable.

2. Although the patient's ABCs are fine and she is alert, her skin signs are a big concern. In addition, your intuition is telling you something is wrong. Caregiver intuition can be one of your best diagnostic tools in patient assessment. This patient is potentially unstable.

3. Assuming the patient's ABCs are fine and her level of hydration is normal, this patient is stable.

4. The steps should be performed first for each of the following patients are as follows:
   - For a patient who is unresponsive with arterial bleeding from his neck: Begin with bleeding control. This bleeding will be fatal in a very short time. You will learn later in the text how to apply an occlusive dressing.
   - For a patient with a broken ankle and no other apparent injury: This patient doesn't appear to have major ABC problems. Do a quick but thorough check of the ABCs to be sure nothing is overlooked.
   - For a patient who is not moving and does not appear to be breathing: This patient would first receive a pulse check and, in the absence of a pulse, begin compressions.
   - For a patient who tells you she has severe difficulty breathing: For this patient, take an ABC approach to check the airway and then position her appropriately. Administration of oxygen or ventilation (as required) would occur next.
   - For a patient who has ingested too much alcohol and is vomiting: Treat the airway first. Suctioning and positioning will be necessary if the patient has an altered mental status and can't control his airway.
   - For a patient who is doubled over and screaming because of abdominal pain: The screaming indicates that the patient is moving air in and out. As part of a thorough airway check, you will need to make sure there has been no vomiting that would require suctioning. This patient likely has a pulse, but you should check the rate and the patient's skin color, temperature, and condition to assess for possible shock from internal bleeding.

Pathophysiology to Practice

1. Unless the level of consciousness improved, administering oxygen would not in itself lead you to change an unresponsive patient's priority. All unresponsive patients should be considered unstable, high-priority patients.

2. Because the patient's family is most familiar with his normal mental status, it is important to gather the history from them. This patient is considered a stable, lower priority patient until you can determine what abnormal behavior prompted their call for help today.

3. Be sure to take Standard Precautions. First, always scan the scene to determine whether it is safe to approach. Because you are alone in the middle of the street, you do not have the benefit of a partner or someone else helping to watch traffic or other hazards for you. Without first taking these precautions, you could become part of the scene yourself. Next, form a general impression to determine how serious the patient's condition is and then call for additional resources to help. If available, enlist a bystander to hold manual stabilization of the patient's head and neck until you can complete full spinal immobilization. Assess the patient's mental status and his ABCs. If during the primary assessment you discover any life-threatening conditions, perform the appropriate interventions immediately. In this case, the patient has gurgling respirations and his airway should be cleared in whatever way is possible. There may not be much more you can do until more help arrives, but remember the saying: "The most important things you can do for your patients are in the ABCs."

Street Scene Questions

1. While rapidly determining responsiveness, you should perform axial in-line stabilization of the spine followed by an assessment of the ABCs.

2. In order to maintain spinal stabilization, the jaw-thrust maneuver is the most appropriate method for securing the airway. It accomplishes two objectives—opening the airway by bringing the tongue and jaw forward while at the same time maintaining in-line stabilization of the spine (in case the spine has been injured).

3. The level of responsiveness is VERBAL because the patient is responding to a verbal stimulus.

4. Primary assessment should always follow the same general steps: form a general impression, assess mental status, assess airway, assess breathing, assess circulation, and determine priority. The cause of Joey's seizures might confirm whether or not he has a medical condition, but you must still identify any immediate life-threatening conditions, correct them, and then decide on the patient's priority for immediate transport or further on-scene interventions. Remember that if the steps in primary assessment are not followed consistently and systematically, it is very possible to overlook and neglect to manage a life-threatening situation.

5. The patient should be positioned on his side (sometimes referred to as the recovery position) if there is no possibility of spinal injury. This will allow for drainage. If cervical-spine trauma is suspected, then the patient should be frequently suctioned. You should only rotate the patient if these conditions are met: full immobilization to a backboard, placement of a cervical collar, and application of the necessary head immobilization devices.

6. The status of the patient was downgraded because of his improved mental status.

7. The value of following a systematic assessment—doing it the same way every time—is that you are less likely to skip a step and overlook something. Failing to check that critical item on a patient could cause you to miss correcting a life-threatening situation.

8. Because the patient is high priority (compromised breathing and diminished circulation), students should understand that you need to spend as little time on the scene as possible. If you have not already done so, you should radio for ALS intervention. The patient's history can be gathered en route.

Chapter 12 Vital Signs and Monitoring Devices

Critical Decision Making

1. First, observe the ease with which the patient speaks. If he speaks long (six-plus-word) sentences without having to catch his breath, the patient is experiencing minimal distress. You can wait a short time for him to stop talking or tell him you'll need him to be quiet so you can listen to his lungs (or heart) while you are really counting respirations through the stethoscope. If patients are aware you are counting their breaths, the results may not be accurate.

2. Obtain the blood pressure once you move the patient to a transportation device and into a more open area. Remember you will have other indicators including mental status, pulse, respirations, and skin color, which are a significant part of the patient picture.

3. In a patient with a serious mechanism of injury, you should next go to the carotid artery to check the pulse. Look for other signs of life including movement, moaning, or respiratory effort. If a patient was responsive and you cannot feel a pulse, you should check the pulse at her other wrist.

Short Answer

1. Vital signs traditionally measured in EMS are respiration; pulse; skin color, temperature, and condition (plus capillary refill in infants and children); pupils; and blood pressure.

2. Vital signs should be taken more than once because the patient's condition may change while in your care. You should repeat vital signs on stable patients every 15 minutes. You should repeat vital signs on unstable patients every 5 minutes. Repeat vital signs after every medical intervention.

Critical Thinking Exercises

1. If you are attempting to assess for a radial pulse and cannot find one, do not spend more than a couple of seconds before checking the other arm or another artery such as the brachial or carotid artery.

2. If you ever question a blood pressure reading, whether the reading came from a blood pressure monitor or was measured by auscultation from another caregiver, always repeat the procedure.

3. Nail polish can cause an inaccurate reading on a pulse oximeter (blue nail polish actually gives the most inaccurate readings). One option is to carry acetone wipes to quickly remove the nail polish from the patient's fingernail before attaching the device. Remove any artificial nail. If the nail is too thick or it is not possible to remove the polish or an artificial nail, you may try attaching a probe to the patient's toe or earlobe.

Pathophysiology to Practice

1. Whenever the heart beats faster than the natural maximum heart rate, the chambers of the heart will fail to completely fill with blood before contracting, leading to poor blood flow from the ventricles and weaker pulses felt in the periphery.

2. The sympathetic nervous system and the hormone epinephrine work to combat blood loss by constricting blood vessels. This causes more blood from the periphery, like the skin, to be shunted toward the core of the body, like the heart and lungs, where it is needed the most. Skin appears pale and sweaty because of the vasoconstrictive properties of epinephrine.

3. The diastolic pressure is the pressure that remains in the arteries when the left ventricle relaxes and refills. Chronically high pressures during this relaxation phase, also known as diastolic hypertension, obviously increase the stress and wear on cardiac structures and put the patient at much greater risk for heart disease, stroke, and kidney disease.

Street Scene Questions

1. After determining scene safety, your primary concern is assessment of the ABCs. In the case of Ms. Alvarez, the airway is patent, but her breathing is a little rapid. This finding warrants further assessment and at least the initial administration of some high-concentration oxygen.

2. Vital signs include number of respirations per minute (including quality), pulse rate per minute (including quality), blood pressure, skin color, and temperature, as well as an evaluation of the pupils.

3. Because Ms. Alvarez is complaining of abdominal pain, questions during the patient interview should be aimed at determining the quality and severity of the pain, the length of time the patient has experienced the pain, what the pain "feels like," and what, if anything brought on the pain.

4. In addition to evaluating the patient's pain, ask if Ms. Alvarez has had previous episodes of the condition and whether she has seen a doctor. If so, find out what the doctor has said about the condition. Inquire about any medications that she might be taking for the abdominal pain or for any other medical conditions.

5. Yes, another set of vital signs should be taken. A patient with rapid respirations and signs and symptoms suggesting possible abdominal bleeding should have vital signs taken approximately every five minutes.

6. In a calm manner, give the patient an honest appraisal of the vital signs and assessment. Point out possible consequences of refusing transport. If the patient still expresses an unwillingness to go to the hospital, you should contact medical direction and perhaps request the patient's permission to contact her personal physician. Also, if you have been unable to convince the patient to go to the hospital, another member of the crew might try to convince her to change her mind.

Chapter 13 Assessment of the Trauma Patient

Critical Decision Making

1. A patient that was found ejected from a vehicle in a rollover collision should receive a rapid trauma exam—even if he appears to have minor injuries—due to the mechanism of injury.

2. A patient who tripped and possibly broke his wrist will receive a focused exam as long as the mechanism of injury doesn't indicate that additional injury is likely. For example, if the patient hit his head during the fall, he will require spinal immobilization.

3. A patient with minor neck pain from a motor vehicle accident with a major mechanism of injury will receive a rapid trauma exam due to the significant mechanism of injury.

4. A patient who fell 6 feet, lost consciousness, and broke an ankle should receive a rapid trauma exam. This may seem like a borderline situation because a fall of 6 feet may not match standards for significant mechanism of injury in an adult, but the loss of consciousness should alert you to potentially serious problems and cause you to be vigilant and complete a rapid trauma exam. You can always slow down if the patient is found to be stable.

Short Answer

1. For the patient without a significant mechanism of injury, it is not necessary to perform a rapid trauma assessment. Instead, you can focus your assessment just on the areas that the patient tells you are painful or that you suspect may be injured. Baseline vital signs and a past medical history must be obtained on all patients.

2. The steps of the rapid trauma assessment are: head, neck, chest, abdomen, pelvis, extremities, and posterior. A patient with a significant mechanism of injury needs a rapid trauma assessment.

3. Remember that the detailed physical exam is a lower priority task and will likely occur en route to the hospital well after you have completed the primary assessment and rapid trauma assessment. The goal is to gather additional information about the patient's injuries and conditions. Repeat the primary assessment before completing the detailed physical exam. The exam will be very similar to the rapid trauma exam you completed on-scene except for a few differences. For example, you'll have to work around much of the equipment (collar and backboard) that has been applied, and reassessing the chest inside a moving ambulance may be more difficult. Otherwise, examine the patient in detail as much as time permits. Managing a high-priority, unstable trauma patient often reduces or eliminates the time you have to complete a detailed physical exam.

Critical Thinking Exercises

1. A patient who fell three stories and is currently bleeding into his airway requires an immediate intervention to correct a life-threatening condition. Bleeding into the airway must be corrected before any further assessment can be completed. Continue suctioning until your partner returns to provide more help.

2. Manage these situations as follows:
   - Cut finger: Although the cut is bleeding profusely, a cut to a finger is not a significant mechanism of injury. Unless you are unable to control the bleeding with direct pressure and other normal methods, you can complete on-scene assessment and care before transporting the patient.
   - Schoolyard shooting: This is a significant mechanism of injury with significant blood loss that has already taken place and caused unknown internal injuries to the patient. Because she is able to speak, assume that her airway and breathing are adequate, at least for the moment. Immediately apply direct pressure to control the bleeding, administer oxygen by nonrebreather mask, provide manual stabilization of the head and neck, apply a cervical collar, immobilize the patient to a backboard, and transport her expeditiously, providing ongoing monitoring and any needed additional care en route.
   - Unconscious on sidewalk: There is no way to know the cause of this patient's condition. Quickly ensure adequate airway and breathing, provide oxygenation or ventilation as needed, provide manual stabilization of the head and neck, apply a cervical collar, immobilize the patient to a backboard, and transport without spending additional time at the scene, monitoring the patient's condition en route.

Pathophysiology to Practice

Lungs produce audible sounds that you can auscultate through a stethoscope whenever air rushes in and out of the lung structures: the lung tubing (bronchi and bronchioles) and the air sacs (alveoli). If a lung collapses, such as in a pneumothorax, air cannot move through these structures and fails to resonate audible sounds.

Street Scene Questions

1. The patient is suffering from multiple trauma. The ABCs are the first priority while protecting the cervical spine. The first treatment priority is securing the airway and assuring adequate respirations (breathing). Due to facial injuries, you must make sure that mucus, blood, and/or teeth are not causing airway obstructions. After applying a cervical collar and placing the patient on a backboard, you should suction as needed and, if necessary, turn the patient on his side to allow for drainage. Next, you should apply occlusive dressing over the stab wound. You should also provide the patient with high-concentration oxygen and, if necessary, assist ventilation. Watch for the potential development of a tension pneumothorax throughout the call.

2. The patient needs rapid transport to a trauma center. After managing the airway and breathing, and controlling any external bleeding, you should package the patient for immediate transport.

3. You should take a baseline set of vital signs as soon as possible. Because the patient has a serious mechanism of injury, vitals should be retaken every 5 minutes.

4. The patient seems to have developed difficulty breathing until you lift part of the occlusive dressing and allow some air to escape. This suggests tension pneumothorax. In this situation, you should raise a corner of the occlusive dressing, which provides some relief. If this is successful, you should then continue to monitor the patient. Be prepared to assist ventilations and, if time allows, consider requesting ALS intercept.

5. The ABCs remain the first priority. However, as time and patient conditions permit, the secondary assessment should include a head-to-toe survey.

Chapter 14 Assessment of the Medical Patient
Critical Decision Making

1. Listening is important, but you will eventually need to focus the history or transport will be delayed. Redirecting the patient politely with phrases such as, "I see, but I need to focus on why you called today. Can you tell me about . . ." may help.

2. You can ask the question while the parents aren't in the room or when bringing the patient out to the ambulance. It may be possible to have a parent leave the room to get something (medications or the patient's coat) so you can ask the question privately.

3. In this case, the patient's behavior may be due to his medical condition. His family may be the best source of information. If he can answer he may do so very slowly, so giving a little time (but not so much as to cause delay in treatment) may help.

4. While ensuring your safety, get down to the patient's level and attempt to establish rapport. Talk slowly and quietly. Ask questions that are easy to answer (e.g., ask the patient's name) to see if the patient is oriented enough to respond.

Short Answer

1. In medical patients, unlike trauma patients, there are not many external sources of information about what is wrong with the patient. For medical emergencies, the most important source of information about the problem is usually what the patient can tell you. So, when the patient is awake and responsive, obtaining the patient's history comes first.

2. For the responsive medical patient, the first step of your secondary assessment is talking with the patient to obtain the history of his present illness and the past medical history, followed by performing the physical exam and gathering the vital signs. In the unresponsive medical patient, the process is turned around. Because you cannot obtain a history from the patient, you will begin with a rapid physical assessment and collection of baseline vital signs. After these procedures, you will gather as much of the patient's history as you can from any bystanders or family members who may be present.

Critical Thinking Exercises

1. To obtain a history of present illness from a patient with chest pain, use OPQRST:
   - Onset—What were you doing when the pain started?
   - Provokes—Can you think of anything that might have triggered this pain?
   - Quality—Can you describe the pain for me?
   - Radiation—Where exactly is the pain? Does it seem to spread anywhere or does it stay right here?
   - Severity—How bad is the pain?
   - Time—When did the pain start? Has it changed at all since it started?

2. Put your hand on his shoulder and say: "I know you are concerned about your father. You can help him by trying to calm down and answer a few questions for me about his medical history. Take a few deep breaths. Good. You look calmer. Are you ready to answer my questions?"

3. Continue to talk to him for a few minutes about unrelated matters, and then say, "Sir, I'm really enjoying our conversation. However, I need to get back into service as soon as possible so that I can take care of other patients. So, I need you to answer a few questions for me related to the problem you're having today. Okay?"

Pathophysiology to Practice

Nicotine present in tobacco products causes increased blood pressure and heart rate, decreased oxygen to the heart, increased blood clotting, and damage to cells that line coronary arteries and other blood vessels. A person's risk of heart attack greatly increases with the number of cigarettes he smokes. People who smoke a pack of cigarettes a day have more than twice the risk of heart attack as non-smokers. About 30 percent of all deaths from heart disease in the United States are directly related to cigarette smoking.

Street Scene Questions

1. The patient presents with difficulty breathing, rapid respirations, and a rapid pulse. Until you can assess her condition further, you should consider her a high-priority patient at this time.

2. You should take a baseline set of vitals, as indicated in the opening part of the scenario. After eliminating any immediate life threats, you should begin to gather a history of the present illness, focusing on questions that pertain to the condition cited by the patient. Administer oxygen, assess for its effect on the patient, and check the patient's pulse oximetry reading (if available).

3. Ask the OPQRST questions and then ask specific questions about her previous medical history. Of particular importance is the use of an inhaler or other medications commonly prescribed to asthma patients.

4. Signs and symptoms of a worsening condition might include: an increase in the level of consciousness, more labored breathing, use of accessory muscles, tripod positioning, increased difficulty talking (e.g., one-word answers), a respiratory rate that is either too fast or too slow, and increased patient anxiety. Signs and symptoms of an improving condition might include: a "normal" respiration rate (e.g., little or no distress), the ability to talk in complete sentences, an alert mental state, absence of cyanosis, and a normal or improved oxygen saturation reading on the pulse oximeter.

Chapter 15 Reassessment

Critical Decision Making

1. A multiple trauma patient who fell 15 feet with a dropping blood pressure is likely deteriorating.

2. A 64-year-old female patient who fell and is complaining of hip pain is having vital signs that are returning to normal.

3. A 19-year-old female with lower extremity injuries that shows a dropping blood pressure and rising pulse is likely deteriorating.

Short Answer

1. The four steps of reassessment are:
   - Repeat the primary assessment—reassess the patient's mental status. Maintain an open airway. Monitor the breathing for rate and quality. Reassess the pulse for rate and quality. Monitor skin color and temperature. Reestablish patient priorities.
   - Repeat and record the vital signs.
   - Repeat the history and physical exam, specifically chief complaints and injuries.
   - Check interventions—assure adequacy of oxygen delivery and artificial ventilation. Assure management of bleeding.

2. By documenting the findings, the EMT can note any changes in the patient's condition, adjust treatment, or begin new treatment. Trending is evaluating and recording changes in a patient's condition, such as slowing respirations or rising pulse rate, that may show improvement or deterioration, and that can be shown by documenting repeated assessments.

Critical Thinking Exercises

If your reassessment turns up these findings, intervene as follows:

1. Gurgling respirations: immediately suction the patient.

2. Bag on nonrebreather mask collapses completely when patient inhales: increase the amount of oxygen being delivered to the patient.

3. Snoring respirations: open or reposition the airway.

Pathophysiology to Practice

Asthma is an obstructive disease resulting from the small bronchioles in the lungs contracting and becoming narrowed while the air sacs (alveoli) in the lungs often overproduce mucus. Air flow becomes severely restricted. Air becomes trapped in the lungs and normal gas exchange, especially the exchange of oxygen with the bloodstream, becomes diminished. Even though your patient's breathing rate may not be affected yet by her asthma attack, the amount of oxygen she's carrying in her blood has been reduced. Measuring the blood oxygen level (SpO_2) with a pulse oximeter tells you how much oxygen is attached to hemoglobin on her red blood cells. Those red blood cells may not have enough oxygen to keep oxygenating her brain, heart, and other tissues. If the SpO_2 number is low, you can help her system facilitate better gas exchange by providing supplemental oxygen.

Street Scene Questions

1. Patients who are less than alert (that are only responding to verbal or painful stimuli) may have difficulty maintaining their airways. These patients may be positioned in such a manner as to occlude their airways through a partial blockage by the tongue—a condition that can be resolved by repositioning. Also, with less-than-alert patients, you need to be prepared for suctioning. You may also need to move these patients into a position that will facilitate drainage. Any patient that is unresponsive or poorly responsive must be monitored constantly. Be prepared to reposition the patient as needed and intervene with airway adjuncts like OPAs (oropharyngeal airways) or NPAs (nasopharyngeal airways) as necessary to control the airway. Have suctioning equipment immediately available.

2. At this point, you should complete a history of the present illness. Questions might include the following: Has the patient had a similar condition in the past? Is the patient taking any blood pressure medication? If so, what is the medication? Is the patient compliant in taking it? In specifically questioning the husband, you might ask: "When was the last time you saw your wife?" "Was she manifesting any of the current signs or symptoms at that point, such as trouble walking, slurred speech, or obvious facial drooping?" In specifically questioning the patient, you might ask: "Are you having any trouble breathing?" "Are you in any pain?"

3. Reassessment includes continually monitoring the patient's airway, breathing, and any changes in her level of consciousness. Periodically reassess the patient's speech and observe for facial drooping. Reassess the patient's pupils and vital signs every five minutes. Periodically reevaluate changes in movement, strength, and sensation in all extremities.

Chapter 16 Critical Thinking and Decision Making

Short Answer

1. Critical thinking is an analytical process that can help someone think through a problem in an organized and efficient manner. It is thinking that is reflective, reasonable, and focused on deciding what to do in a particular situation. It involves the use of facts, principles, theories, and other pieces of information.

2. Different clinicians have different levels of training and experience, time, technology, and other resources. All clinicians begin with the same basic approach: gather information, consider possibilities, and reach a conclusion. How they implement these steps, however, varies significantly. The emergency physician and the EMT are similar in some ways in that they both work under certain time constraints, must quickly rule out or treat immediate threats to life, and they focus much of their questioning and assessment on ruling out the worst case scenario. When settling on a differential diagnosis, they primarily differ in the number of tools and tests available to them. An emergency physician has many more tools available, allowing him or her to focus on a significantly larger number of possible diagnoses compared to the EMT, not to mention the thousands of additional hours of training and clinical exposure physicians have compared to folks working in the prehospital environment.

3. "Search satisfying" means that once you find what you are looking for, you stop looking for other causes or possibilities. If you suspect something is causing the problem and have the slightest inkling it may be true, you may fail to look for a secondary diagnosis. "Confirmation bias" is somewhat similar and means that a clinician looks for evidence to support a particular diagnosis. In doing so, he may overlook evidence that refutes or reduces the probability of that diagnosis.

4. Considering too many possibilities often interferes with developing a coherent and timely treatment plan because it becomes too difficult to organize information, rule out pertinent negatives, and form a conclusion based on the assessment findings. Caregivers that overthink often second guess themselves and worry more about what they've missed than what they've found. In fact, your best approach may be to accept the ambiguity of medicine and not let your endless search for a cause delay treatment of the patient.

Critical Thinking Exercises

1. A 52-year-old man complaining of chest pain while at work who is alert and oriented first needs a calm approach, especially since he tells you he thinks it may "just be stress." Form a general impression and then conduct a quick primary assessment. Use the OPQRST memory aid to gather a history. From a critical thinking perspective, you might ask yourself:
- Does this patient have an obvious problem or do I need to think more critically?
- What other information should I get to confirm or refute the working diagnosis?
- How specific does my field diagnosis have to be to decide the best treatment?

2. A 67-year-old man who is now unresponsive after acting unusually in front of his wife, developing slurred speech, and complaining of an odd feeling in his arm needs an immediate intervention to manage his airway. An unresponsive patient is not likely able to manage his own airway and breathe effectively. While assuring his airway and assessing the rest of his ABCs, you should gather history information from his wife and ask yourself these questions from a critical thinking perspective:
- Have I addressed all potential life threats first before going on with the assessment and diagnostic process?
- Does this patient have an obvious problem or do I need to think more critically?
- Are there other causes besides the obvious one for this patient's condition?
- How specific does my field diagnosis have to be to decide the best treatment?
- What is the best thing I can do for the patient *right now*?

3. An 18-year-old snowboarder who took a fall and thinks he may have broken his ankle mostly needs to be directed to remain still while you conduct a full trauma assessment. Determine the mechanism of injury and the likelihood of any other injuries or the need for spinal immobilization. From a critical thinking perspective, ask yourself:
- Does this patient have an obvious problem or do I need to think more critically?
- What other information should I get to confirm or refute the working diagnosis?

4. A 41-year-old woman with difficulty breathing and pain when she breathes in deeply needs reassurance and a methodical assessment and history gathering. Because she is anxious, she needs a calm approach. The early administration of oxygen may help reduce her anxiety. From a critical thinking perspective, ask yourself:
- Have I addressed life threats first before beginning the assessment and diagnostic process?
- Does this patient have an obvious problem or do I need to think more critically?
- What other information should I get to confirm or refute the working diagnosis?
- How specific does my field diagnosis have to be to decide the best treatment?
- What is the best thing I can do for the patient right now?

Street Scene Questions

1. Once the primary assessment is complete, proceed with a secondary assessment to assess the patient's mental status, check for any pain or discomfort (using the OPQRST memory aid), and consider using the Cincinnati Prehospital Stroke Scale to rule out signs of stroke.

2. Mr. Ronson could be having a diabetic emergency, a neurologic emergency such as a CVA or TIA, or a cardiac emergency such as a heart attack or hypertensive crisis.

3. Knowing the medications patients are taking can often tell you a lot about their history and the illnesses they're being treated for. You might also be able to determine when the patient last took his medication for his diabetic condition.

4. You should complete a full primary and secondary assessment along with an assessment of his mental status and any pain or discomfort. Use the Cincinnati Prehospital Stroke Scale to assess for signs of stroke.

5. This patient should be considered potentially unstable until you can gather more information. Transport should be expedited until you can rule out that he is not having a stroke, heart attack, or serious diabetic emergency.

6. You should call for an ALS intercept anytime the patient needs an ALS intervention such as intravenous dextrose.

Chapter 17 Communication and Documentation

Critical Decision Making—Communication Challenges

1. The Emergency Medical Responders may be busy with a critical patient, they may have forgotten, they could be in danger, or their radio may not work. Call on the radio and ask for an update.

2. Advise the hospital that the patient has apparently ingested a large quantity of alcohol. (Never assume this is the only problem.) Advise of his current level of responsiveness (painful stimuli) and note that it has varied. Recontact the hospital if the patient's condition worsens so they can prepare.

3. Depending on time and resources, you could step away from the chaotic scene to eliminate background noise and try again. Be sure you are talking slowly and clearly. If it appears to be a radio problem, ask the dispatcher if they heard the transmission. If so, they could advise the hospital by radio or phone for you.

4. By stating "The patient is nonverbal but his eyes are open and he localizes pain by looking where painful stimulus is applied," you have painted a picture of the patient's mental status.

Critical Decision Making—Choosing How and What to Document

1. Only information that is medically relevant should be documented. For example, if the patient is addicted to drugs, it may be pertinent to note whether the patient admitted to or denied alcohol or drug use prior to this incident. Alcohol or drug use may also make a patient incapable of providing consent or making an informed patient refusal. Use objective (factual) statements rather than subjective (opinion) statements in your documentation. Use terms like *patient stated* before noting subjective information so anyone reading the report will know the source.

2. You are always allowed to review the call report or PCR before you testify in court or appear in a deposition. This is a legal document that records your observations and actions at the call. It will refresh your memory and not cause bias or interference with the legal proceedings.

3. Cases such as child, elder, and sexual abuse exempt providers from any HIPAA privacy requirements associated with a report to appropriate authorities and relevant health care providers. As a matter of fact, many states specifically provide immunity from lawsuits for those who report these suspected incidents in good faith.

Short Answer

1. The steps of a medical radio report are:
   - Unit identification and level of provider ("Memorial Hospital, this is Community BLS Ambulance 6 en route to your location . . .")
   - Estimated time of arrival (". . . with a 15-minute ETA.")
   - Patient's age and sex ("We are transporting a 68-year-old male patient . . .")
   - Chief complaint (". . . who complains of pain in his abdomen.")
   - Brief, pertinent history of the present illness ("Onset of pain was two hours ago and is accompanied by slight nausea.")
   - Major past illnesses ("The patient has a history of high blood pressure and arthritis.")
   - Mental status ("He is alert and oriented, never lost consciousness.")
   - Baseline vital signs ("His vital signs are pulse 88, regular and full; respirations 20 and unlabored; skin normal; and blood pressure 134 over 88.")
   - Pertinent findings of the physical exam ("Our exam revealed tenderness in both upper abdominal quadrants. They did not appear rigid.")
   - Emergency medical care given ("For care, we have placed him in a position of comfort.")
   - Response to emergency medical care ("The level of pain has not changed during our care. Mental status has remained unchanged. Vital signs are basically unchanged.")
   - If your system requires, or if you have questions, contact medical direction. ("Does medical direction have any orders?")

2. Effective interpersonal communication with patients should include these qualities:
   - Use eye contact.
   - Be aware of your position and body language.
   - Use language the patient can understand.
   - Be honest.
   - Use the patient's proper name.
   - Listen.

3. Subjective information is that which is from an individual point of view—the patient, bystanders, even the EMT (e.g., patient says, "I feel like I've got the flu."). Objective information is that which is observable, measurable, and verifiable (e.g., vital signs). A pertinent negative is something that is not present but that is important to note (e.g., "The patient states that her chest pain does not radiate.").

4. Written reports that are unclear to others may cause harmful errors in patient care. They also make it hard for the quality improvement team to conduct reviews and research.

5. Important steps to take and important items to document when a patient is refusing care or transportation to the hospital include:
   - Try again to persuade the patient to go to a hospital.
   - Ensure the patient is able to make a rational, informed decision (e.g., not under the influence of alcohol or other drugs, or illness/injury effects).
   - Inform the patient why he should go and what may happen to him if he does not.
   - Consult medical direction as directed by local protocol.
   - If the patient still refuses, document any assessment findings and emergency medical care given, and then have the patient sign a refusal form.
   - Have a family member, police officer, or bystander sign the form as a witness. If the patient refuses to sign the refusal form, have a family member, police officer, or bystander sign the form verifying that the patient refused to sign.

Critical Thinking Exercises

1. The correct sequence for a medical radio report is indicated by the numbers in parentheses that precede the information items:
   - (5) Chest pain radiating to the shoulder
   - (3) 56 years old
   - (13) Oxygen applied at 15 liters per minute via nonrebreather
   - (9) Alert and oriented
   - (4) Female
   - (7) Came on 20 minutes ago while mowing the lawn
   - (8) History of high blood pressure and diabetes
   - (2) ETA 20 minutes
   - (10) Pulse 86, respirations 22, skin cool and moist, blood pressure 110/66, SpO_2 96 percent
   - (14) Oxygen relieved the pain slightly
   - (6) Denies difficulty breathing
   - (15) You are requesting orders from medical direction
   - (1) You are on Community BLS Ambulance 4
   - (11) Lung sounds equal on both sides
   - (12) Placed in a position of comfort

2. A sample narrative might say: 56 y.o. female c/o chest pain radiating to the shoulder. Onset 20 minutes prior to our arrival while mowing lawn. Physical exam: alert and oriented, BP 110/66, pulse 86, resp. 22, SpO_2 96 percent, skin cool and moist, lungs equal bilaterally, denies dyspnea. History: HTN and diabetes. Treatment: O_2 15 lpm NRB, placed in POC. Response: some pain relief with O_2.

Street Scene Questions

1. The following information should be included in a prehospital care report: run data (agency name, unit number, date, times, run call number, names and certification levels of crew members); patient data (nature of call, mechanism of injury, location of patient, treatment, signs and symptoms, baseline vitals, level of consciousness, history of present

illness, care administered and the effects of each care step, changes in the patient's condition throughout the call, insurance and billing information); and narrative (objective and pertinent subjective information, pertinent negatives).

2. An accurate and thorough prehospital care report is important because the document is not only included in the patient's permanent medical record, but it is often used as a legal document in civil and criminal cases. In addition, the data from the PCR is used for administrative purposes, education, and quality improvement.

3. Having your partner review your prehospital care report before submitting it is a great way to ensure it gets completed effectively. It is always possible to overlook information or to see situations from a personal perspective. After all, both of you were present on the call and it's important to have consensus about what occurred.

4. All copies of the prehospital care report must be the same and must accurately reflect the care rendered. If the version of events in the medical record were to differ from a version located at the provider or EMS agency, legal questions could arise about the care provided to the patient.

Chapter 18 General Pharmacology

Critical Decision Making—We Are Really Close to the Hospital. Should I Give Aspirin?

Absolutely. The one medication that has been found to reduce mortality in the event of a myocardial infarction (heart attack) is aspirin. The sooner it is administered, the sooner it begins to take effect. As long as protocols allow and there are no medical reasons to avoid administration, you should definitely give the aspirin. Remember that although transport is an important part of your job, EMS was conceived with the idea of bringing therapy to the patient. Aspirin therapy is just such an example.

Critical Decision Making—ALS Is on the Way. Should I Assist the Patient with Her Inhaler?

You should absolutely contact medical direction for permission to assist with the medication. Although ALS is close, early administration of bronchodilator medications like albuterol is important to the overall success of treatment. The arriving paramedics may carry bronchodilators, but even in the five to eight minutes you wait, your patient may progress to a stage of respiratory distress that will be less responsive to the medications the paramedics carry. Your immediate actions may dictate how effective early treatments are. Always follow local protocols, but remember that you have been granted those protocols for important reasons.

Critical Decision Making—How or Whether to Assist with Medications

1. If you are on-scene with a patient experiencing cardiac-type chest pain and he suggests that he take some of his wife's prescription of nitroglycerin, tell him that it is contraindicated. The patient has not been screened for other drug interactions and may be taking a medication that might negatively interact with the nitroglycerin. Consider contacting medical control.

2. A diabetic patient that only responds to loud stimuli and is very sleepy is unlikely able to control her own airway. Administering oral glucose, which is the consistency of thick pancake syrup, will only further compromise the patient's ability to breathe effectively. Oral glucose is limited only to patients who can self-administer it and swallow well.

3. A COPD patient breathing 48 times per minute with shallow tidal volume is in moderate to severe distress. Administering his prescribed inhaler may improve your delivery of oxygen to the patient and could provide temporary relief to the patient until he can be further evaluated in the emergency department.

Short Answer

1. Aspirin, oxygen, and oral glucose are medications that are commonly carried on ambulances and may, in certain circumstances, be administered by an EMT.

2. Bronchodilator inhalers, nitroglycerin, and epinephrine auto-injectors are medications for which EMTs can commonly assist with patient administration.

3. Other forms of medications are powder, liquids, gels, sublingual sprays, and inhaled gases.

4. On-line medical direction implies speaking directly to a physician, as in calling a doctor on the radio from an emergency scene. Off-line medical direction indicates physician involvement "behind the scenes," such as in the development of guidelines and protocols.

5. Medications may be administered orally, administered sublingually, inhaled, injected, or even absorbed through the skin.

Critical Thinking Exercises

Although nitroglycerin may be helpful for chest pain, administering medication that was not specifically prescribed to the patient is never a good idea. You should thank the family member for being willing to help, but you should not administer the non-prescribed medication.

Pathophysiology to Practice

Reassessment should include the primary assessment and vital signs. Certain medications will cause predictable side effects (for example, epinephrine causes an increased heart rate), but in general you should look for any signs of improvement or deterioration in the patient's condition.

Street Scene Questions

1. Additional patient history questions might include:
- How long has the pain been going on?
- Have you ever had this pain before?
- Do you have any medical history?
- Do you take any medications?
- When was your last meal?

2. Nitroglycerin might be helpful if the patient has it prescribed to him. Depending on your local protocol, you may need to contact medical control before making the decision. Always consider the five rights of medication administration before administering it.

3. Assessing the patient's vital signs before administering a medication is essential. Nitroglycerin, especially, can cause a drop in the patient's blood pressure, so it is very important to assure the patient's pressure is not already low before giving the medication.

4. You want to know that the medication is prescribed to the patient, that it is not expired, and that the correct dose can be safely administered.

5. When administering nitroglycerin in tablet form, one tablet should be placed under the patient's tongue until it dissolves. The tablet should not be chewed or swallowed. When administering the spray, do not shake the canister before use; hold it upright, ask the patient to open his mouth, and press the button once with your index finger. Ask the patient to close his mouth and avoid swallowing.

6. Vital signs should be reassessed shortly after administration and every five minutes thereafter.

Chapter 19 Respiratory Emergencies
Critical Decision Making

1. A 14-year-old patient with difficulty breathing and a history of asthma will benefit from the use of an inhaler. Always follow local protocols and medical direction for use of medications.

2. Do not use the inhaler because it isn't prescribed to the patient. Additionally, wheezes may be present in conditions other than asthma. Nothing says the wheezes in the patient are from the same disease as the wheezes experienced by the daughter.

3. Although the inhaler is indicated for the patient's asthma, it won't do much good here because the patient isn't breathing adequately. The reason you don't hear wheezes is that she isn't breathing enough to move air through the constricted airways. The medication in the inhaler won't get deep into the lungs where it is needed. Ventilate the patient with a BVM connected to oxygen, transport promptly, and request an ALS intercept if available in your area.

Short Answer

1. All patients (adults, children, and infants) that become hypoxic will see an increase in their respiratory rate. Sensors in the brainstem and heart constantly detect how much oxygen is being carried in the blood. If it is too low, signals from the brain are sent to breathing muscles to increase the respiratory rate.

2. The effect of hypoxia on the patient's pulse rate may vary depending on the patient's age. In an adult, hypoxia will increase the heart rate, cardiac output, and blood pressure. This is due to the direct stimulation of the sensors in the heart (aortic bodies) that detect low oxygen levels in the bloodstream. In children and infants, the heart rate may briefly increase but often falls sharply to become very slow (bradycardic).

3. Signs of inadequate breathing include a breathing rate above or below normal; irregular rhythm; diminished, unequal, or absent breath sounds; labored or increased respiratory effort; use of accessory muscles (may be pronounced in infants and children and involve nasal flaring, seesaw breathing, grunting, and retractions between the ribs and above the clavicles and sternum); and shallow respiratory depth.

4. A patient in heart failure can also suffer from bronchoconstriction and wheezes. If bronchoconstriction is apparent and the patient's physician has prescribed the inhaler's use during such a situation, then it is indicated. The medication will have the side effect of increasing heart rate, so be sure to monitor vital signs and limit repeated doses of the medication.

5. Differences between adult and child/infant respiratory systems include:
   - Mouth and nose—In general, all structures are smaller and more easily obstructed in children than in adults.
   - Pharynx—Infants' and children's tongues take up proportionally more space in the mouth than do adults'.
   - Trachea—The trachea is narrower and obstructed more easily by swelling; it is also softer and more flexible. Like other cartilage in the infant and child, the cricoid cartilage is less developed and less rigid.
   - Diaphragm—The chest wall is softer; infants and children tend to depend more heavily on the diaphragm for breathing.

6. Signs and symptoms of breathing difficulty include altered level of consciousness, dizziness, fainting, restlessness, anxiety, confusion, combativeness, cyanosis, straining neck and facial muscles, tightness in the chest, straining intercostal muscles, numbness or tingling in the hands and feet, flaring nostrils, pursed lips, coughing, crowing, high-pitched barking, respiratory noises such as wheezing or rattling, and the patient sitting in a tripod position.

Critical Thinking Exercises

1. A 45-year-old male with severe difficulty breathing, rapid rate of respirations, shallow breaths, minimal chest expansion, and difficulty speaking has <u>inadequate</u> breathing. Reasoning: The rapid, shallow breaths and minimal chest expansion do not permit adequate filling of the alveoli of the lungs.

2. A 65-year-old female with a normal rate and regular rhythm of respirations with good chest expansion and slightly labored breathing is breathing <u>adequately</u>. Reasoning: Although the patient perceives that she is having trouble breathing, the normal rate and rhythm and good chest expansion indicate that her respirations are presently able to fill the alveoli of her lungs.

3. A drowsy 3-year-old patient with retractions, nasal flaring, and a rapid rate of respiration is breathing <u>inadequately</u>. Reasoning: The patient's muscle retractions and nasal flaring indicate that the child is working very hard to draw air into her lungs. The rate is too fast to permit adequate filling of the alveoli. The child's drowsiness is an alarming sign of hypoxia.

Pathophysiology to Practice

1. Yes, a patient can develop pulmonary edema without developing peripheral edema. Depending upon how the patient is positioned most of the time, such as lying down, edema may not form in the lower extremities. In addition, if the pulmonary edema is acute—if it has developed quickly and not chronically—peripheral edema will not be a component of the illness.

2. The expiratory phase will be prolonged because asthma is an obstructive disease where air becomes trapped in the lungs due to bronchoconstriction and excessive mucus production. During exhalation, the patient must exhale more forcefully because of the stale, trapped air taking longer to exit the lungs.

3. The SpO_2 simply measures the amount of oxygen being carried on red blood cells in the bloodstream; this is just one measure of what's going on in the body. The patient may be in moderate to severe distress and yet be showing a "normal" pulse oximetry reading. In fact, the patient's tissues might be quite hypoxic if oxygen molecules are not being released from red blood cells when they reach, for example, the brain. There are even some conditions, like a low body temperature of low acid level in the body, that cause oxygen to stay attached to red blood cells instead of oxygenating tissues, leading to hypoxia. This is why you must assess the whole patient—all vital signs including the SpO_2 reading.

For each of these patients, the following conditions are most likely:

4. A 10-year-old patient is more likely to have <u>asthma</u>. The other respiratory diseases do not affect children.

5. An 82-year-old patient who recently discovered she can't sleep lying down is most likely experiencing <u>heart failure</u>. Her "nocturnal dyspnea" or inability to lie flat while sleeping is likely due to fluid accumulating in her lungs during sleep.

6. A 76-year-old patient who reports difficulty breathing with fever and increased mucus production is likely suffering from <u>COPD</u>. This disease is characteristic of mucus production.

7. A patient who has had a prior heart attack with difficulty breathing who reports gaining 5 pounds in the past 2 to 3 days is likely suffering from <u>heart failure</u> and an accumulation of fluids from his weakened heart.

8. A very skinny elderly man who is constantly on a nasal cannula at 2 liters per minute at home is likely suffering from a chronic disease like <u>COPD</u>.

9. A 35-year-old man who has difficulty breathing while playing racquetball is likely suffering an <u>asthma</u> attack because of the sudden onset and no history of chronic illnesses.

Street Scene Questions

1. As with any patient, you should protect the airway and evaluate the patient's breathing. Make sure that the airway is clear and then provide ventilations as necessary. Although the patient is speaking, the tongue or secretions could still be a potential problem.

2. You should ask the husband the questions in a SAMPLE history, except for "E" (event). You should elicit that part of the history from the neighbor. Examples of questions you might ask the neighbor include: "What type of activity was Mrs. Bartolone performing at the onset of her breathing problem?" "When did you first observe the episode?" "What posture was the patient in at that time?" "Was her breathing fast or slow?" "Could she speak in complete sentences?" "Was she working to breathe?" "Was her breathing noisy?" "Did you notice any peculiar skin color—especially around the lips?"

3. The medical history reveals that Mrs. Bartolone had to be intubated and placed on a ventilator during an episode 6 months earlier. This information, coupled with the patient's long smoking history, indicates that you should consider her a high medical emergency.

4. The patient should receive high-concentration oxygen, since her normal 2 liters per minute are obviously insufficient in this situation.

5. No, the patient is not a good candidate for use of an inhaler. Signs and symptoms in the scenario indicate that the patient is in immediate need of oxygen. Also, as later paragraphs indicate, local protocols require that a patient be alert to receive help with a ventilator. Mrs. Bartolone, however, demonstrates signs of drowsiness.

6. This patient should probably be considered a high priority with lights and siren for transport to the hospital. Everything in the case study points toward rapid transport. In most systems, this usually means use of a red light and siren.

Chapter 20 Cardiac Emergencies
Critical Decision Making

1. You should not give nitroglycerin to this 84-year-old patient with chest pain. The drug might make his low blood pressure even lower, which would be harmful to him.

2. You should give nitroglycerin to this 68-year-old patient. He has a history of cardiac problems, he is having chest pain, and his blood pressure is high enough.

3. This patient is trickier to determine than the first two. The confounding factor is that the pain is atypical (in his "stomach"), especially when compared to what he experienced with a prior heart attack, although the pain could still have a cardiac origin. His first nitroglycerin spray didn't work. His vital signs are still within acceptable limits. Get a more detailed history and contact medical direction for additional advice. If for some reason you are unable to contact medical direction, since upper abdominal pain in a patient at risk for heart disease is considered an "angina equivalent," you would be justified in providing nitroglycerin and treating the pain as presumed cardiac pain.

Short Answer

1. Best positions for the following patients are:
   a. For the patient with difficulty breathing and blood pressure 100/70, a sitting-up position as long as the patient tolerates it. If he becomes hypotensive, complains of dizziness, or has diminished mental status, lay the patient back as much as needed.
   b. For the patient with chest pain and blood pressure of 180/90, sitting up.

2. To "clear" a patient before administering a shock, say "Clear!" in a loud voice. In addition, look carefully at the patient from head to toe to ensure no one is touching the patient and no one is touching anything conductive that is touching the patient.

3. Three safety measures to keep in mind when using an AED are: (1) Do not touch the patient or anything conductive that is touching the patient when you are analyzing the rhythm or delivering a shock. (2) If the patient's chest is wet, dry it before applying the pads or delivering a shock. (3) Be sure the patient has no signs of life and no definite pulse before delivering a shock.

4. Steps in the application of the AED are: (1) Use the appropriate-size pads and AED (adult or pediatric). (2) Bare the patient's chest and quickly shave the area where the pads will be placed, if necessary. (3) Turn on the AED. (4) Attach the monitoring/defibrillation electrode pads to the cables and then to the patient. (5) Advise all rescuers, "Stop CPR; we are analyzing." (6) Once the AED is charged and ready and you have ensured everyone is clear of the patient, deliver the shock as directed by the AED.

Critical Thinking Exercises

1. The question asks you to evaluate the system where you work with respect to the chain of survival: links that are strong and links that need work. Answers will vary, depending on the particular system where you are working or studying.

2. The question asks how successful your system is in resuscitating patients from cardiac arrest. Answers will vary, depending on the particular system where you are working or studying.

Pathophysiology to Practice

1. The patient with central chest pain radiating to his back, a "bubble" on a blood vessel in his chest, and normal vital signs has an aortic aneurysm. If the aneurysm ruptures, his chance of survival is low, and if the blood is unable to clot because of aspirin, that would decrease his chance of survival even more. This patient has a normal blood pressure. If he were hypotensive, nitroglycerin would likely decrease his blood pressure to dangerous levels, which would obviously be bad for the patient. If he were hypertensive, lowering his blood pressure with nitroglycerin might reduce the amount of force pushing against the weakened area of the blood vessel, which might help the patient. Contact medical direction for advice regarding nitroglycerin for this patient and, if it is advised, monitor his blood pressure to be sure it does not drop too much.

2. The patient with CHF who has run out of his "water pill," has gained weight, and has wakened short of breath needs to be propped up on two pillows. Because he stopped taking the pill that helps him eliminate excess fluid, he now has too much fluid in his circulatory system for his heart to handle, and the excess fluid is leaking out of his blood vessels. When he is upright during the day, that fluid is likely to leak into his abdominal cavity and/or lower legs. At night, when he lies flat, the capillaries surrounding the alveoli of his lungs leak fluid into the lungs, which causes shortness of breath.

Street Scene Questions

1. The equipment you should take to the side of every potential cardiac patient includes the following: nonrebreather mask, oxygen, a nasal cannula (in the event the patient will not accept the nonrebreather mask), a suction unit, equipment to take vital signs, a defibrillator (AED) in case of cardiac arrest, and a bag-valve mask with oxygen reservoir. (_Note to Instructor:_ Some students may mention a stair chair if, as in the case study, the patient must be carried down stairs.)

2. As with any other patient, treatment priorities include the ABCs. At present, the patient's airway is open, but if she becomes unconscious or vomits, you should become immediately concerned. You should continually monitor the patient for rate of respirations and quality of breathing. If needed, respirations can be supported with a bag-valve mask and supplemental oxygen. (_Note to Instructor:_ Although cardiac patients are usually most comfortable sitting up to breathe, this may affect circulation if the patient is in cardiogenic shock. Remind students that it is not appropriate to lay a patient flat if it impairs breathing and/or makes the patient anxious. Stress the importance of continually monitoring the patient for changes in pain, level of consciousness, breathing, and vital signs.)

3. The assessment information you need to obtain next would be a set of vital signs and a history. Data you solicit should include the following: any relevant medical history, current treatment by a physician, prescribed medications (particularly nitroglycerin), presence of an implanted device (pacemaker or defibrillator), and so on. Additionally, you should ask the patient about the signs and symptoms that led her to summon EMS. Using the OPQRST model, you might ask these questions:
   * **O**nset: When did the signs and symptoms begin?
   * **P**rovocation: What was the patient doing when the symptoms started? Does anything cause the pain to lessen or intensify?
   * **Q**uality: Can the patient describe what the pain feels like?
   * **R**adiation: Where does she feel the pain, and does it radiate to other parts of the body such as the neck or arms?
   * **S**everity: How would she rate her pain on a scale of 1 to 10? Has the severity of the pain changed after the administration of nitroglycerin and/or oxygen?
   * **T**ime: How long has the patient had these particular signs and symptoms?

4. Next, you should immediately connect the patient to the AED. While you are doing this, another crew member should ventilate her with a bag-valve mask and supplemental oxygen. Once the AED is connected, push the "analyze" button and follow the instructions issued by the device, making sure that everyone is clear of the patient. (_Note to Instructor_: Some students may go on to list the care steps described in the scenario.)

Chapter 21 Diabetic Emergencies and Altered Mental Status
Critical Decision Making

1. This patient appears to be responsive and able to protect her airway. Her altered mental status and diabetic history round out the facts needed to decide glucose is appropriate at this time.

2. Although this patient has a diabetic history, there is nothing that says his seizure is related to his diabetes (as opposed to his head injury). Additionally, his mental status isn't alert enough to administer an oral medication. If he comes out of his seizure and becomes alert, you can obtain a further history.

3. Although this patient was involved in a collision, a diabetic emergency may have caused it. His altered mental status and diabetic history is enough to administer the glucose. Ensure that he is able to control his own airway before administering the medication.

Short Answer

1. Signs of a diabetic emergency include altered mental status, seizures, pale skin, diaphoresis, tachycardia, rapid breathing, frequent urination, and increased thirst.

2. A history of diabetes can most easily be obtained by questioning the patient, family, or other bystanders. Other indicators include medic alert bracelets; medications such as insulin or oral antidiabetics; and the presence of syringes, glucose meters, and/or an insulin pump.

3. After assuring scene safety, treatment of a diabetic emergency must include a thorough assessment. Treat immediate life threats such as airway or breathing issues and attempt to determine if the emergency is the result of hyper- or hypoglycemia (if possible). If you cannot make this determination, or if the patient is hypoglycemic, consider administering oral glucose (if it can be done safely and appropriately). Oral glucose will replenish absent sugar stores in the bloodstream and potentially reverse hypoglycemia.

4. Unless local protocols dictate otherwise, baseline vitals should be obtained prior to administration of any medication.

5. Treatment of a seizure patient should include protecting him from trauma related to the seizure, airway and breathing support if necessary, supplemental oxygen, and a thorough assessment to possibly identify the cause of the seizure.

6. For either a conscious or an unconscious stroke patient, conduct a thorough assessment that includes identification of when the stroke began. Care for a conscious stroke patient should include reassuring the patient, monitoring the airway, and administering high-concentration oxygen. Transport the conscious stroke patient in a semi-sitting position. Care for an unconscious stroke patient should include maintaining an open airway and providing high-concentration oxygen. For transport, the unconscious stroke patient should be positioned lying on the affected side. Transport any stroke patient to a hospital with the capabilities to manage a stroke patient or as guided by local stroke care protocol.

7. Care for dizziness and/or syncope should include supplemental oxygen, a request for ALS assistance, laying the patient flat, and loosening tight clothing.

Critical Thinking Exercises

Oral glucose is not appropriate in an unconscious patient. Contact ALS, support the airway and breathing if necessary, provide supplemental oxygen, and initiate transport.

Pathophysiology to Practice

1. A seizure associated with hypoxia may be identified in the primary assessment. Airway and breathing problems make hypoxia a likely etiology. Consider also events leading up to the seizure. Did the patient have trouble breathing or choke? Epilepsy is typically identified through patient history. Does the patient have a history of seizures?

2. The history should reveal an event such as choking that would cause hypoxia or a history of epilepsy (or multiple seizures over a period of years, which would indicate epilepsy even if the patient has not been diagnosed with epilepsy). Vital signs assessment that includes SpO_2 readings would indicate if the patient's blood oxygen level is low (below 95 percent for mild hypoxia, below 90 percent for severe hypoxia). The history and physical assessments would also help to pinpoint other possible causes of a seizure such as stroke, head trauma, toxic exposure or ingestion, hypoglycemia, infection, heat exposure, pregnancy, or others. Some seizures, including those associated with epilepsy, are of unknown origin.

Street Scene Questions

1. Every patient deserves a thorough patient assessment, particularly a patient with an altered mental status.

2. Scene safety is always the first concern, but immediately following safety is the concern for primary assessment-related problems. Always rule out issues with the ABCs first.

3. Many medical problems and traumatic injuries can make a patient seem intoxicated. Brain injuries, stroke, diabetic emergencies, and seizures can all make patients act like they are drunk.

4. Patient assessment should be consistent in most situations. The most important element is to be thorough. If you discover more information, your assessment may be adjusted based on the newfound clues.

5. Obtaining a previous medical history may be difficult in an altered or uncooperative patient. Try asking questions. If that is not possible, consider taking clues from the scene such as medic alert bracelets, patient medications, and other scene findings.

6. Any altered mental status patient is a high priority. Changes in mental status can indicate critical life threats. ALS is certainly warranted here.

Chapter 22 Allergic Reaction

Critical Decision Making

For the patients described below, allergic reaction or anaphylaxis is indicated by their presentation as follows:

1. A patient with a history of allergic reactions to bee stings reporting that she feels her throat "closing up" after a bee sting is likely starting to have an <u>anaphylactic reaction</u> because of the impending compromise of her airway. She needs immediate intervention.

2. A patient who reports an unknown allergy and feels like his skin is "just itching all over" is likely having an <u>allergic reaction</u>. Because there is no respiratory distress or signs or symptoms of shock, you would not consider this anaphylaxis.

3. A patient who has an "allergy" to dairy products and reports a stomach upset and diarrhea is likely having an <u>allergic reaction</u>. Because there is no respiratory distress or signs or symptoms of shock, you would not consider this anaphylaxis.

4. A patient who is allergic to peanuts and has swelling of the face and neck, difficulty breathing, and a rapid pulse is likely having <u>anaphylaxis</u> because of the difficulty breathing. She needs immediate intervention.

5. A patient who is allergic to penicillin, accidentally took a medication containing penicillin, and is reporting to be dizzy with stable vital signs is likely having an <u>allergic reaction</u>. Because there is no respiratory distress or signs or symptoms of shock, you would not consider this anaphylaxis.

Short Answer

1. The indications for the administration of an epinephrine auto-injector include the following: patient exhibits the signs of an allergic reaction, medication is prescribed for the patient by a physician, and medical direction authorizes its use for the patient.

2. Some of the more common causes of allergic reactions include:
   - Insect bites and stings from bees, yellow jackets, and wasps.
   - Foods such as nuts, eggs, shellfish, and milk.
   - Plants such as poison ivy, poison oak, and plant pollen.
   - Medications such as penicillin and other antibiotics.
   - Other things like dust, chemicals, soaps, and makeup.

3. Signs and symptoms of an anaphylactic reaction involving the skin, respiratory system, and cardiovascular system might include:
   - Skin: itching; hives; red skin; swelling of the face; warm, tingling feeling in the face, mouth, chest, feet, and hands.

- Respiratory system: tightness in the throat or chest; cough; rapid breathing; labored, noisy breathing; hoarseness, muffled voice, or loss of voice; stridor; wheezing.
- Cardiovascular system: increased heart rate, decreased blood pressure.

Critical Thinking Exercises

1. This patient does not have respiratory or circulatory compromise but he may be on his way in that direction. His vital signs and adequate breathing indicate this is not the time to give epinephrine. However, the nature of shellfish allergies is that they can become severe. This is a good case to report to medical direction for advice.

2. This is not an anaphylactic reaction. Epinephrine is not appropriate at this time. Transport the patient and observe her for signs of allergic reaction.

3. This is a prime candidate for the epinephrine auto-injector. He has signs of airway compromise and shock. Follow local protocols to give the medication.

Pathophysiology to Practice

Any patients who are awake, whether they are experiencing an anaphylactic reaction or an anxiety attack, will experience similar effects from the administration of epinephrine. Remember that it's a very powerful drug that's primarily used in patients in cardiac arrest to try to save their life. Using it in a conscious patient is very risky because it causes anxiety, difficulty breathing, rapid heart rate, palpitations, sweating, headache, nausea and vomiting, dizziness, and high blood pressure. However, you consider these side effects to be "acceptable trade-offs" when a patient is having anaphylaxis because of the life-threatening nature of the condition and the effectiveness of epinephrine in treating it. Administering epinephrine to a patient having an anxiety attack is a significant—and reportable—drug error.

Street Scene Questions

1. Mr. Meeker is showing signs and symptoms of an anaphylactic reaction. He is using accessory muscles to breathe, and his face and neck look flushed. In addition, he cannot speak in complete sentences. He seems potentially unstable and needs to be monitored closely for what may be a life-threatening condition.

2. He has obviously developed an allergy to bee venom. Physiologically, his immune system's antibodies are responding, but they are getting way out of hand. The over-response of his immune system is causing histamine and other chemicals to be dumped into the bloodstream. This causes blood vessels to dilate, his blood pressure to fall, and many of his tissues to swell, including those surrounding the respiratory system. Thick mucus might be produced in the airways and he might develop urticaria (hives).

3. From the information gathered thus far, it appears that Mr. Meeker is developing severe respiratory distress, which could in turn lead to respiratory arrest. Even if he gets definitive care (an injection of epinephrine), he will probably need ventilatory support and supplemental oxygen.

4. The patient needs immediate control of his airway and breathing by administration of high-concentration oxygen through a bag-valve mask. Monitor the patient for shock and arrange for quick ALS intercept or rapid transport to the nearest hospital.

Chapter 23 Poisoning and Overdose Emergencies

Critical Decision Making

1. Look for prescription bottles and nonprescription meds. Look throughout the house, including the kitchen, bedroom, and bath. Check garbage cans for empty containers. Look for loose pills anywhere in the house. Be sure to ask the patient what he took and what medications he knows of around the house.

2. After ensuring your safety and getting the patient extricated from the hazardous environment, you should attempt to determine how long the patient was in the garage with the car running. You may get this information from the patient (if he is conscious) or from family or neighbors.

3. Look for any chemicals the patient may have been using in the garden. Do not become overcome by the same thing that overcame the patient. Look around the garden, in garages or sheds, and even in garbage cans for chemical containers.

Short Answer

1. Poison can be ingested, inhaled, absorbed, and injected into the body.

2. The sequence of assessment steps in cases of poisoning is: detect and treat immediately life-threatening problems in the primary assessment, perform a history and physical exam, assess baseline vital signs, consult medical direction, and transport the patient with all containers and labels from the substance. Reassess the patient en route.

3. Gather the following information about a poisoning case before contacting medical direction:
   - What substance was involved?
   - When did the exposure occur?
   - How much was ingested?
   - Over how long a period did the ingestion occur?
   - What interventions have the patient, family, or well-meaning bystanders taken?
   - What is the patient's estimated weight?
   - What effects is the patient experiencing from the ingestion?

4. Emergency care steps for an ingested poisoning include gathering whatever information is available about the poison and contacting medical direction on the scene or en route. Administer activated charcoal as directed by medical control, and position the patient for vomiting. Have suction equipment readily available and never discard vomitus until it can be inspected by the receiving facility personnel or physician.

5. Emergency care steps for an inhaled poisoning include removing the patient from the source of the poison, establishing an open airway, and inserting an OPA or NPA. Administer high-concentration oxygen by nonrebreather mask. Gather the patient's history, take vital signs, expose the chest for auscultation, and contact medical direction. Transport. Emergency care steps for an absorbed poisoning include removing the patient from the source of the poison while avoiding your own cross-contamination. Always brush powders from the patient, being careful not to abrade the patient's skin. Remove contaminated clothing. Irrigate with clear water for at least 20 minutes while catching contaminated water and disposing of it safely. Contact medical direction and transport.

Critical Thinking Exercises

Prevent the patient from brushing at his jeans. Making sure that you are wearing protective gloves, brush off as much of the powder that remains on his hands and other body areas as possible. *Do not* try to rinse contaminated areas with water or any other "neutralizing" substance. Remove the patient's jeans and any other clothing or jewelry that might be contaminated with the pesticide. Transport him immediately, bringing along the pesticide container and its labels.

Pathophysiology to Practice

1. The poison control center's information that rattlesnake venom primarily affects the cardiovascular system should help you anticipate signs and symptoms you may see in the patient, like a rapid, weak pulse; a low blood pressure; skin color changes; and weakness. These bites tend to be very painful when they first occur and symptoms develop quickly.

2. The poison control center's information that coral snake venom primarily affects the nervous system should help you anticipate signs and symptoms in the patient like blurred vision, confusion, headache, slurred speech, numbness, paralysis, and coma. These bites may be painless at first and major symptoms may not develop for hours. That's why these patients should always be further evaluated in the emergency department even when they might describe feeling fine right after the bite.

Street Scene Questions

1. Sample questions might include: "Do you have the original container?" "Do you know how much oil was previously in the lamp?" "Did you see your child drink the oil?" "What clues

convinced you that she actually swallowed the oil?" "When do you think your daughter might have drunk the oil?" "Have you provided any treatment for your daughter?" "Has your daughter vomited?" "How much did she vomit?" "Did you save the vomit?"

2. Signs and symptoms for this substance can vary depending upon a number of factors such as the weight of the patient, amount ingested, stomach contents, and whether or not the patient has vomited. Determine the level of consciousness and establish a baseline set of vitals. Observe skin color and temperature. As with any patient, it is important to ensure that the child can maintain her own airway and breathing. Monitor for changes that might alert you to the seriousness of the poisoning. Check the patient's pupils to determine whether they are equal and reactive; some poisons cause the pupils to constrict or dilate. The pupils may or may not react to light. Remember that seizure activity can also occur with an ingested poison.

3. Most of the care should be focused on the ABCs. Consider the need for immediate transport. Depending upon local or state protocols, contact poison control en route to the hospital. Because the ingested substance is a petroleum-based product, the use of both activated charcoal and syrup of ipecac is contraindicated. The lamp, or at least some of the oil, should be transported to the hospital along with the patient.

4. Consider contacting poison control and discuss supportive care with medical direction. Remember that your local, state, and regional protocols will determine many of your actions here.

Chapter 24 Abdominal Emergencies

Critical Decision Making

1. For all patients with abdominal pain, you should get a history of oral intake as well as a history of recent vomiting, urination, and bowel movements. Females should also be asked about their obstetric and gynecologic history and the possibility of pregnancy. You will also perform a physical examination including palpation of the abdominal quadrants.

2. You have the oral intake history, but ask specifically about recent bowel and bladder activity. Palpate the abdomen. Ask about vomiting and fever.

3. As with the first two questions, ask about vomiting and recent bowel and bladder activity. Determine the oral intake. Palpate the abdomen.

Short Answer

1. Some of the signs and symptoms seen with abdominal distress are nausea, vomiting, and diarrhea; pain with palpation and guarding; distention and bloating; discoloration of the abdomen; vomiting blood or coffee ground-like emesis; black, tarry stools; tearing pain that radiates around to the back; and shock.

2. Visceral pain is described as dull and persistent and usually originates from the hollow organs; parietal pain is sharp and localized and may change with body position. Visceral pain may be symptomatic of a person who has a kidney stone, and parietal pain is seen with patients having internal abdominal bleeding.

3. Treat the ABCs, administer 15 lpm of oxygen by nonrebreather mask, place the patient in a position of comfort, and transport promptly. As part of the reassessment, you should monitor vital signs during transport.

4. The abdominal quadrants are the right upper quadrant (RUQ), left upper quadrant (LUQ), right lower quadrant (RLQ), and left lower quadrant (LLQ). The quadrants are determined by dividing the abdomen into four equal parts with imaginary lines drawn both vertically and horizontally through the umbilicus (the navel). The right and left sides of the quadrants are the patient's right and left.

Critical Thinking Exercises

Use the OPQRST memory aid to build a complete picture of the patient's present illness. Ask questions about each of the OPQRST factors (e.g., Provocation/Palliation—What makes the pain better or worse? Quality—Can you describe what the pain is like? Region/Radiation—Can you point to where you feel the pain?). Then continue questioning the patient about the rest of his past medical history (Allergies, Medications, Pertinent Past History, Last Oral Intake, and Events Leading to the Emergency). If the patient is female, you would also ask questions about the patient's menstrual cycle, possible vaginal bleeding, and other questions that might indicate a possible ectopic pregnancy. This patient would probably be most comfortable on her side with her knees drawn up. ·

Pathophysiology to Practice

Elderly patients with abdominal pain must be carefully assessed since research has shown they are up to nine times more likely to die than younger patients with the same cause of the abdominal pain. Compared to younger patients, elderly patients are more likely to present with life-threatening internal bleeding from causes like gastrointestinal bleeding and abdominal aortic aneurysm. GI bleeding can occur anywhere from the esophagus to the rectum and may be gradual or acutely massive. These patients often develop signs of profound hypoperfusion. Abdominal aortic aneurysm (AAA) is a ballooning or weakening in the wall of the aorta as it passes through the abdomen. Blood can leak between the layers of the vessel and the affected area may grow or even rupture. This is a surgical emergency and requires prompt transportation to an appropriate hospital.

Street Scene Questions

1. This patient seems to be showing signs of a medical emergency. Her skin color is pale and sweaty, she is breathing rapidly, and the pulse is fast. You should consider this patient unstable based on this information, and consider rapid intervention and transport.

2. The symptoms reportedly came on suddenly. The rapid breathing, fast pulse, and pale/sweaty skin are initial "clues" that this patient has a potential medical emergency. Consider requesting ALS intervention unless transporting directly to the hospital will take less time.

3. The vomit can provide a number of important pieces of information for the hospital. Some of the helpful information is quantity, contents, presence of blood, coffee ground-looking material, color, and consistency.

4. This patient may require IV therapy in order to replace the fluid and possible blood loss. Also, if she has a breathing emergency that requires a protected airway (and you are unable to perform endotracheal intubation), then ALS will be able to protect the airway, if necessary, and prevent aspiration if the patient vomits again.

5. Yes, this patient seems to be having a potentially life-threatening event that requires definitive care, possibly surgery, and/or blood replacement. The need to get her to a hospital rapidly is important.

6. Yes, the patient seems to be in compensated shock at present and possibly deteriorating into decompensated shock. She has a rapid pulse, pale and sweaty skin, and her breathing is becoming rapid. The patient's blood pressure may be dropping (we don't know her baseline normal given the medication she is taking).

7. It is always important to take notice of something as significant as a "mini-stroke." Also note that she is taking blood pressure medication; this may be the reason for her low blood pressure readings, rather than her presenting problem today. The aspirin she is taking may also be responsible for abdominal bleeding.

8. The patient should be placed in a position of comfort. Additional pain will cause more discomfort and aggravate her condition to the point where vital signs will become affected and the ability to complete a reassessment will also be affected.

Chapter 25 Behavioral and Psychiatric Emergencies and Suicide

Critical Decision Making

1. In this case, a stroke or diabetic emergency could cause similar symptoms. Obtain a history from the patient and observe for medical alert identification. If you have the ability to perform blood glucose measurement, do so. A stroke scale may be helpful if the

patient is cooperative. A history of head injury or other cause of altered mental status should be explored.

2. Alcohol may have caused the emergency, but it isn't the only potential cause. Perform a thorough history and a blood glucose measurement. Stroke isn't as likely in a 21-year-old. Consider drug use in addition to alcohol and diabetes. Also look for evidence of head injury or seizure history.

3. Depression won't normally cause aggressive behavior. Dementia or Alzheimer's may. Look for a history of this as well as compliance with her medications. Look for evidence of seizure, head injury, or diabetes. You may not be able to perform a stroke scale, but observe for signs of asymmetry in speech or for movement that is new to the patient.

Short Answer

1. A number of medical conditions can alter a person's mental status and behavior, including low blood sugar, lack of oxygen, inadequate blood to the brain or stroke, head trauma, mind-altering substances, excessive cold, excessive heat, and psychological conditions.

2. A number of methods will help calm a patient suffering from a behavioral or psychiatric emergency. Always speak slowly and calmly. Use a calm and reassuring tone. Listen to the patient and make him aware of this. Do not be judgmental. Show compassion, not pity. Use positive body language; avoid crossing one's arms or looking disinterested. Acknowledge the patient's feelings. Do not enter the patient's personal space; instead, stay at least 3 feet away.

3. Some of the signs and symptoms of behavioral or psychiatric emergency include panic or anxiety; unusual appearance, disordered clothing, and poor hygiene; agitated or unusual activity; and unusual speech patterns or inability to carry on a coherent conversation.

4. When your scene size-up reveals that it is too dangerous to approach a patient, *always* call for the police and wait for them. Do not leave the patient alone. Try to talk to the patient from a safe distance.

5. A number of factors can help you assess a patient's risk for suicide, including previous threats of suicide; depression; high current or recent stress levels; previous attempts or suicide threats; a suicide plan; recent emotional trauma; age (15 to 25 and over 40 at greater risk); alcohol and drug abuse; sudden improvement from depression.

6. Answers will vary depending on your state laws. In most states, a patient cannot be transported against his will without a legal document or "psychiatric hold" authorizing the transport. In some cases, these can only be signed by a judge; in other cases, they can be signed by law enforcement and physicians.

Critical Thinking Exercises

1. This could be a case of excited delirium, a very dangerous situation in which a patient will act extremely agitated or psychotic. This situation is thought to be due to drug intoxication or elevated temperature. The patient will suddenly cease struggling; often within minutes, the patient begins breathing inadequately and subsequently dies. Meanwhile, law enforcement and rescuers think the patient finally just "calmed down" and may fail to reassess. Always be alert for this sequence of events if patients exhibit this behavior and monitor the patient closely throughout the call. Have plenty of help, plan your activities, and always place the patient face up.

2. Be aware of your state laws regarding involuntary restraint and transportation of minors. Most states have laws that allow a patient to be transported against his will if he is a danger to himself or others. If the parents do not give permission to transport the patient, it will be helpful to contact medical direction and call for a law enforcement response for the safety of yourself, the patient, and the parents, and to help avoid liability problems if you attempt transport on your own.

3. Whether or not someone "thinks" the patient is just seeking attention is completely irrelevant. Statistics show that a person who has attempted suicide in the past is more likely to commit suicide than one who has not. This patient must be assessed and transported.

Pathophysiology to Practice

1. A patient with an imbalance in his blood sugar can cause the rapid onset of erratic and hostile behavior that has nothing to do with the patient's psychological health. It's simply a matter of having too little or too much sugar available in his blood.

2. A patient with head trauma can experience vast personality changes ranging from irritability to irrational behavior, as well as altered mental status, amnesia, or confusion.

3. A lack of oxygen (hypoxia) can cause restlessness, confusion, and altered mental status. The brain is a very sensitive organ that needs a constant supply of oxygen in order to function effectively and remain stable.

Street Scene Questions

1. Your first and foremost concern is scene safety. If the scene is known to be unsafe or if the patient is believed to have violent tendencies, you should not even get close to the scene until law enforcement officials have secured it. Remember that you cannot provide care if you become hurt. In fact, if you become injured in this type of situation, the event is compounded by the need to summon other units. Be safe! Be cautious!

2. In this case, scene safety should be handled by the appropriate law enforcement agency. Police officers are trained and equipped to handle these situations. As indicated in the scenario, you should make sure that all EMS personnel and bystanders are in a safe area in case the patient exits the building prior to the arrival of police officers. You should then await and follow law enforcement directives.

3. You should approach the patient after police declare the scene safe. In addition, a police officer might need to remain in the area until everybody is confident that the patient will not attempt to harm himself or others. In this scenario, you decide to approach without a partner to minimize patient agitation. However, a police officer remains in the area. In some cases, a police officer might accompany EMS personnel to the hospital. As emphasized in the chapter, physical restraints are used cautiously and only in select situations after contact with medical direction.

4. Rules for approaching a patient with a behavior disorder include:
   - Identify yourself.
   - Speak slowly and clearly.
   - Listen to the patient.
   - Do not be judgmental.
   - Use positive body language.
   - Acknowledge the patient's feelings.
   - Do not enter the patient's personal space.
   - Be alert to the patient's emotional status.

5. Guidelines for dealing with agitated patients include:
   - Be alert and remain concerned with scene safety.
   - Treat life-threatening problems during the initial survey.
   - Remember that some medical or traumatic injuries may mimic behavioral emergencies.
   - Be prepared to spend time talking with the patient.
   - Encourage the patient to discuss the problem; then listen.
   - Never play along with visual or auditory hallucinations.
   - If it appears that it might help, involve a family member or friend.
   - Only consider physical restraints as a last resort. If used, make every attempt not to cause additional harm to the patient. Pay very close attention to airway and breathing throughout the entire transport to the hospital.

6. Yes, all patients need to be assessed. In cases of behavioral emergencies, you should never assume the absence of an underlying medical or trauma-related condition. If behavioral patients will cooperate, you have an ethical and legal responsibility to take a full set of vital signs and to conduct a focused and/or detailed assessment. Don't underestimate how important communication skills are in the management of behavioral emergencies.

Chapter 26 Hematologic and Renal Emergencies

Critical Decision Making

1. A 29-year-old patient with sickle cell anemia and severe pain in his arms and chest could be suffering from acute chest syndrome. Chest syndrome is characterized by shortness of breath and chest pain associated with hypoxia when blood vessels in the lungs become blocked. This patient will benefit from an ALS transport.

2. A 42-year-old patient who recently completed his peritoneal dialysis and complains of severe abdominal pain that is worsened by movement likely does not require an ALS transport unless he develops priority signs and symptoms. He may have developed an infection or infiltration of his peritoneum or catheter. He still requires transport and evaluation in the emergency department.

3. A 55-year-old female who refused to leave her house to go to her hemodialysis appointments and now complains of severe difficulty breathing, tachycardia, and anxiety definitely needs ALS intervention because of her priority signs and symptoms. She may be suffering from an electrolyte imbalance or kidney failure; the patient could even go into ventricular fibrillation or other lethal rhythm.

4. A 37-year-old sickle cell anemia patient complaining of extreme fatigue likely does not need an ALS transport as long as he does not develop signs of acute chest syndrome, high fever, hypoperfusion, or stroke.

Short Answer

1. Sickle cell anemia is an inherited disease in which patients have a genetic defect in their hemoglobin that results in an abnormal structure of the red blood cells.

2. Patients with sickle cell disease have red blood cells composed of defective hemoglobin that causes them to lose their ability to have a normal shape and compressibility. Instead of normal, donut-shaped red blood cells, sickle cell patients have red blood cells that resemble a sickle, or crescent, when observed under a microscope. When these misshapen red blood cells move throughout the bloodstream, they often become blocked in capillaries and organs because of their shape. This is known as sludging.

3. Because hemodialysis patients must have intravenous access established so often for their daily or weekly dialysis treatments, they will typically have a surgeon create a specialized site in their body to allow frequent, trouble-free catheterization. Many of these sites are simply the surgical connection between an artery and a vein, known as a fistula. Because arteries maintain a much higher pressure than veins, the site will create turbulent blood flow and enlarge slightly. The palpable vibration of this turbulent blood flow is known as a "thrill."

4. In hemodialysis, a patient is connected to a dialysis machine that pumps his blood through specialized filters to remove toxins and excess fluid. This is almost always completed in a local or regional dialysis center. Peritoneal dialysis, in contrast, is typically completed at home. The patient has a permanent catheter implanted through the abdominal wall and into the peritoneal cavity. Several liters of a specially formulated dialysis solution are run into the abdominal cavity and left in place for several hours, where it absorbs waste material and excess fluid; then the fluid is drained back out into the bag and is discarded.

5. A patient who misses a dialysis appointment is at risk for fluid and toxin build-up in his system. This can manifest with symptoms similar to heart failure. The patient may develop shortness of breath, peripheral edema, and even cardiac rhythm disturbances.

Critical Thinking Exercises

1. It is critical that patients with end-stage renal disease maintain their regularly prescribed schedule of dialysis. Their kidneys simply have no other way of balancing fluids and electrolytes and removing toxins. Missing even a single treatment can be deadly for some patients, who could very quickly develop pulmonary edema and shortness of breath.

2. Unfortunately, it can be very easy to classify patients as "drug-seekers" when you encounter so many different individuals complaining of pain and seeking relief. But doing so in this case is irresponsible. Reviewing the pathophysiology of sickle cell disease

should prompt you to remember that these patients can develop severe pain in their arms, legs, chest, and/or abdomen due to sludging of sickled red blood cells in the capillaries. This is known as sickle cell pain crisis. The patient needs high-concentration supplemental oxygen and transportation to the hospital. Monitor for signs of inadequate breathing, hypoperfusion, and stroke symptoms.

Pathophysiology to Practice

1. A patient with sickle cell disease who starts to show signs and symptoms of stroke is a huge concern. Because sickled cells are more likely to become blocked—or sludge—in capillaries and organs throughout the bloodstream, the risk of stroke in these patients is much higher. This patient should be transported to a designated stroke center if available.

2. One area where sickle cell patients often have problems is with their spleen. This organ is extremely vascular, filters a large percentage of blood, and has infection-fighting functions. Because sickled cells become sludged here, the spleen is impacted and fails to perform its function of fighting infections. This places these patients at a higher risk for severe, life-threatening infections.

Street Scene Questions

1. Initially, you should complete a primary assessment of the patient and evaluate her mental status. Ask the staff members what the patient's normal level of consciousness is and how her presentation today differs from her norm. The patient's color is not good, so get the pulse oximeter attached.

2. The history of the patient's dialysis is significant because any patient with end-stage renal disease has the potential to develop complications with the neurological, respiratory, and cardiovascular system, as well as an increased risk of infection.

3. You should complete a full set of vital signs and a secondary assessment. Listen to her lungs. Test the patient's blood sugar. Because the patient is not really following your commands appropriately, you should assess her for stroke by using the Cincinnati Prehospital Stroke Scale.

4. Because the patient has difficulty breathing and some wet-sounding lung sounds, you should be concerned about pulmonary edema and congestive heart failure. Furthermore, she also has peripheral edema. You can probably rule out a diabetic or stroke emergency at this point given the results of her blood sugar and stroke assessments.

5. Given the patient's deteriorated mental status and respiratory impairment, it is in the patient's best interest to be transported to the hospital where she can be treated for the pulmonary edema and further evaluated by the emergency department physician. Although she will still need dialysis, the hospital will be able to provide it. If the staff on the scene disagrees with your decision, you can always contact medical direction, run the situation by them, and follow their guidance about where to transport the patient.

Chapter 27 Bleeding and Shock

Critical Decision Making

1. You should expedite this patient because of the potential for internal injuries, such as injuries to the chest or lungs. Since his vitals are elevated, this could be a serious situation.

2. Just because the bleeding is from hemorrhoids doesn't mean the patient isn't in shock. His appearance screams shock. His feeling when he stands up indicates orthostatic hypotension. Move it!

3. The patient hasn't lost enough blood to have shock. Your bigger concerns are if the patient can't maintain his airway because of blood flow or if the head injury is a concern. Right now there doesn't seem to be a big rush, but he needs transport.

Short Answer

1. The three main blood vessels and the bleeding that might present from each are:
   - Arteries: arterial bleeding is often rapid, spurting with each heartbeat, profuse, and bright red.

- Veins: venous blood is usually a steady flow, can be quite heavy, and is usually dark red or maroon in color.
- Capillaries: capillary bleeding is usually slow, oozing, and red (though not as bright as arterial blood).

2. The patient care steps for external bleeding include performing a scene size-up, taking Standard Precautions, applying direct pressure to the wound, and administering oxygen. If hemostatic dressings are available, they can be applied, you can use a gloved hand to provide pressure. If bleeding fails to stop, you may need to consider a tourniquet. The patient should be assessed and treated for shock.

3. Perfusion is defined as the supply of oxygen to, and removal of wastes from, the body's cells and tissues as a result of the flow of blood through the capillaries. Hypoperfusion is the body's inability to adequately circulate blood to the body's cells to supply them with oxygen and nutrients, similar to what occurs in shock.

4. Signs and symptoms of shock include altered mental status; pale, cool, and clammy skin; nausea and vomiting; and vital sign changes (increased pulse, increased respirations, decreasing blood pressure, and narrow pulse pressure). Late signs of shock include thirst, dilated pupils, and cyanosis around the lips and nail beds.

5. The three major types of shock and their causes are:
- Hypovolemic (hemorrhagic) shock, caused by uncontrolled bleeding.
- Cardiogenic shock, caused by inadequate pumping of blood by the heart.
- Neurogenic shock, caused by uncontrolled dilation of blood vessels due to nerve paralysis from spinal cord injury.

6. Managing shock includes maintaining an open airway, administering oxygen by nonrebreather mask, and taking spinal precautions as needed. The patient should be kept warm and transported.

Critical Thinking Exercises

The mechanism of injury suggests the possibility of internal bleeding. Vitals indicate that shock may be starting. Obviously, the first step is to take Standard Precautions. Spinal immobilization is definitely indicated. Treat for shock by maintaining the airway, providing high-concentration oxygen, assisting with ventilations (if necessary), controlling any external bleeding, keeping the patient warm, and providing immediate transport. Only apply and inflate the PASG if approved or ordered by your local medical direction.

Pathophysiology to Practice

Some medications cause vasodilation, leading to decreased venous return and hence decreased cardiac output. Some medications, like aspirin and warfarin, can cause severe internal bleeding when taken in excess. Bleeding does not necessarily need to be present in order for shock to occur. Shock can occur from an overdose of medications like beta blockers (Labetalol, Propranolol) and high blood pressure medications (Norvasc, Captopril). An extra note: "Insulin shock," a hypoglycemic (low blood sugar) condition, can be caused by taking too much insulin (which helps move glucose out of the bloodstream and into the body cells) or by taking insulin without eating to replenish blood glucose. Although insulin shock is not shock in the physiological sense, the condition does resemble shock.

Street Scene Questions

1. The fact that the patient has sustained some type of traumatic injury makes him a candidate for high-priority treatment. Even so, the Emergency Medical Responders still need to perform some kind of primary assessment to determine such information as level of responsiveness, breathing, and signs of internal bleeding, which is always a possibility with trauma.

2. In addition to the mechanism of injury, you will want assessment information such as vital signs (respiration rate, pulse, blood pressure, and skin color). They might also ask about bruising or discoloration over the injured area. These are important signs of possible internal bleeding.

3. Yes, the mechanism of injury is important. In the case of a trauma patient, the mechanism of injury can help determine the location, type, and severity of injuries sustained by a patient.

4. Treatment priorities depend upon the ABCs. Because you suspect internal bleeding, rapid transport is indicated. You should consider administration of high-concentration oxygen by nonrebreather mask. You should also attempt to keep the patient warm and remain alert to signs of shock.

5. Vital signs should be taken every five minutes to determine changes in the patient's condition. In cases of internal bleeding, you can expect that the pulse rate will increase and become more thready. You can also expect the respiratory rate to become more rapid and increasingly labored. The patient's skin will grow paler and become more moist. As the signs and symptoms of shock (hypoperfusion) intensify, you can expect dilated pupils, delayed capillary refill time (although not always a reliable indicator), and cyanosis around the lips and nail beds. The detailed assessment may reveal tenderness in the left upper abdominal quadrant.

Chapter 28 Soft-Tissue Trauma
Critical Decision Making

1. This patient's burns are 45 percent superficial.
2. This patient's burns are approximately 3.25 percent partial thickness.
3. This patient's burns are 36 percent partial thickness (legs), 9 percent full thickness (arms).

Short Answer

1. The three types of closed soft-tissue injuries are contusions, hematomas, and crush injuries.
2. Types of open soft-tissue injuries are abrasions, lacerations, punctures, avulsions, amputations, and crush injuries.
3. An object impaled in the cheek should only be removed if it has already gone through the inside surface of the cheek and can be easily pulled out in the same direction that it entered. If this cannot be done, the object should be stabilized in place.
4. The three classifications of burns are:
   • Superficial burn—a burn that involves only the epidermis.
   • Partial thickness burn—a burn in which the epidermis is burned through and the dermis is damaged.
   • Full thickness burn—a burn in which all the layers of the skin are damaged.
5. The difference between a dressing and a bandage is that a dressing is placed directly on a wound and a bandage holds a dressing in place.
6. The qualities of an effective bandage are that it should hold a dressing snugly in place and cover all four of its edges but not restrict blood supply. If a bandage is too loose, it will slip around. Pain, pale or cyanotic skin, cold skin, numbness, and tingling are all indications that a bandage may be too tight.

Critical Thinking Exercises

It's not uncommon to arrive on-scene to find a patient bandaged up like this. However, *you* are the definitive care provider. Despite the sometimes masterpiece bandaging efforts completed by well-meaning bystanders prior to your arrival, *you* need to view all of the patient's wounds with your own eyes. Failure to do so could cause you to miss something or fail to control bleeding properly. Do not make the mistake of arriving at the hospital without having assessed the severity of every potential injury and wound. If the patient is unstable and needs to be expedited, do not delay transport but assess the wounds en route. This is the only way to know how much the patient is bleeding and which wounds need your direct attention or intervention.

Pathophysiology to Practice

When caring for a burn patient, always think beyond the burn. Try to determine any mechanism of injury that might have occurred with the burn incident. If the patient has a decreased blood pressure or other signs of shock, always assume the potential of other serious injuries. Attempt to determine the patient's problem through standard assessment techniques.

Street Scene Questions

1. The patient seems alert and appears to have walked to the present location after her injury. She has an open airway and is breathing without any obvious distress. Judging from the blood-soaked towel, the immediate focus of care is on "C," or circulation.

2. Until further assessment, the patient might be assigned low-priority transport. However, she has the potential to lose a significant amount of blood, and you should be ready to upgrade the patient's priority as necessary.

3. The bleeding must be controlled. You might apply direct pressure with a sterile dressing, or you might leave the towel in place if the bleeding is being controlled. If necessary, you can consider a tourniquet if bleeding remains uncontrolled. Once the bleeding is controlled, you should assess pulses, motor ability, and sensation in the injured arm. You should also administer high-concentration oxygen and observe for signs of shock.

4. A suspicion of alcohol consumption should not interfere with your assessment and treatment. You must obtain a set of vitals and the patient's history. Based on the pool of blood on the patio and the lack of motion in several of the patient's fingers, the patient appears to have the potential to become unstable. You should consider upgrading her priority from "low" to "high" because of their findings.

5. You must monitor the bleeding and stabilize the patient's arm with some type of splinting device or sling. You should take vital signs every 15 minutes and compare them with the baseline set of vitals. You should then reassess motor function and sensation as well. Because of the potential for shock, the patient should be kept warm and perhaps placed on the cot with her legs elevated.

Chapter 29 Chest and Abdominal Trauma

Critical Decision Making

1. Because the patient has diminished lung sounds on one side and describes sharp pain that changes when he breathes, it's likely that he has suffered a collapsed lung or <u>pneumothorax</u>. These can occur spontaneously in patients of any age, including during physical activity like jogging.

2. Absent lung sounds on one side of the chest accompanied by distended neck veins and hypotension following penetrating trauma likely indicates the development of a <u>tension pneumothorax</u>.

3. A patient that was shot in the chest near the 4th intercostal space with hypotension, distended neck veins, narrowing pulse pressure, and normal lung sounds on both sides of the chest is likely developing a <u>cardiac tamponade</u>. The sac surrounding the heart may have been penetrated by the bullet and is filling with blood or fluid, compressing the heart.

Short Answer

1. Signs and symptoms of a flail chest include paradoxical movement of the chest cavity, difficulty breathing, and pain at the injury site. Signs of shock and hypoxia are likely. The patient may become tired and weak.

2. The difference between a pneumothorax and a tension pneumothorax is one of pressure. A pneumothorax occurs when air enters the chest cavity, possibly causing collapse of a lung. In a tension pneumothorax, the air trapped in the chest cavity can build up such pressure that it puts pressure on the heart, great blood vessels, and the unaffected lung. This can reduce the ability of the heart and lungs to pump and oxygenate blood.

3. Care for an open wound to the chest should include maintaining the patient's open airway and providing basic life support, if necessary. Seal the open chest wound as quickly as possible with your gloved hand, if necessary. Apply an occlusive dressing (depending on local protocols, sealed on all four sides or with a flutter valve). Administer high-concentration oxygen. Provide care for shock and transport as soon as possible.

4. Care for an open abdominal wound should include keeping the airway open; staying alert for vomiting; placing the patient on his back, with legs flexed at the knees; administering high-concentration oxygen; providing care for shock, constantly monitoring vital signs, and

transporting as soon as possible. Never give the patient anything by mouth. An open abdominal wound with evisceration should be covered to maintain warmth. Soak a sterile dressing with sterile saline and place the moist dressing over the wound. Apply occlusive dressing over the moist dressing and secure it.

Critical Thinking Exercises

Absent breath sounds on the side of the injury may indicate a collapsed lung. The nail may also have damaged a major blood vessel or the heart itself. If the occlusive dressing you applied is sealed on all four sides, air building up in the chest cavity will have no way to escape and can cause lung collapse and increase pressure on the heart. An open chest wound is a *true emergency*. Maintain an open airway. Administer oxygen, care for shock, and transport as quickly as possible. Provide basic life support (ventilations or CPR), if necessary. Request ALS intercept if available and if it will not delay the patient's arrival at the hospital.

Pathophysiology to Practice

1. Blunt trauma to the chest always carries with it the potential of damage to underlying structures as well as flail chest. However, oxygenation and ventilation of the patient are critical to his survival. If his breathing is becoming shallow or more difficult, you must assist his breathing with high-concentration oxygen via bag-valve-mask device. Be careful in tracking or assisting his inhalations as there is always a possibility that aggressive assisted ventilations might cause a pneumothorax. However, without knowing the extent of his injuries from the blunt trauma, providing him ventilatory assistance is the priority right now.

2. Blunt trauma to the left lower rib area has the potential to injure solid organs like the liver and spleen. Both organs are very vascular; depending on the amount of force exerted, these organs can bleed profusely or may actually just ooze blood undetected until orthostatic hypotension becomes apparent. Blunt force can actually shatter solid organs like these, which are curiously referred to by surgeons as a "fractured spleen" or "fractured liver."

Street Scene Questions

1. Your general impression of the patient is that he's already exhibiting poor skin signs and guarding his chest due to pain. Because the mechanism of injury and impact was on his side of the vehicle, you should be concerned about blunt force chest and abdominal trauma.

2. Until you can assess him further, his skin signs and breathing difficulty should give you concern. He is potentially unstable, and you should consider him a high priority patient at this point.

3. Once you know the scene is safe to enter and you've taken Standard Precautions, you need to delegate someone to maintain manual in-line stabilization of his head until he can be extricated and placed in full spinal immobilization. Apply a cervical collar and begin administering high-concentration oxygen by nonrebreather mask. Try to continue assessing the patient while you work with the fire department to safely extricate the patient from the vehicle.

4. The patient remains a high priority because his radial pulse is weak and rapid. The pain he's describing on his left side could mean he's suffered damage to any of the very vascular organs in that area like the liver and spleen.

5. Complete spinal immobilization and continue to reassess the patient. Try listening to lung sounds again when you can get into the quieter environment of the ambulance. If one is readily available nearby, the patient should be transferred to an advanced life support ambulance. However, transport should not be delayed. The patient meets the criteria to be transported to a trauma center, which is true definitive care for this patient.

Chapter 30 Musculoskeletal Trauma
Critical Decision Making

1. A local hospital is acceptable for this patient as long as the head injury isn't more severe than the suspected fracture. If his mental status and vitals stay within normal limits, a trauma center may not be necessary. When in doubt, radio the hospital for medical direction.

2. Backboard and transport to a trauma center is appropriate for this patient. He has multiple fractures with an altered mental status and vitals which indicate shock.

3. This patient doesn't have major complaints but his mechanism of injury and vital signs scream trauma center. Backboard your patient and go there promptly.

Short Answer

1. Bones are hard, flexible, complex structures composed of calcium and protein fibers. Bones are covered by a strong, white fibrous material called periosteum through which the blood vessels and nerves pass as they enter and leave the bone. They are the body's framework, providing support and protection for the internal organs. They store salts and metabolic materials and are a site of red blood cell production. With the muscles, ligaments, and tendons, they play a major part in the body's ability to move.

2. The signs and symptoms of musculoskeletal injury are pain and tenderness; deformity or angulation; grating, or crepitus; swelling; bruising; exposed bone ends; joints locked into position; and nerve and blood vessel compromise.

3. Take and maintain all Standard Precautions. Perform the primary assessment. After life-threatening conditions have been addressed, all patients with a painful, swollen, or deformed extremity must be splinted. For a low-priority (stable) patient, splint before transport. For a high-priority (unstable) patient, immobilize the whole body on a long spine board, then load and go. If appropriate, cover open wounds with sterile dressings, elevate the extremity, and apply a cold pack to the area to help reduce swelling. Injured long bones should be realigned using manual traction and then splinted. Injured joints should be splinted in the position found unless the distal extremity is cyanotic or lacks pulses.

4. Angulated and deformed injuries to long bones should be realigned to anatomical position in order to restore effective circulation to the affected extremity and to fit it into a splint.

5. The basic principles of splinting are as follows: expose the area and control bleeding before splinting. Assess pulses, motor, and sensation before and after splinting. Align long-bone injuries with gentle traction if there is severe deformation. Splint to immobilize the injury site and adjacent joints. Splint patients before moving them. Pad splints for patient comfort. Choose a splinting method based on the severity of the patient's condition and priority decision. If the patient is unstable, don't waste time splinting.

6. Some of the hazards of splinting include neglecting life-threatening conditions; applying the splint so tightly that soft tissues are compressed and injury is caused to nerves, blood vessels, and muscles; applying the splint so loosely or inappropriately that further soft-tissue injury occurs.

7. The basic splints carried on ambulances include rigid splints, formable splints, and traction splints.

Critical Thinking Exercises

1. Assessment findings that indicate a patient with a musculoskeletal injury is in shock include vital sign changes; altered mental status; pale, cool, or clammy skin; and nausea and vomiting.

2. Identifying a patient with a rapid pulse and anxiety from *pain* versus a patient with a rapid pulse and anxiety from *shock* really comes down to your ability to conduct a thorough assessment and recognize patients who are stable from patients who are unstable. The patient in shock may have the additional signs and symptoms of low blood pressure, altered mental status, and pale, cool, and clammy skin. Other signs of shock include thirst, dilated pupils, and cyanosis around the lips and nail beds.

Pathophysiology to Practice

1. Bones can cause shock because they are living, vascular structures that contain a rich supply of blood. A bone fracture can interrupt millions of tiny vessels innervating the bone tissue, leading to significant bleeding. For example, a fracture of the femur can lead to 1,000 cc of blood loss or more. In addition, broken bone ends can move around and damage surrounding tissues, causing additional bleeding.

2. When distal circulation is compromised or shut down, tissues beyond the injury become starved for oxygen and die, not unlike a blood vessel being occluded during a stroke or heart attack. The extremity must be repositioned so that circulation can be reestablished in that limb. The patient may have a few moments of pain during the maneuver, but it may mean saving the limb and preventing any possibility of amputation.

3. There are many cases when bones might fracture yet present without obvious deformity. Examples include greenstick fractures and comminuted fractures. In some cases, a bone may just not displace when fractured. This is why you should still splint all suspected musculoskeletal fractures.

Street Scene Questions

1. Because the patient appears stable, this patient is probably a low priority. This priority could change after a complete assessment, however; it's always possible the patient may have some internal bleeding at the injury location.

2. Perform a secondary assessment. Ask the patient about allergies, medications, and her last meal. Take a baseline set of vitals.

3. Signs and symptoms of a broken long bone include pain and tenderness, deformity or angulation, grating (crepitus), swelling, bruising, exposed bone ends, joints locked in one position, and nerve and/or blood-vessel compromise. When assessing a patient with a possible musculoskeletal injury, consider assessing the five Ps: pain, pale skin, pulses diminished, paresthesia (a tingling sensation), and paralysis.

4. The major concern with this type of injury is possible nerve, vessel, or muscle damage below the injury. As part of the assessment, take the following steps: evaluate pedal pulses, look at skin color, feel for temperature, check capillary refill in the foot, ask the patient to move her foot and toes, and see if the patient can feel one of them touch her toes and foot.

5. After assessing the patient, splint the injury, making sure the procedure is done with as little movement as possible. The entire leg should be secured in order to immobilize the joint above and below the injury site. Be sure to apply padding as appropriate and then reassess vitals as well as pulses, motor function, and sensation below the injury site.

Chapter 31 Trauma to the Head, Neck, and Spine

Critical Decision Making

1. If the patient appears to have pain (even if she denies it) and she consents to care, she should be immobilized. Sometimes the shock of the crash masks the pain temporarily.

2. The head injury and significant mechanism of injury indicate that immobilization is necessary here.

3. Without a significant mechanism of injury, complaint of pain, or distracting condition evident, the patient doesn't require immobilization.

Short Answer

1. The two components of the central nervous system are the brain and spinal cord. Messages from all over the body are received by the brain, which decides how to respond to changing conditions both inside and outside the body. The spinal cord functions as a relay between most of the body and the brain.

2. Determining possible skull or brain injury can be very difficult. Therefore, you should always assume skull or brain injury when indicated by mechanism of injury. Signs of brain injury can include visible skull fragments; altered mental status; deep laceration or severe bruise to the head; depression or deformity of the skull; severe pain at the site of a head injury; Battle's sign; raccoon eyes; one eye that appears sunken; bleeding or clear fluid from the ears or nose; personality change; Cushing's syndrome; irregular breathing patterns; temperature increase; blurred or multiple image vision; impaired hearing or ringing in the ears; equilibrium problems; forceful vomiting; posturing; paralysis on one side of the body; seizure activity; or deteriorating vital signs.

3. Appropriate treatment for a patient with a possible head or brain injury includes taking Standard Precautions. Use the jaw-thrust maneuver to open and maintain the patient's airway. Monitor changes in breathing. Apply a rigid collar and immobilize the neck and spine. Administer high-concentration oxygen and artificially ventilate, if necessary. Control the patient's bleeding. Keep the patient at rest. Monitor vital signs every five minutes. Talk to the conscious patient, providing emotional support. Dress and bandage open wounds. Manage the patient for shock. Transport promptly.

4. Any of the following mechanisms of injury will support a suspicion of a spine injury: If a patient was involved in a motor-vehicle or motorcycle collision; was struck by a vehicle; fell to the ground from a height; received blunt trauma to the spine or above the clavicles; sustained penetrating trauma to the head, neck, or torso; was involved in a diving accident; was found hanging by the neck; or was found unconscious due to trauma.

5. The appropriate care for a patient with a possible spine injury includes providing manual in-line stabilization for the head and neck. Apply a rigid cervical collar and maintain manual stabilization. Apply the appropriate immobilization device at the appropriate speed. Administer high-concentration oxygen and evaluate the need for artificial ventilation. Reassess sensory and motor function in all four extremities.

Critical Thinking Exercises

1. This may be neurogenic shock. Injuries to the thoracic or lumbar spine can prevent the sympathetic nervous system from responding as it normally would. Rapid pulse and vasoconstriction may be absent.

2. Hyperventilation is only performed in cases of increasing intracranial pressure indicated by serious neurological signs and symptoms including elevated blood pressure, reduced pulse, unequal pupils, and altered mental status.

3. Go to the patient, identify yourself, and seek consent for treatment. Due to the mechanism of injury, assume the possibility of injuries to the head and spine. Provide manual in-line stabilization for the head and neck. Assess the ABCs. Quickly assess the sensory and motor function in all four extremities. Assess the head and the neck. Apply a rigid collar and maintain manual stabilization. Apply the appropriate immobilization device at the appropriate speed. Administer high-concentration oxygen and reevaluate the need for artificial ventilation. Reassess sensory and motor function in all four extremities. Control bleeding. Dress and bandage open wounds. Keep the patient at rest. Manage the patient for shock, even if shock is not present. Reassure the patient. Monitor vital signs every five minutes.

Pathophysiology to Practice

Nipple level T-4

Navel T-10

Little finger C-8

Big toe S-1

Street Scene Questions

1. The patient appears to be unconscious with a head and possible spine injury. The oozing from the head seems to be from an abrasion but merits closer assessment in case it is an indication of a more significant injury, such as an open skull fracture. Because of the mechanism of injury and the patient's lack of consciousness, the teenager should be considered a high priority for transport.

2. Assessment and protection of the ABCs are always the priority. In order to accomplish these tasks, manual in-line stabilization of the head and neck must be applied. After confirming the source of bleeding (from an abrasion), focus on the patient's level of consciousness. Take a baseline set of vitals and get a history from the patient, bystanders, and mother (when she arrives). Don't forget about specific care steps such as the following: Control bleeding from the head wound and apply a dressing. Keep pressure to a minimum if a skull fracture is suspected. Administer high-concentration oxygen and apply a

cervical collar. Place the patient on a backboard, securing the torso first and then the head. Use head blocks and the appropriate immobilization device to secure the head in place. Reassess the patient's vital signs and level of responsiveness.

3. A good way of monitoring changes in the level of responsiveness is to ask the patient to repeat the number that he was previously told. If he can't remember the number, repeat it and ask him to recall it a minute or two later. Another method might be to ask the patient age-appropriate questions, such as his birthday, name, and so on. The purpose is to ascertain the level of alertness and any changes for the better or worse. It is important to become familiar with the neurological assessment method used in your area and that local hospitals understand this tool. For example, if your EMS system uses the Glasgow Coma Scale (GCS), ensure that the receiving hospitals understand the "scoring" system. The same holds true for AVPU. Evaluation tools have limited effectiveness if they can't be used to communicate information on the patient's neurological status.

Chapter 32 Multisystem Trauma

Critical Decision Making

1. Transportation to a local hospital is likely OK as long as the patient remains stable en route.

2. The mental status is the most alarming issue. The potential for head injury should point you in the direction of prompt transport to the trauma center.

3. This woman has trauma to her extremities—and possibly to her uterus. This is a serious condition. The trauma center is the prudent choice, but consult medical direction. The obstetric surgery capabilities at the local hospital may be warranted.

Short Answer

1. You should consider a number of factors when determining whether to perform an intervention on the scene or en route to the hospital. Life-threatening injuries related to the ABCs of primary assessment must be taken care of immediately. Basically, perform those interventions that, if not done at once, could impact upon patient outcome (e.g., permanent disability or death). Such interventions usually include any procedure required to open the airway (such as suctioning), support ventilations, or control bleeding. In addition, perform in-line stabilization of the cervical spine.

2. Interventions to complete prior to transport for a critical trauma patient include suctioning the airway, inserting an oral or nasal airway, restoring a patent airway by sealing a sucking chest wound, ventilating with a bag-valve-mask device, administering high-concentration oxygen, controlling bleeding, and performing spinal immobilization.

3. The decision to bypass a closer hospital in favor of a more distant trauma center is based upon local, regional, or state protocols. Specialized trauma centers can usually provide the definitive treatment required by the patient with multiple injuries. They usually have surgical specialists available 24 hours a day and can provide lifesaving interventions upon the patient's immediate arrival.

4. Although a fractured femur is a severe injury, it becomes a lesser priority if the patient does not have a patent airway or needs ventilatory support. Life-threatening conditions related to the ABCs must come first. In addition, if application of a traction splint will result in a "significant" delay in transport and if the patient is a high priority, then splinting might be postponed so that the patient can receive definitive care at a trauma center or hospital. Remember to treat the whole patient and avoid distraction by a single injury—even if the injury is as serious as a fractured femur. In other words, interventions must be prioritized while keeping in mind the importance of the "golden hour."

Critical Thinking Exercises

Despite what your partner thinks, this patient has borderline vital signs, suffered a significant mechanism of injury, and complains of pain in his chest where he could easily develop any number of life-threatening conditions. The patient meets criteria to go to a trauma center based on the mechanism of injury and perhaps on anatomic criteria. His vital signs might still be adequate to not strictly meet physiologic criteria—but only barely. The patient should go to a trauma center.

Pathophysiology to Practice

1. Geriatric patients must be prioritized higher because they tend not to compensate for shock as effectively as the rest of the population.

2. Any penetrating injury, especially penetrating abdominal trauma, is considered a surgical emergency and should be prioritized higher.

3. A patient taking anticoagulants should be prioritized higher because his blood clotting mechanism will be diminished.

4. Patients with amputations necessitate higher priority because they require prompt surgical intervention in order to realize the best chance for recovery of the reattached limb.

Street Scene Questions

1. The collision appears to be a high-impact crash involving two vehicles—a full-size pickup truck and a compact car. At least two patients are slumped over inside the smaller vehicle and fluid is draining from under the engine. The scene must be secured for a number of reasons—a potentially unstable vehicle, an unknown (and possibly hazardous) fluid leak, high-speed traffic, curious onlookers, and so on. Heavy extrication equipment may be required, and the patients might be high priority, based upon the mechanism of injury (high-speed collision).

2. Additional resources might include police units to control the traffic, heavy rescue for extrication, a fire department crew to handle the leaking fluid, and additional ambulances (depending upon the severity of the injuries and the final number of patients).

3. The passenger should be transported before the driver, if possible. Unlike the driver, who was found conscious but "dazed," the passenger appears motionless at first. Although responsive to verbal stimuli, she is highly agitated, suggesting possible head injury. Her airway is clear, but she exhibits slightly labored and shallow breathing. Patient complaints of right arm pain point to a possible fracture. The patient's radial pulse (strong and rapid) and skin (warm and dry) suggest that her body may be compensating for some blood loss (although the signs do not yet point to a critical situation). The patient is also unrestrained, which means easier removal than the fully restrained driver. Remember not to discount the driver of the pickup truck even though he is ambulatory and reports no immediate life threats.

4. Given the mechanism of injury and the primary assessment findings listed in the preceding answer, you might conclude that the passenger has sustained multiple-system trauma and requires rapid transport to the nearest trauma center and/or hospital. This decision necessitates rapid extrication, as described in the scenario.

5. Examples of critical interventions include in-line stabilization, assurance of an open airway, application of a cervical collar, rapid extrication based on local protocols, a rapid neurological assessment (for pain, sensation, and movement) both before and after extrication, placement and immobilization on a backboard (with proper use of head immobilizers), careful monitoring of the airway, suctioning and application of high-concentration oxygen as necessary, provision for possible ventilatory support (bag-valve mask), immobilization of the right arm (possibly en route to the hospital), and reassessment (vitals every five minutes).

6. If you have not already taken a baseline set of vitals, do so now (to monitor changes in the patient's condition). Although the patient is only alert to verbal stimuli, you can still gather a partial history. For example, you might question the husband or driver of the pickup truck, and take down information on the patient's medic alert bracelet. Perform a focused head-to-toe assessment, paying close attention to lung sounds, pain upon palpation, and signs/symptoms of head trauma (fluid from the nose and ears, deformity, sluggish/nonreactive pupils). Try to elicit information pertinent to the

pregnancy, which should be communicated to medical direction and the receiving hospital as soon as possible.

7. Local, regional, or state protocols usually establish guidelines for transport to a trauma center or hospital. Medical direction, if available, can advise you on the most appropriate action. As previously stated, the assessment findings indicate rapid transport to a trauma center, if available, within an appropriate time frame.

Chapter 33 Environmental Emergencies

Critical Decision Making

1. The patient is several hundred feet out in the water. This is a long distance to swim. Even if you can swim out there, the patient might inadvertently pull you under. Call for help and look for a way to safely rescue the swimmer.

2. Someone has fallen through the ice and the obvious risk is the one you should be worried about: you and the others breaking through and falling in as well. Clear the ice. Call for help. Look for devices such as ropes or sticks that can be used for a rescue.

3. If there are reports that someone has already been bitten by a snake, then the snake (or other snakes) might still be around, especially around the rocks. The patient should be moved to a clearing where both you and the patient will have less chance of further bites.

Short Answer

1. Passive rewarming is always permitted. Active rewarming may be permitted if the patient is alert and responsive, medical direction orders it, and transport time will be great.

2. Situations in which a patient may be suffering from hypothermia in addition to another condition include alcohol ingestion, underlying illness, overdose or poisoning, major trauma, outdoor resuscitation, and decreased ambient temperature.

3. Initially, the skin of the affected area appears white and waxy. As the condition progresses to actual freezing, the skin turns mottled or blotchy, the color turns from white to grayish-yellow, and finally changes to grayish-blue. Swelling and blistering may occur.

4. A patient suspected of having a heat emergency with moist, pale, and cool skin should be managed as follows:
   • Remove the patient to a cooler environment.
   • Administer oxygen.
   • Remove clothing and cool the patient by fanning.
   • Put the patient in supine position, keeping him at rest.
   • If responsive and not nauseated, give the patient water.
   • Apply moist towels over muscle cramps.
   • Transport.

5. A patient suspected of having a heat emergency with hot, dry skin should be managed as follows:
   • Remove the patient to the ambulance with the air conditioner on high.
   • Remove the patient's clothing; apply cool packs to the neck, groin, and armpits. Fan aggressively.
   • Administer oxygen.
   • Transport immediately.

6. The proper care for a patient with a snakebite includes:
   • Call medical direction.
   • Treat for shock and conserve body heat.
   • Keep the patient calm.
   • Control bleeding at the bite marks, if any. Clean the fang marks with soap and water.
   • Remove jewelry on the bitten extremity.
   • Immobilize the bitten extremity, perhaps using a splint.
   • Apply light constricting bands above and below the bite if ordered to do so by medical direction.
   • Transport and continually monitor the patient's vital signs.

Critical Thinking Exercises

1. First of all, always assess the patient's level of consciousness early so you have a baseline upon which to compare changes if they occur during later reassessments of the patient. A hypothermic patient developing an altered mental status may become difficult to manage. The patient may become drowsy, difficult to arouse, and unwilling or unable to follow commands or do even the simplest activities. The patient may become irrational, drift into a stuporous state, or actually start removing his blankets or clothing. A patient that is not alert will not be able to take warm fluids. Transporting a patient in this condition by snowmobile may be too risky and needs to be weighed against the risks of staying on-scene and performing passive rewarming.

2. A patient suffering from a heat emergency that exhibits hot skin rather than cool skin is in serious trouble. The body's temperature-regulating mechanism has failed; therefore, the body can no longer rid itself of excessive heat. This is sometimes known as heat stroke. Normally, temperature is regulated by a number of mechanisms, including perspiration and evaporative heat loss. However, if the patient begins to exhibit hot skin—whether dry or moist—the potential for a true emergency exists.

3. As you first observe the scene of the capsized boat, you must immediately take a number of things into consideration including your own safety and the safety of the others who have started swimming out to the site. Without delay, conduct a scene size-up to include the following:

   - Check for scene safety. If you are not a trained rescuer in water safety, it is probably not prudent for you to attempt the rescue. You won't be any good to those at the scene if you become a victim yourself.
   - Take Standard Precautions, if possible.
   - Try to determine the mechanism of injury.
   - Try to determine the number of patients. You should probably include the people swimming out to the boat who are acting as rescuers since they may become victims themselves.
   - Decide what resources you want to call for. Since you're at a public lake and others are around (and screaming), you may not be the only one calling for help. Think quickly about how you want to frame your report before making the call. Aside from asking for additional help, think also about the equipment you might need including oxygen, backboards, or blankets.

Pathophysiology to Practice

1. Altered mental status results when the electrical system of the brain malfunctions. This occurs when the body temperature falls to about 92°F—which indicates significant hypothermia. Rapid active rewarming in these patients can cause serious cardiac and circulatory complications. Therefore, an altered mental status in a patient who may be hypothermic is a contraindication to active rewarming. Passive rewarming is indicated instead.

2. About 65 percent of the body's cooling mechanisms involve the skin. When the skin is hot, you know that the cooling mechanisms have failed and the patient is in serious condition. He must be cooled rapidly and aggressively to prevent long-term neurological damage and death.

Street Scene Questions

1. Besides the obvious (ABCs, etc.), you should suspect hypothermia as well as other underlying problems such as malnutrition or untreated medical conditions. Because of the patient's situation, he is at risk of pneumonia and respiratory infections as well as medical conditions suggested by the signs and symptoms (stroke, trauma from a fall, and so on).

2. Basically, the patient needs complete primary and secondary assessments. As with all patients, assess the ABCs, make sure the patient's minute volume for breathing is adequate, and consider the use of supplemental oxygen. Once the primary assessment is complete and immediate care is initiated, take a complete set of baseline vital signs. Because the patient was found outside on a cold night, he needs to be assessed for hypothermia. Try

to determine the patient's orientation to time and place and other items in a past medical history. You should utilize a detailed head-to-toe survey to determine whether the patient has other medical problems or has sustained a traumatic fall.

3. Active rewarming in the field is not recommended. However, you can initiate passive rewarming. For example, remove all the patient's wet clothing and wrap the patient in one or more blankets. Consider a thermal (space) blanket as an outer shell. The patient's head should be covered to prevent additional heat loss. Unless recommended by medical direction and/or local protocol, do not apply hot packs or administer warm fluids in the prehospital setting. The exceptions include rare cases of long or delayed transport time and then only with approval from medical direction. Reassess the patient frequently because, even with passive warming, an unresponsive patient or patient suffering from extreme hypothermia can downgrade rapidly.

4. Take the patient's vital signs as often as every 5 minutes. Realize that the more hypothermic the patient, the harder it is to take vital signs. Heart rate and respirations can fall "below normal," but the patient may still sustain the rate and respirations needed to survive. As the saying goes, "Hypothermic patients should not be considered dead until they are warm and dead." When a person becomes hypothermic, he can sometimes survive neurologically intact for a significant period of time after vital signs have become depressed.

5. Hypothermic patients should be handled gently. "Rough" handling can result in ventricular fibrillation. Always keep a defibrillator (AED) close to the patient throughout transport.

Chapter 34 Obstetric and Gynecologic Emergencies
Critical Decision Making

1. This baby is coming—and quickly. Prepare for delivery at the scene.

2. This baby will likely wait. Ask the mother about feeling the need to push and if she feels like she must move her bowels. In the absence of either of these, you should make it to the hospital.

3. Transport this patient. Since there has been no significant change over 8 hours and there are no signs of imminent delivery, transport is the correct decision.

Short Answer

1. The anatomical structures associated with pregnancy are:
   - The ovaries–produce the ova.
   - The fallopian tubes–transport the ova to the uterus and are the site of fertilization.
   - The uterus–the muscular structure that houses the fetus during pregnancy.
   - The placenta–the vascular organ that perfuses and nourishes the fetus during pregnancy.
   - The vagina–the birth canal.

2. The three stages of labor are:
   - Stage 1–start of contractions to full dilation of the cervix.
   - Stage 2–full dilation of the cervix to birth of the fetus.
   - Stage 3–birth to expulsion of the placenta.

3. Prepare the mother for delivery by controlling the scene and the mother's privacy. Ask bystanders to leave. In addition to gloves, put on a gown, cap, mask, and eye protection. Place the mother on the floor, elevate the buttocks with a blanket or pillow, and have the mother lie with her knees drawn up and spread apart. Use sterile sheets or towels to drape the area and position the obstetric kit within easy reach.

4. To resuscitate a newly born infant, the baby should initially be dried, warmed, and stimulated. If that is not enough, administer supplemental oxygen. Positive pressure ventilation and chest compressions follow immediately if other initial measures are unsuccessful.

5. Complications of delivery include breech presentations such as a foot, hand, or buttocks presenting first. Prolapsed cord occurs when the umbilical cord presents prior to the baby. Placenta previa occurs when the placenta blocks the birth canal and can be harmed by the presenting fetus.

6. Predelivery emergencies include eclampsia, where seizures occur, and placental abruptions, where the placenta prematurely detaches from the uterine wall, causing massive internal bleeding.

Critical Thinking Exercises

Because the patient does not have the urge to push or move her bowels and because she is not crowning, there is likely time to transport her to the hospital (although clearly individual circumstances may dictate different plans). Consider also the fact that this is her first pregnancy, which typically takes longer to progress.

Pathophysiology to Practice

1. Vital sign changes that occur with pregnancy include the following: respirations typically increase slightly, blood pressure drops slightly (but can be high), and pulse generally increases.

2. Shock may be more difficult to recognize as vital signs that typically indicate compensation (fast pulse and increased respirations) may already be present under normal circumstances.

3. The severity of vaginal bleeding may be assessed by asking the patient how many pads she has needed to use. The chief concern with vaginal bleeding is not external hemorrhage, but rather the bleeding that is occurring internally.

4. The priorities of assessing and treating a neonate include maintaining warmth while assuring airway, breathing, and circulation.

Street Scene Questions

1. Once safety has been assured, the first priority is to make contact with the patient and assess the status of what sounded like an imminent delivery.

2. You should request ALS, since assistance in treating what may be multiple patients is never a bad idea.

3. In addition to the traditional SAMPLE history, ask the patient how far along the pregnancy is, whether there have been any problems with the pregnancy, and whether the mother has any previous medical problems.

4. Immediate care for the newborn should include suctioning of the mouth and nose, drying, warming, and stimulating.

5. Important maternal care includes providing emotional support, monitoring for excessive hemorrhage, and assessing vital signs. Allowing the baby to begin breast feeding may also help the uterus to contract and stop bleeding.

Chapter 35 Pediatric Emergencies
Critical Decision Making

1. Serious. The patient's limpness is an immediate flag that something is wrong. This is called poor muscle tone and is a serious finding. The upset mother is also a piece in the puzzle.

2. Less serious. The fact that the little girl is "screaming" means that she can move air in and out. Clinging to her mother indicates muscle tone and an appropriate mental status.

3. Serious (until more information can be obtained). The fact that the child is holding his injured arm and clinging to his mother is good. Look for his mental status and why he is quiet before making a final determination. If you approach him and he turns shyly into his mother, you may upgrade this to less serious.

Short Answer

1. Psychological/social characteristics found with each of the following ages might include:
   - 2 year old–Stranger anxiety and separation anxiety may suggest you allow the parent to hold the child during the exam when possible. Fear and increasing independence require that you explain procedures in simple terms.
   - 6 year old–Separation anxiety suggests you keep a parent present. Fear of punishment and pain requires a simple explanation of the procedures. Allow simple decision making.

- 15 year old–Peer pressure suggests you respect modesty and separate from crowds. Independence allows for an adult-like exam, but expect the patient to regress to earlier stages under duress. Allow for decision making.

2. When trying to calm a child during assessment and treatment, always try to identify yourself simply; let the child know that someone has called his parents; let the child have any nearby toy that he may want; kneel or sit at the child's eye level; smile; touch the child; do not use any equipment on the child without first explaining what you will do with it; stop occasionally to find out if the child understands; and never lie. Parents can be calmed by simply explaining what is going on. Take time to update them on their child's status. When possible, involve them in assessment and treatment.

3. The pediatric general assessment is organized as in the pediatric assessment triangle. It includes observation of appearance, work of breathing, and skin color.

4. Upper airway disorders are typically characterized by stridor, difficulty speaking, and barking coughs. Lower airway disorders typically are characterized by wheezing. It is important to distinguish between these disorders as treatments are very different. For example, lower airway disorders can be treated with inhaled bronchodilators (where protocols allow). This type of medication is typically ineffective in treating upper airway disorders.

5. Pediatric trauma patients should essentially be treated like any other trauma patient. Treatment of primary assessment problems will always take priority. However, anatomical and physiological differences must be accounted for. For example, the large head may require padding under the body to achieve neutral position during spinal immobilization. Since pediatric bones flex more than they break, fractures are less common. Nonetheless, internal injuries may be present.

6. Even if child abuse is suspected, emergency medical treatment is always the first priority. Do not let other concerns interfere with providing immediate, necessary care. Once care has been provided, contact law enforcement and/or your local child protective services (always follow local guidelines and protocols). Objectively document all your findings.

Critical Thinking Exercises

First and foremost, consider that any motor vehicle vs. pedestrian collision may be serious. Assume the worst. With a child, you must consider that the vehicle is capable of impacting more body surface area (considering the large car and the small child). Consider also the child's relatively exposed abdominal organs and the flexible chest wall. There exists a massive potential for serious injury. When approaching the child, consider stranger anxiety. This child will be afraid. You will also need to think about the need to reach out to the parents.

Pathophysiology to Practice

The key differences in the anatomy and physiology of infants and children with regard to the following include:

1. Head–Infants and children have heads that are much heavier relative to the rest of their body and their neck muscles are less developed. Brain tissue is thinner and softer. In addition, the fontanelles (the cranial sutures) may still be present in children up to 18 months old.

2. Airway and respiratory system–The tongue is proportionally larger, there are more abundant secretions in the mouth and airway, and the baby (deciduous) teeth are temporary. The nose and face are more flat than in adults. In infants and children, the trachea is shorter, narrower, and more flexible. Kids also have much shorter necks. Respiratory rates tend to be much faster. Infants and children are "nose breathers," meaning that they primarily rely on their most upper airways for ventilation.

3. Chest–Infants and children have more flexible ribs.

4. Abdomen–Infants and children tend to be abdominal breathers. In addition, some abdominal organs like the spleen and liver protrude forward, forming a characteristic "pot belly."

5. Body surface–Kids have more surface area, meaning that they have a larger body surface relative to their body mass. For example, their head is twice the size (as a percentage of surface area) as an adult.

6. Blood volume–The blood volume in infants and children is significantly less than those of larger people.

For the previous elements, you might have to adjust your assessment and/or treatment to account for the differences as follows:

7. Head–There is a higher incidence of head trauma in infants and children because of the disproportion between their heavier head and the rest of the body. Their weaker neck muscles also contribute to them not being able to control their head as well when they fall. Because brain tissue is thinner and softer, kids are often susceptible to serious brain injury. A sunken fontanelle may be a sign of dehydration, whereas a bulging fontanelle may be a sign of intracranial pressure. However, a bulging fontanelle might be perfectly normal in a screaming or crying child.

8. Airway and respiratory system–Because of their larger tongue and abundant secretions, maintaining an open, patent airway in these patients at all times is essential. In addition, the portion of the airway you can't visualize may be even more problematic. Because their trachea is more flexible, any flexion or extension of their head in any direction can actually crimp their trachea closed; sometimes a more neutral but slightly tilted head position works best. Also, their teeth can become easily dislodged and block the airway. Because they are nose breathers, a nasal obstruction can also impair breathing. The shape of their face and nose often makes it difficult to obtain an adequate mask seal when ventilating. Because the respiratory rates of infants and children are much faster, they often fatigue easily and will progress into respiratory failure much quicker. Any child who appears tired from breathing is exhibiting a very ominous sign.

9. Chest–Because infants and children have more flexible ribs, they can be susceptible to traumatic forces to underlying organs (like the lungs) even if the ribs may not show obvious signs of fracture.

10. Abdomen Kids are very reliant on their diaphragm to breathe. This can make it harder to assess breathing difficulty because it is often challenging to assess a child's abdominal area. In addition, many of the abdominal organs protrude forward and are susceptible to trauma.

11. Body surface–Because infants and children have a larger surface area, they become cold faster. Heat loss through their head is especially significant.

12. Blood volume–Because of the smaller blood volume in infants and children, any bleeding can become life-threatening if not immediately controlled.

Street Scene Questions

1. Your assessment plan must include scene safety, general impression (using the pediatric assessment triangle), and a thorough primary assessment.

2. Necessary equipment for a child who is not breathing includes airway and breathing equipment, suction, oxygen, and an AED. Many EMS providers also carry a pediatric bag containing pediatric-specific equipment. If available, this bag is important to bring in. Consider other equipment as local guidelines and protocols recommend.

3. Yes. ALS should be dispatched immediately.

4. Administration of oxygen is important in a patient that was previously not breathing. At this time, a thorough assessment is essential.

5. Assessment of this patient should include a primary assessment, a baseline set of vital signs, and a detailed assessment aimed at determining the nature of her apnea. Consider also conducting a SAMPLE history.

6. The incoming ALS unit should be notified that the patient is breathing. Detail primary assessment findings and a baseline set of vital signs. You might also include any other pertinent information obtained in your assessment.

Chapter 36 Geriatric Emergencies

Critical Decision Making

1. The patient may be taking medications that lower her heart rate. Beta blockers and calcium channel blockers may be the culprits here.

2. Temperature regulation and response in the elderly are diminished. The elderly patient with flu may not spike a fever as would a younger patient with a similar condition.

3. The elderly don't perceive pain the same as younger adults and children. It is more common than not for an elderly patient to have a silent (without chest pain) heart attack.

Short Answer

1. Place yourself where the patient can see you. Try to be at the same level as the patient, even if it means crouching or kneeling. Speak loudly, slowly, clearly, and distinctly. Ask just one question at a time. Give the patient plenty of time to respond to your questions.

2. Ask how the patient is different compared to a week ago.

3. The most common medical conditions include cardiac and respiratory problems and neurological problems like stroke. Falls are the most common mechanism of injury.

4. Some causes of altered mental status in geriatric patients include adverse medication effects, hypoglycemia, stroke, infection, and hypothermia.

Critical Thinking Exercises

1. Assess and care for the patient as you would any patient with a suspected hip fracture. Immobilize the patient to a backboard, taking care to pad the board to accommodate any skeletal abnormalities. Handle the patient carefully to avoid causing further injuries.

2. Your first priority is assessing the patient, providing treatment, and preparing him for transport. Follow any mandatory reporting laws that apply in your area, but at a minimum, report the conditions in which the patient was found to hospital staff.

Pathophysiology to Practice

1. Elderly patients may not be able to increase their heart rate or respiratory rates, or vasoconstrict to improve perfusion. The expected signs of tachycardia and tachypnea may not be present. The patient may not be diaphoretic as expected. Preexisting high blood pressure results in what appears to be a normal measurement, despite inadequate perfusion.

2. The patient's story does not seem plausible, but her ability to give accurate information should not be completely discounted. She will likely be able to tell you her current symptoms, but may be confused about medications and medical history. Confirm the information with another source.

3. The combination of fever, increased respiratory and heart rate, decreased blood pressure, and decreased oxygenation, along with diminished lung sounds in the right lower lung, make pneumonia the most likely cause of the patient's condition. Infection, hypoxia, and hypoperfusion can all contribute to confusion in this patient.

4. For each of the following patients, these conditions are most likely:
   - A 75-year-old complaining of weakness and tiredness that has worsened for three days and who sleeps in a recliner at night likely has congestive heart failure.
   - A 72-year-old complaining of tiredness and dyspnea that has worsened for one week and who takes ibuprofen for arthritis likely has gastrointestinal bleeding.
   - A 65-year-old diabetic complaining of nausea, vomiting, weakness, and not feeling well since this morning may be having a heart attack.
   - An 80-year-old who becomes confused intermittently during the day with a history of hypertension and prostate cancer may have congestive heart failure.
   - A 77-year-old taking aspirin daily with a history of heart attack and vomiting "dark stuff" today is likely having gastrointestinal bleeding.

Street Scene Questions

1. The ABCs are the first concern in regard to care and treatment for this patient. Because the patient is showing signs and symptoms of respiratory distress, the first priority is to ensure that the patient has a patent airway. Although the patient is talking, there may be problems with airway position, mucous blockage, and dentures. Therefore, the airway must be checked and monitored (take vital signs frequently) with corrective action taken as required. In regard to breathing, the patient needs oxygen immediately. Be prepared to assist with ventilations. If ALS is not immediately available, then consider prompt transport.

2. After the initial exam, perform the history and physical exam. Ask the patient about his previous history. Because he is having trouble talking, this may not work well and you may need to search the apartment for information that is written down somewhere, or call a relative or neighbor who can provide more information. It's important to remember that either diverting attention from the "sick" patient or delaying transport too long is probably not in the patient's best interest and the remainder of the patient's history needs to be obtained at the hospital. Make sure that patient doesn't have any other presenting problems that require your immediate attention. Continued monitoring of his vital signs should also occur during this part of the assessment. Complete a detailed assessment as time permits.

3. The fact that the apartment is messy may indicate that this patient may not be taking very good care of his own medical needs, such as diet and medication compliance. In addition, the messiness may mean that it is not regularly cleaned, which could trigger episodes of asthma. This information is important to pass on to the hospital to help in making decisions about discharge planning when they decide to send this patient home, as he may need some type of support services.

4. The assessment indicates that this patient may worsen; therefore, you need to provide ventilatory assistance with a bag-valve mask (BVM) with supplemental oxygen. The vital signs and level of consciousness need to be monitored closely and the BVM prepared so ventilatory assistance can be offered immediately, if indicated. Prepare the patient for immediate transport. Monitor closely so you know when the nonrebreather mask is no longer adequate and the BVM must be used.

5. In addition to vital signs, see if the patient has more ease speaking. If the patient seems more alert and can answer questions better than before, try to elicit some history from the patient. Ask whether he has any pain or discomfort and any other complaints besides the breathing difficulty. Repeat the vital signs every five minutes.

6. Because the patient's living situation appears to be in disarray, he may lack family, friends, or sufficient social support to care for himself adequately. It's important to share this information with the appropriate personnel in the emergency department so that referrals to social services can be generated and a plan for his discharge can be coordinated.

Chapter 37 Emergencies for Patients with Special Challenges
Critical Decision Making

1. The patient's family is the first place to look for answers. You may also contact medical direction for advice. Many devices have an obvious switch to turn it off.

2. In this case, the patient may be the best source of information. Although you should be considerate of the pain she is in, she will be able to answer your questions about how the dialysis works and also give you information on how best to move her with minimal pain.

3. The parents or visiting health care workers are the best source of information. Since health care workers aren't always present, parents are trained in operation and troubleshooting the devices. If the ventilator can't be transported, transport the patient without the ventilator and ventilate the patient through the trach tube en route. Be sure to alert the hospital that you are about to arrive with a patient who needs a ventilator.

Short Answer

1. The following are advanced medical devices that may be found in homes of patients with special challenges:
   - Respiratory devices
     - Continuous positive airway pressure (CPAP)
     - Tracheostomy tube
     - Home ventilator
   - Cardiac devices
     - Implanted pacemaker
     - Automatic implanted cardiac defibrillator (AICD)
     - Left ventricular assist device (LVAD)

- Gastro-urinary devices
  - Nasogastric (NG) tube
  - Gastric tube (G-tube)
  - Urinary catheters
  - Ostomy bags
  - Peritoneal dialysis
- Central IV catheters
  - Peripherally inserted central catheter (PICC) lines
  - Central venous lines (Groshong®, Hickman®, Broviac®)
  - Implanted port (Port-a-Cath®, Mediport®)
- Devices to assist physical impairment
  - TDD/TTY phone
  - Computer that speaks words
  - Cane, walker, or brace
  - Wheelchair

2. Obesity is associated with an increased risk for cancer, diabetes, hypertension, heart attack, stroke, liver and gallbladder disease, arthritis, sleep apnea, and respiratory problems.

3. To clear a blockage in a tracheostomy tube, carefully insert a whistle-tip suction catheter. Determine the correct depth of insertion by measuring the suction tubing against the length of the obturator, which is the same length as the trach tube itself. If you can't locate the obturator for measurement, stop insertion of the catheter when you feel resistance. Suction as the catheter is being withdrawn, using a twisting motion as it is slowly removed. If the patient requires further suctioning (indicated by visible or audible mucus), insert the suction tip into a container of sterile water to remove any mucus left in the catheter, and then repeat. If the patient is on a ventilator, he may need to be ventilated by BVM between suctioning.

4. In the case of a mechanical failure, or during transport of the patient, a bag-valve-mask device can take over the function of the ventilator. During this procedure, you should adjust the rate, volume, and pressure of the BVM to the patient's comfort level. This can be done with guidance from the patient. If the patient can't provide guidance, observe for adequate chest rise and improving skin color. (*NOTE:* If the BVM does not fit the tube attachment, use the face mask from the BVM to cover the stoma and secure the mask to provide a good seal against the neck, then ventilate as normal.)

5. Homelessness can be associated with mental health problems, malnutrition, substance abuse, HIV/AIDS, tuberculosis, bronchitis and pneumonia, environmental emergencies, wounds, and skin infections.

6. A mnemonic to use when dealing with patients who have autism is ABCS: awareness, basic, calm, and safety. These mean:
   - **A**wareness: be aware that ASD patients behave and react differently from most patients.
   - **B**asic: keep instructions, questions, treatments, and the environment simple.
   - **C**alm: be calm and patient; don't lose your temper, yell, or try to force the patient.
   - **S**afety: as much as possible, interact with the patient in his familiar surroundings where he feels safe.

7. The first thing that should be done when approaching the patient is to determine his ability to hear and/or speak. If a hearing loss patient can read lips, then use this approach. If not, then communicate by writing questions and information on a piece of paper. TDD/TTY phones, if available, can be used to relay information. These approaches will also work for patients who are unable to speak. In addition, some patients who are aphasic (unable to speak) may have a computer that speaks words they type into the device.

Critical Thinking Exercises

1. The fistula may be ruptured, causing significant blood loss, which is indicated by swelling at the site. Apply direct pressure and do not release it until advised by a physician to do so.

2. The patient's signs, symptoms, and circumstances likely indicate an infection that may be leading to septic shock. The initial patient care concerns are the patient's airway, breathing, oxygenation, and circulation. The nursing home staff can assist you in preparing the feeding tube, colostomy bag, and urinary catheter for transport. The urinary catheter can be temporarily placed at the patient's level to move her, but should be positioned lower than the patient for transport.

3. If an airway or ventilation device has failed, provide an open airway (use suction as necessary) and use a bag-valve-mask device to ventilate. If a pacemaker or AICD has failed, provide CPR and use the AED as indicated by the patient's condition.

4. If at all possible, you must allow the dog to accompany the patient. You may refuse only if the dog is a threat to you or others.

5. Understanding that this young patient has autism, think about how you can implement the *ABCS* mnemonic. First, simply have an *awareness* that the patient will likely react differently than most. Second, keep your instructions and questions *basic* and your treatment simple. Third, be as *calm* as possible and avoid adding to the patient's level of anxiety. Finally, try to keep the patient in an environment that is *safe* and comfortable, preferably a place she recognizes and is used to.

Pathophysiology to Practice

1. The homeless and poor may be malnourished, live in unsanitary conditions, and may not have been able to seek help for health problems early in their course.

2. A congenital condition is one that is present at birth, such as certain heart defects. An acquired disease occurs after birth and may be the result of exposure to an infectious disease, another medical condition, or trauma. Acquired diseases include AIDS and atherosclerotic heart disease.

3. The lack of sensation means that the patient cannot feel pain associated with excess pressure on the skin, or with developing sores. If he is not properly cared for, he may not be moved often enough to relieve pressure on the tissues to prevent development of bedsores. Weakness of the chest muscles can impair the cough reflex, making it difficult to clear infectious material from the airway, resulting in respiratory infections.

Street Scene Questions

1. The ABCs are the first concern in regard to the care and treatment of this patient. Ensure the patient has a patent airway and assess for problems with positioning or mucous blockage. The airway must be checked and monitored (take vital signs frequently), with corrective action taken as necessary. In regard to breathing, the patient needs oxygen immediately. Be prepared to assist with ventilations. If ALS is not immediately available, then consider prompt transport.

2. After the initial exam, perform the history and physical exam. Ask the patient's aunt about Amber's past medical history. If possible, determine the onset of the problem, including whether it was sudden or gradual, and any associated observations made by the caregiver. Information about the facility that normally treats Amber may allow you to contact them directly, if needed, for guidance.

3. Continue to reassess the patient's skin color, airway, respiratory status, and pulse.

4. If Amber has special equipment that you cannot provide (such as extra suction catheters in the appropriate size), you should take them with you. Ask the aunt whether the parents left instructions about equipment that needs to accompany Amber.

Chapter 38 EMS Operations
Critical Decision Making

1. Park uphill and upwind at potential chemical incidents. You must also be aware of the risk of explosion (e.g., a propane car) and park a significant distance away until the hazards are dealt with. Patients may be brought to you in a safe zone.

2. Park past the collision. On an interstate scene you should have a blocking vehicle (e.g., a fire engine or highway department barricade truck) between you and oncoming traffic. By parking past the scene, you will be able to load the patient with the safety of the blocking vehicles behind you.

3. Stage out of sight from the residence and far enough away so any dangerous persons won't come from the scene to you. Drive to the scene only when advised the police have secured it.

Short Answer

1. The five phases of an ambulance call are:
- Preparing for the ambulance call.
- Receiving and responding to a call.
- Transferring the patient to the ambulance.
- Transporting the patient to the hospital.
- Terminating the call.

2. At the beginning of each shift, spend the time to be sure that you, your vehicle, and your equipment are ready to respond. Talk with the off-going crew, get a brief shift report, and learn about any issues that might have come up with the ambulance or equipment during their shift. Complete a thorough bumper-to-bumper inspection of the ambulance using a checklist provided by your service. Inspect the vehicle and the equipment.

3. There are a number of very effective ways to reduce your chances of having a collision when driving an emergency vehicle. Come to a complete stop at intersections against a red light, minimize lights-and-siren responses whenever possible, and become familiar with your response area so you know where you're going when you receive an emergency dispatch. In addition, work to minimize all possible distractions when driving. Leave the radio communications, navigation, and mapping to your partner, and avoid eating, drinking, talking on the cell phone, or listening to music during an emergency response.

4. A patient-carrying device should have a minimum of three straps for holding the patient securely. The first strap is placed at the chest level, the second strap is placed at the hip or waist level, and the third strap is placed around the lower extremities. Sometimes there is a fourth strap if two are crossed at the chest. Newer stretchers have straps that act as a harness to restrain the upper body.

5. Utilizing air rescue resources comes with some critical responsibilities for those responders on the scene, who must ensure a safe environment exists upon which the aircraft can land and re-launch. Prior to the arrival of the aircraft, set up a landing zone:
- The landing zone should be a minimum of 100-by-100 feet on a flat surface that is clear of wires, towers, vehicles, people, and loose objects that might fly up when the aircraft lands (responders often underestimate the power of the helicopter's down force). Once a site has been chosen, place one flare in an upwind position to allow the pilot to judge wind direction. During night operations, keep emergency lights on and shine headlights onto the landing zone (never skyward toward the pilot).
- Once the helicopter has landed, only approach the aircraft when escorted by flight personnel, and allow the helicopter crew to direct the loading of the patient. It is critical that all personnel be aware of their position compared to the tail rotor of the aircraft and avoid this area at all times.

Critical Thinking Exercises

1. Equipment that should be available to carry onto a scene includes:
- Two-way radio
- Portable oxygen
- Oxygen administration equipment, BVM, airways, and masks
- Pulse oximeter
- Automatic external defibrillator (AED)
- Cervical collars, head immobilization device, backboards, and splints

- Dressings, gauze, bandages, tape, cold packs, and burn sheets
- Obstetrical kit
- Blood pressure cuff, stethoscope, shears, flashlight, blanket, towels, triage tags, bedpan, and urinal
- Infection control equipment such as gloves, eye protection, face protection, gowns, shoe covers, and N-95 or N-100 masks
- Protective helmet for highway operations, reflective outerwear, fire extinguisher, and hazmat guide

2. Items that are retrieved regularly (like the blood pressure cuff, stethoscope, and oxygen masks) for routine calls should be placed in a bag or "jump kit" in the vehicle near the rear or side door (or on top of the stretcher) so that, upon arrival on the scene, your crew can exit the vehicle, retrieve the bag(s), and enter the scene quickly with the most essential equipment in hand. Equipment that is used infrequently (like the obstetrical kit, traction splint, and burn sheets) can be placed inside the vehicle in a more secure location where it can be retrieved under those special circumstances.

3. Special items that may be dictated by local requirements include:
- Advanced or alternative airways
- Glucose meter
- Specialized pediatric equipment like smaller blood pressure cuffs, stethoscopes, spinal immobilization equipment, and oxygen masks and airways
- Medications such as oral glucose, albuterol, nitroglycerin, and auto-injector Epi-Pens
- Specialty equipment related to specific interfacility transfer work
- Cellular telephone

Street Scene Questions

1. The first precaution is to make sure the vehicle has had a proper "pre-flight" check to ensure everything is in safe working order. Next, the driver needs to get into the driver seat with a "safety mindset" and drive defensively, which means driving cautiously and anticipating what other motorists will do. The driver must also drive with "due regard" for the safety of others. Although the laws may grant special privileges to emergency vehicle drivers, they don't excuse a driver from negligence.
- Control your speed and be mindful of road conditions.
- Stop at stop signs and traffic signals.
- Avoid driving with lights and sirens unless it's absolutely necessary.
- Unless the patient is critical, drive to the hospital "cold."
- Remember that the patient and EMTs in the patient compartment need a smooth ride.
- Remember that even with lights and sirens, motorists may not see or hear the ambulance in time. Drive accordingly.

2. Most medical conditions will not be adversely affected by an additional few minutes. It's often said that 95 percent of EMS responses do not require speed or lights and siren, so slow down. Ask yourself this: Is it really worth taking all this risk for a patient with a minor injury or illness to save a few minutes when he might wait in the ED for a few hours? "Hot" responses typically only save a few minutes. Is this really necessary?

3. Slow down and stop at intersections. Drive defensively, "cover the brake," and be prepared to stop! Most ambulance crashes occur at intersections. Proceeding through a traffic signal without stopping is very risky and likely to cause a crash. After the call, have a conversation with the driver about stopping at intersections and slowing down. In addition, have the driver let you operate the siren so he can concentrate on the driving.

4. Make sure the scene is safe, carry in the equipment needed for a possible cardiac arrest, take Standard Precautions, and begin with the ABCs.

5. Give the dispatcher an arrival report. The patient is alert, breathing, and in minimal distress. Advise whether other resources should be cancelled, upgraded, or downgraded in their response. A good arrival report lets the dispatcher and responding units understand the true nature of an incident.

Chapter 39 Hazardous Materials, Multiple-Casualty Incidents, and Incident Management

Critical Decision Making

1. Activate your MCI plan. Based on the fact that you see "dozens" of people, you may be looking at 25+ patients and more may still be inside. This is a large-scale multiple-casualty incident and must be treated as such. It is a bigger issue than simply calling for additional ambulances. This will require prolonged operations and resources. Be sure the hazmat team is activated.

2. Assume that you will need an ambulance and crew for each of the four critical patients. You may also need to call for fire department response for extrication or personnel assistance.

3. This may be a carbon monoxide situation. Assume that there are four patients—and you and your crew may now also fall into the patient category. Exit the building, taking the patients with you. Immediately call for additional ambulances and the fire department.

Short Answer

1. When giving an initial report of a hazardous materials incident, be sure to alert the dispatcher to the fact that you are dealing with a hazmat incident and then request appropriate support services. Try to identify the hazardous material by using binoculars to look for identifying signs, labels, or placards. If possible, try to report:
   - The material involved
   - Wind direction
   - Safe staging location
   - The number of fire and hazmat resources you think you will need
   - Who has information on the substance involved such as MSDS sheets

2. When involved in transportation, vehicles are required to have placards that can be referenced in the yellow emergency response guide. This not only helps identify the substance but also guides the medical care, evacuation, and emergency actions. Buildings may use the NFPA 704 system, which can advise responders about the flammability, danger, and reactivity of the substances inside. The real gold standard though is for the building owner, shipper, or keeper of the substance to provide responders with the MSDS or material safety data sheet. The biggest challenge in dealing with a hazmat situation is in accurately identifying the substance. The most complicated situations can often involve unknown substances or chemicals. In this situation, the hazmat team may have to do extensive work to determine the substance involved.

3. Care of a patient with a hazardous materials injury always starts with a scene size-up, scene safety, and the ABCs. In a hazmat situation, the critical determination is whether the patient poses a risk of secondary contamination to the rescuers. Any patient with a hazardous materials injury must be fully decontaminated by a qualified hazmat team before being turned over to the EMS personnel, regardless of the severity of his medical condition.

4. The major components and benefits of the Incident Management System are interoperability between responding agencies, clear lines of authority, and a management structure conducive to managing a large incident.

5. Overall, the role of EMS in a multiple-casualty incident is triage, treatment, and transportation. The role of the first arriving EMTs is to initiate their agency's incident management plan. Establish Command, do a scene size-up, give an arrival report to dispatch, request or cancel resources, and then begin triage-treatment-transportation activities.

6. Assigning priorities during triage allows limited resources to focus efforts on patients with the greatest needs. The process is focused on saving lives by putting effort into patients who are the most serious first. This gives the greatest number of people the greatest chance of survival.

7. The four priority categories of triage are:
   - Priority-1 (RED)—Treatable life-threatening conditions
   - Priority-2 (YELLOW)—Serious but non-life-threatening conditions

- Priority-3 (GREEN)—Walking wounded
- Priority-4 or 0 (BLACK)—Dead or expected to die

Critical Thinking Exercises

Establish a perimeter around the danger area and keep people out. Radio an arrival report to dispatch and request additional resources such as the power company, fire department, extrication, and additional EMS units. Put on personal protective equipment and position your vehicle in order to protect the scene and create a safe working area. This should be performed in a manner consistent with your local procedures.

Street Scene Questions

1. Given the complexity of the scene, it's important to "unify" the Command with both police and fire service supervisors when they arrive. Another approach might be to transfer overall "Incident Command" to either police or fire. This may allow EMS to better focus on the tactics needed for triage-treatment-transportation. However, when first on the scene and Command is established:
   - Put on an ICS bib and use ICS radio identifiers
   - Size-up the incident
   - Give an arrival report to dispatch
   - Develop a mental "incident action plan"
   - Request any additional resources that are needed
   - Determine how responding units will be used when they arrive
   - Position/stage the resources
   - Assign tactical roles such as extrication, treatment, and transportation

2. The triage officer is responsible to report back on exactly how many patients there are and their priority level. They also must ensure that patients have been properly tagged by priority: RED-YELLOW-GREEN-BLACK.

3. Depending on the number of EMS system resources available, this could be deemed a major incident. Once the number of patients and priority are known, dispatch should call the hospitals and determine how many patients each hospital can take by priority. In an urban area, it may be possible to distribute the patients to multiple hospitals. In rural settings, all the patients may be transported to the same hospital. In any case, notify them early to allow the hospitals as much time as possible to prepare for the surge of patients that will be arriving.

4. There is always a need for a safety officer, especially in this case. There are wires down, a fuel spill, fire hazard, extrication, and multiple casualties. If there isn't a dedicated person to assume the role of safety officer, then Command must assume that function and safety may suffer.

5. The method by which information is transmitted during an MCI depends on the local EMS system. Some systems limit radio traffic by relaying minimal information through dispatch to the hospital. Other systems establish a direct link and call the hospitals from the scene. It's important to understand how your local/regional procedure for MCI management works so that you can follow it effectively.

6. Cooperation with fire and police is essential. Coordinate resource requests to minimize radio traffic and dispatch overload. Share overall incident action plans and tactical objectives.

Chapter 40 Highway Safety and Vehicle Extrication

Critical Decision Making

1. A patient involved in a head-on crash who is unresponsive with a rapid pulse is an <u>unstable patient</u> and requires a <u>quick extrication</u>.

2. A patient who was rear-ended, alert, and oriented with stable vital signs is a <u>stable patient</u> with <u>time available</u> for the extrication.

3. A patient thrown from the front to the back seat during a collision with a rapid pulse and clammy skin is an <u>unstable patient</u> and requires a <u>quick extrication</u>.

Short Answer

1. Your role is the scene size-up, which involves scanning the scene for hazards, the number of patients, degree of entrapment, vehicle instability, and any risks to the rescuers posed by traffic. Although the EMS focus should be on triage-treatment-transportation, all ICS roles must be carried out by the first arriving EMTs if establishing Command. Whoever establishes Command must maintain it until it can be transferred to another agency or a higher-ranking official.

2. ANSI safety vests and helmets should be worn at the scene of a highway incident to improve your visibility to others.

3. EMS or firefighter turnout clothing, including a helmet and eye protection, should be worn during a vehicle extrication. Match the protective gear worn by others at the scene.

4. To deactivate the automobile air bags, disconnect the battery.

5. First try simple access methods like opening the door or rolling down a window. If those are unsuccessful, use complex access methods involving tools such as a spring-loaded punch, axes, or saws designed for window glass to gain access to your patient or patients. Protect patients from breaking glass.

Critical Thinking Exercises

1. Types of rescue specialty teams include vehicle rescue, water rescue, ice rescue, high-angle rescue, hazardous materials response, trench rescue, dive rescue, back country or wilderness rescue, farm rescue, and confined space rescue. One or more of these may be active in your area, depending on the characteristics of your community.

2. After considering the safety of yourself and others, your primary goal at the scene of a vehicle collision is assessment and care of the patient.

Street Scene Questions

1. Scene safety issues deal with both seen and unseen hazards. Although vehicle instability is an obvious safety issue for both the patient and the rescuers, you should suspect possible gasoline leaks and/or problems with the vehicle's electrical system.

2. The first and foremost concerns are checking for any leaking fluids, particularly gasoline, and stabilizing the vehicle. You might also consider disconnecting the battery. Once the vehicle is stabilized, you should look for the safest way of accessing the patient, making sure to safeguard both yourself and the injured driver. Before breaking a window, always check that the door on the less damaged side of the vehicle cannot be opened. If a window must be broken, make every effort to protect the patient from shards of glass, perhaps by using padding or insulating material for protection.

3. Yes, rapid extrication should be considered. Based upon the primary assessment of snoring respirations and level of responsiveness (response only to painful stimuli), the patient appears to be unstable. There is every indication for the need of respiratory assistance. The use of rapid extrication, of course, depends upon the ETA of the rescue team and advice from medical direction.

4. The assessment follows in ABC order. The snoring respirations must be corrected. In most cases, this will require a jaw-thrust maneuver (in a trauma patient) to move the tongue forward, while a second EMT applies a cervical collar. Next, evaluate the patient's respirations. At the very least, this patient should receive high-concentration oxygen by nonrebreather mask. Be prepared to assist ventilations with a bag-valve mask with an oxygen reservoir. Next, check the patient's circulation for external hemorrhage and overt signs and symptoms of internal bleeding. Because this is a trauma patient, you should then initiate a head-to-toe neurological assessment. Once this is completed, obtain a set of vital signs. A SAMPLE history can be taken if the patient regains consciousness. When these steps are completed, conduct a focused and detailed assessment as indicated by patient conditions.

Chapter 41 EMS Response to Terrorism

Critical Decision Making

1. Do not enter the area. The hazmat team should bring decontaminated patients to you. Do not allow contaminated patients or rescuers into your ambulance nor take contaminated patients to the hospital.

2. Do not enter the area until the area has been secured for stability and additional undetonated explosive devices. Terrorists may place secondary devices designed to harm rescuers.

Short Answer

1. The five most common types of terrorist incidents are chemical, biological, radiological, nuclear, and explosive. A chemical event is usually a gaseous material that is released into the atmosphere. This substance has properties that are very toxic or potentially fatal when inhaled. A biological substance is a bacteria, virus, or toxin that can cause immediate illness or death or a substance that can take time to incubate, making people sick in the process. A radiological event is when radiological material is released into the atmosphere. Depending on a number of factors such as proximity, quantity of the material, and potency, it can have an immediate or long-range impact on humans or animals. Nuclear devices can be very similar to radiological devices, but may have the added concern of incendiary potential that may do immediate harm to a large area depending on its size. An explosive device, such as a bomb, can cause injury from the initial explosion as well as the secondary damage caused by destruction from the explosion. In addition, these devices sometimes contain materials (e.g., nails) that are shot into the area of the explosion that can also cause harm.

2. A secondary device is one that goes off after the first device. For example, a device may be set off inside a building, and a secondary device is then set to explode in an area where people might congregate after exiting the building. EMS responders need to be alert to the fact that in a terrorist event there may be more than one device. Scene safety, including being alert to this fact, is a priority. Responders must try to stay clear from the area until it is deemed safe. When establishing staging and triage areas, make sure these areas have been secured and, if necessary, guarded during the entire event.

3. Some of the types of events that should trigger the EMT to be suspicious are symbolic and historical targets, public buildings or places of assembly, controversial businesses, and infrastructure systems.

4. The seven types of harm from an incendiary system are thermal, radiological, asphyxiation, chemical, etiological, mechanical, and psychological. The acronym for these is TRACEM-P.

5. The concept of time, distance, and shielding suggests you minimize the time you are in the area of possible risk at a dangerous scene, maximize the distance from the hazardous area, and use as much shielding as possible whether it be a vehicle, structure, or use of specialized protective clothing and protective breathing apparatus. The more shielding the better, so more than one method should be used when available.

6. Distance can be a helpful self-protection measure for biological incidents. The farther away from the immediate area of danger, the better (also pay attention to wind direction). Use of appropriate protective equipment may be another effective protection technique, particularly if a responder intends to get near or within the contaminated area. This may include use of specialized protective breathing equipment. Limiting the time in the contaminated area should also be a consideration.

7. Isolation can take on many forms at an incident where terrorism is suspected. Make sure that emergency responders and civilians don't get hurt by a secondary device; only permit those that have a need to be there and are wearing proper protective gear to enter inside the perimeter. This also allows for control in an area that is apt to be very chaotic. Notification is alerting the appropriate agencies that there is an event. Many times EMS is one of the first to arrive at an act of terrorism. Notifying additional resources and specialized

response units needs to occur quickly. Identification refers to the agent or material that might be involved. This is important information for protecting responders and making decisions on the types of protective equipment and barriers that are required. In addition, knowing the agent will help in determining how to handle decontamination. Therefore, determining what agents are involved needs to be a priority. Protection is done to shield critical assets from additional harm and damage. Responders must first ensure that they are protected. Once that is done, they must try to protect vehicles, equipment, and supplies.

Critical Thinking Exercises

1. The scene may not have been deemed safe yet. Emergency Medical Responders are often principal targets of a terrorist attack and it's possible that law enforcement wants to ensure there is no secondary device planted somewhere that might injure EMS responders.

2. Treating patients exposed to a nerve agent is delicate work as it is, but to see your own colleagues potentially become victims themselves is terrifying. Stop what you are doing, evacuate immediately, request help for your colleagues, and then report to the hazmat team for decontamination and treatment.

3. The ethnic background of the suspicious man is really irrelevant since many past terrorist incidents on American soil have been the responsibility of U.S. citizens. However, this gentleman appears very suspicious and your intuition tells you something is wrong. You should definitely report your observations immediately to the nearest authority since a suitcase could easily conceal any of the CBNRE agents intended to cause widespread harm to the travelling public.

Street Scene Questions (#1)

1. Indicators that this may be a suspicious incident include the multiple casualties, a "funny smell," and a radical group that has opposed construction.

2. The area should immediately have a perimeter established, for which law enforcement usually takes the primary responsibility. This process should also include determining an inner and outer perimeter. Notify other responding units of the danger in the area and instruct them not to enter.

3. Attempt to determine the mechanism of injury by starting with the initial clues of the smell, numerous victims, and symptoms of the victims. Ask if there is any construction material that might cause these symptoms when talking with the construction manager. See if there is a container that may have markings that can be called in to CHEMTREC for possible identification of the substance. If no container can be identified, then study the signs/symptoms of the ill/injured for possible clues that can be provided to Poison Control, which is a good resource for identification and specific cases.

4. Those who need to be in the inner perimeter (hot zone) need to have full protective equipment (specifically rated for hazmat), which includes proper protective breathing apparatus. Until the substance is identified and specific hazards and risks are known, nobody should enter without proper personal protective equipment (PPE).

Street Scene Questions (#2)

1. The first indicator that this is a suspicious event is the location of the incident (headquarters of a militant group), the next is that the fire is in a dead-end of an alley, and another is the wire that is observed stretched across the alley.

2. Everyone should retreat from the immediate area to a safe distance and shield themselves. Until the possible secondary device (wire across the alley) is deactivated by experts, the scene remains dangerous and unsafe. Another possibility is that there may be an explosive device in the car.

3. The first support agency is the police, who will establish a perimeter and protect civilians and responders. Then experts in explosive devices who can deactivate the device(s) are needed. Certain federal law enforcement agencies may also be needed to investigate.

GLOSSARY

abandonment leaving a patient after care has been initiated and before the patient has been transferred to someone with equal or greater medical training.

ABCs airway, breathing, and circulation.

abdominal quadrants four divisions of the abdomen used to pinpoint the location of a pain or injury: the right upper quadrant (RUQ), the left upper quadrant (LUQ), the right lower quadrant (RLQ), and the left lower quadrant (LLQ).

abortion spontaneous (miscarriage) or induced termination of pregnancy.

abrasion (ab-RAY-zhun) a scratch or scrape.

abruptio placentae (ab-RUPT-si-o plah-SENT-ta) a condition in which the placenta separates from the uterine wall; a cause of prebirth bleeding.

absorbed poisons poisons that are taken into the body through unbroken skin.

acetabulum (AS-uh-TAB-yuh-lum) the pelvic socket into which the ball at the proximal end of the femur fits to form the hip joint.

acromioclavicular (ah-KRO-me-o-klav-IK-yuh-ler) joint the joint where the acromion and the clavicle meet.

acromion (ah-KRO-me-on) process the highest portion of the shoulder.

activated charcoal a substance that adsorbs many poisons and prevents them from being absorbed by the body.

active rewarming application of an external heat source to rewarm the body of a hypothermic patient.

acute coronary syndrome (ACS) a blanket term used to represent any symptoms related to lack of oxygen (ischemia) in the heart muscle. Also called *cardiac compromise*.

acute myocardial infarction (AMI) (ah-KUTE MY-o-KARD-e-ul in-FARK-shun) the condition in which a portion of the myocardium dies as a result of oxygen starvation; often called a heart attack by laypersons.

adolescence stage of life from 13 to 18 years.

advance directive a DNR order; instructions written in advance of an event.

aerobic (air-O-bik) metabolism the cellular process in which oxygen is used to metabolize glucose. Energy is produced in an efficient manner with minimal waste products.

afterbirth the placenta, membranes of the amniotic sac, part of the umbilical cord, and some tissues from the lining of the uterus that are delivered after the birth of the baby.

agonal breathing irregular, gasping breaths that precede apnea and death.

air embolism an air or gas bubble in the bloodstream. The plural is air emboli. The more accurate term is *arterial gas embolism (AGE)*.

airway the passageway by which air enters or leaves the body. The structures of the airway are the nose, mouth, pharynx, larynx, trachea, bronchi, and lungs. *See also* patent airway.

allergen something that causes an allergic reaction.

allergic reaction an exaggerated immune response.

alveolar (al-VE-o-ler) ventilation the amount of air that reaches the alveoli.

alveoli (al-VE-o-li) the microscopic sacs of the lungs where gas exchange with the bloodstream takes place.

amniotic (am-ne-OT-ik) sac the "bag of waters" that surrounds the developing fetus.

amputation (am-pyu-TAY-shun) the surgical removal or traumatic severing of a body part, usually an extremity.

anaerobic (AN-air-o-bik) metabolism the cellular process in which glucose is metabolized into energy without oxygen. Energy is produced in an inefficient manner with many waste products.

anaphylaxis (an-ah-fi-LAK-sis) a severe or life-threatening allergic reaction in which the blood vessels dilate, causing a drop in blood pressure, and the tissues lining the respiratory system swell, interfering with the airway. Also called *anaphylactic shock*.

anatomical position the standard reference position for the body in the study of anatomy. In this position, the body is standing erect, facing the observer, with arms down at the sides and the palms of the hands forward.

anatomy the study of body structure.

anemia lack of a normal number of red blood cells in the circulation.

aneurysm (AN-u-rizm) the dilation, or ballooning, of a weakened section of the wall of an artery.

angina pectoris (AN-ji-nah [or an-JI-nah] PEK-to-ris) pain in the chest, occurring when blood supply to the heart is reduced and a portion of the heart muscle is not receiving enough oxygen.

angulated fracture fracture in which the broken bone segments are at an angle to each other.

anterior the front of the body or body part.

antidote a substance that will neutralize the poison or its effects.

aorta (ay-OR-tah) the largest artery in the body. It transports blood from the left ventricle to begin systemic circulation.

apnea (AP-ne-ah) no breathing.

appendix a small tube located near the junction of the small and large intestines in the right lower quadrant of the abdomen, the function of which is not well understood. Its inflammation, called appendicitis, is a common cause of abdominal pain.

arterial bleeding bleeding from an artery, which is characterized by bright red blood that is rapid, profuse, and difficult to control.

arteriole (ar-TE-re-ol) the smallest kind of artery.

artery any blood vessel carrying blood away from the heart.

artificial ventilation forcing air or oxygen into the lungs when a patient has stopped breathing or has inadequate breathing. Also called *positive pressure ventilation*.

aspirin a medication used to reduce the clotting ability of blood to prevent and treat clots associated with myocardial infarction.

assault placing a person in fear of bodily harm.

asystole (ay-SIS-to-le) a condition in which the heart has ceased generating electrical impulses.

atria (AY-tree-ah) the two upper chambers of the heart. There is a right atrium (which receives unoxygenated blood returning from the body) and a left atrium (which receives oxygenated blood returning from the lungs).

aura a sensation experienced by a seizure patient right before the seizure, which might be a smell, sound, or general feeling.

auscultation (os-kul-TAY-shun) listening. A stethoscope is used to auscultate for characteristic sounds.

autism spectrum disorders (ASD) developmental disorders that affect, among other things, the ability to communicate, report medical conditions, self-regulate behaviors, and interact with others.

auto-injector a syringe preloaded with medication that has a spring-loaded device that pushes the needle through the skin when the tip of the device is pressed firmly against the body.

automatic implanted cardiac defibrillator (AICD) a device implanted under the skin of the chest to detect any life-threatening dysrhythmia and deliver a shock to defibrillate the heart.

automatic transport ventilator (ATV) a device that provides positive pressure ventilations. It includes settings designed to adjust ventilation rate and volume, is portable, and is easily carried on an ambulance.

automaticity (AW-to-muh-TISS-it-e) the ability of the heart to generate and conduct electrical impulses on its own.

autonomic (AW-to-NOM-ik) nervous system the division of the peripheral nervous system that controls involuntary motor functions.

AVPU a memory aid for classifying a patient's level of responsiveness or mental status. The letters stand for alert, verbal response, painful response, unresponsive.

avulsion (ah-VUL-shun) the tearing away or tearing off of a piece or flap of skin or other soft tissue. This term also may be used for an eye pulled from its socket or a tooth dislodged from its socket.

bag-valve mask (BVM) a handheld device with a face mask and self-refilling bag that can be squeezed to provide artificial ventilations to a patient. It can deliver air from the atmosphere or oxygen from a supplemental oxygen supply system.

bandage any material used to hold a dressing in place.

bariatric having to do with patients who are significantly overweight or obese.

bariatrics the branch of medicine that deals with the causes of obesity, as well as its prevention and treatment.

base station a two-way radio at a fixed site such as a hospital or dispatch center.

battery causing bodily harm to or restraining a person.

behavior the manner in which a person acts.

behavioral emergency when a patient's behavior is not typical for the situation; when the patient's behavior is unacceptable or intolerable to the patient, his family, or the community; or when the patient may harm himself or others.

bilateral on both sides.

bladder the round sac-like organ of the renal system used as a reservoir for urine.

blood pressure monitor machine that automatically inflates a blood pressure cuff and measures blood pressure.

blood pressure the pressure caused by blood exerting force against the walls of blood vessels. Usually arterial blood pressure (the pressure in an artery) is measured. There are two parts: *diastolic blood pressure* and *systolic blood pressure*.

blunt-force trauma injury caused by a blow that does not penetrate the skin or other body tissues.

body mechanics the proper use of the body to facilitate lifting and moving and prevent injury.

bonding the sense that needs will be met.

bones hard but flexible living structures that provide support for the body and protection to vital organs.

brachial (BRAY-key-al) artery artery of the upper arm; the site of the pulse checked during infant CPR.

brachial pulse the pulse felt in the upper arm.

bradycardia (BRAY-duh-KAR-de-uh) a slow pulse; any pulse rate below 60 beats per minute.

Braxton-Hicks (braks-tun-hiks) contractions irregular prelabor contractions of the uterus.

breech presentation when the baby's buttocks or both legs appear first during birth.

bronchi (BRONG-ki) the two large sets of branches that come off the trachea and enter the lungs. There are right and left bronchi. *Singular* bronchus.

bronchoconstriction (BRON-ko-kun-STRIK-shun) the contraction of smooth muscle that lines the bronchial passages that results in a decreased internal diameter of the airway and increased resistance to air flow.

calcaneus (kal-KAY-ne-us) the heel bone.

capillary (KAP-i-lair-e) a thin-walled, microscopic blood vessel where the oxygen/carbon dioxide and nutrient/waste exchange with the body's cells takes place.

capillary bleeding bleeding from capillaries, which is characterized by a slow, oozing flow of blood.

cardiac conduction system a system of specialized muscle tissues that conducts electrical impulses that stimulate the heart to beat.

cardiac muscle specialized involuntary muscle found only in the heart.

cardiac output the amount of blood ejected from the heart in 1 minute (heart rate × stroke volume).

cardiogenic shock shock, or lack of perfusion, brought on not by blood loss, but by inadequate pumping action of the heart. It is often the result of a heart attack or congestive heart failure.

cardiopulmonary resuscitation (CPR) actions taken to revive a person by keeping the person's heart and lungs working.

cardiovascular (KAR-de-o-VAS-kyu-ler) system the system made up of the heart (cardio) and the blood vessels (vascular); the *circulatory system*.

carotid (kah-ROT-id) arteries the large neck arteries, one on each side of the neck, that carry blood from the heart to the head.

carotid pulse the pulse felt along the large carotid artery on either side of the neck.

carpals (KAR-pulz) the wrist bones.

cartilage tough tissue that covers the joint ends of bones and helps to form certain body parts such as the ear.

cell phone a phone that transmits through the air instead of over wires so that the phone can be transported and used over a wide area.

cellular respiration the exchange of oxygen and carbon dioxide between cells and circulating blood.

central IV catheter a catheter surgically inserted for long-term delivery of medications or fluids into the central circulation.

central nervous system (CNS) the brain and spinal cord.

central pulses the carotid and femoral pulses, which can be felt in the central part of the body.

central rewarming application of heat to the lateral chest, neck, armpits, and groin of a hypothermic patient.

cephalic (se-FAL-ik) presentation when the baby appears head first during birth. This is the normal presentation.

cerebrospinal (suh-RE-bro-SPI-nal) fluid (CSF) the fluid that surrounds the brain and spinal cord.

cervix (SUR-viks) the neck of the uterus at the entrance to the birth canal.

chemoreceptors (ke-mo-re-cept-erz) chemical sensors in the brain and blood vessels that identify changing levels of oxygen and carbon dioxide.

chief complaint in emergency medicine, the reason EMS was called, usually in the patient's own words.

clavicle (KLAV-i-kul) the collarbone.

closed extremity injury an injury to an extremity with no associated opening in the skin.

closed wound an internal injury with no open pathway from the outside.

cold zone area where the Incident Command post and support functions are located.

combining form a word root with an added vowel that can be joined with other words, roots, or suffixes to form a new word.

Command the first on the scene to establish order and initiate the Incident Command System.

comminuted fracture a fracture in which the bone is broken in several places.

compartment syndrome injury caused when tissues such as blood vessels and nerves are constricted within a space as from swelling or from a tight dressing or cast.

compensated shock when the patient is developing shock but the body is still able to maintain perfusion. *See* shock.

compound a word formed from two or more whole words.

concussion mild closed head injury without detectable damage to the brain. Complete recovery is usually expected.

conduction the transfer of heat from one material to another through direct contact.

confidentiality the obligation not to reveal information obtained about a patient except to other health care professionals involved in the patient's care, or under subpoena, or in a court of law, or when the patient has signed a release of confidentiality.

congestive heart failure (CHF) the failure of the heart to pump efficiently, leading to excessive blood or fluids in the lungs, the body, or both.

consent permission from the patient for care or other action by the EMT.

constrict (kon-STRIKT) get smaller.

contamination contact with or presence of a material (contaminant) that is present where it does not belong and that is somehow harmful to persons, animals, or the environment.

continuous ambulatory peritoneal dialysis (CAPD) a gravity exchange process for peritoneal dialysis in which a bag of dialysis fluid is raised above the level of an abdominal catheter to fill the abdominal cavity and then lowered below the level of the abdominal catheter to drain the fluid out.

continuous cycler-assisted peritoneal dialysis (CCPD) a mechanical process for peritoneal dialysis in which a machine fills and empties the abdominal cavity of dialysis solution.

continuous positive airway pressure (CPAP) a form of noninvasive positive pressure ventilation (NPPV) consisting of a mask and a means of blowing oxygen or air into the mask to prevent airway collapse or to help alleviate difficulty breathing.

contraindications (KON-truh-in-duh-KAY-shunz) specific signs or circumstances under which it is not appropriate, and may be harmful, to administer a drug to a patient.

contusion (kun-TU-zhun) a bruise. In brain injuries, a bruised brain caused when the force of a blow to the head is great enough to rupture blood vessels.

convection carrying away of heat by currents of air, water, or other gases or liquids.

coronary (KOR-o-nar-e) arteries blood vessels that supply the muscle of the heart (myocardium).

coronary artery disease (CAD) diseases that affect the arteries of the heart.

cranium (KRAY-ne-um) the bony structure making up the forehead, top, back, and upper sides of the skull.

crepitation (krep-uh-TAY-shun) the grating sound or feeling of broken bones rubbing together.

crepitus (KREP-i-tus) a grating sensation or sound made when fractured bone ends rub together.

cricoid (KRIK-oid) cartilage the ring-shaped structure that forms the lower portion of the larynx.

cricoid pressure pressure applied to the cricoid ring to minimize air entry into the esophagus during positive pressure ventilation. Also called *Sellick maneuver.*

crime scene the location where a crime has been committed or any place that evidence relating to a crime may be found.

critical incident stress management (CISM) a comprehensive system that includes education and resources to both prevent stress and to deal with stress appropriately when it occurs.

critical thinking an analytical process that can help someone think through a problem in an organized and efficient manner.

crowning when part of the baby is visible through the vaginal opening.

crush injury an injury caused when force is transmitted from the body's exterior to its internal structures. Bones can be broken; muscles, nerves, and tissues damaged; and internal organs ruptured, causing internal bleeding.

cyanosis (SIGH-uh-NO-sis) a blue or gray color resulting from lack of oxygen in the body.

danger zone the area around the wreckage of a vehicle collision or other incident within which special safety precautions should be taken.

dead air space air that occupies the space between the mouth and alveoli but that does not actually reach the area of gas exchange.

decompensated shock when the body can no longer compensate for low blood volume or lack of perfusion. Late signs such as decreasing blood pressure become evident. *See* shock.

decompression sickness a condition resulting from nitrogen trapped in the body's tissues, caused by coming up too quickly from a deep, prolonged dive. A symptom of decompression sickness is "the bends," or deep pain in the muscles and joints.

decontamination a chemical and/or physical process that reduces or prevents the spread of contamination from persons or equipment; the removal of hazardous substances from employees and their equipment to the extent necessary to preclude foreseeable health effects.

defibrillation delivery of an electrical shock to stop the fibrillation of heart muscles and restore a normal heart rhythm.

dehydration (de-hi-DRAY-shun) an abnormally low amount of water in the body.

delirium tremens (duh-LEER-e-um TREM-uns) (DTs) a severe reaction that can be part of alcohol withdrawal, characterized by sweating, trembling, anxiety, and hallucinations. Severe alcohol withdrawal with the DTs can lead to death if untreated.

dermatome (DERM-uh-tohm) an area of the skin that is innervated by a single spinal nerve.

dermis (DER-mis) the inner (second) layer of skin, rich in blood vessels and nerves, found beneath the epidermis.

designated agent an EMT or other person authorized by a Medical Director to give medications and provide emergency care. The transfer of such authorization to a designated agent is an extension of the Medical Director's license to practice medicine.

detailed physical exam an assessment of the head, neck, chest, abdomen, pelvis, extremities, and posterior of the body to detect signs and symptoms of injury. It differs from the rapid trauma assessment only in that it also includes examination of the face, ears, eyes, nose, and mouth during the examination of the head. It may be done less rapidly, and it may be done en route to the hospital after earlier on-scene assessments and interventions are completed.

diabetes mellitus (di-ah-BEE-tez MEL-i-tus) also called "sugar diabetes" or just "diabetes," the condition brought about by decreased insulin production or the inability of the body cells to use insulin properly. The person with this condition is a diabetic.

diabetic ketoacidosis (di-ah-BET-ic KEY-to-as-id-DO-sis) (DKA) a condition that occurs as the result of high blood sugar (hyperglycemia), characterized by dehydration, altered mental status, and shock.

diagnosis a description or label for a patient's condition that assists a clinician in further evaluation and treatment.

dialysis the process by which toxins and excess fluid are removed from the body by a medical system independent of the kidneys.

diaphragm (DI-uh-fram) the muscular structure that divides the chest cavity from the abdominal cavity. A major muscle of respiration.

diastolic (di-as-TOL-ik) blood pressure the pressure remaining in the arteries when the left ventricle of the heart is relaxed and refilling.

differential diagnosis a list of potential diagnoses compiled early in the assessment of the patient.

diffusion a process by which molecules move from an area of high concentration to an area of low concentration.

digestive system system by which food travels through the body and is digested, or broken down into absorbable forms.

dilate (DI-late) get larger.

dilution (di-LU-shun) thinning down or weakening by mixing with something else. Ingested poisons are sometimes diluted by drinking water or milk.

direct carry a method of transferring a patient from bed to stretcher, during which two or more rescuers curl the patient to their chests, then reverse the process to lower the patient to the stretcher.

direct ground lift a method of lifting and carrying a patient from ground level to a stretcher in which two or more rescuers kneel, curl the patient to their chests, stand, then reverse the process to lower the patient to the stretcher.

disability a physical, emotional, behavioral, or cognitive condition that interferes with a person's ability to carry out everyday tasks, such as working or caring for oneself.

disaster plan a predefined set of instructions for a community's emergency responders.

dislocation the disruption or "coming apart" of a joint.

dissemination spreading.

distal farther away from the torso.

distention (dis-TEN-shun) a condition of being stretched, inflated, or larger than normal.

do not resuscitate (DNR) order a legal document, usually signed by the patient and his physician, which states that the patient has a terminal illness and does not wish to prolong life through resuscitative efforts.

domestic terrorism terrorism directed against the government or population without foreign direction.

dorsal referring to the back of the body or the back of the hand or foot. A synonym for posterior.

dorsalis pedis (dor-SAL-is PEED-is) artery artery supplying the foot, lateral to the large tendon of the big toe.

downers depressants, such as barbiturates, that depress the central nervous system, which are often used to bring on a more relaxed state of mind.

draw-sheet method a method of transferring a patient from bed to stretcher by grasping and pulling the loosened bottom sheet of the bed.

dressing any material (preferably sterile) used to cover a wound that will help control bleeding and prevent additional contamination.

drop report (or transfer report) an abbreviated form of the PCR that an EMS crew can leave at the hospital when there is not enough time to complete the PCR before leaving.

drowning the process of experiencing respiratory impairment from submersion/immersion in liquid, which may result in death, morbidity (illness or other adverse effects), or no morbidity

duty to act an obligation to provide care to a patient.

dyspnea (DISP-ne-ah) shortness of breath; labored or difficult breathing.

dysrhythmia (dis-RITH-me-ah) a disturbance in heart rate and rhythm.

early adulthood stage of life from 19 to 40 years.

eclampsia (e-KLAMP-se-ah) a severe complication of pregnancy that produces seizures and coma.

ectopic (ek-TOP-ik) pregnancy when implantation of the fertilized egg is not in the body of the uterus, occurring instead in the fallopian tube (oviduct), cervix, or abdominopelvic cavity.

edema (eh-DEE-muh) swelling associated with the movement of water into the interstitial space causing a buildup of fluid in the tissues.

electrolyte (e-LEK-tro-lite) a substance that, when dissolved in water, separates into charged particles.

embolism (EM-bo-lizm) blockage of a vessel by a clot or foreign material brought to the site by the blood current.

embryo (EM-bree-o) the baby from fertilization to 8 weeks of development.

EMS diagnosis/EMT diagnosis a description or label for a patient's condition, based on the patient's history, physical exam, and vital signs, that assists the EMT in further evaluation and treatment. An EMS diagnosis is often less specific than a traditional medical diagnosis.

end-stage renal disease (ESRD) irreversible renal failure to the extent that the kidneys can no longer provide adequate filtration and fluid balance to sustain life; survival with ESRD usually requires dialysis.

endocrine (EN-do-krin) system system of glands that produce chemicals called hormones that help to regulate many body activities and functions.

enteral (EN-tur-al) referring to a route of medication administration that uses the gastrointestinal tract, such as swallowing a pill.

epidermis (ep-i-DER-mis) the outer layer of the skin.

epiglottis (EP-i-GLOT-is) a leaf-shaped structure that prevents food and foreign matter from entering the trachea.

epilepsy (EP-uh-lep-see) a medical condition that causes seizures.

epinephrine (EP-uh-NEF-rin) a hormone produced by the body. As a medication, it constricts blood vessels and dilates respiratory passages and is used to relieve severe allergic reactions.

ethical regarding a social system or social or professional expectations for applying principles of right and wrong.

evaporation   the change from liquid to gas. When the body perspires or gets wet, evaporation of the perspiration or other liquid into the air has a cooling effect on the body.

evidence-based   description of medical techniques or practices that are supported by scientific evidence of their safety and efficacy, rather than merely on supposition and tradition.

evisceration (e-vis-er-AY-shun)   an intestine or other internal organ protruding through a wound in the abdomen.

exchange   one cycle of filling and draining the peritoneal cavity in peritoneal dialysis.

excited delirium   bizarre and/or aggressive behavior, shouting, paranoia, panic, violence toward others, insensitivity to pain, unexpected physical strength, and hyperthermia, usually associated with cocaine or amphetamine use. Also called *agitated delirium*.

exhalation (EX-huh-LAY-shun)   a passive process in which the intercostal (rib) muscles and the diaphragm relax, causing the chest cavity to decrease in size and air to flow out of the lungs. Also called *expiration*.

expiration   *see* exhalation.

exposure   the dose or concentration of an agent multiplied by the time, or duration.

expressed consent   consent given by adults who are of legal age and mentally competent to make a rational decision in regard to their medical well-being.

extremities (ex-TREM-i-teez)   the portions of the skeleton that include the clavicles, scapulae, arms, wrists, and hands (upper extremities) and the pelvis, thighs, legs, ankles, and feet (lower extremities).

extremity lift   a method of lifting and carrying a patient during which one rescuer slips hands under the patient's armpits and grasps the wrists, while another rescuer grasps the patient's knees.

fallopian (fu-LO-pe-an) tube   the narrow tube that connects the ovary to the uterus. Also called the *oviduct*.

feeding tube   a tube used to provide delivery of nutrients to the stomach. A nasogastric feeding tube is inserted through the nose and into the stomach; a gastric feeding tube is surgically implanted through the abdominal wall and into the stomach.

femoral (FEM-o-ral) artery   the major artery supplying the leg.

femur (FEE-mer)   the large bone of the thigh.

fetus (FE-tus)   the baby from 8 weeks of development to birth.

fibula (FIB-yuh-luh)   the lateral and smaller bone of the lower leg.

FiO$_2$ fraction of inspired oxygen; the concentration of oxygen in the air we breathe.

flail chest   fracture of two or more adjacent ribs in two or more places that allows for free movement of the fractured segment.

flow-restricted, oxygen-powered ventilation device (FROPVD)   a device that uses oxygen under pressure to deliver artificial ventilations. Its trigger is placed so that the rescuer can operate it while still using both hands to maintain a seal on the face mask. It has automatic flow restriction to prevent overdelivery of oxygen to the patient.

flowmeter   a valve that indicates the flow of oxygen in liters per minute.

fontanelle (FON-ta-nel)   a soft spot on an infant's anterior scalp formed by the joining of not yet fused bones of the skull.

foramen magnum (FOR-uh-men MAG-num)   the opening at the base of the skull through which the spinal cord passes from the brain.

Fowler position   a sitting position.

fracture (FRAK-cher)   any break in a bone.

gag reflex   vomiting or retching that results when something is placed in the back of the pharynx. This is tied to the swallow reflex.

gallbladder   a sac on the underside of the liver that stores bile produced by the liver.

general impression   impression of the patient's condition that is formed on first approaching the patient, based on the patient's environment, chief complaint, and appearance.

generalized seizure   a seizure that affects both sides of the brain.

glucose (GLU-kos)   a form of sugar, the body's basic source of energy.

Good Samaritan laws   a series of laws, varying in each state, designed to provide limited legal protection for citizens and some health care personnel when they are administering emergency care.

greenstick fracture   an incomplete fracture.

hallucinogens (huh-LOO-sin-uh-jens)   mind-affecting or mind-altering drugs that act on the central nervous system to produce excitement and distortion of perceptions.

hazardous material   any substance or material in a form which poses an unreasonable risk to health, safety, and property when transported in commerce.

hazardous material incident   the release of a harmful substance into the environment.

head-tilt, chin-lift maneuver   a means of correcting blockage of the airway by the tongue by tilting the head back and lifting the chin. Used when no trauma, or injury, is suspected.

hematoma (hem-ah-TO-mah)   a swelling caused by the collection of blood under the skin or in damaged tissues as a result of an injured or broken blood vessel. In a head injury, a collection of blood within the skull or brain.

hemorrhage (HEM-o-rej)   bleeding, especially severe bleeding.

hemorrhagic (HEM-or-AJ-ik) shock   shock resulting from blood loss.

hemostatic (HEM-o-STAT-IK) agents substances applied as powders, dressings, gauze, or bandages to open wounds to stop bleeding.

herniation (her-ne-AY-shun) pushing of a portion of the brain through the foramen magnum as a result of increased intracranial pressure.

HIPAA the Health Insurance Portability and Accountability Act, a federal law protecting the privacy of patient-specific health care information and providing the patient with control over how this information is used and distributed.

history of the present illness (HPI) information gathered regarding the symptoms and nature of the patient's current concern.

hives red, itchy, possibly raised blotches on the skin that often result from allergic reactions.

hot zone area immediately surrounding a hazmat incident; extends far enough to prevent adverse effects outside the zone.

humerus (HYU-mer-us) the bone of the upper arm, between the shoulder and the elbow.

humidifier a device connected to the flowmeter to add moisture to the dry oxygen coming from an oxygen cylinder.

hydrostatic (HI-dro-STAT-ik) pressure the pressure within a blood vessel that tends to push water out of the vessel.

hyperglycemia (HI-per-gli-SEE-me-ah) high blood sugar.

hypersensitivity an exaggerated response by the immune system to a particular substance.

hyperthermia (HI-per-THURM-e-ah) an increase in body temperature above normal, which is a life-threatening condition in its extreme.

hypoglycemia (HI-po-gli-SEE-me-ah) low blood sugar.

hypoperfusion (HI-po-per-FEW-zhun) inability of the body to adequately circulate blood to the body's cells to supply them with oxygen and nutrients. Also called *shock*. *See also* perfusion.

hypothermia (HI-po-THURM-e-ah) generalized cooling that reduces body temperature below normal, which is a life-threatening condition in its extreme.

hypovolemic (HI-po-vo-LE-mik) shock shock resulting from blood or fluid loss.

hypoxia (hi-POK-se-uh) an insufficiency of oxygen in the body's tissues.

ilium (IL-e-um) the superior and widest portion of the pelvis.

implied consent the consent it is presumed a patient or patient's parent or guardian would give if they could, such as for an unconscious patient or a parent who cannot be contacted when care is needed.

in loco parentis in place of the parents, indicating a person who may give consent for care of a child when the parents are not present or able to give consent.

Incident Command the person or persons who assume overall direction of a large-scale incident.

Incident Command System (ICS) a subset of the National Incident Management System (NIMS) designed specifically for management of multiple-casualty incidents.

index of suspicion awareness that there may be injuries.

indications specific signs or circumstances under which it is appropriate to administer a drug to a patient.

induced abortion expulsion of a fetus as a result of deliberate actions taken to stop the pregnancy.

infancy stage of life from birth to 1 year of age.

inferior away from the head; usually compared with another structure that is closer to the head (e.g., the lips are inferior to the nose).

ingested poisons poisons that are swallowed.

inhalation (IN-huh-LAY-shun) an active process in which the intercostal (rib) muscles and the diaphragm contract, expanding the size of the chest cavity and causing air to flow into the lungs. Also called *inspiration*.

inhaled poisons poisons that are breathed in.

inhaler a spray device with a mouthpiece that contains an aerosol form of a medication that a patient can spray into his airway.

injected poisons poisons that are inserted through the skin; for example, by needle, snake fangs, or insect stinger.

inspiration *see* inhalation.

insulin (IN-suh-lin) a hormone produced by the pancreas or taken as a medication by many diabetics.

international terrorism terrorism that is foreign-based or directed.

interventions actions taken to correct or manage a patient's problems.

intracranial (IN-truh-KRAY-ne-ul) pressure (ICP) pressure inside the skull.

involuntary muscle muscle that responds automatically to brain signals but cannot be consciously controlled.

irreversible shock when the body has lost the battle to maintain perfusion to vital organs. Even if adequate vital signs return, the patient may die days later due to organ failure.

ischium (ISH-e-um) the lower, posterior portions of the pelvis.

jaw-thrust maneuver a means of correcting blockage of the airway by moving the jaw forward without tilting the head or neck. Used when trauma, or injury, is suspected to open the airway without causing further injury to the spinal cord in the neck.

joint the point where two bones come together.

jugular (JUG-yuh-ler) vein distention (JVD) bulging of the neck veins.

kidneys   organs of the renal system used to filter blood and regulate fluid levels in the body.

labia (LAY-be-uh)   soft tissues that protect the entrance to the vagina.

labor   the three stages of the delivery of a baby that begin with the contractions of the uterus and end with the expulsion of the placenta.

laceration (las-er-AY-shun)   a cut. In brain injuries, a cut to the brain.

large intestine   the muscular tube that removes water from waste products received from the small intestine and moves anything not absorbed by the body toward excretion from the body.

larynx (LAIR-inks)   the voice box.

late adulthood   stage of life from 61 years and older.

lateral   to the side, away from the midline of the body.

left ventricular assist device (LVAD)   a battery-powered mechanical pump implanted in the body to assist a failing left ventricle in pumping blood to the body.

liability   being held legally responsible.

libel   false or injurious information in written form.

ligament   tissue that connects bone to bone.

lightening   the sensation of the fetus moving from high in the abdomen to low in the birth canal.

limb presentation   when an infant's limb protrudes from the vagina before the appearance of any other body part.

liver   the largest organ of the body, which produces bile to assist in breakdown of fats and assists in the metabolism of various substances in the body.

local cooling   cooling or freezing of particular (local) parts of the body.

lungs   the organs where exchange of atmospheric oxygen and waste carbon dioxide take place.

malar (MAY-lar)   the cheek bone, also called the *zygomatic bone*.

malleolus (mal-E-o-lus)   protrusion on the side of the ankle. The *lateral malleolus*, at the lower end of the fibula, is seen on the outer ankle; the *medial malleolus*, at the lower end of the tibia, is seen on the inner ankle.

mandible (MAN-di-bul)   the lower jaw bone.

manual traction   the process of applying tension to straighten and realign a fractured limb before splinting. Also called *tension*.

manubrium (man-OO-bre-um)   the superior portion of the sternum.

maxillae (mak-SIL-e)   the two fused bones forming the upper jaw.

mechanism of injury   a force or forces that may have caused injury.

meconium staining   amniotic fluid that is greenish or brownish-yellow rather than clear as a result of fetal defecation; an indication of possible maternal or fetal distress during labor.

medial   toward the midline of the body.

medical direction   oversight of the patient-care aspects of an EMS system by the Medical Director.

Medical Director   a physician who assumes ultimate responsibility for the patient-care aspects of the EMS system.

medical patient   a patient suffering from one or more medical diseases or conditions.

mental status   level of responsiveness.

metabolism (meh-TAB-o-lizm)   the cellular function of converting nutrients into energy.

metacarpals (MET-uh-KAR-pulz)   the hand bones.

metatarsals (MET-uh-TAR-sulz)   the foot bones.

mid-axillary (mid-AX-uh-lair-e) line   a line drawn vertically from the middle of the armpit to the ankle.

mid-clavicular (mid-clah-VIK-yuh-ler) line   the line through the center of each clavicle.

middle adulthood   stage of life from 41 to 60 years.

midline   an imaginary line drawn down the center of the body, dividing it into right and left halves.

minute volume   the amount of air breathed in during each respiration multiplied by the number of breaths per minute.

miscarriage   *see* spontaneous abortion.

mobile radio   a two-way radio that is used or affixed in a vehicle.

mons pubis   soft tissue that covers the pubic symphysis; area where hair grows as a woman reaches puberty.

moral   regarding personal standards or principles of right and wrong.

Moro reflex   when startled, an infant throws his arms out, spreads his fingers, then grabs with his fingers and arms.

multiple birth   when more than one baby is born during a single delivery.

multiple trauma   more than one serious injury.

multiple-casualty incident (MCI)   any medical or trauma incident involving multiple patients.

multisystem trauma   one or more injuries that affect more than one body system.

muscles   tissues or fibers that cause movement of body parts and organs.

musculoskeletal (MUS-kyu-lo-SKEL-e-tal) system   the system of bones and skeletal muscles that support and protect the body and permit movement.

narcotics   a class of drugs that affect the nervous system and change many normal body activities. Their legal use is for the relief of pain. Illicit use is to produce an intense state of relaxation.

nasal (NAY-zul) bones the bones that form the upper third, or bridge, of the nose

nasal cannula (NAY-zul KAN-yuh-luh) a device that delivers low concentrations of oxygen through two prongs that rest in the patient's nostrils.

nasopharyngeal (NAY-zo-fah-RIN-jul) airway a flexible breathing tube inserted through the patient's nose into the pharynx to help maintain an open airway.

nasopharynx (NAY-zo-FAIR-inks) the area directly posterior to the nose.

National Incident Management System (NIMS) the management system used by federal, state, and local governments to manage emergencies in the United States.

nature of the illness what is medically wrong with a patient.

negligence a finding of failure to act properly in a situation in which there was a duty to act, that needed care as would reasonably be expected of the EMT was not provided, and that harm was caused to the patient as a result.

neonate (NEE-oh-nate) a newly born infant or an infant less than 1 month old.

nervous system the system of brain, spinal cord, and nerves that govern sensation, movement, and thought.

neurogenic shock a state of shock (hypoperfusion) caused by nerve paralysis that sometimes develops from spinal cord injuries.

911 system a system for telephone access to report emergencies. A dispatcher takes the information and alerts EMS or the fire or police departments as needed. *Enhanced 911* has the additional capability of automatically identifying the caller's phone number and location.

nitroglycerin (NYE-tro-GLIS-uh-rin) a drug that helps to dilate the coronary vessels that supply the heart muscle with blood.

nonrebreather (NRB) mask a face mask and reservoir bag device that delivers high concentrations of oxygen. The patient's exhaled air escapes through a valve and is not rebreathed.

obesity a condition of having too much body fat, defined as a body mass index of 30 or greater.

occlusion (uh-KLU-zhun) blockage, as of an artery by fatty deposits.

occlusive dressing any dressing that forms an airtight seal.

off-line medical direction standing orders issued by the Medical Director that allow EMTs to give certain medications or perform certain procedures without speaking to the Medical Director or another physician.

on-line medical direction orders given directly by the on-duty physician to an EMT in the field by radio or telephone.

open extremity injury an extremity injury in which the skin has been broken or torn through from the inside by an injured bone or from the outside by something that has caused a penetrating wound with associated injury to the bone.

open wound an injury in which the skin is interrupted, exposing the tissue beneath.

OPQRST a memory aid in which the letters stand for questions asked to get a description of the present illness: onset, provokes, quality, radiation, severity, time.

oral glucose (GLU-kos) a form of glucose (a kind of sugar) given by mouth to treat an awake patient (who is able to swallow) with an altered mental status and a history of diabetes.

orbits the bony structures around the eyes; the eye sockets.

organ donor a person who has completed a legal document that allows for donation of organs and tissues in the event of death.

oropharyngeal (OR-o-fah-RIN-jul) airway a curved device inserted through the patient's mouth into the pharynx to help maintain an open airway.

oropharynx (OR-o-FAIR-inks) the area directly posterior to the mouth.

ostomy bag an external pouch that collects fecal matter diverted from the colon or ileum through a surgical opening (colostomy or ileostomy) in the abdominal wall.

ovaries egg-producing organs within the female reproductive system.

ovulation (ov-U-LA-shun) the phase of the female reproductive cycle in which an ovum is released from the ovary.

oxygen a gas commonly found in the atmosphere. Pure oxygen is used as a drug to treat any patient whose medical or traumatic condition may cause him to be hypoxic, or low in oxygen.

oxygen cylinder a cylinder filled with oxygen under pressure.

oxygen saturation (SpO_2) the ratio of the amount of oxygen present in the blood to the amount that could be carried, expressed as a percentage.

pacemaker a device implanted under the skin with wires implanted into the heart to modify the heart rate as needed to maintain an adequate heart rate.

palmar referring to the palm of the hand.

palmar reflex when you place your finger in an infant's palm, he will grasp it.

palpation touching or feeling. A pulse or blood pressure may be palpated with the fingertips.

pancreas a gland located behind the stomach that produces insulin and juices that assist in digestion of food in the duodenum of the small intestine.

paradoxical (pair-uh-DOCK-si-kul) motion movement of ribs in a flail segment that is opposite to the direction of movement of the rest of the chest cavity.

parenteral (pair-EN-tur-al) referring to a route of medication administration that does not use the gastrointestinal tract, such as an intravenous medication.

parietal pain a localized, intense pain that arises from the parietal peritoneum, the lining of the abdominal cavity.

partial rebreather mask a face mask and reservoir oxygen bag with no one-way valve to the reservoir bag so that some exhaled air mixes with the oxygen; used in some patients to help preserve carbon dioxide levels in the blood to stimulate breathing.

partial seizure a seizure that affects only one part or one side of the brain.

partial thickness burn a burn in which the epidermis (first layer of skin) is burned through and the dermis (second layer) is damaged. Burns of this type cause reddening, blistering, and a mottled appearance. Also called a *second-degree burn*.

passive rewarming covering a hypothermic patient and taking other steps to prevent further heat loss and help the body rewarm itself.

past medical history (PMH) information gathered regarding the patient's health problems in the past.

patella (pah-TEL-uh) the kneecap.

patent (pay-tent) open and clear; free from obstruction.

patent airway an airway (passage from nose or mouth to lungs) that is open and clear and will remain open and clear, without interference to the passage of air into and out of the body.

pathogens the organisms that cause infection, such as viruses and bacteria.

pathophysiology (path-o-fiz-e-OL-o-je) the study of how disease processes affect the function of the body.

patient outcomes the long-term survival of patients.

pedal edema accumulation of fluid in the feet or ankles.

pediatric (pee-dee-AT-rik) of or pertaining to a patient who has yet to reach puberty.

pelvis the basin-shaped bony structure that supports the spine and is the point of proximal attachment for the lower extremities.

penetrating trauma injury caused by an object that passes through the skin or other body tissues.

penis the organ of male reproduction responsible for sexual intercourse and the transfer of sperm.

perfusion (pur-FEW-zhun) the supply of oxygen to, and removal of wastes from, the cells and tissues of the body as a result of the flow of blood through the capillaries.

perineum (per-i-NE-um) the surface area between the vagina and anus.

peripheral nervous system (PNS) the nerves that enter and leave the spinal cord and travel between the brain and organs without passing through the spinal cord.

peripheral pulses the radial, brachial, posterior tibial, and dorsalis pedis pulses, which can be felt at peripheral (outlying) points of the body.

peritoneum the membrane that lines the abdominal cavity (the *parietal peritoneum*) and covers the organs within it (the *visceral peritoneum*).

peritonitis bacterial infection within the peritoneal cavity.

permeation the movement of a substance through a surface or, on a molecular level, through intact materials; penetration, or spreading.

personal protective equipment (PPE) equipment that protects the EMS worker from infection and/or exposure to the dangers of rescue operations.

phalanges (fuh-LAN-jiz) the toe bones and finger bones.

pharmacodynamics (FARM-uh-KO-die-nam-ICS) the study of the effects of medications on the body.

pharmacology (FARM-uh-KOL-uh-je) the study of drugs, their sources, their characteristics, and their effects.

pharynx (FAIR-inks) the area directly posterior to the mouth and nose. It is made up of the oropharynx and the nasopharynx.

physiology the study of body function.

placenta (plah-SEN-tah) the organ of pregnancy where exchange of oxygen, nutrients, and wastes occurs between a mother and fetus.

placenta previa (plah-SEN-tah PRE-vi-ah) a condition in which the placenta is formed in an abnormal location (low in the uterus and close to or over the cervical opening) that will not allow for a normal delivery of the fetus; a cause of excessive prebirth bleeding.

plane a flat surface formed when slicing through a solid object.

plantar referring to the sole of the foot.

plasma (PLAZ-mah) the fluid portion of the blood.

plasma oncotic (PLAZ-ma on-KOT-ik) pressure the pull exerted by large proteins in the plasma portion of blood that tends to pull water from the body into the bloodstream.

platelets components of the blood; membrane-enclosed fragments of specialized cells.

pneumothorax air in the chest cavity.

pocket face mask a device, usually with a one-way valve, to aid in artificial ventilation. A rescuer breathes through the valve when the mask is placed over the patient's face. It also acts as a barrier to prevent contact with a patient's breath or body fluids. It can be used with supplemental oxygen when fitted with an oxygen inlet.

poison any substance that can harm the body by altering cell structure or functions.

portable radio a handheld two-way radio.

positional asphyxia inadequate breathing or respiratory arrest caused by a body position that restricts breathing.

positive pressure ventilation *See* artificial ventilation.

posterior the back of the body or body part.

posterior tibial (TIB-ee-ul) artery artery supplying the foot, behind the medial ankle.

postictal (post-IK-tul) phase the period of time immediately following a tonic-clonic seizure in which the patient goes from full loss of consciousness to full mental status.

power grip gripping with as much hand surface as possible in contact with the object being lifted, all fingers bent at the same angle, and hands at least 10 inches apart.

power lift a lift from a squatting position with weight to be lifted close to the body, feet apart and flat on the ground, body weight on or just behind the balls of the feet, and the back locked-in. The upper body is raised before the hips. Also called the *squat-lift position*.

preeclampsia (pre-e-KLAMP-se-ah) a complication of pregnancy in which the woman retains large amounts of fluid and has hypertension. She may also experience seizures and/or coma during birth, which is very dangerous to the infant.

prefix word part added to the beginning of a root or word to modify or qualify its meaning.

premature infant any newborn weighing less than 5 1/2 pounds or born before the 37th week of pregnancy.

preschool age stage of life from 3 to 5 years.

pressure dressing a bulky dressing held in position with a tightly wrapped bandage, which applies pressure to help control bleeding.

pressure regulator a device connected to an oxygen cylinder to reduce cylinder pressure so it is safe for delivery of oxygen to a patient.

priapism (PRY-ah-pizm) persistent erection of the penis that may result from spinal injury and some medical problems.

primary assessment the first element in a patient assessment; steps taken for the purpose of discovering and dealing with any life-threatening problems. The six parts of primary assessment are: forming a general impression, assessing mental status, assessing airway, assessing breathing, assessing circulation, and determining the priority of the patient for treatment and transport to the hospital.

priority the decision regarding the need for immediate transport of the patient versus further assessment and care at the scene.

prolapsed umbilical cord when the umbilical cord presents first and is squeezed between the vaginal wall and the baby's head.

prone lying face down.

protocols lists of steps, such as assessments and interventions, to be taken in different situations. Protocols are developed by the Medical Director of an EMS system.

proximal closer to the torso.

pubis (PYOO-bis) the medial anterior portion of the pelvis.

pulmonary (PUL-mo-nar-e) arteries the vessels that carry deoxygenated blood from the right ventricle of the heart to the lungs.

pulmonary edema accumulation of fluid in the lungs.

pulmonary respiration the exchange of oxygen and carbon dioxide between the alveoli and circulating blood in the pulmonary capillaries.

pulmonary veins the vessels that carry oxygenated blood from the lungs to the left atrium of the heart.

pulse the rhythmic beats caused as waves of blood move through and expand the arteries.

pulse oximeter an electronic device for determining the amount of oxygen carried in the blood, known as the oxygen saturation or SpO_2.

pulse quality the rhythm (regular or irregular) and force (strong or weak) of the pulse.

pulse rate the number of pulse beats per minute.

pulseless electrical activity (PEA) a condition in which the heart's electrical rhythm remains relatively normal, yet the mechanical pumping activity fails to follow the electrical activity, causing cardiac arrest.

puncture wound an open wound that tears through the skin and destroys underlying tissues. A *penetrating puncture wound* can be shallow or deep. A *perforating puncture wound* has both an entrance and an exit wound.

pupil the black center of the eye.

quality improvement a process of continuous self-review with the purpose of identifying and correcting aspects of the system that require improvement.

radial (RAY-de-ul) pulse the pulse felt at the wrist.

radial artery artery of the lower arm. It is felt when taking the pulse at the wrist.

radiation sending out energy, such as heat, in waves into space.

radius (RAY-de-us) the lateral bone of the forearm.

rapid trauma assessment a rapid assessment of the head, neck, chest, abdomen, pelvis, extremities, and posterior of the body to detect signs and symptoms of injury.

reactivity (re-ak-TIV-uh-te) in the pupils of the eyes, reacting to light by changing size.

reassessment a procedure for detecting changes in a patient's condition. It involves four steps: repeating the primary assessment, repeating and recording vital signs, repeating the physical exam, and checking interventions.

recovery position lying on the side. Also called *lateral recumbent position*.

red blood cells components of the blood. They carry oxygen to, and carbon dioxide away from, the cells.

red flag a sign or symptom that suggests the possibility of a particular problem that is very serious.

referred pain pain that is felt in a location other than where the pain originates.

rem roentgen equivalent (in) man; a measure of radiation dosage.

renal failure loss of the kidneys' ability to filter the blood and remove toxins and excess fluid from the body.

renal system the body system that regulates fluid balance and the filtration of blood. Also called the *urinary system*.

repeater a device that picks up signals from lower-power radio units, such as mobile and portable radios, and retransmits them at a higher power. It allows low-power radio signals to be transmitted over longer distances.

reproductive system the body system that is responsible for human reproduction.

res ipsa loquitur a Latin term meaning "the thing speaks for itself."

respiration (RES-pir-AY-shun) the diffusion of oxygen and carbon dioxide between the alveoli and the blood (pulmonary respiration) and between the blood and the cells (cellular respiration). Also used to mean, simply, breathing.

respiratory arrest when breathing completely stops.

respiratory distress increased work of breathing; a sensation of shortness of breath.

respiratory failure the reduction of breathing to the point where oxygen intake is not sufficient to support life.

respiratory rate the number of breaths taken in 1 minute.

respiratory rhythm the regular or irregular spacing of breaths.

respiratory (RES-puh-ruh-tor-e) quality the normal or abnormal (shallow, labored, or noisy) character of breathing.

respiratory (RES-pir-ah-tor-e) system the system of nose, mouth, throat, lungs, and muscles that brings oxygen into the body and expels carbon dioxide.

reticular (ruh-TIK-yuh-ler) activating system (RAS) series of neurologic circuits in the brain that control the functions of staying awake, paying attention, and sleeping.

retractions pulling in of the skin and soft tissue between the ribs when breathing. This is typically a sign of respiratory distress in children.

retroperitoneal space the area posterior to the peritoneum, between the peritoneum and the back.

root foundation of a word that is not a word that can stand on its own.

rooting reflex when you touch a hungry infant's cheek, he will turn his head toward the side touched.

routes of entry pathways into the body, generally by absorption, ingestion, injection, or inhalation.

rule of nines a method for estimating the extent of a burn. For an adult, each of the following areas represents 9 percent of the body surface: the head and neck, each upper extremity, the chest, the abdomen, the upper back, the lower back and buttocks, the front of each lower extremity, and the back of each lower extremity. The remaining 1 percent is assigned to the genital region. For an infant or child, the percentages are modified so that 18 percent is assigned to the head, 14 percent to each lower extremity.

rule of palm a method for estimating the extent of a burn. The palm of the patient's own hand, which equals about 1 percent of the body's surface area, is compared with the patient's burn to estimate its size.

safe haven law a law that permits a person to drop off an infant or child at a police, fire, or EMS station or to deliver the infant or child to any available public safety personnel. The intent of the law is to protect children who may otherwise be abandoned or harmed.

SAMPLE a memory aid in which the letters stand for elements of the past medical history: signs and symptoms, allergies, medications, pertinent past history, last oral intake, and events leading to the injury or illness.

scaffolding building on what one already knows.

scapula (SKAP-yuh-luh) the shoulder blade.

scene size-up steps taken when approaching the scene of an emergency call: checking scene safety, taking Standard Precautions, noting the mechanism of injury or nature of the patient's illness, determining the number of patients, and deciding what, if any, additional resources to call for.

school age stage of life from 6 to 12 years.

scope of practice a set of regulations and ethical considerations that define the scope, or extent and limits, of the EMT's job.

secondary devices destructive devices, such as bombs, placed to be activated after an initial attack and timed to injure emergency responders and others who rush in to help care for those targeted by an initial attack.

seizure (SEE-zher) a sudden change in sensation, behavior, or movement. The most severe form of seizure produces violent muscle contractions called convulsions.

shock the body's inability to adequately circulate blood to the body's cells to supply them with oxygen and nutrients, which is a life-threatening condition. Also known as *hypoperfusion*.

sickle cell anemia (SCA) an inherited disease in which a genetic defect in the hemoglobin results in abnormal structure of the red blood cells.

side effect any action of a drug other than the desired action.

single incident command command organization in which a single agency controls all resources and operations.

skeleton the bones of the body.

skin the layer of tissue between the body and the external environment.

skull the bony structure of the head.

slander false or injurious information stated verbally.

small intestine the muscular tube between the stomach and the large intestine, divided into the duodenum, the jejunum, and the ileum, which receives partially digested food from the stomach and continues digestion. Nutrients are absorbed by the body through its walls.

sphygmomanometer (SFIG-mo-mah-NOM-uh-ter) the cuff and gauge used to measure blood pressure.

spinous (SPI-nus) process   the bony bump on a vertebra.

spleen   an organ located in the left upper quadrant of the abdomen that acts as a blood filtration system and a reservoir for reserves of blood.

spontaneous abortion   when the fetus and placenta deliver before the 28th week of pregnancy; commonly called a *miscarriage*.

sprain   the stretching and tearing of ligaments.

staging area   the area where ambulances are parked and other resources are held until needed.

staging supervisor   person responsible for overseeing ambulances and ambulance personnel at a multiple-casualty incident.

standard of care   for an EMT providing care for a specific patient in a specific situation, the care that would be expected to be provided by an EMT with similar training when caring for a patient in a similar situation.

Standard Precautions   a strict form of infection control that is based on the assumption that all blood and other body fluids are infectious.

standing orders   a policy or protocol issued by a Medical Director that authorizes EMTs and others to perform particular skills in certain situations.

status epilepticus (STAY-tus or STAT-us ep-i-LEP-ti-kus)   a prolonged seizure or situation when a person suffers two or more convulsive seizures without regaining full consciousness.

sternum (STER-num)   the breastbone.

stillborn   born dead.

stoma (STO-ma)   a permanent surgical opening in the neck through which the patient breathes.

stomach   muscular sac between the esophagus and the small intestine where digestion of food begins.

strain   muscle injury resulting from overstretching or overexertion of the muscle.

strategies   broad general plans designed to achieve desired outcomes.

stress   a state of physical and/or psychological arousal to a stimulus.

stretch receptors   sensors in blood vessels that identify internal pressure.

stridor (STRI-dor)   a high pitched sound generated from partially obstructed air flow in the upper airway.

stroke   a condition of altered function caused when an artery in the brain is blocked or ruptured, disrupting the supply of oxygenated blood or causing bleeding into the brain. Formerly called a *cerebrovascular accident (CVA)*.

stroke volume   the amount of blood ejected from the heart in one contraction.

subcutaneous (SUB-ku-TAY-ne-us) layers   the layers of fat and soft tissues found below the dermis.

sucking chest wound   an open chest wound in which air is "sucked" into the chest cavity.

sucking reflex   when you stroke a hungry infant's lips, he will start sucking.

suctioning (SUK-shun-ing)   use of a vacuum device to remove blood, vomitus, and other secretions or foreign materials from the airway.

sudden death   a cardiac arrest that occurs within 2 hours of the onset of symptoms. The patient may have no prior symptoms of coronary artery disease.

suffix   word part added to the end of a root or word to complete its meaning.

superficial burn   a burn that involves only the epidermis, the outer layer of the skin. It is characterized by reddening of the skin and perhaps some swelling. A common example is a sunburn. Also called a first-degree burn.

superior   toward the head (e.g., the chest is superior to the abdomen).

supine   lying on the back.

supine hypotensive syndrome   dizziness and a drop in blood pressure caused when the mother is in a supine position and the weight of the uterus, infant, placenta, and amniotic fluid compress the inferior vena cava, reducing return of blood to the heart and cardiac output.

syncope (SIN-ko-pee)   fainting.

systemic vascular resistance (SVR)   the pressure in the peripheral blood vessels that the heart must overcome in order to pump blood into the system.

systolic (sis-TOL-ik) blood pressure   the pressure created when the heart contracts and forces blood out into the arteries.

tachycardia (TAK-uh-KAR-de-uh)   a rapid pulse; any pulse rate above 100 beats per minute.

tactics   specific operational actions to accomplish assigned tasks.

tarsals (TAR-sulz)   the ankle bones.

tearing pain   sharp pain that feels as if body tissues are being torn apart.

temperament   the infant's reaction to his environment.

temporal (TEM-po-ral) bone   bone that forms part of the side of the skull and floor of the cranial cavity. There is a right and a left temporal bone.

temporomandibular (TEM-po-ro-mand-DIB-yuh-lar) joint   the movable joint formed between the mandible and the temporal bone, also called the TMJ.

tendon   tissue that connects muscle to bone.

tension pneumothorax   a type of pneumothorax in which air that enters the chest cavity is prevented from escaping.

terrorism   the unlawful use of force or violence against persons or property to intimidate or coerce a government, the civilian population, or any segment thereof, in furtherance of political or social objectives (U.S. Department of Justice, FBI, definition).

testes (TES-tees) the male organ of reproduction used for the production of sperm.

thorax (THOR-ax) the chest.

thrill a vibration felt on gentle palpation, such as that which typically occurs within an arterial-venous fistula.

thrombus (THROM-bus) a clot formed of blood and plaque attached to the inner wall of an artery or vein.

thyroid (THI-roid) cartilage the wing-shaped plate of cartilage that sits anterior to the larynx and forms the Adam's apple.

tibia (TIB-e-uh) the medial and larger bone of the lower leg.

tidal volume the volume of air moved in one cycle of breathing.

toddler phase stage of life from 12 to 36 months.

tonic-clonic (TON-ik-KLON-ik) seizure a generalized seizure in which the patient loses consciousness and has jerking movements of paired muscle groups.

torso the trunk of the body; the body without the head and the extremities.

tort a civil, not a criminal, offense; an action or injury caused by negligence from which a lawsuit may arise.

tourniquet (TURN-i-ket) a device used for bleeding control that constricts all blood flow to and from an extremity.

toxin a poisonous substance secreted by bacteria, plants, or animals.

trachea (TRAY-ke-uh) the "windpipe"; the structure that connects the pharynx to the lungs.

tracheostomy (TRAY-ke-OS-to-me) a surgical incision held open by a metal or plastic tube.

tracheostomy mask a device designed to be placed over a stoma or tracheostomy tube to provide supplemental oxygen.

traction splint a splint that applies constant pull along the length of a lower extremity to help stabilize the fractured bone and to reduce muscle spasm in the limb. Traction splints are used primarily on femoral shaft fractures.

transportation supervisor person responsible for communicating with sector officers and hospitals to manage transportation of patients to hospitals from a multiple-casualty incident.

trauma patient a patient suffering from one or more physical injuries.

trauma score a system of evaluating trauma patients according to a numerical rating system to determine the severity of the patient's trauma.

treatment area the area in which patients are treated at a multiple-casualty incident.

treatment supervisor person responsible for overseeing treatment of patients who have been triaged at a multiple-casualty incident.

Trendelenburg (trend-EL-un-berg) position a position in which the patient's feet and legs are higher than the head.

trending changes in a patient's condition over time, such as slowing respirations or rising pulse rate, that may show improvement or deterioration, and that can be shown by documenting repeated assessments.

triage the process of quickly assessing patients at a multiple-casualty incident and assigning each a priority for receiving treatment; from a French word meaning "to sort."

triage area the area where secondary triage takes place at a multiple-casualty incident.

triage supervisor the person responsible for overseeing triage at a multiple-casualty incident.

triage tag color-coded tag indicating the priority group to which a patient has been assigned.

trust vs. mistrust concept developed from an orderly, predictable environment versus a disorderly, irregular environment.

ulna (UL-nah) the medial bone of the forearm.

umbilical (um-BIL-i-kal) cord the fetal structure containing the blood vessels that carry blood to and from the placenta.

unified command command organization in which several agencies work independently but cooperatively.

universal dressing a bulky dressing.

untoward (un-TORD) effect an effect of a medication in addition to its desired effect that may be potentially harmful to the patient.

uppers stimulants such as amphetamines that affect the central nervous system to excite the user.

ureters (YER-uh-terz) the tubes connecting the kidneys to the bladder.

urethra (you-RE-thra) tube connecting the bladder to the vagina or penis for excretion of urine.

urinary catheter a tube inserted into the bladder through the urethra to drain urine from the bladder.

uterus (U-ter-us) the muscular female abdominal organ where the fetus develops; the womb.

vagina (vuh-JI-na) the female organ of reproduction used for both sexual intercourse and as an exit from the uterus for the fetus.

valve a structure that opens and closes to permit the flow of a fluid in only one direction.

vein any blood vessel returning blood to the heart.

venae cavae (VE-ne KA-ve) the superior vena cava and the inferior vena cava. These two major veins return blood from the body to the right atrium. (Venae cavae is plural, vena cava singular.)

venom a toxin (poison) produced by certain animals such as snakes, spiders, and some marine life forms.

venous bleeding bleeding from a vein, which is characterized by dark red or maroon blood and a steady, easy-to-control flow.

ventilation the process of moving gases (oxygen and carbon dioxide) between inhaled air and the pulmonary circulation of blood.

ventilator a device that breathes for a patient.

ventral referring to the front of the body. A synonym for anterior.

ventricles (VEN-tri-kulz) the two lower chambers of the heart. There is a right ventricle (which sends oxygen-poor blood to the lungs) and a left ventricle (which sends oxygen-rich blood to the body).

ventricular fibrillation (VF) (ven-TRIK-u-ler fib-ri-LAY-shun) a condition in which the heart's electrical impulses are disorganized, preventing the heart muscle from contracting normally.

ventricular tachycardia (V-tach) (ven-TRIK-u-ler tak-i-KAR-de-uh) a condition in which the heartbeat is quite rapid; if rapid enough, ventricular tachycardia will not allow the heart's chambers to fill with enough blood between beats to produce blood flow sufficient to meet the body's needs.

Venturi mask a face mask and reservoir bag device that delivers specific concentrations of oxygen by mixing oxygen with inhaled air.

venule (VEN-yul) the smallest kind of vein.

vertebrae (VERT-uh-bray) the bones of the spinal column (singular vertebra).

visceral pain a poorly localized, dull, or diffuse pain that arises from the abdominal organs, or viscera.

vital signs outward signs of what is going on inside the body, including respiration; pulse; skin color, temperature, and condition (plus capillary refill in infants and children); pupils; and blood pressure.

volatile chemicals vaporizing compounds, such as cleaning fluid, that are breathed in by the abuser to produce a "high."

voluntary muscle muscle that can be consciously controlled.

V/Q match ventilation/perfusion match. This implies that the alveoli are supplied with enough air and that the air in the aveoli is matched with sufficient blood in the pulmonary capillaries to permit optimum exchange of oxygen and carbon dioxide.

warm zone area where personnel and equipment decontamination and hot zone support take place; it includes control points for the access corridor and thus assists in reducing the spread of contamination.

water chill chilling caused by conduction of heat from the body when the body or clothing is wet.

watt the unit of measurement of the output power of a radio.

weaponization packaging or producing a material, such as a chemical, biological, or radiological agent, so that it can be used as a weapon; for example, by dissemination in a bomb detonation or as an aerosol sprayed over an area or introduced into a ventilation system.

weapons of mass destruction (WMD) weapons, devices, or agents intended to cause widespread harm and/or fear among a population.

white blood cells components of the blood. They produce substances that help the body fight infection.

wind chill chilling caused by convection of heat from the body in the presence of air currents.

withdrawal referring to alcohol or drug withdrawal in which the patient's body reacts severely when deprived of the abused substance.

xiphoid (ZI-foid) process the inferior portion of the sternum.

zoonotic able to move through the animal-human barrier; transmissible from animals to humans.

zygomatic (ZI-go-MAT-ik) arches bones that form the structure of the cheeks.

INDEX

Page numbers followed by f indicate figures; those followed by t indicate tables.

Artificial ventilation (*continued*)
  negative side effects, 208
  noninvasive positive pressure, 209–10, 959
  in patient with rapid ventilation, 209
  in patient with slow ventilation, 209
  in pediatric patient, 449, 902–5, 903t, 904f, 905f
Asherman Chest Seal, 684, 684f
Asphyxia/asphyxiation
  positional, 597
  in terrorism incident, 1069
  traumatic, 686, 686f, 687
Aspirin
  for acute coronary syndrome, 426, 426f, 475, 477f
  bleeding risk with, 620
  poisoning with, 547t, 915
Assault, 78
Assessment
  primary (*See* Primary assessment)
  rapid trauma (*See* Rapid trauma assessment)
  reassessment (*See* Reassessment)
  of scene (*See* Scene size-up)
  secondary
    in medical patient (*See* Medical patient, secondary
      assessment)
    in trauma patient (*See* Trauma patient, secondary
      assessment)
Asthma, 431t, 457
Asystole, 487
Atria, 112
Atropine, 430
Aura, 516
Auscultation
  in blood pressure measurement, 301–2, 301f, 304, 304f
  chest, 335, 337f, 452
  defined, 302, 320
Autism spectrum disorders (ASD), 952t, 954–56, 954t
Auto-injector, 536 (*See also* Epinephrine,
      auto-injector)
Auto-Pulse, 501, 501f
Automated external defibrillator (AED)
  advantages, 499–00
  biphasic, 486
  contraindications, 497–98, 499f
  coordinating CPR with, 488f, 489, 492
  coordinating with ALS personnel, 496
  coordinating with first responders, 496
  electricity dose for, 492
  general principles, 495
  mechanisms of action, 486–87
  monophasic, 486
  in pediatric patient, 497
  post-resuscitation care, 496
  procedure overview, 489–92f
  safety considerations, 498–99, 499f
  shockable rhythms, 487
  single rescuer, 497
  treatment sequence, 488f
  types, 486, 486f

Automatic implanted cardiac defibrillator (AICD),
      962–63
Automatic transport ventilator (ATV), 218–19, 218f
Automaticity, 109
Autonomic nervous system, 122, 748
Availability, as diagnostic trap, 388
Avian flu, 30
AVPU, 272 (*See also* Mental status assessment)
Avulsion, 648, 648f, 657
Axial skeleton, 698f, 699f

B

Backboards (*See* Spine boards/immobilizing devices)
Bacteria, as biologic agents, 1072, 1080–81t, 1082–85 (*See
      also* Biological agents/incidents)
Bag-valve mask (BVM)
  cricoid pressure with, 215
  defined, 212
  equipment, 212f
  mechanics, 213, 213t
  one rescuer, 215, 216f
  patient with stoma, 215–16
  for pediatric patient, 905f
  two rescuer, 214–15, 214f
Balloon angioplasty/catheterization, 481
Bandage
  application, 672f, 674f
  defined, 672, 672f
  for open wounds, 676
Bariatric, 58
Bariatrics, 953
Base station, 395
Basket stretcher, 57f, 62
Battery, 78
Battle's sign, 332, 334f, 755, 755f
Behavior, 588
Behavioral and psychiatric emergencies, 588–98
  aggressive or hostile patient, 594–95
  defined, 588
  medical/legal considerations, 597–98
  patient assessment, 591
  patient care, 591
  physical causes, 589, 590f
  psychiatric, 588–89
  reasonable force and restraint in, 595–97, 596f
  situational stress reactions, 590
  suicide, 592–94
  transport to appropriate facility, 597
Bell's palsy, 523f
Beta blocker, 481
Bias, 1145
Bilateral, defined, 97
Biological agents/incidents, 1071–74, 1079
  bacteria, 1072, 1080–81t, 1082–85
  considerations, 1079–81
  contamination, 1073
  exposure, 1072

Laryngopharynx (hypopharynx), 174, 175f
Larynx, 109
Late adulthood, 166–67, 166f (*See also* Geriatric patient)
Lateral, defined, 97, 97f
Lateral malleolus, 107
Lateral recumbent position, 99, 99f
Latex allergy, 532, 534
Lead poisoning, 916
Left atrium, 112
Left ventricle, 112
Left ventricular assist device (LVAD), 963, 964f
Legal issues
  in behavioral emergencies, 597–98
  confidentiality, 83–84, 84t, 411–12, 412f
  crime scenes, 87–88
  do not resuscitate orders, 80–81, 81f
  duty to act, 82, 83
  error correction in documentation, 415–16, 416f
  falsification in documentation, 413, 415
  Good Samaritan laws, 83
  in infection control, 30–35
  involuntary transportation, 77
  medical identification devices, 85, 85f
  negligence, 81–83, 82f
  organ donor, 85, 86f
  patient consent and refusal, 76–80, 79f, 412–13, 414f, 415f
  special crimes and reporting, 88
  testifying in court, 84, 84f
Lethality, biological agent, 1081
Leukocytes, 116
Levels of evidence, in research, 1147–48
Levine's sign, 272f
Liability, 78
Libel, 85
Lifting and moving
  body mechanics, 49–51
  emergency moves, 52, 53f–55f
  non-urgent moves, 56–69
  patient-carrying devices (*See* Patient-carrying devices)
  transfer to hospital stretcher, 69, 70f
  urgent moves, 52, 55
Ligaments, 100, 702, 704f
Lightening, 843
Limb presentation, 862, 862f
Liver, 122, 572t, 934t
Liver injuries, 689
Lividity, 1136
Living wills, 80
Local cooling, 811
Log roll, 52, 55f
Long spine board, 60, 63f, 64f, 775, 775f, 777
"Look test," 270–71
Lower airway, 175–76, 176f
Lower extremity, 107, 700f
Lower extremity injuries (*See also* Wounds)
  amputation, 649, 649f
  ankle or foot, 726–27, 727f
  closed, 706

dressing and bandaging, 673f, 676
femoral shaft fracture, 723–24
in geriatric patient, 939
hip (*See* Hip injuries)
knee (*See* Knee injuries)
open, 706
pelvis (*See* Pelvic injuries)
rapid trauma assessment, 338, 340f
splinting methods, 712, 713–14f
  bipolar traction, 735–36f
  one-splint—leg injuries, 743f
  one-splint—straight knee, 739–40f
  Sager traction, 737f
  two-splint—bent knee, 738f
  two-splint—leg injuries, 742f
  two-splint—straight knee, 741f
  tibia or fibula, 725–26, 725f
Lung(s), 109, 142, 1089
Lung sounds (*See* Breath sounds)

M

Malaise, in geriatric patient, 943
Malar, 748
Male reproductive system
  structures and functions, 105t, 127, 128f
  trauma to external genitalia, 658–59, 659f
Mandated reporters, 924
Mandible, 105, 748, 750f
Mandible injuries, 757, 758f
Manual traction, 710
Manubrium, 106
Marine life, poisoning from, 830–31
Masks, 27, 27f
Material Safety Data Sheets (MSDS), 1011
Maxillae, 105, 748, 750f
MCI (*See* Multiple-casualty incident)
MDMA, 565
Mechanical harm, in terrorism incident, 1070
Mechanism of injury, 253–54, 253f
  blunt-force trauma, 259–60
  bullets, 259, 259f
  falls, 258, 258f
  motor vehicle collisions (*See* Motor vehicle collisions)
  penetrating trauma, 258–59, 259f
  spine, 761–64, 763f
Meconium staining, 845, 866
Medial, defined, 97, 97f
Medial malleolus, 107
Median plane, 96
Medical direction, 15–16
Medical Director, 15
Medical identification devices, 85, 85f, 362–64, 362f
Medical patient
  defined, 351
  primary assessment, 280–81t, 281–82, 352f (*See also* Primary assessment)
  reassessment in responsive patient, 376–77

Volatile chemicals, 564f, 565, 565t, 566
Voluntary muscle, 108
Voluntary (skeletal) muscle, 702, 704f
Vomiting (*See* Nausea and vomiting)

W

Warfarin, 603, 620
Warm zone, 1010
Water
  in body, 148–49
  in cells, 137
Water chill, 805–6
Water moccasin, 829f
Water-related emergencies, 816–26
  diving accidents, 822
  drowning
    care for possible spinal injuries in the water, 819, 820–21f
    defined, 818
    patient care, 819
    rescue breathing in or out of the water, 818–19
  ice rescues, 825–26, 825f
  patient assessment, 817–18
  scuba-diving accidents, 822–24
  water rescues, 824–25, 824f
Water rescues, 824–25, 824f
Watt, 395
Weakness, in geriatric patient, 943
Weaponization, 1077

Weapons of mass destruction (WMD), 1066
West Nile virus, 30
Wheeled stretcher, 56, 57f, 58
Wheeze/wheezing, 296t, 452
White blood cells (WBCs), 116, 117f, 602
Whooping cough (pertussis), 29t
Wind chill, 806, 807
Withdrawal, 562, 566
Woolsorter's disease, 1082
Wounds
  abdominal (*See* Abdominal injuries)
  ambulance supplies for care of, 977t
  bandaging (*See* Bandage)
  blast injuries, 649–50, 650f
  burn (*See* Burns)
  chest (*See* Chest injuries)
  closed (*See* Closed wounds)
  dressing (*See* Dressings)
  open (*See* Open wounds)
Wrist injuries, 733f

X

Xiphoid process, 106

Z

Zoonotic, defined, 1082
Zygomatic arches, 105
Zygomatic bone, 748, 750f